Physical Examination and Health Assessment

Physical Examination and Health Assessment

Carolyn Jarvis, RN, C, MSN, FNP
Family Nurse Practitioner
Chestnut Health Systems
Bloomington, Illinois

and

Adjunct Assistant Professor of Nursing
School of Nursing
Illinois Wesleyan University
Bloomington, Illinois

W. B. SAUNDERS COMPANY
Harcourt Brace Jovanovich, Inc.
Philadelphia ■ London ■ Toronto ■ Montreal ■ Sydney ■ Tokyo

W. B. SAUNDERS COMPANY
Harcourt Brace Jovanovich, Inc.
The Curtis Center
Independence Square West
Philadelphia, Pennsylvania 19106

Library of Congress Cataloging-in-Publication Data
Jarvis, Carolyn.
Physical examination and health assessment / Carolyn Jarvis.
p. cm.
1. Physical diagnosis. 2. Nursing assessment. I. Title.
[DNLM: 1. Nursing Assessment. 2. Physical Examination—methods—nurses' instruction. WB 205 N37p]
RC76.J37 1992
616.07'54—dc20
DNLM/DLC 91-45018

Editor: Michael J. Brown
Developmental Editor: Robin Richman
Designer: W. B. Saunders Staff
Cover Designer: Joan Wendt
Production Manager: Linda R. Garber
Manuscript Editor: Carol DiBerardino
Illustration Specialist: Lisa Lambert
Indexer: Helene Taylor

Original illustrations by Pat Thomas
Assessment photographs by Kevin Strandberg

Physical Examination and Health Assessment ISBN 0-7216-1116-8

Printed in the United States of America.

Last digit is the print number: 9 8 7 6 5 4 3 2 1

To Paul, for love, support, and encouragement

To Sarah and Julia, for hope and joy

To Frances and Donald, for education and inspiration

Contributors

Margaret M. Andrews, PhD, RN, CTN (Certified by the Transcultural Nursing Society), who contributed most of the sections marked Transcultural Considerations, is Chairperson and Professor in the Department of Nursing at Nazareth College of Rochester, New York. In addition to her teaching experience, she is the author of many articles and books on transcultural nursing, has practiced nursing worldwide, and is a respected authority in that field.

Joyce K. Keithly, DNSc, RN, FAAN, the contributor for Chapter 6: Nutritional Assessment, is Chairperson, Department of O.R. and Surgical Nursing at Rush-Presbyterian—St. Luke's Medical Center and Professor at Rush University College of Nursing in Chicago. Because she has worked in both clinical and instructional settings, she is an experienced and well-known practitioner, teacher, researcher, and author in the area of clinical nutrition.

About the Author

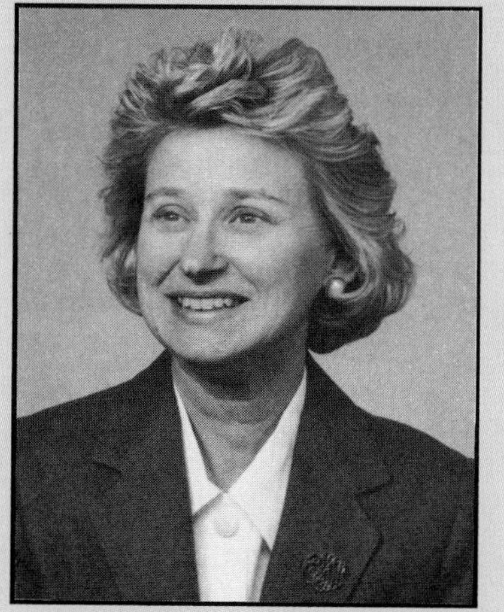

Carolyn Jarvis received her B.S.N. cum laude from the University of Iowa in 1968 and her M.S.N. from Loyola University (Chicago) in 1974. She has taught physical assessment and critical care nursing at Rush University (Chicago), University of Missouri (Columbia), and University of Illinois (Urbana), and she currently serves as Adjunct Assistant Professor at Illinois Wesleyan University in Bloomington.

Ms. Jarvis is a recipient of the University of Missouri's Superior Teaching Award and has taught physical assessment to hundreds of baccalaureate students and nursing professionals, has held 150 continuing education seminars, and is the author of numerous articles and textbook contributions.

Ms. Jarvis has maintained a clinical practice for over 20 years in advanced practice roles—first as a cardiovascular clinical specialist in various critical care settings and, for the last 12 years, as a certified family nurse practitioner in primary care. She is currently a nurse practitioner at Chestnut Health Systems, Bloomington, Illinois.

Preface

Physical Examination and Health Assessment is a textbook of interviewing techniques, approaches to health history taking, physical examination skills, and clinical assessment tools. It provides an excellent foundation to these subjects and serves as a reference in your professional life.

CONCEPTUAL APPROACH

Physical Examination and Health Assessment reflects the belief that nurses must have a current and thorough knowledge of health assessment and highly developed skills in order to function effectively in a demanding, multidisciplinary inpatient setting as well as in an independent, sometimes isolated, outpatient setting.

A commitment to **holism** is the touchstone of nursing. Therefore, this book focuses on the individual as a whole, both in **wellness needs** and **illness needs.**

Nursing has a unique orientation to people seeking health care. Thus, assessment factors cover **physical** parameters and are expanded to include **self-care** behaviors and **health promotion, culture and values, family and social roles,** and **developmental tasks.**

Nurses have a commitment to the **client as an active participant** in health care. Therefore, this book encourages you to elicit what the person already is doing to promote health, and it highlights teaching that you can present to enhance self-care.

This is a global society in which people from many cultures and ethnic backgrounds seek health care. Therefore, **transcultural considerations** are presented in each chapter.

A person's health state must be considered in light of that person's **developmental stage.** An early chapter presents developmental theory and a baseline of developmental tasks and topics expected for each age group. Subsequent chapters integrate relevant developmental content. Developmental anatomy, modifications of examination technique, and expected findings are given for infants and children, adolescents, pregnant females, and aging adults.

Assessment is the first step of a decision-making process, and assessment leads to a diagnosis. Therefore, **nursing diagnoses boxes** are included in the chapters, and you are encouraged to study the interrelation of medical and nursing diagnoses.

BEGINNING TEXT AND CONTINUING REFERENCE

Physical Examination and Health Assessment is a text for beginning learners of physical examination and health assessment as well as a reference for more sophisticated practitioners. The chapter progression and the chapter format permit this scope without sacrificing one use for the other.

Early chapters focus on health assessment and its place in the clinical decision-making process. Physical examination chapters are divided into four major sections: Structure and Function, Subjective Data (history questions), Objective Data (examination and findings), and Abnormal Findings. The beginning student can focus on reviewing anatomy and physiology in the Structure and Function sections, and on learning the skills, expected findings, and common variations for generally healthy people and selected abnormal findings in the Objective Data sections.

Students will continue to use this text in subsequent courses throughout their undergraduate education. As each course demands more detailed skills and techniques, students can review the detailed presentation and the Additional Techniques in the Objective Data sections as well as variations for age levels.

Also, students can study the extensive pathology illustrations and detailed tables in Abnormal Findings sections.

This text is a valuable reference for advanced students and experienced clinicians because it is so comprehensive. It can serve to refresh the memory, to review a specific examination technique when confronted with an unfamiliar clinical situation, or to compare and label a diagnostic finding.

This text is effective with continuing education students who are learning or refining assessment techniques. The clear and orderly presentation, excellent full-color artwork, and generous use of space lend themselves to busy professionals who are balancing full-time employment with continuing education.

ORGANIZATION

Unit 1—Assessment of the Whole Person

The first two chapters present the scope of assessment, its place in the decision-making process, and its application to individuals at each age level. Chapter 1 describes assessment factors, types of data base, concepts of health, clinical decision-making, nursing models, the interrelation of medical and nursing diagnoses, and an introduction to transcultural concepts. Chapter 2 presents the developmental stages for all age groups and expected developmental findings in four aspects: physical, psychosocial, cognitive, and behavioral.

The next two chapters focus on talking with clients. Chapter 3 has the most complete discussion available on the process of communication, interviewing skills, techniques and traps, and transcultural considerations (for example, how nonverbal behavior varies crossculturally, and the use of an interpreter). Chapter 4 presents the complete health history for all age groups. A Functional Assessment subsection reviews activities of daily living and the Comprehensive Older Person Evaluation (COPE), an excellent functional assessment tool.

The next two chapters are detailed assessments that are gathered mainly through interviewing and history questions. Chapter 5 describes the mental health assessment for emotional and cognitive functioning. It includes the Mini-Mental State, a fine clinical tool for concise and repeated mental status assessments. Chapter 6 describes components of nutritional assessment for hospitalized people and those seeking ambulatory care.

Unit 2—Physical Examination

In Unit 2, the focus turns to physical data-gathering techniques. Chapter 7 describes the assessment techniques of inspection, palpation, percussion, and auscultation as well as the equipment needed, the physical setting, and the preparation of examiner and client, with considerations for the person's physical condition and developmental stage. Chapter 8 presents the initial assessment, or the general survey, and a complete description of measurements and vital signs.

Chapters 9 through 23 present the physical examination and the related health history in a body systems approach. This is the most efficient method of performing the examination and, thus, is the most logical method for student learning and retrieval of data. Each chapter has four major sections: Structure and Function, Subjective Data (History), Objective Data (Examination and Findings), and Abnormal Findings. Each of these divisions first presents its material for the prototype of the adult, then presents developmental considerations for infants and children, adolescents, pregnant females, and aging adults.

Unit 3—Integration of the Health Assessment

Chapter 24 is a photo-essay on the integration of the complete physical examination for the adult, the infant, and the child. This format puts all the examination steps together so the student can study and learn the choreography. This chapter also has a case history of a complete write-up of a health history and physical examination.

SPECIAL FEATURES

Physical Examination and Health Assessment is designed with specific learning aids to engage students and enhance learning.

1. **Method of examination** (Objective Data section) is clear and orderly. Hundreds of original examination photos are placed directly with the text to demonstrate the physical examination in a step-by-step format.
2. **Superior full-color art program** has hundreds of pieces of original art showing detailed human anatomy, physiology examination techniques and abnormal findings.
3. **Chapter outlines** on the first page of each chapter show the contents at a glance.
4. **Frequent subheadings** and **instructional headings** assist in easy retrieval of material.
5. An **easy-to-read two-column format** begins in the Subjective Data section, where the running column highlights the rationale for asking health history questions. In the Objective Data section, the running

column highlights selected abnormal findings to show the student a clear relationship between normal and abnormal findings.

6. **Tables of Abnormal Findings** organize and expand on the material in the examination section to help the student recognize, sort and describe abnormal findings. An extensive collection of pathology photographs and original art illustrate these tables.

7. A **developmental approach** in each chapter presents prototype content on the adult, then presents age-specific content for the infant, child, adolescent, pregnant female, and aging adult.

8. **Extensive transcultural content** shows the student expected variations for culturally diverse people and cultural customs to consider when planning the interview and examination.

9. **Relevant health history questions** (Subjective Data) are repeated and expanded in each regional examination chapter to help students understand the relationship between subjective and objective data. Each regional examination chapter could stand on its own if the person had a specific problem related to that body system.

10. **Summary checklists** provide the student with cue-card reviews of examination steps to help develop a mental checklist.

11. **Sample recording** of normal findings shows the written language students should use so that their charting is complete yet succinct.

12. **Sample clinical problems** of frequently encountered situations show the student the application of assessment techniques to the clinical situation. These case histories culminate in diagnoses, and they are presented in language the student actually would use in recording.

13. **Nursing diagnoses boxes (in NANDA format)** show the student how nursing diagnoses are derived from assessment data and present a reference of nursing diagnoses commonly used with function or dysfunction of each body system.

14. A current and extensive **bibliography** for each chapter includes the best of clinical practice readings as well as basic science research and nursing research.

SUPPLEMENTS

The *Instructor's Manual* includes annotated learning objectives, teaching strategies for the classroom, skills for laboratory and independent study, case studies, and a complete test bank of questions.

The *Pocket Companion to Physical Examination and Health Assessment* is a handy clinical reference that includes pertinent material and 100 illustrations from the big book.

CAROLYN JARVIS

Acknowledgments

The difficult task of writing this book was made easier by a tenacious team of colleagues and friends.

I extend my thanks to Pat Thomas, who prepared the stunningly precise artwork and made helpful, original suggestions for the orientation of each piece. Kevin Strandberg took the clear, instructional examination photographs. I appreciate his fine focus and his patience in shooting hundreds of proofs.

I am grateful for the expertise of my colleagues. Joyce Keithly, RN, DNSc, contributed the chapter on nutritional assessment, giving of her clinical experience and knowledge. Margaret Andrews, PhD, RN, contributed most sections of the entitled Transcultural Considerations. She not only shared a wealth of pertinent knowledge, but also a global, objective perspective.

Other colleagues were particularly helpful. Laura Koppenhoefer, RN, MS, contributed much of the nursing diagnoses boxes, lending her background and experience on the application of the topic. Donna Hartweg, RN, PhD, read draft after draft of an early chapter, giving salient advice and careful insight. I am grateful to colleagues who reviewed or provided advice on specific topics in the manuscript: Rene Clark, RN, EdD; Linda Heffernan, RN, MSN, JD; Gail Lamb, MA; Annette Lueckenotte, RN, MSN; Paul Jarvis, PhD; James Butt, MD; Joleen Baum, MA; Lawrence Raines, MD; John Randolph, MD; Mary Evelyn Moore, PhD; Margo Tennis, RN, MSN.

I am grateful to my helpful and supportive colleagues at Illinois Wesleyan University and at Chestnut Health Systems, Bloomington, Illinois, and to the many fine students of physical examination and health assessment, especially to those at the University of Missouri (Columbia) where I first started to teach this topic. Their hunger for knowledge and enthusiasm for learning were an inspiration and a reward.

A host of people at W. B. Saunders Company are responsible for taking on my project, having the dedication to stick with it, and having the skill to transpose it to an impressive product. I am grateful to Michael J. Brown, Editor in Chief, Nursing Books, for his insight and regard; Linda R. Garber, Production Manager, for skillfully coordinating all the elements once this very complicated project was in production; Joan Wendt, Designer, for the creative design; Lisa Lambert, Illustration Coordinator, for the careful attention to detail on hundreds and hundreds of figures; Carol DiBerardino, Manuscript Editor, for meticulous attention to stage after stage of the manuscript; and to Ilze Rader, Acquisitions Editor, for her faith in the germ of a project. I am particularly grateful to Robin Levin Richman, Developmental Editor, for her patience, firm support, and calm determination in piloting this project through all its steps. I could not have wished for a finer author-advocate.

The computer age finds me with no loyal secretary to thank for typing the mounds of manuscript. Rather, I am grateful to my husband Paul Jarvis, who first taught me the computer skills I needed so that I could do it myself. For his skill in choosing hardware, trouble-shooting software, and finding a solution to every question, I am forever grateful.

My deepest debt of gratitude is to my family for their loyal and steadfast support. Even when I felt bogged down and bereft of the muses, they were always encouraging and always proud.

CAROLYN JARVIS

Contents

UNIT 2 Physical Examination ▶ 163

UNIT

1 Assessment of the Whole Person

CHAPTER

1 Assessment for Health and Illness

Ellen K. is a 23-year-old white unemployed female who entered a substance abuse treatment program because of numerous drug-related driving offenses. After her admission, the examiner collected a health history and performed a complete physical examination. The actual preliminary list of significant findings looked like this:

- high school academic record strong (A−/B+) in first 3 years, grades fell senior year but did graduate
- alcohol abuse, started age 16, heavy daily usage × 3 years PTA (prior to admission), last drink 4 days PTA
- cigarette use, 2 PPD (packs per day) × 2 years, prior use 1 PPD × 4 years
- elevated B/P (142/100 at end of exam today)
- diminished breath sounds, with moderate expiratory wheeze and scattered rhonchi at both bases
- grade ii/vi systolic murmur, loudest at left lower sternal border
- resolving hematoma, 2 to 3 cm, R infraorbital ridge
- missing R lower 1st molar, gums receding on lower incisors, multiple dark spots all teeth
- well-healed scar, 28 cm long × 2 cm wide, R lower leg, with R leg 3 cm shorter than L, sequela auto accident age 12
- nutrition—omits breakfast, daily intake has no fruits, no vegetables
- oral contraceptives for birth control × 3 years, last pelvic exam 1 year PTA
- unemployed × 6 months, previous work as cashier, bartender
- physically abusive relationship with boyfriend, orbital hematoma result of being hit. States, "It's OK, I probably deserved it."
- history of sexual abuse by father when Ellen was aged 12 to 16
- relationships—estranged from parents, no close women friends, significant relationship with boyfriend of 2 years whom Ellen describes as physically abusive and alcoholic

The examiner analyzed all the data, sorting out which data to refer and which to treat. Although the diagnostic process is discussed later (p. 5), it is interesting now to note how many significant findings are derived from data the examiner collected. Not just physical data but cognitive, psychosocial, and behavioral data are significant for an analysis of Ellen's health state. Also, the findings are interesting when considered from a life cycle perspective, i.e., a young adult who normally should be concerned with the developmental tasks of emancipation from parents, building an independent lifestyle, establishing a vocation, and choosing a mate (see Chapter 2, p. 36) Many factors are important for a complete health assessment.

THE CONCEPT OF HEALTH DETERMINES ASSESSMENT

Assessment is the collection of data about an individual's health state. A clear idea of health is important because it determines which assessment data to collect. In general, the list of data that must be collected has lengthened as our concept of health has broadened.

The biomedical model of Western tradition views health as the absence of disease. Health and disease are opposites, extremes on a linear continuum. Disease is due to specific agents or pathogens. Thus, the physician's focus is the diagnosis and treatment of those pathogens. Assessment factors are a list of biophysical symptoms and signs. The person is certified as healthy when these symptoms and signs have been eliminated. When disease does exist, medical diagnosis is worded to identify and explain the cause of disease.

The accurate diagnosis and treatment of illness is an important part of health care. But the public's concept of health has expanded since the 1950s. Now we view health in a wider context. We have an increasing interest in lifestyle, personal habits, exercise and nutrition, and the social and natural environment.

Halpert Dunn's view of health is *wellness* (Dunn, 1959, 1980). Wellness is a dynamic process, a move toward optimal functioning. There are different levels of wellness; optimal health is high-level wellness. Wellness is a direction of progress. Health care providers serve to maximize the person's potential, to assist the person to grow toward high-level wellness.

Consideration of the whole person is the essence of *holistic health.* (Dunn, 1959, 1980; Travis, 1986). Holistic health views the mind, body and spirit as interdependent and functioning as a whole within the environment. Health depends on all these factors working together. The basis of disease is multifaceted, originating both from within the person and from the external environment. Thus, the treatment of disease requires the services of numerous providers.

Nursing includes many aspects of the holistic model—the interaction of the mind and body, the oneness and unity of the individual. Both the individual human and the external environment are open systems, which are dynamic and continually changing and adapting to each other. Each person is responsible for his or her own personal health state, and should be considered an active participant in health care.

In a holistic model, assessment factors must be expanded to include such things as culture and values, family and social roles, health maintenance behaviors, job-related stress, developmental tasks, and failures and frustrations of life. All are significant to health.

The nursing model of health care delivery fits nicely with the expanded view of health because nurses have long considered the whole person rather than just separate biologic systems. The consideration of the complete person in the nursing model is illustrated in the list of assessment factors nurses use to judge health (Table 1–1).

Table 1–1 ▶ Standard Assessment Factors for General Professional Nursing Practice

Standard: The collection of data about the health status of the client/patient is systematic and continuous. The data are accessible, communicated, and recorded.

Rationale: Comprehensive care requires complete and ongoing collection of data about the client/patient to determine the nursing care needs of the client/patient. All health status data about the client/patient must be available for all members of the health care team.

1. Health status data include
   growth and development
   biophysical status
   emotional status
   cultural, religious, socioeconomic background
   performance of activities of daily living
   patterns of coping
   interaction patterns
   client's/patient's perception of and satisfaction with his or her health status
   client/patient health goals
   environment (physical, social, emotional, ecological)
   available and accessible human and material resources
2. Data are collected from
   client/patient, family, significant others
   health care personnel
   individuals within the immediate environment and/or the community
3. Data are obtained by
   interview
   examination
   observation
   reading records, reports
4. There is a format for the collection of data that
   provides for a systematic collection of data
   facilitates the completeness of data collection
5. Continuous collection of data is evident by
   frequent updating
   recording of changes in health status
6. The data are
   accessible from the client/patient records
   retrievable from record-keeping systems
   confidential when appropriate

Reprinted with permission from *Standards of Nursing Practice*, ©1973 American Nurses' Association, Kansas City, MO.

ASSESSMENT AS A PART OF DECISION-MAKING

Assessment is the collection of data about the individual's health state. These data include *subjective* data, what the person *says* about himself or herself during history-taking; *objective* data, what the health professional observes by inspecting, percussing, palpating, and auscultating during the physical examination; and the client's record and laboratory studies. These elements form the *data base.*

From the data base, the health professional makes a judgment or diagnosis about the individual's health state. Thus, the *purpose* of assessment is to make a judgment or diagnosis.

The Nursing Process

Assessment is the first step of the nursing process. The nursing process is a sequential method of problem-solving that was formalized in the 1960s. It now includes five steps: assessment, diagnosis, planning, implementing, and evaluating. Assessment starts with the first greeting of the client and ends with the actual or potential nursing diagnosis.

The nursing process is a "clear step-by-step linear approach to nursing judgments" (Tanner, 1988). Tanner believes that the formalization of the nursing process in the 1960s was a revolutionary development because it demonstrated the application of the scientific method to nursing practice (Tanner, 1988).

Diagnostic Reasoning

A way of collecting and analyzing information that is similar to the nursing process is the model of diagnostic reasoning described by Elstein and associates (Elstein et al, 1972, 1978). It has four major components: (1) attending to initially available cues, (2) formulating diagnostic hypotheses, (3) gathering data relative to the tentative hypotheses, and (4) evaluating each hypothesis with the new data collected, thus arriving at a final diagnosis. A cue is a piece of information, a sign or symptom, or a piece of laboratory data. A hypothesis is a tentative explanation for a cue or a set of cues that can be used as a basis for further investigation.

For example, Ellen K. presents with a number of initial cues, one of which is the hematoma under her eye. (1) The nurse recognizes this cue even before history-taking starts. Is it significant? (2) Ellen says she ran into a door, although she mumbles as she speaks and avoids eye contact. At this point, one formulates a hypothesis of trauma. (3) During the history and physical examination, the nurse gathers data to support or reject the tentative hypothesis. (4) The nurse synthesizes the new data collected, which supports the hypothesis of trauma but eliminates the accidental cause. The nurse reaches a final diagnosis.

Elstein found that diagnostic hypotheses were activated very early in the reasoning process. This helps diagnosticians adapt to large amounts of information because it clusters cues into meaningful groups and directs subsequent data collection. Diagnostic reasoning has been studied further with medical students and physicians (Ekwo, 1977; Kassirer, 1978; Neufeld, 1981).

Tanner studied diagnostic reasoning among nurses and nursing students and found that they too generated early hypotheses (Tanner, 1988). Tanner believes the process of diagnosis and planning is not as linear as was originally thought and that the nursing process alone does not explain the dynamic and interactive processes that actually occur in arriving at a diagnosis and planning treatment.

Intuition in Decision-Making

Although the nursing process is a logical step-by-step approach to clinical judgments, it seems that some expert nurses vault over the steps and arrive at a judgment in one leap (Putzier et al, 1985; Rew, 1988; Gruber and Benner, 1989). This is true particularly with expert nurses in critical care situations in which client status changes rapidly and accurate decisions are paramount. The stakes are high, and nursing autonomy is strong. In these cases, the nurse does not settle on the obvious diagnosis if it conflicts with her or his feelings, but acts out of intuition, out of subjective feeling.

Intuition is knowledge received as a whole. The awareness of knowledge is immediate, and it is not acquired through analytical reasoning (Rew, 1988). Benner's study (1984) of skill acquisition showed an evolution of the nurse from novice to expert. The more advanced nurses used intuitive judgment derived from clinical knowledge. Novices operate from a set of rules (such as the nursing process).

Intuition is characterized by pattern recognition—expert nurses learn to attend to a pattern of assessment data and act without consciously labeling it (Tanner, 1988). Action precedes analytic thought. Intuition also has a sense of salience—some assessment data are more important than others.

USING A CONCEPTUAL FRAMEWORK TO GUIDE NURSING PRACTICE

The assessment data listed on p. 5 are the standard set by the American Nurses' Association. But the *organization* of assessment data—the data base—varies depending on the conceptual model of the nurse. A model provides the framework for the nurse in determining what to observe, how to organize the observations or data, and how to interpret and use the information. There are many different nursing models, but they all deal with the same concepts: human beings, environment and society, health and illness, and nursing.

Although all nursing models describe the same four concepts, each one has a different focus or emphasis. For example, the focus of Orem's model (1985) is self-care. The focus of Roy's model (1984) is adaptation. The focus of Leininger's model (1988) is cultural diversity.

The nurse using Orem's model to collect data would focus on the abilities and limitations of the individual for self-care. In using Roy's model, the nurse would focus on data about stimuli in the environment and the individual's adaptation to those stimuli. In using Leininger's model, the nurse would focus on factors that influence care and health patterns for individuals, families, and cultural groups. Although each route is different, all three nursing models should lead to similar nursing diagnoses.

This does not mean nurses must ignore the medical model. According to Feild (1985), a nursing model is used with, not in place of, a medical model. Nurses still use the medical model when they work interdependently with the physician in the diagnosis and treatment of disease. A concurrent nursing model is needed to focus assessment on core nursing concerns, such as skin problems, coping problems, or self-care limitations (Feild, 1985).

There is no *one particular* model that is the hallmark of the entire profession. There are multiple models, some of which are more appropriate in various settings, or with certain types of clients. Nursing models currently are being tested in clinical practice and refined. Although subject to refinement, a model is still useful as a framework for assessment and useful because it leads to the formulation of nursing diagnoses.

As long as there is no consensus on one nursing model, how can we reconcile the various assessment tools called for in each case? Physicians have a standardized format to assess people, whereas nurses do not. Yet, nurses from many institutions must be able to communicate with each other. They must speak a common language so that the health care consumer is assured of consistently efficient care. While the various models are being studied and utilized, nurses can rally around two points.

1. The list of assessment data deemed standard by the American Nurses' Association. This list provides a consistent data base that is adaptable to any nursing model and allows for nursing diagnoses. Whatever format nurses do use should be holistic, systematic and orderly, and practical. Also, the nurse should understand the format and enjoy using it (Guzzetta and Dossey, 1983).
2. The use of nursing diagnoses. These diagnoses give nurses a common language with which to communicate nursing findings. The most recent approved NANDA list is given in Table 1–2.

FOCUS OF ASSESSMENT SKILLS AND DIAGNOSIS IN MEDICINE AND NURSING

Health professionals need a common foundation of knowledge and many shared skills so we can collaborate in health care (Field, 1987). Most of the history-taking and physical examination skills taught in this book are shared by nurses and physicians in providing health care. The history-taking skills described in the mental health assessment are shared not only by physicians and nurses but by psychologists and psychiatric social workers. The physical examination skill of auscultating lung sounds may be shared by physicians, nurses, and respiratory therapists. Although health professionals share knowledge and many skills, what differs is the *purpose* for which the knowledge and skills are used.

The medical diagnosis is used to evaluate the cause and the etiology of disease. The nursing diagnosis is used to evaluate the response of the whole person to actual or potential health problems. For example, both the admitting nurse and later the physician auscultate Ellen's lung sounds and determine that they are diminished and that wheezing is present. This is both a medical and a nursing clinical problem. The physician listens to diagnose the cause of the abnormal sounds (in this case, asthma) and to order specific drug treatment. The nurse listens to detect abnormal sounds early, to monitor Ellen's response to treatment, and to initiate supportive measures and teaching such as advising on behavioral measures to quit smoking and recommending that Ellen initiate a walking program.

The physicians's diagnostic focus is on the function and malfunction of a specific organ system; the nurse's diagnostic focus is on the response of the whole person to the health problem (Feild, 1985).

The medical and nursing diagnoses are independent but are interrelated; they should not be seen as isolated from each other (Field, 1987). It makes sense that the medical diagnosis of asthma be reflected in the nursing diagnoses, as interpreted by the nurse's knowledge of the person's response to asthma. In this book, Chapters 2 and 5 and the chapters in Unit 2 present common nursing diagnoses along with medical diagnoses to illustrate common abnormalities. Please observe how these two types of diagnoses are interrelated.

COLLECTING FOUR TYPES OF DATA

Although the list of data is standard, the *amount* of the data varies depending on the client's needs, the health care setting, and the nurse's role in that setting. There are four kinds of data base every examiner needs to collect: complete, episodic or problem-centered, follow-up, and emergency.

Complete or Total Health Data Base

This includes a complete health history and a full physical examination. It describes the current and past health state and forms a baseline against which all future changes can be measured. It yields the first diagnoses.

In primary care, the complete data base is collected in a primary care setting, such as a pediatric or family practice clinic, independent or group private practice, college health service, women's health care agency, visiting nurse agency, or community health agency. In these settings the nurse is the first health professional to see the client and has primary responsibility for monitoring the person's health care. For the well person, this data base must describe the person's health state, perception of health, strengths or assets such as health maintenance behaviors, individual coping patterns, support systems, current developmental tasks, and any risk factors or lifestyle changes. For the ill person, the data base also includes a description of the person's health problems, perception of illness, and response to the problems.

For well and ill clients, the complete data base must screen for pathology as well as determine the ways peo-

Table 1-2 ▶ NANDA-Approved Nursing Diagnostic Categories (1990)

- Activity Intolerance
- Activity Intolerance, Potential
- Adjustment, Impaired
- Airway Clearance, Ineffective
- Anxiety
- Aspiration, Potential for
- Body Image Disturbance
- Body Temperature, Potential Altered
- Breast-feeding, Effective
- Breast-feeding, Ineffective
- Breathing Pattern, Ineffective
- Communication, Impaired Verbal
- Constipation
- Constipation, Colonic
- Constipation, Perceived
- Decisional Conflict (Specify)
- Decreased Cardiac Output
- Defensive Coping
- Denial, Ineffective
- Diarrhea
- Disuse Syndrome, Potential for
- Diversional Activity Deficit
- Dysreflexia
- Family Coping: Compromised, Ineffective
- Family Coping: Disabling, Ineffective
- Family Coping: Potential for Growth
- Family Processes, Altered
- Fatigue
- Fear
- Fluid Volume Deficit
- Fluid Volume Deficit, Potential
- Fluid Volume Excess
- Gas Exchange, Impaired
- Grieving, Anticipatory
- Grieving, Dysfunctional
- Growth and Development, Altered
- Health Maintenance, Altered
- Health Seeking Behaviors (Specify)
- Home Maintenance Management, Impaired
- Hopelessness
- Hyperthermia
- Hypothermia
- Incontinence, Bowel
- Incontinence, Functional
- Incontinence, Reflex
- Incontinence, Stress
- Incontinence, Total
- Incontinence, Urge
- Individual Coping, Ineffective
- Infection, Potential for
- Injury, Potential for
- Knowledge Deficit (Specify)
- Noncompliance (Specify)
- Nutrition: Less than Body Requirements, Altered
- Nutrition: More than Body Requirements, Altered
- Nutrition: Potential for More than Body Requirements, Altered
- Oral Mucous Membrane, Altered
- Pain
- Pain, Chronic
- Parental Role Conflict
- Parenting, Altered
- Parenting, Potential Altered
- Personal Identity Disturbance
- Physical Mobility, Impaired
- Poisioning, Potential for
- Post-Trauma Response
- Powerlessness
- Protection, Altered
- Rape-Trauma Syndrome
- Rape-Trauma Syndrome, Compound Reaction
- Rape-Trauma Syndrome, Silent Reaction
- Role Performance, Altered
- Self-Care Deficit
  - Bathing/Hygiene
  - Feeding
  - Dressing/Grooming
  - Toileting
- Self-Esteem, Chronic Low
- Self-Esteem, Situational Low
- Self-Esteem Disturbance
- Sensory/Perceptual Alterations (Specify) (visual, auditory, kinesthetic, gustatory, tactile, olfactory)
- Sexual Dysfunction
- Sexuality Patterns, Altered
- Skin Integrity, Impaired
- Skin Integrity, Potential Impaired
- Sleep Pattern Disturbance
- Social Interaction, Impaired
- Social Isolation
- Spiritual Distress
- Suffocation, Potential for
- Swallowing, Impaired
- Thermoregulation, Ineffective
- Thought Processes, Altered
- Tissue Integrity, Impaired
- Tissue Perfusion, Altered (Specify Type) (renal, cerebral, cardiopulmonary, gastrointestinal, peripheral)
- Trauma, Potential for
- Unilateral Neglect
- Urinary Elimination, Altered
- Urinary Retention
- Violence, Potential for: Self-directed or Directed at Others

ple respond to that pathology or to any health problem. The nurse must screen for pathology because the nurse is the first, and often the only, health professional to see the client. The nurse screens for pathology to refer the client to another professional, to help the client make decisions, and to perform appropriate treatments within protocols. But this data base also notes the human responses to health problems. This factor is important because it provides additional information about the person that leads to nursing diagnoses.

In acute hospital care, the complete data base also is gathered following admission to the hospital. In the hospital, data related specifically to pathology already may have been collected by the physician. It makes little sense for the nurse to ask the same questions; the nurse can use the data the physician has collected. The nurse collects additional information on the client's perception of illness, functional ability or patterns of living, activities of daily living, health maintenance behaviors, response to health problems, coping patterns, interaction patterns, and health goals. This approach completes the data base from which the nursing diagnoses can be made.

Episodic or Problem-Centered Data Base

This is for a limited or short-term problem. Here, the nurse collects a "mini" data base, smaller in scope than the complete data base. It concerns mainly one problem, one cue complex, or one body system. It is used in all settings—hospital, primary care, or long-term care. For example, 2 days following surgery, a hospitalized person suddenly has a congested cough, shortness of breath, and fatigue. The history and examination focuses primarily on the respiratory and cardiovascular systems. Or, in an outpatient clinic, a person presents with a rash. The history and examination follow the direction of this presenting concern, such as whether the rash had an acute or chronic onset, was associated with a fever, and was localized or generalized, and must include a clear description of the rash.

Follow-Up Data Base

The status of any identified problems should be evaluated at regular and appropriate intervals. What change has occurred? Is the problem getting better or worse? What coping strategies are used? This type of data base is used in all settings to follow up short-term or chronic health problems.

Emergency Data Base

This calls for a rapid collection of the data base, often compiled concurrently with lifesaving measures. Diagnosis must be swift and sure. For example, in a hospital emergency department, a person is brought in with suspected substance overdose. One of the first history questions is "What did you take?" The person is questioned simultaneously while his or her airway, breathing, and circulation are being assessed. Clearly, the emergency data base requires more rapid collection of data than the episodic data base.

TRANSCULTURAL CONSIDERATIONS

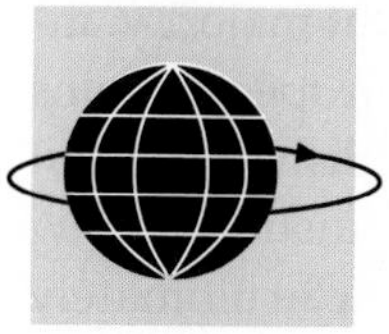

In a holistic model of health care, assessment factors must include culture. An introduction to transcultural concepts follows. These concepts are developed throughout the text as they relate to the specific chapters.

According to the United States Census Bureau, one third of the U.S. population consists of individuals from racial, ethnic, and cultural subgroups, which are sometimes referred to as minorities. By the early part of the next century, individuals from culturally diverse backgrounds will account for 51.1 percent of the total population. For the first time in United States history, the nation's racial and ethnic subgroups will compose a majority of the total population. If current demographic trends continue, the following cultural diversity is expected in the twenty-first century: Hispanics, 23.4 percent; blacks, 14.7 percent; and Asians, 12 percent (United States Census Bureau, 1983). At the same time, the Native American population is projected to remain at 0.6 percent or perhaps decrease slightly because of intermarriage (United States Census Bureau, 1983).

As the twenty-first century approaches, there is projected to be a continued increase in the number of immigrants and refugees in the United States. At the same time, people from around the world seek treatment in American hospitals, particularly for cardiovascular, neurologic, and cancer care, while United States health care providers go abroad to work in a wide variety of health care settings in the international market place. During one's professional nursing career, one may be expected to assess short-term foreign visitors, international university faculty, students studying abroad in United States high schools and universities, family members of foreign diplomats, immigrants, refugees, members of more than 130 different ethnic groups, and Native Americans from more than 200 tribes. A serious conceptual problem exists within nursing in that nurses are expected to know, understand, and meet the health needs of people from culturally diverse backgrounds, without any formal preparation for doing so.

The inclusion of cultural considerations in health assessment is of paramount importance to gather data that are accurate and meaningful and to intervene with culturally sensitive and appropriate care. Members of some cultural groups, most notably blacks and Hispanics, are demanding culturally relevant health care that incorporates their specific beliefs and practices. There is an increasing expectation among members of certain cultural groups that health care providers will respect their "cultural health rights," an expectation that frequently conflicts with the unicultural, Western, biomedical world view taught in American educational programs preparing nurses and other health care providers.

Given the multicultural composition of the United States and the projected increase in the number of individuals from diverse cultural backgrounds anticipated in the future, a concern for the cultural beliefs and practices of people is becoming increasingly important. Nursing is inherently a transcultural phenomenon in that the context and process of helping people involves at least two persons generally having different cultural orientations or intracultural lifestyles.

Culture

Culture has four basic characteristics. Culture is (1) *learned* from birth through the processes of language acquisition and socialization; (2) *shared* by all members of the same cultural group; (3) *adapted* to specific conditions related to environmental and technical factors and to the availability of natural resources; and (4) *dynamic* and ever-changing.

Culture is an all-pervasive, universal phenomenon, without which no human person exists. Yet, the culture that develops in any given society is always specific and distinctive, encompassing all the knowledge, beliefs, customs, and skills acquired by members of the society. Within cultures, groups of individuals share different beliefs, values, and attitudes. Differences occur because of ethnicity, religion, education, occupation, age, and sex. When such groups function within a large culture, they are referred to as subcultural groups.

The term *subculture* is used for fairly large aggregates of people who have shared characteristics that are not common to all members of the culture and that enable them to be thought of as a distinguishable subgroup. Ethnicity, religion, occupation, health-related characteristics, age, and sex and gender are frequently used to identify subcultural groups. Examples of subcultures based on *ethnicity* (those having common traits such as physical characteristics, language, or ancestry) include blacks, Hispanics, Native Americans, Korean-Americans, Eskimos; those based on *religion* include members of the more than 1200 recognized religions such as Catholics, Jews, Mormons, Muslims, and Buddhists; those based on *occupation* include individuals involved in health care professions, such as nursing or medicine, as well as the military; those based on a *health-related characteristic* include the blind, hearing impaired, or mentally retarded; those based on *age* include groups such as adolescents and the elderly; and those based on *sex and gender* or *sexual preference* include women, men, lesbians, and homosexuals.

The term *minority* refers to "a group of people, who because of their physical or cultural characteristics, are singled out from the others in the society in which they live for differential and unequal treatment, and who therefore regard themselves as objects of collective discrimination" (Wirth, 1945). The concept of minority varies widely and is contextual. For example, males may perceive themselves to be a minority group within nursing, a profession in which the majority is female, whereas females are minorities in the more male-dominated professions such as engineering. The federal government recognizes the following four minority groups: blacks (African, Haitian, and Dominican Republican decent); Hispanics (those of Spanish-speaking origins such as Mexican, Cuban, and Puerto Rican descent); Asians (Japanese, Chinese, Filipino, Korean, Vietnamese, Hawaiian, Guamian, Samoan, and East Indian descent); and Native Americans (Eskimos and more than 200 American Indian tribes). Because the term minority is perceived to connote inferiority, members of some of the groups mentioned object to its use and prefer terms such as ethnicity or cultural diversity.

Culture and the Formation of Values

Every society has what is called a *dominant value orientation,* a basic value orientation that is shared by the majority of its members as a result of early common experiences. The dominant value orientations of the United States include individuality, material wealth, comfort, humanitarianism, physical beauty, democracy, newness, cleanliness, education, science, achievement, free enterprise, punctuality, rationality, independence, respectability, self-discipline, effort, and progress (Herberg, 1989). In the United States, the dominant value orientation is embraced by the dominant cultural group, which consists of white, middle-class Protestants, typically those who came to this country at least two generations ago from Northern Europe. Because many members of the dominant cultural group are of Anglo-Saxon descent, they are sometimes referred to as WASPs (white, Anglo-Saxon Protestants).

Although there is sometimes an assumption that the term white refers to a homogenous group of Americans, there is a rich diversity of ethnic variation among the many groups that constitute the dominant majority, including those of Eastern and Western European origins (e.g., Irish, Polish, Italian, French, Swedish, and Russian), as well as those from Canada, Australia, New Zealand, and South Africa (whose origins can ultimately be traced to Western Europe). Appalachians, Amish, and other subgroups are also examples of whites having cultural roots that are recognizably different from the dominant majority group, i.e., WASP origins.

One aspect of a society's value orientation concerns time dimension. According to Kluckhohn and Strodtbeck (1961), there are three major ways in which people can perceive time: (1) The focus may be on the *past* with traditions and ancestors playing an important role in the person's life. For example, many Asians, American Indians, East Indians, and Africans hold beliefs about ancestors and tend to value long-standing traditions. In times of crisis, such as illness, individuals with a value orientation emphasizing the past may consult with ancestors or ask for their guidance or protection during the illness. (2) The focus may be on the *present,* with little attention being paid to the past or the future. These individuals are concerned with "now" and the future is perceived as vague or unpredictable. You may have difficulty encouraging these individuals to prepare for the future, e.g., for discharge from the hospital, for future side effects or adverse reactions from the medication, and so forth. (3) For some people, the focus is on the *future* with progress and change being highly valued. These individuals may express discontent with both the past and the present. In terms of health care, these individuals may inquire about the "latest treatment" and most modern equipment available for a particular problem and may express concern with nurses or physicians whom they perceive to be old-fashioned.

Another aspect of a person's cultural value orientation concerns the relationships that exist with others. There are three ways in which relationships may be categorized: (1) *Lineal* relationships refer to those that exist by virtue of heredity and kinship ties. Lineal relationships follow an ordered succession and have continuity through time. (2) *Collateral* relationships focus primarily on group goals and the family orientation is all-important. For example, many Asian people describe family honor and the importance of working together toward achievement of a group (versus personal) goal. (3) *Individual* relationships refer to personal autonomy and independence. Individual goals dominate, whereas group goals become secondary.

When making health-related decisions, people from culturally diverse backgrounds rely on relationships with others in various ways. If the cultural value orientation is lineal, the person may seek assistance from other members of the family and allow a relative (e.g., parent, grandparent, elder brother) to make decisions about important health-related matters. If collateral relationships are valued, decisions about the person may be interrelated with the impact of illness on the entire family or group. For example, among the Amish, the entire community is affected by the illness of a member because the community pays for health care from a common fund, members join together to meet the needs of both the person and his or her family throughout the illness, and the roles of dozens in the community are likely to be affected by the illness of a single member. The individual value orientation concerning relationships is predominant among the dominant cultural majority in America. Decision-making about health and illness is often an individual matter, with the person being the sole decider, although members of the nuclear family may participate to varying degrees.

Family

Despite the alarmingly high rate of divorce in the United States, the family remains the basic social unit. The essence of family consists of individuals living together as a unit. There are three major categories of family: (1) *nuclear* (husband, wife, and child(ren); (2) *single parent* (either mother or father and at least one child); and (3) *extended family* (which may include grandparents, aunts, uncles, cousins, and even individuals who are not biologically related).

Relationships that may seem apparent sometimes warrant further exploration when interviewing people from culturally diverse backgrounds. For example, the dominant cultural group defines siblings as two persons with either the same mother, the same father, the same mother and father, or the same adoptive parents. In some Asian cultures, a sibling relationship is defined as one in which any infants are breast-fed by the same woman. In other cultures, certain kinship patterns, such as maternal first cousins, are defined as sibling relationships. In some African cultures, anyone from the same village or town may be called "brother" or "sister." Certain subcultures, such as members of the Roman Catholic religion (who may be further subdivided by ethnicity such as Italians, Polish, Spanish, Mexican, and so forth) recognize relationships such as "godmother" or "godfather" in which an individual who is not the biologic parent promises to assist with the moral and spiritual development of an infant and agrees to care for the child in the event of parental death. The godparent makes these promises during the religious ceremony of baptism.

When assessing infants and children, it is important to identify the primary provider of care because this individual may or may not be the biologic parent. Among some Hispanic groups, for example, female members of the nuclear or extended family such as sisters and aunts are primary providers of care. In some black families, the grandmother may be the decision-maker and primary caretaker of children.

FREQUENCY OF ASSESSMENT

The interval of assessment varies with the person's illness and wellness needs. Most ill people seek care because of pain or some abnormal signs and symptoms they have noticed. This prompts an assessment—gathering a complete, an episodic, or emergency data base.

But for the well person, opinions are changing about assessment intervals. In the United States in 1861, a periodic examination was recommended for early detection of disease. In 1922, the American Medical Association passed a resolution urging people to have a periodic health examination. In succeeding years, this became standard and each person was exhorted to have an annual checkup. A physician certified a clean bill of health, which meant the person was free of signs and symptoms of disease. One problem was that little attention was paid to the individual once he or she left the physician's office. There was little or no time spent on lifestyle management, risk assessment, or health promotion.

Also, the term annual checkup is vague. What does it constitute? In practice, its extent varies considerably among physicians, nurses, and agencies. Is the annual checkup necessary? Is it cost effective? Does it sometimes give an implicit promise of health and thus provide false security? Many health professionals are aware of the classic situation of a person suffering a heart attack 2 weeks after a routine checkup and normal findings on ECG. The timing of some formerly accepted procedures is now being questioned. The annual Papanicolaou test for cervical cancer in women, once recommended yearly, now may be performed less frequently at the physician's discretion following three negative tests that are a year apart, unless the person has had intercourse at an early age or has multiple partners, which places the woman in a high-risk group (American Cancer Society, 1990). The annual routine physical examination is no longer recommended for all ages of adults (Breslow and Somers, 1977; Spitzer, 1979; Rose, 1980; Douglass, 1981).

The Lifetime Health Monitoring Program is one example of a positive approach to health assessment (Breslow and Somers, 1977; Somers, 1979). The Lifetime Health Monitoring Program defines a lifetime schedule of health care, organized into packages for 10 specific age levels. For each age group, the Lifetime Health Monitoring Program describes a set of health goals, health professional activities related to the goals, and steps of consumer participation. The Lifetime Health Monitoring Program focuses on *major risk factors specific for each age group* based on lifestyle, health needs, and problems. It moves away from an annual ritual and toward rational and varying periodicity. It includes

1. education and counseling in order to influence health-related behaviors,
2. specific testing procedures to screen early onset of disease, and
3. screening for specific risk factors associated with development of disease.

For example, an adult in Ellen K.'s age group (18 to 24 years old) would have these health goals: (1) to facilitate the transition from dependent adolescent to mature independent adult with maximum physical, mental, and emotional resources; (2) to achieve useful employment and maximum capacity for a healthy marriage, parenthood, and social relations. For preventive health care, Ellen would be recommended to have

1. at least once between the ages of 18 and 24: history and counseling on smoking, unwanted pregnancy, problem drinking, alcoholism, drug abuse, accidents, lack of exercise; eye screening for refractive errors; tetanus-diphtheria booster injection; urinalysis for diabetes, proteinuria, bacteriuria; Tb skin test; blood test for hematocrit, syphilis, serum cholesterol/triglyceride
2. every 2 to 4 years: history and weight assessment, and counseling for obesity
3. every 2 to 3 years: Papanicolaou's smear (assuming no special risk)
4. every 1 to 2 years: dental examination and cleaning; breast examination and counseling about self-examination (Somers, 1979)

Obviously, Ellen's individual health problems demand immediate intervention, and preclude a strict adherence to this preventive list.

ASSESSMENT THROUGHOUT THE LIFE CYCLE

It makes good sense to consider health assessment from a life cycle approach. First, the health professional must be familiar with the usual and expected developmental tasks for each age group (*see* Chapter 2). This alerts one to which physical, psychosocial, cognitive, and behavioral tasks are currently important for each person.

Next, once assessment skills are learned, they are more meaningful when considered from a developmental perspective. One's knowledge of communication skills and health history content is enhanced as one considers how they apply to individuals throughout the life cycle. The physical examination also is more relevant when one considers age-specific data about anatomy, method of examination, normal findings, and abnormal findings.

For each age group, a holistic approach to health assessment arises from an orientation toward wellness and health maintenance. One learns to capitalize on the person's strengths. What is the person already doing that promotes health? What other areas are ripe for health teaching so that the person can further build his or her potential for health?

This attention to life cycle and holism does not detract from the importance of assessment skills themselves. Assessment skills must be practiced and refined to a high level. Nurses no longer can fall back on other professionals for advice on certain findings. In many community settings, the nurse is the first and often the only health professional to see an individual. In the hospital, the nurse is the only health professional continually present at the bedside. Current efforts of cost containment result in a hospital population composed of people who have increased acuity, a shorter stay, and an earlier discharge than in the past. This situation requires faster, more efficient assessments from the nurse. Procedures that used to have a standard hospital stay of several days (e.g. surgery for inguinal hernia) now are done on an outpatient basis. As a result, nurses go to people's homes for follow-up assessment and diagnosis. These situations require first-rate assessment skills, grounded in a holistic approach, with knowledge of age-specific problems.

Bibliography

American Cancer Society: Cancer Facts & Figures—1990. Atlanta GA, American Cancer Society, 1990.

American Nurses' Association: Nursing—a social policy statement. Kansas City, MO, The Association, 1980.

American Nurses' Association: Standards of nursing practice. Kansas City, MO, The Association, 1985.

Andersen JE, Briggs LL: Nursing diagnosis: A study of quality and supportive evidence. Image 20(3):141–144, 1988.

Benner P: From Novice to Expert. Menlo Park, Addison-Wesley, 1984.

Brennan PR, Romano CA: Computers and nursing diagnosis: Issues in implementation. Nurs Clin North Am 22:935–941, 1987.

Breslow L, Somers A: The lifetime health monitoring program. N Engl J Med 296:601–608, 1977.

Dunn H: High-level wellness for man and society. Am J Public Health 49:786–792, 1959.

Dunn H: High Level Wellness. Thorofare, NJ, Charles B Slack, 1980.

Ekwo EE: An analysis of the problem-solving process of third-year medical students. *In* Proceedings of the 16th Annual Conference on Research in Medical Education. Washington, DC, Association of American Medical Colleges, 1977.

Elstein A, Kagan M, Shulman L, et al: Method and theory in the study of medical inquiry. J Med Educ 47:85, 1972.

Elstein A, Shulman L, Sparfka S. Medical Problem-Solving: An Analysis of Clinical Reasoning. Cambridge, Harvard University Press, 1978.

Feild L, Winslow E: Moving to a nursing model. Am J Nurs 85:1100–1101, 1985.

Field PA: The impact of nursing theory on the clinical decision making process. J Advanced Nurs 12:563–571, 1987.

Fitzmaurice JB: Nurses' use of cues in the clinical judgment of activity intolerance. *In* McLane AM (Ed): Classification of Nursing Diagnoses: Proceedings of the Seventh Conference. St. Louis, CV Mosby, 1987.

Gordon M: Implementation of nursing diagnoses: An overview. Nurs Clin North Am 22:875–879, Dec 1987.

Gordon M: Nursing Diagnosis—Process and Application. New York: McGraw-Hill, 1986.

Gruber M, Benner P: The power of certainty. Am J Nursing 89(4):502–503, 1989.

Guzzetta CE, Bunton SD, Prinkey LA, et al. Unitary person assessment tool: Easing problems with nursing diagnoses. Focus Crit Care 15:12, 1988.

Guzzetta CE, Bunton SD, Prinkey LA, et al. Clinical Assessment Tools for Use with Nursing Diagnoses. St. Louis, CV Mosby, 1989.

Guzzetta CE, Dossey BM: Nursing diagnosis: Framework, process, and problems. Heart Lung 12(3):281–291, 1983.

Guzzetta CE, Kinney MR: Mastering the transition from medical to nursing diagnosis. Prog Cardiovasc Nurs 1:41, 1986.

Herberg P: Theoretical foundations of transcultural nursing. *In* Boyle JS, Andrews, MM (Eds): Transcultural Concepts in Nursing Care. Glenview, IL, Scott, Foresman and Company, 1989, pp 3–65.

Kassirer JP, Gorry GA: Clinical problem-solving: A behavioral analysis. Ann Intern Med 89:245–255, 1978.

Kluckhohn F, Strodtbeck O: Variations in Value Orientations. Evanston, IL, Row, Peterson & Company, 1961.

Lee HA, Frenn MD: The use of nursing diagnoses for health promotion in community practice. Nurs Clin North Am 22(4):981–986, 1987.

Leininger M: Transcultural Nursing: Concepts, Theories, and Practice. 2nd ed. New York, John Wiley & Sons, 1988.

Neufeld VR, Norman GR, Feightner JW, Barrows HS: Clinical problem-solving by medical students: A cross-sectional and longitudinal analysis. Med Educ 15:315, 1981.

North American Nursing Diagnosis Association: 21 New diagnoses and a Taxonomy. Am J Nursing 82(12):1414–1415, 1986.

Orem DE: Nursing: Concepts of Practice. 3rd ed. New York: McGraw-Hill, 1985.

Pender N: Health Promotion in Nursing Practice. 2nd ed. Norwalk, CT, Appleton & Lange, 1987.

Putzier DJ, Padrick K, Westfall UE, Tanner CA. Diagnostic reasoning in critical care nursing. Heart Lung 14(5):430–437, 1985.

Redeker NS: Health beliefs and adherence in chronic illness. Image 20(1):31–35, 1988.

Rew L: Intuition in decision-making. Image 20(3):150–154, 1988.

Rose S: The periodic health examination. Primary Care 7:653–665, 1980.

Roy C: Introduction to Nursing: An Adaptation Model. 2nd ed. Englewood Cliffs, NJ, Prentice-Hall, 1984.

Somers A: Lifetime health monitoring—preventive care for the child in utero. Patient Care 13(3):162–178, 1979.

Somers A: Lifetime health monitoring—preventive care—age 1 through adolescence. Patient Care 13(8):201–216, 1979.

Somers A: Lifetime health monitoring—a whole life plan for well patient care. Patient Care 13(11):83–153, 1979.

Spitzer W, Bayne J, Charron KC, et al. The periodic health examination—Canadian task force. CMA J 121:1193–1246, 1979.

Tanner C: Curriculum revolution: The practice mandate. Nursing Health Care 9:427–430, 1988.

Thiele JE, et al. An investigation of decision theory: What are the effects of teaching cue recognition? J Nurs Educ 25(8):319–324, 1986.

Travis JW, Ryan RS: Wellness Workbook. 2nd ed. Berkeley, CA, Ten Speed, 1986.

Westfall UF, Tanner CA, Putzier D, Padrick KP. Activating clinical inferences: A component of diagnostic reasoning in nursing. Res Nurs Health 9:269–277, 1986.

Wirth L: The problem of minority groups. *In* Linton R (Ed): The Science of Man in the World. New York, Columbia University Press, 1945, pp 347–372.

Yura H, Walsh MB: The Nursing Process. 5th ed. New York, Appleton & Lange, 1988.

CHAPTER

2 Developmental Tasks Across the Life Cycle

Much of this book details the method of collecting subjective and objective data about a person in order to construct a data base. The data base is used to assess the health state, to applaud health strengths and assets, and to uncover, diagnose, and treat health problems. In order to fit this data base into a meaningful frame, one must consider the developmental stage of that individual at that particular time. Appraising the life tasks that currently absorb the individual lets one appreciate the holistic frame of reference.

Consider a 66-year-old man who seeks health care for recurrent early morning insomnia: He falls asleep easily at night but awakens around 3:00 AM and spends hours staring out from his armchair. Among the data revealed in the interview is that 7 months ago this man was forced to retire because of his age from a powerful position as sales director for an appliance firm. The diagnosis and treatment of this presenting symptom are affected by the knowledge that the suicide rate among forced retirees is 12 times greater than that for others in the same age group (Kanin, 1978). What interventions would one use had this same symptom been presented by a 38-year-old man who is considering whether to stay with his company or to set up his own business?

Growth is continuous and change is perpetual throughout the life cycle. A person progresses through a series of stages, not only in biologic growth but also in maturation of the physiologic systems, in cognitive development, and in personality development. During each of the stages, certain issues are dominant and consume more of the individual's attention and energy. The stages are not precisely distinct; there are transitions and there is overlap between stages.

How the stages are defined is the bailiwick of the developmental theorists. Only four major theorists are cited in the following sections; there are many more. The reader must refer to texts on personality development for a complete overview of the field. However, it helps the student of health assessment to consider a few of the major frameworks of developmental theory in order to construct a holistic view of health assessment.

THEORIES OF DEVELOPMENT

Cognitive Development

Jean Piaget (1896 to 1980) described stages of cognitive development in the growing child. Cognition is defined as how the individual perceives and processes information about the world; it is the ability to know. Piaget believed that a child's thinking develops progressively from simple reflex behavior into complex logical and abstract thought. This development is biologically inherent in each maturing child and occurs independently of any special training.

The child's cognitive development proceeds through four definite and sequential stages. Each stage demonstrates a *qualitative* change, representing a new way of thinking and behaving. Although the ages of reaching the stages are approximate, the sequence of stages never varies. All children move through the same stages in the same order; no stage is skipped. Each stage is the foundation for the next, and the next stage builds on the stage before it. At each stage, the child's *scheme* (how the child views the world) becomes more intricate and complex. The stages are highlighted here and are expanded in the life cycle portraits to follow.

Sensorimotor Skills (Birth to 2 Years): The infant progresses from responding only through reflexes (crying, rooting, sucking, grasping) to associating symbols with people and events (to think).

Preoperational Skills (2 to 7 Years): The child is highly egocentric, able to view world *only* from his or her own perspective. Thinking is concrete and literal. The child grows in the use of symbols (words) to represent people, objects, and actions in environment.

Concrete Operations (7 to 11 Years): The child is now able to consider others' points of view. Thinking is more logical and systematic. The child is able to reason and understand and is beginning to understand and use concepts and to understand conservation of matter.

Formal Operations (12 or 15 to Adulthood): The child is now able to think in abstract terms, deal with hypothetical situations, and make logical conclusions from reviewing evidence.

Psychoanalytic Theory

Sigmund Freud (1856 to 1939) was an early and long-dominant theorist in the field of personality development. He believed that people experience conflict between their natural instincts and society's restrictions on them. The type of conflict that an individual undergoes is specific to the person's current developmental stage. All people progress through these sequential stages of *psychosexual* development. How the conflict is experienced in the childhood stages has a profound influence on the individual's adult personality. Freud believed that infants and children experience sexual and aggressive drives. Thus, his earlier stages are named for the body areas in which these drives are focused and that are the primary source of gratification.

Oral Stage (Birth to 18 Months): The mouth, lips, and tongue are the center of existence. Sucking and swallowing give pleasure and reduce tension.

Anal Stage (18 Months to 3 Years): The anus is source of gratification. Control of urination and defecation (toilet training) is a source of conflict between child and parent.

Phallic Stage (3 to 5 or 6 Years): Genital stimulation is source of gratification. The conflict is sexual desire for the opposite-sex parent and rivalry and ambivalence toward the same-sex parent (Oedipus/Electra complex).

Latency (5 or 6 Years to Puberty): Oedipal/Electra complexes have been resolved, so this is a time of sexual dormancy. The child directs his or her energy to intellectual and physical quests and seeks pleasure from outside world through peer, school, and adult relationships.

Genital Stage (Puberty through Adulthood): Hormones stimulate sexual development. Sexual urges reawaken but now are directed toward socially acceptable heterosexual liaisons outside the family.

Freud's theory has had a vigorous and lasting impact on numerous scientific disciplines. However, some practitioners now view Freud's focus on resolving psychosexual conflict in order to have a healthy development to be somewhat narrow and limited. Also, Freud's Victorian notions of women's limited potential seems patronizing and demeaning today (Papalia and Olds, 1987).

Stages of Ego Development

While Freud focused on the biologic determinants of behavior, Erik Erikson (b. 1902) included cultural and societal influences. Erikson is concerned with the growth of the *ego* and described eight stages of ego development that encompass the life span (Erikson, 1963).

Each stage is characterized by a distinct conflict, or *crisis,* relating to the person's physiologic maturation and to what society expects of a person at that age (Table 2–1). Each crisis is a bipolar issue, a point at which personality development may go one way or another through the choices made by the individual. The bipolar aspect means the crisis can have a positive or a negative outcome. The crisis must be resolved in order to continue on to the next stage.

If the crisis is resolved in a positive way, the person has adapted and has a solid foundation to tackle and succeed at the next stage. If the resolution is negative,

Table 2–1 ▶ Erikson's Stages of Ego Development

STAGE	AGE	BIPOLAR CRISIS	SUCCESSFUL RESOLUTION	UNSUCCESSFUL RESOLUTION
1	Infancy (birth to 1 year)	Trust versus mistrust	Hope and drive	Fear
2	Early childhood (1 to 3 years)	Autonomy versus shame and doubt	Will power and self-control	Self-doubt
3	Early childhood (4 to 5 years)	Initiative versus guilt	Purpose and direction	Unworthiness
4	Middle childhood (6 to 11 years)	Industry versus inferiority	Competency and method	Incompetency
5	Adolescence (12 to 20 years)	Ego identity versus role confusion	Fidelity and devotion	Uncertainty
6	Early adulthood 20 to 24 years)	Intimacy versus isolation	Love and affiliation	Promiscuity
7	Middle adulthood (25 to 65 years)	Generativity versus stagnation	Care and production	Selfishness
8	Late adulthood (65 on)	Integrity versus despair	Wisdom and acceptance	Meaninglessness and despair

(Modified from Phares EJ: Introduction to Personality. Columbus, Charles E. Merrill, 1984.)

this will impede the person in resolving the next stage. But no outcome is *absolutely* positive or negative. Rather, healthy personality growth comes from a mixture of the two alternatives where the outcome tilts *more* toward the positive solution.

Erikson accepted Freud's idea of stages of personality development with a conflict in each stage, but there are important differences between the concepts of the two theorists. Erikson thought the conflicts had a broader *psychosocial* base rather than the limiting *psychosexual* interpretation of Freud. Also, Erikson expanded the number of stages to include developmental tasks through adolescence and adulthood. Now, however, Erikson is criticized for presenting the male life cycle as the adult life cycle (Sheehy, 1984).

Eras of Adult Development

After Erikson's early writing, little was added to the field of adult development. Daniel Levinson believes the study of adult development is still in its infancy (Levinson, 1986). Through his research Levinson believes that the life cycle progresses through a sequence of *eras* (Fig. 2-1). Each era has a distinct biopsychosocial character within the whole life. The eras are each about 25 years long and partly overlap. The overlap occurs during the cross-era *transition,* lasting about 5 years. The transition ends the existing life structure, clearing the way for a new one. The eras and transitions provide an order or general framework for assessing human development that crosses the boundaries of gender, culture, social class, and time in history and that allows for many variations in each individual (Levinson, 1986).

Childhood and Adolescence (Preadulthood, Birth to 22 Years)

During these formative years, a person lives in a family or its social equivalent. The family gives the support for the person to grow from a highly dependent being into an independent, responsible adult. This era has the most rapid biopsychosocial growth. During the first few years, the child learns the distinction between "me" and "not me," while separating biologically and psychologically from the mother. This is the first step in *individuation* (Levinson, 1986).

EARLY ADULT TRANSITION (17 TO 22 YEARS)

This is a developmental bridge between the closing of preadulthood and the dawning of early adulthood. A new step in individuation commences as the budding

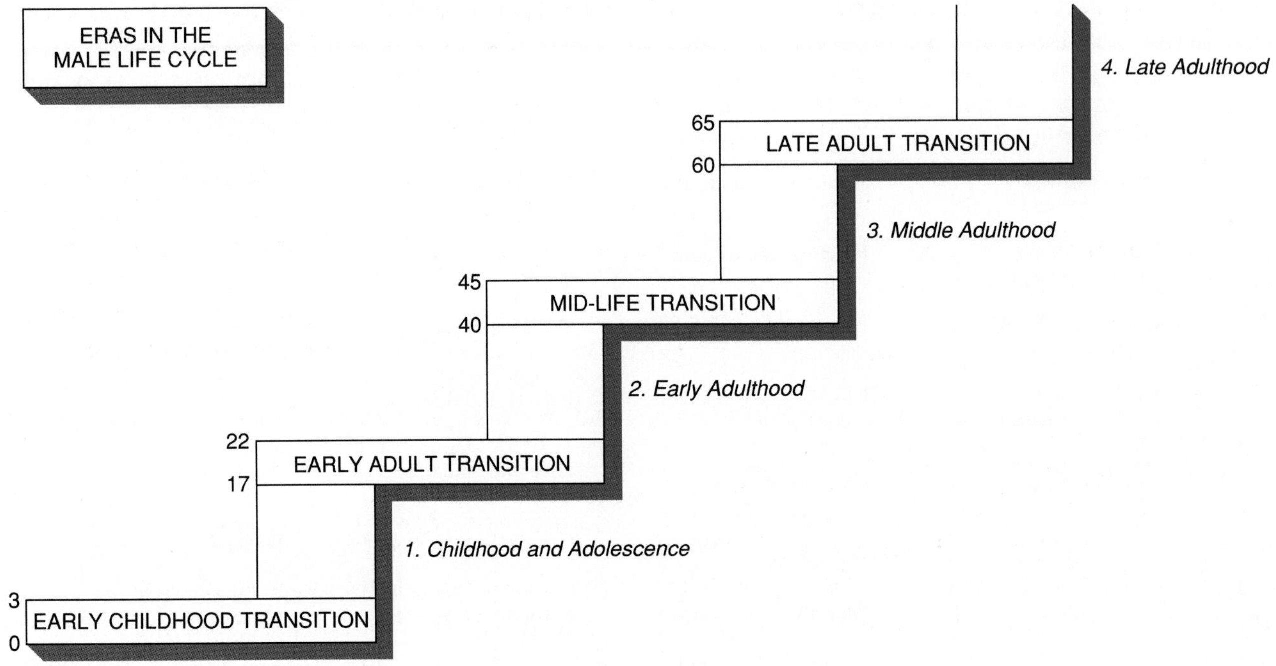

adult modifies his or her relationship with the family and takes a place in an adult world. The choices made now determine the initial adult role.

Early Adulthood (17 to 45 Years)

Levinson believes this is the most dramatic era because it juxtaposes a time of abundant energy and potential with a time of crushing external pressure. The 20s and 30s are a person's biologic peak in the life cycle. This surging energy feeds the drives of the pursuit of love, marriage, raising a family, starting an occupation, and finding a niche in society. Heavy stress results because these major events (e.g., starting a family and starting a career) occur simultaneously. The early adult makes important far-reaching choices (marriage partner, job, parenting, style of living) without the life experience or maturity that would help him or her choose wisely (Levinson, 1986).

MIDLIFE TRANSITION (40 TO 45 YEARS)

This is an important link that ends early adulthood while allowing the start of middle adulthood. The person questions the existing life structure by asking, "What have I done with my life? What do I really get from and give to my spouse, children, friends, work, community—and self?" (Levinson et al, 1986). The person questions nearly every aspect of life, a process that can involve great personal struggle.

People vary as to the extent they experience this transition as a crisis and as to how much they change as a result of it. Levinson believes that one developmental task that is accomplished during this period is a new step in individuation. A person can become "less tyrannized by inner conflicts and external demands" and can become "more compassionate, more reflective, . . . and more genuinely loving" of the self and others (Levinson, 1986). Without this change, a person can lead a trivial and stagnant life.

Middle Adulthood (40 to 65 Years)

Biologically, this person has passed the peak of early adulthood but has sufficient energy and stamina for an active and satisfying life. During the 40s and 50s, a person becomes a senior member of his or her own particular world. This means a person's occupation often has some managerial functions, and he or she is now responsible for others' work. Now viewed as a full generation above the younger worker, the middle adult helps those who are currently young adults (Levinson, 1986).

LATE ADULT TRANSITION (60 TO 65 YEARS)

During this transition, fundamental changes reshape the life structure. Physical stamina and capacity are somewhat decreased. An experience with serious illness or death of a loved one or colleague is a harbinger of one's own mortality. Often the prospect of entering the next era instills anxiety because society equates old age with negative connotations.

Late Adulthood (60 to 80 Years)

The focus of life shifts during late adulthood. The person must move off center stage, and relinquish power and authority to those who follow him or her. An important task to accomplish now is to strike a new balance between one's self and society (Levinson et al, 1986). Purpose and direction shift away from garnering recognition and rewards of society and toward pursuit of one's own inner resources.

Since much of one's life work has been attempted or accomplished, another important task is conducting a life appraisal. No one emerges from this appraisal satisfied that *all* of life's goals have been met. Each person experiences some moment of despair; by moving through this and reconciling the losses and achievements, the person builds a sense of integrity.

LATE LATE ADULTHOOD (80+ YEARS)

Since many people are living long lives, Levinson proposes a new era beginning around age 80. Biologically, the person has experienced numerous ailments and is likely to have chronic illness. Daily life often is preoccupied with the pursuit of physical comfort. Socially, the world has shrunk to a few significant relationships. This is the final period of making peace with one's self and the meaning of life, as well as dealing with the prospect of dying.

DEVELOPMENTAL STAGES

This section combines data from biologic growth and development and from the developmental theories to give a general portrayal of the individual in each stage of the life cycle. Each portrayal considers the physical, psychosocial, cognitive, and behavioral development of the person. Although they are not intended to be limiting, these portrayals offer a general framework. The stages are

1. Infancy (birth to 1 year),
2. Early childhood, toddler (1 to 3 years),
3. Early childhood, preschooler (3 to 6 years),
4. School child (6 to 10 or 12 years),
5. Preadolescent (10 to 12 years),
6. Adolescent (13 to 19 years),
7. Early adult (20 to 40 years),
8. Middle adult (40 to 60 years), and
9. Late adult (60+ years).

Infancy (Birth to 1 Year)

The first year is the most dramatic and rapid period of growth and development. The baby changes from a totally dependent being into a person who interacts with the environment, and forms close relationships with other people.

Physical Development

Growth. Weight, height, and head circumference reflect physical growth and are sensitive indicators of the infant's general health (See Chapter 8, General Assessment.)

The average normal term infant weighs 3.4 kg (7½ lbs) and is 50 cm (20 in) long. During the first few days, the baby loses a little weight but regains the birth weight by 10 days. Growth spurts double the birth weight by 4 to 6 months and triple the birth weight by 1 year. Length increases 50 percent by 1 year.

Head circumference reflects brain size; head growth shows brain growth. At birth, the average head circumference is 35 cm (13 ½ in). Most of the brain growth (90 percent) occurs during the first 2 years. Most infants have no teeth at birth. The first teeth erupt between 5 and 9 months. About six teeth erupt by 1 year, and usually all 20 deciduous teeth have erupted by age 2.

Physiologic Development. The development of each organ system through the life cycle is described in the corresponding physical examination chapter. But the central nervous system (CNS) is worth mentioning here because, during infancy, it makes the most dramatic gains. The tremendous brain growth that occurs during this period already has been mentioned. Also, the baby has numerous primitive reflexes that are present at birth or soon after and persist for specific time periods. These are under subcortical control; as the cerebral cortex grows and matures, it inhibits their expression. In a normal infant, these reflexes should disappear at specific times during the first year (see Chapter 20, Nervous System). Certain protective reflexes (cough, gag, sneeze, eye-blink) are always present. Visual acuity also develops rapidly during the first years—from 20/150 at birth to 20/40 by age 2.

Psychosocial Development

According to Freud, an infant's first year is considered the oral stage. The infant takes pleasure in rooting, sucking, and eating. After teething, additional oral gratification comes through biting. Throughout the oral stage, the erogenous zone is the mouth and lips; the infant derives pleasure from objects contacted there. Most sensory exploration of the world comes through the mouth. The nipple, thumb, fingers, toes, toys, anything that can be reached—it all goes into the mouth.

Erikson's Theory of Trust versus Mistrust. This stage corresponds to Freud's oral stage, but the focus broadens to a more psychosocial dimension. Erikson views the mother as the primary care giver. The crucial element in this stage, then, is the *quality* of the mother-child relationship. The infant is completely helpless and depends on the mother for food, warmth, comfort, and companionship. When the mother is responsive and consistent in her nurturing, the infant learns *trust.* The security from this trust extends to trust in others and in the self. The infant learns the world is a safe and reliable place and that he or she is welcome in it. If the mother is unresponsive, cold, haphazard, or abusing, the infant learns mistrust. Since the infant never feels secure, he or she experiences anxiety and alienation. Without a trusting foundation, this individual will flounder in attempts to resolve future crises.

Absolute trust actually is not the healthy goal of this conflict. When resolution of this crisis is successful, the infant holds *relatively* more trust than mistrust. Total trust would impede survival in later years, because not everyone or everything in the world *should* be trusted.

Cognitive Development

According to Piaget, the sensorimotor period (birth to 2 years) lasts longer than the first year of infancy. It is a time of intelligent activity, even though full language skill has not yet developed. Infants perceive information through the five senses and learn to modify their behavior in response to these environmental stimuli. At birth, the only response is an array of reflexes (crying, rooting, sucking, grasping) that occur automatically. Gradually, the infant learns the important concept of *object permanence,* that objects and people continue to exist even though they are no longer in sight. This starts around 7 months when the infant searches for an object that is partly hidden, but does not search for one completely out of sight. By 9 to 10 months, the infant looks behind a screen for an object, but only if it was seen to be hidden there. By 18 to 24 months, the concept is fully developed and the child conducts a true search in many places for objects hidden from sight. As this concept develops, the infant also learns that he or she is *separate* from objects in the environment.

Last, by age 2 the infant has acquired *mental representation* (or thought) and can think of an external event without actually experiencing it.

Behavioral Development

The behaviors discussed in the following sections develop concurrently, so the infant increasingly can respond to the environment (Whaley and Wong, 1990).

Gross Motor Skills. These skills include posture, head balance, sitting, crawling, and walking. Their development is predictable because it follows the direction of maturation in the nervous system; cephalocaudal (head-to-foot direction) and proximodistal (central-to-peripheral direction, or midline before extremities).

Table 2–2 provides a complete list of these milestones. Consider the following points as highlights. Some head balance already is present at birth for protection; when prone, the baby can turn the head to the side to avoid suffocation. Otherwise there is marked head lag, as when pulled to a sitting position from a lying position. By 3 months of age, the baby can raise the head *and* chest from a prone position with the arms extended for support. By 4 months of age, the head and chest are raised 90 degrees, and only slight head lag is demonstrated when the child is pulled to a sitting position. Sitting alone without support occurs at 6 to 7 months of age.

At 8 months, the baby ventures from the sitting position to explore the environment. Crawling usually begins around 9 to 10 months. At 9 months, the baby pulls to a stand and stands while holding onto an object for support. Between 9 and 11 months, the baby starts to "cruise" the room, walking upright while holding onto the furniture. Usually, the child can stand independently between 12 and 15 months, and the child walks alone.

Fine Motor Skills. The development of fine motor skills involves using the hands and fingers for *prehension,* or the act of grasping. The infant is born with a grasp reflex; it fades at 2 months of age and is absent at 3 months of age. At 3 months, it seems the infant wants to grasp objects, but expresses interest in an object more with the eyes than with the hands (Whaley and Wong, 1990). At 4 months, the infant seems to realize what hands are for: the child inspects his or her hands, looks from object to hands and back, and may try to grasp an object with the hands but overshoots the mark. The voluntary two-handed grasp is present at 5 months.

Further distal refinement follows at 8 to 10 months with a crude pincer grasp using the index, fourth, and fifth fingers. By 10 months, the index finger is in apposition with the thumb for a neat pincer grasp, and the baby is absorbed in picking up raisins and finger foods. By 11 months the baby puts objects into a container and removes them. And at 12 months the baby tries to build a tower of two blocks but fails.

Language Skills. Crying is the infant's first communication. It sounds all the same at first, but by 1 month of age, the crying is differentiated. That means the infant alters the pitch and intensity of the cry to communicate different needs, such as hunger, discomfort, or loneliness. Vocal sounds build rapidly; the baby laughs out loud at 3 months, coos when awakens or when someone talks to him or her at 4 months, and babbles at 4 months. At 9 to 10 months, the baby can imitate the sounds of others, although he or she may not necessarily understand them. At 12 months, a baby usually can say 2 to 3 words with meaning.

Personal-Social Skills. Throughout the first year, the infant learns more and more social ties that bind her or him to other people. Early on, the baby shows a visual preference for the human face, and at 1 week watches the mother intently. The social smile erupts at 6 to 8 weeks, to the family's delight and continual reinforcement. At 4 months, the baby laughs and enjoys other people, and at 6 months extends arms to the parent to be picked up. At 7 months, the baby imitates others' actions, at 9 months their sounds, and at 10 months waves bye-bye and enjoys interactive games like pat-a-cake and peek-a-boo. At 11 months, the baby can help with

Table 2-2 ▶ Summary of Infant Growth and Development

AGE (MOS)	PHYSICAL COMPETENCY	INTELLECTUAL COMPETENCY	EMOTIONAL-SOCIAL COMPETENCY
1 to 2	Holds head in alignment when prone; Moro reflex to loud sound; follows objects; smiles	Reflex activity; vowel sounds produced	Gratification through sucking and basic needs being promptly met; smiles at people
2 to 4	Turns back to side; raises head and chest 45–90 degrees off bed and supports weight on arms; reaches for objects; follows object through midline; drools; begins to localize sounds; prefers configuration of face	Reproduces behavior initially achieved by random activity; imitates behavior previously done. Visually studies objects; locates sounds; makes cooing sounds; does not look for objects removed from presence	Social responsiveness; awareness of those who are not primary care giver; smiles in response to familiar face
4 to 6	Birth weight doubled; teeth eruption may begin; sits with stable head and back control; rolls from abdomen to back; picks up object with palmar grasp	Some intentional actions; some sense of object permanence, looks on same path for vanished object; recognizes partially hidden objects; more systematic in imitative behavior; babbles	Prefers primary care giver; sucking needs decrease; laughs in pleasure
6 to 8	Turns back to stomach; sits alone; crawls; transfers objects hand to hand; turns to sound behind	Continued development as in 4 to 6 months	Differentiated response to nonprimary care takers; evidence of "stranger" or "separation" anxiety
8 to 10	Creeps; pulls to stand; pincer grasp	Actions more goal directed; able to solve simple problems by using previously mastered responses. Actively searches for an object that disappears	Attachment process complete
10 to 12	Birth weight tripled; cruises; stands by self; may use spoon	Begins to imitate behavior done before by others but not by self. Understands words being said; may say 1 to 4 words. Intentionality is present	Begins to explore and separate briefly from parent
	NUTRITION	**PLAY**	**SAFETY**
1 to 2	Breastfed or fortified formula	Variety of positions. Care taker should hold and talk to infant, large, brightly colored objects	Car carrier; proper use of infant seat
2 to 4	As for 1 to 2 months	Talk to and hold. Musical toys; rattle, mobile. Variety of objects of different color, size and texture; mirror, crib toys, variety of settings	Do not leave unattended on couch, bed, etc. Remove any small objects that infant could choke on
4 to 6	Introduction of solids; initial store of iron depleted	Talk to and hold. Provide open space to move and objects to grasp	Keep environment free of safety hazards; check toys for sharp edges and small pieces that might break
6 to 8	As for 4 to 6 months	Provide place to explore. Stack toys, blocks; nursery rhymes	Check infant's expanding environment for hazards
8 to 10	As for 4 to 6 months	Games: hide and seek, peek-a-boo, pat-a-cake, looking at pictures in a book	Keep: electrical outlets plugged, cords out of reach, stairs blocked, coffee and end tables cleared of hazards Do not leave alone in bathtub Keep poisons out of reach and locked up Continue use of safety seat in car
10 to 12	More solids than liquids; increasing use of cup; begin to wean	Increase space; read to infant. Name and point to body parts. Water; sand play; ball	As for 8 to 10 months

(Modified from Foster R, Hunsberger M, Anderson JJ: Family-Centered Nursing Care of Children. Philadelphia, WB Saunders, 1989, pp 222–223. Used with permission.)

feeding and dressing and follows simple directions. Emotions show at 12 months, and the baby will give a hug or kiss and show jealousy, fear, or anger.

Early Childhood (1 to 6 Years)

Toddler (1 to 3 Years)

With successful completion of first-year tasks, the child enters the second year secure in a basic sense of trust. That security plus maturing muscles and developing language enable the child to launch into the process of exploring the environment. The toddler explores everything, inhaling the world with the zeal of all first-time adventurers. Developmental tasks of this next stage include (Whaley and Wong, 1990)

1. differentiating self from others, particularly the mother,
2. tolerating separation from mother or parent,
3. withstanding delayed gratification,
4. controlling bodily functions,
5. acquiring socially acceptable behavior,
6. acquiring verbal communication, and
7. interacting with others in a less egocentric manner.

The child does not master all tasks during the toddler years, but a good foundation at this stage will facilitate successful completion of other tasks later (see Table 2–3).

PHYSICAL DEVELOPMENT

Growth. The rate of growth decelerates during the second year, with the child gaining an average of 2.5 kg (5½ lb) in body weight and 12 cm (4¾ in) in length. Parents are intrigued when told that the child's adult height will equal roughly 2 times what it is at 2 years.

Appearance. Toddler lordosis describes the normal upright posture of the toddler with the potbelly, sway back, and short, slightly bowed legs. The increase in head circumference slows, and the head circumference equals the chest circumference between 1 and 2 years. After the second year, the chest circumference exceeds individual head and abdominal measurements, and the extremities grow faster than the trunk.

Physiologic Systems. Maturation of the physiologic systems is detailed in the corresponding physical examination chapters. Some neurologic advances are cited now because they permit developmental changes during the toddler years. For example, most brain growth occurs during the first 2 years, and changes in certain cortical areas permit language and motor development. In the spinal cord, myelination is almost complete by age 2, matching the gross motor achievements in locomotion. Visual acuity is close to 20/40 at 2 years and close to 20/30 by 3. The maturing convergence-accommodation mechanism matches the toddler's fascination with minute objects.

PSYCHOSOCIAL DEVELOPMENT

Autonomy is the goal of all daily activities. The pursuit of independence occupies the toddler. For example, muscle maturation allows walking, exploring, and some self-care in feeding and dressing; refined visual acuity enhances close scrutiny and attention span; and language advances so the child can make known independent demands such as "me do," "mommy 'way," or "me out." Between 12 and 18 months, the toddler ventures away from the parent to explore the immediate environment, still using her or him as a home base to come back to for support. Practice builds confidence, which encourages more exploration. Between 18 months and 3 years, it occurs to the child that he or she really has become quite separate from the parent. This creates some anxiety, which is manifested in the negativism, or the "terrible twos" behavior, normally seen at this age.

Autonomy versus Shame and Doubt (1 to 3 Years). The quest for autonomy characterizes Erikson's second stage. The toddler wants to be autonomous and to govern his or her own body and experiences. The child wants to apply newly attained skills to explore the world. However, the child has not yet attained any sense of discrimination or judgment. The parent lives in the balance of letting the child explore but also firmly protecting the child from experiences that are dangerous or frustrating for the child's current ability level.

Erikson believes toilet training symbolizes this stage. The toddler's muscle maturation has progressed to the "holding on" and "letting go" of things; this naturally extends to the sphincter muscles.

Freud's Anal Stage (18 Months to 3 Years). This corresponds to Erikson's Stage 2. From a psychosexual perspective, the anal stage centers on the buildup and release of tension at the orifices. The child experiences pleasure from expelling urine and, especially, feces. However society, in the form of the parents, insists that

Table 2-3 ▶ Summary of Toddler Growth and Development and Health Maintenance

AGE	PHYSICAL COMPETENCY	INTELLECTUAL COMPETENCY	EMOTIONAL-SOCIAL COMPETENCY
General: 1 to 3 yrs	Gains 5 kg (11 lb). Grows 20.3 cm (8 in). 12 teeth erupt. Nutritional requirements: Energy 100 Kcal/kg/day Fluid 115–125 ml/kg/day Protein 1.8 gm/kg/day See Chapter 6 for vitamins and minerals.	Learns by exploring and experimenting. Learns by imitating. Progresses from a vocabulary of three to four words at 12 months to about 900 words at 36 months.	Central crisis: to gain a sense of autonomy versus doubt and shame. Demonstrates independent behaviors. Exhibits attachment behavior strongly and regularly until third birthday. Fears persist of strange people, objects, and places and of aloneness and being abandoned. Egocentric in play (parallel play). Imitation of parents in household tasks and activities of daily living.
15 mos	Legs appear bowed. Walks alone, climbs, slides downstairs backwards. Stacks two blocks. Scribbles spontaneously. Grasps spoon but rotates it, holds cup with both hands. Takes off socks and shoes.	Trial and error method of learning. Experiments to see what will happen. Says at least three words. Uses expressive jargon.	Shows independence by trying to feed self and helps in undressing.
18 mos	Runs but still falls. Walks upstairs with help. Slides downstairs backwards. Stacks three to four blocks. Clumsily throws a ball. Unzips a large zipper. Takes off simple garments.	Begins to retain a mental image of an absent object. Concept of object permanence fully develops. Has vocabulary of 10 or more words. Holophrastic speech (one word used to communicate whole ideas)	Fears the water. Temper tantrums may begin. Negativism and dawdling predominate. Bedtime rituals begin. Awareness of gender identity begins. Helps with undressing.
24 mos	Runs quickly and with fewer falls. Pulls toys and walks sideways. Walks downstairs hanging on a rail (does not alternate feet). Stacks six blocks. Turns pages of a book. Imitates vertical and circular strokes. Uses spoon with little spilling. Can feed self. Puts on simple garments. Can turn door knobs.	Enters into preconceptual phase of preoperational period: Symbolic thinking and symbolic play. Egocentric thinking, imagination and pretending are common. Has vocabulary of about 300 words. Uses two-word sentences (telegraphic speech). Engages in monologue.	Fears the dark and animals. Temper tantrums may continue. Negativism and dawdling continue. Bedtime rituals continue. Sleep resisted overtly. Usually shows readiness to begin bowel and bladder control. Explores genitalia. Brushes teeth with help. Helps with dressing and undressing.
36 mos	Has set of deciduous teeth at about 30 months. Walks downstairs alternating feet. Rides tricycle. Walks with balance and runs well. Stacks eight to ten blocks. Can pour from a pitcher. Feeds self completely. Dresses self almost completely (does not know front from back). Cannot tie shoes.	Preconceptual phase of preoperational period as for 24 months. Uses around 900 words. Constructs complete sentences and uses all parts of speech.	Temper tantrums subside. Negativism and dawdling subside. Bedtime rituals subside. Self-care in feeding, elimination and dressing enhances self-esteem.

urinating and defecating occur at the proper time and in the proper location. Toilet training is an act of socialization. The child must learn self-control and delayed gratification to be welcome in society. How the parents approach the issue of toilet training and how the child reacts to it have great influence, Freud believed, on the adult personality.

COGNITIVE DEVELOPMENT

During the second year, the toddler is still considered to be in Piaget's sensorimotor period. The readiness for independence is demonstrated between 12 and 18 months as the child now tries out new activities and new experiments to reach a goal. To reach a desired toy in her toybox, a girl at this age may try the various routes of taking out each object one by one, overturning the box and dumping the contents out, or climbing into the box herself. Learning comes by trial and error.

Between 18 and 24 months, the child develops *mental representation* for external events. This is a major achievement because the toddler can *think* through plans to reach a goal rather than merely perform them and observe the results.

Table 2-3 ▶ Summary of Toddler Growth and Development and Health Maintenance *Continued*

	NUTRITION	PLAY	SAFETY
General: 1 to 3 yrs	Milk 16–24 oz. Appetite decreases. Wants to feed self. Has food jags. Never force food; give nutritious snacks. Give iron and vitamin supplementation only if poor intake.	Books at all ages. Needs physical and quiet activities, does not need expensive toys.	Never leave alone in tub. Keep poisons, including detergents and cleaning products, out of reach. Use car seat. Have ipecac in house.
15 mos	Vulnerable to iron deficiency anemia. Give table foods except for tough meat and hard vegetables. Wants to feed self.	Stuffed animals, dolls, music toys. Peek-a-boo, hide and seek. Water and sand play. Stacking toys. Roll ball on floor. Push toys on floor. Read to toddler.	Keep small items off floor (pins, buttons, clips). Child may choke on hard food. Cords and tablecloths are a danger. Keep electrical outlets plugged and poisons locked away. Risk of kitchen accidents with toddler under foot.
18 mos	Negativism may interfere with eating. Encourage self-feeding. Is easily distracted while eating. May play with food. High activity level interferes with eating.	Rocking horse. Nesting toys. Shape-sorting cube. Pencil or crayon. Pull toys. Four-wheeled toy to ride. Throw ball. Running and chasing games. Rough-housing. Puzzles. Blocks. Hammer and peg board.	Falls: from riding toy; in bathtub; from running too fast. Climbs up to get dangerous objects. Keep dangerous things out of wastebasket.
24 mos	Requests certain foods; therefore snacks should be controlled. Imitates eating habits of others. May still play with food and especially with utensils and dish (pouring, stacking).	Clay and Play-Doh. Finger paint. Brush paint. Record player with record and story book and songs to sing along. Toys to take apart. Toy tea sets. Puppets. Puzzles.	May fall from outdoor large play equipment. Can reach farther than expected (knives, razors, and matches must be kept out of reach).
36 mos	Sits in booster seat rather than high chair. Verbal about likes and dislikes.	Likes playing with other children, building toys, drawing and painting, doing puzzles. Imitation household objects for doll play. Nurse and doctor kits. Carpenter kits.	Protect from: turning on hot water; falling from tricycle; striking matches.

(From Foster R, Hunsberger M., Anderson, JJ: Family-Centered Nursing Care of Children. Philadelphia, WB Saunders, pp 262–263. Used with permission.)

The concept of *object permanence* now is fully developed. The toddler comprehends both visible and invisible *displacements.* That means the child can search for an object in several places, even though it was not seen as it was hidden.

Around age 2, Piaget's *pre-operational* stage begins. This use of symbols to represent objects and experiences is discussed in the next section on preschoolers.

BEHAVIORAL DEVELOPMENT

Gross Motor Skills. Locomotion advances as the toddler usually walks alone at 15 months, runs stiffly at 18 months, and runs well without falling at 2 years. At 2 years, the child also can walk up and down stairs. The child jumps with both feet by 2 ½ years.

Fine Motor Skills. Fine motor development shows increasing manual dexterity. At 15 months, the child can drop a pellet into a narrow-neck container, and can hurl and retrieve objects. Fifteen-month-old hands hold a pencil and make scribbles, whereas by 2 years, the child can reproduce a vertical line from a demonstration.

Language Skills. Language progresses from a vocabulary of about four words at 1 year to hundreds of words by 3 years. At 1 year, sentences begin with the one-word *holophrase,* in which one word represents a complete thought, e.g., "out" for "I want to go out." A 2-year-old uses simple two-word phrases—"all gone," "me up," "baby crying." This is called *telegraphic speech,* which is usually a combination of a noun and a verb and includes only words that have concrete meaning. Interest in language is high during the second year, and a 2-year-old seems to understand all that is said to him or her. A 3-year-old uses more complex sentences with more parts of speech.

Personal-Social Skills. Parents often are surprised at the swift transformation of their loving affectionate child into a determined tyrant who exhibits tantrums. Toddlers want their parents' approval but also want to assert themselves and do as many things for themselves as they can. As they test their powers, they sometimes clash with parents' restrictions, and a battle of wills results. "No" seems to be their favorite word.

This *negativism* is a normal part of the quest for autonomy. Although they protest vigorously, toddlers seem to fare better with firm, consistent limits. The thought of a limitless world and of personal untested powers is disabling to the child. Knowing where they stand, even if they disagree, is reassuring to toddlers.

Ritualism emerges along with the negativity. A 2-year-old wants things done in the same way; any change in schedule or habit is upsetting. A consistent routine lets the child feel in control. Ritualism is heightened at age 2½, especially at bedtime, when the child insists on the same order of night-time tasks, or the same order of colored blankets on the bed.

Another mark of the toddler's sensitivity to change is *global thinking.* A change in one small part (such as a minor shift in the room arrangement) changes the whole environment, and the 2-year-old child's equanimity disintegrates.

Although attachment to the parent is still strong, the toddler begins to play alone. Children 1 and 2 years of age venture away to explore, but still need the reassurance of the parent's being there. Play with peers can be comical to the observer. Toddlers engage in "parallel play," i.e., playing the same thing side by side without interaction. The two children seemingly ignore each other yet unobtrusively check the other out to note what is happening. Imitation in play is apparent, especially imitation of parent activities such as sweeping, lawn mowing, or cooking. As the toddler is increasingly able to form mental images, play reveals increased imagination.

Preschool (3 to 5 or 6 Years)

Successful mastery of the toddler tasks plus a highly energized state make the preschooler ready for this time of developing initiative and purpose. Although parental relationships are still the most important, the preschooler begins to turn to other children and adults to broaden learning and play (see Table 2–4). Tasks during this period include

1. realizing separateness as an individual,
2. identifying sex role and its functions,
3. developing a conscience,
4. developing a sense of initiative,
5. interacting with others in socially acceptable ways,
6. learning to use language for social interaction, and
7. developing readiness for school.

PHYSICAL DEVELOPMENT

The rate of growth continues to slow, and the average child gains about 2 kg (4½ lb) in weight and 7 cm (2¾ in) in height per year. The appearance changes as the "baby face" matures, the potbelly slims, and the legs elongate more than the trunk does. The preschooler looks taller, slimmer, and more graceful.

Most physiologic systems are now mature, but the musculoskeletal system is still developing. Muscles are growing and cartilage is changing to bone at a faster rate than before. Nutrition is crucial for bone growth. A serious nutrient loss at this age alters the shape, thickness, and growth of bones.

PSYCHOSOCIAL DEVELOPMENT

Although still primarily egocentric, the preschooler now broadens the scope to include some awareness of other people's interests, needs, and values. As this happens, the *conscience* or superego develops. The child learns right from wrong and their corresponding rewards and punishments.

Identifying the Sex Role—Freud's Phallic Stage. As children become aware of their separateness, they also learn that they belong to a further differentiated category—male or female. They are learning *gender,* or how males and females *do* differ. At this time, Freud believed that children have a romantic attraction to the parent of the opposite sex. This makes them rivals with their same-sex parent, which produces guilt and fear. Realizing the futility of competing with a bigger and more powerful rival, children resolve their fear by identifying with the same-sex parent. They repress sexual urges and imitate the sex-related behaviors, attitudes, and beliefs of the parent of the same sex.

This imitation is *sex typing,* or how society says males and females *should* differ. Children learn the behaviors and attitudes that their culture says are right for a man or a woman. Probably the parents have the greatest influence in sex typing, as is seen, for example, as a preschool girl imitates words and actions she has observed in her mother. But her social circle is enlarging, and the girl picks up messages from peers, teachers, books, and television about how girls and boys should differ.

Learning is from a broader scope, though, than with learning the appropriate sex role. As the girl mentioned earlier identifies with her mother, she assimilates and internalizes her ideals and values. She learns the standards of society presented to her by the words and deeds of the mother. This is the development of the conscience, which now will direct her behavior.

Initiative versus Guilt (4 to 5 Years). This stage corresponds to Freud's phallic stage, although Erikson's interpretation is broader. Erikson believes the child's chief task is to develop a sense of initiative. With increasing locomotor and mental power, the child now has an energy surplus, resulting in determination and enterprise. The child plans and attacks a new task with gusto and wants to stay with it. Any failures are easily forgotten in the quest to test the world. When the parent encourages, reassures, and cheers the child on (while protecting him or her from harm), the child learns self-assertion, spontaneity, self-sufficiency, direction, and purpose. But if the parent ridicules, punishes, or prevents the child from following through on tasks that could be done, the child feels guilty. The guilt exists not only when the child acts inappropriately but occurs even when thinking of goals he or she would like to accomplish.

COGNITIVE DEVELOPMENT

Piaget's *preoperational* stage covers age 2 to 7 years, a longer span than the preschool years. It is characterized by *symbolic function,* because the child now uses symbols to represent people, objects, and events. This process is liberating. Now the child can conjure up thoughts of the father, for example, without actually seeing him or hearing his voice. The symbolic function is revealed in child's play, as in *delayed imitation.* That means a child can witness an event, form a mental representation of it, and imitate it later in the absence of the model. For example, a little boy watches his father dress and leave for work, then later in the day the boy wraps a tie around his neck, packs his "suitcase," and heads for the door.

Although representational thought is a great milestone, the preschooler's thinking continues to be limited. The preschooler focuses on only one aspect of a situation at a time and ignores others, a characteristic known as *centration.* For example, given a pile of blocks, a preschooler will sort by color (red, blue, yellow), or by shape (square, triangle, circle), but not by both. Also, a preschooler is *egocentric.* This child cannot see another's point of view and feels no need to elaborate his or her own point of view, because the child assumes everyone else sees things as he or she does.

Further, the preoperational child uses *transductive reasoning.* When two events occur simultaneously, the preoperational child thinks one *caused* the other, even though they are unrelated. Because of this, the child thinks his or her thoughts are all-powerful. For example, on the same day a little girl breaks a dish, she is taken to a health care facility for a checkup. If this visit involves some pain (as with an injection or a blood test), she assumes it is punishment for her "bad" behavior. Since adults find this thinking so absurd, they often underestimate its seriousness to an egocentric preschooler.

BEHAVIORAL DEVELOPMENT

Motor Skills. The physical bumbling of the toddler fades and the preschool child demonstrates admirable gross motor and fine motor control. A 4-year-old child can hop on one foot. A 5-year-old child can skip on alternate feet and jump rope and has started to swim and skate. Girls often achieve fine motor milestones ahead of boys of the same age. A 3-year-old child can draw a circle; a 4-year-old child can cut on a line with scissors, draw a person, and make crude letters. A 5-year-old can string beads, control a crayon well, and copy a square and letters and numbers, and has demonstrated preference for the right or left hand.

Language Skills. During this stage, language develops from a primarily egocentric mode into the beginnings of a tool for social interaction. Between 3 and 4 years of age, the child uses three- to four-word *telegraphic* sentences containing only essential words. By 5 to 6 years, the sentences are six to eight words long and are fairly grammatical.

Piaget labels the earlier speech pattern as egocentric (Piaget, 1975). Children at this age talk incessantly. They are wrapped up in their own thoughts and talk to themselves merely for the pleasure of hearing their own voices say the words. Speech here is in the form of a *monologue* to the self, or a *collective monologue* between two children, in which they talk at each other but are still absorbed in themselves and no communication has occurred. Often this speech is functional for *wish fulfill-*

Table 2-4 ▶ Growth, Development, and Health Promotion for Preschoolers

AGE (YRS)	PHYSICAL COMPETENCY	INTELLECTUAL COMPETENCY	EMOTIONAL-SOCIAL COMPETENCY
General: 3 to 5	Gains 4.5 kg (10 lb) Grows 15 cm (6 in) 20 teeth present Nutritional requirements: Energy: 1250 to 1600 cal/day (or 90 to 100 Kcal/kg/day) Fluid: 100 to 125 ml/kg/day Protein: 30 g/day (or 3 g/kg/day) Iron: 10 mg/day	Becomes increasingly aware of self and others Vocabulary increases from 900 to 2100 words Plaget's preoperational/intuitive period	Freud's phallic stage Oedipus complex–boy Electra complex–girl Erikson's stage of Initiative vs. Guilt
3	Runs, stops suddenly Walks backward Climbs steps Jumps Pedals tricycle Undresses self Unbuttons front buttons Feeds self well	Knows own sex Desires to please Sense of humor Language—900 words Follows simple direction Uses plurals Names figure in picture Uses adjectives/adverbs	Shifts between reality and imagination Bedtime rituals Negativism decreases Animism and realism: anything that moves is alive
4	Runs well, skips clumsily Hops on one foot Heel-toe walks Up and down steps without holding rail Jumps well Dresses and undresses Buttons well, needs help with zippers, bows Brushes teeth Bathes self Draws with some form and meaning	More aware of others Uses alibis to excuse behavior Bossy Language—1500 words Talks in sentences Knows nursery rhymes Counts to 5 Highly imaginative Name calling	Focuses on present Egocentrism/unable to see the viewpoint of others, unable to understand another's inability to see own viewpoint Does not comprehend anticipatory explanation Sexual curiosity Oedipus complex Electra complex
5	Runs skillfully Jumps 3–4 steps Jumps rope, hops, skips Begins dance Roller skates Dresses without assistance Tie shoelaces Hits nail on head with hammer Draws person—6 parts Prints first name	Aware of cultural differences Knows name and address More independent More sensible/less imaginative Copies triangle, draws rectangle Knows four or more colors Language—2100 words, meaningful sentences Understands kinship Counts to 10	Continues in egocentrism Fantasy and daydreams Resolution of Oedipus/Electra complex, girls identify with mother, boys with father Body image and body boundary especially important in illness Shows tension in nail-biting, nose-picking, whining, snuffling

ment (Papalia and Olds, 1987). That is, if children cannot attain a goal, at least they can speak about it, and in that limited way, they can make it happen.

Socialized speech develops for communication. It happens when a child adapts speech to the words and behavior of a partner (Papalia and Olds, 1982). Between 5 and 6 years, the child is better able to note another's point of view and to share ideas. The development of socialized speech is important for upcoming school years.

Personal-Social Skills. The preschooler is self-assertive, but the negativism of the toddler years has diminished. This child wants to please others. By taking on the values of the family and developing a conscience, the child monitors his or her own behavior to maximize acceptance. The preschooler is proud of his or her self-sufficiency, and accomplishes everyday self-care (dressing, feeding, toileting) almost completely. The world enlarges because the child's anxiety toward strangers and fear of separation decreases; the preschooler is able to tolerate brief separations from the parents to enjoy visiting peers or preschool.

With their growing social regard, preschoolers enjoy *cooperative* play with each other. This means they play the same game and interact while doing it. The child's

Table 2-4 ▶ Growth, Development, and Health Promotion for Preschoolers *Continued*

	NUTRITION	PLAY	SAFETY
General: 3 to 5	Carbohydrate intake approximately 40 to 50 percent of calories Good food sources of essential vitamins and minerals Regular tooth brushing Parents are seen as examples; if parent won't eat it, child won't	Reading books is important at all ages Balance highly physical activities with quiet times Quiet rest period takes the place of nap time Provide sturdy play materials	Never leave alone in bath or swimming pool Keep poisons in locked cupboard; learn what household things are poisonous Use car seats and seatbelts Never leave child alone in car Remove doors from abandoned freezers and refrigerators
3	1250 cal/day Due to increased sex identity and imitation, copies parents at table and will eat what they eat Different colors and shapes of foods can increase interest	Participates in simple games Cooperates, takes turns Plays with group Uses scissors, paper Likes crayons, coloring books Enjoys being read to and "reading" Plays "dress-up" and "house" Likes fire engines	Teach safety habits early Let water out of bathtub; don't stand in tub Caution against climbing in unsafe areas, onto or under cars, unsafe buildings, drainage pipes Insist on seatbelts worn at all times in cars
4	Good nutrition 1400 cal/day Nutritious between-meal snacks essential Emphasis on quality not quantity of food eaten Mealtime should be enjoyable, not for criticism As dexterity improves, neatness increases	Longer attention span with group activities "Dress-up" with more dramatic play Draws, pounds, paints Likes to make paper chains, sewing cards Scrapbooks Likes being read to, records, and rhythmic play "Helps" adults	Teach to stay out of streets, alleys Continually teach safety; child understands Teach how to handle scissors Teach what are poisons and why to avoid Never allow child to stand in moving car
5	Good nutrition 1600 cal/day Encourage regular tooth brushing Encourage quiet time before meals Can learn to cut own meat Frequent illnesses from increased exposure increases nutritional needs	Plays with trucks, cars, soldiers, dolls Likes simple games with letters or numbers Much gross motor activity: water, mud, snow, leaves, rocks Matching picture games	Teach child how to cross streets safely Teach child not to speak to strangers or get into cars of strangers Insist on seatbelts Teach child to swim

(From Foster R, Hunsberger M, Anderson, JJ: Family-Centered Nursing Care of Children. Philadelphia, WB Saunders, 1989, pp 300–301. Used with permission.)

imagination runs rampant, and this factor shows in the play. Preschoolers love to dress up and imitate the sex role behaviors of their parents as well as admired adult models, such as nurses, doctors, media heroes, firefighters, or police officers. Often this make-believe or fantasy play is a coping strategy: a sheltered workshop in which the preschooler can work out conflicts and fears or master life experiences.

It is easy for fantasy and reality to blur. Children experience the greatest number of new fears between 2 and 6 years of age. Visions of ghosts and monsters, fear of the dark, fear of being lost — all arise from the child's increased imagination as well as some frightening experiences the child really has had. Also, beginning around age 2½ or 3 years, children often invent imaginary playmates. The imaginary friend often serves as an alter ego and tries out behaviors the child yearns to try or takes the blame when the child misbehaves. Although it is important for a time, the imaginary friend is easily given up when the child enters school.

Middle Childhood (School-Aged Child, 6 to 10 or 12 Years)

The best preparation for this age is a firm foundation in trust, autonomy, and initiative. Secure in these attributes, the child is able to move into a larger world and tackle these tasks:

1. mastering skills that will be needed later as an adult,
2. winning approval from other adults and peers,
3. building self-esteem and a positive self-concept,
4. taking a place in a peer group, and
5. adopting moral standards.

Physical Development

Physical growth is slow but steady during the school years (see Table 2–5). The average child gains about 3 kg (6½ lb) and grows about 5.5 cm (2 in) per year. The growth rates in boys and girls are basically the same, with boys only slightly heavier and taller than girls. Black children are slightly larger and Asian children slightly smaller than white children of the same age. The preadolescent growth spurt occurs earlier in girls, at about age 10 years, as compared with age 12 for boys.

The physical appearance of the school-aged child is relatively slimmer than that of the younger child because of the older child's proportionately longer legs, diminishing body fat, and a lower center of gravity. Although the cranium achieved most of its growth in the early years, now the bones of the face and jaw grow faster. During these years, primary teeth are lost, which the children hail as a big event and developmental milestone. The eruption of large permanent teeth into a mouth and face that looks too small for them gives this child the ungainly, so-called ugly duckling appearance.

Body carriage is more agile and graceful. Bones continue to ossify during these years, and bone replaces cartilage. Muscles are stronger and more developed though not yet fully mature. Neuromuscular control is more coordinated. All these refinements ready the school child for repetitive pursuit of activities requiring fine motor skills, such as writing, drawing, needlework, small model building, and playing instruments, and large muscle activities such as running, throwing, jumping, biking, and swimming.

Psychosocial Development

Freud used *latency* to describe the relative sexual quiet of the time of middle childhood (age 6 years to puberty). Middle childhood is an island of time between the more sexually turbulent preschool years and upcoming adolescence. Oedipal/Electra conflicts have been resolved, the child has settled into the appropriate sex role, and energy now is channeled into mastering skills in school, activities, hobbies, and sports. Latency does not mean an *absence* of sexuality during this time (Papalia and Olds, 1987). The school child will think and talk about sex with parents and peers, and considers sexual jokes and "bathroom humor" the height of hilarity.

Erikson highlights the directing of energy into learning skills when he characterizes middle childhood as a period focused on *industry versus inferiority*. In this stage, age 6 to 11 years, the child leaves home for school. Now, the approval and esteem of people outside the immediate family become important. The child wins this recognition by working and producing. Play and fantasy give way to mastering the skills the child will need later to compete in the adult world. This child values independence in tackling a new task and takes pleasure in carrying it through to completion. The young worker is eager, diligent, and absorbed. Also, the value of social relationships emerges as the child sees the benefits of working in an organized group. Children learn to divide labor and to cooperate to achieve a common goal.

Real achievement at this stage builds a feeling of confidence, competence, and industry. The child is rewarded by his or her own inner sense of satisfaction in achieving a skill, and more importantly at this age by external rewards such as approval from teachers, parents, and peers in the form of grades, allowance, or special gifts. Problems arise when the child feels inferior. If the child believes that he or she cannot measure up to society's expectations, the child loses confidence and does not take pleasure in the work. A gnawing feeling of inferiority and incompetence grows and will continue to haunt this child.

The reality is that no one can master everything. There is bound to be something at which each child will feel inferior. Caring parents and teachers will try to balance these weaker skills with areas in which the child can excel. The problem is that, in some cultures, success in certain areas has a higher social value, particularly among peers (Whaley and Wong, 1990). For example, in Western cultures, team sports are admired more than playing chess, or success in reading may be rewarded more than that in drawing. The challenge to adults is to provide the successful experiences and positive reinforcement so that each child can achieve.

At this age, peer approval is beginning to be significant. During middle childhood, it is important to belong to a peer group. The peer group is a key socializing agent. Group solidarity is enhanced by secret codes or strict rules. The child conforms to group rules because

Table 2-5 ▶ Competency Development of the School-Aged Child

AGE (YRS)	PHYSICAL COMPETENCY	INTELLECTUAL COMPETENCY	EMOTIONAL-SOCIAL COMPETENCY
General: 6 to 12	Gains an average of 2.5 to 3.2 kg/year (5½ to 7 lbs/year. Overall height gains of 5.5 cm (2 in) per year; growth occurs in spurts and is mainly in trunk and extremities. Loses deciduous teeth; most of permanent teeth erupt. Progressively more coordinated in both gross and fine motor skills. Caloric needs increase with growth spurts.	Masters concrete operations. Moves from egocentrism; learns he or she is not always right. Learns grammar and expression of emotions and thoughts. Vocabulary increases to 3000 words or more; handles complex sentences.	Central crisis: industry vs. inferiority; wants to do and make things. Progressive sex education needed. Wants to be like friends; competition important. Fears body mutilation, alterations in body image; earlier phobias may recur, nightmares; fears death. Nervous habits common.
6 to 7	Gross motor skill exceeds fine motor coordination. Balance and rhythm are good—runs, skips, jumps, climbs, gallops. Throws and catches ball. Dresses self with little or no help.	Vocabulary of 2500 words. Learning to read and print; beginning concrete concepts of numbers, general classification of items. Knows concepts of right and left; morning, afternoon, and evening; coinage. Intuitive thought process. Verbally aggressive, bossy, opinionated, argumentative. Likes simple games with basic rules.	Boisterous, outgoing, and a know-it-all, whiney; parents should sidestep power struggles, offer choices. Becomes quiet and reflective during seventh year; very sensitive. Can use telephone. Likes to make things: starts many, finishes few. Give some responsibility for household duties.
8 to 10	Myopia may appear. Secondary sex characteristics begin in girls. Hand-eye coordination and fine motor skills well established. Movements are graceful, coordinated. Cares for own physical needs completely. Constantly on move; plays and works hard; enforce balance in rest and activity.	Learning correct grammar and to express feelings in words. Likes books he or she can read alone; will read funny papers, scan newspaper. Enjoys making detailed drawings. Mastering classification, seriation, spatial and temporal, numerical concepts. Uses language as a tool; likes riddles, jokes, chants, word games. Rules guiding force in life now. Very interested in how things work, what and how weather, seasons, etc., are made.	Strong preference for same-sex peers; antagonizes opposite-sex peers. Self-assured and pragmatic at home; questions parental values and ideas. Has a strong sense of humor. Enjoys clubs, group projects, outings, large groups, camp. Modesty about own body increases over time; sex conscious. Works diligently to perfect skills he or she does best. Happy, cooperative, relaxed, and casual in relationships. Increasingly courteous and well-mannered with adults. Gang stage at a peak; secret codes and rituals prevail. Responds better to suggestion than dictatorial approach.
11 to 12	Vital signs approximate adult norms. Growth spurt for girls; inequalities between sexes are increasingly noticeable; boys greater physical strength. Eruption of permanent teeth complete except for third molars. Secondary sex characteristics begin in boys. Menstruation may begin.	Able to think about social problems and prejudices; sees others' points of view. Enjoys reading mysteries, love stories. Begins playing with abstract ideas. Interested in whys of health measures and understands human reproduction. Very moralistic; religious commitment often made during this time.	Intense team loyalty; boys begin teasing girls and girls flirt with boys for attention; best friend period. Wants unreasonable independence. Rebellious about routine; wide mood swings; needs some time daily for privacy. Very critical of own work. Hero worship prevails. "Facts of life" chats with friends prevail; masturbation increases. Appears under constant tension.
	NUTRITION	**PLAY**	**SAFETY**
General: 6 to 12	Fluctuations in appetite due to uneven growth pattern and tendency to get involved in activities. Tendency to neglect breakfast owing to rush of getting to school. Though school lunch is provided in most schools, child does not always eat it.	Plays in groups, mostly of same sex; "gang" activities predominate. Books for all ages. Bicycles important. Sports equipment. Cards, board and table games. Most of play is active games requiring little or no equipment.	Enforce continued use of safety belts during car travel. Bicycle safety must be taught and enforced. Teach safety related to hobbies, handicrafts, mechanical equipment.

Table continued on following page

Table 2-5 ▶ Competency Development of the School-Aged Child *Continued*

	NUTRITION	PLAY	SAFETY
6 to 7	Preschool food dislikes persist. Tendency for deficiencies in iron, vitamin A, and riboflavin. 100 ml/kg of water per day. 3 gm/kg protein daily.	Still enjoys dolls, cars and trucks. Plays well alone but enjoys small groups of both sexes; begins to prefer same sex peer during 7th year. Ready to learn how to ride a bicycle. Prefers imaginary, dramatic play with real costumes. Begins collecting for quantity, not quality. Enjoys active games such as hide-and-seek, tag, jumprope, roller skating, kickball. Ready for lessons in dancing, gymnastics, music. Restrict TV time to 1–2 hours/day.	Teach and reinforce traffic safety. Still needs adult supervision of play. Teach to avoid strangers, never take anything from strangers. Teach illness prevention and reinforce continued practice of other health habits. Restrict bicycle use to home ground; no traffic areas; teach bicycle safety. Teach about the harmful use of drugs, alcohol, smoking. Set a good example.
8 to 10	Needs about 2100 calories/day; nutritious snacks. Tends to be too busy to bother to eat. Tendency for deficiencies in calcium, iron, and thiamine. Problem of obesity may begin now. Good table manners. Able to help with food preparation.	Likes hiking, sports. Enjoys cooking, woodworking, crafts. Enjoys cards and table games. Likes radio and records. Begins qualitative collecting now. Continue restriction on TV time.	Stress safety with firearms. Keep them out of reach and allow use only with adult supervision. Know who the child's friends are; parents should still have some control over friend selection. Teach water safety; swimming should be supervised by an adult.
11 to 12	Males needs 2500 calories per day; female needs 2250 (70 cal/kg/day). 75 ml/kg of water per day. 2 gm/kg protein daily.	Enjoys projects and working with hands. Likes to do errands and jobs to earn money. Very involved in sports, dancing, talking on phone. Enjoys all aspects of acting and drama.	Continue monitoring friends; Stress bicycle safety on streets and in traffic.

(From Foster R, Hunsberger M, Anderson, JJ: Family-Centered Nursing Care of Children. Philadelphia, WB Saunders, 1989, pp 346–347. Used with permission.)

acceptance is paramount. The child begins to prefer peer group activities to activities with the parents.

Cognitive Development

Piaget labels the stage of middle childhood, age 7 to 11 years, as the period in which the child focuses on *concrete operations.* At this age, the child can use symbols (mental representations) of objects and events. This means a child can experience mentally what she or he would have had to do physically before. For example, in order to describe the classic hopscotch maneuvers to you, a girl now can articulate them ("first you hop on one foot . . .") rather than merely performing them.

Armed with the ability to use thinking to experience things or events, the school child can

- Use numbers. He or she has the combinational skill to add and subtract, multiply and divide.
- Read. By using printed symbols (words) for objects and events, the child can process a significant amount of information. Also, reading fosters independence in learning.
- Serialize. The child can order objects by an increasing or decreasing scale, such as according to number size (smallest to largest), or weight (lightest to heaviest).
- Classify. This is the ability to sort objects by something they have in common. It shows in the school-age child's penchant for collections: rocks, shells, novelty cards, cars, and dolls. A child spends many hours sorting the collections, and the logic of the classification system gets more complex as the child grows.
- Understand conservation principles. Understanding conservation of matter is the ability to tell the differ-

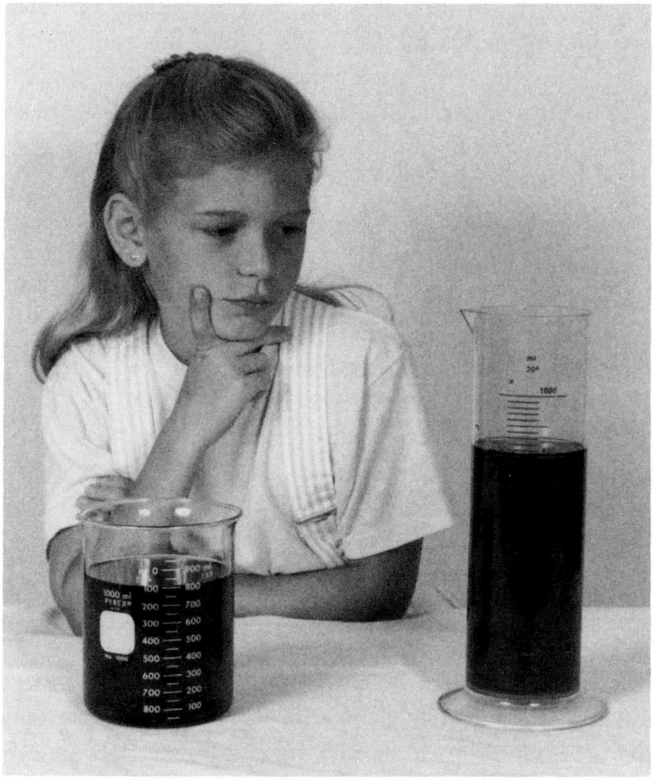

► **Figure 2-2**

ence between how things seem and how they really are. It is the ability to see that mass or quantity stays constant even though shape or position is transformed. For example the child who can conserve sees that two equal amounts of water remain the same even if one is poured into a different-shaped beaker (see Fig. 2-2).

At this age, thinking is more stable and logical. The school child can *decenter* and consider all sides of a situation to form a conclusion. The rigid egocentrism that characterized the early years is diminishing. The school-aged child knows that not everyone sees things as he or she does, and can begin to consider another's point of view. The school-aged child is able to reason, but this reasoning capacity still is limited because he or she cannot yet deal with abstract ideas.

Preadolescence (10 to 12 or 13 Years)

This period covers 5th to 8th grades, ending with puberty. Although this stage is still part of childhood, children in this group have common skills and interests that set them apart. It becomes more difficult now to typify characteristics of a single year. Because of rapid growth, the age levels start to blend and overlap. A child may be at one level physically and intellectually but at another level socially. Children of the same age show diverse development levels.

Physical Development

Physical growth is markedly different at this stage; boys show slow and steady growth, whereas girls have rapid growth. On the average, the growth spurt begins in girls at age 10 years and reaches its greatest velocity at 12, whereas in boys the growth spurt begins at 12 and attains its maximum velocity at 14 years.

Even among girls, growth is varied. In a group of 11-year-old girls, each girl looks different from the others. Some look like children, and some are starting to look like adolescents. At 11 years, some girls have begun their growth spurt and have begun to grow pubic hair and to have breast development. At age 12 years, girls demonstrate the most rapid growth in height and weight. The breasts enlarge, the areolae darken, growth of axillary hair begins, and menarche occurs.

Physical size among 11-year-old boys is fairly uniform. At 12 years, boys show a wider range of growth. Most demonstrate the onset of secondary sex characteristics with initial genital growth, appearance of pubic hair, and the occurrence of erections and nocturnal emissions.

Boys and girls both exhibit a great amount of physical restlessness. Their activity is well directed into individual and team sports. Their percolating energy makes it hard for them to sit still, and it shows by tapping the foot or drumming the finger.

Psychosocial Development

Parent-child ties exhibit some strain as the child gradually starts to drift away from the family. The parents continue to set standards and values, but the child begins to challenge authority and to reject their standards. Parents decrease in stature in the child's eyes as the child learns parents are not perfect and do not know everything. Yet the child loves the parents. He or she needs and wants some restrictions. Making up one's own rules is too frightening.

At 9 to 10 years, the child demonstrates a new ability to love by establishing a relationship with a best friend. This is important because the best friend is the first one outside the family the child loves as being as important as himself or herself. By sharing interests, goals, and secret ideas with the best friend, the child learns a lot about himself or herself. This is comforting because the child realizes he or she is not so different from other children after all. This yields a valuable lesson in self-acceptance (Murray and Zentner, 1989).

Preadolescents demonstrate social interest outside the family. There is strong identity with the peer group by clique or "gang" formation. Girls and boys stay within their own sex group. The gang has an exclusive membership, and one is privileged to belong. The code of the gang is more important than other outside rules or authority. The child merges his or her identity with that of the peer group. The child is substituting conformity with the family to that with the peers because he or she still is not socially stable enough to be independent (Whaley and Wong, 1990).

Despite the fact that peer groupings are composed of the same sex, some preadolescents show an emerging interest in the opposite sex, an interest that will flourish in adolescence.

Adolescence (12 or 13 to 19 Years)

This is a transition stage between childhood and adulthood. Beginning at puberty and extending through the teenage years, the most important task of adolescence is the search for identity, "who I really am" (see Table 2–6). With successful mastery of skills from the previous stage, childhood ends. Now, the adolescent must process the information from earlier stages and assume a personal identity that is more than just the sum of childhood experiences. The search for identity is the motive behind all the other tasks of the period

1. searching for one's identity,
2. appreciating one's achievements,
3. growing independent from parents,
4. forming close relationships with peers,
5. developing analytic thinking,
6. evolving one's own value system,
7. developing a sexual identity, and
8. choosing a career.

Physical Development

Adolescence begins with puberty. Puberty is a time of dramatic physiologic change. It includes the growth spurt—rapid growth in height, weight, and muscular development; development of primary and secondary sex characteristics; and maturation of the reproductive organs. In girls, puberty takes about 3 years, from age 10 to 11 years until about 14 years. Menarche occurs at 12 to 13 years on the average, just after the peak of growth velocity. In boys, puberty lasts about 4 years, from age

Table 2-6 ▶ Characteristics of Adolescents

EARLY ADOLESCENCE (12 TO 14 YR)	MIDDLE ADOLESCENCE (15 TO 16 YR)	LATE ADOLESCENCE (17 TO 21 YR)
Becomes comfortable with own body; egocentric Difficulty solving problems; thinks in present; cannot use past experience to control behavior; sense of invulnerability—society's rules do not apply to him or her Struggle between dependent and independent behavior; begins forming peer alliance Parent-child conflict begins; teen argues but without logic	"Tries out" adult-like behavior Begins to solve problems, analyze, and abstract Established peer group alliance with associated risk-taking behavior Peak turmoil in child-family relations; able to debate issues and use some logic but not continuously	Aware of own strengths and limitations; establishes own value system Able to verbalize conceptually: deals with abstract moral concepts; makes decisions re future Peer group diminishes in importance; may develop first intimate relationship Turbulence subsides. May move away from home. More adult-like friendship with parents

(From Foster R, Hunsberger M, Anderson, JJ: Family-Centered Nursing Care of Children. Philadelphia, WB Saunders, 1989, p 359. Used with permission.)

12 to 16 years. (See Chapters 14 and 21 for the developmental sequence of puberty.)

A changing body affects a person's self-concept. With bodies that are changing so rapidly, it is difficult for boys and girls to adjust. Their self-awareness peaks; they continually compare how their body looks with that of their peers and to some ideal standard of attractiveness. They are keenly attuned to the appearance of secondary sex characteristics but are embarrassed if these appear too early or too late. It is best when their own development parallels that of close friends and peers. Being an early maturer or, especially, a late maturer adds to normal self-doubts they experience.

Physical health is generally good. Childhood illnesses are behind them and the risks of adult illnesses have not occurred yet. What does place their health at risk are episodes of poor or immature judgment resulting in accidents, drug or alcohol abuse, sexually transmitted disease, and unwanted pregnancy. Psychologic dysfunction may occur, such as anorexia nervosa or depression. Suicide acts and attempts affect an increasing number of adolescents. Suicide is the second leading cause of death in this age group. Its incidence would probably be higher if more accidental deaths were investigated.

Psychosocial Development

Theoretical views of adolescence vary. Psychologist G. Stanley Hall (1916) saw adolescence as a transitional stage fraught with turbulence and vacillating emotions. He called it in German *Sturm und Drang,* or storm and stress. In contrast, anthropologists Ruth Benedict (1934) and Margaret Mead (1935, 1953, 1961) saw the importance of cultural influences on adolescence. They observed that in simpler societies in which the child had meaningful, responsible work to do and could see clearly the upcoming adult role, adolescence is smooth and serene.

Freud described the *genital stage* for adolescents. The sexual urges reawaken and can no longer be repressed as they were during latency. Now sexual gratification comes with finding a heterosexual partner in the more socially acceptable realm outside the family. Problems arise in cultures that have strong moral codes against intercourse between unmarried people, particularly adolescents. If the youth decides to conform to the rules prohibiting intercourse, he or she may use *sublimation.* Sublimation is a substitute way of expressing the sex drive. This is done indirectly through artistic or philanthropic activities such as writing poetry, singing, or caring for children or the handicapped (Thomas, 1985).

Erikson believes the main conflict of the fifth stage in his theory to be *ego identity versus role diffusion.* The adolescent is preoccupied with how he or she looks to others, and how that image fits with his or her own view of the self. If this process is successful, a sense of ego identity emerges, culminating in what Erikson terms a career choice. If unsuccessful, if the teen is unsure of his or her skills, self worth, or sexual identity, role confusion results and the adolescent cannot make a career choice. The adolescent feels cut adrift and experiences anxiety about being a social outcast.

Finding one's own identity is stressful. In the search for identity, teens often form cliques, wear fad clothing, and follow rock singers, movie stars, or charismatic heroes in an attempt to siphon identity from them. Falling in love also feeds the quest for personal identity; the teen projects his or her own ego qualities onto another person, and tries to understand them as they are reflected by the loved one.

Cognitive Development

Adolescence corresponds to Piaget's fourth stage in which the person focuses on *formal operations* and the ability to develop abstract thinking. Now, thinking is no longer confined to the concrete or the real but encompasses all that is possible. Abstract thinking is liberating. The adolescent is no longer limited to the present but can ponder the lessons of the past and the possibilities of the future. The adolescent now can analyze and use scientific reasoning. One can imagine hypotheses and then set up experiments to test them. One learns to use logic, and solves problems by methodically eliminating each possibility, one by one. This opens the doors to new academic achievements such as mastering advanced mathematical concepts, chemistry, physics, or logic.

This analytic thinking extends to values. Developing personal values is a part of the search for identity. The adolescent does not accept packaged values of parents or institutions but can reason through his or her inconsistencies and recognize injustices. The adolescent is sensitive to hypocrisy and notes when an adult professes a value (such as honesty) and then acts counter to it (such as cheating on income tax).

Behavioral Development

Socially, the adolescent is in limbo, because he or she rejects identity with the parents but is not yet sure of his or her own individual identity. The perfect solution to this dilemma is immersion in a peer group. Pressure to belong to a peer group intensifies at this age. The adolescent is influenced strongly by the group's norms for dress and behavior. By identifying with peers, the adolescent joins a sheltered workshop in which he or she feels safe and can experiment with various roles. Group members are allies in the universal goal of seeking freedom from parental domination.

Group identity means the adolescent spends more time away from home and the parents. Adolescents often feel ambivalent toward the parents. They desperately want to be independent from the parents but realize that economically, and even emotionally, this is impossible. Their stated desire to escape from parental dominance conceals their anxiety about leaving the "sanctuary of the family" (Gould, 1975). The conflict is exacerbated when the parents try to maintain rigid control and use the protective stance that worked before. Often, things go smoother when the parents are not as strict, allow privacy, respect the adolescent's budding identity, and above all, take the adolescent seriously.

Developing close friendships is important to personal identity. In preadolescence, the experience of the relationship with the best friend is valuable in teaching intimacy, trust, and regard for another person. These lessons become a link in the new quest of developing close relationships with the opposite sex. Finding a girlfriend or boyfriend enables the adolescent to learn his or her own sex role identity. In many settings, group dating (youth groups, teen dances) is the norm, at first. This decreases stress from paired dating. When adolescents do pair off, they usually have a monogamous relationship involving affection and fidelity.

Most adolescents worry that an occasional homosexual thought or act means they are homosexual. These adolescent experiences are very common and cannot turn a person into a permanent homosexual (Masters and Johnson, 1988). Of course, some adults do discover that they have a homosexual orientation and that this lifestyle feels natural for them.

The end of adolescence is more difficult to define. Some societies have recognized rites of passage, usually at puberty, when the young person earns a place in the adult world with its attendant responsibilities. But in complex Western societies, the adolescent remains dependent on the parents through the teen years and into the 20s for economic and educational reasons. This extends the period of adolescence. Consequently, the role is not well defined in our society, and this is a source of conflict.

Early Adulthood (20 to 45 Years)

The young adult is concerned with emancipation from his or her parents and building an independent lifestyle. The young adult has finished most formal schooling and is ready to embark on a chosen path. The tasks of this era include

1. growing independent from the parents' home and care,
2. establishing a career or vocation,
3. forming an intimate bond with another and choosing a mate,
4. learning to cooperate in a marriage relationship,
5. setting up and managing one's own household,
6. making friends and establishing a social group,
7. assuming civic responsibility and becoming a citizen in the community,
8. beginning a parenting role, and
9. forming a meaningful philosophy of life.

Physical and cognitive developments now are steady and do not affect the young adult as much as they have before. Rather, sociocultural factors and values buffet the novice adult.

Physical Development

By early adulthood, the body reaches its maximum potential for growth and development. All body systems now operate at peak efficiency. The young adult enjoys maximum muscle tone and coordination, a high energy level, and optimum mental power. This person exudes freshness and vitality.

Since growth is finished, nutritional needs depend on maintenance and repair requirements and on activity levels. If activity decreases from its level during adolescence, calories must be reduced. Sensible nutrition is a major problem for many adults, and this is not confined to persons with low-level incomes. The American diet has changed from one high in fruits, vegetables, and grain to one now high in sugar, salt, and fat. A sedentary lifestyle adds further problems. However, more adults are learning that frequent steady exercise maintains weight, muscle strength, and joint flexibility; builds heart and lung capacity; and reduces stress.

Cognitive Development

During adolescence, cognitive functioning reached the new level of formal operations, or the capacity for abstract thinking. This level continues, but the young adult's thinking is different from the adolescent's. The young adult is less egocentric now and operates in a more realistic and objective manner (Wadsworth, 1988). Now, the young adult is close to maximum ability to acquire and use knowledge. The potential for sophisticated problem-solving and creative thinking is at a new height.

Education continues through early adulthood, from formal courses in college and graduate schools to on-the-job training, military service, and continuing education classes. Usually, this education prepares the young adult to do some type of work. Work is an important factor in the young adult's life because it is tied closely with ego identity. A person with job satisfaction feels challenged, rewarded, and fulfilled. One who is frustrated with work feels bored and apathetic.

Psychosocial Development

Erikson's sixth stage covers the first years of early adulthood, from 20 to 24 years. He believes the major crisis to be resolved is that of *intimacy versus isolation.* Once self-identity is established after adolescence, it can be merged with another's in an intimate relationship. During the early 20s, the adult seeks the love, commitment, and intimacy of an intense lasting relationship. This mature relationship includes mutual trust, cooperation, sharing of feelings and goals, and complete acceptance of the other person. Although Erikson had a heterosexual union in mind, this intimacy could be satisfied through a homosexual relationship or through a bond with a cause or an institution.

Erikson believes that without a secure personal identity, a person cannot form a love relationship. The result is a person who is isolated, withdrawn, and lonely. This person may fill the void through numerous transient liaisons or promiscuity, but Erikson believes these experiences will be found to be shallow and the person will feel remote and alone.

Levinson's time frame of early adulthood is much broader than Erikson's. It encompasses 22 to 40 years, after the transition at age 17 to 22 years from the preadult era. Levinson believes an adult's life alternates between periods of *structure building,* in which a lifestyle is fashioned, and periods of *transition,* in which this lifestyle is evaluated, appraised, and modified.

The era of Early Adulthood has two structure-building periods. In the 20s (about 22 to 28 years), the novice adult establishes the "entry structure," a first provisional lifestyle linking him or her to adult society. He or she is building a home base. The first set of important choices are made during this time concerning a mate, friends, an occupation, values, and lifestyle. In making these choices, the person must juggle the conflicting drives of (1) *exploring* many possibilities and keeping options open on the one hand and (2) securing some *stability* on the other hand (Levinson et al, 1986). Others characterize the 20s as a time of advancing one's career (Sheehy, 1984), and choosing a pathway that at this time one believes to be the one true course in life, not wasting energy wondering if this general commitment is the right one (Gould, 1972).

The Age Thirty Transition, age 28 to 33 years, is a time of self-reflection. Questions asked include "Where am I going?" and "Why am I doing these things?" This is the first major reassessment in life. A person ponders aspects he or she wants to add, exclude, or modify in life. The person feels, "If there is anything I want to change I better start now, or it will be too late" (Levinson et al, 1986). Sometimes, this is easy and reaffirms what one was doing. But this self-questioning can reach crisis proportions if the person realizes the pathway carved out in the 20s does not fit as well as one thought it would and may even be intolerable. Should one now get married, change jobs, get divorced, have children, stay home, or go back to work?

According to Levinson, the rest of the 30s (33 to 40 years) is characterized by settling down. A person takes the reforms or the reaffirmations established during the transitional period of the 30s and fashions a culminating life structure, one that realizes his or her youthful aspirations. During these years, the adult strives to establish a niche in society and to build a better life in all the choice points. This person is building a nest, using deliberation and seeking order and stability. Sheehy (1984) describes this as the time to make a financial and emotional investment in a home, and to advance a career by striving for promotion or tenure.

Sometimes, the reforms include having children. Whether children are chosen now or when the couple is in their 20s, the addition of children brings a major readjustment to the couple's relationship. Roles are reshaped in the new family unit. The father is more involved in child care than he was in the past. Often, the mother's role includes a choice between full-time parenting or a return to employment outside the home. There are more women in the work force now. Though the opportunities are wider, the risk for stress exists because there are choices. The tension shifts from having no choice in a former traditional role to whether or not the right decision is being made now.

Middle Adulthood (40 to 65 Years)

At some point around or after age 40, the realization dawns and grows that life is half over. No longer does the dream of young adulthood seem fully attainable. To some, it seems there is more time to look back on than to see ahead. How the person deals with these feelings and builds a meaningful life structure is the task of middle adulthood. Its composite tasks include

1. accepting and adjusting to the physical changes of middle age,
2. reviewing and redirecting career goals,
3. achieving desired performance in career,
4. developing hobby and leisure activities,
5. adjusting to aging parents,
6. helping adolescent children in their search for identity,
7. accepting and relating to the spouse as a person, and
8. coping with an empty nest at home.

Physical Development

A look in the mirror brings rueful recognition of the beginning of aging effects on the body. The skin loses its taut surface and forms wrinkles around the eyes, mouth, and forehead. Some notice pouches under the eyes and sagging jowls. The hair thins a little, starts to lose pigment, and turns gray, and in men the hairline often recedes. An abdominal paunch grows from increased fat deposits and decreased physical activity. Internally, most organ systems hold constant, with some small decrease in respiratory capacity and cardiac function. Sensory function remains intact except for some visual changes, e.g., decreased accommodation for near vision, or presbyopia.

In the late 40s and early 50s, females experience the *menopause,* the decreasing frequency and finally the cessation of menstruation. This involves a decrease in the female hormones, estrogen and progesterone, which brings attendant symptoms such as atrophy of reproductive organs, vasomotor disturbances, and mood swings. (See Chapter 22.) Although men do not have such an abrupt halt to reproductive ability, they experience a decrease in the production of testosterone, which causes decreased sperm and semen production and less intense orgasms.

Middle-aged adults are suddenly aware of the occasional death of their peers. This is a rude reminder of their own mortality. The leading causes of death during middle adulthood are cardiovascular disease, cancer, and stroke. Morbidity also is increased, probably caused most often by obesity. Obesity is associated primarily with hypertension and also with cardiovascular disease, diabetes, and mobility dysfunction such as arthritis. Chronic smoking leads to health problems that arise for the first time in middle adulthood.

Cognitive Development

Intelligence levels remain generally constant during middle adulthood. Intelligence is further enhanced by the knowledge that comes with life experience, self-confidence, a sense of humor, and flexibility. The middle-aged adult is interested in how new knowledge is applied, not just in learning for learning's sake. Continuing education courses meet the need to keep knowledge current in occupational and personal interest areas. Many middle-aged adults are seeking college degrees for the first time or are pursuing advanced degrees.

Psychosocial Development

The era of middle adulthood is a clear example of the way developmental factors blend (Turner and Helms, 1987). Physical, personal, and social forces all interact at this time. How a person reacts to the physical cues of aging affects the personality and his or her self-perception. A success or disappointment in the career affects a person's self-image, stress level, and interpersonal relationships.

Erikson believes the most important task for personality development is resolution of the crisis of *generativity versus stagnation.* During the middle years, Erikson believes that adults have an urge to contribute to the next generation. This need can be fulfilled either by producing the next generation or by producing something to pass on to the next generation. Thus, middle-aged adults want to rear their own children or engage in other creative, socially useful work. The motivation is to create and/or nurture those who will follow.

The middle-aged adult needs to be needed, to leave something behind, to leave one's mark on the world.

Generativity is sharing, giving, contributing to the growth of others. If this need is not fulfilled, the adult stagnates. Stagnation means experiencing boredom and a sense of emptiness in life, which leads to being inactive, self-absorbed, self-indulgent, a chronic complainer.

Levinson (1986) describes the era of middle adulthood as beginning with a mid-life transition. Roughly between 40 and 45 years, the person starts a major reassessment, "What have I done with my life?" Levinson's research on men's lives revealed that some do very little searching, that others search but do not find it too painful, but that most men have a crisis, a significant struggle with the self. These people questioned every aspect of life and believed that life could not proceed on the track it was taking.

The rest of the 40s, according to Levinson, involves making choices and building a new life structure. For those who have come through the mid-life transition and have found inner meaning, life will be "less tyrannized by the ambitions, passions, and illusions of youth" (Levinson et al, 1986). There is another transitional period, the Age Fifty Transition, in which the person works further on the tasks of the mid-life transition. If rejuvenation occurs during this transition, the 50s find the adult settling into the established life structure and experiencing great fulfillment.

Since "crisis" can have a negative connotation, and since not all adults experience a crisis, "mid-life transition" better describes this period of reassessment (Turner and Helms, 1987). The person confronts reality; some goals simply cannot be met. This must be accepted and goals adjusted. The person takes stock and emerges with a new perception of the self and the environment.

There are sex differences in mid-life transition (Turner and Helms, 1987). Men seem more involved in career assessment because their traditional role has been focused on becoming established in the career world. Women, even those employed, see the family as the central issue. This does not mean that family is not important to men, nor that career issues are not important to women. But many women have experienced the problem of children who are growing in independence and leaving home. This affects the women's identity. They feel that they are no longer needed in the same way. On the other hand, some see this as liberating, because they now can attend to their own needs.

Sheehy believes that women enter the mid-life transition earlier than men, at 35 (Sheehy, 1984). This is the age at which the average woman sees her youngest child enter school, at which the average married woman reenters the work force, and at which the biologic boundary of childbearing is now in sight. Women feel a time pinch that forces an "all-points survey" of their life. Aging and biology force women to review options that were set aside and that will be closed off in the now foreseeable future. Even those satisfied with the number of children or without children will face this review.

Whatever the central issue, all those in mid-life transition explore the meaning of their career, their family, and their personal identity. In terms of career, a person who spent the 30s searching for power and responsibility now may crave inner meaning (Levinson, 1986). Also, the middle-aged adult is aware of the time left until retirement; the question most often asked is "Am I on schedule or behind with my career goals" (Kimmel, 1980). This may result in a reordering of goals or in a new career path. A new career path may be a shift of emphasis within the same career cluster (Turner and Helms, 1987), such as the critical care nurse who heads up the outpatient program in cardiac rehabilitation. Or it may be a dramatic and complete career switch, as the business person who starts up a yacht chartering service in a warmer climate.

Career reassessment is intertwined with personal and family reassessment. New roles emerge as the middle-aged adult deals with growing children and aging parents. The adult often is caught in a "squeeze" between the simultaneously changing needs of adolescent children and aging parents (Aizenberg, 1982).

Role realignment occurs in the individual's relationship with aging parents. Even if the parents are healthy and active, there is a role reversal (Gould, 1979). The middle-aged adult gradually starts to take the parent's place as the one in charge. When one of the parents dies, the middle-aged adult is confronted with loss of the protective myth, "Death cannot happen to me or my loved ones" (Gould, 1979). The parent was a shield between the self and death. Once the parent dies, the middle-aged adult is more vulnerable and realizes the limited quantity of time left.

Another family task facing the middle-aged adult is to help the adolescent child in his or her search for identity. The parent must adjust to the adolescent's desire to be independent and less involved in the family activities and the need for increased responsibility. Some parents nurture the independence and delight in the budding individual. Others tend to be overprotective and controlling. They may feel their adolescent is too immature. Or they do not want the adolescent to make the same mistakes they did. The adolescent resents this attempt to relive the parent's life through his or her own. Also, some parents dread the empty nest.

Once the youngest child does leave home, the parent faces the empty nest. If the parent, often the mother, has focused only on the children, she may feel left with little to live for. Will she find something as important as the children to replace them? This dilemma is more poignant now than it was in the past when adult children stayed pretty close to home. With society's current mobility, the grown child often starts a new nuclear family at a far-away location.

The empty nest leaves parents alone as a couple again. They may face a relationship that is devoid of meaning apart from their children. They may find themselves dissatisfied, that they do not know each other, that they have drifted apart. Divorce may result and loom as a major crisis. Other couples find this a positive phase. Their marriage is happier with shared activities, increased freedom, and more time to travel. They look back on the shared memories of parenting with a satisfied smile.

Late Adulthood (60+ Years)

Although negative stereotypes exist for each age group, none is more prevalent than the one for aging adults. *Ageism* means discrimination based on age. It is a derogatory attitude that characterizes older adults as sick, senile, and useless and as a burden on the economy. It reveals our society's anxiety about aging. The attitude stems in part from our cultural emphasis on youth, beauty, and vigor. Other cultures respect and revere their aging members.

This ageist attitude is changing, partly because late adulthood now is the fastest-growing segment of our population and its members command attention. Older adults should be seen not as a homogeneous group with predictable reactions but as individuals with specific needs and widely divergent responses.

Developmental tasks of this group include

1. adjusting to changes in physical strength and health;
2. forming a new family role as an in-law and/or grandparent;
3. affiliating with one's age group;
4. adjusting to retirement and reduced income;
5. developing post-retirement activities that enhance self-worth and usefulness;
6. arranging satisfactory physical living quarters;
7. adjusting to the death of spouse, family members, and friends;
8. conducting a life review; and
9. preparing for the inevitability of one's own death.

Physical Development

Everyone does not age at the same rate. One person at 60 years can look older and feel weaker than another at 75 years. The widely divergent response depends on subjective attitude, physical activity, nutrition, personal habits, and the occurrence of physical illness. Though aging is known to be a lifelong process, its mechanism is not fully understood. There is an inevitable decline in body functions that seems to occur independently of stress, trauma, and disease (Turner and Helms, 1987). The degenerative effects of normal aging are described for each organ system in the corresponding chapter on physical examination.

Illness affects aging people more than those in other age groups. There is an increased incidence of chronic disease, a decrease in resistance to illness, and a decrease in recuperative power. That is, after an acute illness an aging person does not recover as quickly or as completely as a younger person. There is an increase in everyday body aches and pains. Some older people become preoccupied with their physical discomfort, whereas others adjust to a few aches with equanimity. All these events mean the aging person is increasingly dependent on the health care system for advice, health teaching, and physical care.

Cognitive Development

Aging does not have a predictable effect on intelligence. Intellectual function depends on various factors, such as motivation, interest, sensory impairment, educational level, how far in the past that school learning occurred, deliberate caution, and a tendency to conserve time and emotional energy rather than acting assertively (Murray and Zentner, 1989). Older adults do have a slower reaction time. They often have decreased ability for complex decision-making and decreased speed of performance, but there is no decrease in general knowledge. There is little or no loss in verbal comprehension, or in the application of experience (Kalish, 1982). Memory may be affected. If so, the effect is usually on short-term memory rather than on long-term memory (Turner and Helms, 1987).

Psychosocial Development

Levinson proposes a transitional period in the late adult stage from about 60 to 65 years. The study by Levinson and associates (1986) suggests a relationship between physical changes of the body and personality. By 60 years, most people are aware of some body decline. Although variations exist, most aging persons have at least one serious illness or limiting condition and are aware of the increasing frequency of death in peers. These issues, coupled with society's negative connotation of aging, lead to a fear that the person has lost all vestiges of youth, even those to which one had a tenuous hold during middle adulthood. The person fears ". . . that the youth within him is dying and that only the old man — an empty, dry structure devoid of energy, interests or inner resources — will survive for a brief and foolish old age" (Levinson et al, 1986). The task, then, is to look for a new form of youthfulness, a new force of inner growth to sustain the last era.

The era of late adulthood directs this inner youthfulness toward new creative endeavors. The older adult has stepped off center stage both in formal employment and in the family clan. This can be traumatic because it means a loss of recognition and authority. But now the person can direct energy inward. When financially and socially secure, the older adult can pursue whatever activity is important. One has paid one's dues to society and now can pursue whatever is pleasing. The person creates a new balance with society; he or she is less interested in society's extrinsic rewards and more interested in using inner resources.

Confronting Tasks. How an older adult responds to retirement depends largely on job satisfaction. If the job was rote and meaningless, the person may welcome the release provided by retirement. But if the job signified power and status, retirement may have a devastating effect. The retired person feels the loss of title and authority. There is also a loss of professional associates who had common interests and were intellectually stimulating. Also, there is a lost social outlet when coworkers had become a friendship group.

It is important to develop post-retirement activities that enhance self-worth and give a feeling of usefulness. These activities may include developing a new "semi-retired" career, or a hobby, sport interest, or community service activity. The transition to retirement is eased if these activities are well in place before the last formal day on the job.

Having the retired person spend more time at home affects the marriage relationship. Traditionally, it was the husband who was suddenly at home and "under foot." Now there are more employed women who face the same retirement adjustment. Some couples do find that having one or both at home more means an invasion of previously held "turf," such as the kitchen, garden, or workshop. Other couples develop a more egalitarian relationship. They are now free of earlier sex role definitions and are able to share household tasks and leisure activities equally.

Family roles also are adjusted with the marriage of grown-up children and the addition of in-laws. How the sons- or daughters-in-law are absorbed into the family affects the older adult. This often involves a new role as grandparent. Being able to indulge and provide moral support to a grandchild is usually positive for all, unless the care-taking becomes a burden to the grandparent.

Retirement often involves financial adjustment. This may involve a reduced income, perhaps only social security and a small pension. This may be hard if the person is used to a higher standard of living. Even if the retired person owns his or her own home, the cost of maintaining it may exceed the income.

Establishing suitable living arrangements has both financial and family significance. In our culture, the extended family mostly has disappeared today. No longer do three generations live under one roof. In the past, the older adult contributed light household tasks that gave a sense of personal worth (Murray and Zentner, 1989). Now, the contributions to the extended family that were made by the older family member have been replaced by advances in household mechanization, food processing, and day care centers.

Thus, most older adults choose to live independently, either as couples or alone. When it becomes difficult to manage self-care, they face the choice of moving in with grown children or moving into a retirement home or nursing home. All of these choices involve some disbursement of personal belongings and relinquishing some privacy.

Through the late adult years, each person is reminded of one's own limited time left by the increasing frequency of death and serious illness of friends, colleagues, siblings, or other family members or perhaps the spouse.

The Life Review. One important task of late adulthood is performing a life review. Older adults have finished all or most of their life's work. Their contribution to society and to their own immortality are mostly completed (Levinson et al, 1986). The life review is a cataloging of life events, a considering of one's successes and failures with the perspective of age. The objective of the task is to gain a sense of integrity in reviewing one's life as a whole.

This period relates to Erikson's last ego stage, with its key polarity of *integrity versus despair.* A successful resolution to this final conflict occurs when the adult accepts "one's one and only life cycle as something that had to be and that, by necessity, permitted of no substitutions" (Erikson, 1963). The adult feels content with his or her one life on earth, satisfied that if it were possible to do it over again, he or she would live it the same way. The older adult reviews events, experiences, and relationships and realizes that these have been mostly good. There are cherished memories. The person has had a meaningful part in human history, and can meet death with equanimity.

Failure to resolve this last crisis leaves the person with a sense of despair, resentment, futility, hopelessness, and a fear of death. However, a successful outcome completes a cycle. The contented older adult who does not fear death serves as a role model for younger adults that life can be trusted.

Levinson believes everyone has a sense of utter despair at some point during this time. To gain a sense of integrity, one has to confront the *lack* of integrity (Levinson et al, 1986). Some goals were not achieved, and what is worse, the damage is done and it is too late to set it right. The person realizes that whatever values were held, he or she cannot fully live up to them. This must be reconciled; it is an imperfect world. The task is to make peace with the self.

This final sense of what life is about is a close parallel of Erikson's last stage. Levinson likens the person's perspective at this time as a "view from the bridge" at the end of the life cycle (Levinson et al, 1986). One "must come finally to terms with the self—knowing it and loving it reasonably well, and being ready to give it up."

DEVELOPMENTAL SCREENING TESTS

The Denver II—Revision and Restandardization of the Denver Developmental Screening Test (DDST)

Age range: Birth to 6 years

Time required: 10 to 25 minutes

Authors: W. Frankenburg, J. Dodds, P. Archer, B. Bresnick, H. Shapiro

Available from: Denver Developmental Materials, Inc.
P.O. Box 6919
Denver, Colo. 80206

This is a simple screening instrument designed to detect developmental delays in infants and preschoolers. It tests four functions: gross motor, language, fine motor-adaptive, and personal-social skills.

The Denver II is not an IQ test; it does not predict current or future intellectual ability. It is not diagnostic; it does not suggest treatment regimens. What the Denver II does do is screen; it helps identify children who may be slow in development. This is important because early detection increases the opportunities for effective treatment.

The Denver II was revised in 1989 and restandardized for a sample including three ethnic groups, three residence categories (rural, suburban, and urban), and three levels of maternal education (less than high school, high school, and more than high school). These norms should ameliorate the limitations of the earlier DDST concerning its relevance to various population groups (Frankenburg, 1981; O'Pray, 1980). The Denver II also appears to address the limitations experienced by Olade (1984) in using the earlier DDST in developing countries. Olade's study of African children in Nigeria suggested language differences (naming certain colors, limited use of plurals and parents' last names) and unfamiliar interactive games (peek-a-boo) affected DDST results. These items are omitted or adjusted in the Denver II. However, the culture of developing countries still must be considered when using screening tests.

The Denver II easily is incorporated into the daily professional regimen of nurses, physicians, and teachers. The 125 items are arranged in chronologic order and are displayed in groupings corresponding to recommended ages for health maintenance visits (see Fig. 2–3). The clear pictorial charts make it easy to administer, score, and interpret. It is reliable and economical. The materials are few in number, attractive to children, and easily maintained and replaced. The scoring avoids diagnostic labeling (such as mental retardation, language disorder, and cerebral palsy). Instead, the child's performance is scored either "normal," "abnormal," or "questionable," and includes an adjustment in scoring for premature infants.

Uses of the Denver II include (Frankenburg and Camp, 1975)

- Screening of infants, whose rapid rate of development

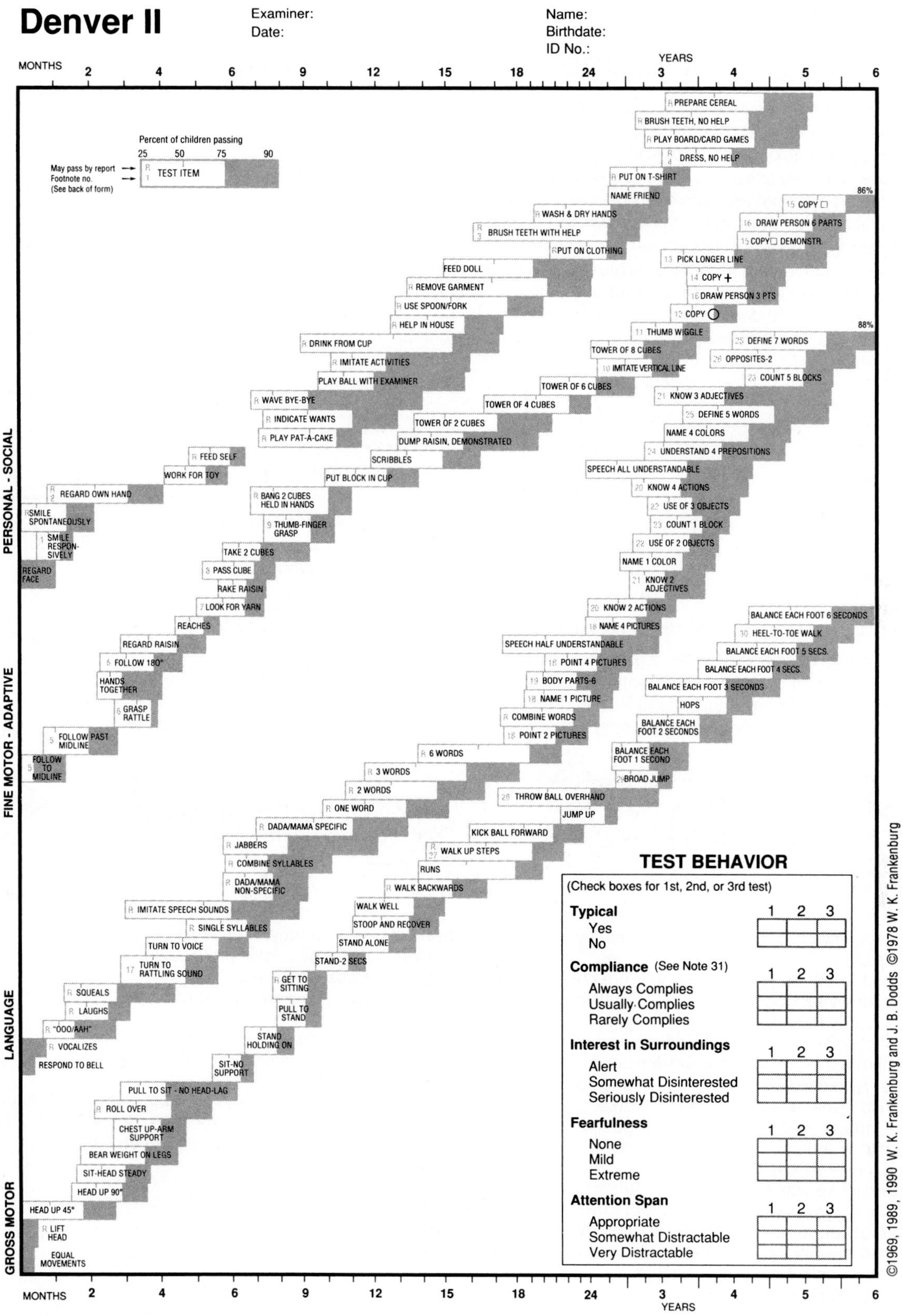

► **Figure 2-3**

Illustration continued on following page

DIRECTIONS FOR ADMINISTRATION

1. Try to get child to smile by smiling, talking or waving. Do not touch him/her.
2. Child must stare at hand several seconds.
3. Parent may help guide toothbrush and put toothpaste on brush.
4. Child does not have to be able to tie shoes or button/zip in the back.
5. Move yarn slowly in an arc from one side to the other, about 8" above child's face.
6. Pass if child grasps rattle when it is touched to the backs or tips of fingers.
7. Pass if child tries to see where yarn went. Yarn should be dropped quickly from sight from tester's hand without arm movement.
8. Child must transfer cube from hand to hand without help of body, mouth, or table.
9. Pass if child picks up raisin with any part of thumb and finger.
10. Line can vary only 30 degrees or less from tester's line. ∕
11. Make a fist with thumb pointing upward and wiggle only the thumb. Pass if child imitates and does not move any fingers other than the thumb.

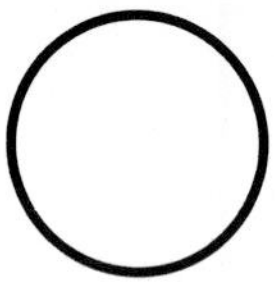

12. Pass any enclosed form. Fail continuous round motions.

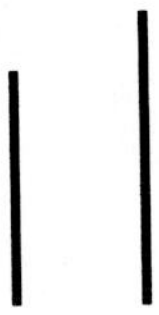

13. Which line is longer? (Not bigger.) Turn paper upside down and repeat. (pass 3 of 3 or 5 of 6)

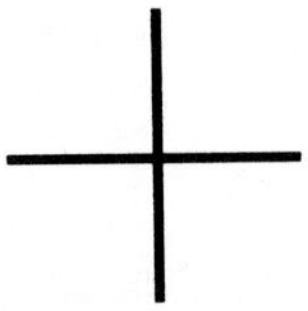

14. Pass any lines crossing near midpoint.

15. Have child copy first. If failed, demonstrate.

When giving items 12, 14, and 15, do not name the forms. Do not demonstrate 12 and 14.

16. When scoring, each pair (2 arms, 2 legs, etc.) counts as one part.
17. Place one cube in cup and shake gently near child's ear, but out of sight. Repeat for other ear.
18. Point to picture and have child name it. (No credit is given for sounds only.)
 If less than 4 pictures are named correctly, have child point to picture as each is named by tester.

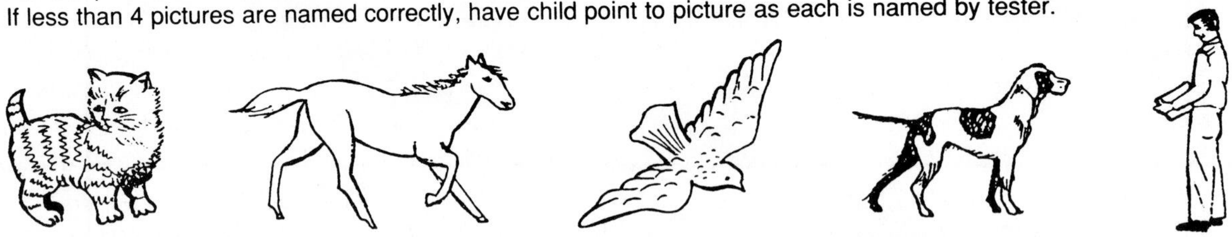

19. Using doll, tell child: Show me the nose, eyes, ears, mouth, hands, feet, tummy, hair. Pass 6 of 8.
20. Using pictures, ask child: Which one flies?... says meow?... talks?... barks?... gallops? Pass 2 of 5, 4 of 5.
21. Ask child: What do you do when you are cold?... tired?... hungry? Pass 2 of 3, 3 of 3.
22. Ask child: What do you do with a cup? What is a chair used for? What is a pencil used for?
 Action words must be included in answers.
23. Pass if child correctly places <u>and</u> says how many blocks are on paper. (1, 5).
24. Tell child: Put block **on** table; **under** table; **in front of** me, **behind** me. Pass 4 of 4.
 (Do not help child by pointing, moving head or eyes.)
25. Ask child: What is a ball?... lake?... desk?... house?... banana?... curtain?... fence?... ceiling? Pass if defined in terms of use, shape, what it is made of, or general category (such as banana is fruit, not just yellow). Pass 5 of 8, 7 of 8.
26. Ask child: If a horse is big, a mouse is __? If fire is hot, ice is __? If the sun shines during the day, the moon shines during the __? Pass 2 of 3.
27. Child may use wall or rail only, not person. May not crawl.
28. Child must throw ball overhand 3 feet to within arm's reach of tester.
29. Child must perform standing broad jump over width of test sheet (8 1/2 inches).
30. Tell child to walk forward, ⊂○⊃⊂○⊃⊂○⊃➔ heel within 1 inch of toe. Tester may demonstrate.
 Child must walk 4 consecutive steps.
31. In the second year, half of normal children are non-compliant.

OBSERVATIONS:

Table 2-7 ▶ Denver Articulation Screening Examination (DASE)

Denver Articulation Screening Examination

(For children 2.5 to 6 years of age)

NAME

HOSPITAL NO.

ADDRESS

Instructions: Have child repeat each word after you. Circle the underlined sounds that he or she pronounces correctly. Total number of correct sounds is the raw score. Use charts below to score results.

Date: __________ Child's age: ________ Examiner: ______________________ Raw score: __________

Percentile: __________ Intelligibility: ____________ Result: ____________________

1. table	6. zipper	11. sock	16. wagon	21. leaf
2. shirt	7. grapes	12. vacuum	17. gum	22. carrot
3. door	8. flag	13. yarn	18. house	
4. trunk	9. thumb	14. mother	19. pencil	
5. jumping	10. toothbrush	15. twinkle	20. fish	

Intelligibility (circle one): 1. Easy to understand
2. Understandable half of the time
3. Not understandable
4. Cannot evaluate

Comments:

makes it difficult to rely on professional opinion or on parent history alone

- Longitudinal following of a single child in health care or educational setting
- Follow-up in clinics, where a child may be seen briefly, infrequently, or by different examiners
- Prekindergarten screening

The Denver Articulation Screening Examination (DASE)

Age range: 2.5 to 6 years

Time required: 5 minutes

Author: Amelia F. Drumwright

Available from: LADOCA Project and Publishing Co.
East 51st Avenue and Lincoln St.
Denver, Colo. 80216

This is a screening test of articulation skill. Its purpose is (1) to reliably detect disorders in a disadvantaged population of children between the ages of 2.5 and 6 years, (2) to be acceptable to speech pathologists, and yet (3) to be easily understood by nonspeech professionals who work with children (e.g., physicians, nurses, teachers, and paraprofessionals) (Drumwright et al, 1973).

The child repeats 22 words that represent 30 speech sounds (Table 2-7). The examiner judges the accuracy of articulation, the intelligibility of the child's speech, and the presence of any abnormal voice disorders (Frankenburg and Camp, 1975). The scoring forms are understandable and easy to use.

Trainers are nonspeech professionals who have had a training program.

Uses of the DASE include identification of young, economically disadvantaged children who may have communication problems (Frankenburg and Camp, 1975).

Adult Life Stress Measures

Some tools are available that attempt to quantify the impact of life change on a person's health. They are based on the assumption that there is a relationship between marked life stress and a person's susceptibility to physical and psychologic problems (Sarason et al, 1978). Many of the life change events are the developmental tasks discussed earlier in the chapter.

Table 2–7 ▶ Denver Articulation Screening Examination (DASE) *Continued*

To score DASE words: Note raw score for child's performance. Match raw score line (extreme left of chart) with column representing child's age (to the closest *previous* age group). Where raw score line and age column meet denotes percentile rank of child's performance when compared with other children that age. Percentiles above heavy line are *abnormal,* below heavy line are *normal.*

PERCENTILE RANK

Raw Score	2.5 yr	3.0 yr	3.5 yr	4.0 yr	4.5 yr	5.0 yr	5.5 yr	6 yr
2	1							
3	2							
4	5							
5	9							
6	16							
7	23							
8	31	2						
9	37	4	1					
10	42	6	2					
11	48	7	4					
12	54	9	6	1	1			
13	58	12	9	2	3	1	1	
14	62	17	11	5	4	2	2	
15	68	23	15	9	5	3	2	
16	75	31	19	12	5	4	3	
17	79	38	25	15	6	6	4	
18	83	46	31	19	8	7	4	
19	86	51	38	24	10	9	5	1
20	89	58	45	30	12	11	7	3
21	92	65	52	36	15	15	9	4
22	94	72	58	43	18	19	12	5
23	96	77	63	50	22	24	15	7
24	97	82	70	58	29	29	20	15
25	99	87	78	66	36	34	26	17
26	99	91	84	75	46	43	34	24
27		94	89	82	57	54	44	34
28		96	94	88	70	68	59	47
29		98	98	94	84	84	77	68
30		100	100	100	100	100	100	100

To score intelligibility:

	NORMAL	ABNORMAL
2.5 years	Understandable half of the time or easy to understand	Not understandable
3 years and older	Easy to understand	Understandable half of the time or not understandable

Test result: 1. Normal on DASE and intelligibility = *normal*
2. Abnormal on DASE or intelligibility = *abnormal**

* If abnormal on initial screening, rescreen within 2 weeks. If abnormal again, child should be referred for complete speech evaluation.

(Reprinted with permission from NK Frankenburg, University of Colorado Medical Center, Denver, 1971. Copyright © 1971, Amelia F. Drumwright.)

Recent Life Changes Questionnaire

Age range: adult

Author: R.H. Rahe

This is a 55-item self-administered questionnaire whose purpose is to assess life stress (Table 2–8). The respondent considers a list of events, and checks those experienced in the prior 6 months to 2 years. Items have been rated as to the average amount of social readjustment required, with marriage given an arbitrary standard value. The amount of social readjustment is the number of *life change units* for each event. These are added to yield a total life stress score. A high recent life change score correlates with the development of health problems (Rahe, 1975).

The life stress score combines both desirable and undesirable life events. This tool considers life change, per se, as stressful whether events experienced are desirable or undesirable.

Life Experiences Survey (LES)

Age range: adult

Authors: I.G. Sarason, J.H. Johnson, J.M. Siegel

This is a 47-item self-administered questionnaire that considers events that occurred over the past year. Unlike the Rahe instrument, this test weighs the desirability or undesirability of life experiences. The assumption is that events considered *negative* by the respondent are more likely to be associated with stress. Also the respondent is allowed to rate the personal impact of the events experience.

The respondent weighs the desirability or undesirability of each event on a 7-point scale, from extremely negative (−3) to extremely positive (+3) (see Table 2–9). The negative and positive subscores are added to determine a total change score.

This test suggests a relationship between negative life changes and psychologic problems. The effect of stress differs depending on individual characteristics, the degree of perceived control over the events, and the degree of psychosocial assets (Sarason et al, 1978).

Table 2–8 ▶ Recent Life Changes Questionnaire

I. INSTRUCTIONS FOR MARKING YOUR RECENT LIFE CHANGES

To answer the questions below, mark an "X" in one or more of the columns to the right of each question. If the event in question has occurred to you within the past two years, indicate when it occurred by marking the appropriate column: 0-6 months ago, 7-12 months ago, etc. It may be the case with some of the events below that you experienced them over more than one of the time periods listed for the past two years. If so, mark all the appropriate columns. If the event has not occurred to you during the last two years (or has never occurred to you) leave all the columns empty.

Now go through the questionnaire and mark your recent life changes. The column marked "Your Adjustment Score" will be explained at the end of the questionnaire.

A. HEALTH *Within the time periods listed, have you experienced:*	*19 to 24 mo. ago*	*13 to 18 mo. ago*	*7 to 12 mo. ago*	*0 to 6 mo. ago*	*Your Adjust. Score*
1. an illness or injury which:					
(a) kept you in bed a week or more, or took you to to the hospital?	____	____	____	____	____
(b) was less serious than described above?	____	____	____	____	____
2. a major change in eating habits?	____	____	____	____	____
3. a major change in sleeping habits?	____	____	____	____	____
4. a change in your usual type and/or amount of recreation?	____	____	____	____	____
5. major dental work?	____	____	____	____	____
B. WORK					
Within the time periods listed, have you:					
6. changed to a new type of work?	____	____	____	____	____
7. changed your work hours or conditions?	____	____	____	____	____

Table continued on following page

Table 2-8 ▶ Recent Life Changes Questionnaire *Continued*

	19 to 24 mo. ago	*13 to 18 mo. ago*	*7 to 12 mo. ago*	*0 to 6 mo. ago*	*Your Adjust. Score*
8. had a change in your responsibilities at work:					
(a) more responsibilities?	___	___	___	___	___
(b) less responsibilities?	___	___	___	___	___
(c) promotion?	___	___	___	___	___
(d) demotion?	___	___	___	___	___
(e) transfer?	___	___	___	___	___
9. experienced troubles at work:					
(a) with your boss?	___	___	___	___	___
(b) with co-workers?	___	___	___	___	___
(c) with persons under your supervision?	___	___	___	___	___
(d) other work troubles?	___	___	___	___	___
10. experienced a major business readjustment?	___	___	___	___	___
11. retired?	___	___	___	___	___
12. experienced being:					
(a) fired from work?	___	___	___	___	___
(b) laid off from work?	___	___	___	___	___
13. taken courses by mail or studied at home to help you in your work?	___	___	___	___	___
C. HOME AND FAMILY					
Within the time periods listed, have you experienced:					
14. a change in residence:					
(a) a move within the same town or city?	___	___	___	___	___
(b) a move to a different town, city or state?	___	___	___	___	___
15. a change in family "get-togethers"?	___	___	___	___	___
16. a major change in the health or behavior of a family member (illnesses, accidents, drug or disciplinary problems, etc.)?	___	___	___	___	___
17. major change in your living conditions (home improvements or a decline in your home or neighborhood)?	___	___	___	___	___
18. the death of a spouse?	___	___	___	___	___
19. the death of a:					
(a) child?	___	___	___	___	___
(b) brother or sister?	___	___	___	___	___
(c) parent?	___	___	___	___	___
(d) other close family member?	___	___	___	___	___
20. the death of a close friend?	___	___	___	___	___
21. a change in the marital status of your parents:					
(a) divorce?	___	___	___	___	___
(b) remarriage?	___	___	___	___	___

Table 2-8 ▶ Recent Life Changes Questionnaire *Continued*

NOTE: (Questions 22–33 concern marriage. For persons never married, go to Item 34)	*19 to 24 mo. ago*	*13 to 18 mo. ago*	*7 to 12 mo. ago*	*0 to 6 mo. ago*	*Your Adjust. Score*
22. marriage?	____	____	____	____	____
23. a change in arguments with your spouse?	____	____	____	____	____
24. in-law problems?	____	____	____	____	____
25. a separation from spouse:					
(a) due to work?	____	____	____	____	____
(b) due to marital problems?	____	____	____	____	____
26. a reconciliation with spouse?	____	____	____	____	____
27. a divorce?	____	____	____	____	____
28. a gain of a new family member:					
(a) birth of a child?	____	____	____	____	____
(b) adoption of a child?	____	____	____	____	____
(c) a relative moving in with you?	____	____	____	____	____
29. wife beginning or ceasing work outside the home?	____	____	____	____	____
30. wife becoming pregnant?	____	____	____	____	____
31. a child leaving home:					
(a) due to marriage?	____	____	____	____	____
(b) to attend college?	____	____	____	____	____
(c) for other reasons?	____	____	____	____	____
32. wife having a miscarriage or abortion?	____	____	____	____	____
33. birth of a grandchild?	____	____	____	____	____
D. PERSONAL AND SOCIAL					
Within the time periods listed, have you experienced:					
34. a major personal achievement?	____	____	____	____	____
35. a change in your personal habits (your dress, friends, life-style, etc.)?	____	____	____	____	____
36. sexual difficulties?	____	____	____	____	____
37. beginning or ceasing school or college?	____	____	____	____	____
38. a change of school or college?	____	____	____	____	____
39. a vacation?	____	____	____	____	____
40. a change in your religious beliefs?	____	____	____	____	____
41. a change in your social activities (clubs, movies, visiting)?	____	____	____	____	____
42. a minor violation of the law?	____	____	____	____	____
43. legal troubles resulting in your being held in jail?	____	____	____	____	____
44. a change in your political beliefs?	____	____	____	____	____
45. a new, close, personal relationship?	____	____	____	____	____

Table continued on following page

Table 2-8 ▶ Recent Life Changes Questionnaire *Continued*

	19 to 24 mo. ago	*13 to 18 mo. ago*	*7 to 12 mo. ago*	*0 to 6 mo. ago*	*Your Adjust. Score*
46. an engagement to marry?	___	___	___	___	___
47. a "falling out" in a close personal relationship?	___	___	___	___	___
48. girlfriend (or boyfriend) problems?	___	___	___	___	___
49. a loss or damage of personal property?	___	___	___	___	___
50. an accident?	___	___	___	___	___
51. a major decision regarding your immediate future?	___	___	___	___	___
E. FINANCIAL					
Within the time periods listed, have you:					
52. taken on a moderate purchase, such as a T.V., car, freezer, etc.?	___	___	___	___	___
53. taken on a major purchase or a mortgage loan, such as a home, business, property, etc.?	___	___	___	___	___
54. experienced a foreclosure on a mortgage or loan?	___	___	___	___	___
55. experienced a major change in finances:					
(a) increased income?	___	___	___	___	___
(b) decreased income?	___	___	___	___	___
(c) credit rating difficulties?	___	___	___	___	___
6-month LCU totals	___	___	___	___	
6-month SLCU totals	___	___	___	___	

II. INSTRUCTIONS FOR SCORING YOUR ADJUSTMENT TO YOUR RECENT LIFE CHANGES

Persons adapt to their recent life changes in different ways. Some people find the adjustment to a residential move, for example, to be enormous, while others find very little life adjustment necessary. You are now requested to "score" each of the recent life changes that you marked with an "X" as to the amount of adjustment you needed to handle the event.

Your scores can range from 1 to 100 "points." If, for example, you experienced a recent residential move but felt it required very little life adjustment, you would choose a low number and place it in the blank to the right of the question's boxes. On the other hand, if you recently changed residence and felt it required a near maximal life adjustment, you would place a high number, toward 100, in the blank to the right of that question's boxes. For intermediate life adjustment scores you would choose intermediate numbers between 1 and 100.

Please go back through your questionnaire and for each recent life change you indicated with an "X," choose your personal life change adjustment score (between 1 and 100) which reflects what you saw to be the amount of life adjustment necessary to cope with or handle the event. Use both your estimates of the intensity of the life change and its duration to arrive at your scores.

LCU, life change units; SLCU, subjective life change units.

(From Rahe RH: Epidemiological studies of life change and illness. Int J Psychiatry 6:133–146, 1975. Reprinted with permission.)

Table 2-9 ▶ Life Experiences Survey

Listed below are a number of events which sometimes bring about change in the lives of those who experience them and which necessitate social readjustment. *Please check those events which you have experienced in the recent past and indicate the time period during which you have experienced each event.* Be sure that all check marks are directly across from the items they correspond to.

Also, for each item checked below, *please indicate the extent to which you viewed the event as having either a positive or negative impact on your life* at the time the event occurred. That is, *indicate the type and extent of impact that the event had.* A rating of −3 would indicate an extremely negative impact. A rating of 0 suggests no impact either positive or negative. A rating of +3 would indicate an extremely positive impact.

	0 TO 6 MO	7 MO TO 1 YR	EXTREMELY NEGATIVE	MODERATELY NEGATIVE	SOMEWHAT NEGATIVE	NO IMPACT	SLIGHTLY POSITIVE	MODERATELY POSITIVE	EXTREMELY POSITIVE
1. Marriage			−3	−2	−1	0	+1	+2	+3
2. Detention in jail or comparable institution			−3	−2	−1	0	+1	+2	+3
3. Death of spouse			−3	−2	−1	0	+1	+2	+3
4. Major change in sleeping habits (much more or much less sleep)			−3	−2	−1	0	+1	+2	+3
5. Death of close family member:									
a. Mother			−3	−2	−1	0	+1	+2	+3
b. Father			−3	−2	−1	0	+1	+2	+3
c. Brother			−3	−2	−1	0	+1	+2	+3
d. Sister			−3	−2	−1	0	+1	+2	+3
e. Grandmother			−3	−2	−1	0	+1	+2	+3
f. Grandfather			−3	−2	−1	0	+1	+2	+3
g. Other (specify)			−3	−2	−1	0	+1	+2	+3
6. Major change in eating habits (much more or much less food intake)			−3	−2	−1	0	+1	+2	+3
7. Foreclosure on mortgage or loan			−3	−2	−1	0	+1	+2	+3
8. Death of close friend			−3	−2	−1	0	+1	+2	+3
9. Outstanding personal achievement			−3	−2	−1	0	+1	+2	+3
10. Minor law violations (traffic tickets, disturbing the peace, etc.)			−3	−2	−1	0	+1	+2	+3
11. *Male:* Wife/girlfriend's pregnancy			−3	−2	−1	0	+1	+2	+3
12. *Female:* Pregnancy			−3	−2	−1	0	+1	+2	+3
13. Changed work situation (different work responsibility, major change in working conditions, working hours, etc.)			−3	−2	−1	0	+1	+2	+3
14. New job			−3	−2	−1	0	+1	+2	+3
15. Serious illness or injury of close family member:									
a. Father			−3	−2	−1	0	+1	+2	+3
b. Mother			−3	−2	−1	0	+1	+2	+3
c. Sister			−3	−2	−1	0	+1	+2	+3
d. Brother			−3	−2	−1	0	+1	+2	+3
e. Grandfather			−3	−2	−1	0	+1	+2	+3
f. Grandmother			−3	−2	−1	0	+1	+2	+3
g. Spouse			−3	−2	−1	0	+1	+2	+3
h. Other (specify)			−3	−2	−1	0	+1	+2	+3
16. Sexual difficulties			−3	−2	−1	0	+1	+2	+3
17. Trouble with employer (in danger of losing job, being sus-			−3	−2	−1	0	+1	+2	+3

Table continued on following page

Table 2-9 ▶ Life Experiences Survey *Continued*

	0 TO 6 MO	7 MO TO 1 YR	EXTREMELY NEGATIVE	MODERATELY NEGATIVE	SOMEWHAT NEGATIVE	NO IMPACT	SLIGHTLY POSITIVE	MODERATELY POSITIVE	EXTREMELY POSITIVE
pended, demoted, etc.)									
18. Trouble with in-laws			−3	−2	−1	0	+1	+2	+3
19. Major change in financial status (a lot better off or a lot worse off)			−3	−2	−1	0	+1	+2	+3
20. Major change in closeness of family members (increased or decreased closeness)			−3	−2	−1	0	+1	+2	+3
21. Gaining a new family member (through birth, adoption, family member moving in, etc.)			−3	−2	−1	0	+1	+2	+3
22. Change of residence			−3	−2	−1	0	+1	+2	+3
23. Marital separation from mate (due to conflict)			−3	−2	−1	0	+1	+2	+3
24. Major change in church activities (increased or decreased attendance)			−3	−2	−1	0	+1	+2	+3
25. Marital reconciliation with mate			−3	−2	−1	0	+1	+2	+3
26. Major change in number of arguments with spouse (a lot more or a lot less arguments)			−3	−2	−1	0	+1	+2	+3
27. *Married male:* Change in wife's work outside the home (beginning work, ceasing work, changing to a new job, etc.)			−3	−2	−1	0	+1	+2	+3
28. *Married female:* Change in husband's work (loss of job, beginning new job, retirement, etc.)			−3	−2	−1	0	+1	+2	+3
29. Major change in usual type and/or amount of recreation			−3	−2	−1	0	+1	+2	+3
30. Borrowing more than $10,000 (buying home, business, etc.)			−3	−2	−1	0	+1	+2	+3
31. Borrowing less than $10,000 (buying car, TV, getting school loan, etc.)			−3	−2	−1	0	+1	+2	+3
32. Being fired from job			−3	−2	−1	0	+1	+2	+3
33. *Male:* Wife/girlfriend having abortion			−3	−2	−1	0	+1	+2	+3
34. *Female:* Having abortion			−3	−2	−1	0	+1	+2	+3
35. Major personal illness or injury			−3	−2	−1	0	+1	+2	+3
36. Major change in social activities, e.g., parties, movies, visiting (increased or decreased participation)			−3	−2	−1	0	+1	+2	+3

Table 2-9 ▶ Life Experiences Survey *Continued*

	0 TO 6 MO	7 MO TO 1 YR	EXTREMELY NEGATIVE	MODERATELY NEGATIVE	SOMEWHAT NEGATIVE	NO IMPACT	SLIGHTLY POSITIVE	MODERATELY POSITIVE	EXTREMELY POSITIVE
37. Major change in living conditions of family (building new home, remodeling, deterioration of home, neighborhood, etc.)			−3	−2	−1	0	+1	+2	+3
38. Divorce			−3	−2	−1	0	+1	+2	+3
39. Serious injury or illness of close friend			−3	−2	−1	0	+1	+2	+3
40. Retirement from work			−3	−2	−1	0	+1	+2	+3
41. Son or daughter leaving home (due to marriage, college, etc.)			−3	−2	−1	0	+1	+2	+3
42. Ending of formal schooling			−3	−2	−1	0	+1	+2	+3
43. Separation from spouse (due to work, travel)			−3	−2	−1	0	+1	+2	+3
44. Engagement			−3	−2	−1	0	+1	+2	+3
45. Breaking up with boyfriend/girlfriend			−3	−2	−1	0	+1	+2	+3
46. Leaving home for the first time			−3	−2	−1	0	+1	+2	+3
47. Reconciliation with boyfriend/girlfriend			−3	−2	−1	0	+1	+2	+3
Other recent experiences which have had an impact on your life. List and rate.									
48. ________________.			−3	−2	−1	0	+1	+2	+3
49. ________________.			−3	−2	−1	0	+1	+2	+3
50. ________________.			−3	−2	−1	0	+1	+2	+3

(From Sarason IG, Johnson JH, Siegal JM: Assessing the impact of life changes: development of life experiences survey. J Consulting Clinical Psychol 46(5):932–946, 1971. Used with permission.)

NURSING DIAGNOSES COMMONLY ASSOCIATED WITH DEVELOPMENTAL DISORDERS

Diagnosis	Related Factors (Etiology)	Defining Characteristics (Symptoms and Signs)
CHILDHOOD		

Altered growth and development	Effects of physical disability
	Environmental and stimulation deficiencies
	Inadequate care-taking
	  Indifference
	  Inconsistent responsiveness
	  Multiple care takers
	Prescribed dependence
	Separation from significant others
		Altered physical growth
		Decreased responses
		Delay or difficulty in performing skills that are typical of age group
		  Motor
		  Social
		  Expressive
		Flat affect

Table continued on following page

Diagnosis	Related Factors (Etiology)	Defining Characteristics (Symptoms and Signs)
		Inability to perform self-care or self-control activities appropriate for age
ADOLESCENCE Decisional conflict	Unclear personal values/beliefs Peer pressure Lack of experience or interference with decision-making Support system deficit	Verbalized uncertainty about choices Verbalized undesired consequences of alternative actions being considered Vacillation among alternative choices Delayed decision-making
ADULTHOOD Ineffective family coping: compromised	Isolation of family members from one another Lack of support for family members Temporary family disorganization and role changes Effects of acute or chronic illness Incompatible or differing values, beliefs, or goals Unrealistic expectations	Ineffective responses to illness, disability, or situational crises Inability to demonstrate supportive behaviors Expressed concern about significant other's response to health problem Impaired intimacy or closeness Attempted assistive behaviors with less than satisfactory results
LATE ADULTHOOD Anticipatory grieving	Expected loss of Friends Occupation Function Home Multiple crises Lack of social support system	Expressed distress at potential loss Denial Guilt Sorrow Change in eating habits Change in sleep patterns Change in social patterns Decreased libido

Bibliography

Aizenberg R, Harris R: Family demographic changes: The middle generation squeeze. Generations 7(2):6–7, 1982.

Berk LE: Child Development. 2nd ed. Boston, Allyn and Bacon, 1991.

Benedict R: Patterns of Culture. Boston, Houghton Mifflin, 1934.

Blair KA: Aging: Physiological aspects and clinical implications. Nurse Pract 15(2):14–28, 1990.

Brazelton TB: The Neonatal Behavioral Assessment Scale. Philadelphia, JB Lippincott, 1984.

Carey WB, McDevitt SC: Revision of the infant temperament questionnaire. Pediatrics 61:735, 1978.

Comfort A: A Good Old Age. New York, Crown, 1976.

DeAngelis C: Pediatric Primary Care. 3rd ed. Boston, Little, Brown, 1984.

Drumwright A, Van Natta P, Camp B, Frankenburg W: The Denver articulation screening exam. Speech Hearing Dis 38:3–14, 1973.

Erikson EH: Childhood and Society. New York WW Norton, 1963.

Erikson EH: Identity—Youth and Crisis. New York, WW Norton, 1968.

Foster R, Hunsberger M, Anderson JJ: Family-Centered Nursing Care of Children. Philadelphia, WB Saunders, 1989.

Frankenburg WK, Dodds JB: The Denver Developmental Screening Test. J Pediatr 71(2):181–191, 1967.

Frankenburg WK, Camp BW: Pediatric Screening Tests. Springfield, IL, Charles C Thomas, 1975.

Frankenburg WK, Fandal AW, Sciarillo W: The newly abbreviated and revised Denver Developmental Screening Test. J Pediatr 99(6):995–999, 1981.
Gould R: The phases of adult life: A study in developmental psychology. Am J Psychiatry 129:33–43, 1972.
Gould R: Adult life stages—growth toward self-tolerance. Psychology Today 8:74–81, 1975.
Gould RL: Transformations: Growth and Change in Adult Life. New York, Simon and Schuster, 1979.
Hall GS: Adolescence. New York, Appleton, 1916.
Johnson TR, Moore WM (Eds): Children Are Different—Developmental Physiology. 2nd ed. Columbus, OH, Ross Laboratories, 1978.
Kalish RA: Late Adulthood: Perspectives on Human Development. 2nd ed. Monterey, CA, Brooks Cole, 1982.
Kanin G: It Takes a Long Time to Become Young. New York, Doubleday, 1978.
Kimmel DC: Adulthood and Aging: An Interdisciplinary Development View. 3rd ed. New York, John Wiley, 1989.
Levinson DJ: A conception of adult development. Am Psychol 41:3–13, 1986.
Levinson DJ, Darrow CN, Klein EB: The Seasons of a Man's Life. 2nd ed. New York, Ballantine, 1986.
Martin AC, Starling BP: Managing common marital stresses. Nurs Pract 14(10):11–18, 1989.
Masters W, Johnson V, Kolodny R: Human Sexuality. 3rd ed. Glenview, IL, F Scott, 1988.
McElmurry BJ, LiBrizzi SJ: The health of older women. Nurs Clin North Am 21(1):161–171, 1986.
Mead M: Sex and Temperament in Three Primitive Societies. New York, Morrow, 1935.
Mead M: Growing Up in New Guinea. New York, Mentor, 1953.
Mead M: Coming of Age in Samoa. New York, Morrow, 1961.
Murray RB, Zentner JP: Nursing Assessment and Health Promotion Strategies Through the Life Span. 4th ed. Englewood Cliffs, NJ, Prentice Hall, 1989.
Olade RA: Evaluation of the Denver Developmental Screening Test as applied to African children. Nurs Res 33(4):204–207, 1984.
O'Pray M: Developmental screening tools: Using them effectively. Maternal Child Nursing 5:126–130, 1980.
Papalia D, Olds S: A Child's World—Infancy Through Adolescence. 4th ed. New York, McGraw-Hill, 1987.
Phares EJ: Introduction to Personality. 2nd ed. Glenview, IL, F Scott, 1988.
Piaget J: Judgment and Reasoning in the Child. Totowa, NJ, Littlefield, Adams, 1968.
Piaget J: The Construction of Reality in the Child. New York, Balantine, 1975.
Rahe RH: Epidemiological studies of life changes and illness. Int J Psychiatry 6(1/2):133–146, 1975.
Rebenson-Piano M: The physiologic changes that occur with aging. Crit Care Nurs Q 12(1):1–14, 1989.
Sarason EG, Johnson JH, Siegal JM: Assessing the impact of life changes—development of life experiences survey. J Consulting Clinical Psychologist 45(5):932–946, 1978.
Sheehy G: Passages. New York, Bantam, 1984.
Stokes SA, Gordon SE: Development of an instrument to measure stress in the older adult. Nurs Res 37(1):16–19, 1988.
Thomas RM: Comparing Theories of Child Development. 2nd ed. Belmont, CA, Wadsworth, 1985.
Turner JS, Helms DB: Lifespan Development. 3rd ed. New York, Holt, Rinehart and Winston, 1987.
Wadsworth B: Piaget's Theory of Cognitive and Affective Development. 4th ed. White Plains, NY, Longman, 1988.
Whaley L, Wong D: Nursing Care of Infants and Children. 4th ed. St. Louis, CV Mosby, 1990.

CHAPTER

3 The Interview

The interview is a meeting between yourself and your client. The meeting's goal is your record of a complete health history. The health history is important in beginning to identify the person's health strengths and problems and as a bridge to the next step in data collection, the physical examination.

The interview is the first and really the most important part of data collection. It collects *subjective data,* what the person says about himself or herself. The interview is the first and the best chance a person has to tell you what *he or she* perceives the health state to be. Once people enter the health care system, they may relinquish some control. At this point the person is still in charge. The individual knows everything about his or her own health state, and you know nothing. Your skill in interviewing will glean all the necessary information as well as build rapport for a successful working relationship.

When you have a successful interview, you

1. gather complete and accurate information about the person's health state, including the description and chronology of any symptoms,
2. establish rapport and trust so the person feels accepted and thus free to share all relevant data,
3. give the person an understanding about the health state so that the person can begin to participate in identifying problems,
4. build rapport to establish a continuing working relationship. This rapport will facilitate future diagnoses, planning, and treatment.

Consider the interview is similar to forming a contract between you and your client. A contract consists of spoken or unspoken rules for behavior. In this case, the contract concerns what the person needs and expects from health care and what you, the health professional, have to offer. Your mutual goal is optimal health for the client. The contract's terms include

- time and place of the interview and succeeding physical examination;
- introduction of yourself and a brief explanation of your role,
- the purpose of the interview;
- how long it will take;
- expectation of participation for each person;
- presence of any other people, e.g. client's family, other health professionals, students;
- confidentiality and to what extent it may be limited; and
- any costs that the client must pay.

Although the client already may know some information through telephone contact with receptionists or the admitting office, the remaining points need to be stated explicitly. If the terms are not understood clearly at the outset, someone will be confused. This could produce resentment and anger, which is hardly the openness and trust you need to facilitate the interview.

THE PROCESS OF COMMUNICATION

The vehicle that carries you and your client through the interview is communication. Communication is exchanging information so that each person clearly understands the other. Understanding is the difficult part. If you do not understand each other, if you have not *conveyed meaning,* there has been no communication.

It is challenging to teach the skill of interviewing because initially, most students think there is little to be learned. If they can talk and hear, they assume they can communicate. But there is much more than talking and hearing. Communication is all behavior, conscious and unconscious, verbal and nonverbal. *All behavior has meaning.*

Sending

The following section details verbal and nonverbal communication. Likely, you are most aware of *verbal* communication—the words you speak, vocalizations, the tone of voice, even what you do *not* say. *Nonverbal* communication also occurs—through posture, gestures, facial expression, eye contact, touch, even where you place your chair. Since nonverbal communication is under less conscious control than verbal communication, nonverbal communication probably is more reflective of your true feelings.

Receiving

Being aware of the messages you send is only part of the process. Your words and gestures are merely symbols. They must be interpreted in a *specific context* to have meaning (Cassell, 1980c). You have a specific context in mind when you send your words. The receiver puts his or her own interpretation on them. The receiver attaches meaning determined by his or her past experiences, culture, self-concept, as well as current physical and emotional state. Sometimes these contexts do not coincide. Remember how frustrating it was to try to communicate something to a friend, only to have your message totally misunderstood? Your message was sabotaged by the listener's bias. It takes mutual understanding by the sender and receiver to have successful communication.

There is even greater risk for misunderstanding in the health care setting than in a social setting. The client usually has a health problem, and this factor emotionally charges your professional relationship. It intensifies the communication, because the person feels dependent on you to get better.

Communication is not an art that only can be polished with years of experience. It is a *basic skill* that can be learned and perfected when you are a beginning practitioner. It is a tool, as basic to quality health care as the tools of inspection or palpation. To maximize your communicating skill, first you need to be aware of internal and external factors and their influence.

Internal Factors

Internal factors are those inside the examiner, what you bring in to the interview. Cultivate the three inner factors of liking others, empathy, and the ability to listen.

Liking Others. One essential factor for an examiner's "goodness of fit" into a helping profession is a genuine liking of other people. This means a generally optimistic view of people; an assumption of their strengths and a tolerance for their weaknesses (Benjamin, 1980). An atmosphere of warmth and caring is necessary. The client must feel that he or she is accepted unconditionally.

The respect for other people extends to respect for their own control over their health. Your goal is *not* to make your clients dependent on you, but to be increasingly responsible for themselves. You wish to promote their growth. You have the health care resources to offer clients. They must choose how to apply those resources to their own lives.

Empathy. A Native American legend encourages one person not to judge another "until you have walked two moons in his moccasins." Empathy means this—viewing the world from the other's inner frame of reference while remaining yourself. Empathy means recognizing and accepting the other person's feelings without criticism. It is described as "feeling *with* the person rather than feeling *like* the person" (Bernstein, 1985). It does not mean you become lost in the other person at the expense of your own self. If this occurred you would cease to be helpful. Rather, it is to *understand with* the person how *he or she* perceives his or her world (Rogers, 1951).

The Ability to Listen. To have empathy you need to listen. Listening is not a passive role in the communication process; it is active and demanding. Listening requires your complete attention. You cannot be preoccupied with your own needs or the needs of other clients or you will miss something important. For the time of this interview, no one is more important than this person. This person's needs are your sole concern. This is the highest compliment you can give.

Active listening is the route to understanding. You cannot be thinking of what you are going to say as soon as the person stops for breath. Listen to *what* the person says. The story may not come out in the order you would ask it or will record it later. Let the person talk from his or her own outline; nearly everything that is said will be relevant. Listen to the way things are said, the tone of the person's voice, and even to what the person is leaving out.

Sandra B., 32, sought care for headaches she had during the last 3 months, which were unresponsive to aspirin and were interfering with her job. She was interviewed for 30 minutes. Through this time she never mentioned her husband, though they had been married only 5 months before. Finally the examiner asked, "I haven't heard you mention your husband. Tell me about him." It unfolded that Sandra's husband lost his job a few months after they were married because of alcohol-related work errors. Though Sandra related extreme personal stress and worry, she never thought that her headaches might be related to the stressful situation.

External Factors

Before you meet your client, prepare the physical setting. The setting may be in a hospital room, an examination room in an office or clinic, or in the person's home (where you will have less control). In any location, optimal conditions are important to have a smooth interview.

Ensure Privacy. Aim for geographic privacy—a private room in the hospital, clinic, office, or home. This may involve asking an ambulatory roommate to step out for a while or finding an unoccupied room or an empty lounge. If geographic privacy is not available, "psychologic privacy" by curtained partitions may suffice as long as the person feels sure no one can overhear the conversation or interrupt (Bernstein and Bernstein, 1985).

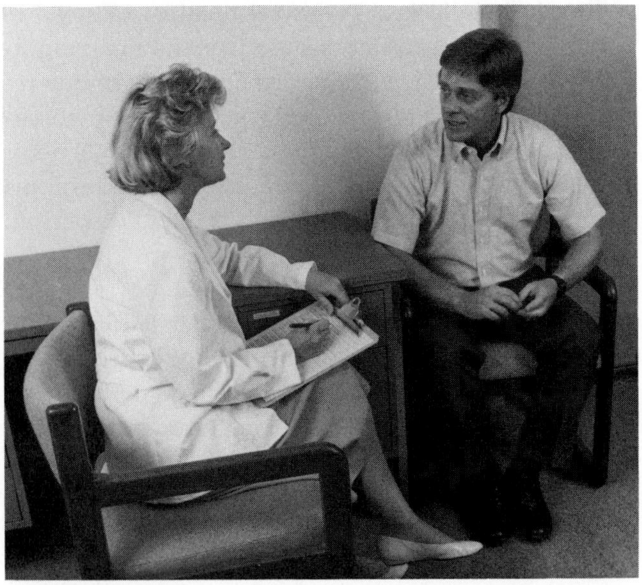

▶ **Figure 3-1**

Refuse Interruptions. Most people resent interruptions except in cases of an emergency. Inform any support staff of your interview, and ask that they not interrupt you during this time. Discourage other health professionals from interrupting you with *their* need for access to the client. You need to concentrate and to establish rapport. An interruption can destroy in seconds what you have spent many minutes building up.

Physical Environment

- Set the room temperature at a comfortable level.
- Provide sufficient lighting so that each party can see the other clearly. Avoid facing the client directly toward you when there is a lighted window behind you. The client must squint into the full light, as if on stage.
- Reduce noise. Multiple stimuli are confusing. Turn off the television, radio, and any unnecessary equipment.
- Remove distracting objects or equipment. It is appropriate to leave some professional equipment (microscope, B/P manometer) in view. However, clutter, stacks of mail, files of other clients, or your lunch should not be seen. The room should advertise the professional nature of the interviewer.
- Place the distance between you at 4 to 5 feet (twice arm's length). If you place the client any closer, you may invade his or her private space and you may create anxiety. If you place the client farther away, you seem distant and aloof. (See the section on Cultural Considerations for more information.)
- Arrange equal-status seating. Both you and the client should be comfortably seated, at eye level, and place the desk or table so that it does not look like a barrier. Placing the chairs at 90 degrees is good because it allows the person either to face you or to look straight ahead from time to time. Most important, avoid standing. Standing does two things: (1) it communicates your haste, and (2) it assumes superiority. Standing makes you loom over the client as an authority figure. When you are sitting, the person feels some control in the setting.

Dress

- The client should remain in street clothes except in the case of an emergency.
- Your appearance and clothing should be appropriate to the setting and should meet conventional professional standards.

Note-Taking. Some use of history forms and note-taking may be unavoidable. When you sit down later to record the interview, you cannot rely completely on memory to furnish details of previous hospitalizations or review of body systems, for example. But be aware that note-taking during the interview has disadvantages:

- It breaks eye contact too often.
- It shifts your attention away from the client, diminishing his or her sense of importance.
- It can interrupt the client's narrative flow. You may say "Please slow down, I'm not getting it all." Or, the client sees you recording furiously, and in an effort to please you, adjusts his or her tempo to your writing. Either way, the client's natural mode of expression is lost.
- It impedes your observation of the client's nonverbal behavior.

So keep note-taking to a minimum, and try to focus your attention on the person. Any recording you do should be secondary to the dialogue and should not interfere with the person's spontaneity. With experience, you will not rely on note-taking as much.

Tape and Video Recording. An audio tape documents a complete record of what was said in the interview. You cannot refer to it as easily as you can to your notes, but the tape is an excellent teaching tool to study objectively your performance as a beginning interviewer. After listening, other students have said,

"I never realized how much I talked. I really dominated the client."

"I have to watch my interrupting. I cut her off that time."
"There. That response really worked. She opened up. I want to be that effective more often."

Tapes demonstrate how you can improve your communication. And, as you gain experience, the tapes also document ways you have improved. This process is very rewarding.

A video recording takes the teaching-learning tool one step further because you can study both verbal and nonverbal communication at the same time.

"I must have crossed and uncrossed my legs 20 times! I never realized I did that. My fidgeting sure made Mr. J. look distracted."
"It was good that I leaned toward her when she paused that time. I think it helped her continue."

If you use any tape recording, some ethical considerations are necessary. Explain to the person the purpose of the recording (whether for teaching, supervision, research), exactly who will hear it (you, supervisor), and that it will then be destroyed. Obtain consent before you start. Be thoroughly familiar with the equipment; fumbling with the controls is distracting. Arrange the microphone between you and place the rest of the recording equipment out of sight. It is likely that after a few moments, neither of you will be aware of the recording.

TECHNIQUES OF COMMUNICATION

Introducing the Interview

The client is here and you are ready for the interview. If you are nervous about how to begin, remember to keep the beginning short. Probably, the client is nervous, too, and is anxious to start. Address the person, using his or her surname. Introduce yourself and state your role in the agency (if you are a student, say so). If you are gathering a complete history, give the reason for this interview:

"Ms. Taft, I want to ask you some questions about your health so that we can identify what is keeping you healthy and explore any problems."
"Mr. Craig, I want to ask you some questions about your health and your usual daily activities so that we can plan your care here in the hospital."

If the person is in the hospital, more than one health team member may be collecting a history. People will not feel exasperated because they believe they are repeating the same thing if you give a reason for this interview.

After this brief introduction, ask an open-ended question (see the following section) and then let the person proceed. You do not need friendly small talk to build rapport. This is not a social visit; the person has some concern to talk about and wants to get on with it. You will build rapport best by letting him or her discuss the concern early.

Verbal Skills

Verbal skills include questions and responses. There are two types of questions: open-ended and closed. Each type has a different place and function in the interview.

Open-Ended Questions

The open-ended question asks for narrative information. It states the topic to be discussed but only in general terms. Use it to begin the interview, to introduce a new section of questions, and whenever the person introduces a new topic.

"What brings you to the hospital?"
"Tell me why you have come here today."
"How have you been getting along?"
"You mentioned shortness of breath. Tell me more about that."

The open-ended question is unbiased; it leaves the person free to answer in any way. This question encourages the person to respond in paragraphs and to give a spontaneous account in any order chosen. It lets the person express herself or himself fully.

As the person answers, stop and *listen.* What usually happens is that the person answers with a short phrase or sentence, pauses, and then looks at you expecting some direction of how to go on. What you do next is the key to the direction of the interview. If you pose new questions on other topics, you may lose much of the initial story. Instead, respond to the first statement with "Tell me about it," or, "Anything else?" The person then will tell the story.

Closed or Direct Questions

Closed or direct questions ask for specific information. They elicit a short, one or two word answer, a yes or no, or a forced choice. Whereas the open-ended question allows the client to have free rein, the direct question limits his or her answer (see Table 3–1).

Use the direct questions after the person's narrative to fill in any details he or she left out. Also use direct questions when you need many specific facts, such as

Table 3–1. ▶ Comparison of Closed and Open-Ended Questions

OPEN-ENDED	DIRECT, CLOSED
Use for narrative information	Use for specific information
Calls for long paragraph answers	Calls for short one- to two-word answers
Elicits feelings, opinions, ideas	Elicits cold facts
Builds and enhances rapport	Limits rapport and leaves interaction neutral

when asking about past health problems or during the review of systems. You need direct questions to speed up the interview. Asking all open-ended questions would be unwieldy and may take hours. But be careful not to overuse closed questions. Follow these guidelines:

1. Ask only one question at a time. Avoid bombarding the person with long lists: "Have you ever had pain, double vision, watering or redness in the eyes?" The person does not know which question to answer. And if the person answers "yes," you do not know which question the person has answered.

2. Choose language the person understands. You may need to use regional phrases or colloquial expressions. For example, "running off" means running away in standard English, but it means diarrhea to Appalachian mountain people. They use dialects that are different from standard English, both in vocabulary and pronunciation (Tripp-Reimer, 1977).

Responses—Assisting the Narrative

You have asked the first open-ended question, and the person answers. As the person talks, your role is to encourage free expression, but to not let the person wander off course. Your responses help the teller amplify the story.

Some people seek health care for short-term or relatively simple needs. Their history is direct and uncomplicated; for these people, two responses (facilitation and silence) may be all you need to get a complete picture. Other people have a complex story, a long history of a chronic condition, or accompanying emotions. Additional responses help you gather data without cutting them off.

There are 9 types of verbal responses in all. In addition to facilitation and silence, you may choose reflection, empathy, clarification, confrontation, interpretation, explanation, and providing a summary. The first five responses involve your *reactions* to the facts or feelings the person has communicated. Your response focuses on the client's frame of reference. Your own frame of reference does not enter into the response. You start to express yourself in the last four responses. The frame of reference shifts from the client's perspective to yours (Benjamin, 1980). In the first five responses, the client leads; in the last four responses, you lead. These responses include your own thoughts and feelings. Use the last four responses only when merited by the situation. If you use them too often, you take over at the client's expense.

Facilitation. These responses encourage the client to say more, to continue with the story ("mm-hmm, go on, continue, uh-huh"). Also called general leads, these responses show the person you are interested and will listen further. Simply maintaining eye contact, shifting forward in your seat with increased attention, nodding "Yes," or using your hand to gesture, "Yes, go on, I'm with you," encourage the person to continue talking.

However, notice your tone of voice when you say "Mm-hmm." It should indicate "Go on." When said a different way, "Mm-hmm" can indicate "Good," meaning that you approve of *what* the person is saying. Avoid this, because it sounds like a judgment and can influence what the person says next.

Silence. Silent attentiveness is effective after open-ended questions. It communicates that the person has time to think, to organize what he or she wishes to say without interruption from you. This "thinking silence" is the one health professionals interrupt most often. The interruption destroys the person's train of thought (Benjamin, 1980). The client is often interrupted because silence is uncomfortable for beginning examiners. They feel responsible for keeping the dialogue going and feel at fault if it stops. But silence has advantages. One advantage is letting the person collect his or her thoughts. Also, silence gives you a chance to observe the person unobtrusively and to note nonverbal cues. Finally, silence gives you time to plan your next approach.

Reflection. This response echoes the client's words. It repeats part of what the person has just said. In this example, it focuses further attention on a specific phrase and helps the person continue in his own way:

Client: I'm here because of my water. It was cutting off.
Response: It was cutting off?

Client: Yes, yesterday it took me 30 minutes to pass my water. Finally I got a tiny stream, but then it just closed off.

Reflection also can help express feeling behind a person's words. The feeling is already in the statement. You focus on it and encourage the person to elaborate:

Client: It's so hard having to stay flat on my back in the hospital with this pregnancy. I have two more little ones at home. I'm so worried they are not getting the care they need.
Response: You feel worried and anxious about your children?

Think of yourself as a mirror reflecting the person's words or feelings. This helps the person to elaborate on the problem.

Empathy. A physical symptom, condition, or illness often has accompanying emotions. Many people have trouble expressing these feelings, perhaps because of confusion or from embarrassment. In the reflecting example above, the person already had stated her feeling and you echo it. But in the following example, he has not said it yet. An empathic response recognizes a feeling and puts it into words. It names the feeling and allows the expression of it. When the empathic response is used, the client feels accepted and can deal with the feeling openly.

Client (sarcastically): This is just great. I have my own business, I direct 20 employees everyday, and now here I am having to call you for every little thing.
Response: It must be hard—one day having so much control, and now feeling dependent on someone else.

Your response does not cut off further communication as would happen by giving false reassurance ("Oh, you'll be back to work in no time"). Also, it does not deny the feeling and indicate that it is not justified ("Now I don't do *every*thing for you. Why, you are feeding yourself"). An empathic response recognizes the feeling, accepts it, and allows the person to express it without embarrassment. It strengthens rapport. An empathic response does not criticize. It shows you accept even those feelings you personally believe are wrong. Other empathic responses are, "This must be very hard for you," or just placing your hand on the person's arm.

Clarification. Use this when the person's word choice is ambiguous or confusing, e.g., "Tell me what you mean by 'bad blood.'" Clarification also is used to summarize the person's words, simplify the words to make them clearer, then ask if you are on the right track. You are asking for agreement, and the person can then confirm or deny your understanding.

Response: Now as I understand you, this heaviness in your chest comes when you shovel snow or climb stairs, and it goes away when you stop doing those things. Is that correct?
Client: Yes, that's pretty much it.

Confrontation. Recall that in these last four responses, the frame of reference shifts from the client's perspective to yours. In this case, you have observed a certain action, feeling, or statement and you now focus the person's attention on it. You give your honest feedback about what you see or feel. This may focus on a discrepancy: "You say it doesn't hurt, but when I touch you here, you grimace." Or, it may focus on the person's affect: "You look sad" or "You sound angry." Or, you may confront the person when you notice parts of the story are inconsistent: "Earlier you said you were laying off alcohol and just now you said you had a few drinks after work."

Interpretation. This statement is not based on direct observation as is confrontation, but it is based on your inference or conclusion. It links events, makes associations, or implies cause: "It seems that every time you feel the stomach pain, you have had some kind of stress in your life." Interpretation also ascribes feelings and helps the person understand his or her own feelings in relation to the verbal message.

Client: I have decided I don't want to take any more treatments. But I can't seem to tell my doctor that. Every time she comes in, I tighten up and can't say any thing.
Response: Could it be that you're afraid of her reaction?

You do run a risk of making the wrong inference. If this is the case, the person will correct it. But even if the inference is corrected, interpretation helps to prompt further discussion of the topic.

Explanation. With these statements, you inform the person. You share factual and objective information. This may be for orientation to the agency setting: "Your dinner comes at 5:30 PM." Or, it may be to explain cause: "The reason you cannot eat or drink before your blood test is that the food will change the test results."

Summary. This is a final review of what you understand the person has said. It condenses the facts and presents a survey of how you perceive the health problem or need. It is a type of validation in that the person can agree with it or correct it. Both you and the client should participate. When the summary occurs at the end of the interview, it signals that termination of the interview is imminent.

Ten Traps of Interviewing

The verbal skills discussed above are productive and enhance the interview. Now take time to consider nonproductive, defeating verbal messages such as providing misleading assurance or reassurance, giving unwanted advice, using authority, using avoidance language, engaging in distancing, using professional jargon, using leading or biased questions, talking too much, interrupting, and using "why" questions. It is easy to fall into these traps because you are anxious to help. The danger is that they restrict the client's response. They are obstacles to obtaining complete data and to establishing rapport.

Providing Assurance or Reassurance. A woman says, "Oh I just know this lump is going to turn out to be cancer." What happens inside you? The automatic response of many health professionals is to say, "Now don't worry. I'm sure you will be all right." This "courage builder" relieves *your* anxiety and gives you the false sense of having provided comfort. But for the woman it closes off communication. It trivializes her anxiety and effectively denies any further talk of it. Consider instead these responses:

"You are really worried about the lump, aren't you?"
"It must be hard to wait for the biopsy results."

These responses acknowledge the feeling and open the door for more communication.

Giving Advice. Know when to give it and when to refrain from giving it. Often, people seek health care because they want your professional advice and opinion on the management of a health problem: "My child has chicken pox. How should I take care of him?" This is a straightforward request for information that you have that the parent needs. You respond by giving a health prescription, a constructive plan based on your knowledge and experience.

In other situations, advice is different; it is based on a hunch or feeling. Consider the woman who has just left a meeting with her consultant physician: "Dr. Kline just told me my only chance of getting pregnant is to have an operation. I just don't know. What would you do?" Does the woman really want your advice? If you answer, "If I were you, I'd . . ." then you would be making a mistake. You are not her. If you give your answer, you have shifted the accountability for decision-making from her to you. She has not worked out her own solution. She has learned nothing about herself.

Does the woman really want to know what you would do? Probably not. Instead, a better response is reflection:

Response: Have an operation?
Woman: Yes, and I'm terrified of being put to sleep. What if I don't wake up?

Now you know her *real* concern and can help her deal with it. She will have grown in the process and may be better equipped to meet her next decision.

In order to accept advice, it has to be meaningful and appropriate for the person (Bernstein and Bernstein, 1985). For example, in planning cardiac rehabilitation for a man who has had a recent heart attack, you advise him to undertake a planned walking program. However, he has not asked you for help and he does not particularly see the need for your advice. He can treat your advice in two ways: either to follow it or not. He may ignore it, thinking it not appropriate for him ("I get plenty of exercise at work anyway").

If he does follow your advice, two outcomes are possible: the situation improves or it worsens. If the walking strengthens him, the situation has improved. But if he felt no input in arriving at the decision, the psychological reward is limited because it was not his solution. This promotes further dependency. If walking does not help his situation and angina returns, the advice did not work. Since it was not his idea anyway, he can avoid responsibility for the failure ("Look, I did what you wanted, and I still get chest pain. What did you tell me to do this for anyway?").

Although it is quicker just to give advice, take the time to involve the client in a problem-solving process. When he participates, he is more likely to learn and to change behavior.

Using Authority. "Your doctor/nurse knows best" is a response that promotes dependency and inferiority. Although you and the client cannot have equality of professional skill and experience, you are equally worthy human beings, each respecting the other (Benjamin and Benjamin, 1985).

Using Avoidance Language. People use euphemisms such as "passed on" to avoid reality or to hide their feelings. They think if they just say the word "death," it might really happen. So to protect themselves, they evade the issue. Although it seems this will make comfortable potentially fearful topics, it does not. Not talking about the fear does not make it go away; it just suppresses the fear and makes it even more frightening (Cassell, 1980a). Using direct language is the best way to deal with frightening topics.

Engaging in Distancing. This is the use of impersonal speech to put space between a threat and the self. "My friend has a problem. She is afraid she . . ." Or, "There is a lump in the left breast." By using "the" instead of "my," the woman can deny any association with her breast and protect herself from it (Cassell, 1980a). Health professionals use distancing, too, to soften reality. This does not work because it communicates to the other person that you also are afraid of the procedure. The use of blunt specific terms actually is preferable to defuse anxiety.

Using Professional Jargon. What is called a myocardial infarction in the health profession is called a heart attack by most laypeople. Use of jargon sounds exclusionary and paternalistic. You need to adjust your vocabulary to the person, but avoid sounding condescending.

If a client uses medical jargon, do not assume he or she always knows the correct meaning. For example, some people think "hypertensive" means that they are very tense. As a result, they take their medication only when feeling stressed and not when they feel relaxed. This misinformation must be corrected. They need to understand that hypertension is a chronic condition that needs consistent medication to avoid side effects. On the other hand, you do not need to feel that it is a moral imperative to correct all misstatements. Many people say "prostrate" for prostate; just leave the obvious ones alone.

Using Leading or Biased Questions. Asking a man, "You don't smoke, do you?" implies that one answer is "better" than another. If the person wants to please you, either he is forced to answer in a way corresponding to your values or he feels guilty when he must admit the other answer. He risks your disapproval. And if he feels dependent on you for care, the last thing he wants to do is alienate you.

Talking Too Much. Some examiners associate helpfulness with verbal productivity (Bernstein and Bernstein, 1985). If the air has been thick with their oratory and advice, these examiners leave thinking they have met the client's needs. Just the opposite is true. Anxious to please the examiner, the client lets the professional talk at the expense of his need to express himself. A good rule for every interviewer is to *listen more than you talk.*

Interrupting. Often, when you think you know what the person will say, you interrupt and cut the person off. This does not show you are clever. Rather, it signals you are impatient or bored with the interview.

A related trap is thinking of your next remark while the person is talking. You cannot fully understand what the person says. You are so preoccupied with your own role as the interviewer that you are not really listening (Benjamin, 1980). Aim for a second of silence between the person's statement and your next response.

Using "Why" Questions. A young child asks, "Why does the moon look like the end of my fingernail?" The motive behind this question is an innocent search for information. This is quite different from that of an adult's "why" question, such as "*Why* were you carrying so many dishes?" The adult's use of why questions usually implies blame and condemnation; it puts the person on the defensive (Benjamin, 1980).

Consider your use of "why" questions in the health care setting. "Why did you take so much medication?" Or, let's say you ask a man who has just come to the emergency department, "Why did you wait so long before coming to the hospital?" The only possible answer to a "why" question is "because . . ." and the man may not know the answer. He may not have worked it out. You sound whining, accusatory, and judgmental. And the man now must produce an excuse to rationalize his own behavior. To avoid this trap say, "I noticed you didn't come to the hospital until dinner time, even though you had been having chest pains all day. I'd like to find out what was happening during that time."

Nonverbal Skills

Learn to listen with your eyes as well as with your ears (Dirckx, 1985). Nonverbal modes of communication include physical appearance, posture, gestures, facial expression, eye contact, voice, and touch. Nonverbal messages are very important in establishing rapport and in conveying information, especially about feelings. Nonverbal messages provide clues to understanding feelings. When nonverbal and verbal messages are congruent, the verbal is reinforced. When they are incongruent, the nonverbal message tends to be the true one, because it is under less conscious control. Thus, it is important to study the nonverbal messages of clients and examiners and to understand their meanings.

Physical Appearance. Hans Selye (1956) reports his interest in the body's total response to stress began as a student. Unbiased as yet by medical knowledge, he noted that some patients just "looked sick," even though they did not exhibit the specific characteristic signs that would lead to a precise medical diagnosis. Such people simply felt and looked ill or feverish. The same view can work for you. Inattention to dressing or grooming suggests the person is too sick to maintain self-care or has an emotional dysfunction such as depression. Choice of clothing also sends a message, projecting such varied images as role (student, worker, or professional) or attitude (casual, suggestive, or rebellious).

Your own appearance sends a message to the client. Professional dress varies among agencies and settings. Depending on the setting, the use of a professional uniform may create a positive stereotype (comfort or ease of identification) or a negative stereotype (distance, authority, or formality) (Purtilo, 1984). Whatever your personal choice in clothing or grooming, the aim should be to convey a competent, professional image.

Posture. Note the client's position. An open position with extension of large muscle groups shows relaxation, physical comfort, and a willingness to share information. A closed position with arms and legs crossed looks defensive and anxious. Note any change in posture. If a person in a relaxed position suddenly tenses, it suggests discomfort with the new topic.

Your own calm relaxed posture creates a feeling of warmth and trust and conveys an interest in the client. Standing and hastily filling out a history form with periodic peeks at your watch communicates you are busy with many more important things than interviewing this person. Even when your time is limited, appear calm and unhurried. Sit down, even if it is only for a few minutes, and look as if nothing else mattered except this person.

Gestures. Gestures send messages. For example, nodding or an open turning out of the hand shows acceptance, attention, or agreement. A wringing of the hands often indicates anxiety. Pointing a finger occurs with anger and vehemence. Also, hand gestures can reinforce a person's description of pain. When a crushing substernal chest pain is described, the person often holds the hand twisted into a fist in front of the sternum. Or, pain that is bright and sharply localized is shown by pointing one finger to the exact spot: "It hurts right here."

Facial Expression. The face reflects a wide variety of relevant emotions and conditions. The expression may look alert, relaxed, and interested or it may look anxious, angry, and suspicious. Physical conditions such as pain or shortness of breath also show in the expression.

Your own expression should reflect a professional who is attentive, sincere, and interested in the client. Any expression of boredom, distraction, disgust, criticism, or disbelief is picked up by the other person, and rapport will dissolve.

Eye Contact. Lack of eye contact suggests that the person is shy, withdrawn, confused, bored, intimidated, apathetic, or depressed. This applies to examiners, too. You should aim to maintain eye contact but do not stare down the person. Do not have a fixed, penetrating look but rather an easy gaze toward the person's eyes, with occasional glances away. One exception to this is when you are interviewing someone from a culture that avoids direct eye contact (see the section on Cultural Considerations).

Voice. Beside the spoken words, meaning comes through the tone of voice, the intensity and rate of speech, the pitch, and any pauses. These are just as important as words in conveying meaning. For example, the tone of a person's voice may show sarcasm, disbelief, sympathy, or hostility. An anxious person often speaks in a loud, fast voice. A whining voice is similar; it has a high-pitched wavering quality and long, drawn-out syllables. A soft voice may indicate shyness or fear. A hearing-impaired person may use a loud voice.

Even the use of pauses conveys meaning (Cassell, 1980e). When your question is easy and straightforward, a client's long unexpected pause indicates the person is taking time to think of an answer. This raises some doubt as to the honesty of the answer. Unusually frequent and long pauses, when combined with speech that is slow and monotonous and a weak breathy voice, indicates depression.

Touch. The meaning of physical touch is influenced by the person's age, sex, cultural background, past experience, and current setting. The meaning of touch is easily misinterpreted. In most Western cultures, physical touch is reserved for expressions of love and affection or for rigidly defined acts of greeting (see the section on Cultural Considerations). Do not use touch during the interview unless you know the person well and are sure how it will be interpreted. When appropriate, touch communicates effectively, such as a touch of the hand or arm to signal empathy.

In sum, an examiner's nonverbal messages that are productive and enhancing to the relationship are those that show attentiveness and unconditional acceptance. Defeating, nonproductive nonverbal behaviors are those of inattentiveness, authority, and superiority (see Table 3–2).

Table 3-2. ▶ Nonverbal Behaviors of the Interviewer

POSITIVE	NEGATIVE
Appropriate professional appearance	Appearance objectionable to client
Equal status seating	Standing
Close proximity to client	Sitting behind desk, far away, turned away
Relaxed open posture	Tense posture
Leaning slightly toward person	Slouched back
Occasional facilitating gestures	Critical or distracting gestures: pointing finger, clenched fist, finger-tapping, foot-swinging, looking at watch
Facial animation, interest	Bland expression, yawning, tight mouth
Appropriate smiling	Frowning, lip biting
Maintain appropriate eye contact	Shifty, avoiding eye contact, focusing on notes
Moderate tone of voice	Strident, high-pitched tone
Moderate rate of speech	Rate too slow or too fast
Appropriate touch	Too frequent or inappropriate touch

Closing the Interview

The session should end gracefully. An abrupt or awkward closing can destroy rapport and leave the person with a negative impression of the whole interview. To ease into the closing, ask the person,

"Is there anything else you would like to mention?"
"Are there any questions you would like to ask?"
"Are there any other areas I should have asked about?"

This gives the person the final opportunity for self-expression. Then, to indicate closing is imminent say, "Our interview is just about over." No new topic should be introduced now. This is a good time to give your summary or a recapitulation of what you have learned during the interview. This is a final statement of what you and the client agree the health state to be. It should include positive health aspects, any health problems that have been identified, any plans for action, or an explanation of the following physical examination. As you part from clients thank them for the time spent and for their cooperation.

DEVELOPMENTAL CONSIDERATIONS

Consider these additional points when interviewing people of different age groups.

The Younger Person

When your client is a child, you must build rapport with two people—the child and the accompanying parent. Greet both by name, but with a younger child (1 to 6 years old), focus more on the parent. By ignoring the child temporarily, the child can size you up from a safe distance. The child can observe your interaction with the parent, see that the parent accepts and likes you, and relax.

Begin by interviewing the parent and child together. If any sensitive topics arise (e.g., the parents' troubled relationship or the child's problems at school or with peers), explore them later when the parent is alone. Provide toys to occupy the child as you and the parent talk. This frees the parent to concentrate on the history. And it indicates the level of attention span or independent play of the child. Through the interview, be alert to ways the parent and child interact.

For younger children, the parent will provide all or most of the history. Thus you are collecting the child's health data from the parent's frame of reference. Usually, this viewpoint is reliable because most parents have the child's well-being as a priority and see cooperation with you as a way to enhance this well-being. But the possibility exists for parental bias. Bias can occur

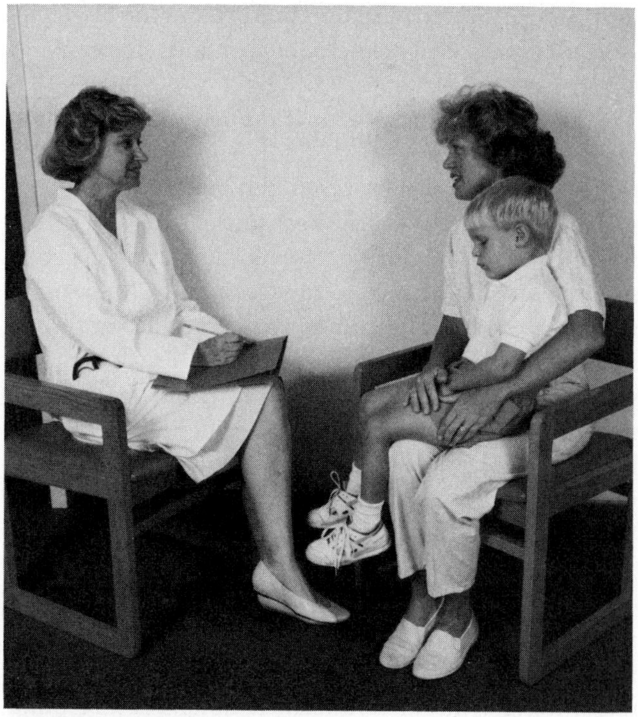

▶ **Figure 3-2**

when asked to describe the child's achievements, or whenever their own parenting ability seems called into question. For example, if you ask, "His fever was 103 and you did not bring him in?" you are implying a lack of parenting skill. This puts the parent on the defensive and increases anxiety. Instead, use open-ended questions that increase description and defuse threat, e.g., "What happened when the fever went up?"

A parent with more than one child has more than one set of data to remember. Be patient as the parent sorts through his or her memory to pull out facts of developmental milestones or past history.

In collecting developmental data, avoid being judgmental about the age of achievement of certain milestones. Parents are understandably proud of their child's achievements and are sensitive to inferences that these milestones may occur late.

Refer to the child by name, not as "the baby." Also, be clear when identifying the parents. The mother's present husband may not necessarily be the child's father. Instead of asking about "your husband's" health ask, "Is Joan's father in good health?"

Although most of your communication is with the parent, do not ignore the child completely. You need to make contact to ease into the physical examination later. Begin by asking about the toys the child is playing with or about a special doll or teddy bear brought from home: "Does your doll have a name?" or, "What can your truck do?" Stoop down to meet the child at his or her eye level. Adult size can be overwhelming to young children and emphasize their smallness.

Nonverbal communication is even more important to children than it is to adults. Children are quick to pick up feelings, anxiety, or comfort from nonverbal cues. Keep your physical appearance neat and clean, and avoid formal uniforms that distance you. Keep any gestures slow, deliberate, and close to your body. Children are frightened by quick or grandiose gestures. Do not try to maintain constant eye contact; this feels threatening to a small child. Use a quiet, measured voice, and choose simple words in your speech. Considering the child's level of language development is valuable in planning your communication (Pontious, 1982; Whaley and Wong, 1990).

The Infant. Nonverbal communication is the primary method. Most infants look calm and relaxed when all their needs are met, and they cry when they are frightened, hungry, tired, or uncomfortable. They respond best to firm, gentle handling and a quiet, calm voice. Your voice is comforting, even though they do not understand the words. Older infants have anxiety toward strangers. They are more cooperative when the parent is kept in view.

The Preschooler. A 2- to 6-year-old is completely egocentric. He or she sees the world only from their own point of view. Everything revolves around them. It is useless to cite the example of another child's behavior to get them to cooperate. It has no meaning. Only their own experience is relevant.

Their communication is direct, concrete, literal, and set in the present. Avoid expressions such as "climbing the walls," because they are easily misinterpreted by young children. Use short, simple sentences with a concrete explanation. Take time to give a short simple explanation for any unfamiliar equipment that will be used on the child. Preschoolers are *animistic;* they imagine inanimate objects can come alive and have human characteristics. Thus a blood pressure cuff can wake up and bite or pinch.

The School-Age Child. A child 7 to 12 years old can tolerate and understand others' viewpoints. This child is more objective and realistic. He or she wants to know functional aspects—how things work and why things are done.

Children of this age group have the verbal ability to add important data to the history. Interview the parent and child together, but when there is a presenting symptom or sign, ask the child about it first, then gather data from the parent. For the well child seeking a checkup, pose questions about school, friends, or activities directly to the child.

The Adolescent. Adolescents want to be adults, but they do not have the cognitive ability to achieve their goal. They are between two stages. Sometimes they are capable of mature actions, and other times fall back on childhood response patterns, especially in times of stress. You cannot treat adolescents as children, yet you cannot overcompensate and assume their communication style, learning ability, and motivation are consistently at an adult level.

Adolescents value their peers. They crave acceptance and sameness with their peers. Adolescents think no adult can understand them. Because of this, some act with aloof contempt, answering only in monosyllables. Others make eye contact and tell you what they think you want to hear, but inside they are thinking "You'll never know the full story about me."

This knowledge about adolescents is apt to paralyze you in communicating with them. However, successful communication is possible, and rewarding. The guidelines are simple.

The first consideration is your attitude, which must be one of respect. Respect is the most important thing you can communicate to the adolescent. The adolescent needs to feel validated as a human being, accepted, and worthy.

Second, your communication must be totally honest. The adolescent's intuition is highly tuned and can detect phoniness or when information is withheld. Always give them the truth. Play it straight or you will lose them. They will cooperate if they understand your rationale.

Stay in character. Avoid using language that is absurd for your age or professional role. It is helpful to understand some of the jargon used by adolescents, but you cannot use those words yourself simply to try to bond with the adolescent. Do not try to be his or her peer. You are not, and they will not accept you as such.

Use icebreakers. Focus first on the adolescent, not on the problem. Although an adult just wants to get on with it and talk about the health concern immediately, the adolescent responds best when the focus is on him or her as a person. Show an interest in the adolescent. Ask open friendly questions about school, activities, hobbies, friends. Refrain from asking questions about parents and family for now — these issues can be emotionally charged during adolescence.

Do not assume adolescents know *anything* about a health interview or a physical examination. Explain every step and give the rationale. They need direction. They will cooperate when they know the reason for the questions or actions.

Keep your questions short and simple. "Why are you here?" sounds brazen to you, but it is effective with the adolescent. Be prepared for the adolescent who does *not* know why he or she is there. Some adolescents are pushed into coming to the examination by a parent.

The communication responses described for the adult need to be reconsidered when talking with the adolescent. Silent periods usually are best avoided. Giving adolescents a little time to collect their thoughts is acceptable, but a silence for other reasons is threatening. Also, avoid reflection. If you use reflection, the adolescent is likely to answer, "What?" They just do not have the cognitive skills to respond to that indirect mode of questioning. Also, adolescents are more sensitive to nonverbal communication than are adults. Be aware of your expressions and gestures.

If confidential material is uncovered during the interview, consider what can remain confidential and what you feel you must share for the well-being of the adolescent. For example, if the adolescent talks about an abusive home situation, state that you must share this information with other health professionals for his or her own protection. Ask the adolescent, "Do you have a problem with that?" and, "You will have to trust that I will handle this information professionally and in your best interest."

The Older Adult

The aging adult has the task of finding the meaning of life and the purpose of his or her own existence, and adjusting to the inevitability of death. Some people have developed comfortable and satisfying answers and greet you with a calm demeanor and self-assurance. Be alert for the occasional person who sounds hopeless and despairing about life at present and in the future.

Address the person always by the last name. Some older adults resent being called by their first name by younger persons, and almost all cringe at the ignominious "Grandma," or "Pop."

The interview usually takes longer with older adults because they have a longer story to tell. You may need to break up the interview into more than one visit, collecting the most important historical data first. Or certain portions of the data, such as past history or the review of systems, can be provided on a form that is filled out at home, as long as the person's vision and handwriting are adequate. Take time to review these parts with the person during the interview.

It is important to adjust the pace of the interview to

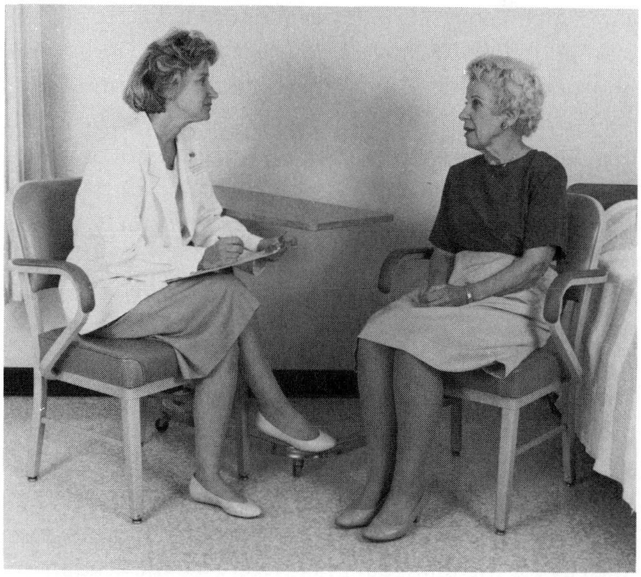

▸ **Figure 3-3**

the aging person. The older person has a great amount of background material to sort through, and this takes some time. Also, some aging persons need a greater amount of response time to interpret the question and process their answer. Avoid trying to hurry them along. This approach only affirms their stereotype of younger persons in general and health care providers in particular, i.e., people who are merely interested in numbers of clients and filling out forms. Any urge from you to get on with it will surely make them retreat. You will lose valuable data, and their needs will not be met.

Consider physical limitations when planning the interview. An aging person may fatigue earlier and may require that the interview be broken up into shorter segments. For the person with impaired hearing, face directly so that your mouth and face are fully visible. Do not shout; it does not help and actually distorts speech.

Touch is a nonverbal skill that is very important to older persons. Their other senses may be diminished, and touch grounds you in reality. Also, a hand on the arm or shoulder is an empathic message that communicates you empathize with the person and want to understand his or her problem (see section on Cultural Considerations for exceptions).

INTERVIEWING PEOPLE WITH SPECIAL NEEDS

Hearing-Impaired People

Although many people will tell you in advance that they have a hearing deficit, others must be recognized by clues such as staring at your mouth and face, not attending unless looking at you, or speaking in a voice unusually loud or with guttural or garbled sounds. The deaf person may be familiar with some equipment in the hospital or office setting, or may have had previous experience with health care settings. But without full communication, the hearing impaired person is sure to feel isolated and anxious. Ask the deaf person the preferred way to communicate—by signing, lip reading, or writing.

A complete health history requires a sign language interpreter. Since most health care professionals are not proficient in signing, try to find an interpreter through a social service agency or the person's own social network. You may use family members, but be aware that they sometimes edit for the person. Use the same guidelines as for the bilingual interpreter (see the section on Cultural Considerations).

If the person prefers lip reading, be sure to face him or her squarely and have good lighting on your face. Examiners with a beard, moustache, or foreign accents are less effective. Do not exaggerate your lip movements because this distorts your words. Similarly, shouting distorts the reception of a hearing aid the person may wear. Speak slowly and supplement your voice with appropriate hand gestures or pantomime. Nonverbal cues are important adjuncts because the lip reader only understands at best 50 percent of your speech when relying solely on vision (Hipskind, 1989). Be sure the person understands your questions. Many hearing-impaired people nod "yes" just to be friendly and cooperative but really do not understand.

Written communication is efficient in sections such as past health history or review of systems. For the present history of illness, writing is very time consuming and laborious. The syntax of the person's written words will read normally if the hearing impairment occurred after speech patterns developed. If the deafness occurred before speech patterns developed, the written syntax follows that of signing, which is different from that of English.

Acutely Ill People

An emergency demands your prompt action. You must combine interviewing with physical examination skills to determine lifesaving actions. Although life support measures may be paramount, still try to interview the person as much as possible. Subjective data are crucial to determine the cause and course of the emergency. Abbreviate your questioning. Identify the main area of distress and question about that. Often family or friends can provide important data.

A hospitalized person with a critical or severe illness usually is too weak, too short of breath, or in too much pain to talk. First attend to the comfort of the person. Then establish a priority; find out immediately what parts of the history are the most relevant. Explore the first concern the person mentions. Begin to use closed, direct questions earlier. Finally, watch that your statements are very clear. When a person is very sick, he or she can misconstrue even the simplest sentence. The person will react according to preconceived ideas about what a serious illness means, so anything you say should be direct and precise.

People Under the Influence of Street Drugs or Alcohol

It is common for persons under the influence of alcohol or other drugs to be admitted to a hospital; alcohol depresses the central nervous system, putting the person at great risk for accidents and injuries. Also, chronic use creates complex medical problems that require increasing care.

When interviewing a person currently under the influence of alcohol or other drugs, ask simple and direct questions. Take care to make your manner and questions nonthreatening. Avoid confrontation at this point. Further, avoid any display of scolding or disgust, because this person may become belligerent. One priority is to find out the time of the person's last drink and how much he or she drank at this episode as well as the name and amount of other drugs taken. This information will help assess any withdrawal patterns.

Once he or she is sober, the hospitalized substance abuser should be assessed for the extent of the problem and the meaning of the problem for the person and family. Initially you encounter the use of denial and increased defensiveness; special interview techniques are needed (Kinney, 1990).

Personal Questions

Occasionally, people will ask you questions about *your* personal life or opinions, such as "Are you married?" "Do you have children?" or "Do you smoke?" You do not need to answer every question. You may supply brief information when you feel it is appropriate, but be sensitive to the possibility that there may be a motive behind the personal questions. Try directing your response back to the person's frame of reference (Benjamin, 1980). You might say, "No, I don't have children. I wonder if your question is related to how I can help you care for little Jamie?"

Sexually Aggressive People

On rare occasions, these personal questions extend to flirtatious compliments, seductive innuendo, or advances. Some people experience serious or chronic illness as a threat to their self-esteem and sexual adequacy. This creates anxiety that makes them act out in sexually aggressive ways.

Your response must make it clear that you are a health professional who can best care for the person by maintaining a professional relationship. At the same time, you should communicate that you accept the person and you understand the need to be self-assertive but that you cannot tolerate sexual advances. This may be difficult, considering that the words or gestures may have left you shocked, embarrassed, or angry. Your feelings are normal. A response that would open communication would be, "Your behavior makes me uncomfortable. I wonder if it relates to your illness or to being in the hospital?"

Crying

A beginning examiner usually feels horrified when the client starts crying. But crying actually is a big relief to a person. Health problems come with powerful emotions. Worries about illness, death, or loss take a great amount of energy to keep bottled up inside. When you say something that "makes the person cry," do not think you have hurt the person. You have just hit on a topic that is important. Do not go on to a new topic. Just let the person cry and express his or her feelings fully. You can offer a tissue and wait until the crying subsides to talk. The person will regain control soon.

Sometimes your client looks as if he or she is on the verge of tears but is trying hard to suppress them. Again instead of moving on to something new, acknowledge the expression ("You look sad"). Do not worry that you will open an uncontrollable floodgate. The person may cry but will be relieved, and you will have gained insight to a serious concern.

Anger

Occasionally you will try to interview a person who is already angry. Try not to personalize this anger; usually it does not relate to you. The person is showing aggression as a response to his or her own feelings of anxiety or helplessness. Do ask about the anger and hear the person out. Deal with the angry feelings before you ask anything else. An angry person cannot be an effective participant in a health interview.

Maybe *you* are angry when you come into the interview. When you are angry, say so and tell the client that you are angry at something or someone else. Otherwise the client, unusually vulnerable and dependent on you, thinks you are angry at him or her.

Anxiety

Finally, take it for granted that nearly all sick people have some anxiety (Dirckx, 1985). This is a normal response to being sick. It makes some people aggressive and others dependent. Remember that the person is not reacting as typically as when he or she is healthy.

TRANSCULTURAL CONSIDERATIONS

CROSS-CULTURAL COMMUNICATION

Verbal and nonverbal communication are influenced by the cultural background of both the health care professional and the client. *Cross-cultural* or *intercultural communication* refers to the communication process occurring between a health care professional and a client, each with different cultural backgrounds, in which both attempt to understand the other's point of view from a cultural perspective.

The Professional Relationship

From your initial introduction to the client through the termination of the relationship, you will be in a continuous process of communication. Because beginning impressions are so important in all human relationships, cross-cultural considerations concerning introductions warrant a few brief remarks. In order to ensure that a mutually respectful relationship is established, introduce yourself and indicate how you prefer to be called, i.e., by first name, last name, or title. Ask the client to do the same. This enables you to address the person in a manner that is culturally appropriate and could actually spare you embarrassment. For example, it is the custom among some Asian and European cultures to write the last name first; thus, you will be sure to have a very basic piece of data, the person's name, correct.

Both you and your client are likely to bring cultural stereotypes to the professional relationship. For example, when Ragucci (1981) studied the views of Italian Americans toward nurses, she found a very traditional expectation with respondents generally expecting nurses to carry out physicians' orders without making independent health care judgments. Similarly, a study of Asian clients reveals that nurses are expected to provide medications, including injections, and to perform treatments ordered by physicians (Gould-Martin and Ngin, 1981) but not to provide psychosocial care. In Asia, as well as in many parts of Africa, family members perform all support tasks such as bathing, feeding, and other comfort measures, whereas nurses engage in strictly procedural activities such as changing dressings or administering medications.

One of the major challenges you will face in assessing people from culturally diverse backgrounds is overcoming your own *ethnocentrism.* Ethnocentrism is the tendency to view your own way of life as the most desirable, acceptable, or best and to act in a superior manner to another culture's lifeways. A related admonition is to beware of *cultural imposition,* the tendency to impose your beliefs, values, and patterns of behavior on individuals from another culture. These admonitions are more easily stated than practiced.

Space, Distance, and Intimacy

Both the client's and your own sense of spatial distance are significant throughout the interview and physical examination, with culturally appropriate distance zones varying widely. For example, you may find yourself backing away from people of Hispanic, East Indian, or Middle Eastern origins who invade your personal space with regularity in an attempt to bring you closer into the space that is comfortable to them. Although you are uncomfortable with their close physical proximity, they are perplexed by your distancing behaviors and may perceive you as aloof and unfriendly. Summarized in Table 3–3 are the four distance zones identified for the functional use of space that are embraced by the dominant cultural group, including that of most health care professionals.

Table 3-3. ▶ Functional Use of Space

ZONE	REMARKS
Intimate zone (0 to $1\frac{1}{2}$ feet)	Visual distortion occurs Best for assessing breath and other body odors
Personal distance ($1\frac{1}{2}$ to 4 feet)	Perceived as an extension of the self similar to a bubble Voice is moderate Body odors inapparent No visual distortion Much of the physical assessment occurs at this distance
Social distance (4 to 12 feet)	Used for impersonal business transactions Perceptual information much less detailed Much of the interview will occur at this distance
Public distance ($12+$ feet)	Interaction with others impersonal Speaker's voice must be projected Subtle facial expressions imperceptible

(From Hall E: Proxemics: The study of man's spatial relations. *In* Galdston I (Ed): Man's Image in Medicine and Anthropology. New York: International University Press, pp 109–120, 1963.)

Interactions between clients and health care professionals may also depend on the client's desired degree of intimacy, which may range from very formal interactions to close personal relationships. For example, some Southeast Asians expect those in authority, i.e., nurses or physicians, to be authoritarian, directive, and detached. In seeking health care, some Asians may expect the health care provider to intuitively know what is wrong with them, and you may actually lose some credibility by asking a fairly standard interview question such as, "What brings you here?" The Asian may be thinking, "Don't you know why I'm here? You're supposed to be the one with all the answers."

The emphasis on social harmony among Asians and Native Americans may prevent the full expression of concerns or feelings during the interview. Such reserved behavior may leave you with the impression that the person agrees with or understands your explanation. Nodding or smiling by Asians may only reflect their cultural value for interpersonal harmony, not agreement with you. You may distinguish between socially compliant client responses aimed at maintaining harmony and genuine concurrence by obtaining validation of your assumptions. This may be accomplished by inviting the person to respond frankly to your suggestions or by giving the person "permission" to disagree.

In contrast, Appalachians traditionally have close family interaction patterns that often lead them to expect close personal relationships with health care providers. The Appalachian may evaluate your effectiveness on the basis of interpersonal skills rather than professional competencies. Appalachians are likely to be uncomfortable with the impersonal, bureaucratic orientation of most health care institutions. Those of Latin American or Mediterranean origins often expect an even higher degree of intimacy and may attempt to involve you in their family system by expecting you to participate in personal activities and social functions. These individuals may come to expect personal favors that extend beyond the scope of your professional practice and may feel it is their privilege to contact you at home during any time of the day or night for care (Lipson and Meleis, 1983).

Overcoming Communication Barriers

Health care providers tend to have stereotypical expectations of the client's behavior during the interview and physical examination. In general, they expect behavior to consist of undemanding compliance, an attitude of respect for the health care provider, and cooperation with requested behavior throughout the examination. Although clients may ask a few questions for the purpose of clarification, slight deference to recognized authority figures, i.e., health care providers, is expected. Individuals from culturally diverse backgrounds, however, may have significantly different perceptions about the appropriate role of the individual and his or her family when seeking health care. If you find yourself becoming annoyed that a client is asking too many questions, assuming a defensive posture, or otherwise feeling uncomfortable, you might pause for a moment to examine the source of the conflict from a cross-cultural perspective.

During illness, culturally acceptable sick role behavior may range from aggressive, demanding behavior to silent passivity. According to Hartog and Hartog (1983), complaining, demanding behavior during illness is often rewarded with attention among American Jewish and Italian groups, whereas Asians and Native Americans are likely to be quiet and compliant during illness. During the interview, Asians may provide you with the answers they think you want to hear, behavior consistent with the dominant cultural value for harmonious relationships with others. Thus, you should attempt to phrase questions or statements in a neutral manner that avoids foreshadowing an expected response. Appalachians may reject an interviewer whom they perceive as prying or nosey owing to a cultural ethic of neutrality that mandates minding one's own business and avoiding assertive or argumentative behavior.

Nonverbal Communication

Unless you make an effort to understand the client's nonverbal behavior, you may overlook important information such as that which is conveyed by facial expressions, silence, eye contact, touch, and other body language. Communication patterns vary widely cross-culturally even for seemingly innocent behaviors such as smiling and handshaking. Among many Hispanics, for example, smiling and handshaking are considered an integral part of sincere interactions and essential to establishing trust, whereas a Soviet might perceive the same behavior as insolent and frivolous (Tripp-Reimer and Lauer, 1987). Sex and gender issues also become significant; e.g., among some women of Middle Eastern origins men and women simply do not shake hands or touch each other in any other manner outside of the marital relationship. If the health care provider and client are both female, however, a handshake is generally acceptable.

Wide cultural variation exists when interpreting silence. Some individuals find silence extremely uncomfortable and make every effort to fill conversational lags with words. In contrast, Native Americans consider silence essential to understanding and respecting the other person. A pause following your question signifies that what you have asked is important enough to be given thoughtful consideration. In traditional Chinese and Japanese cultures, silence may mean that the speaker wishes the listener to consider the content of what has been said before continuing. Other cultural meanings of silence may be found. The English and Arabs may use silence out of respect for another's privacy, whereas the French, Spanish, and Soviets may interpret it as a sign of agreement. Asian cultures often use silence to demonstrate respect for elders (Boyle and Andrews, 1989; Tripp-Reimer and Lauer, 1987).

Eye contact is perhaps among the most culturally variable nonverbal behaviors. Although most health care providers have been taught to maintain eye contact while interviewing clients, individuals from culturally diverse backgrounds may misconstrue this behavior. Asian, Native American, Indochinese, Arab, and Appalachian people may consider direct eye contact impolite or aggressive, and they may avert their own eyes during the interview. Native Americans often stare at the floor during the interview, a culturally appropriate behavior indicating that the listener is paying close attention to the speaker.

In some cultures, including Arab, Hispanic, and black groups, modesty for women is interrelated with eye contact. For Muslim-Arab women, modesty is, in part, achieved by avoiding eye contact with males (except for one's husband) and keeping eyes downcast when encountering members of the opposite sex in public situations. In many cultures, the only woman who smiles and establishes eye contact with men in public is a prostitute! Hasidic Jewish males also have culturally based norms concerning eye contact with females. You may observe the male avoiding direct eye contact and turning his head in the opposite direction when walking past or speaking to a woman. The preceding examples are intended to be illustrative, not exhaustive.

Touch

Without a doubt, touching the client is a necessary component of a comprehensive assessment. While recognizing the benefits reported by many health care providers in establishing rapport with clients through touch, including the promotion of healing through therapeutic touch, physical contact with clients conveys various meanings cross-culturally. In many cultures, e.g., Arab and Hispanic, male health care providers may be prohibited from touching or examining either all or certain parts of the female body. During pregnancy the woman may prefer female health care providers or may actually refuse to be examined by a male. Be aware that the client's significant others may also exert pressure on health care providers by enforcing these culturally meaningful norms in the health care setting.

Touching children may also have associated meaning cross-culturally. For example, Hispanics may believe in "mal ojo," meaning "evil eye," in which the individual becomes ill as a result of excessive admiration by another. Many Asians believe that one's strength resides in the head and touching the head is considered disrespectful. Thus, palpating the fontanel of an infant from Southeast Asian descent should be approached with sensitivity. You may find it necessary to rely on alternative sources of information (e.g., assessing for clinical manifestations of increased intracranial pressure or signs of premature fontanel closure). Or you alter your assessment technique and place your own hand over the mother's while asking for a description of what she feels.

Gender

Violating norms related to appropriate male-female relationships among various cultures may jeopardize your therapeutic professional relationship. Among Arab-Americans, you may find that an adult male is never alone with a female (except his wife) and is generally accompanied by one or more other males when interacting with females. This behavior is culturally very significant and failure to adhere to the *cultural code* (set of rules or norms of behavior used by a cultural group to guide their behavior and to interpret situations) is viewed as a serious transgression, often one in which the lone male will be accused of sexual impropriety. The best way to ensure that cultural variables have been considered is to ask the person about culturally relevant aspects of male-female relationships, preferably at the beginning of the interview, before you have an opportunity to violate any culturally based practices.

Language

When assessing non-English-speaking people, you may find yourself in one of two situations—either choosing an interpreter or communicating effectively when there is no interpreter.

Interviewing the non-English-speaking person requires a bilingual interpreter for full communication. Even the person from another culture or country who has a basic command of English may need an interpreter when faced with the anxiety-provoking situation of entering a hospital, encountering a strange symptom, or discussing a sensitive topic such as birth control and gynecologic or urologic concerns. It is tempting to ask a relative, friend, or even another client to interpret because this person is readily available and probably would like to help. This is disadvantageous because it violates confidentiality for the client, who may not want personal information shared with another. Furthermore, the friend or relative, though fluent in ordinary language usage, is likely to be unfamiliar with medical terminology, hospital or clinic procedures, and medical ethics.

Whenever possible, work with a bilingual team member or a trained medical interpreter. This person knows interpreting techniques, has a health care background, and understands patients' rights. The trained interpreter also is knowledgeable about cultural beliefs and health practices. This person can help you bridge the cultural gap and can advise you concerning the cultural appropriateness of your recommendations.

Although you will be in charge of the focus and flow of the interview, view yourself and the interpreter as a team. Ask the interpreter to meet the client beforehand to establish rapport and to garner the client's age, occupation, educational level, and attitude toward health care. This enables the interpreter to communicate on the client's level.

Allow more time for this interview. With the third person repeating everything, it can take considerably longer than interviewing English-speaking people. You need to focus on priority data.

There are two styles of interpreting—line-by-line and summarizing. Translating line-by-line takes more time, but it ensures accuracy. Use this for most of the

Table 3-4. ▶ Overcoming Language Barriers: Use of an Interpreter

Before locating an interpreter, be sure that you know what language the person speaks at home because it may be different from the language spoken publicly (e.g., French is sometimes spoken by aristocratic or well-educated people from certain Asian or Middle Eastern cultures).

Avoid interpreters from a rival tribe, state, region, or nation (e.g., a Palestinian who knows Hebrew may not be the best interpreter for a Jewish client).

Be aware of sex and gender differences between interpreter and client (to avoid violation of cultural mores related to modesty).

Be aware of age differences between interpreter and client

Be aware of socioeconomic differences between interpreter and client

Ask interpreter to translate as closely to verbatim as possible

An interpreter who is a nonrelative may seek compensation for services rendered

Recommendations for institutions:

Maintain a computerized list of interpreters who may be contacted as the situation warrants

Set up a network with area hospitals, colleges, universities, and other organizations that may serve as resources for interpreters

Table 3-5. ▶ Overcoming Language Barriers: What to Do When There is No Interpreter

1. Be polite and formal
2. Greet the person using the last or complete name. Gesture to yourself and say your name. Offer a handshake or nod. Smile.
3. Proceed in an unhurried manner. Pay attention to any effort by the patient or family to communicate.
4. Speak in a low, moderate voice. Avoid talking loudly. Remember that there is a tendency to raise the volume and pitch of your voice when the listener appears not to understand. The listener may perceive that you are shouting and/or angry.
5. Use any words that you might know in the person's language. This indicates that you are aware of and respect their culture.
6. Use simple words, such as "pain" instead of "discomfort." Avoid medical jargon, idioms, and slang. Avoid using contractions, e.g., don't, can't, and won't. Use nouns repeatedly rather instead of pronouns.
   Example:
   Do not say: "He has been taking his medicine, hasn't he?"
   Do say: "Does Juan take medicine?"
7. Pantomime words and simple actions while you verbalize them.
8. Give instructions in the proper sequence.
   Example:
   Do not say: "Before you rinse the bottle, sterilize it."
   Do say: "First wash the bottle. Second, rinse the bottle."
9. Discuss one topic at a time. Avoid using conjunctions.
   Example:
   Do not say: "Are you cold and in pain?"
   Do say: "Are you cold (while pantomiming)? Are you in pain?"
10. Validate if the person understands by having him or her repeat instructions, demonstrate the procedure, or act out the meaning.
11. Write out several short sentences in English and determine the person's ability to read them.
12. Try a third language. Many Indo-Chinese speak French. Europeans often know two or more languages. Try Latin words or phrases.
13. Ask who among the person's family and friends could serve as an interpreter.
14. Obtain phrase books from a library or bookstore, make or purchase flash cards, contact hospitals for a list of interpreters, and use both a formal and an informal network to locate a suitable interpreter.

interview. Both you and the client should speak only a sentence or two, then allow the interpreter time. Use simple language yourself, not medical jargon that the interpreter must simplify before it can be translated. Summary translation progresses faster and is useful for teaching relatively simple health techniques with which the interpreter is already familiar. Be alert for nonverbal cues as the client talks. These cues can give valuable data. A good interpreter also notes nonverbal messages and passes them on to you. Summarized in Table 3–4 are suggestions for the selection and use of an interpreter.

Although use of an interpreter is the ideal, you may find yourself in a situation with a non-English-speaking client when no interpreter is available. Table 3–5 summarizes some suggestions for overcoming language barriers when there is no interpreter.

Bibliography

Avila DL, Combs AW, Purkey WW: The Helping Relationship Source Book. 2nd ed. Boston, Allyn and Bacon, 1977.

Benjamin A: The Helping Interview. 3rd ed. Boston, Houghton Mifflin, 1980.

Bernstein L, Bernstein RS: Interviewing—A Guide for Health Professionals. 4th ed. Norwalk, CT, Appleton-Century-Crofts, 1985.

Boyle JS, Andrews MM: Transcultural Concepts in Nursing Care. Glenview, IL, Scott, Foresman, and Company, 1989.

Bradley JC, Edinberg MA: Communication in the Nursing Context. 2nd ed. New York, Appleton & Lange, 1986.

Cassell EJ: Changing the Words Changes the World. Patient Care 14:126–142, 1980a.

Cassell EJ: Exploring thoughts that underlie speech. Patient Care 14:148–160, 1980b.

Cassell EJ: Hear what the patient means, say what you mean. Patient Care 14:80–90, 1980c.

Cassell EJ: Listen: "Illogical" patients often make sense. Patient Care 14:91–106, 1980d.

Cassell EJ: Untwisting the fibers of "paralanguage." Patient Care 14:186–204, 1980e.

Combs AW, Avila DL: Perspectives on Helping Relationships. Boston, Allyn and Bacon, 1985.

Diaz-Duque OF: Advice from an interpreter. Am J Nurs 82:1380–1382, 1982.

Dirckx JH: Talking with patients, the art of history-taking. Clin Nurse Practitioner 3:13–14, 1985.

Drew N: Exclusion and confirmation—a phenomenology of patients' experiences with caregivers. Image 18:39–43, 1986.

Gonzalez-Swafford MJ, Gutierrez MG: Ethno-medical beliefs and practices of Mexican-Americans. Nurse Practitioner 8:29–34, 1983.

Gould-Martin K, Ngin C: Chinese Americans. *In* Harwood A (Ed): Ethnicity and Medical Care. Cambridge, Harvard University Press, 1981.

Grasska MA, McFarland T: Overcoming the language barrier—problems and solutions. Am J Nurs 82:1376–1379, 1982.

Hartog J, Hartog FA: Cultural aspects of health and illness in hospitals. West J Med 139:911–918, 1983.

Hipskind NM: Visual stimuli in communication. *In* Schow RL, Nerbonne MA (Eds): Introduction to Aural Rehabilitation. 2nd ed. Austin, Tx PRO-ED, 1989.

Kasch CR: Toward a theory of nursing action: Skills and Competency in nurse-patient interaction. Nurs Res 35(4):226–230, 1986.

Kinney J: Loosening the Grip. 4th ed. St. Louis, C.V. Mosby, 1990.

Lipson J, Meleis A: Issues in health care of Middle Eastern patients. West J Med 139:854–861, 1983.

Miller EL: Interviewing the sexually abused child. Maternal Child Nurs 10:103–105, 1985.

Okun BF: Effective helping: Interviewing & Counseling Techniques. 3rd ed. Monterey, CA, Brooks/Cole, 1986.

Pontious SL: Practical Piaget—helping children understand. Am J Nurs 82:114–117, 1982.

Purtilo, R: Health Professional/Patient Interaction. 3rd ed. Philadelphia, W.B. Saunders, 1984.

Ragucci AT: Italian Americans. *In* Harwood A (Ed): Ethnicity and Medical Care. Cambridge, Harvard University Press, 1981, pp 56–84.

Rogers CR: Client-Centered Therapy. Boston, Houghton Mifflin, 1951.

Selye, Hans: The stress of Life. New York, McGraw-Hill, 1956.

Spector RE: Cultural Diversity in Health and Illness. New York, Appleton-Century-Crofts, 1985.

Tripp-Reimer T, Friedl MC: Appalachians—a neglected minority. Nurs Clin North Am 12:41–54, 1977.

Tripp-Reimer T, Lauer GM: Ethnicity in families with chronic illness. *In* Wright LM, Leahey M (Eds): Families and Chronic Illness. Springhouse, PA, Springhouse, 1987, pp 77–99.

Whaley LP, Wong DL: Nursing Care of Infants and Children. 4th ed. St. Louis, CV Mosby, 1990.

CHAPTER

4 The Complete Health History

The purpose of the health history is to collect *subjective* data, what the person *says* about himself or herself. The history is combined with the objective data from the physical examination and laboratory studies to form the data base. The data base is used to make a judgment or a diagnosis about the health status of the individual.

The following health history is a complete picture of the person's past and present health. It describes the individual as a whole and how the person interacts with the environment. It records health strengths and coping skills. The history should recognize and affirm what the person is doing right; what he or she is doing to help stay well. For the well person, the history is used to assess his or her lifestyle such as exercise, diet, risk reduction, and health promotion behaviors. For the ill person, it includes a detailed and chronologic record of the health problem. For all, the health history is a screening tool for abnormal symptoms, health problems, and concerns, and it records ways of responding to the health problems.

In many settings, the client fills out a printed history form or checklist. This allows the person ample time to recall and consider such items as dates of health landmarks and relevant family history. The interview is then used to validate the written data and to collect more data on lifestyle management and current health problems.

Although history forms vary, most contain information in this sequence of categories:

1. biographical data
2. reason for seeking care
3. present health or history of present illness
4. past history
5. family history
6. review of systems
7. functional assessment or activities of daily living

The health history discussed in the following section follows this format and includes all data listed in the American Nurses' Association (ANA) Standards of Practice. Because of the diversity of roles, practice settings, and conceptual frameworks in use, this history presents a generic data base for all practitioners. Those in primary care settings may use all of it, whereas the nurse in a hospital may focus primarily on the history of present illness and the functional, or patterns of living, data.

THE HEALTH HISTORY—THE ADULT

Biographical Data

Name, address and phone number, age and birthdate, birthplace, sex, marital status, race, ethnic origin, occupation, usual and present. (Alteration in health state may have prompted change in occupation.)

Source of History

Supply a record of:

1. Who furnishes the information. This is usually the person herself or himself, although the source may be a relative or friend.
2. Your judgment of how reliable the informant seems and how willing he or she is to communicate. A reliable person always gives the same answers, even when questions are rephrased, or are repeated later in the interview.
3. Any special circumstances, such as the use of an interpreter. Sample statements include:

Client herself who seems reliable
Client's son, John Ramirez, who seems reliable
Mrs. R. Fuentes, interpreter for Theresa Castillo who does not speak English

Reason for Seeking Care

This is a brief spontaneous statement in the person's own words that describes the reason for the visit. Think of it as the "title" for the story to follow. It states one (possibly two) signs or symptoms and their duration. It is enclosed in quotation marks to indicate the person's exact words.

"Chest pain" for 2 hours.
"Earache and fussy all night."
"Need yearly physical for work."
"Want to start jogging and need checkup."

[In the past, this statement was called the "Chief Complaint" (CC). This title is avoided now because it labels the person a "complainer," and more importantly, does not include wellness needs.]

The reason for seeking care is not a diagnostic statement. Avoid translating it into the terms of a medical diagnosis. For example, Mr. J. Schmidt enters with shortness of breath, and you ponder writing "emphysema." Even if he is known to have emphysema from previous visits, it is not the chronic emphysema which prompted *this visit,* but rather the "increasing shortness of breath" for 4 hours.

Some people try to self-diagnose based on similar signs and symptoms in their relatives or friends, or based on conditions they know they have. Rather than record a woman's statement that she has "strep throat," ask her what symptoms she has that makes her think this is true and record those symptoms.

Occasionally, a person may list *many* reasons for seeking care. The most important reason to the person may not necessarily be the one stated first. Try to focus on which is the most pressing concern by asking the person which one prompted him or her to seek help *now*.

Present Health or History of Present Illness

For the well person, this is a short statement about the general state of health.

For the ill person, this section is a chronologic record of the reason for seeking care, from the time of the onset of the symptom until now. Isolate each reason for care identified by the person and say, for example, "Please tell me all about your headache, from the time it started, until the time you came to the hospital." If the concern started months or years ago, record what occurred during that time and find out why the person is seeking care *now*.

Although you want the person to respond in a narrative format without interruption from you, your final summary of any symptom the person has should include these *eight critical characteristics:*

1. Location. Be specific, ask the person to point to it. If it is pain, note the precise site. "Head pain" is vague, whereas descriptions like "pain behind the eyes," "jaw pain," and "occipital pain" are more precise and are diagnostically significant. Is the pain localized to this site or radiating? Is the pain superficial or deep?
2. Character or quality. This calls for specific descriptive terms as burning, sharp, dull, aching, gnawing, throbbing, shooting, viselike. Use similies—does blood in the stool look like sticky tar, or blood in vomitus look like coffee grounds?
3. Quantity or severity. Attempt to quantify the sign or symptom such as "profuse menstrual flow soaking five pads per hour." The symptom of pain is difficult to quantify because of individual interpretation. What one person may identify as "terrible pain," another may feel that it is "not too bad." With pain, avoid adjectives and ask how it affects daily activities. Then the person might say, "I was so sick I was doubled up and couldn't move," or "I was able to go to work, but then I came home and went to bed."
4. Timing (onset, duration, frequency). When did the symptom first appear? Give the specific date and time, or state specifically how long ago the symptom started prior to arrival (PTA). "The pain started yesterday" will not mean much when you return to read the record in the future. The report must include questions such as: How long did the symptom last (duration)? Was it steady or did it come and go during that time (constant or intermittent)? Did it resolve completely, and reappear days or weeks later (cycle of remission and exacerbation)?
5. Setting. Where was the person or what was the person doing when the symptom started? What brings it on? For example, "Did you notice the chest pain after shoveling snow, or did the pain start by itself?"
6. Aggravating or relieving factors. What makes the pain worse? Is it aggravated by weather, activity, food, medication, standing bent over, fatigue, time of day, season, and so on. What relieves it, e.g., rest, medication, or ice pack? What is the effect of any treatment? Ask, "What have you tried?" or, "What seems to help?"
7. Associated factors. Is this primary symptom associated with others, e.g., urinary frequency and burning associated with fever and chills? Review the body system related to this symptom now rather than wait for the review of systems.
8. Client's perception. Find out the meaning of the symptom by asking how it affects daily activities. Also ask directly, "What do you think it means?" This is crucial because it alerts you to potential anxiety if the person thinks the symptom may be ominous.

As the person talks, do not jump to conclusions and bias the story by adding your professional opinion. Collect all the data first.

Past Health

Past health events may have residual effects on the current health state. Also, the previous experience with illness may give clues as to how the person responds to illness and to the significance of illness for him or her.

Childhood Illnesses. Record the occurrence of measles, mumps, rubella, chicken pox, pertussis, and strep throat. Avoid recording "usual childhood illnesses," because an illness common in the person's childhood may be unusual today, e.g., measles. Ask about serious illnesses which may have sequelae for the person in later years, e.g. rheumatic fever, scarlet fever, and poliomyelitis.

Accidents or Injuries. Record auto accidents, fractures, penetrating wounds, head injuries (especially if associated with unconsciousness), and burns.

Serious or Chronic Illnesses. Indicate, for example, the presence of diabetes, hypertension, heart disease, sickle cell anemia, cancer, and seizure disorder.

Hospitalizations. Record the cause, name of hospital,

how the condition was treated, how long the person was hospitalized, and name of the physician.

Operations. Record the type of surgery, date, name of the surgeon, name of hospital, and how the person recovered.

Obstetric History. Record the number of pregnancies (gravity), number of deliveries in which the fetus reached viability (parity), and number of abortions. For each complete pregnancy, note the course of pregnancy; labor and delivery; sex, weight, and condition of each infant; and postpartum course. For any incomplete pregnancies, record the duration and whether the pregnancy resulted in spontaneous (S) or induced (I) abortion.

Immunizations. Record all childhood immunizations (measles/mumps/rubella, polio, diphtheria/pertussis/tetanus). Were they kept up to date? Note the date of the last tetanus immunization, last tuberculosis skin test, and last flu shot.

Last Examination Date. Record the most recent physical, dental, vision, hearing, ECG, chest x-ray examinations.

Allergies. Note both the allergen (medication, food, or contact agent, such as fabric or environmental agent) and the reaction (rash, itching, runny nose, watery eyes, difficulty breathing). With a drug, this symptom should not be a side effect but a true allergic reaction.

Current Medications. Note all prescription and over-the-counter medications. Ask specifically about vitamins, birth control pills, aspirin, antacids, because many people do not consider these to be medications. For each medication, give the name, dose, schedule, "How often do you take it each day," "What is it for?" Record the duration of the prescription.

Family History

Ask about the age and health or the age and cause of death of blood relatives, such as parents, grandparents, and siblings. These data may have genetic significance for the client. Also ask about close family members, such as spouse and children. You need to know about the person's prolonged contact with any communicable disease or the effect of a family member's illness on this person.

Specifically ask for any family history of: heart disease, high blood pressure, stroke, diabetes, blood disorders, cancer, sickle cell anemia, arthritis, allergies, obesity, alcoholism, mental illness, seizure disorder, kidney disease, and tuberculosis. Construct a family tree, or genogram, to show this information clearly and concisely (See Fig. 4–1).

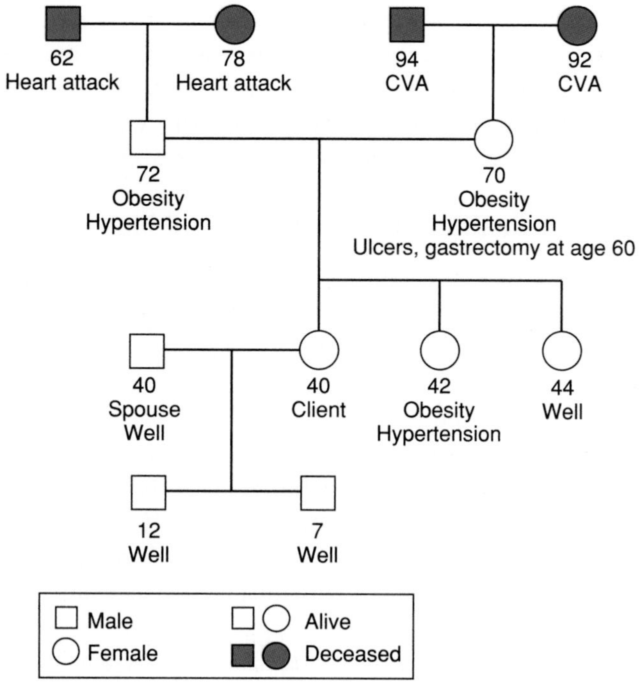

► **Figure 4–1**

Review of Systems

The purposes of this section are (1) to evaluate the past and present health state of each body system, (2) to double check in case any significant data were omitted in the present illness section, and (3) to evaluate health promotion practices. The order of the examination of body systems is roughly head-to-toe. The items within each system are not inclusive and only the most common symptoms are listed. If the present illness section covered one body system, you do not need to repeat all the data here. For example, if the reason for seeking care is earache, the present illness section describes most of the symptoms listed for the auditory system. Just ask now what was not asked in the present illness. Medical terms are listed here, but these need to be translated for the client. (Note that only symptoms and health promotion activities are listed here. These terms are repeated and expanded in each related physical examination chapter, along with suggested ways to pose questions and a rationale for each system.)

When recording information, avoid writing "negative" after the system heading. You need to record the *presence or absence* of all symptoms, otherwise the reader does not know which factors you asked.

A common mistake made by beginning practitioners is to record some physical finding, or objective data here, e.g. "skin warm and dry." The history should be limited to client responses, or subjective data—factors that the person *says* were or were not present.

General Overall Health State. Ask about the person's present weight (gain or loss, period of time, by diet or other factors), fatigue, weakness or malaise, fever, chills, and sweats or night sweats.

Skin. Record any history of skin disease (eczema, psoriasis, hives), pigment or color change, change in mole, excessive dryness or moisture, pruritis, excessive bruising, and rash or lesion.

Hair. Ask about recent loss, change in texture. Nails: Ask about change in shape, color, or brittleness.

Health Promotion. Amount of sun exposure; how does person care for skin and hair?

Head. Record any history of unusually frequent or severe headache, any head injury, dizziness (syncope) or vertigo.

Eyes. Ask about difficulty with vision (decreased acuity, blurring, blind spots), eye pain, diplopia (double vision), redness or swelling, watering or discharge, and glaucoma or cataracts.

Health Promotion. Ask if the person wears glasses or contacts; last vision check or glaucoma test; and how the person copes with loss of vision if any.

Ears. Ask about earaches, infections, discharge and its characteristics, tinnitis, and vertigo.

Health Promotion. Ask about hearing loss, hearing aid use, how loss affects the person's daily life, any exposure to environmental noise, and how the person cleans ears.

Nose and Sinuses. Inquire about discharge and its characteristics, any unusually frequent or severe colds, sinus pain, nasal obstruction, nosebleeds, allergies or hay fever, or change in sense of smell.

Mouth and Throat. Ask about mouth pain, frequent sore throat, bleeding gums, toothache, lesion in mouth or tongue, dysphagia, hoarseness or voice change, tonsillectomy, and altered taste.

Health Promotion. Ask about pattern of daily dental care, use of prostheses (dentures, bridge), and last dental checkup.

Neck. Ask about pain, limitation of motion, lumps or swelling, enlarged or tender nodes, and goiter.

Breast. Ask about pain, lump, nipple discharge, rash, history of breast disease, and any surgery on the breasts.

Health Promotion. Ask whether the woman performs breast self-exam including its frequency and method used.

Axilla. Ask about tenderness, lump or swelling, and rash.

Respiratory System. Inquire about history of lung diseases (asthma, emphysema, bronchitis, pneumonia, tuberculosis), chest pain with breathing, wheezing or noisy breathing, shortness of breath, how much activity produces shortness of breath, cough, sputum (color, amount), hemoptysis, and toxin or pollution exposure.

Health Promotion. Note last chest x-ray study.

Cardiovascular. Ask about precordial or retrosternal pain, palpitation, cyanosis, dyspnea on exertion (specify amount of exertion, e.g., walking one flight stairs, walking from chair to bath, or just talking), orthopnea, paroxysmal nocturnal dyspnea, nocturia, edema, history of heart murmur, hypertension, coronary artery disease, and anemia.

Health Promotion. Note date of person's last ECG or other heart tests. (Alternatively, information on coping and stress maintenance can be placed here.)

Peripheral Vascular. Ask about coldness, numbness and tingling, swelling of legs (time of day, activity), discoloration in hands or feet (bluish red, pallor, mottling, associated with position, especially around feet and ankles), varicose veins or complications, intermittent claudication, thrombophlebitis, and ulcers.

Health Promotion. Does the person's work involve long-term sitting or standing? Does the person avoid crossing legs at the knees or wear support hose?

Gastrointestinal. Ask about appetite, food intolerance, dysphagia, heartburn, indigestion, pain (associated with eating), other abdominal pain, pyrosis (esophageal and stomach burning sensation with sour eructation), nausea and vomiting (character), vomiting blood, history of abdominal disease (ulcer, liver or gallbladder, jaundice, appendicitis, colitis), flatulence, frequency of bowel movement, any recent change, stool characteristics, constipation or diarrhea, black stools, rectal bleeding, and rectal conditions (hemorrhoids, fistula).

Health Promotion. Indicate the person's use of antacids or laxatives. (Alternatively, diet history and substance habits can be placed here.)

Urinary System. Inquire about frequency; urgency; nocturia (the number of times the person awakens at night to urinate, recent change); dysuria; polyuria or oliguria; hesitancy or straining; narrowed stream; urine color (cloudy or presence of hematuria); incontinence; history of urinary disease (kidney disease, kidney stones, urinary tract infections, prostate); and pain in flank, groin, suprapubic region, or low back.

Health Promotion. After childbirth, does woman perform Kegel exercises and use measures to avoid or treat urinary tract infections.

Male Genital System. Ask about any penis or testicular pain, sores or lesions, penile discharge, lumps, hernia.

Health Promotion. Does the man perform testicular self-examination? Record its frequency.

Female Genital System. Ask about the woman's menstrual history (age at menarche, last menstrual period, cycle and duration, any amenorrhea or menorrhagia, premenstrual pain or dysmenorrhea, intermenstrual spotting), vaginal itching, discharge and its characteristics, age at menopause, menopausal signs or symptoms, and postmenopausal bleeding.

Health Promotion. Record the woman's last gynecologic checkup and last Papanicolaou smear.

Sexual Health. Indicate whether the person is presently in a relationship involving intercourse. Are the aspects of sex satisfactory to the client and his or her partner? Record any dyspareunia (for female), any changes in erection or ejaculation (for male), and use of contraceptive. Is the contraceptive method satisfactory? Is the person aware of contact with a partner who has any sexually transmitted disease (gonorrhea, herpes, chlamydia, venereal warts, AIDS, or syphilis)?

Musculoskeletal System. Note any history of arthritis, or gout. In the joints, is there pain, stiffness, swelling (location, migratory nature), deformity, limitation of motion, noise with joint motion? In the muscles, is there any pain, cramps, weakness, gait problems or problems with coordinated activities. In the back, is there any pain (location and radiation to extremities), stiffness, limitation of motion, or history of back pain or disc disease.

Health Promotion. How much walking does the person do per day? What is the effect of limited range of motion on daily activities, such as on grooming, feeding, toileting, dressing. Are any mobility aids used.

Neurologic System. Indicate history of seizure disorder, stroke, fainting, blackouts. In motor function, ask about weakness, tic or tremor, paralysis, or coordination problems. In sensory function, ask about numbness and tingling (paresthesia). In cognitive function, ask about memory disorder (recent or distant, disorientation). In mental status, ask about nervousness, mood change, depression, or any history of mental health dysfunction or hallucinations.

Health Promotion. Alternatively, data about interpersonal relationships, coping patterns placed here.

Hematologic System. Ask about bleeding tendency of skin or mucous membranes, excessive bruising, lymph node swelling, exposure to toxic agents or radiation, and blood transfusion and reactions.

Endocrine System. Record any history of diabetes or diabetic symptoms (polyuria, polydipsia, polyphagia), history of thyroid disease, intolerance to heat and cold, change in skin pigmentation or texture, excessive sweating, relationship between appetite and weight, abnormal hair distribution, nervousness, tremors, and need for hormone therapy.

Functional Assessment (Activities of Daily Living)

Functional assessment measures a person's self-care ability in the areas of physical health, activities of daily living, nutritional status, and psychosocial status. This may mean organizing the entire assessment around functional "pattern areas" (Gordon, 1987). Or, the health history may be supplemented by a standardized instrument on functional assessment. These instruments objectively measure a person's present functional status and monitor any changes over time. (Granger, 1979; Mahoney and Barthel, 1965; Katz, 1963; Linn and Linn, 1982; Pearlman, 1987). Whether or not you use any of these formalized instruments, the following section lists questions to be included in the standard health history. These questions provide data on the lifestyle and type of living environment to which the person is accustomed. Since some of the data may be judged private by the individual, the questions are best asked now after you have had time to establish rapport.

Self-Esteem, Self-Concept. Include information on the person's education (last grade completed, other significant training), financial status (whether he or she believes income is adequate for lifestyle and/or health concerns), value-belief system (ask about the person's religious practices and perception of personal strengths).

Activity-Exercise. Include a daily profile reflecting usual daily activities ("Tell me how you spend a typical day"). Is the person able to perform activities of daily living (ADL): whether the person is independent or needs assistance with feeding, setting up food, hygiene; whether the person is able to bathe, brush his or her teeth, comb his or her hair, shave, apply deodorant, dress self, use toilet, get out of bed or chair. Any problem walking, standing, or climbing stairs? If the person uses a wheelchair, is he or she able to propel it? How does the person tolerate activity, use prostheses, or mobility aids? Record leisure activities enjoyed and exercise pattern (type, amount per day or week, whether a warm-up session is included, how the person monitors the body's response to exercise).

Sleep/Rest. Record the person's sleep patterns and any sleep aids used.

Nutrition. Record the diet by asking the person to recall all food and beverages taken over the last 24 hours. Ask, "Is that menu typical of most days?" Describe eating habits and current appetite. (Who buys food and prepares food? Are the person's finances adequate for food? Who is present at mealtimes?) Indicate any food allergy or intolerance. Record habits such as the person's daily intake of caffeine (coffee, tea, cola drinks), alcohol ("When was your last drink of alcohol?" "How much did you drink that time?" "Have you ever had a drinking problem?"), smoking ("Do you smoke?" "At what age did you start?" "How many packs do you smoke per day?" "How many years have you smoked?"), and street drugs ("Have you ever tried any drugs, such as marijuana, cocaine, amphetamines, barbiturates?" "How often do you use these drugs?" and "How has usage affected your work or social relationships?")

Interpersonal Relationships. Include information on the person's social roles ("How would you describe your role in the family?" "How would you say you get along with family, friends, and co-workers?") and support systems composed of family and significant others ("To whom could you go for support with a problem at work, with your health, or a personal problem?")

Coping and Stress Management. Inquire about the person's housing and neighborhood (whether the person lives alone and knows neighbors; whether the area is safe; whether the person has adequate heat and utilities and access to transportation; whether the person is involved in community services) and environmental health (ask about hazards in workplace, hazards at home, use of seatbelts, geographic or occupational exposures, travel or residence in other countries including time spent abroad during military service). What kinds of stresses does the person identify in life and in the last year? Has there been any change in the person's lifestyle or any current stress? What steps has the person tried to relieve stress? Has this helped?

Perception of Health

Ask the person questions, such as: "How do you define health?" "How do you view your situation now?" "What are your concerns?" "What do you think will happen in the future?" "What are your health goals?" "What do you expect from us as nurses, physicians, (other health care providers)?"

DEVELOPMENTAL CONSIDERATIONS

The Younger Person (From Birth to Adolescence)

The health history is adapted to include information specific for the age and developmental stage of the child, e.g., the mother's health during pregnancy, labor and delivery, and the perinatal period. Note that the developmental history and nutritional data are listed as separate sections because of their importance for current health.

Biographical Data

Include the child's name, nickname, address and phone number, parents' names and work numbers, child's age and birthdate, birthplace, sex, race, ethnic origin, and information on other children and family members at home.

Source of History

1. Who is providing information and their relation to child?
2. What is your impression of reliability of information?
3. Are there any special circumstances, e.g., the use of an interpreter?

Reason for Seeking Care

Record the parent's spontaneous statement. Because of the frequency of well child visits for routine health care, there will be more reasons such as "time for the child's checkup" or "she needs the next baby shot." Reasons for health problems may be initiated by the child, parent, or by a third party such as the classroom teacher.

Sometimes the reason stated may not be the real reason for the visit. A parent may have a "hidden agenda," such as the mother who brought her 4-year-old child in because "she looked pale." Further questioning brought out that the mother had heard recently from a former college friend whose own 4-year-old child had just been diagnosed with leukemia.

Present Health or History of Present Illness

If the parent or child seeks routine health care, include a statement about the usual health of the child and any common health problems or major health concerns.

Describe any presenting symptom or sign with the same format as for the adult. Some additional considerations include:

- Severity of pain. "How do you know the child is in pain," e.g., pulling at ears alerts parent to ear pain. Note effect of pain on usual behavior, e.g., does it stop child from playing?
- Associated factors, such as relation to activity, eating, and body position.
- The parent's intuitive sense of a problem. As the constant care giver, this intuitive sense is often very accurate. Even if proved otherwise, this factor gives you an idea of parent's area of concern.
- Parent's coping ability and reaction of other family members to child's symptoms or illness.

Past Health

Prenatal Status. How was this pregnancy spaced? Was it planned? What was the mother's attitude toward the pregnancy? What was the father's attitude? Was there medical supervision for the mother? At what month was the supervision started? What was the mother's health during pregnancy? Were there any complications (bleeding, excessive nausea and vomiting, unusual weight gain, high blood pressure, swelling of hands and feet, infections—rubella or sexually transmitted diseases, falls)? During what month were diet and medications prescribed and/or taken during pregnancy (dose and duration)? Record the mother's use of alcohol, street drugs or cigarettes and any x-ray studies taken during pregnancy.

Start with an open-ended question, "Tell me about your pregnancy." If she questions the relevancy of the statement, mention that these questions are important to gain a complete picture of the child's health.

Labor and Delivery. Indicate the parity of the mother, the duration of the pregnancy, name of the hospital, the course and duration of labor, use of anesthesia, type of delivery (vertex, breech, cesarean section), birth weight, Apgar scores, onset of breathing, any cyanosis, need for resuscitation, and use of special equipment or procedures.

Postnatal Status. Note any problems in the nursery, length of hospital stay, neonatal jaundice, whether the baby was discharged with the mother, whether the baby was breast- or bottle-fed, weight gain, any feeding problems, "blue spells," colic, diarrhea, patterns of crying and sleeping, the mother's health postpartum, and the mother's reaction to the baby.

Childhood Illnesses. Note age and any complications of measles, mumps, rubella, chicken pox, whooping cough, strep throat, and frequent ear infections. Also, indicate any recent exposure to illness.

Serious Accidents or Injuries. Record age of occurrence, extent of injury, how the child was treated, and complications of auto accidents, falls, head injuries, fractures, burns, and poisonings.

Serious or Chronic Illnesses. Note age of onset, how the child was treated, and complications of meningitis or encephalitis; seizure disorders; asthma, pneumonia, and other chronic lung conditions; rheumatic fever; scarlet fever; diabetes; kidney problems; sickle cell anemia; high blood pressure; and allergies.

Operations or Hospitalizations. Record reason for care, age at admission, name of surgeon or primary care providers, name of hospital, duration of stay, how child reacted to hospitalization, and any complications. (If child reacted poorly, he or she may be afraid now and will need special preparation for the examination that is to follow.)

Immunizations. Note age when administered, date administered, and any reactions following immunizations. Tables 4–1 and 4–2 list suggested immunization schedules. Because of recent outbreaks of measles across the United States, the American Academy of Pediatrics

Table 4-1. ▶ Immunization Schedule Suggested for Normal Infants and Children

AGE	IMMUNIZING AGENTS
2 months	DTP, TOPV
4 months	DTP, TOPV
6 months	DTP, TOPV*
15 months	MMR
18 months	DTP, TOPV
24 months	Hib
4 to 6 years	DTP, TOPV
14 to 16 years and every 10 years thereafter	Td

DTP = Diphtheria and tetanus toxoids combined with pertussis vaccine. Diphtheria and tetanus toxoid combination (DT) should be used if pertussis vaccine is contraindicated.

TOPV = Trivalent oral polio vaccine.

MMR = Combined measles, mumps, rubella vaccine.

Hib = *Haemophilus influenzae*, type b polysaccharide vaccine.

Td = Combined tetanus and diphtheria toxoids (adult type) for those 7 years of age and older; diphtheria and tetanus toxoid (DT) and DTP contain larger amounts of diphtheria antigen and should be used only in children less than 7 years of age.

* This dose of TOPV is necessary only for infants in areas of high endemicity.

(From Feigin RD, Cherry JD: Textbook of Pediatric Diseases, vol. II. 2nd ed. Philadelphia; W.B. Saunders, 1987, p. 2266.)

Table 4-2. ▶ Primary Immunization Schedule Suggested for Children Not Immunized in Early Infancy

SCHEDULE	IMMUNIZING AGENTS
Less Than 7 Years of Age	
Initial visit	DTP, TOPV, MMR
Interval following initial visit	
2 months	DTP, TOPV
4 months	DTP, TOPV*
10 to 16 months	DTP, TOPV
Age 4 to 6 years†	DTP, TOPV
Age 14 to 16 years and every 10 years thereafter	Td
7 Years of Age and Older	
Initial visit	Td, TIPV,‡ MMR
Interval following initial visit	
2 months	Td, TOPV
8 to 14 months	Td, TOPV
Every 10 years after last Td	Td

DTP = Diphtheria and tetanus toxoids combined with pertussis vaccine. DTP (or DT, diphtheria and tetanus toxoids combined for pediatric use, if a contraindication to pertussis vaccine exists) may be used until age 7; thereafter diphtheria and tetanus toxoids combined (Td, for adult use) should be used.

TOPV = Trivalent oral polio vaccine.

MMR = Combined measles, mumps, rubella vaccine. Measles vaccine should not be routinely given before 15 months of age.

Td = Diphtheria and tetanus toxoids combined for adult use.

* This TOPV dose is necessary only for infants in areas of high endemicity.

† These doses not necessary if the fourth DTP and third TOPV doses are received after the fourth birthday.

‡ Inactivated polio vaccine (IPV) preferred for those 18 years and older.

(From Feigin RD, Cherry JD: Textbook of Pediatric Diseases, vol II. 2nd ed. Philadelphia; W.B. Saunders, 1987, p. 2266. [Originally appeared in: Centers for Disease Control; General recommendations on immunization. M.M.W.R. 32(1):1–17, 1983.])

now is recommending two doses of MMR, one at 15 months and one at age 11 or 12 when the child enters middle school or junior high school. (American Academy of Pediatrics, 1989).

Allergies. List any drugs, foods, contact agents, and environmental agents to which the child is allergic. Record reaction to allergen. Note allergic reactions particularly common in childhood, such as allergic rhinitis, insect hypersensitivity, eczema, and urticaria.

Medications. List any prescription and over-the-counter medications (vitamins) the child takes, including the dose, daily schedule, why the medication is given, and any problems.

Developmental History

Growth. Record height and weight at birth and at 1, 2, 5, and 10 years. Indicate periods of rapid gain or loss. Record process of dentition (age of tooth eruption and pattern of loss).

Milestones. Indicate age when child first held head erect, rolled over, sat alone, walked alone, cut his or her first tooth, said his or her first words with meaning, spoke in sentences, was toilet trained, tied shoes, dressed without help. Does the parent believe this development has been normal? How does this child's development compare with siblings or peers?

Current Development (Children 1 Month Through Preschool). Record information on gross motor skills (rolls over, sits alone, walks alone, skips, climbs), fine motor skills (inspects hands, brings hands to mouth, pincer grasp, stacks blocks, feeds self, uses crayon to draw, uses scissors), language skills (vocalizes, first words with meaning, sentences, persistance of baby talk, speech problems), and personal-social skills (smiles, tracks movement with eyes to midline, past midline, attends to sound by turning head, recognizes own name). If the child is undergoing toilet training, indicate the method used, age of bladder/bowel control, parents' attitude toward toilet training, and terms used for toileting.

School-Aged Child. Record gross motor skills (runs, jumps, climbs, rides bicycle, general coordination), fine motor skills (ties shoelace, uses scissors, writes name and numbers, draws pictures), and language skills (vocabulary, verbal ability, able to tell time, reading level).

Nutritional History

The amount of needed information on this topic depends on the child's age; the younger the child, the more detailed and specific the data. For the infant, record whether breast- or bottle-feeding is used. If the child is breast-fed, record nursing frequency and duration, any supplements (vitamin, iron, fluoride, bottles), family support for nursing, and age and method of weaning. If the child is bottle-fed, record type formula used, frequency and amount, any problems with feeding (spitting up, colic, diarrhea), supplements used, and any bottle propping. Record introduction of solid foods (age when the child began eating solids, which foods, whether foods are home or commercially made, amount given, child's reaction to new food, parent's reaction to feeding).

For preschool and school-aged children and adolescents, record the child's appetite, 24-hour diet recall (meals, snacks, amounts), vitamins taken, how much junk food is eaten, who eats with the child, food likes and dislikes, and parent's perception of child's nutrition.

A week-long diary of food intake may be more accurate than a spot 24-hour recall. Also, consider cultural practices in assessing child's diet (see the section on cultural considerations).

Family History

As with the adult, diagram a family tree for the child, including siblings, parents, grandparents. Give the age, health, or age and cause of death of each. Ask specifically for the family history of heart disease, high blood pressure, diabetes, blood disorders, cancer, sickle cell anemia, arthritis, allergies, obesity, cystic fibrosis, alcoholism, mental illness, seizure disorder, kidney disease, mental retardation, learning disabilities, birth defects, and sudden infant death. (When interviewing the mother, ask about the "child's father," not "your husband," in case of the separation of child's biologic parents.)

Review of Systems

General. Ask about significant gain or loss of weight, failure to gain weight appropriate for age, frequent colds, ear infections, illnesses, energy level, fatigue, overactivity, and behavior change (irritability, increased crying, nervousness).

Skin. Ask about birthmarks, skin disease, pigment or color change, mottling, change in mole, pruritus, rash, lesion, acne, easy bruising or petechiae, easy bleeding, and changes in hair or nails.

Head. Ask about headache, head injury, and dizziness.

Eyes. Ask about strabismus, diplopia, pain, redness, discharge, cataracts, vision changes, reading problems. Is the child able to see the board at school? Does the child sit too close to the television?

Health Promotion. Does the child wear glasses? When was his or her last vision screening?

Ears. Ask about earaches, frequency of ear infections, myringotomy tubes in ears, discharge (characteristics), cerumen, ringing or crackling, and whether parent perceives any hearing problems.

Health Promotion. How does the child clean his or her ears?

Nose and Sinuses. Ask about discharge and its characteristics, frequency of colds, nasal stuffiness, nosebleeds, and allergies.

Mouth and Throat. Ask about cleft lip or palate, frequency of sore throats, toothache, caries, sores in mouth or tongue, tonsils present, mouth breathing, difficulty chewing, difficulty swallowing and hoarseness or voice change.

Health Promotion. Inquire about the child's pattern of brushing teeth and last dental checkup.

Neck. Ask about swollen or tender glands, limitation of movement, or stiffness.

Breast. For preadolescent and adolescent girls, when did they notice that their breasts were changing? What is the girl's self-perception of development? For older adolescents, does the girl perform breast self-examination? (See Chapter 14 for suggested phrasing of questions.)

Respiratory System. Record history of croup or asthma, wheezing or noisy breathing, shortness of breath, and chronic cough.

Cardiovascular System. Inquire about congenital heart problems, history of murmur, and cyanosis (what prompts this condition). Is there any limitation of activity, or can the child keep up with peers? Is there any dyspnea on exertion, palpitations, high blood pressure, or coldness in the extremities?

Gastrointestinal System. Ask about abdominal pain, nausea and vomiting, history of ulcer, frequency of bowel movements, stool color and characteristics, diarrhea, constipation or stool-holding, rectal bleeding, anal itching, history of pinworms, and use of laxatives.

Urinary System. Ask about painful urination, polyuria/oliguria, narrowed stream, urine color (cloudy, dark), history of urinary tract infection, whether toilet trained, when toilet training was planned, any problems, bed wetting (when the child started, frequency, associated with stress, how child feels about it).

Male Genital System. Ask about penis or testicular pain, whether told if testes are descended, any sores or lesions, discharge, hernia or hydrocele, or swelling in scrotum during crying. For the preadolescent and adolescent male, has the boy noticed any change in the penis and scrotum? Is the boy familiar with normal growth patterns, nocturnal emissions, and sex education? Screen for sexual abuse. (See Chapter 21 for suggested phrasing of questions.)

Female Genital System. Has girl noted any genital itching, rash, vaginal discharge? For the preadolescent and adolescent girl, when did menstruation start? Was the girl prepared? Screen for sexual abuse. (See Chapter 22 for suggested phrasing of questions.)

Sexual Health. What is the child's attitude toward the opposite sex? Who provides sex education? How does the family deal with sex education, masturbation, dating patterns? Is the adolescent in a relationship involving intercourse? Does he or she have information on birth control and sexually transmitted diseases? (See Chapters 21 and 22 for suggested phrasing of questions.)

Musculoskeletal System. In bones and joints, ask about arthritis, joint pain, stiffness, swelling, limitation of movement, gait strength and coordination. In muscles, ask about pain, cramps, and weakness. In the back, ask about pain, posture, spinal curvature, and any treatment.

Neurologic System. Ask about numbness and tingling. (Behavior and cognitive issues are covered in the sections on development and interpersonal relationships.)

Hematologic Systems. Ask about excessive bruising, lymph node swelling, and exposure to toxic agents or radiation.

Endocrine System. Indicate any history of diabetes or thyroid disease, excessive hunger or thirst or urinating, abnormal hair distribution, and precocious or delayed puberty.

Functional Assessment (Activities of Daily Living)

Interpersonal Relationships. Within the family constellation, record the child's position in family; whether the child is adopted; who lives with the child; who is the primary care taker; who is the care taker if both parents work outside of the home; any support from relatives, neighbors, or friends; and the ethnic or cultural milieu.

Indicate family cohesion. Does the family enjoy activities as a unit? Has there been a recent family change or crisis (death, divorce, move)? Record information on child's self image and level of independence. Does the child use a security blanket or toy? Is there any repetitive behavior (bed-rocking, head-banging), pica, thumb-sucking, or nail-biting? Note method of discipline used. Indicate type used at home. How effective is it? Who disciplines the child? Is there any occurrence of negativism, temper tantrums, withdrawal, or aggressive behavior.

Provide information on the child's friends: whether the child makes friends easily. How does the child get along with friends? Does he or she play with same age or older or younger children.

Home Environment. Where does family live (house, apartment)? Is the size of the home adequate? Is there access to an outdoor play area? Does the child share a room, have is or her own bed, and have toys appropriate for his or her age?

Activity and Rest. Record the child's play activities. Indicate amount of active and quiet play, outdoor play, time watching TV, and special hobbies or activities. Record sleep and rest. Indicate pattern and number of hours at night and during the day and the child's routine at bedtime. Is the child a sound sleeper, or is he or she wakeful? Does the child have nightmares, night terrors, or somnambulation? How does the parent respond? Does the child have naps during the day?

Record school attendance. Has the child had any experience with day care or nursery school? What grade is the child in in school? Has the child ever skipped a grade or been held back? Does the child seem to like school?

What is his or her school performance? Are the parent and child satisfied with the performance? Were days missed in school? Provide a reason for the absence. (These questions give an important index to child's functioning outside the home.)

Economic Status. Ask about the mother's occupation and father's occupation. Indicate the number of hours each parent is away from home. Do parents perceive their income as adequate? What is the effect of illness on financial status?

Coping/Stress Management. Does the child have the ability to adapt to new situations? Record recent stressful experiences (death, divorce, move, loss of special friend). How does the child cope with stress? Has there been any recent change in behavior or mood? Has counseling ever been sought?

Environment. Inquire about home safety (precautions for poisons, medications, household products, presence of gates for stairways, and safe yard equipment). Provide information on the child's residence (adequate heating, ventilation, bathroom facilities), neighborhood (residential or industrial, age of neighbors, safe play areas, playmates available, distance to school, amount of traffic, is area remote or congested and overcrowded, is crime a problem, presence of air or water pollution), and automobile (child safety seat, seat belts).

Habits. Has the child ever tried cigarette smoking? How much did he or she smoke? Has the child ever tried alcohol? How much alcohol did he or she drink weekly or daily? Has the child ever tried other drugs (marijuana, cocaine, amphetamines, barbiturates)?

Health Promotion. Who is the primary health care provider? When was the child's last checkup? Who is the dental care provider, and when was the last checkup? Provide date and result of screening for vision, hearing, urinalysis, phenylketonuria, hematocrit, tuberculosis skin test, sickle cell trait, blood lead, and other tests specific for high-risk population.

The Older Adult

This health history includes the same format as described for the younger adult, as well as some additional questions. These questions address ways the activities of daily living may have been affected by normal aging processes or by the effects of chronic illness or disability. There is no specific age at which to ask these additional questions. Use them when it seems appropriate.

It is important for you to recognize positive health measures; what the person has been doing to help him or her stay well and to live to an older age. Older people have spent a lifetime with a traditional health care system that searches only for pathology and what is wrong with their health. It may be a pleasant surprise to have a health professional affirm the things that they are "doing right" and to note health strengths.

As you study the following, keep in mind the format for the "younger" adult. Only *additional* questions or a varying focus are addressed here.

Reason for Seeking Care

It may take time to figure out the reason the older person has come in for an examination. An aging person may shrug off a symptom as evidence of growing old, and may be unsure whether it is "worth mentioning." Also, some older people have a conservative philosophy toward their health status; "if it isn't broken, don't fix it." These people come for care only when something blatantly is wrong.

Another older person may have many chronic problems, such as diabetes, hypertension, or constipation. It is challenging to filter out what brought the person in this time. The final statement should be the *person's* reason for seeking care, not your assumption of what the problem is.

Past Health

General Health. Health state in the last 5 years.

Accidents or Injuries, Serious or Chronic Illnesses, Hospitalizations, Operations. These areas may produce lengthy responses, and probably, the person will not relate them in chronologic order. Let the person talk freely; you can reorder the events later when you do the writeup. The amount of data included here can indicate the amount of stress the person has faced during his or her lifetime. This section of the history can be filled out at home or before the interview, if the person's vision and writing ability are adequate. Then you can concentrate remaining time of the interview on reviewing pertinent data and on the present health of the person.

Last Examination. Ask about most recent mammography, proctoscopy, and tonometry.

Obstetric Status. It is *not* necessary to collect a detailed account of each pregnancy and delivery if the woman has passed menopause and has no gynecologic symptoms. Merely record the number of pregnancies and the health of each newborn.

Current Medications. For each medication, record the name, purpose, and daily schedule. Does the person have a system to remember to take the medicine? Does medicine seem to work? Are there any side effects? If so, does the person feel like skipping medicine because of them? Also consider the following issues:

- Some older persons take a large number of drugs, prescribed by different physicians.
- The person may not know drug name or purpose. When this occurs, ask the person to bring in the drug to be identified.
- Is cost a problem? When the person is unable to afford a drug, he or she may decrease the dosage, take one pill instead of two, or not refill the empty bottle immediately.
- Is traveling to the pharmacy to refill a prescription a problem?
- Is the person taking any over-the-counter medications? Some people use local pharmacist for self-treatment.
- Has the person ever shared medications with neighbor or friends? Some establish "lay referral" networks by comparing symptoms and thus medications.

Family History

This is not as useful in predicting which familial diseases the person may contract, because most of those will have occurred at an earlier age. But this data is useful to assess which diseases or causes of death of relatives the person has experienced. Also it describes the person's existing social network.

Review of Systems

Remember, these are *additional* items to question. Refer to the history for the young adult for the basic list.

General. Ask the present weight and what the person would like to weigh (gives idea of body image).

Skin. Ask about change in sensation to pain, heat, or cold.

Eyes. Does the person wear bifocals? Is there any trouble adjusting to far vision (problems with stairs)?

Ears. Ask about increased sensitivity to background noise and whether conversation sounds garbled or distorted.

Mouth. If the person has dentures, does he or she wear them? When does the person wear them (always, all day, only at meals, only at social occasions, never)? How does the person clean them? Any difficulty wearing the dentures (loose, pain, makes whistling or clicking noise)? Are there cracks at corners of the mouth (indicates poorly fitting dentures or that the person is edentulous)?

Respiratory System. Ask about shortness of breath and level of activity that produces it. Shortness of breath often is an early sign of cardiac dysfunction, but many older people dismiss it as "a cold," or getting "winded" because of old age.

Cardiovascular System. If chest pain occurs, the person may not feel it as intensely as a younger person. Instead, he or she notes dyspnea on exertion.

Peripheral Vascular System. Ask whether the person wears constrictive clothing, garters, or rolls stockings at knees, and if the person has noted color change at feet or ankles.

Urinary System. Ask about urinary retention, incomplete emptying, straining to urinate, change in force of stream. If a weakened stream occurs, men may note the need to stand closer to toilet. Women may note incontinence when coughing, laughing, or sneezing.

Sexual Health. Ask about any changes in sexual relationship the person has experienced. Note for men, it is normal for an erection to develop slowly. (See Chapter 21.) Note for women, is there any vaginal dryness or pain with intercourse? Note for all, are aspects of sex satisfactory and is there adequate privacy for sexual relationship?

Musculoskeletal System. Ask about gait change (balance, weakness, difficulty with steps, fear of falling), use of any assistive device (cane, walker). Does the person know how to work the device? Is there any joint stiffness? During what part of the day does the stiffness occur? Does the pain occur with activity or rest?

Neurologic System. Inquire about cognitive problems, such as memory dysfunction (recent or remote) and disorientation (time of day, in what settings).

Functional Assessment (Activities of Daily Living)

Self-Concept, Self-Esteem

Education. When the aging person was an adolescent, educational opportunities were not as available as they

Table 4-3. ▶ Comprehensive Older Persons' Evaluation

Name (print): ______________________ Date of visit: ________

Chief complaint: ______________________

Today I will ask you about your overall health and function and will be using a questionnaire to help me obtain this information. The first few questions are to check your memory.

Preliminary Cognition Questionnaire: *Record if answer is correct with (+); if answer is incorrect with (−). Record total number of errors.*

(+, −)

1) What is the date today? ____
2) What day of the week is it? ____
3) What is the name of this place? ____
4) What is your telephone number or rm. no.? (*record answer:* ______) ____
   If subject does not have phone, ask:
   What is your street address?
5) How old are you? (*record answer:* ______) ____
6) When were you born? (*record answer from records if patient cannot answer:* ______) ____
7) Who is the president of the United States now? ____
8) Who was the president just before him? ____
9) What was your mother's maiden name? ____
10) Subtract 3 from 20 and keep subtracting from each new number you get, all the way down. ____

Total errors ____

If more than 4 errors, ask 11. If more than 6 errors, complete questionnaire from informant.

11) Do you think you would benefit from a legal guardian, someone who would be responsible for your legal and financial matters? Do you have a living will? Would you like one?
   a) No
   b) Has functioning legal guardian for sole purpose of managing money (*describe:* ______)
   c) Has legal guardian
   d) Yes

Demographic Section

1) Patient's race or ethnic background (*record:* ______)
2) Patient's gender (*circle*) Male Female
3) How far did you go in school?
   a) Post-graduate education
   b) Four-year degree
   c) College or technical school
   d) High school complete
   e) High school incomplete
   f) 0–8 years

Social Support Section: Now there are a few questions about your family and friends.

4) Are you married, widowed, separated, divorced, or have you never been married?
   a) Now married
   b) Widowed
   c) Separated
   d) Divorced
   e) Never married
5) Who lives with you? (*circle all responses*)
   a) Spouse
   b) Other relative or friend (*specify:* ______)
   c) Group living situation (non-health)
   d) Lives alone
   e) Nursing home, no. years ______
6) Have you talked to any friends or relatives by phone during the last week?
   a) Yes
   b) No
7) Are you satisified by seeing your relatives and friends as often as you want to, or are you somewhat dissatisfied about how little you see them?
   a) Satisfied (*skip to #8*)
   b) No (*ask A*)
      A) Do you feel you would like to be involved in a Senior Citizens Center for social events, or perhaps meals?
         1) No
         2) Is involved (*describe:* ______)
         3) Yes
8) Is there someone who would take care of you for as long as you needed if you were sick or disabled?
   a) Yes (*skip to C*)
   b) No (*ask A*)
      A) Is there someone who would take care of you for a short time?
         1) Yes (*skip to C*)
         2) No (*ask B*)
      B) Is there someone who could help you now and then?
         1) Yes (*ask C*)
         2) No (*ask C*)
      C) Who would we call in case of an emergency? (*record name and telephone:* ______)

Financial Section

9) Do you own, or are you buying, your own home?
   a) Yes (*skip to #10*)
   b) No (*ask A*)
      A) Do you feel you need assistance with housing?
         1) No
         2) Has subsidized or other housing assistance
         3) Yes (*describe:* ______)
      B) What type of housing did you have prior to coming here?
10) Are you covered by private medical insurance, Medicare, Medicaid, or some disability plan? (*circle all that apply*)
   a) Private insurance (*specify and skip to #11:* ______)
   b) Medicare
   c) Medicaid
   d) Disability (*specify and ask A:* ______)
   e) None
   f) Other (*specify:* ______
      A) Do you feel you need additional assistance with your medical bills?
         1) No
         2) Yes
11) Which of these statements best describes your financial situation?
   a) My bills are no problem to me (*skip to #12*)
   b) My expenses make it difficult to meet my bills (*ask A*)
   c) My expenses are so heavy that I cannot meet my bills (*ask A*)

Table 4-3. ▶ Comprehensive Older Persons' Evaluation *Continued*

A) Do you feel you need financial assistance such as: (*circle all that apply*)
1) Food stamps
2) Social Security or disability payments
3) Assistance in paying your heating or electrical bills
4) Other financial assistance? (*describe:* ______________)

Psychological Health Section: The next few questions are about how you feel about your life in general. There are no right or wrong answers, only what best applies to you. Please answer yes or no to each question.

	Yes	No
12) Is your daily life full of things that keep you interested?	_____	_____
13) Have you, at times, very much wanted to leave home?	_____	_____
14) Does it seem that no one understands you?	_____	_____
15) Are you happy most of the time?	_____	_____
16) Do you feel weak all over much of the time?	_____	_____
17) Is your sleep fitful and disturbed?	_____	_____

18) Taking everything into consideration, how would you describe your satisfaction with your life in general at the present time—good, fair, or poor?
a) Good
b) Fair
c) Poor

19) Do you feel you now need help with your mental health; for example, a counselor or psychiatrist?
a) No
b) Has (*specify:* ______________________________)
c) Yes

Physical Health Section: The next few questions are about your health.

20) During the past month (30 days), how many days were you so sick that you couldn't do your usual activities, such as working around the house or visiting with friends?__________

21) Relative to other people your age, how would you rate your overall health at the present time: excellent, good, fair, poor or very poor?
a) Excellent (*skip to #22*)
b) Very good (*skip to #22*)
c) Good (*ask A*)
d) Fair (*ask A*)
e) Poor (*ask A*)
A) Do you feel you need additional medical services such as a doctor, nurse, visiting nurse or physical therapist? (*circle all that apply*)
1) Doctor
2) Nurse
3) Visiting nurse
4) Physical therapist
5) None

22) Do you use an aid for walking, such as a wheelchair, walker, cane or anything else? (*circle aid usually used*)
a) Wheelchair
b) Other (*specify:* ______________________________)
c) Visiting nurse
d) Walker
e) None

23) How much do your health troubles stand in the way of your doing things you want to do: not at all, a little or a great deal?
a) Not at all (*skip to #24*)
b) A little (*ask A*)
c) A great deal (*ask A*)
A) Do you think you need assistance to do your daily activities; for example, do you need a live-in aide or choreworker?
1) Live-in aide
2) Choreworker
3) Has aide, choreworker or other assistance (*describe:* ______________________________)
4) None needed

24) Have you had, or do you currently have, any of the following health problems? (*If yes, place an "X" in appropriate box and describe; medical record information may be used to help complete this section.*)

	HX	CURRENT	DESCRIBE
a) Arthritis or rheumatism?			
b) Lung or breathing problem?			
c) Hypertension?			
d) Heart trouble?			
e) Phlebitis or poor circulation problems in arms or legs?			
f) Diabetes or low blood sugar?			
g) Digestive ulcers?			
h) Other digestive problem?			
i) Cancer?			
j) Anemia?			
k) Effects of stroke?			
l) Other neurological problem? (*specify:* ______________)			
m) Thyroid or other glandular problem? (*specify:* ______________)			
n) Skin disorders such as pressure sores, leg ulcers, burns?			
o) Speech problem?			
p) Hearing problem?			
q) Vision or eye problem?			
r) Kidney or bladder problems, or incontinence?			
s) A problem of falls?			
t) Problem with eating or your weight? (*specify:* ______________)			
u) Problem with depression or your nerves? (*specify:* ______________)			
v) Problem with your behavior? (*specify:* ______________)			
w) Problem with your sexual activity?			
x) Problem with alcohol?			
y) Problem with pain?			
z) Other health problems? (*specify:* ______________)			

Immunizations: ______________________________

25) What medications are you currently taking, or have been taking, in the last month? (May I see your medication bottles?) (*If patient cannot list, ask categories a-r and note dosage and schedule, or obtain information from medical or pharmacy records and verify accuracy with the patient.*)

Table continued on following page

Table 4-3. ► Comprehensive Older Persons' Evaluation *Continued*

Allergies:

	Rx (DOSAGE AND SCHEDULE)
a) Arthritis medication	
b) Pain medication	
c) Blood pressure medication	
d) Water pills or pills for fluid	
e) Medication for your heart	
f) Medication for your lungs	
g) Blood thinners	
h) Medication for your circulation	
i) Insulin or diabetes medication	
j) Seizure medication	
k) Thyroid pills	
l) Steroids	
m) Hormones	
n) Antibiotics	
o) Medicine for nerves or depression	
p) Prescription sleeping pills	
q) Other prescription drugs	
r) Other non-prescription drugs	

26) Many people have problems remembering to take their medications, especially ones they need to take on a regular basis. How often do you forget to take your medications? Would you say you forget often, sometimes, rarely or never?
a) Never
b) Rarely
c) Sometimes
d) Often

Activities of Daily Living: The next set of questions asks whether you need help with any of the following activities of daily living.

27) I would like to know whether you can do these activities without any help at all, or if you need assistance to do them. Do you need help to: (*If yes, describe, including patient needs.*)

	YES	NO	DESCRIBE (INCLUDE NEEDS)
a) Use the telephone?			
b) Get to places out of walking distance (using transportation)			
c) Shop for clothes and food?			
d) Do your housework?			
e) Handle your money?			
f) Feed yourself?			
g) Dress and undress yourself?			
h) Take care of your appearance?			
i) Get in and out of bed?			
j) Take a bath or shower?			
k) Prepare your meals?			
l) Do you have any problem getting to the bathroom on time?			

28) During the past six months, have you had any help with such things as shopping, housework, bathing, dressing and getting around?
a) Yes (*specify:* ________________)
b) No

Signature of person completing the form:

____

(From Pearlman R: Development of a functional assessment questionnaire for geriatric patients: COPE. J Chronic Dis 40:85S–94S, 1987. Reprinted with permission.)

are today, nor were they equally available for women. The aging person may be sensitive to having achieved the level of only elementary school education or less.

Occupation. Ask about past positions, volunteer activities, and community activities. Many people continue to work past the age of 65; they grew up with strong work ethic and are proud to continue. If the person is retired, how has he or she adjusted to the change in role? It may mean loss of social role or social status, loss of personal relationships formed at work, and reduced income.

Activity and Exercise

Daily Profile. How does the person spend a typical day in work, hobbies, and leisure activities? Is there any day this routine changes, e.g., Sunday visits from family? Note that the person suffering from chronic illness or disability may have a self-care deficit, musculoskeletal changes such as arthritis, and mental confusion. For all older adults, the Comprehensive Older Persons' Evaluation (Table 4–3) helps assess the activities or daily living as well as physical, social, psychological, demographic, financial, and legal issues.

Leisure activities. List significant hobbies, sports, community activities. Is there a community senior citizen center available for nutrition, social network, and screening of health status?

Exercise. What is the type, amount, and frequency of the exercise? Is a warm-up included? How does the person's body respond?

Sleep and Rest. Note the person's sleep pattern. Does he or she feel rested during day? Is his or her energy sufficient to carry out daily activities? Does the person need naps? Is there a problem with night wakenings (nocturia, shortness of breath, light sleep, insomnia [difficulty falling asleep, awakening during night, early morning wakening])? If the person has no routine, does he or she tend to nap all afternoon? Does insomnia worsen with lack of a daily schedule?

Nutrition. Record a 24-hour recall. Is this typical of most days? (Nutrition may vary greatly. Ask the person to keep a weekly log to bring in.) What are the meal patterns? Are there three full meals or five to six smaller meals per day? How much convenience foods and soft foods does the person use? Who prepares meals? Does the person eat alone? Who shops for food? How does the person transport groceries home? Is the person's income adequate for groceries? Is there a problem preparing meals (adequate vision, motor deficit, adequate energy)? Are the person's appliances and water and utilities adequate for meal preparation? Is there any difficulty chewing or swallowing? What are the person's food preferences (aging persons often eat high amounts of carbohydrates because these foods are cheaper, easier to make, and easier to chew).

Interpersonal Relationships. Does the person live alone? Is this satisfactory? Does the person have a pet? How close does the person live to family or friends? How often does the person see family or friends? Does the person live with family, such as a spouse, children, or a sibling? Is this a satisfactory arrangement? What is the person's role in family for preparation of meals, housework, and other activities? Are there any conflicts? If the person lives far from family, how often does he or she see them? Does he or she experience this as a loss? Who does the person depend on for emotional support? Who helps the person cope with problems? Who meets the person's affection needs?

Coping and Stress Management. Has there been a recent change in lifestyle, such as loss of occupation, spouse, friends, move from home, illness of self or family member, or has income been decreased? How does the person deal with stress? If a loved one has died, how is the person responding to the loss? How does the person feel about being "alone" and having to take on unfamiliar responsibilities now?

Environment. Inquire about the person's home (safety, one floor or are there stairs, state of repair, is money adequate to maintain home, exits for fire, heating and utilities adequate, how long the person has lived in the present home), transportation (auto, last driver's test, does the person consider self a safe driver, income adequate for maintenance; public transportation access, receive drives from community resources, friends), and neighborhood (secure in personal safety at day or night; danger of loss of possessions; amount of noise and pollution; access to family and friends, grocery store, drug store, laundry, church, temple, mosque, health care facilities).

TRANSCULTURAL CONSIDERATIONS

HEALTH-RELATED BELIEFS AND PRACTICES

One aspect of a comprehensive health history concerns the collection of data related to culturally based beliefs and practices about health and illness. Before determining whether cultural practices are helpful, harmful, or neutral, you must first understand the logic of the belief system underlying the practice and then be certain that you fully grasp the nature and meaning of the practice from the person's cultural perspective.

Health and Culture

The first step in understanding the health care needs of others is to understand your own culturally based values, beliefs, attitudes, and practices. Sometimes this requires considerable introspection and may necessitate that you confront your own biases, preconceptions, and prejudices about specific racial, ethnic, religious, sexual, or socioeconomic groups. Secondly, you need to identify the meaning of health to the client, remembering that concepts are derived, in part, from the way in which members of their cultural group define health. Considerable research has been conducted on the various definitions of health that may be held by various groups. For example, Jamaicans define health as having a good appetite, feeling strong and energetic, performing activities of daily living without difficulty, and being sexually active and fertile (Mitchell, 1983). In a study of Italian women, Ragucci (1981) observed that health means the ability to interact socially and to perform routine tasks such as cooking, cleaning, and caring for self and others. On the other hand, some individuals of Hispanic origins believe that coughing, sweating, and diarrhea are a normal part of living, not symptoms of ill health — perhaps because of their high frequency of these conditions in the country of origin. Thus, individuals may define themselves or others in their group as healthy even though you identify them as having symptoms of disease.

Illness and Culture

For clients, symptom labeling and diagnosis depends on the degree of difference between the individual's behaviors and those the group has defined as normal, beliefs about the causation of illness, level of stigma attached to a particular set of symptoms, prevalence of the pathology, and the meaning of the illness to the individual and his or her family.

Throughout history, humankind has attempted to understand the cause of illness and disease. Theories of causation have been formulated based on religious beliefs, social circumstances, philosophical perspectives, and level of knowledge.

Causes of Illness

There are three major ways in which disease causation may be viewed: from a biomedical or scientific, naturalistic or holistic, and magicoreligious perspective. The first, called the *biomedical* or *scientific* theory of illness causation, is based on the assumption that all events in life have a cause and effect, that the human body functions more or less mechanically (i.e., the functioning of the human body is analogous to the functioning of an automobile), that all life can be reduced or divided into smaller parts (e.g., the reduction of the human person into body, mind, and spirit) and that all of reality can be observed and measured (e.g., intelligence tests and psychometric measures of behavior). Among the biomedical explanations for disease is the germ theory, which posits that microscopic organisms such as bacteria and viruses are responsible for specific disease conditions. Most educational programs for physicians, nurses, and other health care providers embrace the biomedical or scientific theories that explain the causes of both physical and psychologic illnesses.

The second way in which clients explain the cause of illness is from the *naturalistic* or *holistic* perspective, a viewpoint that is found most frequently among Native Americans, Asians, and others who believe that human life is only one aspect of nature and a part of the general order of the cosmos. Individuals from these groups believe that the forces of nature must be kept in natural balance or harmony.

Among many Asians there is a belief in the *yin/yang theory,* in which health is believed to exist when all aspects of the person are in perfect balance. Rooted in the ancient Chinese philosophy of *Tao,* the yin/yang theory states that all organisms and objects in the universe consist of *yin* and *yang energy forces.* The seat of the energy forces are within the autonomic nervous system where balance between the opposing forces is maintained during health. Yin energy represents the female and negative forces, such as emptiness, darkness, and cold; whereas yang forces are male and positive, emitting warmth and fullness. Foods are classified as hot and cold in this theory and are transformed into yin and yang energy when metabolized by the body. Yin foods are cold and yang foods are hot. Cold foods are eaten with a hot illness, and hot foods are eaten with a cold illness. The yin/yang theory is the basis for *Eastern* or *Chinese* medicine and is commonly embraced by Asian-Americans.

The naturalistic perspective posits that the laws of nature create imbalances, chaos, and disease. Individuals embracing the naturalistic view use metaphors such as the healing power of nature, and they call the earth "Mother." From the perspective of the Chinese, for example, illness is not seen as an intruding agent but as a part of life's rhythmic course and as an outward sign of disharmony within.

Many Hispanic, Arab, Black, and Asian groups embrace the *hot/cold theory* of health and illness, an explanatory model having its origins in the ancient Greek humoral theory. The four humors of the body — blood, phlegm, black bile, and yellow bile — regulate basic bodily functions and are described in terms of temperature, dryness, and moisture. The treatment of disease consists of adding or subtracting cold, heat, dryness, or wetness to restore the balance of the humors.

Beverages, foods, herbs, medicines, and diseases are classified as hot or cold according to their perceived effects on the body, not on their physical characteristics. Illnesses believed to be caused by cold entering the body include earache, chest cramps, paralysis, gastrointestinal discomfort, rheumatism, and tuberculosis. Among those illnesses believed to be caused by overheating are abscessed teeth, sore throats, rashes, and kidney disorders.

According to the hot/cold theory, the individual as a whole, not just a particular ailment, is significant. Those who embrace the hot/cold theory maintain that health consists of a positive state of total well-being, including physical, psychological, spiritual, and social aspects of the person. Paradoxically, the language used to describe this artificial dissection of the body into parts is itself a reflection of the biomedical/scientific perspective, not a naturalistic or holistic one.

The third major way in which people view the world and explain the causation of illness is from a *magico-religious* perspective. The basic premise of this explanatory model is that the world is seen as an arena in which supernatural forces dominate. The fate of the world and those in it depends on the action of supernatural forces for good or evil. Examples of magical causes of illness include belief in voodoo or witchcraft among some Blacks and others from circum-Caribbean countries. *Faith healing* is based on religious beliefs and is most prevalent among certain Christian religions, including Christian Scientists, whereas various healing rituals may be found in many other religions such as Roman Catholicism, Mormonism (Church of Jesus Christ of Latter-Day Saints), and others.

Culture and Healing

When self-treatment is unsuccessful, the individual may turn to the lay or folk healing systems, to spiritual or religious healing, or to scientific biomedicine. All cultures have their own preferred lay or popular healers, recognized symptoms of ill health, acceptable sick role behavior, and treatments. In addition to seeking help from you as a biomedical/scientific health care provider, clients may also seek help from folk or religious healers. Some people, such as those of Hispanic or Native American origins, may believe that the cure is incomplete unless healing of body, mind, and spirit are all carried out, although the division of the person into parts is itself a Western concept. For example, an Hispanic person with a respiratory infection may take the antibiotics prescribed by a physician or nurse practitioner, herbal teas recommended by a "curandero," and may say prayers for healing suggested by a Catholic priest.

The variety of healing beliefs and practices used by the many subcultural groups found in this country far exceeds the limitations of this chapter. It is important, however, that you be aware of the existence of alternative practices and recognize that, in addition to folk practices, there are many other alternative healing practices. Although it is dangerous to assume that all indigenous approaches to healing are innocuous, the majority of practices are quite harmless, whether or not they are effective.

Folk Healers

Although there are numerous folk healers, you may find Hispanics turning to a "curandero," "espiritualista" (spiritualist), "yerbo" (herbalist), or "sabador" (equivalent to a chiropractor). Blacks may mention having received assistance from a "hougan" (a voodoo priest or priestess), spiritualist, or old lady (an older woman who has successfully raised a family and who specializes in child care and folk remedies). Native Americans may seek assistance from a shaman or medicine man. People of Asian descent may mention that they have visited herbalists, acupuncturists, or bone setters. Each culture has its own healers, most of whom speak the native tongue of the client, make house calls, and cost significantly less than healers practicing in the biomedical/scientific health care system. In addition to folk healers, many cultures have lay midwives (e.g., "parteras" for Hispanic women) or other health care provider available for meeting the needs of pregnant women.

In some religions, spiritual healers may be found among the ranks of the ordained and official religious hierarchy, and may be known by a variety of names such as priest, bishop, elder, deacon, rabbi, brother, sister, and so forth. In other religions, a separate category of healer may be found, e.g., Christian Science "nurses" (not licensed by states) or practitioners.

TRANSCULTURAL EXPRESSION OF ILLNESS

There is wide cultural variation in the manner in which certain symptoms and disease conditions are perceived, diagnosed, labeled, and treated. The same disease that is considered grounds for social ostracism in one culture may be reason for increased status in another. For example, epilepsy is seen as contagious and untreatable among Ugandans; as a cause for family shame among Greeks; as a reflection of a physical imbalance among Mexican Americans; and as a sign of having gained favor by enduring a trial by a God among the Hutterites (Tripp-Reimer, 1984).

Bodily symptoms are also perceived and reported in a variety of ways. For example, individuals of Mediterranean descent tend to report common physical symptoms more often than persons of Northern European or Asian heritage. Among Chinese, there is no translation for the English word "sadness," yet all people experience the feeling of sadness at sometime in life. To express emotion, Chinese sometimes somaticize their symptoms, e.g., complain of cardiac symptoms because the center of emotion in the Chinese culture is the heart. You may collect in-depth data about the cardiovascular system only to learn subsequently that all diagnostic tests are negative. On further assessment, you may determine that the person has experienced a loss and is grieving, e.g., has experienced the death of a close friend or relative, or has been divorced or separated. Although some biomedical/scientific clinicians may refer to this as a psychosomatic illness, others recognize it as a culturally acceptable somatic expression of emotional disharmony.

A discussion of pain follows to illustrate the cultural variability that may occur with a symptom of significant concern.

Transcultural Expression of Symptoms: Pain

To illustrate the manner in which symptom expression may reflect the person's cultural background, an extensively studied symptom, pain, is used. Pain is a universally recognized phenomenon and is an important aspect of assessment for people of various ages. Pain is a very private, subjective experience that is greatly influenced by cultural heritage. Expectations, manifestations, and management of pain are all embedded in a cultural context. The definition of pain, like that of health or illness, is culturally determined.

The term pain is derived from the Greek word for penalty, which helps explain the long association between pain and punishment in Judeo-Christian thought. The meaning of painful stimuli for individuals, the way people define their situation, and the impact of personal experience all help determine the experience of pain.

Much cross-cultural research has been conducted on pain. Pain has been found to be a highly personal experience, depending on cultural learning, the meaning of the situation, and other factors unique to the individual. Silent suffering has been identified as the most valued response to pain by health care professionals. The majority of nurses have been socialized to believe that in virtually any situation, self-control is better than open displays of strong feelings.

In a study of nurses' attitudes toward pain by Davitz and Davitz (1981), it was discovered that the ethnic background of patients is important in the nurses' assessment of both physical and psychological pain. Nurses preconceive that Jewish and Spanish patients suffer the most and that Anglo-Saxon and German patients suffer the least. In addition, nurses who infer relatively greater patient pain tended to report their own experiences as more painful. In general, nurses from Eastern and Southern European or African backgrounds tend to infer greater suffering than do nurses of Northern European backgrounds. Years of experience, current position, and area of clinical practice are unrelated to inferences of suffering.

In addition to expecting variations in pain perception and tolerance, you should also expect variations in the expression of pain. It is a well-known fact that individuals turn to their social environment for validation and comparison. A first important comparison group is the family, which transmits cultural norms to its children.

The anthropologist Zborowski (1952, 1969) found that the meaning of pain and behavioral responses to the painful stimulus are culturally learned and culturally specific. Zborowski studied pain in four groups of men admitted to a veterans' hospital. "Old American" patients, defined as third-generation Americans, were found to be unexpressive—they reported pain but emotional behavior was controlled. Complaining, crying, or screaming was viewed as useless or unnecessary. Both Jewish and Italian men were expressive in their pain response and asked for immediate pain relief by any means possible. Lastly, Irish men saw pain as a private event to be endured alone. This group was unemotional and nonexpressive of pain. In addition, when in pain, the "Old American" and Irish groups tended to withdraw socially, whereas the Jewish and Italian groups preferred the company of friends and relatives.

HEALTH-RELATED RELIGIOUS BELIEFS AND PRACTICES

As an integral component of the individual's culture, religious beliefs may influence the person's explanation of the cause(s) of illness, perception of its severity, and choice of healer(s). In times of crisis, such as serious illness and impending death, religion may be a source of consolation for the person and his or her family and may influence the course of action believed to be appropriate.

Religion and Spirituality

Religious concerns evolve from and respond to the mysteries of life and death, good and evil, and pain and suffering. In health care settings, you frequently encounter people who find themselves searching for a spiritual meaning to help explain their illness or disability.

Although the religions of the world offer various interpretations to many of life's mysteries, most people seek a personal understanding and interpretation at some time in their lives. Ultimately, this personal search becomes a pursuit to discover a supreme being (called by various names—Allah, God, Yahweh, Jehovah, and so forth), or some unifying truth, that will render meaning, purpose, and integrity to existence (Cluff, 1986).

An important distinction needs to be made between religion and spirituality. *Religion* refers to an organized system of beliefs concerning the cause, nature, and purpose of the universe, especially a belief in or the worship of God or gods. There are more than 1200 religions in the United States. *Spirituality* arises out of each person's unique life experience and his or her personal effort to find purpose and meaning in life.

Illness during childhood may be an especially difficult clinical situation. Children as well as adults have spiritual needs that vary according to the child's developmental level and the religious climate that exists in the family. Parental perceptions about the illness of their child may be partially influenced by religious beliefs. For example, some parents may believe that a transgression against a religious law is responsible for a congenital anomaly in their offspring. Other parents may delay seeking medical care because they believe that prayer should be tried first. Certain types of treatment, e.g., administration of blood; medications containing caffeine, pork, or other prohibited substances; and selected procedures, may be perceived as *cultural taboos,* i.e., to be avoided (by both children and adults).

Values held by the dominant American culture, such as emphasis on independence, self-reliance, and productivity, influence aging members of society. Americans define people as old at the chronologic age of 65 and then limit their work in contrast to other cultures in which persons are first recognized as being unable to work and then are identified as being old.

In adopting a cultural perspective in working with aging individuals from different culturally diverse backgrounds, you should consider that the main task of these persons is to achieve a sense of integrity in accepting responsibility for their own lives and in gaining a sense of accomplishment. Individuals who achieve integrity see aging as a positive experience, make adjustments in their personal space and social relationships, maintain a sense of usefulness, and begin closure and life review.

Older persons may develop their own means of coping with illness through self-care, assistance from family members, and support from social groups. Some cultures have developed attitudes and specific behaviors for older adults that may include humanistic care and identification of family members as care providers. The older adults may have special family responsibilities, e.g., providing hospitality to visitors among Amish cultures and communicating to members of younger generations skills and accrued wisdom among Filipinos.

Older immigrants who have made major lifestyle adjustments in their move from their homeland to the United States or from a rural to an urban area (or vice versa) may not be aware of health care alternatives, preventive programs, health care benefits, and screening programs for which they are eligible. These individuals may also be in various stages of *culture shock,* a term used to describe the state of disorientation or inability to respond to the behavior of a different cultural group because of its sudden strangeness, unfamiliarity, and incompatibility to the stranger's perceptions and expectations (Leininger, 1988).

CULTURE AND TREATMENT

After a symptom is identified, the first effort at treatment is often self-care. In the United States an estimated 70 to 90 percent of all illness episodes are treated first, or exclusively, through self-care (Zola, 1979), often with significant success. The availability of over-the-counter medications, relatively high literacy level of Americans, and influence of the mass media in communicating health-related information to the general population have contributed to the high percentage of cases of self-treatment. Home treatments are attractive for their accessibility, especially when compared with the inconvenience associated with traveling to a physician, nurse practitioner, and pharmacist, particularly for people from rural or sparsely populated areas. Furthermore, home treatment may mobilize the person's social support network and provide the sick individual with a caring environment in which to convalesce. You should be aware, however, that not all home remedies are inexpensive. For example, urban Black populations in the Southeast sometimes use medicinal potions that cost much more than the equivalent treatment with a biomedical intervention (Tripp-Reimer & Lauer, 1987).

A wide variety of so-called nontraditional interventions are gaining the recognition of health care professionals in the biomedical/scientific health care system. Acupuncture, acupressure, therapeutic touch, massage, biofeedback, relaxation techniques, meditation, hypnosis, distraction, imagery, herbal remedies, and others are interventions that clients may use either alone or in combination with other treatments.

CULTURAL ASSESSMENT

A *cultural assessment* refers to a systematic appraisal or examination of individuals, groups, and communities in relation to their cultural beliefs, values, and practices to determine explicit nursing needs and intervention practices within the cultural context of the people being evaluated (Leininger, 1988). Cultural assessments tend to be broad and comprehensive because they deal with cultural values, belief systems, and ways of living now and in the recent past. However, you can learn to appraise segments of these larger areas, such as a particular cultural value, and then relate this finding to other aspects, such as cultural practices. Appendix 4–1. summarizes major data categories pertaining to the culture of clients and offers suggested questions that you might ask the client to elicit the information.

Bibliography

American Academy of Pediatrics: Measles: reassessment of the current immunization policy. Pediatrics 84(6):1110–1113, 1989.

Campbell LA, Thompson BL: Evaluating elderly patients: A critique of comprehensive functional assessment tools. Nurse Pract 15(8):11–18, 1990.

Cluff CB: Spiritual intervention reconsidered. Top Geriatr Rehabil 1(2):77–82, 1986.

Davitz JR, Davitz LJ: Influences of Patients' Pain and Psychological Distress. New York, Springer-Verlag, 1981.

Gordon M: Nursing Diagnosis: Process and Application. New York, McGraw-Hill, 1987.

Granger CV, Albrecht GL, Hamilton BB: Outcome of comprehensive medical rehabilitation: Measures of PULSES profile and the Barthel index. Arch Phys Med Rehabil 60:145–154, 1979.

Gulick EE: The self-assessment of health among the chronically ill. Top Clin Nurs 8(1):74–82, 1986.

Katz S, Ford AB, Moskowitz RS, et al: Studies of illness in the aged. The Index of ADL: A standardized measure of biological and psychosocial function. JAMA 185:94–98, 1963.

Leininger M: Transcultural Nursing: Concepts, Theories, and Practices. 2nd ed. New York, John Wiley & Sons, 1988.

Lenihan AA: Identification of self-care behaviors in the elderly: A nursing assessment tool. J Prof Nurs 4(4):285–288, 1988.

Linn MW, Linn BS: The rapid disability rating scale—2. J Am Geriatr Soc 30(6):378–382, 1982.

Mahoney FI, Barthel DW: Functional evaluation: The Barthel Index. Maryland State Med J 14:61–65, 1965.

Mitchell M: Popular medical concepts in Jamaica and their impact on drug use. West J Med 139:841–847, 1983.

Pearlman R: Development of a functional assessment questionnaire for geriatric patients: The comprehensive older persons' evaluation (COPE). J Chronic Dis 40:85S–94S, 1987.

Ragucci AT: Italian Americans. *In* Harwood A (Ed): Ethnicity and Medical Care. Cambridge, MA, Harvard Press, 1981, pp 56–84.

Speake DL, Cowart ME, Pellet K: Health perceptions and lifestyles of the elderly. Res Nurs Health 12:93–100, 1989.

Tripp-Reimer T, Lauer GM: Ethnicity and families with chronic illness. *In* Wright LM, Leahey M (Eds): Families and Chronic Illness. Springhouse, PA, Springhouse Corporation, 1987, pp 77–99.

Tripp-Reimer T: Cultural assessment. *In* Bellack J, Bamford P (Eds): Nursing Assessment: A Multidimensional Approach. Monterey, CA, Wadsworth Health Sciences, 1984, pp 57–89.

Zborowski M: Cultural components in response to pain. J Social Issues 8:16–30, 1952.

Zborowski M: People in Pain. San Francisco, CA, Jossey-Bass, 1969.

Zola IK: Oh where, oh where has ethnicity gone? *In* Gelfand D, Kutzik A (Eds): Ethnicity and Aging: Theory, Research, and Policy. New York, Springer Publishing, 1979, pp 14–36.

APPENDIX 4–1. CULTURAL ASSESSMENT GUIDE

OBTAIN A BRIEF HISTORY OF THE ETHNIC AND RACIAL ORIGINS OF THE CLIENT'S CULTURAL GROUP

- With what ethnic group do you affiliate (e.g., Hispanic, Polish, Navajo, or a combination)? To what degree do you identify with the cultural group (e.g., do you have a "we" concept of solidarity or a fringe member concept)?
- What is your racial affiliation (e.g., Black, Native American, or Asian)?
- Where were you born?
- Where have you lived (country, city) and when (during what years)? (Note: If a recent relocation to the U.S., knowledge of prevalent diseases in country of origin may be helpful.)

VALUES ORIENTATION

- What are your attitudes, values, and beliefs about birth, death, health, illness, health care providers?
- How do you view work, leisure, and education?
- How do you perceive change?

CULTURAL SANCTIONS AND RESTRICTIONS

- Do you have any restrictions related to sexuality, exposure of body parts, certain types of surgery (e.g., amputation, vasectomy, and hysterectomy)?
- Are there any restrictions against discussion of dead relatives or fears related to the unknown?

COMMUNICATION

- What language do you speak at home? What other languages do you speak or read? In what language would you prefer to communicate?
- Is there a relative or friend who you would like to interpret? Is there anyone you would prefer did not interpret (e.g., member of the opposite sex, a person younger or older than yourself, or a member of a rival tribe or nation)?
- Do you prefer to receive care from a nurse of the same cultural background, gender, and/or age?
- With which language(s) and/or dialect(s) are you most comfortable?

HEALTH-RELATED BELIEFS AND PRACTICES

- To what cause(s) do you attribute illness and disease (e.g., divine wrath, imbalance in hot/cold or yin/yang, punishment for moral transgressions, hex, or soul loss)?
- What do you believe promotes health (eating certain foods; wearing amulets to bring good luck; exercise; prayer; or rituals to ancestors, saints, or intermediate deities)?
- What is your religious affiliation (e.g., Judaism, Islam, Pentacostalism, West African voodooism, Seventh Day Adventism, Catholicism, or Mormonism)?
- Do you rely on cultural healers (e.g., curandero, shaman, spiritualist, priest, minister, monk)? Who determines the type of healer and treatment that should be sought?
- In what types of cultural healing practices do you engage (use of herbal remedies, potions, massage, wearing of talismans or charms to discourage evil spirits, healing rituals, incantations, or prayers)?
- What is appropriate "sick role" behavior for you? Who determines when you are sick and when you are no longer sick? Who cares for you at home?

NUTRITION

- What is the meaning of food and eating to you? With whom do you usually eat? What types of foods do you usually eat? What do you define as food? What do you believe comprises a "healthy" versus an "unhealthy" diet?
- How are foods prepared at home (type of food preparation; cooking oils used; length of time foods are cooked, especially vegetables; amount and type of seasoning added to various foods during preparation)?
- Do religious beliefs and practices influence your diet (e.g., amount, type, preparation or delineation of acceptable food combinations, e.g., kosher diets)? Do you abstain from certain foods at regular intervals, on specific dates determined by the religious calendar, or at other times?
- If your religion mandates or encourages fasting, what does the term "fast" mean (e.g., refraining from certain types or quantities of foods, eating only during certain times of the day)? For what period of time are you expected to fast?
- During fasting, do you refrain from liquids or beverages? Does your religion allow exemption from fasting during illness? If so, do you believe that an exemption applies to you?

SOCIOECONOMIC CONSIDERATIONS

- Who comprises your social network (family, peers, and cultural healers)? How do they influence your health or illness status?
- How do members of your social support network define caring (e.g., being continuously present, doing things for you, looking after your family)? What is the role of various family members during health and illness?
- How does your family participate in your nursing care (e.g., bathing, feeding, touching, being present)?
- Who is the principal wage earner in your family? Is there more than one wage earner? Are there other sources of financial support (extended family, investments)?

EDUCATIONAL BACKGROUND

- What is the highest educational level you have obtained?
- Can you read and write English or is another language preferred?
- What learning style is most comfortable or familiar? Do you prefer to learn through written materials, oral explanation, or demonstration?

RELIGIOUS AFFILIATION

- What is the role of your religious beliefs and practices during health and illness?
- Are there healing rituals or practices that you believe can promote well-being or hasten recovery from illness? If so, who performs these practices?
- What is the role of significant religious representatives during health and illness? Are there recognized religious healers (e.g., Islamic imams, Christian Scientist practitioners or nurses, Catholic priests, Mormon elders, or Buddhist monks)?

CHAPTER

5 Mental Health Assessment

DEFINING MENTAL STATUS

Mental status is a person's emotional and cognitive functioning. Optimal functioning aims toward simultaneous life satisfaction in work, in caring relationships, and within the self. Mental health is relative and ongoing. Everyone has "good" and "bad" days. Usually, mental status strikes a balance, allowing the person to function socially and occupationally.

The stress surrounding a traumatic life event (death of a loved one, serious illness) tips the balance, causing transient dysfunction. This is an expected response to a trauma. Mental status assessment at this time can identify remaining strengths, and can help the individual mobilize resources and use coping skills.

A *mental disorder* is apparent when a person's response is much greater than the expected reaction to a traumatic life event. A mental disorder is defined as a significant behavioral or psychological *pattern* that is associated with distress (a painful symptom) or disability (impaired functioning), and has a significant risk of pain, disability, or death, or a loss of freedom (American Psychiatric Association, 1987). Mental disorders include organic brain disease (due to brain dysfunction of *known* specific organic cause, e.g. delirium or dementia), and psychiatric mental illness (in which organic etiology has not yet been established, e.g., anxiety disorder or schizophrenia). Mental status assessment serves to document a dysfunction and to determine how that dysfunction affects self-care in everyday life.

Mental status cannot be scrutinized directly like the characteristics of skin or heart sounds. Its functioning is *inferred* through assessment of an individual's behaviors:

Consciousness: being aware of one's own existence, feelings, and thoughts and aware of the environment. This is the most elementary of mental status functions.

Language: using the voice to communicate one's thoughts and feelings. This is a basic tool of humans and its loss has a heavy social impact on the individual.

Mood and affect: both of these elements deal with the prevailing feelings: affect is a temporary expression of feelings or state of mind; mood is more durable, a prolonged display of feelings that color the whole emotional life.

Orientation: the awareness of the objective world in relation to the self.

Attention: the power of concentration, the ability to focus on one specific thing without being distracted by many environmental stimuli.

Memory: the ability to lay down and store experiences and perceptions for later recall. *Recent* memory evokes day-to-day events; *remote* memory brings up years' worth of experiences.

Abstract reasoning: pondering a deeper meaning beyond the concrete and literal.

Thought process: the *way* a person thinks, the logical train of thought.

Thought content: *what* the person thinks: specific ideas, beliefs, the use of words.

Perceptions: an awareness of objects through any of the five senses.

DEVELOPMENTAL CONSIDERATIONS

Infants and Children

The maturation of emotional and cognitive functioning is described in detail in Chapter 2. It is difficult to separate and trace the development of just one aspect of mental status. All aspects are interdependent. For example, consciousness is rudimentary at birth because the cerebral cortex is not yet developed; the infant cannot distinguish the self from the mother's body. Consciousness gradually develops along with language, so that by 18–24 months the child learns he or she is separate from objects in the environment and has words to express this. We can trace language development, too: from the differentiated crying at 4 weeks, the cooing at 6 weeks, through one-word sentences at one year to multiword sentences at 2 years. Yet the concept of language as a social tool of communication occurs around 4 to 5 years of age, coincident with the child's readiness to cooperatively play with other children.

Attention gradually increases in span through preschool years so that, by school age, most children are able to sit and concentrate on their work for a period of time. Some children are late in developing concentration. School readiness coincides with the development of the thought process; around age 7, thinking becomes more logical and systematic, and the child is able to reason and understand. Abstract thinking, the ability to consider a hypothetical situation, usually develops between age 12 to 15, though a few adolescents never achieve it.

The Aging Adult

The aging process leaves the parameters of mental status mostly intact. There is no decrease in general knowledge and little or no loss in vocabulary. Response time is slower than in youth; it takes a bit longer for the brain to process information and react to it. Thus, performance on timed intelligence tests may be lower for the aging person, not because intelligence has declined, but because it takes longer to respond to the questions. The slower response time affects new learning; if a new presentation is rapidly paced, the older person does not have time to respond to it (Rossman, 1986).

Recent memory, which requires some processing (e.g., medication instructions, 24 hour diet recall, names of new acquaintances), is somewhat decreased with aging. Remote memory is not affected.

Age-related changes in sensory perception can affect mental status. For example, vision loss (as detailed in Chapter 11) may result in apathy, social isolation, and depression. Hearing changes are common in older adults (see the discussion of presbycusis in Chapter 12). Age-related hearing loss involves high sound frequencies. Consonants are high-frequency sounds, so older people who have difficulty hearing them have problems with normal conversation. This problem produces frustration, suspicion, and social isolation, as well as making the person look confused (Rossman, 1986).

The era of older adulthood contains more potential for loss than do earlier eras, such as loss of loved ones, loss of job status and prestige, loss of income, and the loss of an energetic and resilient body. The grief and despair surrounding these losses can affect mental status. These losses can result in disorientation, disability, or depression.

PURPOSES AND COMPONENTS OF THE MENTAL STATUS EXAMINATION

The full mental status examination is a systematic check of emotional and cognitive functioning. The steps described here, though, rarely need to be taken in their entirety. Usually, you can assess mental status through the context of the health history interview. During that time, keep in mind the four main headings of mental status assessment:

appearance, behavior, cognition, and
thought processes, or
A, B, C, T.

Integrating the mental status examination into the interview is sufficient for most people. You will collect ample data in order to assess mental health strengths and coping skills, and to screen for any dysfunction.

It is necessary to perform a full mental status examination when you discover any abnormality in affect or behavior, and in cases of a person with:

- family members concerned about behavioral changes, e.g., memory loss, inappropriate social interaction.
- brain lesions (trauma, tumor, cerebrovascular accident). A mental status assessment documents any emotional or cognitive change associated with the lesion (Strub & Black, 1985). Not recognizing these changes hinders care planning and creates problems with social readjustment.
- aphasia. A mental status examination assesses language dysfunction as well as any emotional problems associated with it, such as depression or agitation.
- symptoms of psychiatric mental illness, especially with acute onset.

In every mental status examination, note these factors from the health history that could affect your findings:

- any known illnesses or health problems, such as alcoholism, or chronic renal disease;
- current medications, whose side effects may cause confusion or depression;
- the usual educational and behavioral level—note that factor as the normal baseline, and do not expect performance on the mental status examination to exceed it;
- responses to personal history questions, indicating current stress, social interaction patterns, and sleep habits.

In the following examination the sequence of steps form a *hierarchy,* in which the most basic functions (consciousness, language) are assessed first. The first steps must be accurately assessed to ensure validity for the steps to follow. That is, if consciousness is clouded, then the person cannot be expected to have full attention and to cooperate with new learning. Or, if language is impaired, subsequent assessment of new learning or abstract reasoning (anything that requires language functioning) can give erroneous conclusions.

OBJECTIVE DATA

METHOD OF EXAMINATION

Preparation

Equipment—occasionally need pencil, paper, and reading material

PROCEDURE

NORMAL RANGE OF FINDINGS	ABNORMAL FINDINGS
Appearance	
Posture is erect and *position* is relaxed.	Sitting on edge of chair or curled in bed, tense muscles, frowning, darting watchful eyes, occur with anxiety and metabolic disorders. Sitting slumped in chair, slow walk, dragging feet occur with depression and some organic brain diseases.
Body movements are voluntary, deliberate, coordinated, and smooth and even.	Restless, fidgety movements, hyperkinetic appearance occur with anxiety. Apathy and psychomotor slowing occur with depression and organic brain disease. Abnormal posturing and bizarre gestures occur with schizophrenia. Facial grimaces.
Dress is appropriate for setting, season, age, gender, and social group. Clothing fits and is put on appropriately.	Wearing under garments on top of outer clothing can occur with organic brain syndrome. Eccentric dress combination and bizarre make-up occur with schizophrenia or manic syndrome.
Grooming and hygiene should be noted. The person is clean and well groomed, hair is neat and clean, women have moderate or no make-up, men are shaved or beard or moustache are well groomed. Nails are clean (though some jobs leave nails chronically dirty). Note: A disheveled appearance in a previously well-groomed person is significant. Use care in interpreting clothing that is disheveled, bizarre, or in poor repair, because these sometimes reflect the person's economic status or a deliberate fashion trend.	Unilateral neglect (total inattention to one side of body) occurs following some cerebrovascular accidents. Inappropriate dress, poor hygiene, and lack of concern with appearance occur with depression and organic brain syndrome. Meticulously dressed and groomed ap-

NORMAL RANGE OF FINDINGS	ABNORMAL FINDINGS
	pearance and fastidious manner may occur with obsessive-compulsive disorders.
Behavior	
Level of Consciousness. The person is awake, alert, aware of stimuli from the environment and within the self, and responds appropriately to stimuli.	Lethargic, obtunded. See Table 5–3, Levels of Consciousness.
Facial Expression. The look is appropriate to the situation and changes appropriately with the topic. There is comfortable eye contact unless precluded by cultural norm, e.g., Native American.	Flat, mask-like expression occurs with parkinsonism and depression.
Speech. Quality—The person makes laryngeal sounds effortlessly and shares conversation appropriately.	Dysphonia, a problem with volume, pitch. See Table 5–4. Monopolizes interview. Silent, secretive, or uncommunicative.
The pace of the conversation is moderate, and stream of talking is fluent.	Slow, monotonous with parkinsonism, depression. Rapid-fire and loud talking occur with manic syndrome.
Articulation (ability to form words) is clear and understandable.	Dysarthria, see Table 5–4. Misuse of words; omits letters, syllables, or words; transposes words; occurs with aphasia. Circumlocution, or repetitious abnormal patterns: neologism, echolalia, see Tables 5–5 and 5–7.
Word choice is effortless and appropriate to educational level. The person completes sentences, occasionally pausing to think.	Unduly long word-finding or failure in word search occurs with aphasia.
Mood and affect. Judge this by body language and facial expression, and by asking directly, "How do you feel today," or "How do you usually feel?" The mood should be appropriate to the person's place and condition and change appropriately with topics. The person is willing to cooperate with you.	See Table 5–6, Abnormalities of Mood and Affect. Wide mood swings occur with manic syndrome. Bizarre mood is apparent in schizophrenia.
Cognitive Functions	
Orientation. You can discern orientation through the course of the interview, or ask for it directly, using tact. "Some people have trouble keeping up with the dates while in the hospital. Do you know today's date?" Assess:	
Time: day of week, date, year, season *Place: where person lives, present location, type of building, name of city and state* *Person: own name, age, who examiner is, type of worker.* Many hospitalized people normally have trouble with the exact date but are fully oriented on the remaining items.	Disorientation occurs with organic brain disorders. Orientation is usually lost first to time, then to place, and rarely to person (Keller and Manschrek, 1981).

NORMAL RANGE OF FINDINGS	ABNORMAL FINDINGS
Attention Span. Check the person's ability to concentrate by noting whether he or she completes a thought without wandering. Note any distractibility or difficulty attending to you. Or, give a series of directions to follow, and note the correct sequence of behaviors, e.g., "Please take this glass of water with your left hand, drink from it, shift it to your right hand, and set it on the table." Note that attention span commonly is impaired in people who are anxious, fatigued, or drug intoxicated.	Digression from initial thought. Easily distracted; "stimulus bound," i.e., any new stimulus quickly draws attention. Confusion, negativism.
Recent Memory. Assess recent memory in the context of the interview by the 24-hour diet recall, or asking the time the person arrived at the agency. Ask questions you can corroborate. This screens for the occasional person who confabulates or makes up answers to fill in the gaps of memory loss.	Recent memory deficit with the remote memory intact occurs with organic syndromes.
Remote Memory. In the context of the interview, ask the person verifiable past events, e.g., describe past health, the first job, birthday and anniversary dates, and historical events that are relevant for that person.	Remote memory is lost when cortical storage area for that memory is damaged, such as in Alzheimer's dementia or any disease that damages the cortex.
New Learning—the Four Unrelated Words Test. This tests the person's ability to lay down new memories. It is a highly sensitive and valid memory test. It requires more effort than does the recall of personal or historic events. It also avoids the danger of unverifiable material. To the person, say, "I am going to say four words. I want you to remember them. In a few minutes I will ask you to recall them." To be sure the person has understood, have the words repeated. Pick four words with semantic and phonetic diversity: 1. brown — 1. fun 2. honesty — 2. carrot 3. tulip — 3. ankle 4. eyedropper — 4. loyalty	
The normal response is an accurate four-word recall after a 10-minute delay, and at least three words remembered correctly after 30 minutes (Strub and Black, 1985).	Impaired new learning ability occurs with Alzheimer's dementia as well as with anxiety (due to inattention and distractibility) and depression (due to lack of effort mobilized to remember).
Additional Testing for Persons with Aphasia ***Word Comprehension.*** Point to articles in the room, body parts, articles from pockets, and ask the person to name them. ***Reading.*** Ask the person to read available print. Be aware that reading is related to educational level. Use caution that you are not just testing literacy. ***Writing.*** Ask the person to make up and write a sentence. Note coherence, spelling, and parts of speech (the sentence should have a subject and verb).	See Table 5–4, Speech Disorders. This functioning is important in planning health teaching and rehabilitation.
Higher Intellectual Function These tests measure problem solving and reasoning abilities. Results are closely related to the person's general intelligence, and must be assessed considering educational and cultural background. Tests of higher intellec-	

NORMAL RANGE OF FINDINGS	ABNORMAL FINDINGS

tual functioning have been used to discriminate between organic brain disease and psychiatric disorders; errors on the tests indicate organic dysfunction.

Although they have been widely used, there is little evidence that most of these tests are valid in detecting organic brain disease (Keller and Manschrek, 1981). Further, most of these tests have little relevance for daily clinical care. Thus, many time-honored, standard tests of higher intellectual function are not discussed here, such as fund of general knowledge, digit span repetition, calculation, proverb interpretation and similarities to test abstract reasoning, or hypothetical situations to test judgment.

Judgment. A person exercises judgment when he or she can compare and evaluate the alternatives in a situation and reach an appropriate course of action. Rather than testing the person's response to a hypothetical situation (e.g., "What would you do if you found a stamped, addressed envelope lying on the sidewalk?"), you should be more interested in the person's judgment about daily or long-term life goals, the likelihood of acting in response to delusions or hallucinations, and the capacity for violent or suicidal behavior (Keller and Manschrek, 1981).

To assess judgment in the context of the interview, note what the person says about job plans, social or family obligations, and plans for the future. Job and future plans should be realistic, considering the person's health situation. Also, ask the person to describe the rationale for personal health care, and how he or she decided about whether or not to comply with prescribed health regimens. The person's actions and decisions should be realistic.

Impaired judgment (unrealistic or impulsive decisions, wish fulfillment), occurs with mental retardation, emotional dysfunction, schizophrenia, and organic brain disease.

Thought Processes and Perceptions

Thought Processes. Ask yourself, "Does this person make sense? Can I follow what the person is saying?" The *way* a person thinks should be logical, goal directed, coherent, and relevant. The person should complete a thought.

Illogical, unrealistic thought processes. Digression from initial thought. Ideas run together. Evidence of blocking (person stops in middle of thought). See Table 5–7, Abnormalities of Thought Processes.

Thought Content. *What* the person says should be consistent and logical.

Obsessions, compulsions, See Table 5–8, Abnormalities of Thought Content.

Perceptions. The person should be consistently aware of reality. The perceptions should be congruent with yours. Ask the following questions:

- How do people treat you?
- Do other people talk about you?
- Do you feel like you are being watched, followed, or controlled?
- Is your imagination very active?
- Have you heard your name when alone?

Illusions, hallucinations. See Table 5–9, Abnormalities of Perception. Auditory and visual hallucinations occur with psychiatric and organic brain disease and with psychedelic drugs. Tactile hallucinations occur with alcohol withdrawal.

Screen for Suicidal Thoughts. When the person expresses feelings of sadness, hopelessness, despair or grief, it is important to assess any possible risk of physical harm to himself or herself. Begin with more general ques-

NORMAL RANGE OF FINDINGS	ABNORMAL FINDINGS

tions. If you hear affirmative answers, continue with more specific questions:

- Have you ever felt so blue you thought of hurting yourself?
- Do you feel like hurting yourself now?
- Do you have a plan to hurt yourself?
- What would happen if you were dead?
- How would other people react if you were dead?

It is very difficult to question people about possible suicidal wishes, especially for beginning examiners. Examiners fear invading privacy, and may have their own normal denial of death and suicide. However, the risk is far greater if you skip these questions when you have the slightest clue that they are appropriate. You may be the only health professional to pick up clues to suicide risk. You are responsible for encouraging the person to talk about suicidal thoughts. Sometimes you cannot prevent a suicide when someone really wishes to kill himself or herself. However, for the people who are ambivalent, and they are the majority, you can buy time so the person can be helped to find an alternate route to the situation.

Supplemental Mental Status Examination

The Mini-Mental State is a simplified scored form of the cognitive functions of the mental status examination (Folstein, et al, 1975; replicated by Depaulo and Folstein, 1978) (Table 5–1). It is quick and easy, includes a standard set of only 11 questions, and requires only 5 to 10 minutes to administer. It is useful for both initial and serial measurement, so you can demonstrate worsening or improvement of cognition over time and with treatment. It concentrates only on cognitive functioning, not on mood or thought processes. It is a valid detector of organic disease; thus, it is a good screening tool to detect dementia and delirium.

The maximum score on the test is 30; normal people average 27.

Scores below 20 occur with dementia and delirium.

DEVELOPMENTAL CONSIDERATIONS

Infants and Children

The mental status assessment of infants and children covers behavioral, cognitive, and psychosocial development, and examines how the child is coping with his or her environment. Essentially, you will follow the same A-B-C-T guidelines as for the adult, with special consideration for developmental milestones. Your best examination "technique" arises from thorough knowledge of developmental milestones as described in Chapter 2. Abnormalities are often problems of *omission;* the child does not achieve a milestone you would expect.

The parent's health history, especially the sections on the developmental history and personal history, yields most of the mental status data.

In addition, the Denver II screening test (See Chapter 2) gives you a chance to interact directly with the young child to assess mental status. For the child from birth to 6 years of age the Denver II helps identify those who

Table 5-1 ▶ Mini-Mental State Examination

Patient ____________ Examiner ____________ Date ________

Maximum Score	Score	
		ORIENTATION
5	( )	What is the (year) (season) (date) (day) (month)?
5	( )	Where are we: (state) (county) (town) (hospital) (floor).
		REGISTRATION
3	( )	Name 3 objects: 1 second to say each. Then ask the patient all 3 after you have said them. Give 1 point for each correct answer. Then repeat them until he learns all 3. Count trials and record. Trials ________
		ATTENTION AND CALCULATION
5	( )	Serial 7's. 1 point for each correct. Stop after 5 answers. Alternatively spell "world" backwards.
		RECALL
3	( )	Ask for the 3 objects repeated above. Give 1 point for each correct.
		LANGUAGE
9	( )	Name a pencil, and watch (2 points) Repeat the following "No ifs, ands, or buts." (1 point) Follow a 3-stage command: "Take a paper in your right hand, fold it in half, and put it on the floor." (3 points) Read and obey the following: **CLOSE YOUR EYES (1 point)** Write a sentence (1 point) Copy design (1 point)
________		Total Score
		ASSESS level of consciousness along a continuum ________ Alert Drowsy Stupor Coma

Instructions for Administration of Mini-Mental State Examination

ORIENTATION

(1) Ask for the date. Then ask specifically for parts omitted, e.g., "Can you also tell me what season it is?" One point for each correct.
(2) Ask in turn "Can you tell me the name of this hospital?" (town, country, etc.). One point for each correct.

REGISTRATION

Ask the patient if you may test his memory. Then say the names of 3 unrelated objects, clearly and slowly, about one second for each. After you have said all 3, ask him to repeat them. This first repetition determines his score (0–3) but keep saying them until he can repeat all 3, up to 6 trials. If he does not eventually learn all 3, recall cannot be meaningfully tested.

ATTENTION AND CALCULATION

Ask the patient to begin with 100 and count backwards by 7. Stop after 5 subtractions (93, 86, 79, 72, 65). Score the total number of correct answers.

If the patient cannot or will not perform this task, ask him to spell the word "world" backwards. The score is the number of letters in correct order. E.g/ dlrow = 5, dlorw = 3.

RECALL

Ask the patient if he can recall the 3 words you previously asked him to remember. Score 0–3.

LANGUAGE

Naming: Show the patient a wrist watch and ask him what it is. Repeat for pencil. Score 0–2.

Repetition: Ask the patient to repeat the sentence after you. Allow only one trial. Score 0 or 1.

3-Stage command: Give the patient a piece of plain blank paper and repeat the command. Score 1 point for each part correctly executed.

Reading: On a blank piece of paper print the sentence "Close your eyes," in letters large enough for the patient to see clearly. Ask him to read it and do what it says. Score 1 point only if he actually closes his eyes.

Writing: Give the patient a blank piece of paper and ask him to write a sentence for you. Do not dictate a sentence, it is to be written spontaneously. It must contain a subject and verb and be sensible. Correct grammar and punctuation are not necessary.

Copying: On a clean piece of paper, draw intersecting pentagons, each side about 1 in., and ask him to copy it exactly as it is. All 10 angles must be present and 2 must intersect to score 1 point. Tremor and rotation are ignored.

Estimate the patient's level of sensorium along a continuum, from alert on the left to coma on the right.

(From Folstein MF, Folstein SE, McHugh PR: Mini-mental state. J Psychiatric Res 12:189–198, 1975. Reprinted with permission.)

NORMAL RANGE OF FINDINGS | ABNORMAL FINDINGS

Table 5-2 ▶ Behavioral Checklist

1. Prefers to play alone
2. Gets hurt in major accidents
3. Does he/she ever play with fire
4. Has difficulties with teachers
5. Gets poor grades in school
6. Is absent from school
7. Becomes angry easily
8. Daydreams
9. Feels unhappy
10. Acts younger than other children his/her age
11. Does not listen to parents
12. Does not tell the truth
13. Unsure of himself/herself
14. Has trouble sleeping
15. Seems afraid of someone or something
16. Is nervous and jumpy
17. Has a nervous habit
18. Does not show feelings
19. Fights with other children
20. Is understanding of other people's feelings
21. Refuses to share
22. Shows jealousy
23. Takes things that are not his/hers
24. Blames others for his/her troubles
25. Prefers to play with children not his/her age
26. Gets along well with grown-ups
27. Teases others

Scoring is a point system: 0—never; 1—sometimes; 2—often. Scoring is reversed for items 20 and 26.

Scores between 15 to 22 indicate closer following; scores above 22 warrant psychiatric evaluation.

(From Jellinek M, Evans N, Knight R: Use of a behavior checklist on a pediatric inpatient unit. J Pediatr 94:156–158, 1979.)

may be slow in development in behavioral, language, cognitive, and psychosocial areas. An additional language test is the Denver Articulation Screening Exam (DASE, See Chapter 2).

For school-aged children, ages 7 to 11, who have grown beyond the age when developmental milestones are very useful, the "Behavioral Checklist" (Table 5–2) is an additional tool that can be given to the parent along with the history. It covers five major areas: mood, play, school, friends, and family relations. It is easy to administer and lasts about 5 minutes.

For the adolescent, follow the same A-B-C-T guidelines as described for the adult.

The Aging Adult

It is important to conduct even a brief examination on all older people admitted to the hospital. "Confusion" is common in aging people and is easily misdiagnosed.

NORMAL RANGE OF FINDINGS

ABNORMAL FINDINGS

Check sensory status before assessing any aspect of mental status. Vision and hearing changes due to aging may alter alertness and leave the person looking confused. Follow the same A-B-C-T guidelines as described for the younger adult with these *additional* considerations.

Behavior

Level of Consciousness. In a hospital or extended care setting, the Glasgow Coma Scale (see Chapter 20) is a quantitative tool that is useful in testing consciousness in aging persons in whom confusion is common. It gives a numerical value to the person's response in eye-opening, best verbal response, and best motor response. This system avoids ambiguity when numerious examiners care for the same person.

Cognitive Functions

Orientation. Many aging persons experience social isolation, loss of structure without a job, a change in residence, or some short-term memory loss (Hays and Borger, 1985). These factors affect orientation, and this person may not provide the precise date or complete name of agency. You may consider aging persons oriented if they know *generally* where they are and the present period. That is, consider them oriented to time if the year and month are correctly stated. Orientation to place is accepted with the correct identification of the type of setting (e.g., the hospital) and the name of the town (Hays and Borger, 1985)

Supplemental Mental Status Examination

The Set Test was developed specifically for use with an aging population. The original study tested people age 65 to 85. It is a quantifiable test, designed to screen for dementia (Isaacs and Kennie, 1973). The test is easy to administer and takes less than 5 minutes. Ask the person to name 10 items in each of four categories or sets: fruits, animals, colors, and towns (FACT). Do not coach, prompt, or hurry the person. Each correct answer is one point. The maximum total score is 40. No one with a score over 25 has been found to have dementia. (Note: since this is a verbal test, do not use it with persons with hearing impairments or aphasia.)

Set Test scores of less than 15 indicate dementia. Scores between 15 and 24 show less association with dementia and should be evaluated carefully.

The Set Test is a more holistic approach to testing cognitive function (Hays and Borger, 1985). It assesses mental function as a whole instead of examining individual parts of cognitive function. That is, by asking the person to categorize, name, remember, and count the items in the test, you are really assessing this person's alertness, motivation, concentration, short-term memory, and problem-solving ability.

NURSING DIAGNOSES COMMONLY ASSOCIATED WITH MENTAL HEALTH DISORDERS

Diagnosis	Related Factors (Etiology)	Defining Characteristics (Symptoms and Signs)
Powerlessness	Immobility	Anger
	Difficulty in performing self-care	Violent behavior
	Low self-esteem	Anxiety
	Cultural role	Resentment
	Communication barriers	Guilt
	Loss of financial independence	Apathy
	Lifestyle of helplessness	Withdrawal
	Lack of knowledge or skills	Devalues own feelings or opinions
	Health care environment	Reluctance to express true feelings, fearing alienation from care giver
	Illness-related regimen	Verbal expressions of having no control over situation, outcome, or self-care
		Expressions of doubt about self-worth or role performance
Potential for violence (self-directed or directed at others)	Substance abuse or withdrawal	Rage
	Toxic reaction to medication	Overt and aggressive acts
	Explosive, impulsive, immature personality	Self-destructive behavior
	Paranoia	Aggression
	Panic state	Increased motor activity
	Rage reaction	Hostile, threatening verbalizations
	Manic excitement	Body language: clenched fists, facial expressions, rigid posture, tautness
	Loneliness	Provocative behavior
	Perceived threat to self-esteem	
	Response to catastrophic event	

Diagnosis	Related Factors (Etiology)	Defining Characteristics (Symptoms and Signs)
	Suicidal behavior Change in mental or physical health status Feelings of alienation Physical, sexual, or psychological abuse Manipulative behavior Developmental crisis Lack of support systems Actual or potential loss of significant other Significant change in lifestyle	Increasing anxiety level Depression Paranoid ideation Expresses intent to harm self or others Possession of destructive means: gun, knife, or other weapon Hallucination, delusions
Spiritual distress	Loss of significant others Challenged belief and value system Beliefs opposed by family, peers, or health care providers Disruption in usual religious activity Effects of personal and family disasters or major life changes	Feeling separated or alienated from deity Feelings of helplessness or hopelessness Expresses concerns about meaning of life and death and/or belief system Verbalizes inner conflict about beliefs Inability to participate in usual religious practices Regards illness as punishment

Other related nursing diagnoses:
- Ineffective individual coping
- Low self-esteem
- Impaired adjustment
- Anxiety
- Personal identity disturbance
- Altered thought processes

ABNORMAL FINDINGS

Table 5-3 ▸ Levels of Consciousness

These terms are commonly used in clinical practice. They spread over a continuum from full alertness to deep coma. The terms are qualitative and therefore are not always reliable. (A *quantitative* tool that serves the same purpose and eliminates ambiguity is the Glasgow Coma Scale in Chapter 20. These terms are widely accepted, however, and are useful as long as all co-workers agree on definitions and are consistent in their application.

To increase clarity when using these terms, record also:

1. the level of stimulus used, ranging progressively from
   a. name called in normal tone of voice
   b. name called in loud voice
   c. light touch on person's arm
   d. vigorous shake of shoulder
   e. pain applied
2. the person's response
   a. amount and quality of movement
   b. presence and coherence of speech
   c. opens eyes and makes eye contact
3. what the person does on cessation of your stimulus.

ALERT

Awake or readily aroused, oriented, fully aware of external and internal stimuli and responds appropriately, conducts meaningful interpersonal interactions.

LETHARGIC

Somnolent, drifts off to sleep when not stimulated, can be aroused to name when called in normal voice but looks drowsy, responds appropriately to questions or commands but thinking seems slow and fuzzy, inattentive, loses train of thought, spontaneous movements are decreased.

OBTUNDED

(Transitional state between lethargy and stupor; some sources omit this level.)

Sleeps most of time, difficult to arouse—needs loud shout or vigorous shake, acts confused when is aroused, converses in monosyllables, speech may be mumbled and incoherent, requires constant stimulation for even marginal cooperation.

STUPOR OR SEMI-COMA

Spontaneously unconscious, responds only to vigorous shake or pain; has appropriate motor response (i.e., withdraws hand to avoid pain); otherwise can only groan, mumble, or move restlessly; reflex activity persists.

COMA

Completely unconscious, no response to pain nor to any external or internal stimuli (e.g., when suctioned, will not try to push the catheter away), light coma has some reflex activity but no purposeful movement, deep coma has no motor response.

ACUTE CONFUSIONAL STATE (DELIRIUM)

Clouding of consciousness (dulled cognition, impaired alertness); inattentive; incoherent conversation; impaired recent memory and confabulatory for recent events; often agitated and having visual hallucinations; disoriented, with confusion worse at night when environmental stimuli are decreased.

(Adapted from Strub RL, Black FW: The Mental Status Examination in Neurology. 2nd ed. Philadelphia, FA Davis, 1985, with permission.)

Table 5-4 ► Speech Disorders

CONDITION	DISORDER OF	DESCRIPTION
Dysphonia	Voice	Difficulty or discomfort in talking with abnormal pitch or volume, due to laryngeal disease. Voice sounds hoarse or whispered, but articulation and language are intact.
Dysarthria	Articulation	Distorted speech sounds; speech may sound unintelligible; basic language (word choice, grammar, comprehension) intact.
Aphasia	Language comprehension and production	True language disturbance, defect in word choice and grammar, or defect in comprehension; defect is in *higher* integrative language processing.

TYPES OF APHASIA

An earlier dichotomy classified aphasias as expressive or receptive. Since all people with aphasia have some difficulty with expression, beginning examiners tended to classify them all as expressive. The following system is more descriptive.

CONDITION	DESCRIPTION
Global aphasia	The most common and severe form. Spontaneous speech is absent or reduced to a few stereotyped words or sounds. Comprehension is absent or reduced to only the person's own name and a few select words. Repetition, reading, and writing are severely impaired. Prognosis for language recovery is poor.
Broca's aphasia	This is characterized by nonfluent, dysarthric, and effortful speech. The speech is mostly nouns and verbs (high-content words) with few grammatical fillers, termed "agrammatic" or "telegraphic" speech. Repetition and reading aloud are severely impaired. Auditory and reading comprehension are surprisingly intact.
Wernicke's aphasia	The linguistic opposite of Broca's aphasia. Speech is fluent, effortless, and well articulated. Output has many paraphasias (word substitutions that are malformed or wrong) and neologisms (made up words) and often lacks substantive words. Speech can be totally incomprehensible. Often, there is a great urge to speak. Essentially, it is a defect of auditory comprehension. Repetition, reading, and writing also are impaired.

(For a discussion of other types of aphasia [e.g., conduction, anomic, transcortical, and so on], please consult a neurology text.)

(Data on aphasia have been adapted from Strub RL, Black FW: The Mental Status Examination in Neurology. 2nd ed. Philadelphia, FA Davis, 1985.)

Table 5-5 ▶ Variant Speech Patterns

PATTERN	DEFINITION	CLINICAL EXAMPLE
Rhyming	Same terminal sounds of words or sentences regularly interjected into conversation	"mister, sister"
Punning	Clever or humorous play on words, words sound similar but have two different meanings	bear, bare sense, cents
Circumlocution	Round about expression, substituting a phrase when cannot think of name of object	Saying, "the thing you open the door with" for "key."

Table 5-6 ▶ Abnormalities of Mood and Affect

TYPE OF MOOD OR AFFECT	DEFINITION	CLINICAL EXAMPLE
Flat affect (blunted affect)	Lack of emotional response; no expression of feelings; voice monotonous and the face immobile	Topic varies, expression does not
Depression	Sad, gloomy, dejected. Symptoms may occur with rainy weather, after a holiday, or an illness. If the situation is temporary, symptoms fade quickly	"I've got the blues."
Depersonalization (lack of ego boundaries)	Loss of identity, feels estranged, perplexed about own identity and meaning of existence	"I don't feel real;" "I feel like I'm not really here."
Elation	Joy and optimism, over confidence, increased motor activity, not necessarily pathologic	"I'm feeling very happy."
Euphoria	Excessive well-being, unusually cheerful or elated, which is inappropriate considering physical and mental condition, implies a pathologic mood	"I am high." "I feel like I'm flying." "I feel on top of the world."
Anxiety	Worried, uneasy, apprehensive from the anticipation of a danger whose source is unknown	"I feel nervous and high strung." "I worry all the time." "I can't seem to make up my mind."
Fear	Worried, uneasy, apprehensive, external danger is known and identified	Fear of flying in airplanes
Irritability	Annoyed, easily provoked, impatient	Person internalizes a feeling of tension, and a seemingly mild stimulus "sets him off."

Table 5-6 ▶ Abnormalities of Mood and Affect *Continued*

TYPE OF MOOD OR AFFECT	DEFINITION	CLINICAL EXAMPLE
Rage	Furious, loss of control	Person who has expressed violent behavior toward self or others.
Ambivalence	The existence of opposing emotions toward an idea, object, person	A person feels love and hate toward another at the same time
Lability	Rapid shift of emotions	Person expresses euphoric, tearful, angry feelings in rapid succession
Inappropriate affect	Affect clearly discordant with the content of the person's speech	Laughs while discussing admisson for liver biopsy

Table 5-7 ▶ Abnormalities of Thought Process

TYPE OF PROCESS	DEFINITION	CLINICAL EXAMPLE
Blocking	Sudden interruption in train of thought, unable to complete sentence, seems related to strong emotion	"Forgot what I was going to say"
Confabulation	Fabricates events to fill in memory gaps	Gives detailed description of his long walk around the hospital though you know Mr. J. remained in his room all afternoon
Neologism	Coining a new word, invented word has no real meaning except for the person, may condense several words	"I'll have to turn on my thinkilator."
Circumstantiality	Talks with excessive and unnecessary detail, delays reaching point. Sentences have a meaningful connection but are irrelevant. This occurs normally in some people.	"When was my surgery? Well I was 28, I was living with my aunt, she's the one with psoriasis, she had it bad that year because of the heat, the heat was worse then than it was the summer of '82, . . . "
Loosening associations	Shifting from one topic to an unrelated topic. Person seems unaware that topics are unconnected.	"My boss is angry with me and it wasn't even my fault. (pause) I saw that movie too, Lassie. I felt really bad about it. But she kept trying to land the airplane and she never knew what was going on."

Table continued on following page

Table 5-7 ► Abnormalities of Thought Process *Continued*

TYPE OF PROCESS	DEFINITION	CLINICAL EXAMPLE
Flight of ideas	Abrupt change, rapid skipping from topic to topic, practically continuous flow of accelerated speech. Topics usually have recognizable associations or are plays on words.	"Take this pill? The pill is blue. I feel blue. (sings) She wore blue velvet."
Word salad	Incoherent mixture of words, phrases, and sentences; illogical; disconnected; includes neologisms	"Beauty, red based five, pigeon, the street corner, sort-of"
Perseveration	Persistent repeating of verbal or motor response, even with varied stimuli	"I'm going to lock the door, lock the door. I walk every day and I lock the door. I usually take the dog and I lock the door."
Echolalia	Imitation, repeats others' words or phrases, often with a mumbling, mocking, or mechanical tone	Nurse: "I want you to take your pill." Client (mocking): "Take your pill. Take your pill."
Clanging	Word choice based on sound, not meaning, includes nonsense rhymes and puns	"My feet are cold. Cold, bold, told. The bell tolled for me."

Table 5-8 ► Abnormalities of Thought Content

TYPE OF CONTENT	DEFINITION	CLINICAL EXAMPLE
Phobia	Strong, persistent, irrational fear of an object or situation, feels driven to avoid it	Cats, dogs, heights, enclosed spaces
Hypochondriasis	Morbid worrying about his or her own health, feels sick with no actual basis for that assumption	Preoccupied with the fear of having cancer; any symptom or physical sign means cancer
Obsession	Unwanted, persistent thoughts or impulses; logic will not purge them from consciousness; experienced as intrusive and senseless	Violence (parent having repeated impulse to kill a loved child); contamination (becoming infected by shaking hands)
Compulsion	Unwanted, repetitive, purposeful act; driven to do it; behavior thought to neutralize or prevent discomfort or some dreaded event	Hand washing, counting, checking and rechecking, touching
Delusions	Firm, fixed, false beliefs; irrational; person clings to delusion despite objective evidence to contrary	Grandiose – person believes he or she is God; persecution – "They are out to get me."

Table 5-9 ▸ Abnormalities of Perception

TYPE OF PERCEPTION	DEFINITION	CLINICAL EXAMPLE
Hallucination	Sensory perceptions for which there are no external stimuli; may strike any sense: visual, auditory, tactile, olfactory, gustatory	Visual: seeing an image (ghost) of a person who is not there; auditory: hearing voices or music.
Illusion	*Mis*perception of an actual existing stimulus, by any sense	Folds of bedsheets appear to be animated

Table 5-10 ▸ Organic Brain Syndromes*

DELIRIUM

Sudden onset of impaired cognition

Characteristics

1. Difficulty maintaining attention, easily distracted (e.g., questions must be repeated because attention wanders); difficulty in appropriately shifting attention to new stimuli (e.g., perseverates answer to a previous question)
2. Disorganized thinking, as indicated by rambling, irrelevant, or incoherent speech
3. At least TWO of the following:
   a. Reduced level of consciousness, e.g., difficulty keeping awake during examination
   b. Perceptual disturbances: misinterpretations, illusions, or hallucinations
   c. Disturbance of sleep-wake cycle, with insomnia or daytime sleepiness
   d. Increased or decreased psychomotor activity
   e. Disorientation to time and place is common
   f. Memory impairment, e.g., inability to learn new material, such as the names of several unrelated objects after five minutes, or to remember past events such as history of current episode of illness.

Course

Develops over short period of time, and fluctuates during the day, i.e., worse during sleepless nights or in the dark

Age

Especially common in children and after age 60

Etiology

Usually due to an acute medical problem: systemic infections; metabolic disorders such as hypoxia, hypercapnia, hypoglycemia, ionic imbalances, hepatic or renal disease, or thiamine deficiency; postoperative states; psychoactive substance intoxication and withdrawal; following seizures or head trauma.

DEMENTIA

Slow onset of deterioration in cognitive functioning

Characteristics

1. Memory impairment. Impaired short-term memory indicated by inability to remember three objects after five minutes. Impaired long-term memory indicated by inability to remember past personal information (e.g., what happened yesterday, birthplace, occupation) or facts of common knowledge (e.g., past presidents, well-known dates).
2. At least ONE of the following:
   a. impairment in abstract thinking, as indicated by inability to find similarities and differences

Table continued on following page

Table 5-10 ▸ Organic Brain Syndromes* *Continued*

between related words, difficulty in defining words and concepts

b. impaired judgment, as indicated by inability to make reasonable plans to deal with interpersonal, family and job-related problems and issues

c. disturbances of higher cortical function, such as aphasia, apraxia, agnosia (failure to recognize objects despite intact sensory function), and "constructional difficulty" (e.g., inability to copy three-dimensional figures, assemble blocks, or arrange sticks in specific designs)

d. personality change, i.e., alteration or accentuation of previous traits

Severity

Early Signs. Memory loss most marked for recent events; forgets names, telephone numbers, and appointments; loses objects; makes mistakes with money; inefficient at work; tires easily; irritable and anxious; poverty of ideas (repeats cliches and set phrases); bizarre behavior (puts ice cream in oven); poor social judgment and poor impulse control (coarse language, inappropriate sexual advances)

Progressing Signs. Disheveled appearance, neglect of personal hygiene, sloppy eating habits, incontinence, speech choppy and aimed at food or physical needs, disorientation, increasingly flat affect, rigid thinking, paranoid ideation

Late Signs. Unable to feed self or walk, speech limited to a few words, then incoherent or mute; stupor, then coma

For further discussion and discussion of other organic brain syndromes (e.g., amnestic syndrome, organic hallucinosis), please consult DSM-III-R or a neurology text.

(Adapted from American Psychiatric Association: Diagnostic and Statistical Manual of Mental Disorders. 3rd ed. Revised. Washington, DC, American Psychiatric Association, 1987.)

* These diagnostic categories are meant to be illustrative, not inclusive. The reader is referred to DSM-III-R or a psychiatry textbook for further categories, such as personality disorders or somatiform disorders.

Table 5-11 ▸ Substance Use Disorders*

Substances taken nonmedically in order to alter mood or behavior (APA, 1987).

Intoxication: Ingestion of substance produces maladaptive behavior changes

Abuse: Daily use in order to function, inability to stop, impaired social and occupational functioning

Dependence: Physiologic dependence on substance

Tolerance: Requires increased amount of substance to produce same effect

Withdrawal: Cessation of substance produces a syndrome of physiologic symptoms

SUBSTANCE	INTOXICATION	WITHDRAWAL
Alcohol	**Appearance.** Unsteady gait, incoordination, nystagmus, flushed face **Behavior.** Talkativeness, slurred speech, impaired judgment, inattention, impaired memory, irritability, euphoria, depression, emotional lability	**Uncomplicated.** (Shortly after cessation drinking, lasts 5 to 7 days) coarse tremor of hands, tongue, eyelids, anorexia, nausea and vomiting, malaise, autonomic hyperactivity (tachycardia, sweating, elevated blood pressure), headache, insomnia, anxiety, depression or irritability, transient hallucinations or illusions.

Table 5-11 ▸ Substance Use Disorders* *Continued*

SUBSTANCE	INTOXICATION	WITHDRAWAL
		Withdrawal Delirium, "Delirium Tremens:" (Much less common than uncomplicated, occurs within 1 week of cessation) coarse, irregular tremor; marked autonomic hyperactivity (tachycardia, sweating); vivid hallucinations; delusions; agitated behavior; fever
Sedatives Hypnotics	Similar to alcohol **Appearance.** Unsteady gait, incoordination **Behavior.** Talkativeness, slurred speech, inattention, impaired memory, irritability, emotional lability, sexual aggressiveness, impaired judgment, impaired social or occupational functioning	Anxiety or irritability, nausea or vomiting, malaise, autonomic hyperactivity (tachycardia, sweating), orthostatic hypotension, coarse tremor of hands, tongue and eyelids, marked insomnia, grand mal seizures
Cannabis (Marijuana)	**Appearance.** Injected (reddened) conjunctivae, tachycardia, dry mouth, increased appetite, especially for "junk" food **Behavior.** Euphoria, anxiety, slowed time perception, increased perceptions, impaired judgment, social withdrawal, suspiciousness or paranoid ideation	
Cocaine	**Appearance.** Pupillary dilation, tachycardia, elevated blood pressure, sweating, chills, nausea, vomiting **Behavior.** Euphoria, talkativeness, hypervigilance, pacing, psychomotor agitation, impaired judgment, impaired social or occupational functioning, fighting, grandiosity, visual or tactile hallucinations	Dysphoric mood (anxiety, depression, irritability), fatigue, insomnia or hypersomnia, or psychomotor agitation
Amphetamines	Similar to cocaine. **Appearance.** Pupil dilation, tachycardia, elevated blood pressure, sweating or chills, nausea and vomiting **Behavior.** Elation, talkativeness, hypervigilance, psychomotor agitation, fighting, grandiosity, impaired judgment, impaired social and occupational functioning	Dysphoric mood (anxiety, depression, irritability), fatigue, insomnia or hypersomnia, psychomotor agitation

Table continued on following page

Table 5-11 ▶ Substance Use Disorders* *Continued*

SUBSTANCE	INTOXICATION	WITHDRAWAL
Opiates (morphine heroin meperidine)	**Appearance.** Pinpoint pupils decreased blood pressure, pulse, respirations and temperature **Behavior.** Lethargy, somnolence, slurred speech, initial euphoria followed by apathy, dysphoria, and psychomotor retardation, inattention, impaired memory, impaired judgment, impaired social or occupational functioning	Dilated pupils, lacrimation, runny nose, tachycardia, fever, elevated blood pressure, piloerection, sweating, diarrhea, yawning, insomnia. Also restlessness, irritability, depression, nausea, vomiting, malaise, tremor, muscle and joint pains. Symptoms are remarkably similar to clinical picture of influenza

(Adapted from American Psychiatric Association: Diagnostic and Statistical Manual of Mental Disorders. 3rd ed. Revised. Washington, DC, American Psychiatric Association, 1987.)

* These diagnostic categories are meant to be illustrative, not inclusive. The reader is referred to DSM-III-R or a psychiatry textbook for further categories, such as personality disorders or somatiform disorders.

Table 5-12 ▶ Schizophrenia*

CHARACTERISTICS

1. An active phase of psychotic symptoms
   a. bizarre delusions, i.e., involving a phenomenon that the person's culture would regard as totally implausible, e.g., thought broadcasting, being controlled by a dead person
   b. prominent hallucinations, auditory are most common, e.g., voices speaking directly to the person or commenting on his or her ongoing behavior
   c. incoherence or marked loosening of association
   d. catatonic behavior
   e. flat or grossly inappropriate affect
2. Prodromal or residual symptoms (leading up to and following the active phase)
   a. marked social isolation or withdrawal
   b. marked impairment in role functioning, e.g., as wage-earner, student, or homemaker
   c. markedly peculiar behavior (e.g., collecting garbage, talking to self in public, hoarding food)
   d. marked impairment in personal hygiene and grooming
   e. blunted or inappropriate affect
   f. digressive, vague, over elaborate, or circumstantial speech, or poverty of speech, or poverty of coherent speech
   g. odd beliefs or magical thinking, influencing behavior and inconsistent with cultural norms, e.g., superstitiousness, belief in clairvoyance, telepathy, "sixth sense," "others can feel my feelings," overvalued ideas, ideas of reference
   h. unusual perceptual experiences, e.g., recurrent illusions, sensing the presence of a force or person not actually present
   i. marked lack of initiative, interests or energy

(Adapted from American Psychiatric Association: Diagnostic and Statistical Manual of Mental Disorders. 3rd ed. Revised. Washington, DC, American Psychiatric Association, 1987.)

*These diagnostic categories are meant to be illustrative, not inclusive. The reader is referred to DSM-III-R or a psychiatry textbook for further categories, such as personality disorders or somatiform disorders.

Table 5-13 ▶ Mood Disorders*

MANIC EPISODE

Characteristics

1. Distinct period during which the predominant mood is either elevated, expansive, or irritable
2. Associated symptoms during the period of mood disturbance
   a. inflated self-esteem or grandiosity
   b. decreased need for sleep
   c. pressure of speech; speech is loud, rapid, and difficult to interrupt
   d. flight of ideas or feels that thoughts are racing
   e. distractibility, responds easily to various irrelevant external stimuli
   f. increase in goal-directed activity (socially, at work or school, sexually) or psychomotor agitation
   g. excessive involvement in pleasurable activities that have a high potential for painful consequences (e.g., unrestrained buying sprees, sexual indiscretions, foolish business investments)

MAJOR DEPRESSIVE EPISODE

Characteristics

1. Period of at least 2 weeks during which the person shows either depressed mood (or can be irritable mood in children or adolescents) or loss of interest or pleasure in all, or almost all, activities
2. Associated symptoms during same period
   a. appetite disturbance, and can have attendant significant weight loss or weight gain
   b. insomnia or, sometimes, hypersomnia
   c. psychomotor agitation or retardation
   d. fatigue or loss of energy
   e. sense of worthlessness or excessive guilt
   f. difficulty concentrating, slowed thinking, indecisiveness
   g. recurrent thoughts of death

(Adapted from American Psychiatric Association: Diagnostic and Statistical Manual of Mental Disorders. 3rd ed. Revised. Washington, DC, American Psychiatric Association, 1987.)

* These diagnostic categories are meant to be illustrative, not inclusive. The reader is referred to DSM-III-R or a psychiatry textbook for further categories, such as personality disorders or somatiform disorders.

Table 5-14 ▶ Anxiety Disorders*

PANIC DISORDER

Recurrent panic attacks, i.e., discrete periods of intense fear and discomfort that occur unexpectedly

Associated symptoms that develop during the attack:

1. shortness of breath (dyspnea) or smothering sensations
2. dizziness, unsteady feelings, or faintness
3. palpitations or accelerated heart rate (tachycardia)
4. trembling or shaking
5. sweating
6. choking
7. nausea or abdominal distress
8. depersonalization or derealization
9. numbness or tingling sensations (paresthesias)
10. flushes (hot flashes) or chills
11. chest pain or discomfort
12. fear of dying
13. fear of going crazy or of doing something uncontrolled

SOCIAL PHOBIA

Persistent fear of situation(s) in which the person is exposed to possible scrutiny by others and fears that he or she may do something or act in a way that will be humiliating or embarrassing, e.g., unable to continue talking while speaking in public.

SIMPLE PHOBIA

Persistent fear of a specific object or situation that, when the person is exposed to it, almost invariably provokes an immediate anxiety response. Examples include phobias involving animals (dogs, snakes, in-

Table continued on following page

Table 5–14 ▶ Anxiety Disorders* *Continued*

sects, mice), closed spaces (claustrophobia), heights (acrophobia), and air travel.

OBSESSIVE-COMPULSIVE DISORDER

Recurrent obsessions or compulsions (see Table 5–8) that may be severe enough to cause marked distress, may be time consuming, or may interfere significantly with the person's normal routine, occupational functioning, or usual social activities or relationships with others.

GENERALIZED ANXIETY DISORDER

Unrealistic or excessive anxiety and worry about two or more life circumstances, e.g., worry about possible misfortune to one's child (who is in no danger) and worry about finances (for no good reason), for 6 months or longer. In children or adolescents, worry may be over academic, athletic, or social performance. Associated symptoms when the person is anxious include the following elements:

Motor Tension. Trembling, twitching, or feeling shaky; muscle tension and aches or soreness; restlessness; and easy fatigability

Autonomic Hyperactivity. Shortness of breath or smothering sensations; palpitations or tachycardia; sweating or cold clammy hands; dry mouth; dizziness or lightheadedness; nausea, diarrhea, or other abdominal distress; flushes or chills; frequent urination; and trouble swallowing or a lump in the throat.

Vigilance and Scanning. Feeling keyed up or on edge; exaggerated startle response; difficulty concentrating or mind going blank; trouble falling or staying asleep; and irritability.

(Adapted from American Psychiatric Association: Diagnostic and Statistical Manual of Mental Disorders. 3rd ed. Revised. Washington, DC, American Psychiatric Association, 1987.)

* These diagnostic categories are meant to be illustrative, not inclusive. The reader is referred to DSM-III-R or a psychiatry textbook for further categories, such as personality disorders or somatiform disorders.

Bibliography

American Psychiatric Association: Diagnostic and Statistical Manual of Mental Disorders. 3rd ed. Revised. Washington, DC, American Psychiatric Association, 1987.

Birren JE, Schaie KW (Eds): Handbook of the Psychology of Aging. 2nd ed. New York, Van Nostrand Reinhold, 1985.

Bruss CR: Nursing diagnosis of hopelessness. J Psychosocial Nurs 26(3):28–31, 1988.

Bydlon-Brown B, Billman R: At risk for suicide. Am J Nurs 88(10):1358–1361, 1988.

Carpenito LJ: Altered thoughts or altered perceptions? Am J Nurs 85(11):1283, 1985.

Depaulo, JR Jr, Folstein, MF: Psychiatric disturbances in neurological patients: Detection, recognition and hospital course. Ann Neurol 4:225–228, 1978.

Folstein MF, Folstein SE, McHugh PR: "Mini-mental state:" A practical method for grading the cognitive state of patients for the clinician. J Psychiatric Res 12:189–198, 1975.

Hays AM, Borger, F: A test in time. Am J Nurs 85:1107–1110, 1985.

Hays A: The set test to screen mental status quickly. Geriatr Nurs 5:96–97, 1984.

Hoch CC, Reynolds CF, Houck PR: Sleep patterns in Alzheimer, depressed, and healthy elderly. West J Nurs Res 10(3):239–256, 1988.

Isaacs B, Kennie, A: The set test as an aid to the detection of dementia in old people. Br J Psychiatry 123:467–470, 1973.

Jellinek M, Evans N, Knight R: Use of a behavior checklist on a pediatric inpatient unit. J Pediatr 94:156–158, 1979.

Johnson CE: Recognizing borderline personality disorder in the primary care client. Nurs Pract 13(8):11–18, 1988.

Kaplan HI, Sadock BJ: Synopsis of Psychiatry. 5th ed. Baltimore, Williams & Wilkins, 1987.

Keller MB, Manschreck, TC: The bedside mental status examination —reliability and validity. Compr Psychiatry 22(5):500–511, 1981.

Long KA: Are children too young for mental disorders? Am J Nurs 85(11):1254–1257.

Matzo M: Confusion in older adults: Assessment and differential diagnosis. Nurs Prac 15(9):32–46, 1990.

McDougall GJ: A review of screening instruments for assessing cognition and mental status in older adults. Nurs Pract 15(11):18–28, 1990.

McFarland GK, Wasli, EL: Nursing diagnoses and process in psychiatric mental health nursing. Philadelphia, JB Lippincott, 1986.

Morrison E, Fisher LY, Wilson HS, Underwood P: NSGAE: Nursing Adaptation Evaluation: A proposed Axis VI of DSM-III. J Psychosocial Nurs 23(8):10–13, 1985.

Motto JA, Heilbron DC, Juster RP: Development of a clinical instrument to estimate suicide risk. Am J Psychiatry 142(6):680–686, 1985.

Ninos M, Makohon R: Functional assessment of the patient. Geriatric Nurs 6:139–142, 1985.

Overall JE, Rhoades HM, Moreschi E: The nurses evaluation rating scale (NERS). J Clin Psychol 42(3):454–466, 1986.

Puskar KR, Obus NL: Management of the psychiatric emergency. Nurs Prac 14(7):9–26, 1989.

Reich JH: Proverbs and the modern mental status exam. Compr Psychiatry 22(5):528–531, 1981.

Rossman I: Clinical Geriatrics. 3rd ed. Philadelphia, JB Lippincott, 1986.

Shapira J, Schlesinger R, Cummings JL: Distinguishing dementias. Am J Nurs 86:699–702, 1986.

Strub RL, Black FW: The Mental Status Examination in Neurology. 2nd ed. Philadelphia, FA Davis, 1985.

Vincent KG, Coler MS: A unified nursing diagnostic model. Image 22(2):93–95, 1990.

CHAPTER

6 Nutritional Assessment

DEFINING NUTRITIONAL STATUS

Nutritional status refers to the health of an individual as it is affected by the intake, storage, and use of nutrients. Adequate nutrition is essential for normal body functioning, growth, resistance to infection, and repair of tissue. The major nutrients—carbohydrates, proteins, and fats—can be used for energy, converted to structural components of cells, or stored as fat, depending on the level of intake. Vitamins, minerals, and trace elements are required for proper use of the major nutrients and are involved in a wide variety of physiologic functions. They serve as structural materials in bone, teeth, cell membranes, and connective tissue. They also regulate cellular metabolism, maintain acid-base balance and osmotic pressure, and maintain nerve and muscle irritability.

The Recommended Daily Allowances (RDAs) (Appendix 6–1) set forth guidelines for protein, energy, vitamin, and mineral intakes for healthy individuals according to age, sex, height, and weight. Healthy adults require a protein intake of approximately 0.8 g/kg of body weight and a caloric intake of approximately 1800 kcal/day to meet basal energy needs (normal metabolic and physiologic demands of the body).

The classic Harris and Benedict equations (1919) are frequently used to estimate basal energy expenditure (BEE) based on weight, height, and age:

$$\text{BEE (men)} = 66.47 + 13.75W + 5.0H - 6.74A$$

$$\text{BEE (women)} = 655.10 + 9.56W + 1.85H - 4.68A$$

where: W = weight in kg
H = height in cm
A = age in years

Activity factors (Long, 1984) are then multiplied by the BEE to precisely determine resting energy expenditure that allows for minimal activity above BEE:

Activity Factors: confined to bed = 1.2
ambulatory = 1.3

Resting energy expenditure typically ranges from 1,800 to 2,400 kcal in the healthy adult.

Caloric or energy intake in excess of energy expended is stored in body reserves (Table 6–1). In the normal adult, this amounts to about 250 g of carbohydrate, 6000 g of protein, and 15,000 g of fat. Carbohydrate (4 kcal/g) is stored primarily as liver and muscle glycogen, supplies about 1000 kcal, and meets basal energy needs for less than a day. Protein (4 kcal/g) reserves contain approximately 24,000 kcal in two forms—visceral and somatic protein stores. Visceral protein stores include plasma proteins, hemoglobin, several clotting components, hormones, and antibodies; somatic proteins include skeletal and smooth muscle stores. Because these protein stores serve important physiologic functions in the body, use of them to meet energy needs results in loss of essential function. For example, catabolism of antibodies or clotting components can lead to sepsis or bleeding disorders, respectively. Fat (9 kcal/g) is stored as triglycerides in the adipose tissue. It is the largest fuel reserve (135,000 kcal), and is an excellent source of energy because it can be used without affecting essential tissue or function.

DEVELOPMENTAL CONSIDERATIONS

Infants and Children

The time from birth to 4 months of age is the most rapid period of growth of the life cycle. Although infants lose weight during the first few days of life, birth weight is usually regained by the 7th to 10th day after birth. Thereafter, infants double their birth weight by 4 months and triple it by 1 year of age. The number of pounds gained during the second year approximates the birth weight. Infants increase their length by 50 percent during the first year of life, and double it by 4 years of age. Brain size also increases very rapidly during infancy and childhood. By age 2 years, the brain has reached 50 percent of its adult size; by age 4, 75 percent; and by age 8, 100 percent. For this reason, infants and children should not drink skim or low-fat milk—fat is essential for proper central nervous system development.

The RDAs suggest a daily energy intake of 115 kcal/kg during the first 6 months of life, 105 kcal/kg in the

Table 6–1 ► Body Fuel Stores

Carbohydrate (250 g or 1000 kcal)
muscle glycogen
liver glycogen
Protein (6000 g or 24,000 kcal)
Somatic
skeletal muscle
smooth muscle
Visceral
plasma proteins
Fat (15,000 g or 135,000 kcal)

second 6 months, and 100 kcal/kg for ages 12 to 36 months. Energy requirements diminish to 80 kcal/kg/day by age 9 years. Protein requirements during infancy and childhood are higher than those of the older child or adult. Suggested daily protein intakes are 2.2 g/kg for birth to 6 months, 2.0 g/kg for 6 to 12 months, and 1.8 g/kg for 12 to 36 months. Protein intake per kilogram of body weight decreases to 1.2 g by age 9 years.

Adolescence

Following a period of slow growth in late childhood, adolescence is characterized by rapid physical growth and endocrine and hormonal changes. Caloric and protein requirements increase to meet this demand, and because of bone growth and increasing muscle mass (and, in girls, the onset of menarche), calcium and iron requirements also increase. Typically, these increased requirements cannot be met by three meals per day; nutritious snacks play an important role in achieving adequate nutrient intake. The recommended ranges of caloric and protein intakes for adolescence are shown in Appendix 6–1. In general, boys grow taller than girls; the percent of body fat increases in females to about 25 percent and decreases in males (replaced by muscle mass) to about 12 percent. Typically, girls double their body weight between the ages of 8 and 14; boys double their body weight between 10 and 17 years of age.

Pregnancy and Lactation

In order to support the synthesis of maternal and fetal tissues, sufficient calories and protein must be consumed. The RDAs state that, in addition to the 2000 to 2200 kcal/day adult women require, pregnant women need an additional 300 kcal/day. After delivery, and for the duration of lactation, an additional 500 to 800 kcal/day is needed for adequate milk production. Currently, the RDAs recommend 30 g of extra protein per day for pregnancy, and 20 g of extra protein per day during lactation. Iron, B-complex vitamins, and other vitamins and minerals should also be increased to meet the increased requirements of pregnancy and lactation (see Appendix 6–1). Appendix 6–2 illustrates approximate weight gains considered normal for each week of pregnancy.

Adulthood

During adulthood, growth and nutrient needs stabilize. Most adults are in relatively good health. However, unhealthy habits such as cigarette smoking, stressful lifestyles, lack of exercise, excessive alcohol intake, and diets high in saturated fat, cholesterol, salt, and sugar and low in fiber can be factors in the development of hypertension, obesity, atherosclerosis, cancer, osteoporosis, and diabetes mellitus. The adult years, therefore, are an important time for education, to preserve health and prevent or delay the onset of chronic disease. The RDAs for this group (persons aged 23 to 50 years) are shown in Appendix 6–1.

The Aging Adult

As people age, a number of changes occur that make them prone to undernutrition or overnutrition. Tooth loss, decreased sensory acuity (taste, smell, hearing, and touch), chronic disease, loss of spouse, social isolation, alcoholism, medications, reduced income, physical handicaps, impairments, decreased gastrointestinal motility, decreased metabolic rate, and decreased activity are among the many causes of malnutrition in older adults. The most important nutritional feature of the older years is the decrease in energy requirements. Between the ages of 51 and 75, energy needs decrease by approximately 200 kcal/day in both men and women. After age 75, energy needs decrease by 500 kcal and 400 kcal in males and females, respectively. The protein requirement of 0.8 g/kg/day for younger adults is appropriate for the healthy older person. In both men and women, height decreases slowly beginning during the early thirties, leading to an average lifetime height loss of 2.9 cm in men and 4.9 cm in women (Bowman and Rosenberg, 1982).

TRANSCULTURAL CONSIDERATIONS

Because foods and eating customs are culturally distinct, they become long-lasting and deeply rooted in the ethnic identity of individuals and families. Immigrants commonly maintain traditional eating customs long after the language and manner of dress of an adopted country become routine (especially for holidays and observance of religious customs). Occupation, class, religion, gender, and health awareness also have a great bearing on eating customs. Within the last decade, hundreds of thousands of Southeast Asians, Mexicans, and Cubans have immigrated to the United States. Not only do their food habits change to accommodate their new cultures, but their food habits have influence on their adoptive country. The taco is a good example of the Mexican American's influence on American eating habits.

Newly arriving immigrants may be at nutritional risk for a variety of reasons. They frequently come from countries with limited food supplies caused by poverty, poor sanitation, war, or political strife. Malnutrition, hypertension, dental caries, and iron-deficiency anemia are among the problems of new immigrants from developing countries. When immigrants arrive in the United States, other factors contribute to their nutritional problems: they are in a new country with a completely new language, culture, and society. They are faced with unfamiliar foods, food storage, food preparation, and food-buying habits. Many familiar foods are difficult or impossible to obtain. Low income may also limit their access to familiar foods.

Because rapid changes in eating patterns and customs are occurring in all countries, what are considered customs today may not be considered traditional in a few years. The best way to learn about the eating patterns of a people is to talk with them, eat with them, and ask about their dietary customs. It is important to keep in mind that recent immigrant groups, such as the Southeast Asians, are often shorter and weigh less than their Western counterparts, so American standard tables of weight for age, height for age, and weight for height may not be appropriate to evaluate growth and development of immigrant children. At present there are no reliable standards to evaluate every immigrant group.

The cultural factors that must be considered are the cultural definition of food, frequency and number of meals eaten away from home, form and content of ceremonial meals, amount and types of foods eaten, and regularity of food consumption. Because potential inaccuracies may occur, the 24-hour dietary recalls or three-day food records used traditionally for assessment may be inadequate when dealing with people from culturally diverse backgrounds. Standard dietary handbooks may fail to provide you with culture-specific diet information because nutritional content and exchange tables are generally based on Western diets (Pennington, 1976). Another source of error may originate from the cultural patterns of eating, for example, among low income urban black families, in which elaborate weekend meals are frequently eaten while weekday dietary patterns are markedly more moderate.

Although you may assume that the term food is a universal concept, you should have the person clarify what is meant by the term. For example, certain Latin American groups do not consider greens, an important source of vitamins, to be food, and thus fail to list intake of these vegetables on daily records. Among Vietnamese refugees, the dietary intake of calcium may appear inadequate, particularly with the low consumption of dairy products common among members of this group. Pork bones and shells are, however, commonly con-

Table 6-2 ▶ Dietary Practices of Selected Religious Groups—Prohibited Foods and Beverages

HINDUISM
- All meats

ISLAM
- Pork
- Intoxicating beverages

JUDAISM
- Pork
- Predatory fowl
- Shellfish and other water creatures (fish with scales are permissible)
- Mixing milk and meat dishes at same meal
- Blood by ingestion (e.g., blood sausage, raw meat); blood by transfusion is acceptable

Additional Notes:

Foods should be kosher (meaning "properly prepared")

All animals must be ritually slaughtered by a shochet (quickly, with the least pain possible) to be kosher.

MORMONISM (CHURCH OF JESUS CHRIST OF LATTER-DAY SAINTS)
- Alcohol
- Tobacco
- Beverages containing caffeine (coffee, tea, colas, and selected carbonated soft drinks)

SEVENTH DAY ADVENTIST
- Pork
- Certain seafood including shellfish
- Fermented beverages

Additional Note:

A vegetarian diet is encouraged

sumed, thus providing adequate quantities of calcium to meet daily requirements.

Food itself is only one part of eating. In some cultures, social contacts during meals are restricted to members of the immediate or extended family. For example, in some Middle Eastern cultures, men and women eat meals separately, or women may be permitted to eat with their husbands, but not with other males. Among some Hispanic groups, the male breadwinner is served first, then women and children. Etiquette during meals, the use of hands, type of eating utensils (e.g., chopsticks, special flatware), and protocols governing the order in which food is consumed during a meal all vary cross-culturally.

Dietary Practices of Selected Cultural Groups

It is necessary to avoid *cultural stereotyping,* the tendency to view individuals of common cultural backgrounds similarly and according to a preconceived notion of how they "ought" to behave. For example, despite the widely held stereotype, we know that there are Chinese who do not like rice, Italians who despise spaghetti, Irish who dislike corned beef and cabbage, and so forth. Aggregate dietary preferences among people from certain cultural groups, however, can be described (e.g., characteristic ethnic dishes, methods of food preparation), and the reader is referred to nutrition texts on the topic for detailed information about culture-specific diets and the nutritional value of ethnic foods.

Cultural food preferences are often interrelated with religious dietary beliefs and practices. Many religions use foods as symbols in celebrations and rituals. Knowing the person's religious practices related to food enables you to suggest improvements or modifications that will not conflict with dietary laws (see Table 6–2).

Other issues are fasting and other religious observations that may limit a person's food or liquid intake during specified times (e.g., many Catholics fast and abstain from meat on Ash Wednesday and the Fridays of Lent; Muslims refrain from eating during the daytime hours for an entire month called Ramadan in the Islamic calendar but are permitted to eat after sunset; Mormons refrain from all solid foods and liquids on the first Sunday of each month).

EFFECTS OF STARVATION AND STRESS ON NUTRITIONAL REQUIREMENTS

The incidence of malnutrition in the population at-large is estimated to range from 10 to 20 percent (Garn and Clark, 1975); in hospitalized individuals, the incidence may be as high as 50 percent (Bistrian et al, 1974; Mullen et al, 1979). Malnutrition is associated with general debilitation, apathy, increased rates of morbidity (for example, poor wound healing and increased infection) and mortality, and greater medical expenses. The incidence and severity of malnutrition can be prevented or significantly reduced when it is identified and treated early.

Response to Starvation

During starvation, glycogen or carbohydrate stores, which supply about 1000 kcal, are used first, but these stores are small and are usually exhausted within 15 to 20 hours. After that, caloric needs are supplied by conversion of skeletal muscle protein to glucose. But, as discussed earlier, the use of body proteins for energy impairs essential body functions, so the body adapts by using fat, its largest and most dispensable energy store, and by decreasing resting energy expenditure to diminish protein depletion and energy requirements. When fat stores are depleted by prolonged starvation, the entire energy requirement must be met by remaining protein stores. Severe depletion of these proteins causes impaired wound healing, altered immune competence, and the inability to maintain the work of breathing; it eventually leads to multiple organ failure and death.

Response to Stress

The stress of injury, major surgery, and sepsis produces a response that differs markedly from that of starvation. Adaptive mechanisms preserve protein stores and diminish energy expenditure in starvation; in contrast, the stress of injury is characterized by accelerated tissue breakdown, increased energy expenditure, and increased loss of protein.

In the acute phase after injury, there is a release of stress hormones (catecholamines, growth hormone, glucocorticoids, and glucagon), which stimulates accelerated breakdown of protein and fat stores. This phase is also characterized by diminished insulin levels—hyperglycemia results.

The administration of concentrated glucose solutions during the acute phase may exacerbate hyperglycemia and may even lead to nonketotic hyperosmolar coma. The net effect of the acute phase is a highly catabolic hormonal environment that provides vital energy needs at the expense of skeletal muscle.

As secretion of stress hormones abates, usually within 3 to 5 days after injury, hyperglycemia resolves and muscle breakdown is reduced. During this adaptive phase, resistance to insulin diminishes and nutritional support can be effectively instituted to reduce protein loss and to promote protein synthesis.

PURPOSES AND COMPONENTS OF NUTRITIONAL ASSESSMENT

The state of the body's fuel reserves and the effects of starvation or stress on nutritional status can be determined by the application of nutritional assessment techniques. In general, these techniques are noninvasive, inexpensive, and easy to perform.

The purposes of nutritional assessment are to (1) provide data for designing a nutrition plan of care that will prevent or minimize the development of malnutrition; (2) establish baseline data for evaluating the efficacy of nutritional care; and (3) identify individuals who are malnourished or are at risk of developing malnutrition.

Regardless of the clinical setting—primary, acute, or long-term care—the first step in evaluating nutritional status is screening to determine whether or not any potential for nutritional risk exists. Minimal nutritional *screening* involves taking a health history regarding conditions that might interfere with adequate food intake, measurement of height and weight, and routine laboratory tests. Table 6–3 is an example of a form used to compile screening information.

A *comprehensive* nutritional assessment is recom-

Table 6–3 ▶ Screening Nutritional Assessment Form

I. Initial Screening

Age ______ Height ______________ (cm/in)

Current Weight ______________________ (kg/lb) Usual Weight ______________________ (kg/lb)

$$\%\ \text{Ideal Body Weight} = \frac{\text{Current Weight}}{\text{Ideal Body Weight}} \times 100$$

$$\%\ \text{Usual Body Weight} = \frac{\text{Current Weight}}{\text{Usual Weight}} \times 100$$

$$\%\text{Weight Change} = \frac{\text{Usual Weight} - \text{Current Weight}}{\text{Usual Weight}} \times 100$$

II. Risk Factors

Check if person is experiencing any of the following problems.

YES	NO		
______	______	A.	Recent unintentional weight loss. How many pounds ______? Time period ______?
______	______	B.	Recent weight gain. How many pounds ______? Time period ______?
______	______	C.	Decreased appetite. Since ______?
______	______	D.	Taste alterations. Since ______?
______	______	E.	Difficulty ______ chewing and/or ______ swallowing. Since ______?
______	______	F.	Recent surgery/trauma/burns/sepsis. What ______? When ______?
______	______	G.	Chronic conditions ______
______	______	H.	Cancer chemotherapy/radiation therapy ______
______	______	I.	Vomiting ______ times/day
______	______	J.	Diarrhea ______ times/day
______	______	K.	Constipation ______ times/week
______	______	L.	Food allergies or intolerances ______
______	______	M.	Multiple medications ______
______	______	N.	Fad diets ______
______	______	O.	Low income ______
______	______	P.	Immobile ______
______	______	Q.	Unable to feed self ______
______	______	R.	Substance abuse ______
______	______	S.	Social isolation ______

Albumin ______________ Hemoglobin ______________ Hematocrit ______________

Triglycerides ______________________ Cholesterol ______________________

Total lymphocytes ______ Other labs, if abnormal ______________________

III. Screening Summary*

	YES	NO
1. Is person severely underweight (weight 20 percent ≤ideal)?	______	______
2. Is person severely overweight (weight 20 percent ≥ideal)?	______	______
3. Has person unintentionally lost ≥10% of usual body weight?	______	______
4. A. through S. above (3 or more marked yes)?	______	______
5. Is serum albumin ≤3.5 g/dl?	______	______
6. Is total lymphocyte count ≤1200/mm^3?	______	______

* If one or more of these items are present, a comprehensive nutritional assessment is indicated.

Table 6–4 ▶ Comprehensive Nutritional Assessment Form

I. Dietary History/Intake

Current Diet ____

Consistency: ___ Regular ___ Soft ___ Ground ___ Pureed ___ Other

Food Preferences ____

Food Dislikes ____

Food Restrictions ____

Nutritional Supplement (type and amount) ____

Vitamin/Mineral Supplement (type and amount) ____

Facilities for meal preparation:
___none
___hot plate only
___full kitchen facilities
___refrigerator
___other ____

Preparation of meals:
___does own meal preparation
___receives assistance with meal preparation
___someone else prepares meals
___other ____

Transportation to market:
___walks
___takes a bus
___drives
___needs transportation
___other ____

Daily Food Intake

Meal	Time/Location	Kind/Amount of Food
Breakfast		
Snack(s)		
Lunch		
Snack(s)		
Dinner		
Snack(s)		

Summary of Daily Food Intake

	Recommended Number of Servings					
Food Group	**Child**	**Teen**	**Adult**	**Pregnant**	**Lactating**	**Number Eaten**
Milk	3	4	2	4	4	
Meat/protein	2	2	2	3	2	
Fruits/vegetables	4	4	4	4	4	
Breads/cereals	4	4	4	4	4	
Fats/sweets	–	–	–	–	–	

Estimated Level of Nutrient Intake

	Calor	Prot	Fat	CHO	Vit A	Thia	Ribo	Fol	Vit C	Iron	Ca*
Adequate											
Inadequate											

II. Physical Signs

Body Area	Signs	No	Yes	Comments
Skin	dry, flaky, scaly			
	petechiae, ecchymoses			
	cracks, rash			
Hair	dull, dry			
	sparse, shedding			
Eyes	cloudy, pale			
	dry			
	red			
Lips	swollen, red			
	cracks at sides			
Tongue	swollen, red			
	pale			
	fissured			
	magenta			
Gums	bleeding			

Table continued on following page

Table 6-4 ▶ Comprehensive Nutritional Assessment Form *Continued*

Body Area	Signs	No	Yes	Comments
Nails	brittle, ridged			
	spoon-shaped			
	splinter hemorrhages			
Musculoskeletal	pain in calves, thighs			
	osteomalacia, rickets			
	joint pain			
	muscle wasting			
Neurologic	peripheral neuropathy			
	hyporeflexia			
	disorientation/iritability			

General appearance: ____________

III. Anthropometry

Triceps skinfold (TSF)	____________	mm
Mid-upper arm circumferance (MAC)	____________	cm
Mid-upper arm muscle circumference (MAMC)	____________	cm
Mid-arm muscle area (MAMA)	____________	cm^2
Body mass index	____________	
Arm span	____________	cm
Elbow breadth	____________	cm

IV. Laboratory Studies

Serum transferrin	____________	
Response to skin test antigen	____________	mm
Nitrogen balance	____________	
Creatinine height index	____________	%

* Calor, calories; Prot, protein; CHO, carbohydrate; Vit A, vitamin A; Thia, thiamine; Ribo, riboflavin; Fol, folacin; Vit C, vitamin C; Iron, iron; Ca, calcium.

mended for all individuals with confirmed nutritional risk, i.e., with one or more of the following risk factors:

1. Weight < 80 percent or > 120 percent of ideal weight
2. History of unintentional weight loss > 4.5 kg (10 lb) or ≥ 10 percent of usual weight
3. Serum albumin concentration < 3.5 g/dl
4. Total lymphocyte count < 1500 cells/mm^3
5. History of illnesses, symptoms, or factors that are associated with nutritional depletion or interfere with nutrient intake or absorption

In addition to the screening assessment parameters, comprehensive nutritional assessment includes dietary history and dietary intake information, physical examination of clinical signs, anthropometric measures, and laboratory tests. Table 6–4 is an example of a form for compiling comprehensive nutritional assessment data.

Various methods for collecting current dietary intake information are available—24-hour recall, food frequency questionnaire, and food diary. During hospitalization, documentation of nutritional intake can best be achieved through a calorie count of nutrients consumed and/or infused.

The easiest and most popular routine method for obtaining information about dietary intake is the *24-hour recall.* The individual or family member completes a questionnaire or is interviewed and asked to recall everything eaten within the last 24 hours. However, there are several significant sources of error in using this method: (1) the individual or family member may not be able to recall the type or amount of food eaten; (2) intake within the last 24 hours may be atypical of usual intake; (3) the individual or family member may alter the truth for a variety of reasons; and (4) snack items and use of gravies, sauces, and condiments either may not be reported or may be under-reported.

To counter some of the difficulties inherent in the 24-hour recall method, a *food frequency questionnaire* may also be completed. With this tool, information is collected on how many times per day, week, or month the individual eats particular foods. Drawbacks to the use of the food frequency questionnaire are (1) it does not quantify amount of intake and (2) like the 24-hour recall, it relies on the individual's or family member's memory for how often a food was eaten.

Food diaries or records require asking the individual or family member to write down everything consumed for a certain period of time. Three days—two weekdays and one weekend day—are customarily used. A food diary is most complete and accurate if the individual is instructed to record information immediately after eating. Potential problems with the food diary include (1) noncompliance, (2) inaccurate recording, (3) atypical intake on the recording days, and (4) conscious alteration of diet during the recording period.

Direct observation of the feeding and eating process can lead to detection of problems not readily identified through standard nutrition interviews. For example, observing the typical feeding techniques used by a parent or care giver and the interaction between the individual and his or her care giver can be of value when assessing failure to thrive in children or unintentional weight loss in older adults.

The basic four food groups, as shown in the Comprehensive Nutritional Assessment Form (Table 6–4, Section I), and the RDAs (Appendix 6–1) are most often used as a basis for determining nutritional adequacy of diet. The number of servings consumed from each food group is compared with the number of servings suggested (see Table 6–4, Section I). One shortcoming of following the RDAs is that they are not meant to be applied to sick individuals, whose nutrient requirements may be very different from those of healthy individuals, for whom the RDAs were designed. Specific nutrient values of foods can be obtained from several publications (e.g., *Bowes and Church's Food Values of Portions Commonly Used,* 1980; Young et al., 1981) and from nutrition labels and food manufacturers' information.

SUBJECTIVE DATA

Eating Patterns
Usual weight, changes in weight
Changes in appetite, taste, chewing, swallowing
Recent surgery, trauma, burns, infection
Chronic illnesses
Vomiting, diarrhea, constipation
Food allergies and intolerances
Medications and/or nutritional supplements
Alcohol and illegal drug use
Socioeconomic factors
Usual activity, exercise patterns

QUESTIONS FOR ALL CLIENTS

EXAMINER ASKS:	RATIONALE:
1. What are your typical **eating patterns?** How many meals/snacks do you have per day? What kind and amount of food do you eat? Where do you eat? Do you have any food preferences or dislikes? Any religious or cultural food restrictions? Are you able to feed yourself?	Most individuals are knowledgeable about, or interested in, the foods they consume. If misconceptions are present, begin gradual instruction to correct them. Ethnic or religious beliefs may alter intake of certain foods.
2. What is your **usual weight?** Have you experienced any **change in weight** during the past 6 months? How many pounds did you lose or gain? Over what period of time did you lose or gain the weight? What was the reason for your weight gain or loss?	Persons who have had a recent, unintentional weight loss or who are extremely overweight are at nutritional risk. Individuals who are underweight are more vulnerable because somatic and visceral proteins may already be depleted. Frequently, malnutrition is not recognized in overweight persons; they may be protein depleted but appear well nourished.

EXAMINER ASKS:	RATIONALE:
3. Have you experienced any changes in **appetite, taste,** or **smell** or in **chewing** or **swallowing** ability? What was the change? When did you first notice the change?	Poor appetite, taste and smell alterations, as well as chewing and swallowing difficulties interfere with adequate nutrient intake and increase the likelihood of being at nutritional risk.
4. Have you had any recent **surgery, trauma, burns,** or **infection?** What type? When did this occur? How was it treated? Do you have any conditions that cause increased nutrient losses (e.g., draining wounds, fistulae, effusions, blood loss)?	Persons who have had recent surgery, trauma, sepsis, or conditions causing nutrient losses may have caloric and nutrient needs that are two or three times greater than normal
5. Do you have any **chronic illnesses?** What are they? How long have you had them? How are they treated? Have you recently received cancer chemotherapy or radiation therapy?	Individuals with chronic illnesses that affect nutrient use (e.g., diabetes mellitus, pancreatitis, or malabsorption) or those receiving cancer treatment are twice as likely to have nutritional deficits.
6. Have you had any **vomiting, diarrhea,** or **constipation?** What seems to bring this on? How long has it been occurring?	Gastrointestinal symptoms such as vomiting, diarrhea, or constipation may interfere with nutrient intake or absorption.
7. Have you ever experienced any **food allergies** or **intolerances?** Please describe. When did this occur?	Food allergies and intolerances may exacerbate adverse symptoms and result in nutrient deficiencies (e.g., diarrhea after milk ingestion).
8. Do you take any **medication?** Do you use any **vitamin, mineral,** or **nutritional supplements?** What type(s)? How much? For how long?	Analgesics, antacids, anticonvulsants, antibiotics, diuretics, laxatives, antineoplastic drugs, and oral contraceptives are among the drugs that can interact with nutrients, impairing their digestion, absorption, utilization, or metabolism. Nutritional supplements may cause harmful side effects if taken in large amounts.
9. What facilities are available for meal preparation? Who prepares meals? Is your income adequate to buy sufficient food? Who does the shopping? What transportation is available to travel to the market?	**Socioeconomic factors** may interfere with ingestion of adequate amounts of food or usual diet.
10. Do you use **alcohol** or **illegal drugs?** When did you have your last drink of alcohol? How much did you drink at that episode? How much do you drink each day? How much each week? (Repeat questions for each drug used.)	These agents interfere with ingestion of adequate amounts of food or usual diet. Also, pregnant women who smoke, drink alcohol, or use illegal drugs give birth to a disproportionate number of infants with low birth weights, failure to thrive, and other complications.
11. What are your **exercise** and **activity patterns?** Please describe type and amount per day.	Exercise and activity patterns affect nutritional intake. Usually, caloric and nutrient needs increase with increased activity and exercise.

DEVELOPMENTAL CONSIDERATIONS

Additional Questions for Infants and Children

Dietary histories of infants and children are generally obtained from the child's parents, guardian, baby sitter, or day care center. Usually, the person responsible for food preparation is able to provide a fairly accurate dietary history. Having the care givers keep a thorough daily food diary and occasionally requesting 24-hour recalls during clinic visits are the most commonly employed techniques for this population group.

EXAMINER ASKS:	RATIONALE:
1. Is there any history of obesity or heart disease in the family? 2. How many children are in the family? 3. What is the economic level of the parents and care givers? What is the educational level of the parents and care givers?	Conditions such as obesity, atherosclerosis, and possibly hypertension may have their origins in childhood malnutrition — either undernutrition or overnutrition. The Ten-State Nutrition Survey (1968 to 1970) (Garn and Clark, 1975) showed that certain nutritional problems could be predicted by general family characteristics. Among the findings were that the incidence of malnutrition increases as family income levels decrease; the higher the educational level of the family members responsible for purchasing the food, the better the nutritional status of family members under 17 years of age.
4. Is your child willing to eat what you prepare? Any special likes or dislikes? How much will the child eat? 5. How do you control snack foods?	

Additional Questions for the Adolescent

1. What is your present weight? What would you like to weigh? 2. Are you on any special diet to lose weight? Have you been on other diets to lose weight? If so, were they successful? Do you constantly think about "feeling fat?" Do you intentionally vomit or use laxatives or diuretics after eating?	Obesity, particularly in girls, may precipitate fad dieting and malnutrition. Also, because of adolescents' increased body awareness and self-consciousness, they are prone to develop eating disorders such as anorexia nervosa or bulimia, conditions in which the real or perceived body image does not compare favorably to an ideal image — that found in advertisements or pictures of fashion models.
3. What snacks or fast foods do you like to eat? When do you eat them? How much do you eat?	An accurate dietary history may be difficult to obtain from the adolescent because of the frequency of between-meal snacks and

EXAMINER ASKS:	RATIONALE:
	meals eaten on the run. These may be omitted or forgotten during the interview or in a food diary.
4. When did you first start menstruating? What is your menstrual flow like?	Menarche is usually delayed if malnutrition is present. Likewise, amenorrhea or scant menstrual flow is associated with nutritional deficiency.

Additional Questions for the Pregnant Female

1. How many times have you been pregnant? When? Any problems encountered during previous pregnancies? This pregnancy?	If the mother is multiparous, with pregnancies occurring less than a year apart, there is a greatly increased chance that her nutritional reserves are depleted. Previous complications of pregnancy such as excessive vomiting or anemia must also be noted. Slower gastrointestinal motility and pressure from the fetus may cause constipation, hemorrhoids, and indigestion. In the later months of pregnancy, women should be routinely monitored for these conditions. A past history of giving birth to a low-birth-weight infant suggests past nutritional problems. Giving birth to an infant with a birth weight of 4.5 kg (10 lbs) or more may signal the presence of *latent* diabetes in the mother.
2. What foods do you prefer when you are pregnant? What foods do you avoid? Do you crave any particular foods?	The expectant mother may be extremely vulnerable to familial, cultural, and traditional influences for food choices. Cravings for particular foods are usually psychological in origin and should be evaluated for their potential contribution to, or interference with, dietary intake.

Additional Questions for Adults

Is there any family or personal history of heart disease, osteoporosis, cancer, gout, obesity, and/or diabetes mellitus? What effect have they had on eating patterns? What effect have they had on activity patterns?	Long-term nutritional deficiencies or excesses may first become manifest as disease. During the adult years, some common examples of such conditions are heart disease, osteoporosis, cancer, gout, obesity, and dia-

EXAMINER ASKS:	RATIONALE:
	betes mellitus. Early identification of nutritional alterations permits dietary and activity modifications to occur promptly—at a time when the body can more fully recover.

Additional Questions for the Aging Adult

How does your diet differ from when you were in your 40s and 50s? Why? What factors affect the way you eat?	Normal physiologic changes in aging adults that directly affect nutritional status include poor dentition, decreased visual acuity, decreased saliva production, slowed gastrointestinal motility, decreased gastrointestinal absorption, and diminished olfactory and taste sensitivity. Socioeconomic conditions frequently have the greatest effect on the nutritional status of the aging adult; these factors should be closely evaluated. Decline of extended families and increased mobility of families reduce available support systems. Facilities for meal preparation and eating, transportation to grocery stores, physical limitations, income, and social isolation are frequent problems and can obviously interfere with the acquisition of a balanced diet. Medications must also be considered, because aging adults frequently take multiple medications that have a potential for interaction with nutrients and with one another.

OBJECTIVE DATA

CLINICAL SIGNS

Observation of an individual's general appearance—obese, cachectic, or edematous—can also provide clues to overall nutritional status. More specific clinical signs and symptoms suggestive of nutritional deficiencies can be detected through a physical examination. Because clinical signs are late manifestations of malnutrition, only in areas in which there is rapid turnover of epithelial tissue — skin, hair, mouth, lips, and eyes — are the nutritional deficiencies readily detectable. These signs may also be nonnutritional in origin. Therefore, laboratory testing is required in order to make an accurate diagnosis. Laboratory tests for assessment of nutritional status are reviewed later in this chapter. Clinical signs of various nutritional deficiencies are summarized in Table 6–5 and are depicted in the section on abnormalities at the end of this chapter.

Table 6–5 ▶ Clinical Signs of Malnutrition

AREA OF EXAMINATION	NORMAL APPEARANCE	SIGNS ASSOCIATED WITH MALNUTRITION	NUTRIENT DEFICIENCY
Skin	Smooth, no signs of rashes, bruises, flaking	Dry, flaking, scaly	Vitamin A, vitamin B-complex, linoleic acid
		Petechiae/ecchymoses	Vitamins C and K
		Follicular hyperkeratosis (dry bumpy skin)	Vitamin A, linoleic acid
		Cracks in skin, lesions on the hands, legs, face, or neck	Niacin, tryptophan
		Pellagrous dermatosis (hyperpigmentation of skin exposed to sunlight)	Niacin
		Nasolabial seborrhea	Riboflavin, vitamin B_6
		Acneiform forehead rash	Vitamin B_6
		Eczema	Linoleic acid
		Xanthomas (excessive deposits of cholesterol)	Excessive serum levels of LDLs or VLDLs
Hair	Shiny, firm, does not fall out easily, healthy scalp	Dull, dry, sparse	Protein, zinc, linoleic acid
		Color changes	Copper or protein
		Corkscrew hair	Copper
Eyes	Corneas are clear, shiny; membranes are pink and moist; no sores at corners of eyelids	Foamy plaques (Bitot's spots)	Vitamin A
		Dryness (xerophthalmia)	Vitamin A
		Softening (keratomalacia)	Vitamin A
		Pale conjunctivae	Iron
		Red conjunctivae	Riboflavin
		Blepharitis	B-complex, biotin
Lips	Smooth, not chapped or swollen	Cheilosis (vertical cracks in lips)	Riboflavin, niacin
		Angular stomatitis (red cracks at sides of mouth)	Riboflavin, niacin, iron, vitamin B_6
Tongue	Red in apearance; not swollen or smooth, no lesions	Glossitis (beefy red)	Vitamin B-complex
		Pale	Iron
		Papillary atrophy	Niacin
		Papillary hypertrophy	Multiple nutrients
		Magenta/purplish colored tongue	Riboflavin
Gums	Reddish-pink, firm, no swelling or bleeding	Bleeding	Vitamin C
Nails	Smooth, pink	Brittle, ridged, or spoon-shaped (koilonychia)	Iron
		Splinter hemorrhages	Vitamin C
Musculoskeletal	Erect posture, no malformations, good muscle tone, can walk or run without pain	Pain in calves, thighs	Thiamine
		Osteomalacia	Vitamin D, calcium
		Rickets	Vitamin D, calcium
		Joint pain	Vitamin C
		Muscle wasting	Protein, carbohydrate, fat
Neurologic	Normal reflexes, appropriate affect	Peripheral neuropathy	Thiamine, vitamin B_6
		Hyporeflexia	Thiamine
		Disorientation or irritability	Vitamin B

* LDLs, low-density lipoproteins; VLDLs, very-low-density lipoproteins.

NORMAL RANGE OF FINDINGS	ABNORMAL FINDINGS

ANTHROPOMETRIC MEASURES

Anthropometry is the measurement and evaluation of growth and development. The most commonly used anthropometric measures are height, weight, triceps skinfold thickness, elbow breadth, and arm and head circumferences. Measurement of height, weight, and head circumference is described in Chapter 8.

Equipment Needed

- Lange or Harpenden skinfold calipers
- Ross Insertion Tape or other measurement tape
- Anthropometer
- Pen or pencil
- Nutritional assessment data form

Derived Weight Measures

Three derived weight measures are used to depict changes in body weight.

Weight as a Percentage of Ideal Body Weight

Body weight as a percentage of ideal body weight is calculated using the following formula:

$$\text{Percent Ideal Body Weight} = \frac{\text{Current Weight}}{\text{Ideal Weight}} \times 100$$

(Ideal weight is based on the Metropolitan Life Insurance Tables, 1983; see Chapter 8.)

As a general rule, a current weight of 80 to 90 percent of ideal weight is suggestive of mild malnutrition; 70 to 80 percent, of moderate malnutrition; and less than 70 percent is indicative of severe malnutrition.

Current Weight as a Percentage of Usual Weight

The percent usual body weight is calculated as follows:

$$\text{Percent Usual Body Weight} = \frac{\text{Current Weight}}{\text{Usual Weight}} \times 100$$

A current weight of 85 to 95 percent of usual body weight is an indication of mild malnutrition; 75 to 84 percent, of moderate malnutrition; and less than 75 percent, of severe malnutrition.

Recent Weight Change

Recent weight change is calculated using the following formula:

$$\frac{\text{Usual Weight} - \text{Current Weight}}{\text{Usual Weight}} \times 100$$

An unintentional loss of 10 percent of body weight over any time period is considered clinically significant.

Skinfold Thickness

Skinfold thickness measurements provide an estimate of body fat stores or the extent of obesity or undernutrition. Although other sites can be used (biceps, subcapsular, or suprailiac skinfolds), the triceps skinfold (TSF) is

NORMAL RANGE OF FINDINGS	ABNORMAL FINDINGS

most commonly selected because of its easy accessibility and because standards and techniques are most developed for this site. To measure triceps skinfold thickness:

1. Have the ambulatory person stand with arms hanging freely at the sides and back to the examiner. (Nonambulatory persons should lie on one side. The uppermost arm should be fully extended, with the palm of the hand resting on the thigh.)
2. Using the thumb and forefinger of your left hand, gently grasp a fold of skin and fat on the posterior aspect of the person's left upper arm, midway between the acromion process of the scapula and the olecranon process (the tip of the elbow). Gently pull the skinfold away from the underlying muscle (Fig. 6–1).

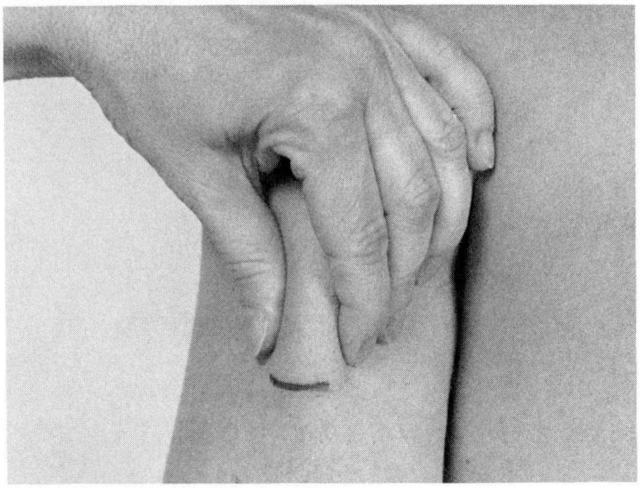

► **Figure 6–1**

3. While grasping the skinfold, pick up the calipers with your right hand and depress the spring-loaded lever. Apply caliper jaws horizontally to the fat fold. Release the lever of the calipers while holding the skinfold. Wait 3 seconds, then take a reading. Repeat three times and average the three skinfold measurements (Fig. 6–2).
4. Record measurements to the nearest 5 mm (0.5 cm) on the nutritional

Triceps skinfold values that are 10 percent below or above standard are suggestive of undernutrition and overnutrition, respectively. Conditions such as edema or subcutaneous emphysema may produce falsely high readings. Nonreproducible readings may be due to instrument malfunction, use of plastic calipers (which are less accurate), or examiner error.

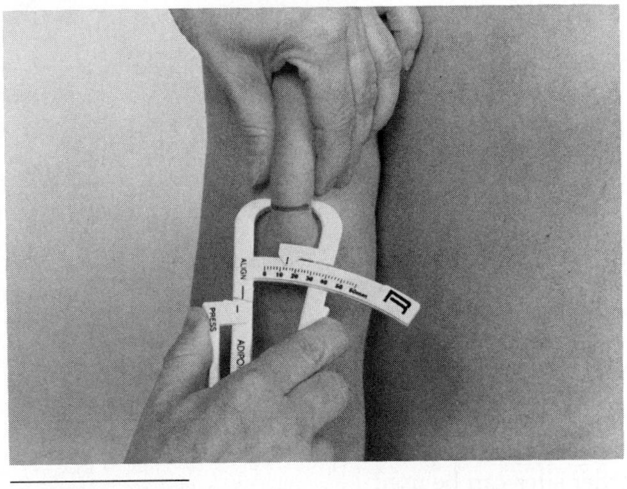

► **Figure 6–2**

NORMAL RANGE OF FINDINGS | **ABNORMAL FINDINGS**

assessment data form. Compare the person's measurements with standards by age and sex (Tables 6–6 and 6–7).

Mid-Upper Arm Circumference

Mid-upper arm circumference (MAC) estimates skeletal muscle mass and fat stores.

Table 6–6 ▶ Selected Percentiles of Triceps Skinfold Thickness and Bone-Free Upper Arm Area by Height in U.S. Men, Age 25 to 54 Years, with Small, Medium, and Large Frames

HEIGHT		TRICEPS (mm)							BONE-FREE MAMA (cm^2)						
		5	10	15	50	85	90	95	5	10	15	50	85	90	95
Small Frame															
in	*cm*														
62	157				11							52			
63	160			6	10	17					32	48	54		
64	163		5	5	10	16	18			37	38	49	58	63	
65	165	4	5	6	11	17	19	21	31	35	37	47	60	63	71
66	168	5	6	6	11	18	18	20	31	36	38	49	60	62	71
67	170	5	6	6	11	18	20	22	35	39	41	49	58	60	62
68	173	5	6	6	10	15	16	20	33	37	40	49	59	62	69
69	175		6	6	11	17	20			36	40	58	61	63	
70	178			7	10	17					35	48	57		
71	180			7	10	16					39	47	52		
72	183				10							45			
73	185														
74	188														
Medium Frame															
in	*cm*														
62	157				15							58			
63	160				11							55			
64	163		6	6	12	18	20			43	47	56	67	71	
65	165	5	7	8	12	20	22	25	40	43	45	56	67	69	70
66	168	5	6	7	11	16	18	22	38	42	44	55	69	72	78
67	170	5	7	7	13	21	23	28	39	42	44	53	66	69	73
68	173	4	5	7	11	18	20	24	41	44	45	55	67	71	76
69	175	5	6	7	12	18	20	24	38	41	44	54	66	69	73
70	178	5	6	7	12	18	20	23	39	42	43	55	65	68	72
71	180	4	5	7	12	19	21	25	37	41	44	54	67	68	73
72	183	5	7	7	12	20	22	26	40	42	44	56	65	67	74
73	185	6	7	8	12	20	24	27	39	42	43	55	67	69	73
74	188		6	9	13	21	23			43	43	55	62	63	
Large Frame															
in	*cm*														
62	157														
63	160														
64	163														
65	165				14							62			
66	168			9	14	30					48	58	76		
67	170		7	7	11	23	27			50	52	61	73	78	
68	173		9	10	14	22	23			51	53	65	78	86	
69	175	6	7	8	15	25	29	31	46	48	49	61	73	78	83
70	178	7	7	7	14	23	25	30	43	47	50	61	75	77	86
71	180	6	8	10	15	25	27	31	47	48	50	62	75	81	83
72	183	5	6	7	12	20	22	25	45	48	50	61	77	80	86
73	185	5	6	7	13	19	22	31	47	49	51	66	79	83	86
74	188			8	12	19					53	66	78		

(Adapted from Frisancho AR: New standards of weight and body composition by frame size and height for assessment of nutritional status of adults and the elderly. Am J Clin Nutr Assoc 40:808–819, 1984 © American Society for Clinical Nutrition.)

NORMAL RANGE OF FINDINGS

ABNORMAL FINDINGS

1. Have the subject stand or sit with arm hanging fully extended and relaxed by the side of the body.
2. Loop the insertion tape or measuring tape around the arm at the midpoint of the upper arm (midway between the acromion and olecranon processes).

Table 6–7 ▶ Selected Percentiles of Triceps Skinfold Thickness and Bone-Free Upper Arm Area by Height in U.S. Women, Age 25 to 54 Years, with Small, Medium, and Large Frames

HEIGHT		TRICEPS (mm)							BONE-FREE MAMA (cm^2)						
		5	10	15	50	85	90	95	5	10	15	50	85	90	95
Small Frame															
in	*cm*														
58	147		12	13	24	30	33			22	24	29	36	44	
59	150	8	11	14	21	29	36	37	17	20	22	28	38	39	43
60	152	8	11	12	21	28	29	33	19	21	22	28	36	40	44
61	155	11	12	14	21	28	31	34	20	21	23	28	38	39	42
62	157	10	12	14	20	28	31	34	20	21	21	27	33	35	37
63	160	10	11	13	20	27	30	36	20	21	22	27	33	35	38
64	163	10	13	13	20	28	30	34	22	23	23	28	34	38	42
65	165	12	13	14	22	29	31	34	21	22	23	28	37	39	47
66	168			12	19	30					23	27	35		
67	170				18							26			
68	173				20							25			
69	175														
70	178														
Medium Frame															
in	*cm*														
58	147			20	25	40					24	35	42		
59	150	15	19	21	30	37	40	40	23	24	26	33	43	45	49
60	152	14	15	17	26	35	37	41	22	25	25	32	42	45	49
61	155	11	14	15	25	34	36	42	21	24	25	31	42	45	51
62	157	12	14	16	24	34	36	40	21	23	25	31	40	43	48
63	160	12	13	15	24	33	35	38	22	23	25	32	41	43	50
64	163	11	14	15	23	33	36	40	21	23	24	31	40	43	48
65	165	12	14	15	22	31	34	38	21	23	24	31	40	43	49
66	168	11	13	14	22	31	33	37	21	23	24	30	39	41	44
67	170	12	13	15	21	29	30	35	22	24	25	30	40	43	48
68	173	10	14	15	22	31	32	36	22	24	25	30	37	38	39
69	175		11	12	19	29	31			23	24	30	36	39	
70	178				19							32			
Large Frame															
in	*cm*														
58	147														
59	150				36							45			
60	152				38							44			
61	155		25	26	36	48	50			29	33	41	62	74	
62	157	16	19	22	34	48	48	50	26	28	31	44	56	63	72
63	160	18	20	22	34	48	48	50	27	30	32	43	60	65	77
64	163	16	20	21	32	43	45	49	26	28	29	39	50	55	63
65	165	17	20	21	31	43	46	48	27	28	29	39	56	59	67
66	168	13	17	18	27	40	43	45	23	24	27	35	49	53	69
67	170	13	16	17	30	41	43	49	25	28	30	37	50	53	55
68	173		16	20	29	37	40			28	30	38	51	54	
69	175			21	30	42					27	35	49		
70	178				20							37			

(Adapted from Frisancho AR: New standards of weight and body composition by frame size and height for assessment of nutritional status of adults and the elderly. Am J Clin Nutr 40:808–819, 1984 © American Society for Clinical Nutrition.)

NORMAL RANGE OF FINDINGS | **ABNORMAL FINDINGS**

3. Position the tape horizontally at the midpoint, then tighten it firmly around the arm, but not so tightly as to cause skin contour indentation or pinching (Fig. 6–3).

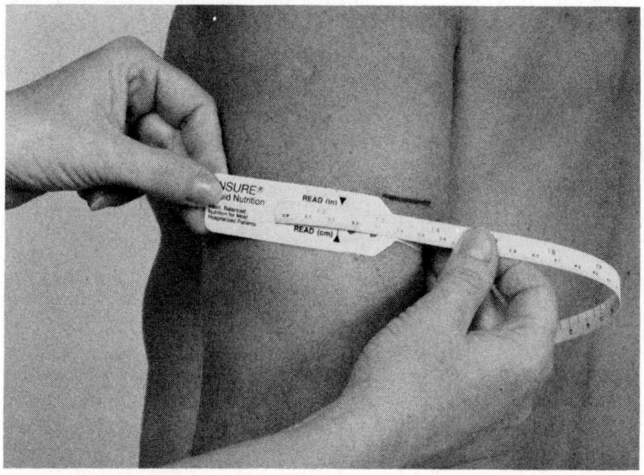

▶ **Figure 6–3**

4. Note and record the measurement (in centimeters) on the appropriate form. Compare with norms (Table 6–8).

Remember that accurate mid-upper arm circumference and triceps skinfold measurements are difficult to obtain and interpret in older adults because of sagging skin, changes in fat distribution, and declining muscle mass.

Individuals whose measurements fall below the 10th percentile or above the 95th percentile warrant further medical and nutritional evaluation. Very high or very low readings may be due to examiner error.

Derived Anthropometric Measures

Although the mid-upper arm circumference is of little value in and of itself, when combined with the triceps skinfold measurement, it is possible to indirectly determine the arm muscle *circumference* and arm muscle *area*.

Mid-Upper Arm Muscle Circumference

Mid-upper arm muscle circumference (MAMC) estimates skeletal muscle reserves or the amount of lean body mass and is derived from the triceps skinfold and mid-upper arm circumference measures using the following formula:

$$\text{MAMC} = \text{MAC} - \frac{\pi \times \text{TSF}}{10}$$

where

$\pi = 3.14$
MAC = mid-upper arm circumference (in cm)
TSF = triceps skinfold (in mm)
MAMC = mid-upper arm muscle circumference (in cm)

Record calculation on data forms. Compare with norms (Table 6–8).

Mid-upper arm muscle circumference is dependent on accurate measurement of the mid-upper arm circumference and triceps skin fold. In general, a mid-upper arm muscle circumference that is 90 percent of standard is suggestive of mild malnutrition; 60 to 90 percent suggests moderate malnutrition; and less than 60 percent is indicative of severe malnutrition.

NORMAL RANGE OF FINDINGS

ABNORMAL FINDINGS

Mid-Arm Muscle Area

Mid-arm muscle area (MAMA) is a good indicator of lean body mass and thus skeletal protein reserves. These reserves are important in growing children, and are especially valuable in evaluating persons who may be malnourished because of chronic illness, multiple surgeries, or inadequate dietary intake.

Table 6-8 ▶ Percentiles of Upper Arm Circumference (mm) and Estimated Upper Arm Muscle Circumference (mm)

	ARM CIRCUMFERENCE (mm)							ARM MUSCLE CIRCUMFERENCE (mm)						
AGE GROUP	5	10	25	50	75	90	95	5	10	25	50	75	90	95
							Males							
1–1.9	142	146	150	159	170	176	183	110	113	119	127	135	144	147
2–2.9	141	145	153	162	170	178	185	111	114	122	130	140	146	150
3–3.9	150	153	160	167	175	184	190	117	123	131	137	143	148	153
4–4.9	149	154	162	171	180	186	192	123	126	133	141	148	156	159
5–5.9	153	160	167	175	185	195	204	128	133	140	147	154	162	169
6–6.9	155	159	167	179	188	209	228	131	135	142	151	161	170	177
7–7.9	162	167	177	187	201	223	230	137	139	151	160	168	177	190
8–8.9	162	170	177	190	202	220	245	140	145	154	162	170	182	187
9–9.9	175	178	187	200	217	249	257	151	154	161	170	183	196	202
10–10.9	181	184	196	210	231	262	274	156	160	166	180	191	209	221
11–11.9	186	190	202	223	244	261	280	159	165	173	183	195	205	230
12–12.9	193	200	214	232	254	282	303	167	171	182	195	210	223	241
13–13.9	194	211	228	247	263	286	301	172	179	196	211	226	238	245
14–14.9	220	226	237	253	283	303	322	189	199	212	223	240	260	264
15–15.9	222	229	244	264	284	311	320	199	204	218	237	254	266	272
16–16.9	244	248	262	278	303	324	343	213	225	234	249	269	287	296
17–17.9	246	253	267	285	308	336	347	224	231	245	258	273	294	312
18–18.9	245	260	276	297	321	353	379	226	237	252	264	283	298	324
19–24.9	262	272	288	308	331	355	372	238	245	257	273	289	309	321
25–34.9	271	282	300	319	342	362	375	243	250	264	279	298	314	326
35–44.9	278	287	305	326	345	363	374	247	255	269	286	302	318	327
45–54.9	267	281	301	322	342	362	376	239	249	265	281	300	315	326
55–64.9	258	273	296	317	336	355	369	236	245	260	278	295	310	320
65–74.9	248	263	285	307	325	344	355	223	235	251	268	284	298	306
							Females							
1–1.9	138	142	148	156	164	172	177	105	111	117	124	132	139	143
2–2.9	142	145	152	160	167	176	184	111	114	119	126	133	142	147
3–3.9	143	150	158	167	175	183	189	113	119	124	132	140	146	152
4–4.9	149	154	160	169	177	184	191	115	121	128	136	144	152	157
5–5.9	153	157	165	175	185	203	211	125	128	134	142	151	159	165
6–6.9	156	162	170	176	187	204	211	130	133	138	145	154	166	171
7–7.9	164	167	174	183	199	216	231	129	135	142	151	160	171	176
8–8.9	168	172	183	195	214	247	261	138	140	151	160	171	183	194
9–9.9	178	182	194	211	224	251	260	147	150	158	167	180	194	198
10–10.9	174	182	193	210	228	251	265	148	150	159	170	180	190	197
11–11.9	185	194	208	224	248	276	303	150	158	171	181	196	217	223
12–12.9	194	203	216	237	256	282	294	162	166	180	191	201	214	220
13–13.9	202	211	223	243	271	301	338	169	175	183	198	211	226	240
14–14.9	214	223	237	252	272	304	322	174	179	190	201	216	232	247
15–15.9	208	221	239	254	279	300	322	175	178	189	202	215	228	244
16–16.9	218	224	241	258	283	318	334	170	180	190	202	216	234	249
17–17.9	220	227	241	264	295	324	350	175	183	194	205	221	239	257
18–18.9	222	227	241	258	281	312	325	174	179	191	202	215	237	245
19–24.9	221	230	247	265	290	319	345	179	185	195	207	221	236	249
25–34.9	233	240	256	277	304	342	368	183	188	199	212	228	246	264
35–44.9	241	251	267	290	317	356	378	186	192	205	218	236	257	272
45–54.9	242	256	274	299	328	362	384	187	193	206	220	238	260	274
55–64.9	243	257	280	303	335	367	385	187	196	209	225	244	266	280
65–74.9	240	252	274	299	326	356	373	185	195	208	225	244	264	279

(From Frisancho AR: New norms of upper limb fat and muscle areas for assessment of nutritional status. Am J Clin Nutr 30:2540–2548, 1981 © American Society for Clinical Nutrition.)

NORMAL RANGE OF FINDINGS | **ABNORMAL FINDINGS**

The equation for calculating MAMA is:

$$\text{MAMA} = \text{MAC} - \frac{\text{MAMC}}{4\pi}$$

where

MAMA = mid-arm muscle area (in cm^2)
MAC = mid-upper arm circumference (in cm)
MAMC = mid-upper arm muscle circumference (in cm)
$4\pi = 4 \times 3.14 = 12.56$

Record calculation on data forms. Compare with norms (Tables 6–6 and 6–7).

Mid-arm muscle area is considered to be a more sensitive measure of long-standing malnutrition than mid-arm muscle circumference. A mid-arm muscle area of 90 percent of standard reflects mild malnutrition; 60 to 90 percent suggests moderate malnutrition; and less than 60 percent indicates severe malnutrition.

Arm Span or Total Arm Length

Measurement of arm span is useful for those situations in which height is difficult to measure, such as in children with cerebral palsy or scoliosis or in aging persons with spinal curvature. Arm span, which is nearly equivalent to height, is sometimes used clinically instead of height (Mitchell and Lipschitz, 1982). Ask the person to hold the arms straight out from the sides of the body. Measure the distance from the tip of the middle finger on one hand to that on the other hand.

Frame Size

Body frame size reflects the sum effects of body width, bone thickness, muscularity, and trunk length relative to height. The Metropolitan Life Insurance Tables of ideal weight for height contain classifications of weight by frame size. Frisancho and Flegel (1983) have proposed measurement of elbow breadth as an index of frame size. To measure it, you must be familiar with the use of skinfold calipers or a broad-blade anthropometer.

1. Instruct the person to extend the right arm forward, perpendicular to the body. Bend the elbow to a 90 degree angle, with the palm of the hand turned laterally.
2. Facing the person, place the skinfold calipers on the condyles of the humerus (a broad-blade anthropometer may be needed if the skinfold calipers do not extend to the breadth of the elbow).
3. Read the distance between the condyles; record measurement (in centimeters) on the appropriate form. Compare with norms (Table 6–9).

Body Mass Index

Body mass index is a simple indicator of total body fat or obesity. In children, adolescent girls, and adults, it provides an especially useful estimate of obesity.

A body mass index of 27 or greater indicates obesity.

$$\text{Body Mass Index} = \frac{\text{Weight}}{\text{Height}^2}$$

where

weight is measured in kilograms
height is measured in meters

NORMAL RANGE OF FINDINGS | **ABNORMAL FINDINGS**

Table 6-9 ▶ Frame Size by Elbow Breadth (cm) of Male and Female Adults in the United States

AGE	FRAME SIZE		
	Small	Medium	Large
yr			
Males			
18–24	≤6.6	>6.6 and <7.7	≥7.7
25–34	≤6.7	>6.7 and <7.9	≥7.9
35–44	≤6.7	>6.7 and <8.0	≥8.0
45–54	≤6.7	>6.7 and <8.1	≥8.1
55–64	≤6.7	>6.7 and <8.1	≥8.1
65–74	≤6.7	>6.7 and <8.1	≥8.1
Females			
18–24	≤5.6	>5.6 and <6.5	≥6.5
25–34	≤5.7	>5.7 and <6.8	≥6.8
35–44	≤5.7	>5.7 and <7.1	≥7.1
45–54	≤5.7	>5.7 and <7.2	≥7.2
55–64	≤5.8	>5.8 and <7.2	≥7.2
65–74	≤5.8	>5.8 and <7.2	≥7.2

(From Frisancho AR: New standards of weight and body composition by frame size and height for assessment of nutritional status of adults and the elderly. Am J Clin Nutr 40:808–819, 1984, 1981 © American Society for Clinical Nutrition.)

DEVELOPMENTAL CONSIDERATIONS

Infants and Children

Weight. As previously mentioned, infants double their birth weight at 4 to 5 months of age and triple it at 1 year. During infancy, childhood, and adolescence, height and weight should be measured at regular intervals, because longitudinal growth is one of the best indices of nutritional status over time.

Skinfold Thickness. Determination of skinfold thickness may be useful in evaluating childhood overnutrition. An estimated 10 percent or more of children in the United States are obese.

Adolescents

Weight. Typically, girls double their body weight between the ages of 8 and 14; boys double their body weight between 10 and 17 years of age.

Skinfold Thickness. If obesity is suspected, measuring skinfold thickness provides an estimate of body fat stores.

The Pregnant Female

Weight. The expectant mother should be considered at nutritional risk if her weight is 10 percent or more below ideal or 20 percent or more above the norm for her height and age group. Appendix 6–2 illustrates approximate weight gain considered normal for each week of pregnancy.

NORMAL RANGE OF FINDINGS | **ABNORMAL FINDINGS**

The Aging Adult

Height. With age, height declines in both men and women very slowly from the early 30s, leading to an average 2.9 cm loss in men and 4.9 cm loss in women (Bowman and Rosenberg, 1982). Height measures may not be accurate in individuals confined to a bed or wheelchair or those over 60 years of age (because of osteoporotic changes). Therefore, arm span, which is correlated with height, may be a better measure for the elderly.

Other Measurements. Mid-arm circumference and triceps skinfold measures may not be accurate and are difficult to obtain in older adults (because of sagging skin, changes in fat distribution, and declining muscle mass) (See Frisancho (1984) for data on weight and triceps skinfold thickness by height in U.S. men and women age 55–74 years.)

LABORATORY STUDIES

Routine laboratory tests are of particular value in nutritional assessment because they are objective, can detect preclinical nutritional deficiencies, and can be used to confirm subjective findings. Use caution, however, when interpreting test results that may be outside normal ranges, because they do not always reflect a nutritional problem and because standards for aging adults have not yet been firmly established.

The best routinely performed laboratory indicators of nutritional status are hemoglobin, hematocrit, cholesterol, triglycerides, total lymphocyte count, and serum albumin. Glucose and total protein levels also provide meaningful information.

Hemoglobin

The hemoglobin determination is used to detect iron deficiency anemia. Normal values include

Infants	
1 to 3 days	14.5 to 22.5 g/dl
2 months	9.0 to 14.0 g/dl
Children	
6 to 12 years	11.5 to 15.5 g/dl
Adults	
Males	14 to 18 g/dl
Females	12 to 16 g/dl

Increased hemoglobin levels are suggestive of hemoconcentration due to polycythemia vera or dehydration.

Decreased hemoglobin levels may indicate anemia, recent hemorrhage, or hemodilution caused by fluid retention.

Hematocrit

Hematocrit, a measure of cell volume, is also an indicator of iron status. Normal values are

Infants	
1 to 3 days	44 to 72 percent
2 months	28 to 42 percent
Children	
6 to 12 years	35 to 45 percent
Adults	
Males	37 to 49 percent
Females	36 to 46 percent

A low value indicates insufficient hemoglobin formation, and for this reason, hematocrit and hemoglobin values should be interpreted together.

NORMAL RANGE OF FINDINGS | **ABNORMAL FINDINGS**

Cholesterol

Total cholesterol is measured to evaluate fat metabolism and to assess the risk of cardiovascular disease. Normal cholesterol concentrations vary with age and sex and may range from 120 mg/dl to 200 mg/dl.

A diet high in saturated fat raises cholesterol levels by stimulating absorption of lipids, including cholesterol from the intestine; a low-saturated-fat diet and/or malnutrition lowers it.

Triglycerides

Serum triglycerides are used to screen for hyperlipidemia and to determine the risk of coronary artery disease. Triglyceride values are age related. Some controversy exists over the most appropriate normal ranges, but the following are fairly widely accepted:

Age	Triglycerides (mg/dl)
0 to 29	10 to 140
30 to 39	10 to 150
40 to 49	10 to 160
50 to 59	10 to 190

Increased serum cholesterol and triglyceride levels lead to increased risk of cardiovascular disease. Decreased serum levels are suggestive of malnutrition.

Total Lymphocyte Count

The most commonly used tests of immune function are total lymphocyte count (TLC) and skin testing, also called delayed cutaneous hypersensitivity testing. Total lymphocyte count is an important indicator of visceral protein status, and therefore, of cellular immune function.

The total lymphocyte count is derived from the white blood cell count (WBC) and the differential count:

$$TLC = WBC \times \frac{\text{Number of Lymphocytes in Differential}}{\text{100 cells}}$$

where TLC is calculated in cells per cubic millimeter.

Normal values for all age categories are between 1800 and 3000 cells/mm^3.

Loss of immunocompetence is strongly correlated with malnutrition in stressed and starving patients.

As standards, Blackburn and associates (1977) recommend using 1500 to 1800 to indicate mild lymphocyte depletion, 900 to 1500 to indicate moderate depletion, and less than 900 to indicate severe depletion.

Skin Testing

Adequate immunity can also be demonstrated by a positive reaction to multiple skin test antigens. In these tests of immune function, antigens are injected intradermally in the forearm area and the response (redness and/or induration) is noted at 24 and 48 hours. A 5 mm or greater response is generally considered to be a positive reaction.

Commonly used antigens in current clinical use are *Candida*, purified protein derivative (PPD), mumps, and tetanus.

Lymphopenia and the lack of a positive response to skin test antigens place the person at increased risk of infection, sepsis, shock, and other complications.

NORMAL RANGE OF FINDINGS | **ABNORMAL FINDINGS**

Serum Albumin

Serum albumin is another common measurement of visceral protein status. Because of its relatively long half-life (17 to 20 days) and large body pool (4.0 to 5.0 g/kg), albumin is not an early indicator of protein malnutrition.

Normal serum albumin concentration in infants and children older than 6 months and adults ranges from 3.5 to 5.5 g/dl.

In general, a serum albumin level of 2.8 to 3.5 g/dl represents moderate visceral protein depletion, and less than 2.8 g/dl denotes severe depletion (Bistrian et al, 1976).

Low serum albumin levels may be caused by reasons other than protein-calorie malnutrition—for example, altered hydration status, blood loss, or blood transfusions.

Serum Transferrin

Levels of serum transferrin, an iron-transport protein, can be measured directly or by an indirect measurement of total iron-binding capacity. Serum transferrin, with a half-life of 8 to 10 days, may be a more sensitive indicator of visceral protein status than albumin.

The most widely used formula for computing serum transferrin is:

$$\text{Serum Transferrin} = (0.8 \times \text{Total Iron-binding capacity}) - 43$$

The normal values for serum transferrin are 170 to 250 mg/dl.

Levels of 150 to 170 mg/dl are considered evidence of mild deficiency; 100 to 150 mg/dl, moderate deficiency; and levels less than 100 mg/dl are indicative of severe deficiency (Rudman, 1987). Because a variety of clinical conditions and incidents can alter serum albumin and transferrin levels, the person's history must be considered in conjunction with these values for accurate interpretation.

Nitrogen Balance

Nitrogen balance is also used as an index of protein nutritional status. Nitrogen is released with the catabolism of amino acids and is excreted in the urine as urea. Nitrogen balance therefore indicates whether the person is anabolic (positive nitrogen balance) or catabolic (negative nitrogen balance).

Nitrogen balance is estimated by a formula based on urine urea nitrogen (UUN) excreted during the previous 24 hours:

$$\begin{aligned}\text{Nitrogen Balance} &= \text{Nitrogen Intake} - \text{Nitrogen Excretion}\\ &= \text{Protein Intake}/6.25 - (\text{24-hr UUN} + 4)\end{aligned}$$

where

Nitrogen balance is determined in grams
24-hr UUN = urinary urea nitrogen; measured in grams
4 = nonurea nitrogen losses via feces, skin, sweat, and lungs; measured in grams

In response to stress and increased protein demand, the body rapidly mobilizes its protein compartments, which results in increased production of urea and excretion of urea in the urine. With infection, an estimated loss of 9 to 11 g/day of UUN can be expected. In patients with major burns, 12 to 18 g/day of urea nitrogen may be expected in the urine (Blackburn et al, 1977).

NORMAL RANGE OF FINDINGS | **ABNORMAL FINDINGS**

Creatinine-Height Index

The creatinine height index (CHI) is a method of estimating the amount of skeletal muscle mass. Creatinine is derived from the breakdown of creatine, an energy-containing complex found in muscle. Creatinine is excreted unchanged in the urine at a constant rate in proportion to the amount of body muscle.

CHI is calculated by first measuring urinary creatinine using a carefully collected 24-hour urine specimen. This value is then compared with ideal urinary creatinine levels from a creatinine for height standard table, by means of the following equation:

$$\text{CHI} = \frac{\text{Actual 24-hr Urine Creatinine}}{\text{Ideal 24-hr Urine Creatinine for Height}} \times 100$$

The person's CHI is then compared with a CHI standard table to determine the degree of skeletal muscle depletion.

The validities of CHI and nitrogen balance studies are dependent on the accuracy of the 24-hour urine collection. Failure to obtain an accurate sample, abnormal renal function, and certain other conditions can result in underestimation of creatinine and nitrogen losses.

Assuming an accurate 24-hour urine specimen has been collected, a CHI of 60 to 80 percent of standard indicates a moderate deficit in body mass. A value of less than 60 percent indicates a severe deficit of body muscle mass (Blackburn, et al, 1977). Stress, fever, and trauma can increase urinary creatinine excretion.

Biocultural Variations in Laboratory Studies

Biocultural variations occur with some laboratory tests, such as measurement of *hemoglobin/hematocrit, serum cholesterol, and serum transferrin.* The normal *hemoglobin level* for blacks is 1 g lower than for other groups, a factor that should be considered in the treatment of anemia. Data indicate that native Americans, Hispanics, Asian Americans, and whites do not differ in this factor.

The difference between blacks and whites with respect to *serum cholesterol* is quite interesting. At birth, blacks and whites have similar serum cholesterol levels but during childhood blacks have higher serum cholesterol levels than whites (5 mg/100 ml). These differences reverse during adulthood when black adults have lower serum cholesterol levels than white adults. The Pima Indians have considerably lower serum cholesterol levels than whites, both during childhood (20 to 30 mg/100 ml lower) and adulthood (50 to 60 mg/100 ml lower).

In a study of children 1 to 3 1/2 years of age, *serum transferrin* levels were found to differ between white and black children. The mean value for white children was 200 to 400 mg/100 ml, whereas the mean of black children was 341.4 (Roode et al, 1975). The higher serum transferrin levels in black children may be due to their lowered hemoglobin/hematocrit levels (Ritchie, 1979). Transferrin levels increase in the presence of anemia. If the hemoglobin and hematocrit levels are normally lower in blacks, then higher transferrin levels should be considered normal (Overfield, 1985).

NORMAL RANGE OF FINDINGS	ABNORMAL FINDINGS

Developmental Considerations

In infancy and childhood, laboratory tests are performed only when undernutrition is suspected or if the child has acute or chronic illnesses that affect nutritional status.

During adolescence, unless overt disease is suspected, laboratory evaluation of hemoglobin and hematocrit levels and urinalysis for glucose and protein levels are adequate.

In pregnancy, hemoglobin and hematocrit values can be used to detect deficiencies of protein, folacin, vitamin B_{12}, and iron. Urine is frequently tested for glucose and protein (albumin), which can signal diabetes, pre-eclampsia, and renal disease.

In older adulthood, all serum and urine data must be interpreted with an understanding of declining renal efficiency and a tendency for aging adults to be overhydrated or underhydrated.

INTERPRETATION OF NUTRITIONAL ASSESSMENT DATA

Based on the findings of the nutritional assessment, the type of malnutrition can be diagnosed. The four major types of malnutrition are obesity, marasmus, kwashiorkor, and marasmus-kwashiorkor mix (Table 6–10). Each type of malnutrition has characteristic clinical and laboratory findings and a distinct cause.

Obesity

In the United States, it is estimated that between 30 and 40 percent of adults are overweight or obese. The term overweight is applied to individuals who are 10 to 20 percent above ideal body weight. Obesity, on the other hand, refers to weights 20 percent or more above ideal body weight. Persons who are 100 percent or more above ideal body weight are categorized as morbidly obese. The causes of overweight and obese conditions are complex and multifaceted; genetic, social, cultural, pathologic, psychological, and physiologic factors have all been implicated. Regardless of its cause, the underlying problem is usually an imbalance of caloric intake and caloric expenditure. In most cases, a small caloric surplus over a long period of time results in the extra pounds. Although visceral protein levels and immunocompetence are generally normal in the obese individual, anthropometric measures are above normal.

Table 6–10 ▶ Classification of Malnutrition

	VISCERAL PROTEINS	ANTHROPOMETRIC MEASURES	IMMUNOCOMPETENCE
Obesity	Normal	Increased	Normal
Marasmus	Normal	Decreased	Normal or Decreased
Kwashiorkor	Decreased	Normal	Decreased
Marasmus/Kwashiorkor Mix	Decreased	Decreased	Decreased

Marasmus

Marasmus (protein-calorie malnutrition) is the result of prolonged starvation or inadequate intake of protein and calories. Anorexia, bowel obstruction, cancer cachexia, and chronic illness are among the clinical conditions leading to marasmus. Marasmus is characterized by decreased anthropometric measures—weight loss and subcutaneous fat and muscle wasting. Visceral protein levels may remain within normal ranges.

Kwashiorkor

Kwashiorkor (protein malnutrition) is associated with diets that may be high in calories but that contain little or no protein. Examples of such diets are low-protein liquid diets, fad diets, and long-term use of dextrose-containing intravenous fluids. Individuals with kwashiorkor, in contrast to those with marasmus, have decreased visceral protein levels and depressed immune function, but generally they have adequate anthropometric measures. These individuals may, therefore, appear well nourished or even obese.

Marasmus-Kwashiorkor Mix

Mixed malnutrition, or marasmus-kwashiorkor mix, combines elements of both marasmus and kwashiorkor. Nutritional assessment findings include muscle, fat, and visceral protein wasting, along with immune incompetence. Individuals with marasmus-kwashiorkor mix are usually those who have undergone acute catabolic stress, such as major surgery, trauma, or burns in combination with prolonged starvation. Without nutritional support, this type of malnutrition is associated with the highest risk of morbidity and mortality.

Serial Assessment

To monitor nutritional status in malnourished individuals or in individuals at risk for malnutrition, serial measurements of nutritional assessment parameters are made at routine intervals. At the minimum, weight, hemoglobin, hematocrit, serum albumin, and total lymphocyte count should be evaluated weekly. Because triceps skinfold thickness, mid-upper arm circumference, and arm muscle circumference measures change more slowly, data on these indicators may be collected biweekly or monthly.

☑ SUMMARY CHECKLIST

1 ▶ Obtain a health history relevant to nutritional status

2 ▶ Elicit dietary history, if indicated

3 ▶ Inspect skin, hair, eyes, oral cavity, nails, and musculoskeletal and neurologic systems for clinical signs and symptoms suggestive of nutritional deficiencies.

4 ▶ Measure height, weight, and other anthropometric parameters, as indicated

5 ▶ Review relevant laboratory tests

SAMPLE RECORDING

Adult

Subjective

▶ No history of diseases or surgery that would alter intake/requirements; no recent weight changes; no appetite changes; socioeconomic history is noncontributory. Does not smoke, drink alcohol, or use illegal, prescription, or OTC drugs; no food allergies. Sedentary lifestyle; plays golf once per week.

Objective

▶ Dietary intake is adequate to meet protein and energy needs. No clinical signs of nutrient deficiencies. Height, weight, and screening laboratory tests within normal ranges.

SAMPLE CLINICAL PROBLEM 1

R.G. is a single, 33-year-old white male high school teacher with a primary diagnosis of acquired immune deficiency syndrome (AIDS).

Subjective

▶ 6 weeks PTA — Diagnosis of AIDS confirmed by positive human immunodeficiency virus antibody (HIV) test. No appetite changes; no anorexia or nausea; no weight loss; occasional "flu-like symptoms" — fever and chills.

1 day PTA — Symptoms include intractable diarrhea (3 to 12 L/day); fever; anorexia; weight loss of 17 kg; and depression. States that he feels helpless and that friends and family are avoiding him. "I would rather just get it over with." Daily caloric intake averages 1000 kcal (usual intake is 2000 kcal).

Objective

- Avoids eye contact and answers questions with short responses during history.

Inspection

- Slightly raised patches resembling milk curds present in mouth. General appearance is pale and cachectic.

Anthropometric

- Height is 166.4 cm (65.5 inches). Current weight is 50.9 kg (112 lbs); usual and ideal body weight is 68 kg (150 lbs). Triceps skinfold measures 8.5 mm (normal value is 12.5).

Laboratory

- Serum albumin (1.86 g/dl) and total lymphocyte count (1000/mm^3) are well below normal ranges. Stool is of watery consistency; stool analysis reveals *Cryptosporidium* infection.

Assessment

- Altered nutrition: less than body requirements R/T anorexia, effects of AIDS, and oral *Candida albicans*
- Malnutrition (marasmus)
- Reactive depression related to diagnosis and future

SAMPLE CLINICAL PROBLEM 2

E.F. is an 87-year-old widow who lives alone in her own home. She has enjoyed good health all of her life.

Subjective

- During the past year, she has experienced declining memory and no longer cooks or drives. Relies on children to take her grocery shopping and prepare occasional meals. Income adequate. Describes her appetite as excellent. Spends her days watching television and reading. Experiences occasional constipation. Eats a well-balanced diet and enjoys high carbohydrate foods such as cookies, candy, and doughnuts because they are easy to chew. Caloric intake is 1800 kcal/day.

Objective

Anthropometric

- Height is 160 cm (63 inches). Current weight is 56.8 kg (125 lbs); usual weight is 56.8 kg (125 lbs), and ideal weight is 56.4 kg (124 lbs).

Laboratory

- Hemoglobin, hematocrit, and albumin values within normal limits. No clinical signs of nutrient deficiencies.

Assessment

- Normal nutriture
- Constipation related to inactivity and diet high in refined carbohydrates

NURSING DIAGNOSES COMMONLY ASSOCIATED WITH NUTRITIONAL DISORDERS

Diagnosis	Related Factors (Etiology)	Defining Characteristics (Symptoms and Signs)
Altered nutrition: less than body requirements	Impaired absorption Alteration in taste or smell Dysphagia Nausea and vomiting Fatigue Inability to chew Decreased level of consciousness Stress Decreased appetite Decreased salivation Effects of hyperanabolic or catabolic states Cancer Burns Infection Effects of aging—decreased sense of taste	Loss of body weight with adequate food intake Body weight 20% or more less than ideal weight for height Aversion to eating Diarrhea and/or steatorrhea Inadequate food intake Triceps skinfold (TSF) <60 percent of standard measurement Midarm circumference (MAC) <60 percent of standard measurement Abdominal pain or cramping Sore, inflamed buccal cavity Pale conjunctival and mucous membranes Poor muscle tone or skin turgor Loss of hair Decreased serum albumin or total protein Decreased serum transferrin or iron binding capacity Metabolic demands in excess of intake Anemia Lack of interest in food Reported or evidence of lack of food
Altered nutrition: more than body requirements	Lack of physical exercise Decreased activity pattern Eating in response to stress or emotional trauma Eating as a comfort measure/substitute gratification Learned eating behaviors Decreased metabolic need Lack of knowledge regarding nutritional needs	Weight 10 percent to 20 percent over ideal for height and frame Reported and observed dysfunctional eating patterns Pairing food with other activities Concentrating food intake at end of day Eating in response to external cues such as time of day Eating in response to internal cues other than hunger, e.g., anxiety

Table continued on following page

Diagnosis	Related Factors (Etiology)	Defining Characteristics (Symptoms and Signs)
	Perceived lack of control Ethnic and cultural values Lack of social support for weight loss Decreased self-esteem Negative body image Feelings of anxiety, depression, guilt, boredom, frustration	Sedentary activity level Triceps skinfold > 15 mm for men and > 25 mm for women

Other related nursing diagnoses:
- Impaired skin integrity (See Chapter 9)
- Fluid volume deficit (See Chapter 9)
- Body image disturbance (See Chapter 10)
- Altered oral mucous membrane (See Chapter 13)
- Fluid volume excess (See Chapter 15)

ABNORMAL FINDINGS

Table 6-11 ► Abnormalities Due to Nutritional Deficiencies

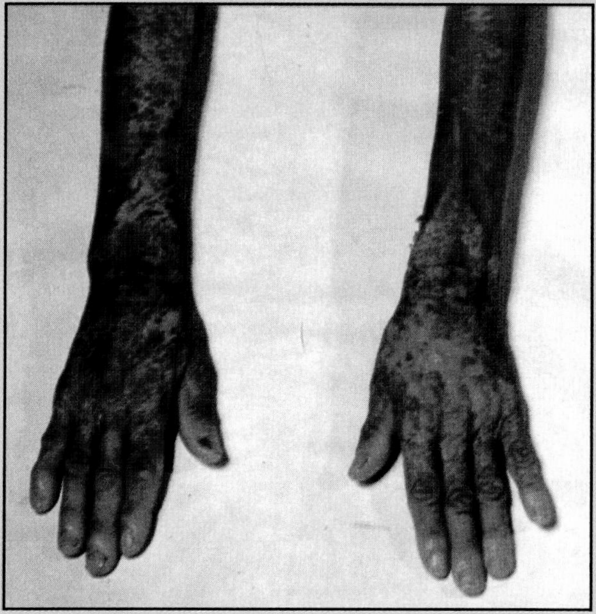

PELLAGRA

Cracks in skin, dermatitis, and lesions resulting from a deficiency of niacin.

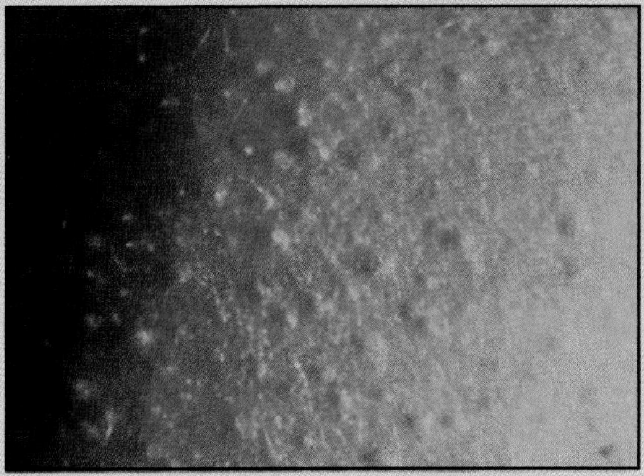

FOLLICULAR HYPERKERATOSIS

Dry, bumpy skin associated with vitamin A and/or linoleic acid (fatty acid) deficiency. Linoleic acid deficiency may also result in eczematous skin, especially in infants.

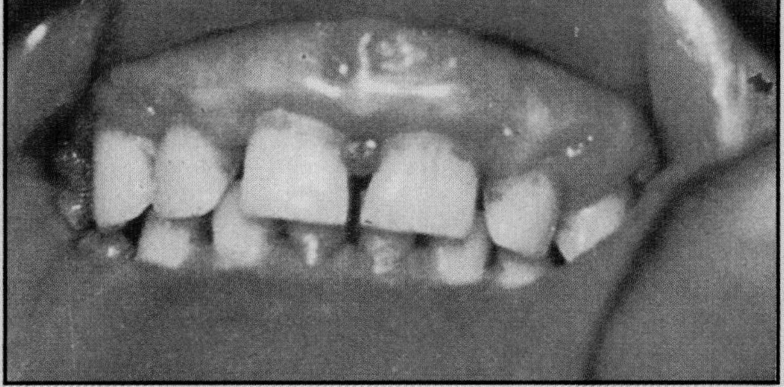

SCORBUTIC GUMS

Deficiency of vitamin C. Gums are swollen, ulcerated, and bleeding.

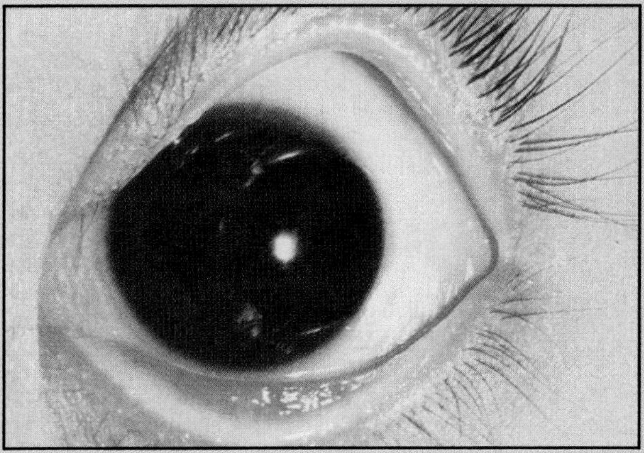

BITOT'S SPOTS

Foamy plaques of the cornea that are a sign of vitamin A deficiency.

Table continued on following page

Table 6-11 ▶ Abnormalities Due to Nutritional Deficiencies *Continued*

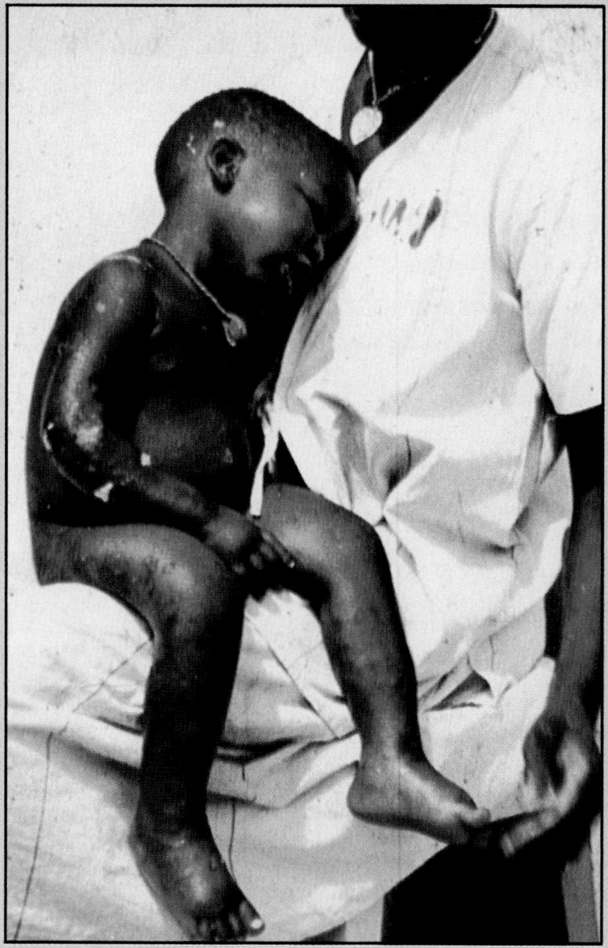

KWASHIORKOR

Occurs in children and adults whose diets contain mostly carbohydrate and are grossly deficient in protein.

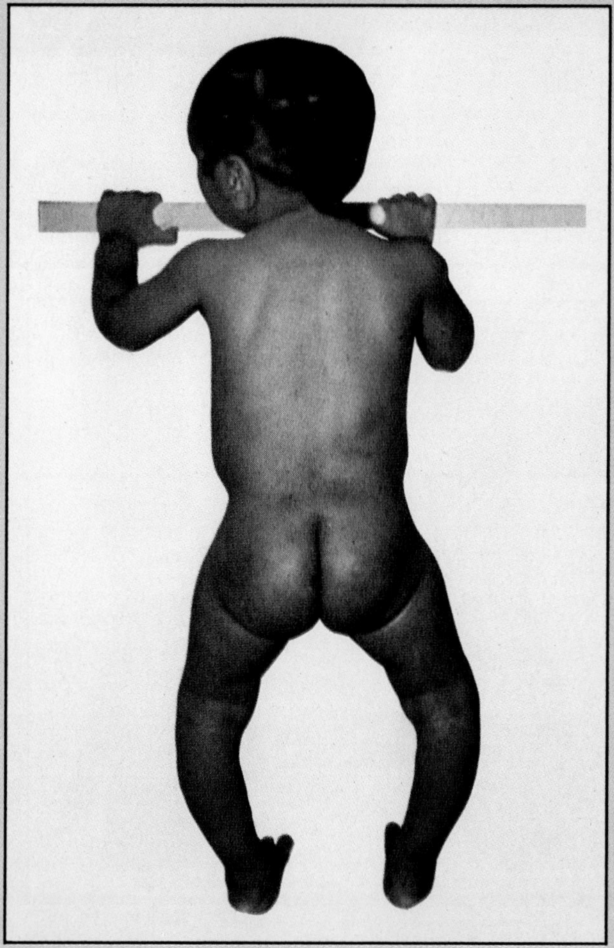

RICKETS

Sign of vitamin D and calcium deficiencies in children and adults (osteomalacia).

TONGUE

"Magenta tongue" is a sign of riboflavin deficiency. In contrast, a pale tongue is probably attributable to iron deficiency; a beefy red-colored tongue is caused by vitamin B-complex deficiency.

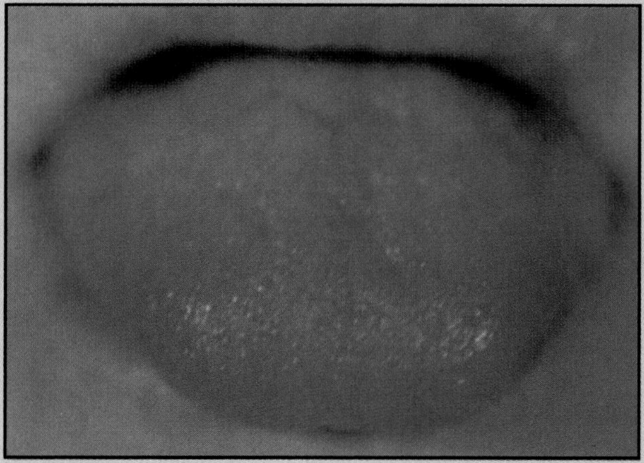

References

Bistrian BR, Blackburn GL, Hallowell EL, Heddle R: Protein status of general surgical patients. J Am Med Assoc 230(6):858–860, 1974.

Blackburn GL, Bistrian BR, Maini BS, Schlamm HT, Smith MF: Nutritional and metabolic assessment of the hospitalized patient. J Parenter Enter Nutr 1(1):11–22, 1977.

Bowman BB, Rosenberg IH: Assessment of nutritional status of the elderly. Am J Clin Nutr 35:1142–1151, 1982.

Frisancho AR, Flegel PN: Elbow breadth as a measure of frame size for U.S. males and females. Am J Clin Nutr 31:311–314, 1983.

Frisancho AR: New standards of weight and body composition by frame size and height for assessment of nutritional status of adults and the elderly. Am J Clin Nutr 40:808–819, 1984.

Garn SM, Clark DC: Nutrition, growth, development, and maturation: Findings from the ten-state nutrition survey of 1968–1970. Pediatrics 56(2):306–319, 1975.

Harris JA, Benedict FG: A Biometric Study of Basal Metabolism in Man. Washington, D.C.: Carnegie Institute Publication, 1919.

Long CL: Energy and protein requirements in stress and trauma. Crit Care Nurs Curr 2(2):7–12, 1984.

Mitchell CO, Lipschitz DA: Arm length measurement as an alternative to height in nutritional assessment of the elderly. J Parenter Enter Nutr 6:226–229, 1982.

Mullen JL, Gertner MH, Buzby GP, et al: Implications of malnutrition in the surgical patient. Arch Surg 114:121–125, 1979.

Pennington JAT, Church HN: Bowes and Church's Food Values of Portions Commonly Used. 13th Edition. Philadelphia, J.B. Lippincott, 1980.

Recommended Daily Dietary Allowances, Revised 1980. Washington, DC, National Academy of Sciences, National Research Council Food and Nutrition Board, 1980.

Roode H, Prinsloo JG, Laubscher NF, et al.: Serum transferrin levels in White and Black toddlers. S Afr Med J 49(9):319–321, 1975.

Rudman D: Assessment of nutritional status. *In* Braunwald E, Isselbacher KJ, Petersdorf RG, et al: (Eds): Harrison's Principles of Internal Medicine. 11th ed. New York, McGraw-Hill, 1987, pp 390–393.

Young EA, Brennan EH, Irving GL: Update: nutritional analysis of fast foods. Diet Curr 8(2):1–12, 1981.

Bibliography

Bray GA, Jordan HA, Sims EAH: Evaluation of the obese patient. I. An algorithm. J Am Med Assoc 235:1487–1491, 1976.

Christakis G (Ed): Nutritional Assessment in Health Programs. Washington, DC, American Public Health Association, 1973.

Fanelli MT, Stevenhagen KJ: Consistency of energy and nutrient intakes of older adults: 24-hour recall vs. 1-day food record. J Am Diet Assoc 86:655–667, 1986.

Fomon SJ, Haschke F, Ziegler EE, Nelson SE: Body composition of reference children from birth to age 10 years. Am J Clin Nutr 35:1169–1175, 1982.

Frisancho AR: Triceps skinfold and upper arm muscle size norms for assessment of nutritional status. Am J Clin Nutr 27:1052–1053, 1974.

Frisancho AR: New norms of upper limb fat and muscle areas for assessment of nutritional status. Am J Clin Nutr 30:2540–2548, 1981.

Gleason C: Nutritional assessment of boys with physical deformities: Stature estimation (abstract). Fed Proc 42:1044, 1983.

Grant JP, Custer PB, Thurlow J: Current techniques of nutritional assessment. Symposium on surgical nutrition. Surg Clin North Am 61:437–463, 1981.

Grant JP: Nutritional assessment in clinical practice. Nutr Clin Pract 1(1):3–11, 1986.

Hamill PV, Drizd TA, Johnson CL, et al: Physical growth: Nutritional Center for Health Statistics Percentiles. Am J Clin Nutr 32:607–629, 1979.

Hattner JAT, Kerner, JA, Jr: Nutritional assessment of the pediatric patient. *In* Kerner JA, Jr (Ed): Manual of Pediatric Parenteral Nutrition. New York, John Wiley & Sons, 1983, pp 19–60.

Jelliffe DB: The assessment of the nutritional status of the community. World Health Organization Monograph, Series 53, 1966.

Karkeck JM: Assessment of nutritional status of the elderly. Nutr Supp Serv 4(10):23–33, 1984.

Keithley JK: Nutritional assessment of the patient undergoing surgery. Heart Lung 14(5):449–456, 1985.

Krey SH, Murray RL (Eds): Dynamics of Nutrition Support: Assessment, Implementation, Evaluation. Norwalk, CT, Appleton-Century-Crofts, 1986.

McLaren DS, Meguid MM: Nutritional assessment at the crossroads. J Parenter Enter Nutr 7(6):575–579, 1983.

Overfield T: Biologic Variation in Health and Illness: Race, Age, and Sex Differences. Menlo Park, CA, Addison-Wesley Publishing, 1985.

Owens G, Lippman G: Nutritional status of infants and young children. Pediatr Clin North Am 24:211–227, 1977.

Parsons HG, Francoeur TE, Howland P, et al: The nutritional status of hospitalized children. Am J Clin Nutr 33:1140–1146, 1980.

Pollack MM, Wiley JS, Kanter R, Holbrook PR: Malnutrition in critically ill infants and children. J Parenter Enter Nutr 6:20–24, 1982.

Ritchie RF: Specific proteins. *In* Henry JB (Ed): Clinical Diagnosis and Management by Laboratory Methods. Philadelphia, WB Saunders Company, 1979.

Roche AF, Himes JH: Incremental growth charts. Am J Clin Nutr 33:2041–2052, 1980.

Russell RM: Evaluating the nutritional status of the elderly. Clin Nutr 2:4–8, 1983.

Spector RE: Cultural Diversity in Health and Illness. 2nd ed. Norwalk, CT, Appleton-Century-Crofts, 1985.

Spencer H, Kramer L, Osis D: Factors contributing to calcium loss in aging. Am J Clin Nutr 36:776–787, 1982.

Sutphen JL: Growth as a measure of nutritional status. J Pediatr Gastroenterol Nutr 4:169–181, 1985.

Taylor KB, Anthony LE: Clinical Nutrition. New York, McGraw-Hill, 1983.

Twomey P, Ziegler D, Rombeau, J: Utility of skin testing in nutritional assessment: A critical review. J Parenter Enter Nutr 6:50–58, 1980.

Appendix 6–1 ▶ Recommended Dietary Allowances*

CATEGORY	AGE (YEARS) OR CONDITION	WEIGHT† (kg)	WEIGHT† (lb)	HEIGHT‡ (cm)	HEIGHT‡ (in)	PROTEIN (g)	FAT-SOLUBLE VITAMINS: Vitamin A (μg RE)‡	Vitamin D (μg)§	Vitamin E (mg α-TE)‖	Vitamin K (μg)
Infants	0.0–0.5	6	13	60	24	13	375	7.5	3	5
	0.5–1.0	9	20	71	28	14	375	10	4	10
Children	1–3	13	29	90	35	16	400	10	6	15
	4–6	20	44	112	44	24	500	10	7	20
	7–10	28	62	132	52	28	700	10	7	30
Males	11–14	45	99	157	62	45	1,000	10	10	45
	15–18	66	145	176	69	59	1,000	10	10	65
	19–24	72	160	177	70	58	1,000	10	10	70
	25–50	79	174	176	70	63	1,000	5	10	80
	51+	77	170	173	68	63	1,000	5	10	80
Females	11–14	46	101	157	62	46	800	10	8	45
	15–18	55	120	163	64	44	800	10	8	55
	19–24	58	128	164	65	46	800	10	8	60
	25–50	63	138	163	64	50	800	5	8	65
	51+	65	143	160	63	50	800	5	8	65
Pregnant						60	800	10	10	65
Lactating	1st 6 months					65	1,300	10	12	65
	2nd 6 months					62	1,200	10	11	65

WATER-SOLUBLE VITAMINS: Vitamin C (mg)	Thiamin (mg)	Riboflavin (mg)	Niacin (mg NE¶)	Vitamin B_6 (mg)	Folate (μg)	Vitamin B_{12} (μg)	MINERALS: Calcium (mg)	Phosphorus (mg)	Magnesium (mg)	Iron (mg)	Zinc (mg)	Iodine (μg)	Selenium (μg)
30	0.3	0.4	5	0.3	25	0.3	400	300	40	6	5	40	10
35	0.4	0.5	6	0.6	35	0.5	600	500	60	10	5	50	15
40	0.7	0.8	9	1.0	50	0.7	800	800	80	10	10	70	20
45	0.9	1.1	12	1.1	75	1.0	800	800	120	10	10	90	20
45	1.0	1.2	13	1.4	100	1.4	800	800	170	10	10	120	30
50	1.3	1.5	17	1.7	150	2.0	1,200	1,200	270	12	15	150	40
60	1.5	1.8	20	2.0	200	2.0	1,200	1,200	400	12	15	150	50
60	1.5	1.7	19	2.0	200	2.0	1,200	1,200	350	10	15	150	70
60	1.5	1.7	19	2.0	200	2.0	800	800	350	10	15	150	70
60	1.2	1.4	15	2.0	200	2.0	800	800	350	10	15	150	70
50	1.1	1.3	15	1.4	150	2.0	1,200	1,200	280	15	12	150	45
60	1.1	1.3	15	1.5	180	2.0	1,200	1,200	300	15	12	150	50
60	1.1	1.3	15	1.6	180	2.0	1,200	1,200	280	15	12	150	55
60	1.1	1.3	15	1.6	180	2.0	800	800	280	15	12	150	55
60	1.0	1.2	13	1.6	180	2.0	800	800	280	10	12	150	55
70	1.5	1.6	17	2.2	400	2.2	1,200	1,200	320	30	15	175	65
95	1.6	1.8	20	2.1	280	2.6	1,200	1,200	355	15	19	200	75
90	1.6	1.7	20	2.1	260	2.6	1,200	1,200	340	15	16	200	75

* The allowances, expressed as average daily intakes over time, are intended to provide for individual variations among most normal persons as they live in the United States under usual environmental stresses. Diets should be based on a variety of common foods in order to provide other nutrients for which human requirements have been less well defined. See text for detailed discussion of allowances and of nutrients not tabulated.

† Weights and heights of Reference Adults are actual medians for the U.S. population of the designated age, as reported by NHANES II. The median weights and heights of those under 19 years of age were taken from Hamill et al. (1979). The use of these figures does not imply that the height-to-weight ratios are ideal.

‡ Retinol equivalents. 1 retinol equivalent = 1 μg retinol or 6 μg β-carotene. See text for calculation of vitamin A activity of diets as retinol equivalents.

§ As cholecalciferol. 10 μg cholecalciferol = 400 IU of vitamin D.

‖ α-Tocopherol equivalents. 1 mg d-α tocopherol = 1 α-TE. See text for variation in allowances and calculation of vitamin E activity of the diet as α-tocopherol equivalents.

¶ 1 NE (niacin equivalent) is equal to 1 mg of niacin or 60 mg of dietary tryptophan.

(From Recommended Dietary Allowances Revised. Washington, D.C., Food and Nutrition Board, National Academy of Sciences, National Research Council, 1989.)

Appendix 6–2 ▶ Pattern of Normal Prenatal Weight Gain

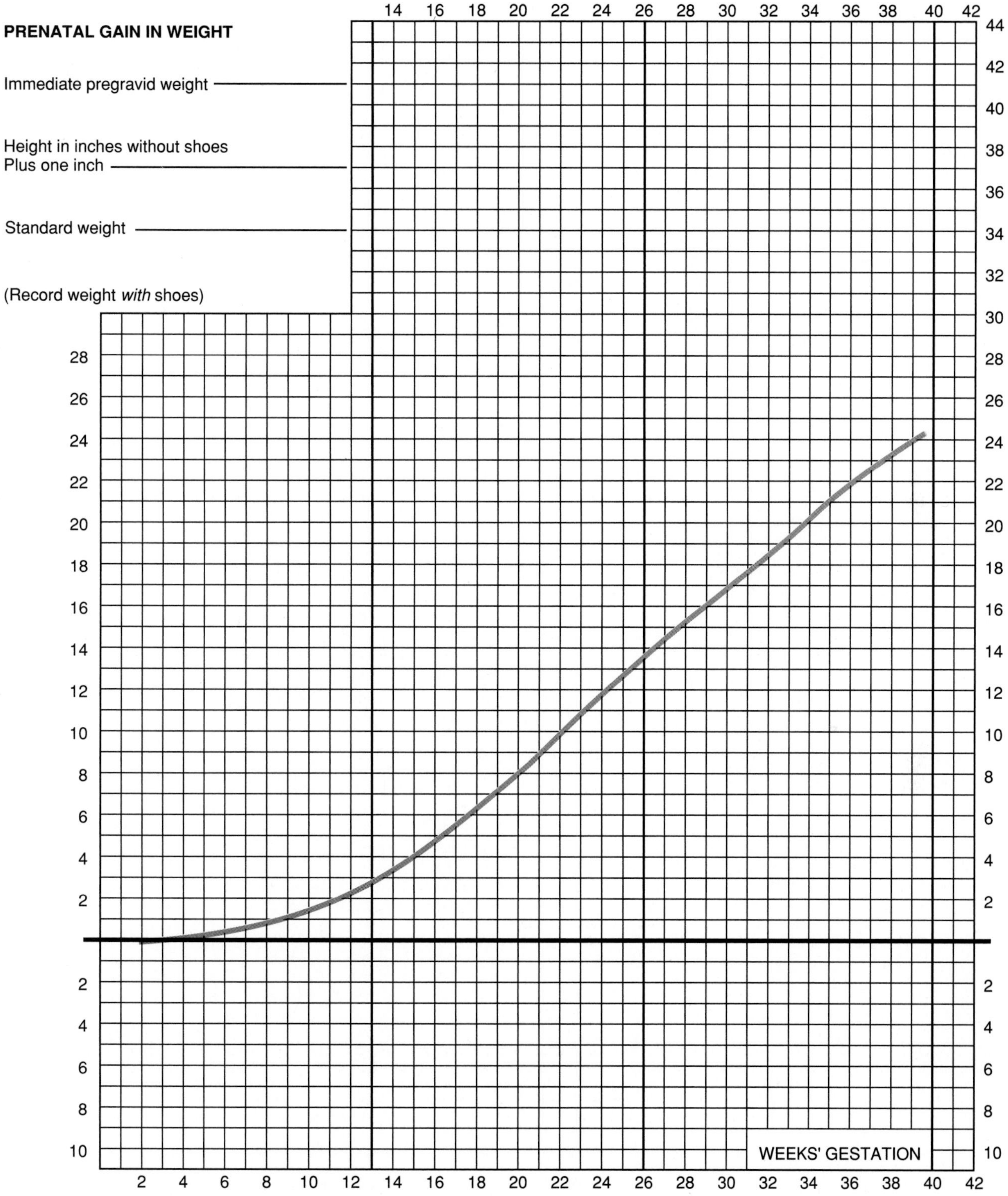

Pattern of normal prenatal weight gain. (From Committee on Maternal Nutrition, Food and Nutrition Board, National Research Council, National Academy of Sciences: *Maternal Nutrition and the Course of Pregnancy.* Washington, D.C.: Government Printing Office, 1970.)

UNIT

2 Physical Examination

CHAPTER

7 Assessment Techniques and Approach to the Clinical Setting

The health history described in the preceding chapters provides *subjective* data for health assessment, the individual's *own* perception of the health state. Unit 2 presents *objective* data, the signs perceived by the examiner through the physical examination.

The physical examination requires that the examiner develop technical skills and a knowledge base. The technical skills are the tools to gather data. You will relate those data to your knowledge base and to your previous experience. A sturdy knowledge base enables you to look *for,* rather than merely look *at.* Consider a statement by the eighteenth century German poet Goethe, "We see only what we know." In order to recognize a significant finding, you need to know what to look for.

CULTIVATING YOUR SENSES

You will use your senses—sight, smell, touch, and hearing—to gather data during the physical examination. You always have perceived the world through your senses, but now they will be focused in a new way. Applying your senses to assess each individual's health state may seem awkward at first, but this will be polished with repetition and tutored practice. The skills requisite for the physical examination are inspection, palpation, percussion, and auscultation. The skills are performed one at a time and in this order.

Inspection

Inspection is concentrated watching. It is close careful scrutiny, first of the individual as a whole and then of each body system. Inspection begins the moment you first meet the individual and develop a "general assessment." (Specific data to consider for the general assessment are presented in the following chapter.) Then as you proceed through the examination, start the assessment of each body system with inspection.

Inspection always comes first. Initially, you may feel embarrassed "staring" at the person without also "doing something." But do not be too eager to touch the person. A focused inspection takes time, and yields a surprising amount of data. Train yourself not to rush through inspection by placing your hands in your pockets or holding them behind your back.

Learn to use each person as his or her own control and compare the right and left sides of the body. The two sides are nearly symmetric. Inspection requires good lighting, adequate exposure, and occasional use of certain instruments (otoscope, ophthalmoscope, penlight, nasal and vaginal specula) to enlarge your view.

Palpation

Palpation follows and often confirms points you noted during inspection. Palpation applies your sense of touch to assess these factors: texture, temperature, moisture, organ location and size, as well as any swelling, vibration or pulsation, rigidity or spasticity, crepitation, presence of lumps or masses, and presence of tenderness or pain. Different parts of the hands are best suited for assessing different factors:

- Fingertips—Best for fine tactile discrimination, such as skin texture, swelling, pulsatility, and determining presence of lumps.
- A grasping action of the fingers—To detect the position, shape, and consistency of an organ or mass.
- The dorsa (backs) of hands and fingers—Best for determining temperature because the skin here is thinner than on the palms.
- Base of fingers (metacarpophalangeal joints) or ulnar surface of the hand—Vibration.

Your palpation technique should be slow and systematic. A person stiffens when touched suddenly, making it difficult for you to feel very much. Use a calm, gentle approach. Warm your hands by kneading them together or holding them under warm water. Identify any tender areas, and palpate them last.

Start with light palpation to detect surface characteristics and to accustom the person to being touched. Then perform deeper palpation, perhaps by helping the person use relaxation techniques such as imagery or deep breathing. Your sense of touch is blunted with heavy or continuous pressure. When deep palpation is needed (as for abdominal contents), intermittent pressure is better than one long continuous palpation. Bimanual palpation requires the use of both of your hands to envelop or capture certain body parts or organs, such as the kidneys, uterus, or adnexa, for more precise delimitation (see Chapters 17 and 22.)

Percussion

Percussion is tapping the person's skin with short, sharp strokes in order to assess underlying structures. The strokes yield a palpable vibration and a characteristic sound that depicts the location, size, and density of the underlying organ. Why learn percussion when an x-ray study is so much more accurate? Because your percussing hands are always available, are easily portable, give instant feedback, and have no radiative side effects. Percussion has the following uses:

- Mapping out the *location* and *size* of an organ by exploring where the percussion note changes between the borders of an organ and its neighbors.
- Signaling the *density* (air, fluid, or solid) of a structure by a characteristic note.
- Detecting an abnormal mass if it is fairly superficial. The percussion vibrations penetrate about 5 cm deep. A deeper mass would give no change in percussion.
- Eliciting pain if the underlying structure is inflamed, as with sinus areas or over the kidney.
- Eliciting a deep tendon reflex using the percussion hammer.

There are two methods of percussion — *direct* (sometimes called immediate) and *indirect* (or mediate). In direct percussion, the striking hand directly contacts the body wall. This produces a sound and is used in percussing the infant's thorax or the adult's sinus areas. *Indirect* percussion is used more often, and involves both hands. The striking hand contacts the stationary hand fixed on the person's skin. This yields a sound and a subtle vibration. This is the procedure.

The Stationary Hand. Hyperextend the middle finger (sometimes called the pleximeter) and place its distal portion, the phalanx and distal interphalangeal joint, *firmly* against the person's skin. Avoid the person's ribs and scapulae. Percussing over a bone yields no data because it always sounds "dull." Lift the rest of the stationary hand up off the person's skin (Fig. 7–1). Otherwise the resting hand will dampen off the produced vibrations, just as a drummer uses the hand to halt a drum roll.

The Striking Hand. Use the middle finger of your dominant hand as the *striking* finger (sometimes called the plexor) (Fig. 7–2). Hold your forearm close to the skin surface with your upper arm and shoulder steady. Scan

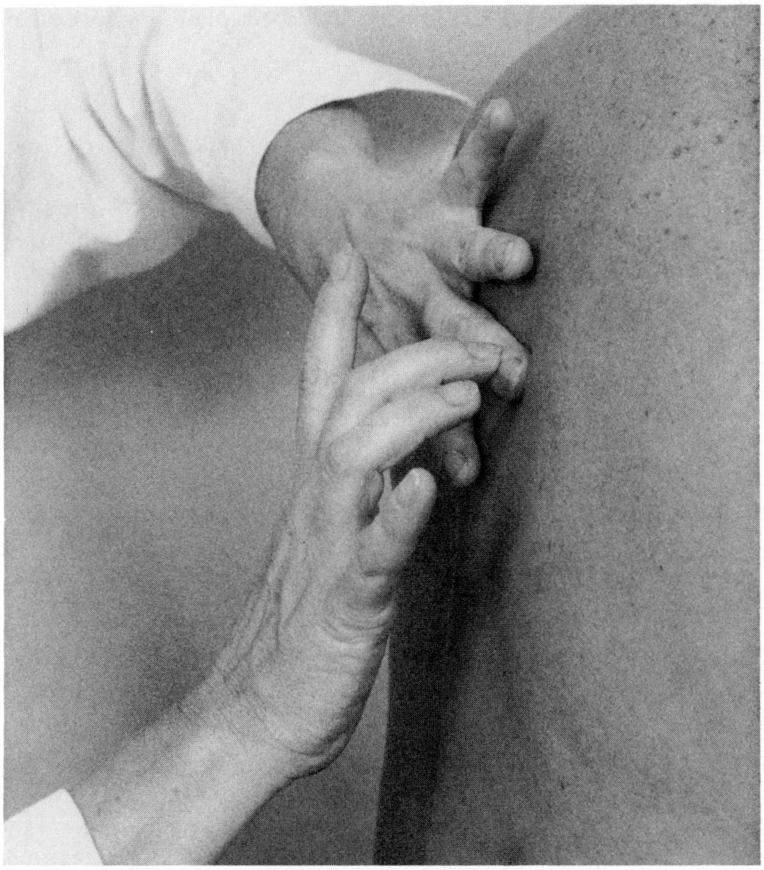

► **Figure 7–1**

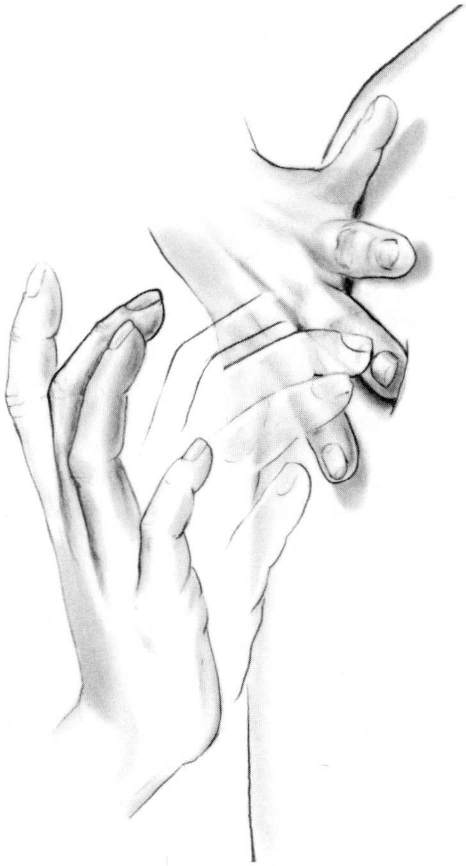

► **Figure 7–2**

your muscles to make sure they are steady but not rigid. The action is all in the wrist and it *must* be relaxed. Spread your fingers, swish your wrist, and bounce your middle finger off of the stationary one. Aim for just behind the nail bed or at the distal interphalangeal joint; the goal is to hit the portion of the finger that is pushing the hardest into the skin surface. Flex the striking finger so that its tip, not the finger pad, makes contact. It hits directly at right angles to the stationary finger.

Percuss two times in this location using even staccato blows. Lift the striking finger off quickly; a resting finger damps off vibrations. Then move to a new body location and repeat, keeping your technique even. The force of the blow determines the loudness of the note. You do not need a very loud sound; use just enough force to achieve a clear note. The thickness of the person's body wall will be a factor. You will need a stronger percussion stroke for persons with obese or very muscular body walls.

Percussion can be an awkward technique for beginning examiners. You may feel surprised and embarrassed when your striking finger misses your stationary hand completely. You may wince when the fingernail of your striking finger is too long and painfully gouges your stationary finger. As with all new skills, refinement follows practice. After a few weeks your hand placement becomes precise and feels natural, and your ears learn to perceive the subtle difference in percussion notes.

Production of Sound. All sound results from vibration of some structure (Fig. 7–3). Percussing over a body structure causes vibrations that produce characteristic waves and are heard as "notes" (Table 7–1). Each of the five percussion notes is differentiated by the following components.

1. **Amplitude** (or intensity), a loud or soft sound. The louder the sound, the greater the amplitude. Loudness depends on the force of the blow and the structure's ability to vibrate.
2. **Pitch** (or frequency), the number of vibrations per second, written as "cps," or cycles per second. More rapid vibrations produce a high-pitched tone, slower vibrations yield a low-pitched tone.
3. **Quality** (timbre), a subjective difference due to a sound's distinctive overtones. A pure tone is a sound of one frequency. Variations within a sound wave produce overtones. Overtones allow you to distinguish a C on a piano from a C on a violin.
4. **Duration,** the length of time the note lingers.

A basic principle is that a structure with relatively more air (such as the lungs) produces a louder, deeper, and longer sound because it vibrates freely. However, a denser, more solid structure (such as the liver) gives a softer, higher, shorter sound, because it does not vibrate as easily. Although Table 7–1 describes five "normal" percussion notes, there are variations in clinical practice. The "note" you hear depends on the nature of the underlying structure, as well as the thickness of the body wall and your correct technique. Do not learn these various notes just from written description. Practice on a willing partner.

Auscultation

Auscultation is listening to sounds produced by the body, such as the heart and blood vessels and the lungs and abdomen. Likely you already have heard certain body sounds with your ear alone, for example the harsh gurgling of very congested breathing. However, most body sounds are very soft and must be channeled through a *stethoscope* for you to evaluate them. The stethoscope does not magnify sound, but does block out extraneous room sounds. Of all the equipment you will use, the stethoscope quickly becomes a very personal

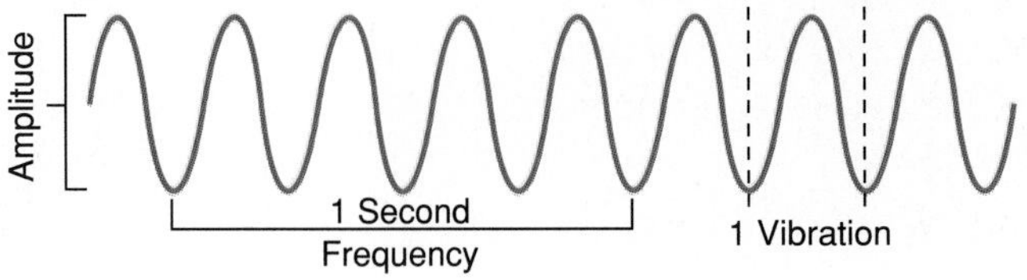

▶ **Figure 7–3**

Table 7-1 ► Characteristics of Percussion Notes

	AMPLITUDE	PITCH	QUALITY	DURATION	SAMPLE LOCATION
Resonant 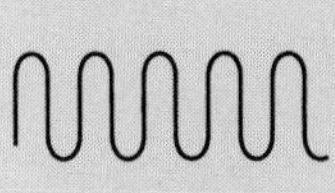	Medium-loud	Low	Clear, hollow	Moderate	Over normal lung tissue
Hyperresonant 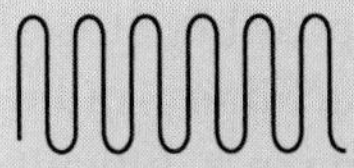	Louder	Lower	Booming	Longer	Normal over child's lung. In the adult, over lungs with abnormal amount of air, as in emphysema
Tympany 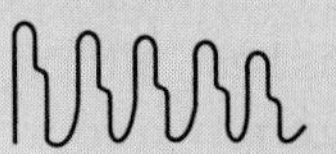	Loud	High	Musical and drumlike (like the kettle drum)	Sustained longest	Over air-filled viscus, e.g., the stomach, the intestine
Dull 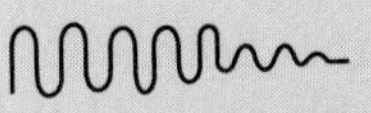	Soft	High	Muffled thud	Short	Relatively dense organ, as liver or spleen
Flat 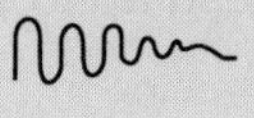	Very soft	High	A dead stop of sound, absolute dullness	Very short	When no air is present, over thigh muscles, bone, or over tumor

instrument. Take time to learn its features and to fit one individually to yourself.

The fit and quality of the stethoscope are important. You cannot assess what you cannot hear through a poor instrument. The slope of the earpieces should point forward toward your nose. This matches the natural slope of your ear canal and efficiently blocks out environmental sound. If necessary, use pliers to parallel the slope of the earpieces with that of your ear canals. The earpieces should fit snugly but if they hurt, they are inserted too far. Adjust the tension and experiment with different rubber or plastic earplugs to achieve the most comfort. The tubing should be of thick material, with an internal diameter of 4 mm (1/8 in), and about 30 to 36 cm (12 to 14 in) long. Longer tubing may distort the sound.

Choose a stethoscope with two endpieces—a diaphragm and a bell (Fig. 7-4). You will use the *diaphragm* most often because its flat edge is best for high-pitched sounds—breath, bowel, and normal heart sounds. Hold the diaphragm firmly against the person's skin, firm enough to leave a slight ring afterward. The *bell* endpiece has a deep, hollow cuplike shape. It is best for soft, low-pitched sounds such as extra heart sounds or

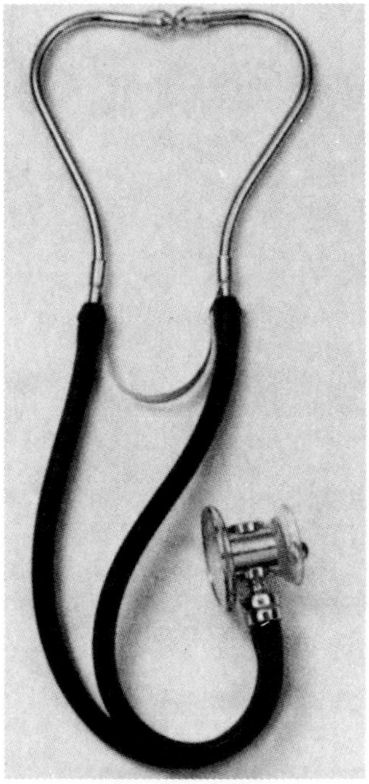

► **Figure 7-4**

murmurs. Hold it lightly against the person's skin; just enough that it forms a perfect seal. Any harder causes the person's skin to act as a diaphragm, obliterating the low-pitched sounds.

Before you can evaluate body sounds, you must eliminate any confusing artifacts. Any extra room noise can produce a "roaring" in your stethoscope, so the room must be quiet. Keep the examination room warm. If the person starts shivering, the involuntary muscle contractions could drown out other sounds. Also warm the endpiece by rubbing it in your palm. This avoids the "chandelier sign" elicited when placing a cold endpiece on a warm chest! Also, the friction on the endpiece from a male's hairy chest causes a crackling sound that mimics an abnormal breath sound called crackles or rales. To minimize this problem, wet the hair before auscultating the area. Finally, avoid your own "artifact," such as breathing on the tubing, or the "thump" from bumping the tubing together.

Auscultation is a skill that beginning examiners are eager to learn, but one that is difficult to master. First, you must learn the wide range of normal sounds. Once you can recognize normal sounds, you can distinguish the abnormal sounds and "extra" sounds. Be aware that in some body locations you may hear more than one sound; this can be confusing. You will need to listen selectively, to only one thing at a time. As you listen, ask yourself: What am I *actually hearing* and what *should* I be hearing at this spot?

SETTING

The examination room should be warm and comfortable, quiet, private, and well lit. When possible, stop any distracting noises, such as humming machinery, radio or television, people talking, that could make it difficult to hear body sounds. Your time with the individual should be secure from interruptions from other health care personnel. Lighting with natural daylight is best, although it is often not available; artificial light from two sources will suffice and will avoid shadows. A gooseneck stand lamp is needed for high-intensity lighting.

Position the examination table so that both sides of the person are easily accessible. The table should be at a height from which you can stand without stooping and should be equipped to raise the person's head up to 45

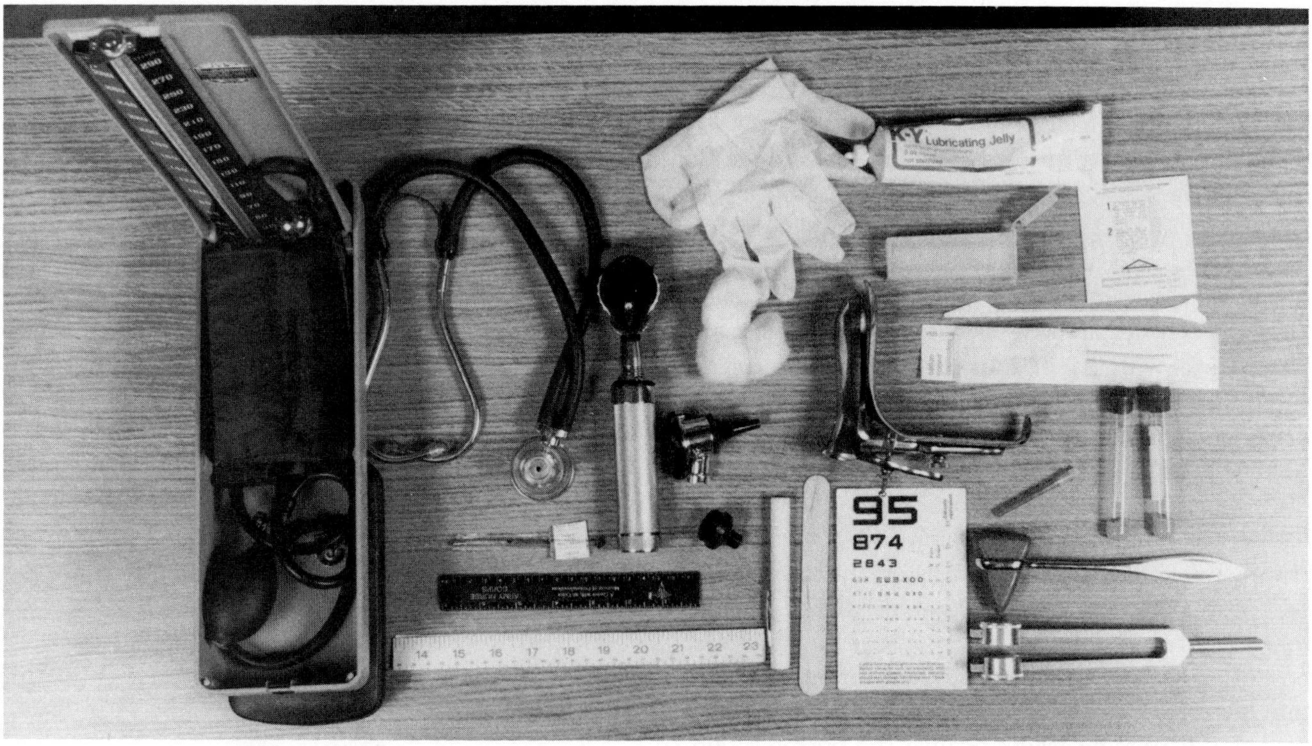

▶ **Figure 7–5**

degrees. A roll-up stool is used for the sections of the examination for which you must be sitting. A bedside stand or table is needed to lay out all your equipment.

EQUIPMENT

During the examination, you do not want to be searching for equipment or to have to leave the room to find an item. Have all your equipment at easy reach and laid out in an organized fashion (Fig. 7–5). These items are usually needed for a screening physical examination:

sphygmomanometer
stethoscope with bell and diaphragm endpieces
thermometer
flashlight or penlight
otoscope/ophthalmoscope
tuning fork
nasal speculum (if a short, broad speculum is not included with the otoscope)
tongue depressor
pocket vision screener
skin marking pen
flexible tape measure and ruler marked in cm
reflex hammer
sharp object (sterile needle or split tongue blade)
cotton balls
bivalve vaginal speculum
clean gloves
materials for cytologic study
lubricant
guaiac test reagents

Most of the equipment is described as it comes into use throughout the text. However, take some time now for introductory comments on the otoscope and ophthalmoscope.

The *otoscope* funnels light into the ear canal and onto the tympanic membrane. The base serves both as the power source by holding a battery and as the handle. To attach the head, press it down onto the male adaptor end of the base and turn clockwise until you feel a stop. To turn the light on, press the red button rheostat down and clockwise. (Always turn it off after use to increase the life of the bulb and battery.) There are five different-sized specula available to attach to the head (Fig. 7–6). (The short broad speculum is for viewing the nares.) Choose the largest one that will fit comfortably into the person's ear canal. See Chapter 12 for technique on use of the otoscope.

The *ophthalmoscope* illuminates the internal eye structures. Its system of lenses and mirrors enables you to look through the pupil at the fundus (background) of the eye, much like looking through a keyhole at a room beyond. The ophthalmoscope head attaches to the base male adaptor just as the otoscope head does (Fig. 7–7). The head has five different parts:

1. Viewing aperture, with 5 different apertures
2. Aperture selector dial on the front
3. Mirror window on the front
4. Lens selector dial
5. Lens indicator

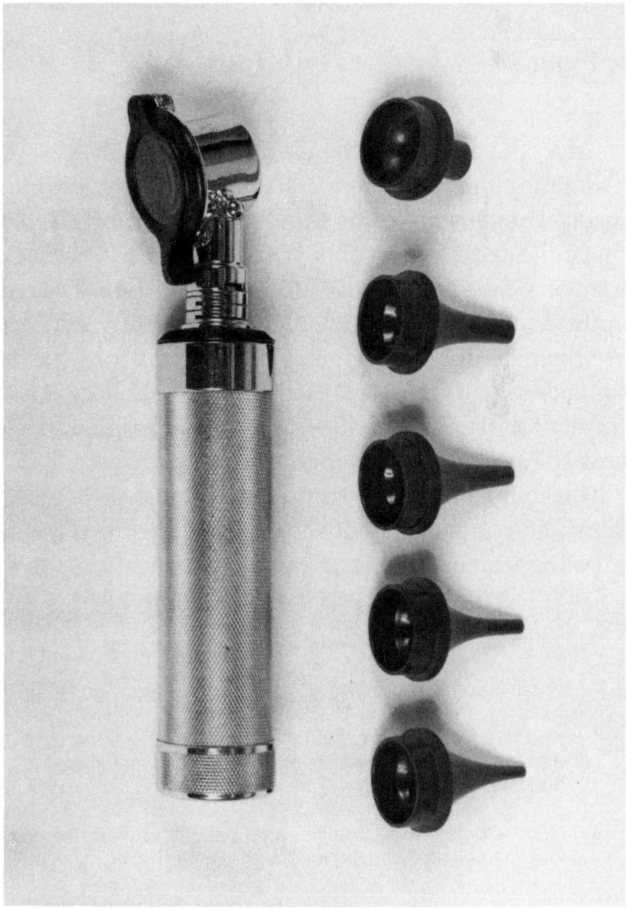

► **Figure 7–6**

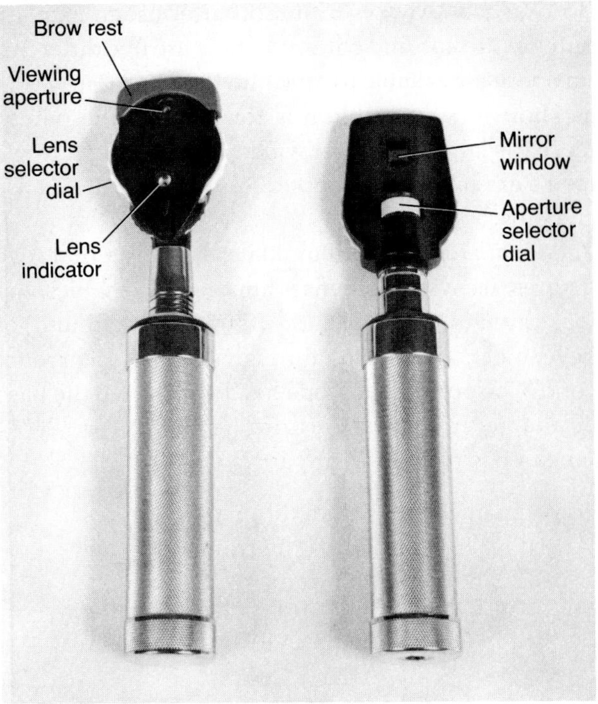

▶ **Figure 7-7**

Select the aperture to be used (Fig. 7-8).

Rotating the lens selector dial brings the object into focus. The lens indicator shows a number, or *diopter,* that indicates the value of the lens in position. The black numbers indicate a positive lens, from 0 to +40. The red numbers indicate a negative lens, from 0 to −20. The ophthalmoscope can compensate for myopia (nearsightedness) or hyperopia (farsightedness) but will not correct for astigmatism. See Chapter 11 for details on how to hold the instrument and what to inspect.

The following equipment occasionally will be used depending on the individual's needs: fetoscope for auscultating fetal heart tones, pelvimeter to measure pelvic width, and a goniometer to measure joint range of motion.

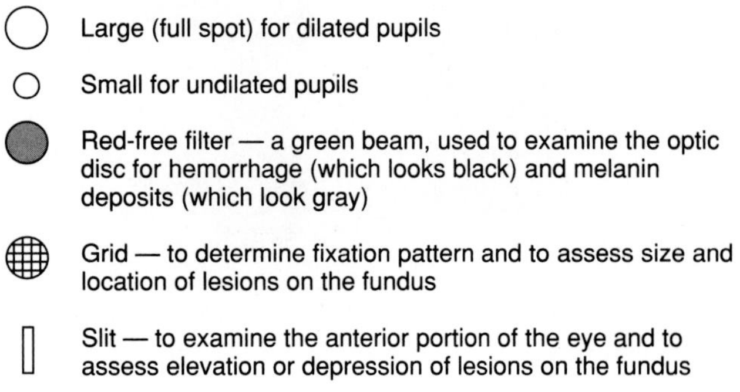

Large (full spot) for dilated pupils
Small for undilated pupils
Red-free filter — a green beam, used to examine the optic disc for hemorrhage (which looks black) and melanin deposits (which look gray)
Grid — to determine fixation pattern and to assess size and location of lesions on the fundus
Slit — to examine the anterior portion of the eye and to assess elevation or depression of lesions on the fundus

▶ **Figure 7-8**

For a child you also will need: appropriate pediatric-sized endpieces for stethoscope and otoscope specula, materials for developmental assessment, appropriate-age toys, and a nipple or pacifier for an infant.

APPROACH TO THE CLINICAL SETTING

General Approach

Consider your emotional state and that of the person being examined. The person is usually anxious, owing to the anticipation of being examined by a stranger and the unknown outcome of the examination. If anxiety can be reduced, the person will feel more comfortable and the data gathered will more closely describe the person's natural state. Anxiety can be reduced by an examiner who is confident and self-assured, as well as considerate and unhurried.

Usually, a beginning examiner feels anything *but* self-assured! Most worry about their technical skill, about missing something significant, or about forgetting a step. Many are embarrassed themselves about encountering a partially dressed individual. All these fears are natural and common. The best way to minimize them is with a lot of tutored practice on a healthy willing subject, usually a fellow student. You have to feel comfortable with your motor skills before you can absorb what you are actually seeing or hearing in a "real" client. This comes with practice under the guidance of an experienced tutor, in an atmosphere in which it is acceptable to make mistakes and to ask questions. Your subject should "act like a real client" so that you can deal with the "real" situation while still in a safe setting. After you feel comfortable with the laboratory setting, accompany your tutor as he or she examines an actual client so that you can observe an experienced examiner.

With this preparation, it is possible to interact with your own client in a confident manner. Begin by measuring the person's height, weight, blood pressure, temperature, pulse, and respirations (see Chapter 8). If needed, measure visual acuity at this time using the Snellen eye chart. All these are familiar, relatively nonthreatening actions; they will gradually accustom the person to the examination. Then ask the person to change into an examining gown, leaving the underpants on. This will feel more comfortable, and the underpants easily can be removed just before the genital examination. Unless your assistance is needed, leave the room as the person undresses.

As you reenter the room, wash your hands in the person's presence. This indicates you are protective of this person and are starting fresh for him or her. Explain each step in the examination and how the person can cooperate. Encourage the person to ask questions. Keep your own movements slow, methodical, and deliberate. Begin by touching the person's hands, checking skin color, nail beds, and metacarpophalangeal joints (see Chapters 9 and 19). Again, this is a less threatening way to ease a person into being touched. Most people are used to having relative strangers touch their hands.

As you proceed through the examination, avoid distractions and concentrate on one step at a time. The sequence of the steps may differ depending on the age of the person and your own preference. However, you should establish a system that works for you and stick to it to avoid omissions. Organize the steps so the person does not change positions too often. Although proper exposure is necessary, use additional drapes to maintain the person's privacy and to prevent chilling.

Do not hesitate to write out the examination sequence and refer to it as you proceed. The client will accept this as quite natural if you explain you are making brief notations to ensure accuracy. Many agencies use a printed form. You will find you will glance at the form less and less as you gain experience. Even with a form, you sometimes may forget a step in the examination. When you realize this, perform the maneuver in the next logical place in the sequence. (See Chapter 24 for the sequence of steps in the complete physical examination.)

As you proceed through the examination, occasionally offer some brief teaching about the person's body. For example, you might say, "This tapping on your back (percussion) is a little like playing different drums. The different notes I hear tell me where each organ starts and stops. You probably can hear the difference yourself from within your body." Or, "Everyone has two sounds for each heartbeat, something like this—lub-dup. Your own beats sound normal." Do not do this with every single step, or you will be hard pressed to make a comment when you do come across an abnormality. But some sharing of information builds rapport and increases the person's confidence in you as an examiner. It also gives the person a little more control in a situation in which it is easy to feel completely helpless.

At some point, you will want to linger in one location to concentrate on some complicated findings. To avoid anxiety, tell the person, "I always listen to heart sounds on a number of places on the chest. Just because I am listening a long time does not necessarily mean anything is wrong with you." And it follows that sometimes you will discover a finding that may be abnormal and you want another examiner to double check. You need to give the person some information, yet you should not alarm the person unnecessarily. Say something like, "I do not have a complete assessment of your heart sounds. I want Ms. Wright to listen to you too."

At the end of the examination, summarize your findings and share the necessary information with the person. Thank the person for the time spent. In a hospital setting, apprise the person of what is scheduled next. Before you leave a hospitalized person, lower the bed, make the person comfortable and safe, and return the bedside table, television, or any equipment to the way it was originally.

Developmental Considerations

The Younger Person

Children are different from adults. Their difference in size is obvious. Their bodies grow in a predictable pattern that is assessed during the physical examination. However, their behavior also is different. Behavior grows and develops through predictable stages, just as the body does. Each examiner needs to know the expected emotional and cognitive features of these stages and to perform the physical examination based on developmental principles (Erikson, 1963; Yoos, 1981; Whaley and Wong, 1990).

With all children, the goal is to increase their comfort in the setting. This approach reveals their natural state as much as possible and will give them a more positive memory of health care providers. Remember that a "routine" examination is anything but routine to the child. You can increase their comfort by attending to the following developmental principles and approaches. The *order* of the stages is more meaningful than the exact chronologic age. Each child is an individual and will not fit exactly into one category. For example, if your efforts to "play games" with the preschooler are rebuffed, modify your approach to the security measures used with the toddler.

THE INFANT

Erikson defines the major task of infancy as establishing trust. An infant is completely dependent on the parent for his or her basic needs. If these needs are met promptly and consistently, the infant feels secure and learns to trust others.

Position

- The parent is always present to understand normal growth and development and for child's feeling of security.
- Place the neonate or young infant flat on a padded examination table. The infant also may be held against the parent's chest for some steps.
- Once the baby can sit without support (around 6 months), as much of the examination as possible should be performed while the infant is in the parent's lap.
- By 9 to 12 months, the infant is acutely aware of the surroundings. Anything outside the infant's range of vision is "lost," so the parent must be in full view.

Preparation

- Timing should be 1 to 2 hours after feeding, when the baby is not too drowsy nor too hungry.
- Maintain a warm environment. A neonate may require an overhead radiant heater.
- An infant will not object to being nude. Have the parent remove outer clothing and leave a diaper on a boy.
- An infant does not mind being touched, though make sure your hands and stethoscope endpiece are warm.
- Use a soft, crooning voice during the examination; the baby responds more to the feeling in the tone of the voice than to what is actually said.
- An infant likes eye contact; lock eyes from time to time.
- Smile; a baby prefers a smiling face to a frowning one. (Often beginning examiners are so absorbed in their technique that they look serious or stern.) Take time to play.
- Keep movements smooth and deliberate, not jerky.
- Use a pacifier for crying or during invasive steps.
- Offer brightly colored toys for a distraction when the infant is fussy.
- Let an older baby touch the stethoscope or tongue blade.

Sequence

- Seize the opportunity with a sleeping baby to listen to heart, lung, and abdomen sounds first.
- Perform least distressing steps first. (See the sequence in Chapter 24.) Save the invasive steps of examination of the eye, ear, nose, and throat until last.
- Elicit the Moro reflex at the end of the examination.

THE TODDLER

This is Erikson's stage of developing autonomy. However, the need to explore the world and be independent is in conflict with the basic dependency on the parent. This often results in frustration and negativism. The toddler may be difficult to examine; do not take this personally. Since he or she is acutely aware of the new environment, the toddler may be frightened and cling to the parent. Also, the toddler has fear of invasive procedures and dislikes being restrained.

Position

- Sitting up on parent's lap for all of examination. When the toddler must be supine (as in the abdominal examination), move chairs to sit knee-to-knee with parent. Have the toddler lie in the parent's lap with the toddler's legs in your lap.
- Enlist the aid of a cooperative parent to help position the toddler during invasive procedures. The child's legs can be captured between the parent's. An arm of the parent can encircle the child's head, holding it against the chest and the other arm can hold the child's arms. (See Figure 13–25 in Chapter 13.)

Preparation

- Children of 1 or 2 years of age can understand symbols, so a security object, such as a special blanket or teddy bear, is helpful.
- Begin by greeting the child and the accompanying parent by name, but with a child 1 to 6 years old, focus more on the parent. By essentially "ignoring" the child at first, you allow the child to adjust gradually and to size you up from a safe distance. Then turn your attention gradually to the child, at first to a toy or object the child is holding, or perhaps to compliment a dress, the hair, or what a big girl or boy the child is. If the child is ready, you will note these signals: eye contact with you, smiling, talking with you, or accepting a toy or a piece of equipment.
- A 2-year-old child does not like to take off his or her clothes; have the parent undress one part at a time.
- Children 1 or 2 years of age like to say "No." Do not offer a choice when there really is none. Avoid saying, "May I listen to your heart now?" When the 1- or 2-year-old child says "No," and you go ahead and do it anyway, you lose trust. Instead, use clear firm instructions, in a tone that expects cooperation, "Now it is time for you to lie down so I can check your tummy."
- Also, 1- or 2-year-old children like to make choices. When possible, enhance autonomy by offering the

limited option, "Shall I listen to your heart next, or your tummy?"
- Demonstrate the procedures on the parent.
- Praise the child when he or she is cooperative.

Sequence
- Collect some objective data during the history, which is a less stressful time. While you are focusing on the parent, note the child's gross motor and fine motor skills and gait.
- Begin with "games," the Denver II test, or cranial nerve testing.
- Start with nonthreatening areas. Save distressing procedures, such as examination of the head, ear, nose, or throat, for last.

PRESCHOOL CHILD

This stage displays developing initiative. The preschooler takes on tasks independently and plans the task and sees it through. A child of this age is often cooperative, helpful, and easy to involve. However, children of this age have fantasies and may see illness as punishment for being "bad." The concept of body image is limited. The child fears any body injury or mutilation, so he or she will recoil from invasive procedures, e.g. tongue blade, rectal temperature, injection, and venipuncture.

Position
- With a 3-year-old child, the parent should be present and may hold the child on his or her lap.
- A 4- or 5-year-old child usually feels comfortable on the examining table, with the parent present.

Preparation
- A preschooler can talk. Verbal communication becomes helpful now, but remember that the child's understanding is still limited. Use short, simple explanations.
- The preschooler is usually willing to undress. Leave underpants on until the genital examination.
- Talk to the child and explain the steps in the examination exactly.
- Do not allow a choice when there is none.
- As with the toddler, enhance the autonomy of the preschooler by offering choice when possible.
- Allow the child to play with equipment to reduce fears.
- A preschooler likes to help; have the child hold the stethoscope for you.
- Use games. Have the child "blow out" the light on the penlight as you listen to the breath sounds. Or, pretend to listen to the heart sounds of the child's teddy bear first. One technique that is absorbing to a preschooler is to trace their shape on the examining table paper (Whaley and Wong, 1990). You can comment on how big the child is, then fill in the outline with a heart or stomach and listen to the paper doll first. After the examination, the child can take the paper doll home as a souvenir.
- Use a slow, patient, deliberate approach. Do not rush.
- During the examination give the preschooler needed feedback and reassurance, "Your tummy feels just fine."
- Compliment the child on his or her cooperation.

Sequence
- Examine the thorax, abdomen, extremities, and genitalia first. Though the preschooler is usually cooperative, continue to assess head, eye, ear, nose, and throat last.

THE SCHOOL-AGED CHILD

During the school-aged period, the major task of the child is developing industry. The child is developing basic competency in school and in social networks and desires the approval of parents and teachers. When successful, the child has a feeling of accomplishment. During the examination, the child is cooperative and is interested in learning about the body. Language is more sophisticated now but do not overestimate and treat the school-aged child as a small adult. The child's level of understanding does not match that of his or her speech.

Position
- Sitting on examination table.
- A 5-year-old child has a sense of modesty. To maintain privacy, let the older child (an 11- or 12-year-old child) decide whether parents or siblings should be present.

Preparation
- Break the ice with small talk about family, school, friends, music, or sports.
- The child should undress himself or herself, leave underpants on, and use a gown and drape.
- Demonstrate equipment—a school-aged child is curious to know how equipment works.
- Comment on the body and how it works. An 8- or 9-year-old child has some understanding of the body and is interested to learn more. It is rewarding to see

the child's eyes light up when he or she hears the heart sounds.

Sequence

- As with the adult, progress from head to toes.

The Adolescent

The major task of adolescence is developing a self-identity. This takes shape from various sets of values and different social roles (son or daughter, sibling, and student). In the end, each person needs to feel satisfied and comfortable with who he or she is. In the process, the adolescent is increasingly self-conscious and introspective. Peer group values and acceptance are important.

POSITION

- Sitting on the examination table.
- Examine the adolescent alone, without parent or sibling present.

PREPARATION

- The body is changing rapidly. During the examination, the adolescent needs feedback that his or her own body is healthy and developing normally.
- The adolescent has keen awareness of body image, often comparing himself or herself to peers. Apprise the adolescent of the wide variation among teenagers on the rate of growth and development (see Sex Maturity Rating, Chapters 14, 21, and 22).
- Communicate with some care. Do not treat the teenager like a child, but do not overestimate and treat him or her like an adult either.
- Since the person is idealistic at this age, the adolescent is ripe for health teaching. Positive attitudes developed now may last through adult life. Focus your teaching on ways the adolescent can promote wellness.

SEQUENCE

- As with the adult, a head-to-toe approach is appropriate. Examine genitalia last, and do it quickly.

The Aging Adult

During later years, the tasks are developing the meaning of life and one's own existence and adjusting to the inevitability of death. Erikson's term is integrity versus despair.

POSITION

- Sitting on the examination table.
- Arrange the sequence to allow as few position changes as possible.
- Allow rest periods when needed.

PREPARATION

- Adjust examination pace to meet possible slowed pace of the aging person. It is better to break the complete examination into a few visits than to rush through the examination and turn off the person.
- Use physical touch (unless there is a cultural contraindication). This is especially important with aging person because other senses, such as vision and hearing, may be diminished.
- Do not mistake diminished vision or hearing for confusion. Confusion of sudden onset may signify a disease state. It is noted by short-term memory loss, diminished thought process, diminished attention span, and labile emotions (see Mental Health Assessment, Chapter 5).
- Be aware that aging years contain more of life's stress. Loss is inevitable, including changes in physical appearance of the face and body, declining energy level, loss of job through retirement, loss of financial security, loss of long-time home, and death of friends or spouse. How the person adapts to these losses significantly affects health assessment.

SEQUENCE

- Use the head-to-toe approach as in the younger adult.

The Ill Person

For the person in some distress, alter the position during the examination. For example, a person with shortness of breath or ear pain may want to sit up, whereas a person with faintness or overwhelming fatigue may want to be supine. Initially, it may be necessary just to examine the body areas appropriate to the problem, collecting a *mini data base.* You may return to finish a complete assessment after the initial distress is resolved.

Bibliography

Blaesing S, Brockhaus J: The development of body image in the child. Nurs Clin North Am 7:597–607, 1972.

Blair KA: Aging: Physiological aspects and clinical implications. Nurse Pract 15(2):14–28, 1990.

Brazelton TB: Infants and Mothers: Individual Differences in Development. New York, Dell Publishing, 1983.
Burggraf V, Donlon B: Assessing the elderly: System by system. AJN 85:974–984, 1985.
Colwell CB, Smith J: Determining the use of physical assessment skills in the clinical setting. J Nurs Educ 24(8):333–337, 1985.
Erikson EH: Childhood and Society. New York, WW Norton, 1963.
Holbrook J, Schneiderman H: Honing physical diagnostic skills. Patient Care 24(7):123–141, 1990.
Ilg FL, Ames LB: Child Behavior. New York, Harper & Row, 1955.
Rebenson-Piano M: The physiologic changes that occur with aging. Crit Care Nurs Q 12(1):1–14, 1989.
Smith J: Big differences in little people. AJN 88(4):459–462, 1988.
Whaley LF, Wong DL: Nursing Care of Infants and Children. 4th ed. St. Louis, CV Mosby Co., 1990.
Yoos L: A developmental approach to physical assessment. MCN 6:168–170, 1981.

CHAPTER

8 General Assessment, Measurement, Vital Signs

THE GENERAL ASSESSMENT

The general assessment is a survey of the whole person, covering the general health state and any obvious physical characteristics. It is an introduction for the physical examination that will follow; it should give an overall impression, a "gestalt," of the person (see sample recording, p. 218) Objective parameters are used to form the general assessment, but these apply to the whole person not just to one body system.

Begin building a general assessment from the moment you first encounter the person. What leaves an immediate impression? Does the person stand promptly as his or her name is called and walk easily to meet you? Or does the person look sick, rising slowly or with effort, with shoulders slumped and eyes without luster or downcast? Is the hospitalized person conversing with visitors, involved in reading or television, or lying perfectly still? Even as you introduce yourself and shake hands, you collect data. Does the person fully extend the arm, shake your hand firmly, make eye contact, or smile? Are the palms dry or wet and clammy? As you proceed through the health history, the measurements, and the vital signs, note the following points that will add up to the general assessment. Consider these four areas: physical appearance, body structure, mobility, and behavior.

NORMAL RANGE OF FINDINGS	ABNORMAL FINDINGS
PHYSICAL APPEARANCE	
Age — The person appears his or her stated age.	Appears older than stated age, as with chronic illness, chronic alcoholism.
Sex — Sexual development is appropriate for gender and age.	Delayed or precocious puberty.
Level of consciousness — The person is alert and oriented, attends to your questions and responds appropriately.	Confused, drowsy, lethargic (see Table 5–3).
Skin color — Color tone is even, pigmentation varying with genetic background, skin is intact with no obvious lesions.	Pallor, cyanosis, jaundice, any lesions (see Chapter 9).
Facial features — Facial features are symmetric with movement.	Immobile, masklike; asymmetric, drooping (see Table 10–5).
There are no signs of acute distress.	Respiratory signs — shortness of breath, wheezing. Pain, indicated by facial grimace, holding body part.
BODY STRUCTURE	
Stature — The height appears within normal range for age, genetic heritage. (See Measuring Height, p. 185.)	Excessively short or tall (see Table 8–8).

NORMAL RANGE OF FINDINGS	ABNORMAL FINDINGS
Nutrition—The weight appears within normal range for height and body build. Body fat distribution is even.	Cachectic, emaciated. Simple obesity, with even fat distribution. Centripetal (truncal) obesity—fat concentrated in face, neck, trunk, with thin extremities, as in Cushing's syndrome (hyperadrenalism).
Symmetry—Body parts look equal bilaterally and are in relative proportion to each other.	Unilateral atrophy or hypertrophy. Asymmetric location of a body part.
Posture—The person stands comfortably erect as appropriate for age. Note the normal "plumb line" through anterior ear, shoulder, hip, patella, ankle. Exceptions are the standing toddler who has a normally protuberant abdomen ("toddler lordosis") and the aging person who may be stooped with kyphosis.	Rigid spine and neck; moves as one unit, e.g., arthritis. Stiff and tense, ready to spring from chair, fidgety movements. Shoulders slumped; looks deflated, e.g., depression.
Position—The person sits comfortably in a chair or on the bed or examination table, arms relaxed at sides, head turned to examiner.	Tripod—leaning forward with arms braced on chair arms, occurs with chronic pulmonary disease. Sitting straight up and resists lying down, e.g., left-sided congestive heart failure. Curled up in fetal position, e.g., acute abdominal pain.
Body build, contour—Proportions are: 1. Arm span (fingertip to fingertip) equals height. 2. Body length from crown to pubis roughly equal to length from pubis to sole.	Elongated arm span, arm span greater than height, e.g., Marfan's syndrome, hypogonadism (see Table 8–8).
Obvious physical deformities—Note any congenital or acquired defects.	Missing extremities or digits; webbed digits.

MOBILITY

NORMAL RANGE OF FINDINGS	ABNORMAL FINDINGS
Gait—Normally, the base is as wide as the shoulder width; foot placement is accurate, the walk is smooth, even, and well-balanced; and associated movements, such as symmetric arm swing, are present.	Exceptionally wide base. Staggered, stumbling. Shuffling, dragging nonfunctional leg. Limping with injury. Propulsion—difficulty stopping (see Table 20–7).
Range of motion—Note full mobility for each joint, and that movement is deliberate, accurate, smooth, and coordinated. (See Chapter 19 for information on more detailed testing of joint range of motion.)	Limited joint range of motion. Paralysis—absent movement. Movement jerky, uncoordinated.
No involuntary movement.	Tics, tremors, seizures (see Table 20–6).

NORMAL RANGE OF FINDINGS	ABNORMAL FINDINGS

BEHAVIOR

Facial expression — The person maintains eye contact (unless there is a cultural taboo), expressions are appropriate to the situation, e.g., thoughtful, serious, or smiling. (Note expressions both while the face is at rest and while the person is talking.)	Flat, depressed, angry, sad, anxious. However, note that anxiety is common in ill people. Also, some people smile when they are anxious.
Mood and affect — The person is comfortable and cooperative with the examiner, and interacts pleasantly.	Hostile, distrustful, suspicious, crying.
Speech — Articulation (the ability to form words) is clear and understandable.	Dysarthria, dysphagia. Speech defect, monotone, garbled speech.
The stream of talking is fluent, with an even pace.	Extremes of few words or constant talking.
The person conveys ideas clearly.	
Word choice is appropriate to culture and education.	
The person communicates in prevailing language easily by himself or herself or with an interpreter.	
Dress — Clothing is appropriate to the climate, looks clean and fits the body, and is appropriate to the person's culture and age group, e.g., normally, Amish women wear clothing from the nineteenth century, Indian women wear saris, Arab men wear long robes. Culturally determined dress should not be labeled as bizarre by Western standards.	Trousers too large and held up by belt suggest weight loss, as does the addition of new holes in belt. If the belt is moved to a looser fit, it may indicate obesity or ascites. Consistent wear of certain clothing may provide clues: neck scarves may conceal thyroidectomy scar; long sleeves may conceal needle marks of drug abuse; broad brimmed hats may reveal sun intolerance of lupus erythematosus; Velcro fasteners instead of buttons may indicate chronic motor dysfunction.
Personal hygiene — The person appears clean and groomed appropriately for his or her age, occupation, and socioeconomic group. (Note that a wide variation of dress and hygiene is "normal." Many cultures do not include use of deodorant or women shaving legs.)	
Hair is groomed, brushed. Women's make-up is appropriate for age and culture.	In a previously carefully groomed woman, unkept hair and absent make-up may indicate malaise or illness.

DEVELOPMENTAL CONSIDERATIONS

The Younger Person

Note the same basic elements as with the adult, with consideration to age and development.

NORMAL RANGE OF FINDINGS	ABNORMAL FINDINGS
Behavior—Note the response to stimuli and level of alertness appropriate for age.	
Parental bonding—Note the child's interactions with parents, that parent and child show a mutual response and are warm and affectionate, appropriate to the child's condition. The parent provides appropriate physical care of child and promotes new learning.	Some signs of child abuse are that the child avoids eye contact; the child exhibits no separation anxiety when you would expect it for age; the parent is disgusted by child's odor, sounds, drooling, or stools. Deprivation of physical or emotional care. Signs of physical abuse (see Chapter 9).

The Aging Adult

Physical appearance—By the eighth and ninth decades, body contour is sharper, with more angular facial features, and body proportions are redistributed. See measuring weight and height, p. 199.

Posture—A general flexion occurs by the 8th or 9th decade.

Gait—Older adults often use a wider base to compensate for diminished balance, arms may be held out to help balance, and steps may be shorter or uneven.

MEASUREMENT

Measurement includes the physical parameters that reflect the individual's general health state such as weight, height, and vital signs (temperature, pulse, respiration and blood pressure).

NORMAL RANGE OF FINDINGS | **ABNORMAL FINDINGS**

WEIGHT

Use a standardized *balance* scale. Instruct the person to remove his or her shoes and heavy outer clothing before standing on the scale. When a sequence of repeated weights is necessary, aim for approximately the same time of day and the same type of clothing worn each time. Record the weight in kilograms and in pounds.

NORMAL RANGE OF FINDINGS

The weight tables from the Metropolitan Life Insurance Company, revised in 1983, give a recommended range for adults aged 25 to 59 years (Table 8–1).

The target weights are higher on the revised tables than on the earlier 1959 tables, reflecting heavier American norms. (The American Heart Association warns this should not be a green light for individuals to gain more weight.)

ABNORMAL FINDINGS

An unexplained weight loss may be a sign of a short-term illness (e.g. fever, infection, disease of the mouth or throat), or a chronic illness (endocrine disease, malignancy, mental health dysfunction).

Table 8–1 ▶ Height and Weight Tables for Men and Women According to Frame, Ages 25-59

HEIGHT*		WEIGHT†		
Feet	Inches	Small Frame	Medium Frame	Large Frame
Men				
5	2	128–134	131–134	138–150
5	3	130–136	133–143	140–153
5	4	132–138	135–145	142–156
5	5	134–140	137–148	144–160
5	6	136–142	139–151	146–164
5	7	138–145	142–154	149–168
5	8	140–148	145–157	152–172
5	9	142–151	148–160	155–176
5	10	144–154	151–163	158–180
5	11	146–157	154–166	161–184
6	0	149–160	157–170	164–188
6	1	152–164	160–174	168–192
6	2	155–168	164–178	172–197
6	3	158–172	167–182	176–202
6	4	162–176	171–187	181–207
Women				
4	10	102–111	109–121	118–131
4	11	103–113	111–123	120–134
5	0	104–115	113–126	122–137
5	1	106–118	115–129	125–140
5	2	108–121	118–132	128–143
5	3	111–124	121–135	131–147
5	4	114–127	124–138	134–151
5	5	117–130	127–141	137–155
5	6	120–133	130–144	140–159
5	7	123–136	133–147	143–163
5	8	126–139	136–150	146–167
5	9	129–142	139–153	149–170
5	10	132–145	142–156	152–173
5	11	135–148	145–159	155–176
6	0	138–151	148–162	158–179

* Shoes with 1-inch heels.
† Weight in pounds. Men: allow 5 lb of clothing. Women: allow 3 lb of clothing.
(Courtesy of Metropolitan Life Insurance Company, 1983.)

NORMAL RANGE OF FINDINGS

Compare the person's current weight with the previous health visit. A recent weight loss may be explained by successful dieting. A weight gain usually reflects overabundant caloric intake, unhealthy eating habits, and sedentary lifestyle.

HEIGHT

Use the measuring pole on the balance scale. Align the extended headpiece with the top of the head. The person should be shoeless, standing straight, and looking straight ahead.

DEVELOPMENTAL CONSIDERATIONS

The Younger Person

Weight

Weigh an infant on a platform-type balance scale (Fig. 8–1). To check calibration, set the weight at zero and observe the beam balance. Guard the baby so that he or she does not fall. Weigh to the nearest 10 g (1/2 oz) for infants and 100 g (1/4 lb) for toddlers. By age 2 or 3 years, use the upright scale. Leave underpants on the child. Some young children are fearful of the rickety standing platform and may prefer sitting on the infant scale. Use the upright scale with preschoolers and school-aged children, maintaining modesty with light clothing (Fig. 8–2).

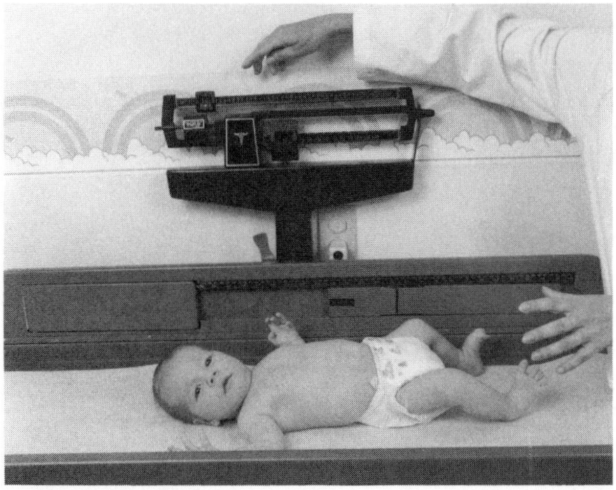

► **Figure 8–1**

ABNORMAL FINDINGS

Obesity occasionally may be due to endrocrine disorders, drug therapy (e.g., corticosteroids), or mental depression.

NORMAL RANGE OF FINDINGS | ABNORMAL FINDINGS

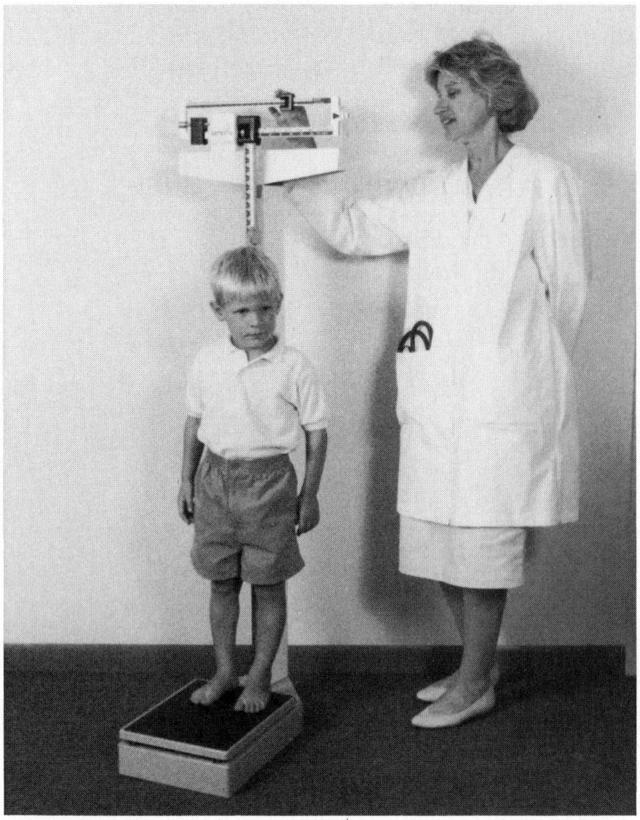

► Figure 8-2

Length

Until age 2 years, measure the infant's body length supine using a horizontal measuring board (Fig. 8-3). Hold the head in the midline. Because the infant normally has flexed legs, extend them momentarily by holding the

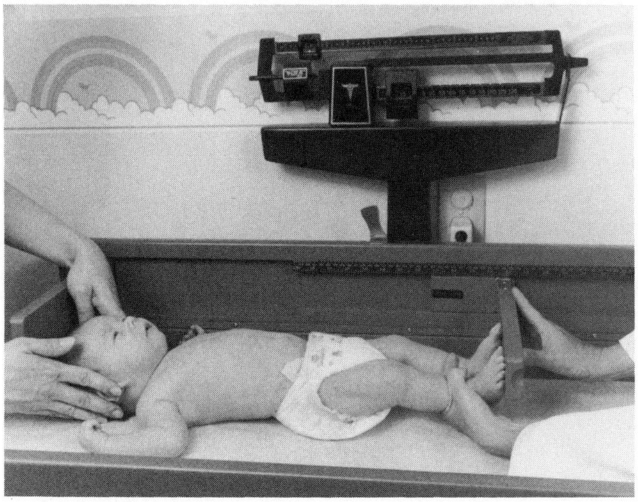

► Figure 8-3

NORMAL RANGE OF FINDINGS

ABNORMAL FINDINGS

knees together and pushing them down until the legs are flat on the table. Avoid using a tape measure along the infant's length because this is inaccurate.

By age 2 or 3 years, measure the child's height by standing the child against the pole on the platform scale or back against a flat ruler taped to the wall (Fig. 8–4). (Sometimes a child will stand more erect against the solid wall than against the narrow measuring pole on the scale.) Encourage the child to stand straight and tall and to look straight ahead without tilting the head. The shoulders, buttocks, and heels should touch the wall. Hold a book or flat board on the child's head at a right angle to the wall. Mark just under the book, noting the measure to the nearest 1 mm (1/8 in).

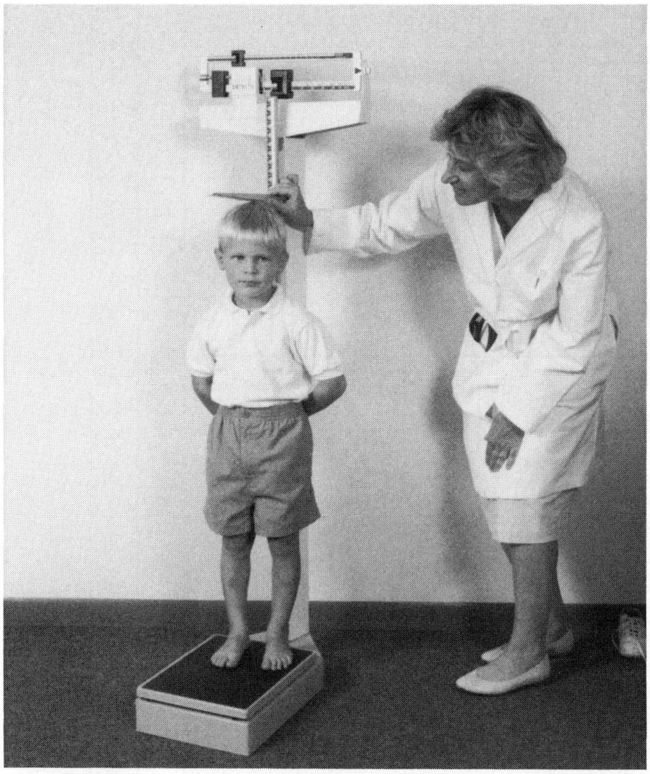

► **Figure 8–4**

Physical growth is perhaps the best index of a child's general health. The child's height and weight are recorded at every health care visit to determine normal growth patterns. The results are plotted on one growth sheet. (See Fig. 8–5 for weight and height charts from birth to 36 months for girls and boys, and from 2 to 18 years for males and females.) Healthy childhood growth is continuous though uneven, with rapid growth spurts occurring during infancy and adolescence. Results are more reliable when comparing numerous growth measures over a long time. These charts also compare the individual child's measurements against the general population. Normal limits range from the 5th to the 95th percentile on the standardized charts.

*Adapted from: Hamill PVV, Drizd TA, Johnson CL, Reed RB, Roche AF, Moore WM: Physical growth: National Center for Health Statistics percentiles. AM J CLIN NUTR 32:607-629, 1979. Data from the Fels Longitudinal Study, Wright State University School of Medicine, Yellow Springs, Ohio.

© 1982 Ross Laboratories

GIRLS: BIRTH TO 36 MONTHS
PHYSICAL GROWTH
NCHS PERCENTILES*

NAME _____ RECORD # _____

Ross
Growth &
Development
Program

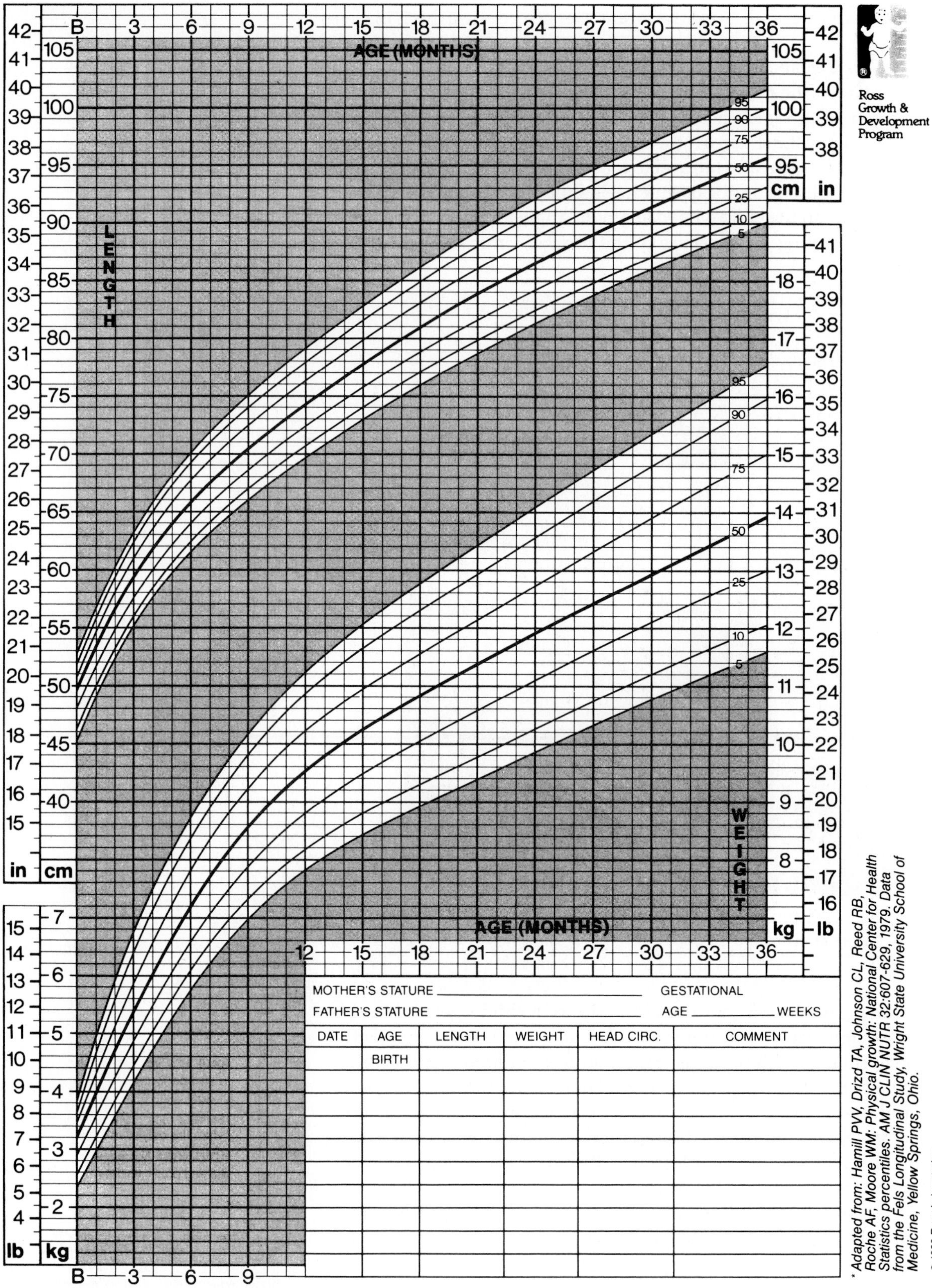

MOTHER'S STATURE _____ GESTATIONAL
FATHER'S STATURE _____ AGE _____ WEEKS

DATE	AGE	LENGTH	WEIGHT	HEAD CIRC.	COMMENT
	BIRTH				

► Figure 8–5A

GIRLS: BIRTH TO 36 MONTHS
PHYSICAL GROWTH
NCHS PERCENTILES*

NAME ______________________ RECORD # ____________

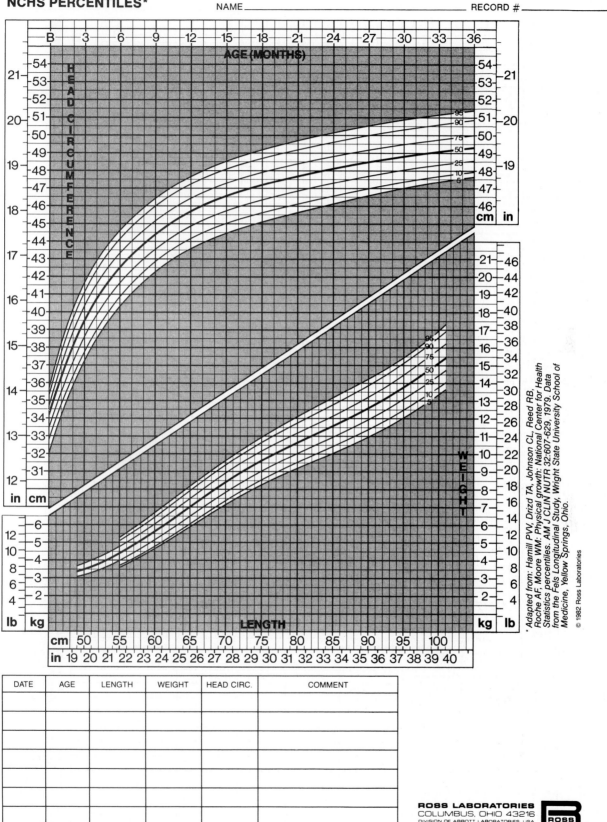

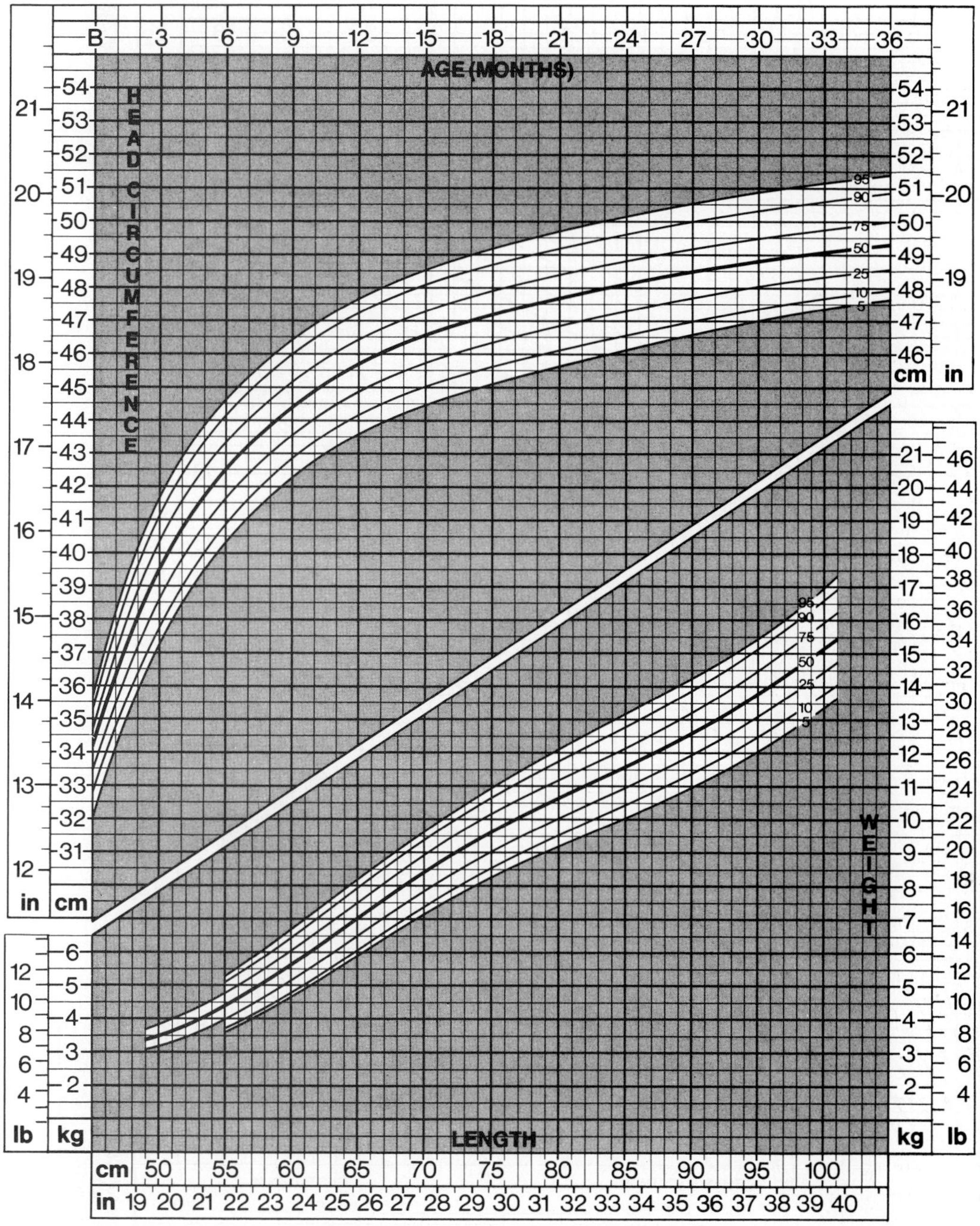

* Adapted from: Hamill PVV, Drizd TA, Johnson CL, Reed RB, Roche AF, Moore WM: Physical growth: National Center for Health Statistics percentiles. AM J CLIN NUTR 32:607-629, 1979. Data from the Fels Longitudinal Study, Wright State University School of Medicine, Yellow Springs, Ohio.

DATE	AGE	LENGTH	WEIGHT	HEAD CIRC.	COMMENT

ROSS LABORATORIES
COLUMBUS, OHIO 43216
DIVISION OF ABBOTT LABORATORIES, USA

G106(0.05)/JANUARY 1986 LITHO IN USA

▶ **Figure 8 – 5*B***

BOYS: BIRTH TO 36 MONTHS
PHYSICAL GROWTH
NCHS PERCENTILES*

NAME ______________________ RECORD # ____________

Ross Growth & Development Program

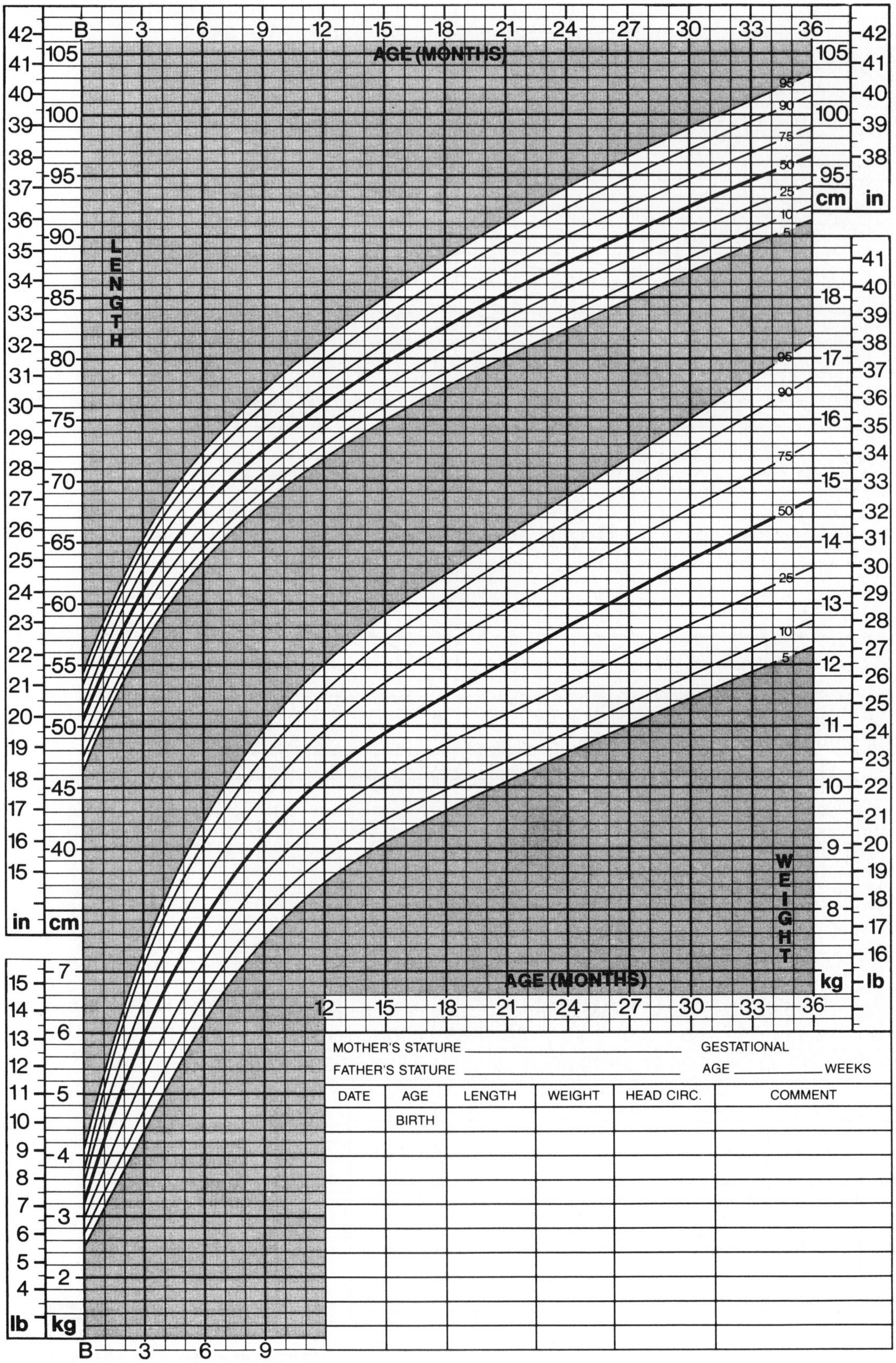

MOTHER'S STATURE ____________ GESTATIONAL
FATHER'S STATURE ____________ AGE ________ WEEKS

DATE	AGE	LENGTH	WEIGHT	HEAD CIRC.	COMMENT
	BIRTH				

*Adapted from: Hamill PVV, Drizd TA, Johnson CL, Reed RB, Roche AF, Moore WM: Physical growth: National Center for Health Statistics percentiles. AM J CLIN NUTR 32:607-629, 1979. Data from the Fels Longitudinal Study, Wright State University School of Medicine, Yellow Springs, Ohio.

► **Figure 8-5C**

BOYS: BIRTH TO 36 MONTHS
PHYSICAL GROWTH
NCHS PERCENTILES*

NAME ______________________ RECORD # ____________

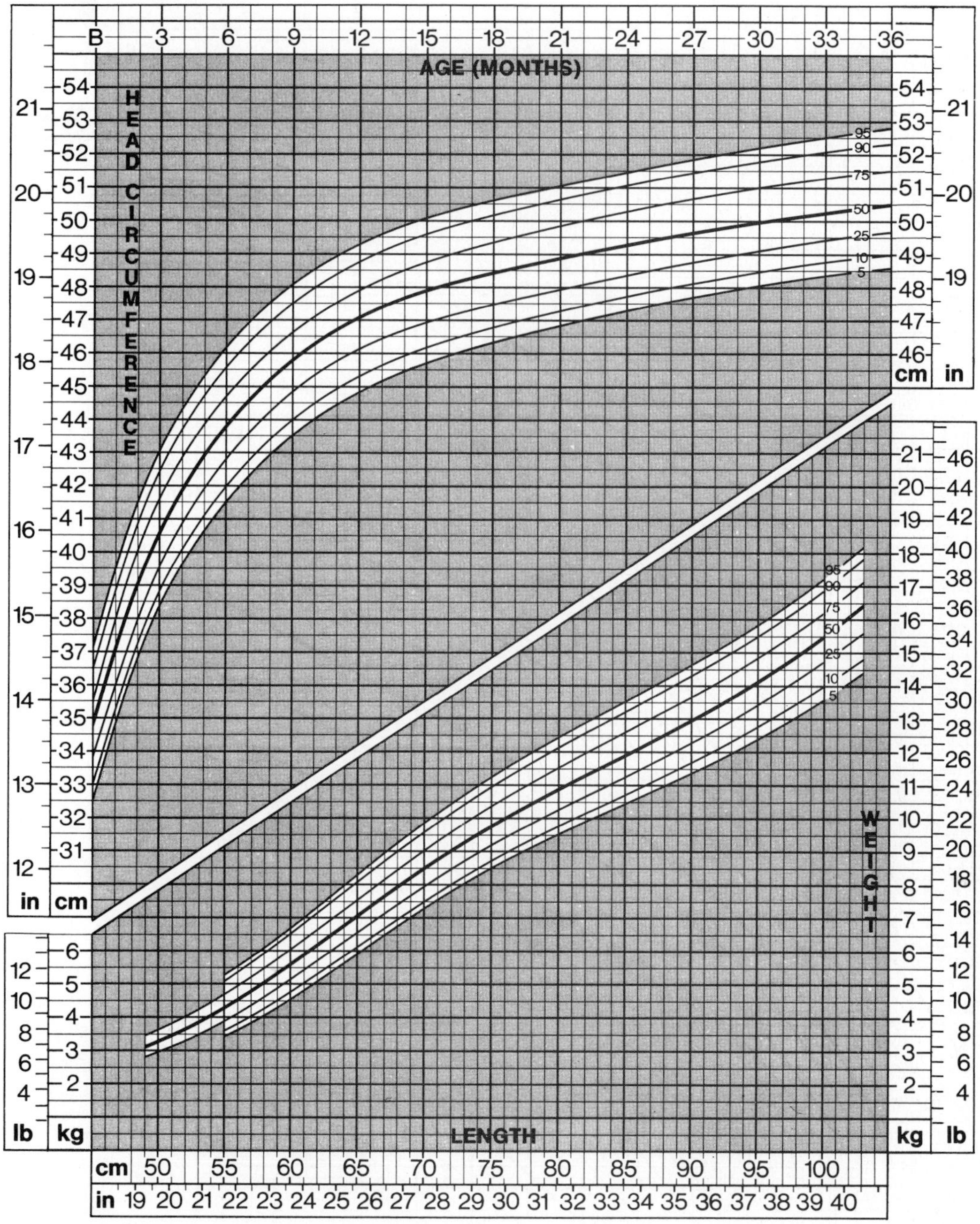

*Adapted from: Hamill PVV, Drizd TA, Johnson CL, Reed RB, Roche AF, Moore WM: Physical growth: National Center for Health Statistics percentiles. AM J CLIN NUTR 32:607-629, 1979. Data from the Fels Longitudinal Study, Wright State University School of Medicine, Yellow Springs, Ohio.

DATE	AGE	LENGTH	WEIGHT	HEAD CIRC.	COMMENT

ROSS LABORATORIES
COLUMBUS, OHIO 43216
DIVISION OF ABBOTT LABORATORIES, USA

G105(0.05)/APRIL 1989 LITHO IN USA

► **Figure 8-5*D***

GIRLS: 2 TO 18 YEARS
PHYSICAL GROWTH
NCHS PERCENTILES*

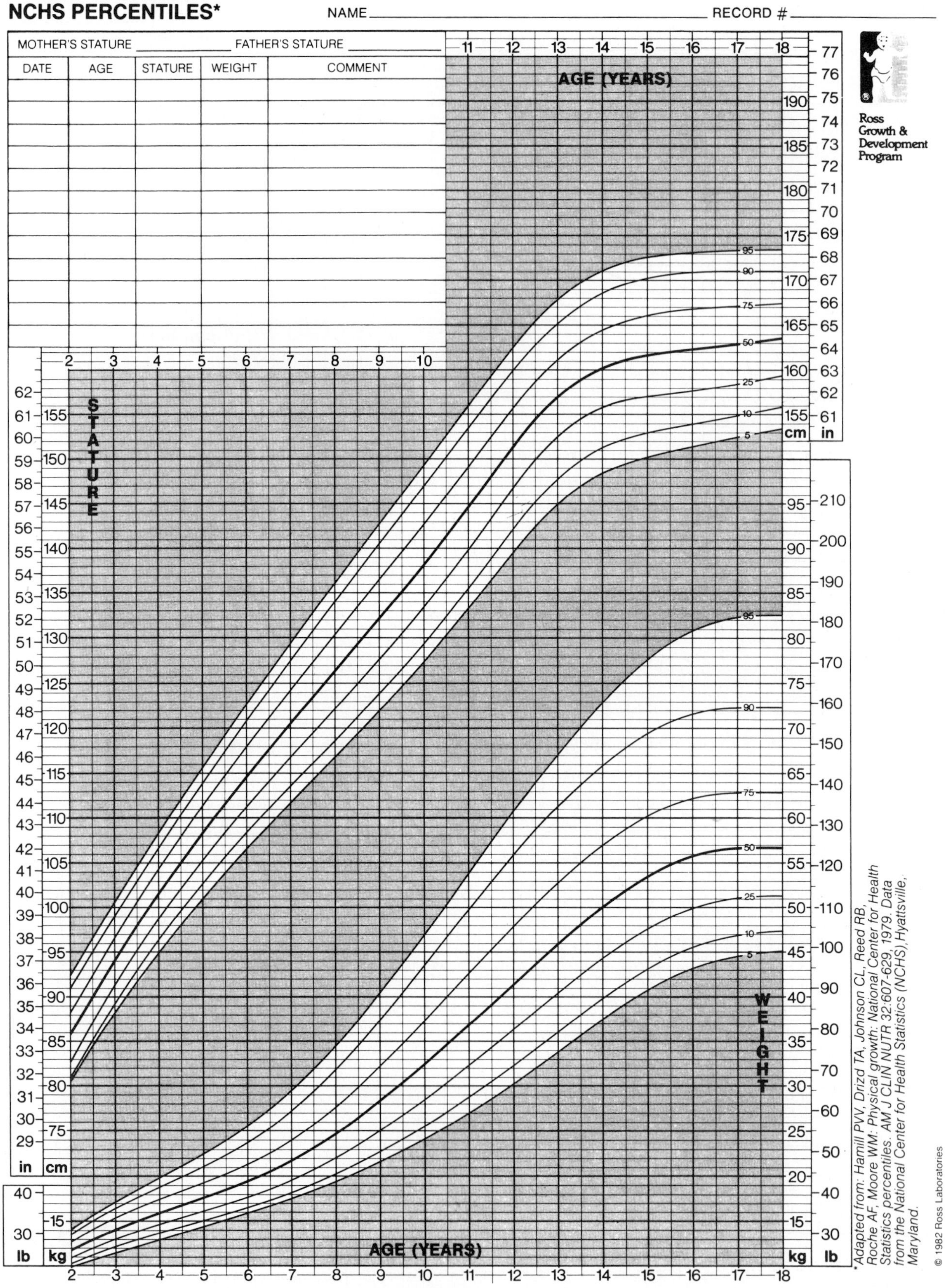

► **Figure 8–5*E***

BOYS: 2 TO 18 YEARS
PHYSICAL GROWTH
NCHS PERCENTILES*

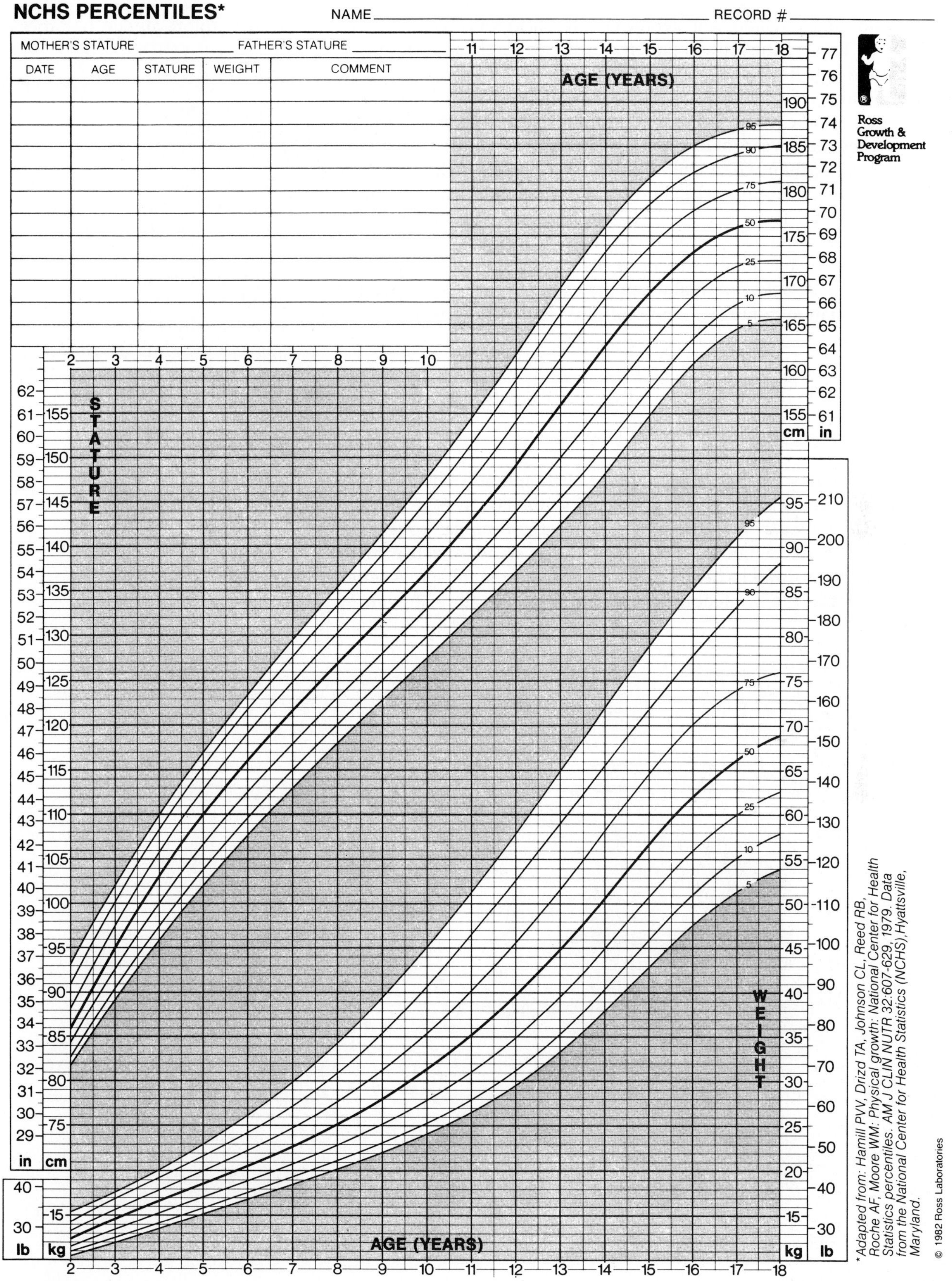

► **Figure 8-5F**

NORMAL RANGE OF FINDINGS

Use your judgment and consider the genetic background of the small-for-age child. Explore the growth patterns of the parents and siblings. Be aware that the statistical averages for the United States charts are based on norms for white children and may not necessarily generalize to other ethnic groups. Studies indicate black children weigh less than white children during the first 2 years of life, but afterward black children tend to be taller and heavier than white children of the same age. Asian children (particularly girls) are found to be shorter and lighter than white counterparts (Robson et al, 1975; Barr et al, 1972). Race-specific standards are needed before making judgments on growth of infants and children. Otherwise an excessive number of young black infants or Asian children may be judged to be below normal when they actually may be normal for their own population group (see Transcultural Considerations, p. 216).

ABNORMAL FINDINGS

Further explore any growth measure that:

- falls below the 5th or above the 95th percentile with no genetic explanation.
- shows a wide percentile difference between height and weight, e.g., a 10th percentile height with a 95th percentile weight.
- shows that growth has suddenly stopped when it had been steady.
- fails to show normal growth spurts during infancy and adolescence (Whaley and Wong, 1990).

Head Circumference

Measure the infant's head circumference at birth and at each well child visit up to age 2 years, then yearly up to age 6 years (Fig. 8-6). Circle the tape around the head at the prominent frontal and occipital bones; the widest span is correct. Plot the measurement on standardized growth charts. Compare the infant's head size with that expected for age. A series of measurements is more valuable than a single figure to show the *rate* of head growth.

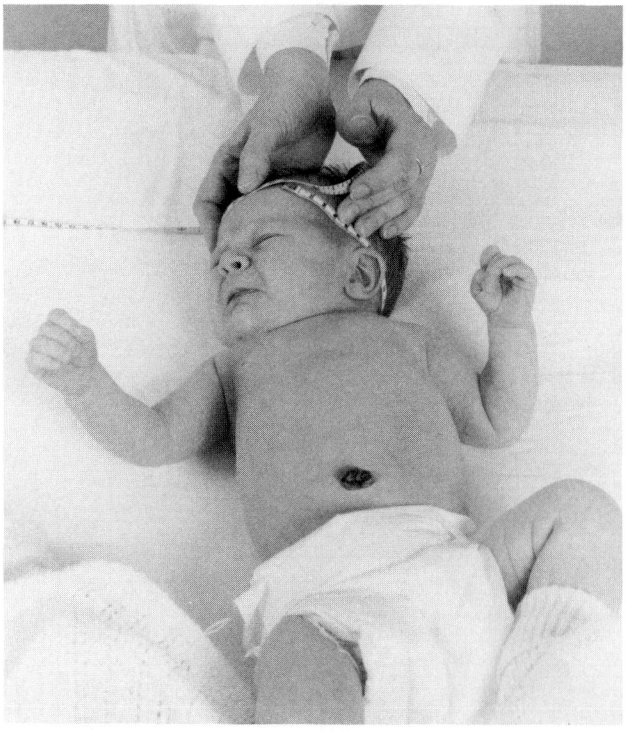

► **Figure 8-6**

NORMAL RANGE OF FINDINGS

The newborn's head measures about 32 – 38 cm (average around 34 cm) and is about 2 cm larger than the chest circumference. The chest grows at a faster rate than the cranium; at some time between 6 months and 2 years, both measurements are about the same, and after age 2, the chest circumference is greater than the head circumference.

Measurement of the chest circumference is valuable in a comparison with the head circumference but not necessarily by itself. Encircle the tape around the chest at the nipple line. It should be snug, but not too tight to leave a mark (Fig. 8–7).

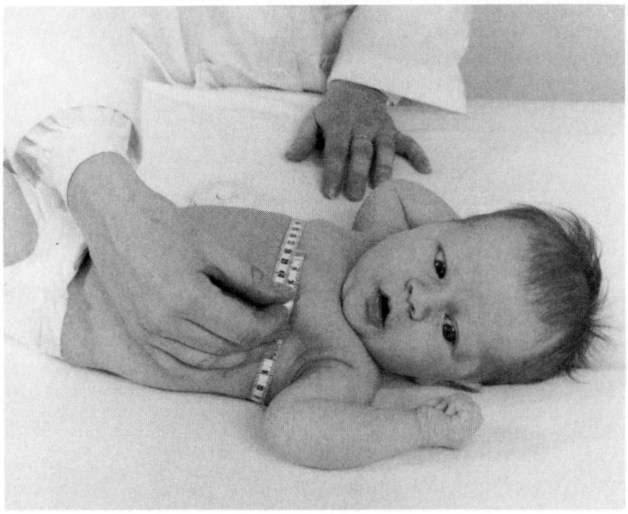

► **Figure 8–7**

Estimation of Gestational Age

Occasionally, you will need to compare these three measurements—weight, length, and head circumference—with a newborn's gestational age (GA) in order to assess maturity. GA is the number of weeks from the first day of the mother's last menstrual period (LMP) to the newborn's date of birth. GA for a full-term newborn is 38 to 42 weeks.

Assume you are examining a small newborn. Is the baby preterm and logically small or is the baby at term but small for his or her gestational age? Estimating the GA is useful to distinguish this. The Dubowitz Clinical Assessment has standardized criteria for this estimate (Dubowitz et al, 1970) (Table 8–2). The scale has 11 external signs to measure physical maturity, and 10 neuromuscular signs to measure neurologic maturity. Physical maturity is measured by progressive tissue development, and neurologic maturity is measured by active and passive muscle tone.

The newborn should be alert and quiet. Wait until the condition is stable but perform the test within 48 hours of birth. After 5 days, the score is less accurate because the passage of time has added tissue and produced neuromuscular maturation. Follow the measures in Table 8–2. Add the score of the external signs (physical maturity) to the score of neurologic maturity to attain the final score. Compare the final score with the maturity rating scale to arrive at the estimated GA. This is accurate within 2 weeks of the actual GA. A normal *term* infant has a GA of 38 to 42 weeks.

ABNORMAL FINDINGS

Enlarged head circumference occurs with increased intracranial pressure (see Chapter 10, Assessment of the Head and Neck).

Preterm—<38 weeks
Post-term—>42 weeks

Table 8-2 ▶ Dubowitz Score Sheet of Gestational Age

External Physical Characteristics

External Sign	Points: 0	1	2	3	4	Score
Edema	Obvious edema of hands and feet; pitting over tibia	No obvious edema of hands and feet; pitting over tibia	No edema			
Skin texture	Very thin, gelatinous	Thin and smooth	Smooth; medium thickness. Rash or superficial peeling	Slight thickening and peeling especially of hands and feet	Thick and parchment like; superficial or deep cracking	
Skin color	Dark red	Uniformly pink	Pale pink; variable over body	Pale; only pink over ears, lips, palms, or soles		
Skin opacity (trunk)	Numerous veins and venules clearly seen, especially over abdomen	Veins and tributaries seen	A few large vessels clearly seen over abdomen	A few large vessels seen indistinctly over abdomen	No blood vessels seen	
Lanugo (over back)	No lanugo	Abundant; long and thick over whole back	Hair thinning especially over lower back	Small amount of lanugo and bald areas	At least 1/2 of back devoid of lanugo	
Plantar creases	No skin creases	Faint red marks over anterior half of sole	Definite red marks over > anterior 1/2; indentations over < 1/3	Indentations over > anterior 1/3	Definite deep indentations over > anterior 1/3	
Nipple formation	Nipple barely visible, no areola	Nipple well defined; areola smooth and flat, diameter < 0.75 cm	Areola stippled, edge not raised, diameter < 0.75 cm	Areola stippled, edge raised, diameter > 0.75 cm		
Breast size	No breast tissue palpable	Breast tissue on one or both sides, < 0.5 cm diameter	Breast tissue both sides; one or both 0.5–1.0 cm	Breast tissue both sides; one or both > 1 cm		
Ear form	Pinna flat and shapeless, little or no incurving of edge	Incurving of part of edge of pinna	Partial incurving whole of upper pinna	Well-defined incurving whole of upper pinna		
Ear firmness	Pinna soft, easily folded, no recoil	Pinna soft, easily folded, slow recoil	Cartilage to edge of pinna, but soft in places, ready recoil	Pinna firm, cartilage to edge; instant recoil		
Genitals						
Male	Neither testis in scrotum	At least one testis high in scrotum	At least one testis right down			
Female (with hips 1/2 abducted)	Labia majora widely separated, labia minora protruding	Labia majora almost cover labia minora	Labia majora completely cover labia minora			
					EXTERNAL TOTAL:	

Neurologic Characteristics

POSTURE: Observed with infant quiet and in supine position. Score 0: Arms and legs extended; 1: beginning of flexion of hips and knees, arms extended; 2: stronger flexion of legs, arms extended; 3: arms slightly flexed, legs flexed and abducted; 4: full flexion of arms and legs.
SQUARE WINDOW: The hand is flexed on the forearm between the thumb and index finger of the examiner. Enough pressure is applied to get as full a flexion as possible, and the angle between the hypothenar eminence and the ventral aspect of the forearm is measured and graded according to diagram. (Care is taken not to rotate the infant's wrist while doing this maneuver.)
ANKLE DORSIFLEXION: The foot is dorsiflexed onto the anterior aspect of the leg, with the examiner's thumb on the sole of the foot and other fingers behind the leg. Enough pressure is applied to get as full flexion as possible, and the angle between the dorsum of the foot and the anterior aspect of the leg is measured.

Table 8-2 ▶ Dubowitz Score Sheet of Gestational Age *Continued*

Neurologic Characteristics

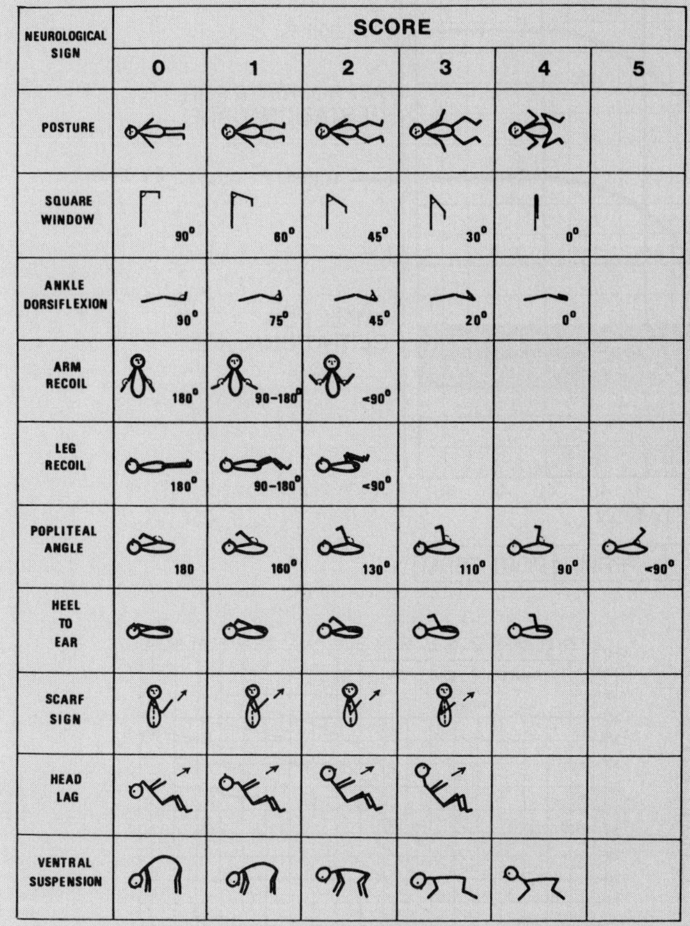
NEUROLOGICAL SIGN
SCORE
0
1
2
3
4
5
POSTURE
SQUARE WINDOW
90°
60°
45°
30°
0°
ANKLE DORSIFLEXION
90°
75°
45°
20°
0°
ARM RECOIL
180°
90–180°
<90°
LEG RECOIL
180°
90–180°
<90°
POPLITEAL ANGLE
180
160°
130°
110°
90°
<90°
HEEL TO EAR
SCARF SIGN
HEAD LAG
VENTRAL SUSPENSION

TOTAL SCORE	GESTATIONAL AGE (IN WEEKS)
0–9	26
10–12	27
13–16	28
17–20	29
21–24	30
25–27	31
28–31	32
32–35	33
36–39	34
40–43	35
44–46	36
47–50	37
51–54	38
55–58	39
59–62	40
63–65	41
66–69	42

ARM RECOIL: With the infant in the supine position the forearms are first flexed for 5 seconds, then fully extended by pulling on the hands, and then released. The sign is fully positive if the arms return briskly to full flexion (Score 2). If the arms return to incomplete flexion or the response is sluggish, it is graded Score 1. If they remain extended or are only followed by random movements, the score is 0.

LEG RECOIL: With the infant supine, the hips and knees are fully flexed for 5 seconds, then extended by traction on the feet and released. A maximal response is one of full flexion of the hips and knees (Score 2). A partial flexion scores 1, and minimal or no movement scores 0.

POPLITEAL ANGLE: With the infant supine and his pelvis flat on the examining couch, the thigh is held in the knee-chest position by the examiner's left index finger and thumb supporting the knee. The leg is then extended by gentle pressure from the examiner's right index finger behind the ankle and the popliteal angle is measured.

HEEL TO EAR MANEUVER: With the baby supine, draw the baby's foot as near to the head as it will go without forcing it. Observe the distance between the foot and the head as well as the degree of extension at the knee. Grade according to diagram. Note that the knee is left free and may draw down alongside the abdomen.

SCARF SIGN: With the baby supine, take the infant's hand and try to put it around the neck and as far posteriorly as possible around the opposite shoulder. Assist this maneuver by lifting the elbow across the body. See how far the elbow will go across and grade according to illustrations. Score 0: Elbow reaches opposite axillary line; 1: Elbow between midline and opposite axillary line; 2: Elbow reaches midline; 3: Elbow will not reach midline.

HEAD LAG: With the baby lying supine, grasp the hands (or the arms if a very small infant) and pull him slowly towards the sitting position. Observe the position of the head in relation to the trunk and grade accordingly. In a small infant the head may initially be supported by one hand. Score 0: Complete lag; 1: Partial head control; 2: Able to maintain head in line with body; 3: Brings head anterior to body.

VENTRAL SUSPENSION: The infant is suspended in the prone position, with examiner's hand under the infant's chest (one hand in a small infant, two in a large infant). Observe the degree of extension of the back and the amount of flexion of the arms and legs. Also note the relation of the head to the trunk. Grade according to diagrams.

If score differs on the two sides, take the mean.

(Adapted with permission from Dubowitz L, et al: Clinical assessment of gestational age in the newborn infant. J Pediatr 77:1, 1970.)

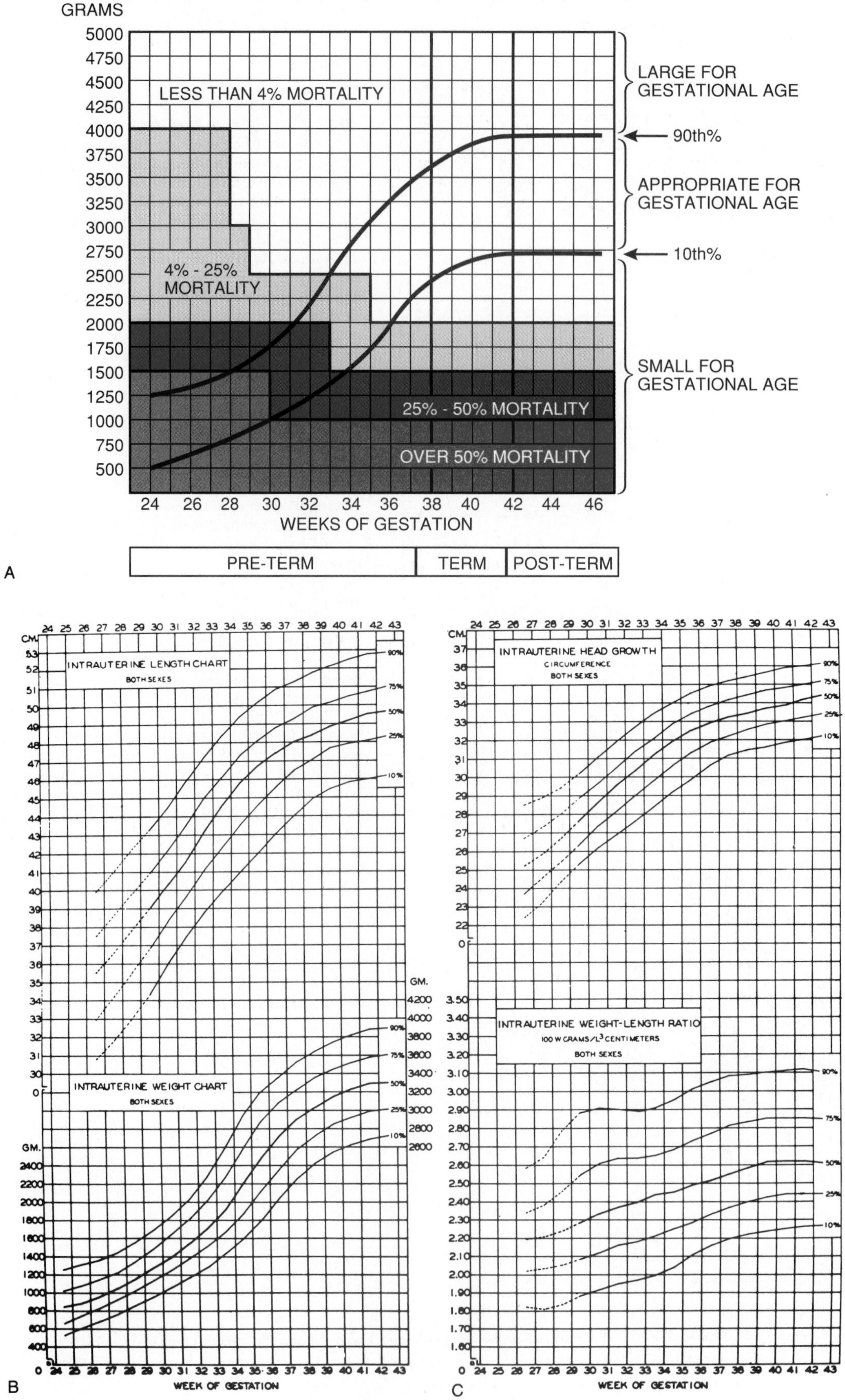
GRAMS
5000
4750
4500
4250
4000
3750
3500
3250
3000
2750
2500
2250
2000
1750
1500
1250
1000
750
500
LESS THAN 4% MORTALITY
4% - 25% MORTALITY
25% - 50% MORTALITY
OVER 50% MORTALITY
LARGE FOR GESTATIONAL AGE
90th%
APPROPRIATE FOR GESTATIONAL AGE
10th%
SMALL FOR GESTATIONAL AGE
24 26 28 30 32 34 36 38 40 42 44 46
WEEKS OF GESTATION
PRE-TERM
TERM
POST-TERM
A
INTRAUTERINE LENGTH CHART
BOTH SEXES
INTRAUTERINE WEIGHT CHART
BOTH SEXES
CM.
GM.
90%
75%
50%
25%
10%
WEEK OF GESTATION
B
INTRAUTERINE HEAD GROWTH
CIRCUMFERENCE
BOTH SEXES
INTRAUTERINE WEIGHT-LENGTH RATIO
100 W GRAMS/L³ CENTIMETERS
BOTH SEXES
WEEK OF GESTATION
C

► **Figure 8-8**

NORMAL RANGE OF FINDINGS

Once you have determined the GA, you can assess the newborn's relative size. Compare the baby's weight, length, and head circumference to the GA in order to tell if the newborn is

AGA—appropriate for gestational age	10–90th percentile
SGA—small for gestational age	<10th percentile
LGA—large for gestational age	>90th percentile

Use the chart on the opposite page to plot percentiles (Lubchenco et al, 1963) (Fig. 8–8).

At the 50th percentile, a baby of average GA (40 weeks) measures an average weight of 3200 g (7 lb 1 oz), an average length of 49 cm (19.3 in), and an average head circumference of 34 cm (13.5 in).

The Aging Adult

Weight

The aging person appears sharper in contour with more prominent bony landmarks than the younger adult. Body weight decreases during the 9th and 10th decades. This factor is more evident in males, perhaps because of greater muscle shrinkage. The distribution of fat also changes during the 80s and 90s. Even with good nutrition, subcutaneous fat is lost from the face and periphery (especially the forearms), whereas additional fat is deposited on the abdomen and hips (Fig. 8–9).

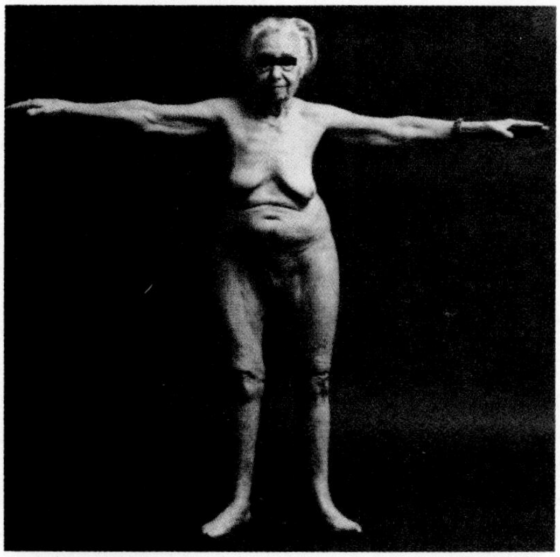

▸ **Figure 8–9**

Height

By the 9th and 10th decades, many people are shorter than they were in their 70s. This results from shortening in the spinal column due to thinning of the vertebral discs and shortening of the individual vertebrae as well as the postural changes of kyphosis and slight flexion in the knees and hips. Since long bones do not shorten with age, the overall body proportion looks different; a shorter trunk with relatively long extremities (Fig. 8–9).

ABNORMAL FINDINGS

SGA and LGA infants have an increased risk of morbidity and mortality.

MEASURING VITAL SIGNS

The vital signs include temperature, pulse, respiration, and blood pressure; they are key physiologic measures of the person's general health state. Compare each value with the normal standard for the person's age and with the normal range for that individual on the earlier health visits.

NORMAL RANGE OF FINDINGS | **ABNORMAL FINDINGS**

TEMPERATURE

Cellular metabolism requires a stable core temperature of 37° C (98.6° F). The body maintains a steady temperature through a thermostat, or feedback mechanism, regulated in the hypothalamus of the brain. The thermostat balances heat production (from metabolism, exercise, food digestion, external factors) with heat loss (through radiation, evaporation of sweat, convection, conduction).

The various routes of temperature measurement reflect the body's core temperature. The normal oral temperature in a resting person is 37° C (98.6° F), with a range of 35.8 to 37.3° C (96.4 to 99.1° F). The rectal temperature measures 0.4 to 0.5° C (0.7 to 1° F) higher. The normal temperature is influenced by:

- A diurnal cycle of 1 to 1.5° F, with the trough occurring in the early morning hours and the peak occurring in late afternoon to early evening.
- The menstruation cycle in women. Progesterone secretion, occurring with ovulation at midcycle, causes a 0.5 to 1.0° F rise in temperature that continues until menses.
- Exercise. Moderate to hard exercise increases body temperature.
- Age. Wider normal variations occur in the infant and young child due to less effective heat control mechanisms. In older adults, temperature is usually lower than in other age groups, with a mean of 36.2° C (97.2° F).

The thermostatic function of the hypothalamus may become scrambled during illness or central nervous system disorders.

Hyperthermia, or fever, occurs due to pyrogens secreted by toxic bacteria during infections or from tissue breakdown such as that following myocardial infarction, trauma, surgery, or malignancy. Neurologic disorders (e.g., a cerebral vascular accident, cerebral edema, brain trauma, tumor, or surgery) also can reset the brain's thermostat at a higher level, resulting in heat production and conservation.

Hypothermia is usually due to accidental, prolonged exposure to cold. It also may be purposefully induced to lower the body's oxygen requirements during heart or peripheral vascular surgery, neurosurgery, amputation, or gastrointestinal hemorrhage.

The *oral* temperature is the most accurate and convenient measure. It responds to changes in arterial temperature faster than the rectal route, because the oral sublingual site has a rich blood supply from the carotid arteries that reflects inner core temperature. Shake the *mercury-in-glass* thermometer down to 35.5° C (96° F) and place it at the base of the tongue in either of the posterior sublingual pockets, *not* in front of the tongue. Instruct the person to keep his or her lips closed. Full registering of a glass thermometer takes 8 minutes. Wait 15 minutes if the person has just taken hot or iced liquids and 2 minutes if he or she has just smoked.

The *electronic thermometer* has the advantages of swift and accurate measurement as well as safe, unbreakable, disposable probe covers. The instrument must be fully charged and correctly calibrated. Most children enjoy watching their temperature numbers advance on the box.

The *axillary* temperature is safe and accurate for infants and young children when the environment is reasonably controlled (see Developmental Considerations, p. 211). Take a *rectal* temperature only when the other routes are not practical, e.g., for comatose or confused persons, for persons

NORMAL RANGE OF FINDINGS	ABNORMAL FINDINGS

in shock, or for those who cannot close the mouth due to breathing or oxygen tubes, wired mandible, or other facial dysfunction. Insert a lubricated rectal thermometer (with a short, blunt tip) only 2–3 cm (1 inch) into the adult rectum, directed toward the umbilicus, and leave in place for 2 1/2 minutes.

Report the temperature in centigrade. Use this conversion:

$$\text{Degrees C} = 5/9\ (\text{degrees F} - 32)$$
$$\text{Degrees F} = 9/5\ (\text{degrees C} + 32)$$

Note that it is far easier to learn to think in the centigrade scale than it is to convert each reading.

PULSE

With every beat, the heart pumps an amount of blood—the *stroke volume*—into the aorta. The force flares the arterial walls and generates a pressure wave, which is felt in the periphery as the **pulse.** Palpating the peripheral pulse gives the rate and rhythm of the heartbeat, as well as local data on the condition of the artery. The *radial* pulse is usually palpated while vital signs are measured.

Using the pads of your first three fingers, palpate the radial pulse at the flexor aspect of the wrist laterally along the radius bone (Fig. 8–10). Push until you feel the strongest pulsation. If the rhythm is regular, count the number of beats in 15 seconds and multiply by 4. Contrary to traditional teaching, using a 15-second interval is found to be *more* accurate than longer intervals. Using longer intervals invites error because you may lose count (Jones, 1970). However, if the rhythm is irregular, count for 1 full minute. As you begin the counting interval, start your count with "zero" for the first pulse felt. The second pulse felt is "one," and so on. Assess the pulse, including (1) rate, (2) rhythm, (3) force, and (4) elasticity.

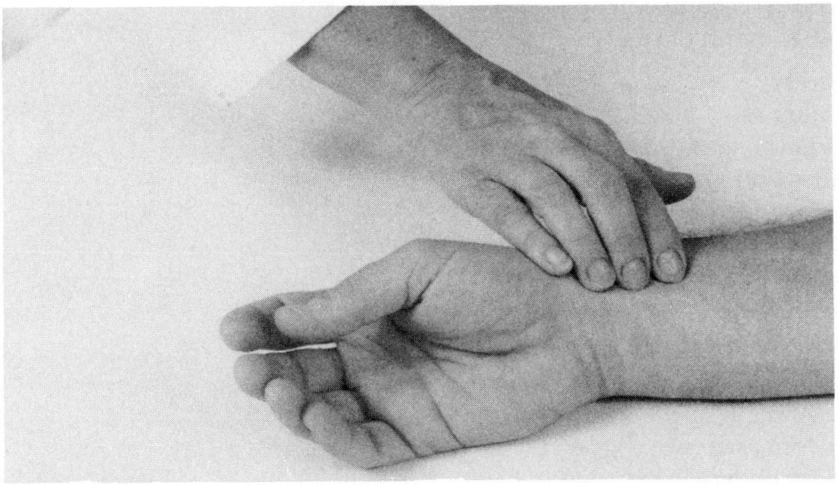

► **Figure 8–10**

Rate. In the resting adult, the normal heart rate range is 60 to 100 beats per minute (bpm). The rate normally varies with age, being more rapid in infancy and childhood and more moderate during adult and older years. The rate also varies with sex; after puberty, females have a slightly faster rate than males (Table 8–3).

NORMAL RANGE OF FINDINGS

Table 8-3 ▶ Normal Resting Pulse Rates—Across Age Groups

AGE	AVERAGE (BEATS PER MINUTE)	NORMAL LIMITS
Newborn	120	70-190
1 year	120	80-160
2 years	110	80-130
4 years	100	80-120
6 years	100	75-115
8 years	90	70-110
10 years	90	70-110
12 years		
Female	90	70-110
Male	85	65-105
14 years		
Female	85	65-105
Male	80	60-100
16 years		
Female	80	60-100
Male	75	55-95
18 years		
Female	75	55-95
Male	70	50-90
Well-conditioned athlete	May be 50-60	50-100
Adult		60-100
Aging		60-100

In the adult, a heart rate less than 60 bpm is called *bradycardia.* This occurs normally in the well-trained athlete whose heart muscle develops along with the skeletal muscles. The stronger, more efficient heart muscle pushes out a larger stroke volume with each beat, thus requiring fewer beats per minute to maintain a stable cardiac output. (Review the equation CO = SV × R, or Cardiac Output = Stroke Volume × Rate, in Chapter 16). A more rapid heart rate, over 100 bpm, is *tachycardia.* It occurs normally with anxiety or with increased exercise to match the body's demand for increased metabolism.

Rhythm. The rhythm of the pulse normally has an even tempo. However, one irregularity that is commonly found in children and young adults is *sinus arrhythmia.* Here the heart rate varies with the respiratory cycle, speeding up at the peak of inspiration and slowing to normal with expiration. Inspiration momentarily causes a decreased stroke volume from the left side of the heart; to compensate, the heart rate increases. (See Chapter 16 for a full discussion on sinus arrhythmia.) If any other irregularities are felt, auscultate heart sounds for a more complete assessment (see Chapter 16).

Force. The force of the pulse shows the strength of the heart's stroke volume. A "weak, thready" pulse reflects a decreased stroke volume, e.g., as occurs with hemorrhagic shock. A "full, bounding" pulse denotes an increased stroke volume, as with anxiety, exercise, and some abnormal conditions. The pulse force is recorded using a three-point scale:

3+—full, bounding

2+—normal

ABNORMAL FINDINGS

For abnormal rates and rhythms, see Table 18-2, Variations in Arterial Pulse.

NORMAL RANGE OF FINDINGS | **ABNORMAL FINDINGS**

1+—weak, thready

0—absent.

Some agencies use a four-point scale; make sure your system is consistent with that used by the rest of your staff. Either scale is somewhat subjective. Experience will increase your clinical judgment.

Elasticity. With normal elasticity, the arterial feels springy, straight, resilient.

Chapter 16 presents assessment of the precordium, including listening to the heart rate and rhythm as well as the quality of heart sounds. Chapter 18, on peripheral vascular assessment, presents further data on other pulse sites.

RESPIRATIONS

Normally, a person's breathing is relaxed, regular, automatic, and silent. Since most people are unaware of their breathing, do not mention that you will be counting the respirations, because sudden awareness may alter the normal pattern. Instead, maintain your position of counting the radial pulse and unobtrusively count the respirations. Count for 30 seconds or for 1 full minute if you suspect an abnormality. Avoid the 15-second interval. The result can vary by a factor of + or − 4, which is significant with such a small number.

Note that respiratory rates presented in Table 8–4 normally are more rapid in infants and children. Also, a fairly constant ratio of pulse rate to respiratory rate exists, which is about 4:1. Normally, both pulse and respiratory rates rise as a response to exercise or anxiety. More detailed assessment on respiratory status is presented in Chapter 15.

Table 8–4 ▶ Normal Respiratory Rates

AGE	BREATHS PER MINUTE
Neonate	30–40
1 year	20–40
2 years	25–32
4 years	23–30
6 years	21–26
8 years	20–26
10 years	20–26
12 years	18–22
14 years	18–22
16 years	16–20
18 years	12–20
Adult	10–20

BLOOD PRESSURE

Blood pressure is the force of the blood pushing against the side of its container, the vessel wall. The strength of the push changes with the event in the cardiac cycle. The *systolic* pressure is the maximum pressure felt on

NORMAL RANGE OF FINDINGS

ABNORMAL FINDINGS

the artery during left ventricular contraction, or systole. The *diastolic* pressure is the elastic recoil, or resting, pressure that the blood exerts constantly in between each contraction. The *pulse pressure* is the difference between the systolic and diastolic and reflects the stroke volume (Fig. 8–11).

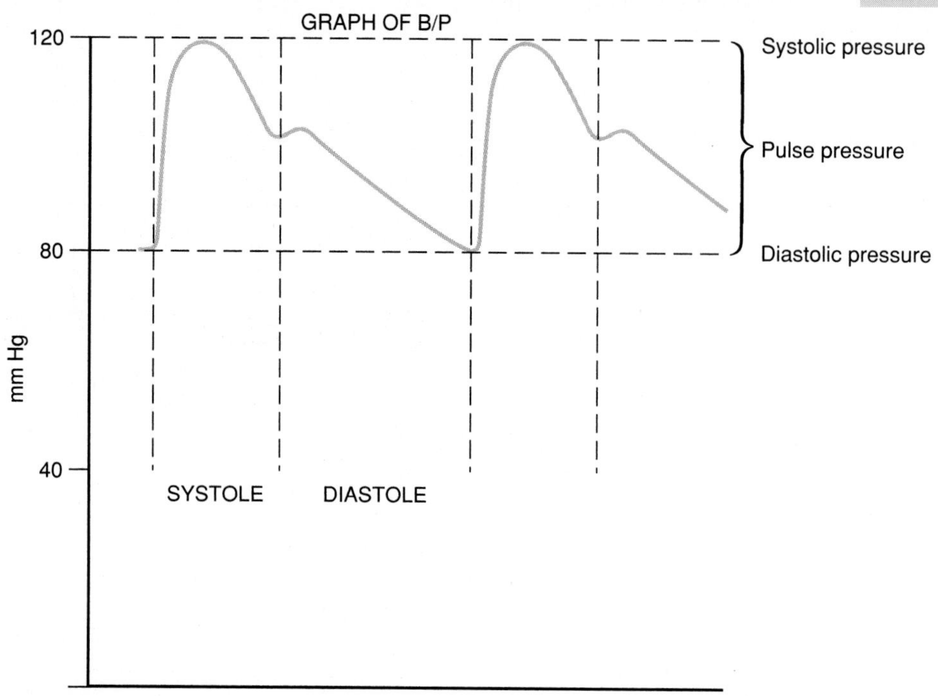

► **Figure 8–11**

The level of blood pressure is determined by five factors:

1. Cardiac output. If the heart pumps more blood into the container (i.e., the blood vessels), the pressure on the container walls increases (Fig. 8–12).
2. Peripheral vascular resistance. This is the opposition to blood flow through the arteries. When the container becomes smaller (e.g., such as with constricted vessels), the pressure needed to push the contents becomes greater.
3. Volume of circulating blood. This is how tightly the blood is packed into the arteries. Increasing the contents in the container increases the pressure.
4. Viscosity. The "thickness" of blood is determined by its formed elements, the blood cells. When the contents are thicker, the pressure increases.
5. Elasticity of vessel walls. When the container walls are stiff and rigid, the pressure needed to push the contents increases.

The average blood pressure in the young adult is 120/80 mm Hg, although this varies normally with many factors, such as:

- Age. Normally, there is a gradual rise through childhood and into adult years (see Fig. 8–19).
- Sex. Before puberty, there is no difference between males and females. After puberty, females usually show a lower blood pressure reading than male counterparts. After menopause, blood pressure in females is higher than in male counterparts.

NORMAL RANGE OF FINDINGS | ABNORMAL FINDINGS

PHYSIOLOGIC FACTORS CONTROLLING BLOOD PRESSURE

FACTOR	CONDITION	RESULT
Cardiac output	↑ with heavy exercise to meet body demand for increased metabolism	↑ B/P
	↓ with pump failure (weak pumping action after myocardial infarction, or in shock)	↓ B/P
Vascular resistance	↑ resistance (vasoconstriction)	↑ B/P
	↓ resistance (vasodilatation)	↓ B/P
Volume	↓ volume (hemorrhage)	↓ B/P
	↑ volume (intravenous fluid overload)	↑ B/P
Viscosity	↑ viscosity (increased hematocrit in polycythemia)	↑ B/P
Elasticity of arterial walls	↑ rigidity, hardening as in arteriosclerosis (heart pumping against greater resistance)	↑ B/P

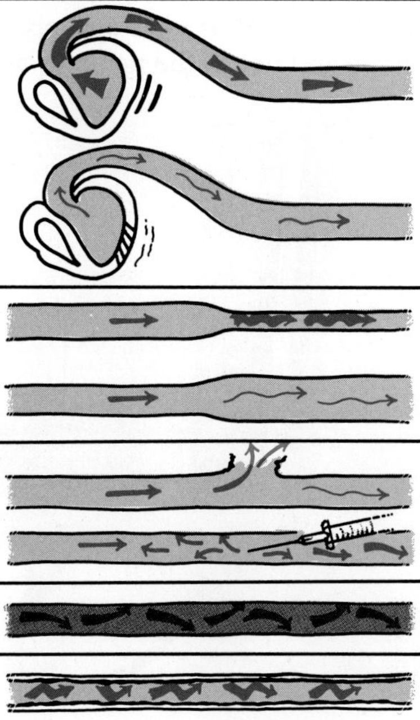

► **Figure 8–12**

- Race. In the United States, a black adult's blood pressure is usually higher than whites of the same age. The incidence of hypertension is twice as high in blacks as in whites. The reasons for this difference are not understood fully but appear to be due to genetic heritage and environmental factors.
- Diurnal rhythm. There is a daily cycle of a peak and a trough: the blood pressure climbs to a high in late afternoon or early evening, and then declines to an early morning low.
- Weight. Blood pressure is higher in obese persons than in persons of normal weight of the same age (including adolescents).
- Exercise. Increasing activity yields a proportionate increase in blood pressure. Within 5 minutes of terminating the exercise, the blood pressure normally returns to baseline (Burch and DePasquale, 1962).
- Emotions. The blood pressure momentarily rises with fear, anger, and pain as a result of stimulation of the sympathetic nervous system.
- Stress. The blood pressure is elevated in persons experiencing continual tension because of their lifestyle, occupational stress, or life problems.

Blood pressure is measured using a stethoscope and a *sphygmomanometer* of either the mercury or the aneroid type. The mercury type is accurate and reliable but not as portable as the aneroid. However, the aneroid gauge is subject to drift, and must be recalibrated at least once each year against a reliable mercury manometer.

The cuff consists of an inflatable rubber bladder inside a cloth cover. The width of the rubber bladder should equal 40 percent of the circumference of the extremity used. The length of the bladder should equal 80 percent of this circumference. The size is important; using a cuff that is too

NORMAL RANGE OF FINDINGS | **ABNORMAL FINDINGS**

narrow yields a falsely high blood pressure because it takes extra pressure to compress the artery. Available cuffs include six sizes that fit newborns to the extra-large adult, as well as tapered cuffs for the cone-shaped obese arm, and thigh cuffs. Match the appropriate size cuff to the person's arm size and shape and not to the person's age (Fig. 8-13).

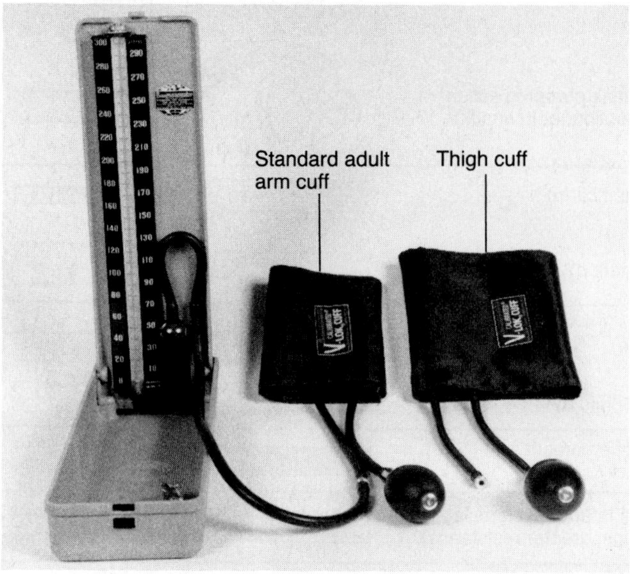

► **Figure 8-13**

Arm Pressure. A comfortable, relaxed person yields a valid blood pressure. Many people are anxious at the beginning of an examination; if this is the case with the person being examined, retake the blood pressure later during the visit. The person may be sitting or lying, with the bare arm supported at heart level. Palpate the brachial artery, which is located just above the antecubital fossa medially. With the cuff deflated, center it about 2.5 cm (1 in) above the brachial artery and wrap it evenly. Now palpate the brachial or the radial artery (Fig. 8-14). Inflate the cuff until

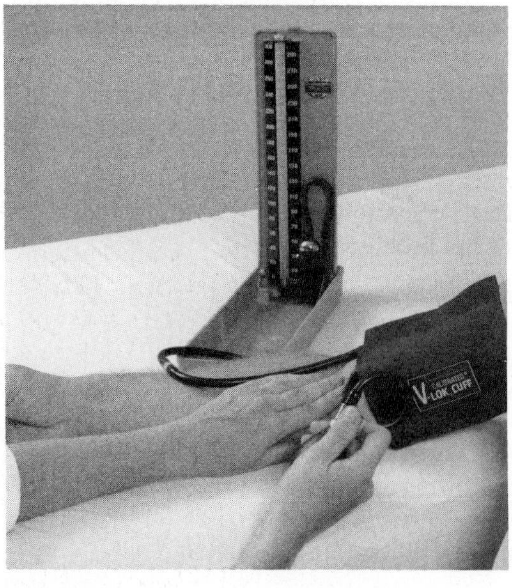

► **Figure 8-14**

NORMAL RANGE OF FINDINGS	ABNORMAL FINDINGS

the artery pulsation is obliterated and then 20 to 30 mm Hg beyond. This will avoid missing an auscultatory gap, which is common with hypertension (Table 8–5).

Place the stethoscope over the site of the brachial artery, making a light but airtight seal (Fig. 8–15). Deflate the cuff slowly and evenly, about

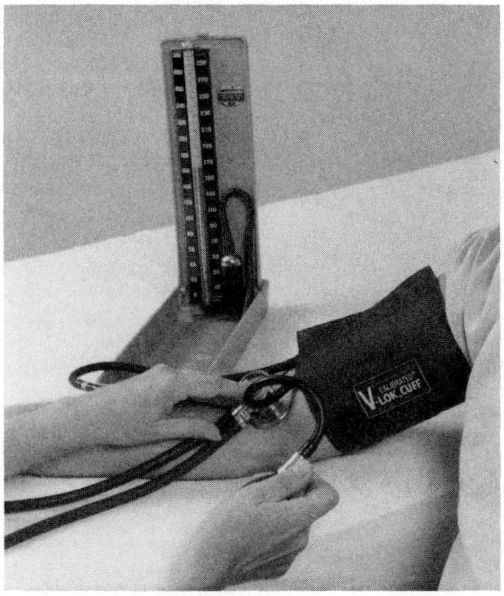

► **Figure 8–15**

2 mm Hg per heartbeat. Note the points at which you hear the first appearance of sound, the muffling of sound, and the final disappearance of sound. These are phases I, IV, and V of *Korotkoff's sounds,* which are the components of a blood pressure reading first described by a Russian surgeon in 1905 (Table 8–5).

In children, phase IV (muffling) is the more accurate measure of diastolic pressure, whereas in adults, phase V (the last audible sound) indicates diastolic pressure best (Frohlich et al, 1988). However, when a variance greater than 10 to 12 mm Hg exists between phase IV and V, record *both* phases along with the systolic reading, e.g., 142/98/80. Clear communication is important because the results significantly affect diagnosis and planning of care. See Table 8–6 for a list of common errors in blood pressure measurement.

See Table 8–9.

If the person is known to have hypertension or is taking antihypertensive medications or if the person reports a history of fainting or syncope, take the blood pressure reading in three positions—lying down, sitting, and standing. When the position is changed from supine to standing, normally there may be a slight decrease (less than 10 mm Hg) in systolic pressure.

Orthostatic hypotension, a drop in systolic pressure of more than 20 mm Hg, occurs with a quick change to a standing position. It is due to abrupt peripheral vasodilatation without a compensatory increase in cardiac output. Aging people have the greatest risk of this problem. It also occurs with prolonged bedrest, hypovolemia, and some drugs.

Thigh Pressure. When blood pressure measured at the arm is excessively high, particularly in adolescents and young adults, compare it with the thigh pressure to check for *coarctation* of the aorta (a congenital form of narrowing). Normally, the thigh pressure is higher than that in the arm. If

With coarctation of the aorta, arm pressures are high. Thigh pressure

NORMAL RANGE OF FINDINGS — ABNORMAL FINDINGS

Table 8-5 ▶ Korotkoff Sounds

PHASE	QUALITY	DESCRIPTION	RATIONALE
Cuff correctly inflated	No sound		Cuff inflation compresses brachial artery. Cuff pressure exceeds heart's systolic pressure, occluding brachial artery blood flow.
I	Tapping	Soft, clear tapping, increasing in intensity.	The SYSTOLIC pressure. As the cuff pressure lowers to reach intraluminal systolic pressure, the artery opens, and blood first spurts into the brachial artery.
Auscultatory gap*	No sound	Silence for 30–40 mm Hg.	Sounds temporarily disappear during end of phase I, then reappear in phase II. Common with hypertension. If undetected, results in falsely low systolic or falsely high diastolic reading.
II	Swooshing	Softer murmur follows tapping.	Turbulent blood flow through still partially occluded artery.
III	Knocking	Crisp, high-pitched sounds.	Artery closes just briefly during late diastole.
IV	Abrupt muffling	Sound mutes to a low-pitched, cushioned murmur; blowing quality.	Artery no longer closes in any part of cardiac cycle. Change in quality, not intensity. American Heart Association proposes this as most accurate level of diastolic pressure in children (Frohlich et al, 1988).
V	Silence		Descreased velocity of blood flow. Streamlined blood flow is silent. The last audible sound (marking the disappearance of sounds is adult DIASTOLIC pressure.)

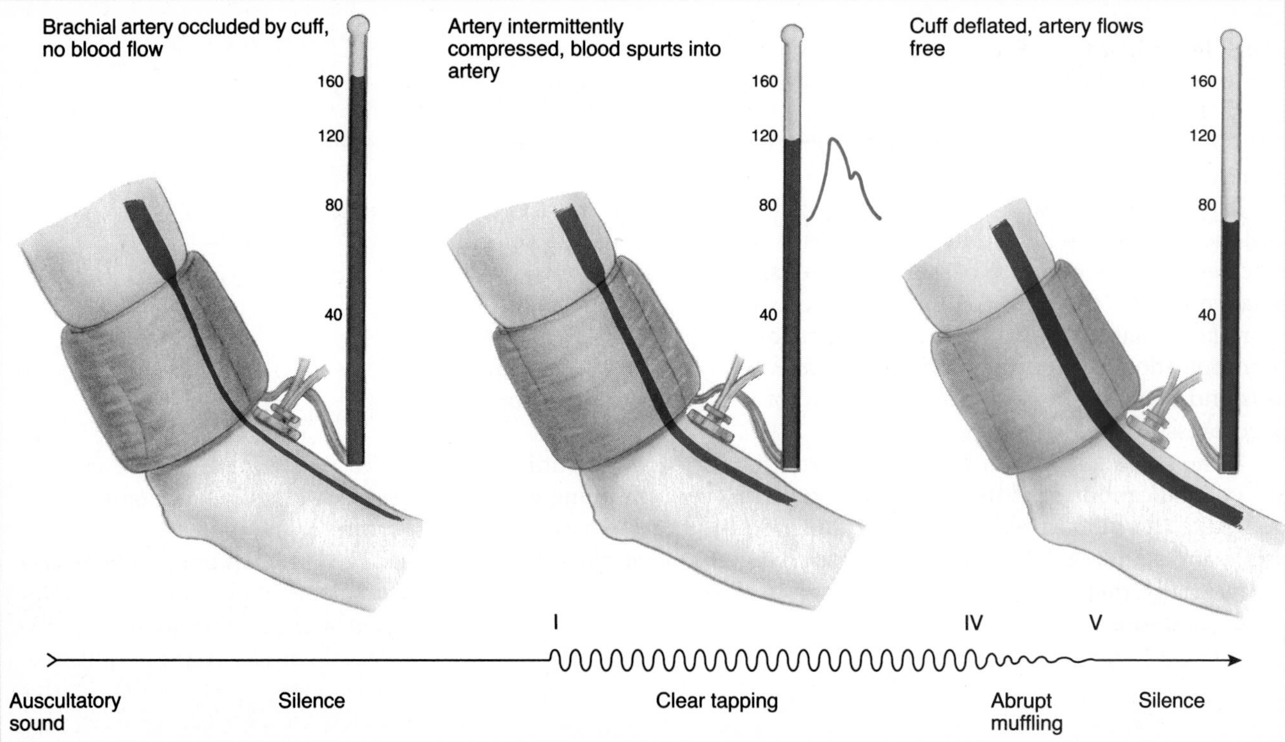

* This is an abnormal finding.

NORMAL RANGE OF FINDINGS

possible, turn the person into the prone position on the abdomen. (If the person must remain in the supine position, bend the knee slightly.) Wrap a large cuff, 18 to 20 cm, around the lower third of the thigh, centered over the popliteal artery on the back of the knee. Auscultate the popliteal artery for the reading (Fig. 8 – 16). Normally, the systolic value is 10 to 40 mm Hg higher than in the arm, and the diastolic pressure is the same.

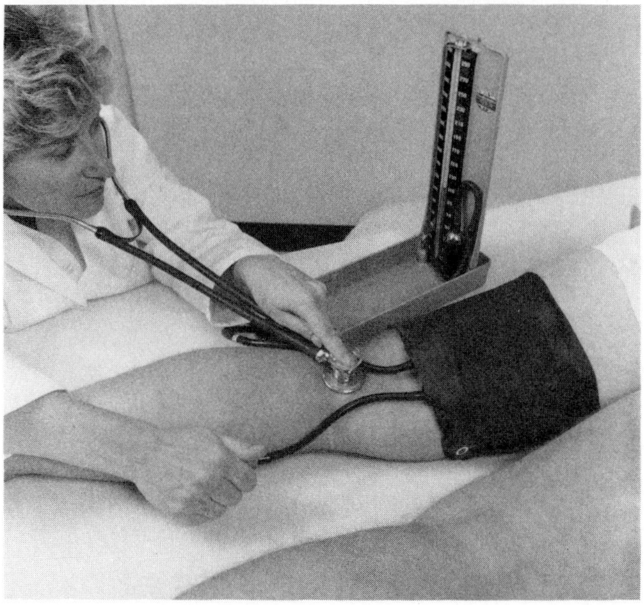

► **Figure 8 – 16**

ABNORMAL FINDINGS

is *lower* because the blood supply to the thigh is below the constriction.

Table 8 - 6 ► Common Errors in Blood Pressure Measurement

FACTOR	RESULT	RATIONALE
Taking blood pressure reading when person is anxious or angry or has just been active.	Falsely high	Sympathetic nervous system stimulation
Faulty arm position:		
above level of heart	Falsely low	Eliminates effect of hydrostatic pressure
below level of heart	Falsely high	Additional force of gravity added to brachial artery pressure
person supports own arm	Falsely high diastolic	Sustained isometric muscular contraction
Examiner's eyes not at level with meniscus of mercury column:		
Looking up at meniscus	Falsely high	Parallax
Looking down on meniscus	Falsely low	
Inaccurate cuff size:*		
cuff too narrow for extremity	Falsely high	Needs excessive pressure to occlude brachial artery.
Cuff wrap is too loose or uneven, or bladder balloons out of wrap.	Falsely high	Needs excessive pressure to occlude brachial artery.
Failure to palpate radial artery while inflating:		
Inflating not high enough	Falsely low systolic	Miss initial systolic tapping. Or, may tune in during *auscultatory gap* (tapping sounds disappear for 10 to 40 mm Hg and then return; common with hypertension)
Inflating cuff too high	Pain	

Table continued on following page

NORMAL RANGE OF FINDINGS | ABNORMAL FINDINGS

Table 8-6 ▶ Common Errors in Blood Pressure Measurement *Continued*

FACTOR	RESULT	RATIONALE
Pushing stethoscope too hard on brachial artery.	Falsely low diastolic	Excessive pressure distorts artery and the sounds continue
Deflating cuff:		
too quickly	Falsely low systolic and/or falsely high diastolic	Insufficient time to hear tapping
too slowly	Falsely high diastolic	Venous congestion in forearm makes sounds less audible.
Halting during descent and reinflating cuff to recheck systolic.	Falsely high diastolic	Venous congestion in forearm
Failure to wait 1-2 minutes before repeating entire reading.	Falsely high diastolic	Venous congestion in forearm
Any observer error:		
Examiner's "subconscious bias"; a preconceived idea of what blood pressure reading *should* be owing to person's age, race, sex, weight, history, or condition.	Error anywhere	
Examiner's haste Faulty technique Examiner's digit preference, "hears" more results that end in zero than would occur by chance alone, e.g., 130/80. Diminished hearing acuity Defective or inaccurately calibrated equipment.	Error anywhere	

* This is the most common error

DEVELOPMENTAL CONSIDERATIONS

The Younger Person

Measure vital signs with the same purpose and frequency as you would in an adult. With an *infant,* reverse the order of vital sign measurement to respiration, pulse, and temperature. Taking a rectal temperature may cause the infant to cry, which will increase the respiratory and pulse rate, thus masking the normal resting values. A *preschooler's* normal fear of body mutilation is increased with any invasive procedure. Whenever possible, avoid the rectal route and take an axillary temperature. When this is not feasible, use the reverse order and measure the rectal temperature last. Promote the cooperation of the *school-aged child* by explaining the procedure completely and encouraging the child to handle the equipment. Your approach to measuring vital signs with the *adolescent* is much the same as with the adult.

Temperature

The choice of route for taking the temperature is important with the younger child.

Oral. Use this route when the child is old enough to keep the mouth closed and does not bite on the glass thermometer. This is usually at age 5

NORMAL RANGE OF FINDINGS	ABNORMAL FINDINGS

or 6, though some 4-year-old children can cooperate. When available, use an electronic thermometer because it is unbreakable and it registers quickly.

Axillary. Whenever possible, use the axillary route with the premature and term newborn because it avoids the risk of rectal perforation. Also, it is preferable with toddlers and preschoolers because it is not intrusive. Place the tip well into the axilla, and hold the child's arm close to the body. An accurate reading will register by 5 minutes (Eoff and Joyce, 1981).

Rectal. Use this route with infants. Use it with other age groups when the other routes are not feasible, such as with the child who is unable to cooperate, agitated, unconscious, critically ill, or seizure prone. An infant may be supine or side lying, with the examiner's hand flexing the knees up onto the abdomen. (When supine, cover the boy's penis with a diaper.) Or, an infant may lie prone across the adult's lap (Fig. 8–17). Separate the

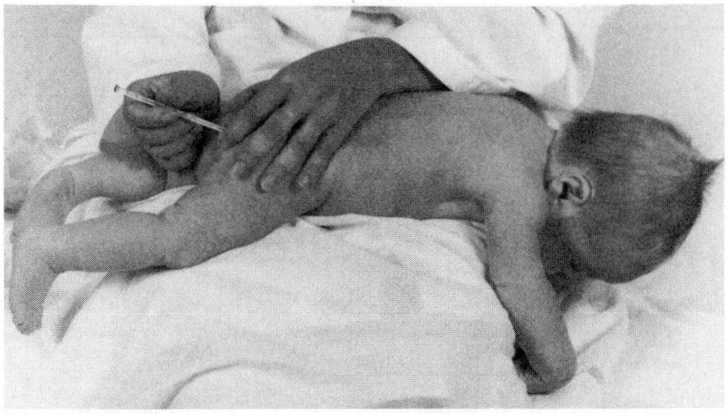

► **Figure 8–17**

buttocks with one hand, and insert the lubricated stubby-tipped thermometer *no farther than* 2.5 cm (1 in). Any deeper insertion risks rectal perforation because the colon curves posteriorly at 3 cm (1 1/4 in). The temperature will register by 3 minutes.

Normally, rectal temperatures measure higher in infants and young children than in adults, with an average of 37.8° C (100° F) at 18 months. Also, the temperature normally may be elevated in the late afternoon, after vigorous playing or after eating.

Up to ages 6 to 8, children have higher fevers with illness than adults do. Even with minor infections, fevers may elevate to 39.5 to 40.5° C (103–105° F).

Pulse

Palpate or auscultate an apical rate with infants and toddlers. (See Chapter 16 for location of apex and technique.) In children older than 2 years of age, use the radial site. Count the pulse for 1 full minute to take into account normal irregularities, such as sinus arrhythmia. The heart rate normally fluctuates more with infants and children than with adults in response to exercise, emotion, and illness.

Respirations

Watch the infant's abdomen for movement, because the infant's respirations are normally more diaphragmatic than thoracic. Count 1 full minute, because the pattern varies significantly from rapid breaths to short periods of apnea. Note the normal rate in Table 8–4.

Periods of apnea > 20 seconds may indicate risk of sudden infant death syndrome (SIDS), even with infants who look healthy.

NORMAL RANGE OF FINDINGS

Blood Pressure

After age 3, a routine blood pressure is measured at least annually. For accurate measurement in children, make some adjustment in the choice of equipment and technique. The most common error is failure to use the correct size cuff. The cuff width must cover two-thirds of the upper arm, and the cuff bladder must completely encircle it. Use a pediatric-sized endpiece on the stethoscope to locate the sounds. If possible, allow a crying infant to become quiet for 5 to 10 minutes before measuring the blood pressure; crying may elevate the systolic pressure by 30 to 50 mm Hg. Finally, *always* use the muffling of sounds (phase IV Korotkoff) for the true diastolic reading. Children have a higher velocity of blood flow than do adults, which prolongs phase V beyond the true diastolic value. Note the normal blood pressure values by age groups in Figure 8–18.

ABNORMAL FINDINGS

Further explore any blood pressure that is greater than the 95th percentile.

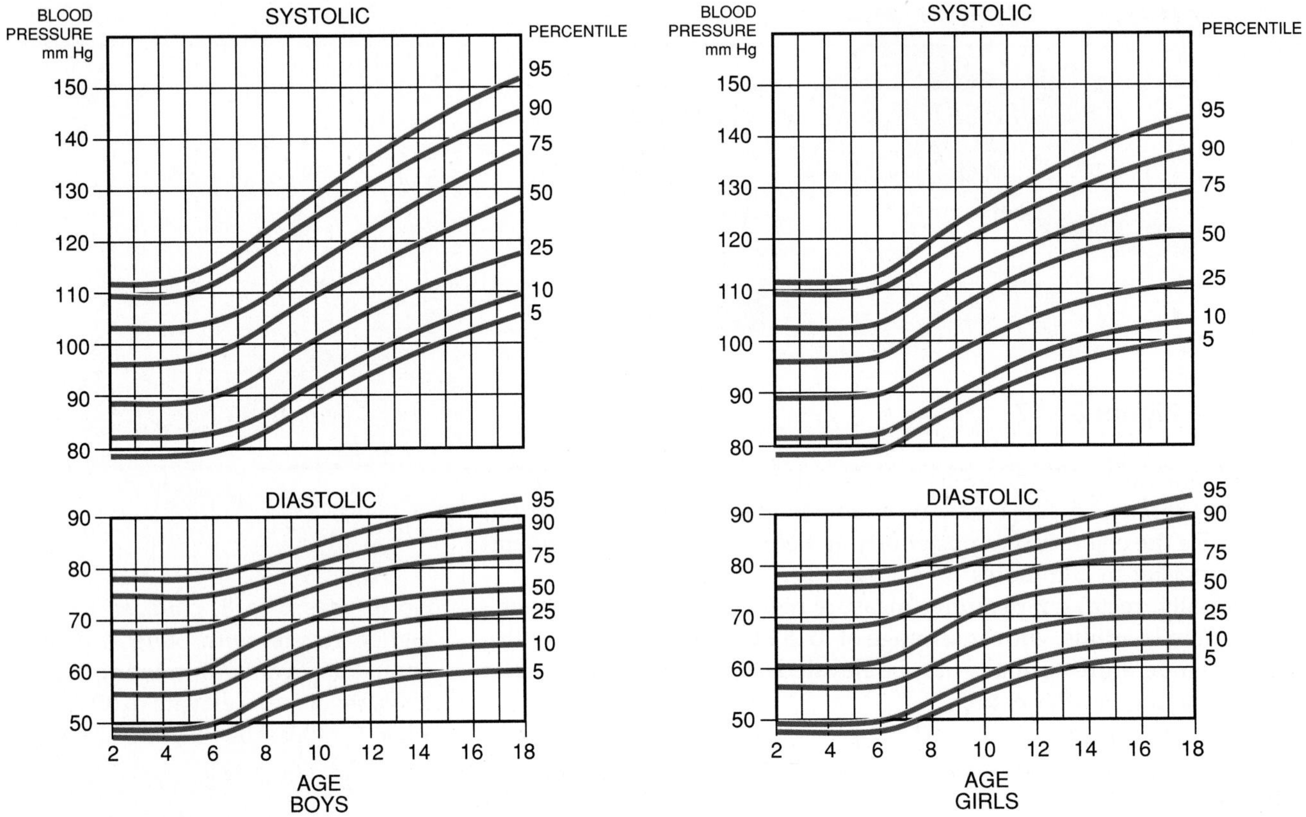

▶ **Figure 8–18**

Children under 2 years of age have such small arms that it is difficult to hear Korotkoff's sounds using a stethoscope. Instead, use a *Doppler* ultrasound device to amplify the sounds. This instrument is easy to use and can be used by one examiner. (Note the technique for using the Doppler on p. 215.)

If no Doppler ultrasound device is available, the flush technique is a fair alternative for a mean pressure:

NORMAL RANGE OF FINDINGS	ABNORMAL FINDINGS

- Use only when the infant is lying quietly.
- Place the manometer gauge close to the baby's extremity (the arm or the leg) so that you can see both together.
- Position the correctly sized neonatal cuff on the infant's leg.
- Elevate the leg to drain venous blood. Further milk the leg by squeezing the foot with your hand or by wrapping an elastic bandage from the toes up toward the cuff. (Bandaging is more accurate than hand compression.) All this will blanch the leg.
- Inflate the cuff to 120 to 140 mm Hg and then lower the leg.
- Unwrap the ace bandage; then deflate the cuff pressure, no faster than 5 mm Hg per second.
- Note the point of the leg's first full flush. This is the mean systolic-diastolic pressure.

Normally, the result is 30 to 60 mm Hg for infants weighing over 2500 g (6.7 lb). Use of the flush technique is limited to the light-skinned infant with a fairly healthy cardiovascular system. A valid result is impossible if you cannot see a flush, as in dark-skinned infants and in infants suffering from cyanosis, severe anemia, peripheral vasoconstriction, marked hypothermia, or edema. Obviously, this limits the usefulness of the flush technique because it is in the latter instances that you need a valid blood pressure.

The Aging Adult

Temperature

Changes in the body's temperature regulatory mechanism leave the aging person less likely to develop fever but at a greater risk of developing hypothermia. Thus, the temperature is a less reliable index of the older person's true health state. Sweat gland activity is also diminished.

Pulse

The normal range of heart rate is 60 to 100 bpm, but the rhythm may be slightly irregular. The radial artery may feel stiff, rigid, and tortuous in an older person, although this condition does not necessarily imply vascular disease in the heart or brain. The increasingly rigid arterial wall needs a faster upstroke of blood, so the pulse actually is easier to palpate.

Respirations

Aging causes a decrease in vital capacity and a decreased inspiratory reserve volume. You may note a shallower inspiratory phase and an increased respiratory rate.

NORMAL RANGE OF FINDINGS

ABNORMAL FINDINGS

Blood Pressure

The aorta and major arteries tend to harden with age. As the heart pumps against a stiffer aorta, the systolic pressure increases, leading to a widened pulse pressure (see Fig. 8 – 19 for mean blood pressure readings in apparently healthy persons from birth to old age). With many older people, both the systolic and diastolic pressures increase, making it difficult to distinguish normal aging values from abnormal hypertension.

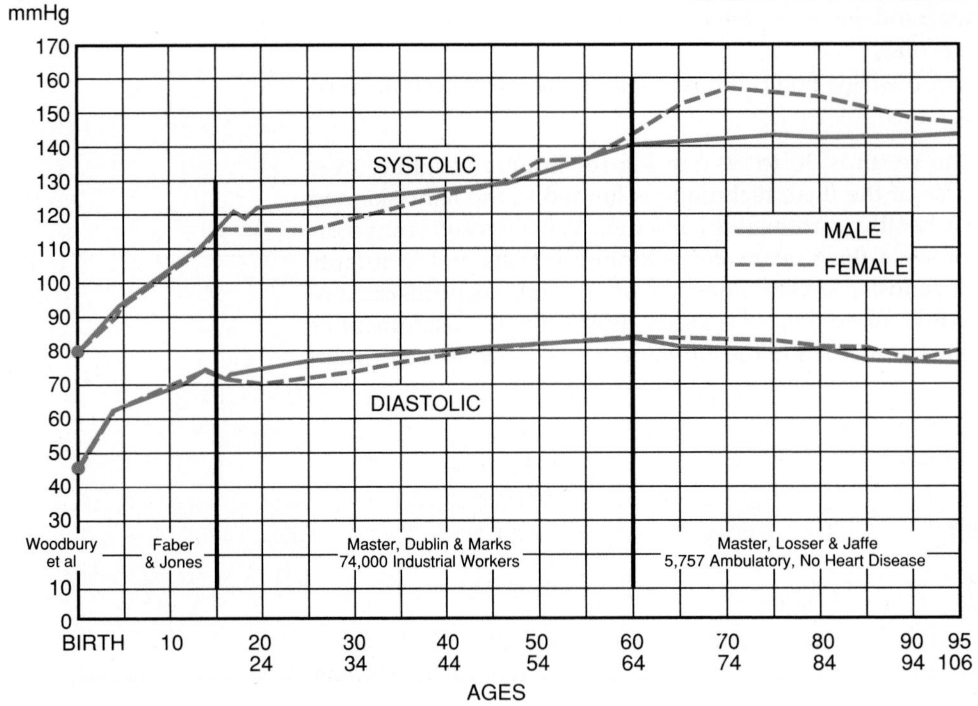

▶ **Figure 8 – 19**

ADDITIONAL TECHNIQUES

The Doppler Technique. In many situations, pulse and blood pressure measurement are enhanced using an electronic device, the *Doppler ultrasonic flowmeter.* The Doppler technique works by a principle discovered in the nineteenth century by an Austrian physicist, Johannes Doppler. Sound varies in pitch in relation to the distance between the sound source and the listener; the pitch is higher when the distance is small, and the pitch lowers as the distance increases. Think of a railroad train speeding toward you; its train whistle sounds higher the closer it gets, and the pitch of the whistle lowers as the train fades away.

Here, the sound source is the blood pumping through the artery in a rhythmic manner. A hand-held transducer picks up changes in sound frequency as the blood flows and ebbs and it amplifies them. The listener hears a whooshing pulsatile beat.

The Doppler technique is used to locate the peripheral pulse sites (see Chapter 18 for further discussion of this technique.) For blood pressure measurement, the Doppler technique will augment Korotkoff's sounds (Fig. 8 – 20). Through this technique, sounds that are hard to hear with a

NORMAL RANGE OF FINDINGS | **ABNORMAL FINDINGS**

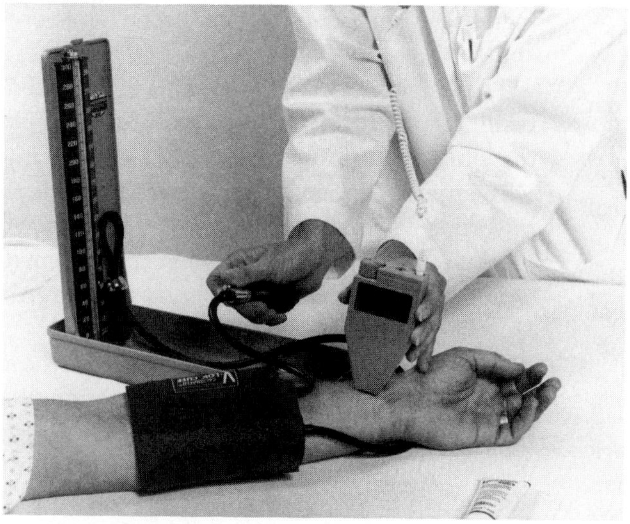

▶ **Figure 8-20**

stethoscope, such as those in infants with small arms and in obese persons in whom the sounds are muffled by layers of fat, may be evaluated. Also, proper cuff placement is difficult on the obese person's cone-shaped upper arm. In this situation, you can place the cuff on the more even forearm and hold the Doppler probe over the radial artery. For either location, use this procedure:

- Apply coupling gel to the transducer probe.
- Turn Doppler on.
- Touch the probe to the skin, holding the probe perpendicular to the artery.
- A pulsatile whooshing sound indicates location of the artery. You may need to rotate the probe, but maintain contact with the skin. Do not push the probe too hard or you will wipe out the pulse.
- Inflate the cuff until the sounds disappear, then proceed another 20 to 30 mm Hg beyond that point.
- Slowly deflate the cuff, noting the point at which the first whooshing sounds appear. This is the systolic pressure.
- A muffling of sounds indicates the diastolic pressure (phase IV of Korotkoff's sounds).

TRANSCULTURAL CONSIDERATIONS

GENERAL APPEARANCE

Cultural differences are found in the body proportions of individuals. In general, white males are 1.27 cm (0.5 in) taller than black males, whereas white and black women are, on the average, the same height. Sitting/standing height ratios reveal that blacks of both sexes have longer legs and shorter trunks than whites. Because proportionately most of the weight is in the trunk, white men appear more obese than black men. Asians are markedly shorter, weigh less, and have smaller body frames.

Despite their longer legs, black women are consistently heavier than white women at every age, with black women carrying an average of 9.1 kg (20 lb) more than white women between the ages of 35 and 64 years (Overfield, 1985).

Bone length, as revealed by stature, shows definite biocultural differences, with blacks having longer legs and arms than whites. Asians and Native Americans have, on the average, longer trunks and shorter limbs than whites. Blacks tend to be wide shouldered and narrow hipped, whereas Asians tend to be wide hipped and narrow shouldered. Shoulder width is largely produced by the clavicle. Because the clavicle is a long bone, this explains why taller people have wide shoulders, whereas shorter people have narrower shoulders.

Although not all groups have been studied, research on selected populations reveals that children of some immigrant groups to the United States are taller than their peers in the country of origin. For example, Japanese Americans residing in Hawaii are taller than those Japanese living in Japan. Although the sitting/standing height ratio is the same, Italians in California are 3.8 cm (1.5 in) taller than those of the same age living in Italy (Hulse, 1968; Overfield, 1985). This indicates that the increase in height occurs in both the long bones and the spine (Brues, 1977).

The height increase in migrants is theorized to be the result of two factors: (1) better nutrition is provided in the United States and (2) there is decreased interference with growth from infectious diseases during the formative years. Furthermore, the overall height of Americans increased 1.8 cm (0.7 in) for men and 1.3 cm (0.5 in) for women during the 10-year period studied (Abraham et al, 1976).

There are also biocultural differences in the amount of body fat and the distribution of fat throughout the body. In general, individuals from the lower class are more obese than those from the middle class, who are more obese than members of the upper class. In addition to socioeconomic considerations, blacks tend to have smaller (1 mm) skinfold thicknesses in their arms than whites but the distribution of fat on the trunk is similar.

CULTURE AND DISEASE PREVALENCE

For the past generation, the United States as a whole has enjoyed improvement in the health status of its people. Despite this fact, there continues to be disparity in deaths and illnesses experienced by racial and ethnic minority populations, and it is well known that diseases are not distributed equally among all segments of the population but rather tend to cluster around certain racial and ethnic subgroups. Abnormal biocultural variations may be genetic or acquired. Summarized in Table 8–7 is a list of selected genetic traits and disorders by

Table 8–7 ▶ Distribution of Selected Genetic Traits and Disorders by Population or Ethnic Group

ETHNIC OR POPULATION GROUP	GENETIC OR MULTIFACTORIAL DISORDER PRESENT IN RELATIVELY HIGH FREQUENCY
Aland Islanders	Ocular albinism (Forsius-Eriksson type)
Amish	Limb-girdle muscular dystrophy (IN—Adams, Allen counties)
	Ellis-van Creveld (PA—Lancaster county)
	Pyruvate kinase deficiency (OH— Mifflin county)
	Hemophilia B (PA—Holmes county)
Armenians	Familial Mediterranean fever
	Familial paroxysmal polyserositis

Table 8-7 ▶ Distribution of Selected Genetic Traits and Disorders by Population or Ethnic Group *Continued*

ETHNIC OR POPULATION GROUP	GENETIC OR MULTIFACTORIAL DISORDER PRESENT IN RELATIVELY HIGH FREQUENCY
Blacks (African)	Sickle cell disease
	Hemoglobin C disease
	Hereditary persistence of hemoglobin F
	G6PD deficiency, African type
	Lactase deficiency, adult
	β-Thalassemia
Burmese	Hemoglobin E disease
Chinese	Alpha thalassemia
	G6PD deficiency, Chinese type
	Lactase deficiency, adult
Costa Rican	Malignant osteopetrosis
Druze	Alkaptonuria
English	Cystic fibrosis
	Hereditary amyloidosis, type III
Eskimos	Congenital adrenal hyperplasia
	Pseudocholinesterase deficiency
	Methemoglobinemia
French Canadians (Quebec)	Tyrosinemia
	Morquio syndrome
Finns	Congenital nephrosis
	Generalized amyloidosis syndrome, V
	Polycystic liver disease
	Retinoschisis
	Aspartylglycosaminuria
	Diastrophic dwarfism
Gypsies (Czech)	Congenital glaucoma
Hopi Indians	Tyrosinase positive albinism
Iceland	Phenylketonuria
Irish	Phenylketonuria
	Neural tube defects
Japanese	Acatalasemia
	Cleft lip/palate
	Oguchi disease
Jews	
Ashkenazi	Tay-Sachs disease (infantile)
	Niemann-Pick disease (infantile)
	Gaucher disease (adult type)
	Familial dysautonomia (Riley-Day syndrome)
	Bloom syndrome
	Torsion dystonia
	Factor XI (PTA) deficiency
Sephardi	Familial Mediterranean fever
	Ataxia-telangiectasia (Morocco)
	Cystinuria (Libya)
	Glycogen storage disease III (Morocco)
Oriental	Dubin-Johnson syndrome (Iran)
	Ichthyosis vulgaris (Iraq, India)
	Werdnig-Hoffmann disease (Karcite Jews)
	G6PD deficiency, Mediterranean type
	Phenylketonuria (Yemen)
	Metachromatic leukodystrophy (Habbanite Jews, Saudi Arabia)
Lapps	Congenital dislocation of hip
Lebanese	Dyggus-Melchior-Clausen syndrome
Mediterranean people (Italians, Greeks)	G6PD deficiency, Mediterranean type
	β-Thalassemia
	Familial Mediterranean fever
Navaho Indians	Ear anomalies
Polynesians	Clubfoot
Polish	Phenylketonuria
Portuguese	Joseph disease
Nova Scotia Acadians	Niemann-Pick disease, type D

Table continued on following page

Table 8-7 ▶ Distribution of Selected Genetic Traits and Disorders by Population or Ethnic Group *Continued*

ETHNIC OR POPULATION GROUP	GENETIC OR MULTIFACTORIAL DISORDER PRESENT IN RELATIVELY HIGH FREQUENCY
Scandinavians (Norwegians, Swedes, Danes)	Cholestasis-lymphedema (Norwegians)
	Sjögren-Larsson syndrome (Swedes)
	Krabbe disease
	Phenylketonuria
Scots	Phenylketonuria
	Cystic fibrosis
	Hereditary amyloidosis, type III
Thai	Lactase deficiency, adult
	Hemoglobin E disease
Zuni Indians	Tyrosinase positive albinism

(From Cohen FI: Clinical Genetics in Nursing Practice. Philadelphia, JB Lippincott Company, 1984.)

population or ethnic group. This information is useful in assessing people from various subgroups because you are able to focus your assessment according to the increased statistical probability that a particular condition may occur. For example, if you are examining a black child with gastrointestinal symptoms, you may focus more on the possibility of lactose intolerance or sickle cell anemia while considering cystic fibrosis, known primarily among white children, a much less likely source of the problem. Thus, in your assessment, you will want to be certain that you have gathered the appropriate data needed to support or refute your suspicions.

SAMPLE RECORDING

A.J. is a 47-year-old black female high school principal, well nourished, well developed, appears stated age. She is alert, oriented, cooperative, with no signs of acute distress. Ht. 163 cm (5′4″), Wt. 57 kg (126 lbs), TPR 37° C — 76 — 14, B/P 146/84 right arm, sitting.

Table 8–8 ► Abnormalities in Body Height and Proportion

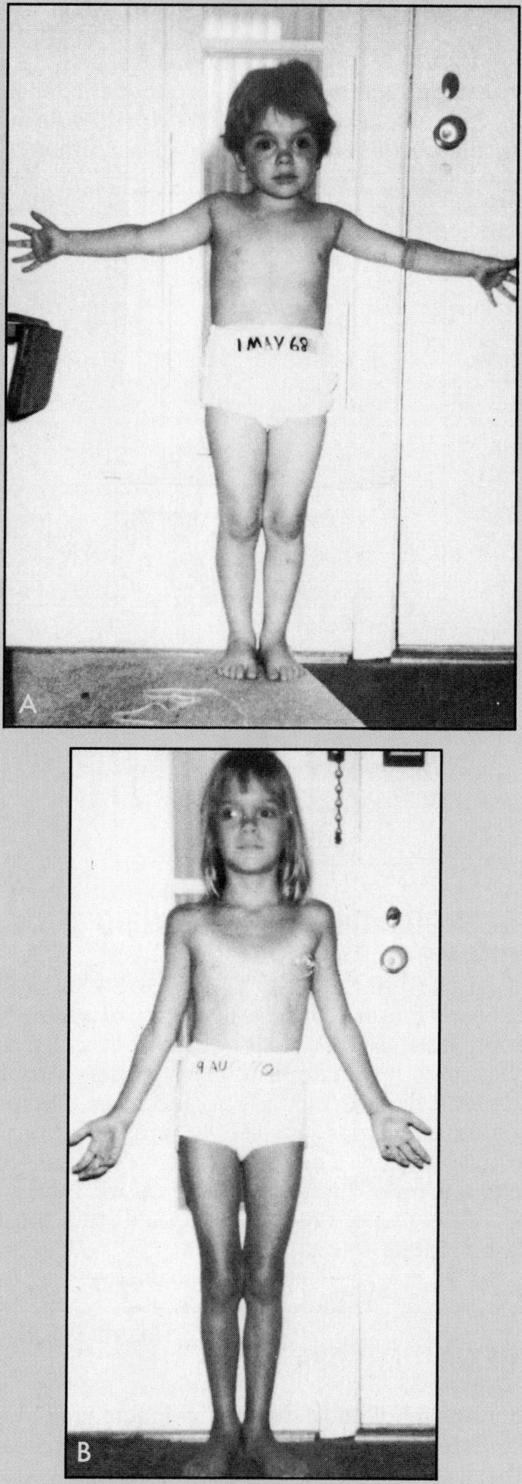

HYPOPITUITARY DWARFISM

Deficiency in growth hormone in childhood results in retardation of growth and delayed puberty. The 6-year-old girl at top appears much younger than her chronologic age with infantile facial features and chubbiness. The same girl at bottom 15 months later after treatment with growth hormone shows increased height, more mature facies, and loss of infantile fat.

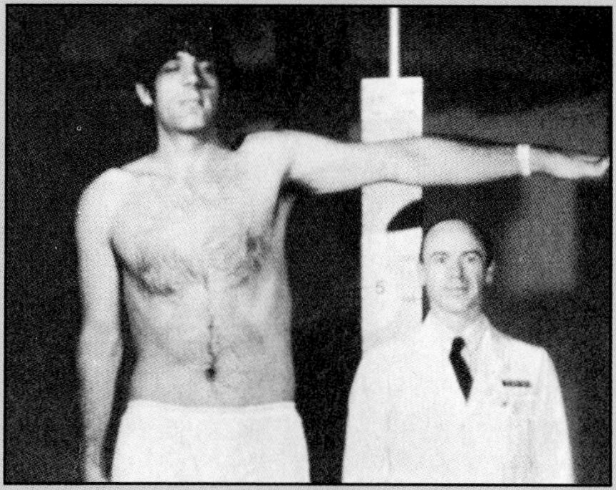

GIGANTISM

Excessive secretion of growth hormone before closure of bone epiphyses in puberty causes increased height and weight and delayed sexual development.

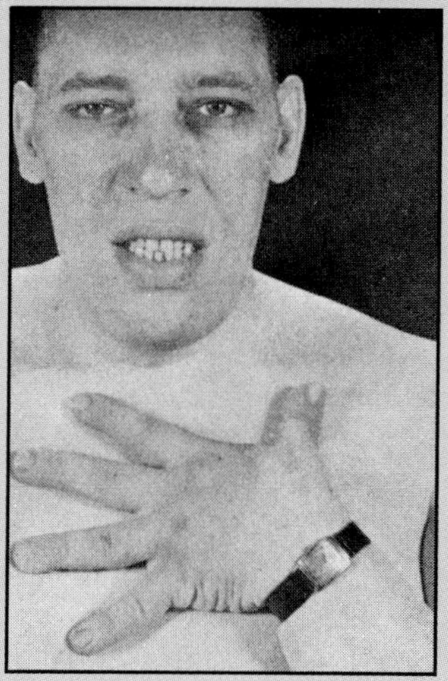

ACROMEGALY (HYPERPITUITARISM)

Excessive secretion of growth hormone after normal completion of body growth causes overgrowth of bone in the face, head, hands and feet.

Table continued on following page

Table 8-8 ▸ Abnormalities in Body Height and Proportion *Continued*

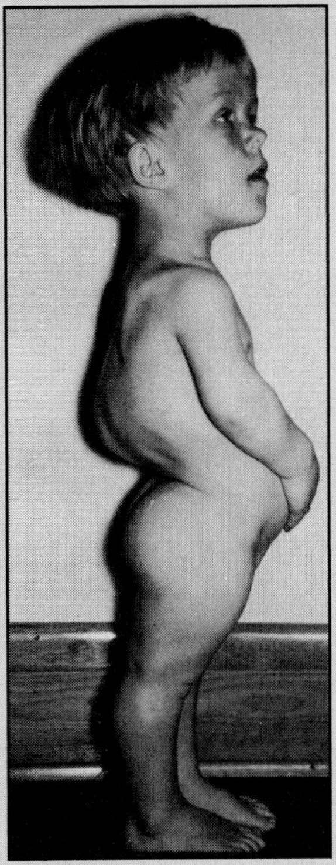

ACHONDROPLASTIC DWARFISM

Congenital skeletal malformation due to genetic disorder characterized by relatively large head, short stature, short limbs, thoracic kyphosis, prominent lumbar lordosis, and abdominal protrusion. The mean adult height in men is about 131.5 cm (51.8 in) and in women about 125 cm (49.2 in).

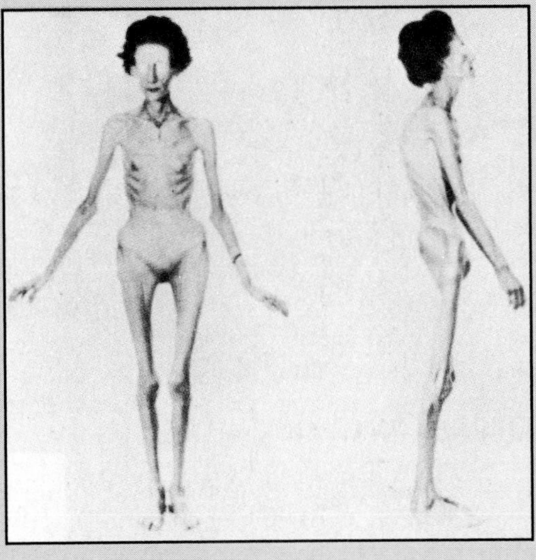

MARFAN'S SYNDROME (not illustrated)

Connective tissue disorder resulting in tall, thin stature with long extremities and long hyperextensible fingers. Arm span exceeds height. Pubis-to-sole measurement exceeds crown-to-pubis measurement.

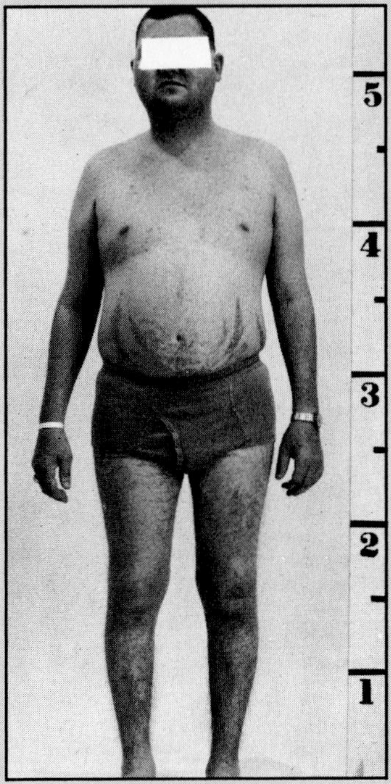

ENDOGENOUS OBESITY—CUSHING'S SYNDROME

Excessive secretion of or administration of adrenocorticotropic hormone (ACTH). Characterized by central obesity with thin arms and legs, muscle atrophy, round plethoric face (moon face), hirsutism, and purple abdominal striae as well as multiple internal organ dysfunction. This is markedly different from *exogenous* obesity due to excessive caloric intake, in which body fat is evenly distributed and muscle strength is intact.

ANOREXIA NERVOSA

A serious psychological disorder characterized by severe and debilitating weight loss and amenorrhea in an otherwise healthy adolescent or young woman. Behavior is characterized by fanatic concern about weight, distorted body image (perceives self as fat despite skeletal appearance), starvation diets, frenetic exercise patterns, and striving for perfection.

Table 8-9 ► Abnormalities in Blood Pressure

HYPOTENSION

In normotensive adults:	below 95/60
In hypertensive adults:	below the person's average reading, but above 95/60
In children:	below expected value for age

Occurs With	Rationale
Acute myocardial infarction	Decreased cardiac output
Shock	Decreased cardiac output
Hemorrhage	Decrease in total blood volume
Vasodilatation	Decrease in peripheral vascular resistance
Addison's disease (hypofunction of adrenal glands)	

HYPERTENSION

In adults under 40:	>140/90
In adults over 40:	>160/95
In children:	>95th percentile expected for age

(Diagnosis follows at least three separate elevated readings, not on one isolated high value.)

Essential or Primary Hypertension

This occurs from no known cause but is responsible for about 95 percent of cases of hypertension in adults.

Secondary Hypertension

This is due to a specific, often curable cause and occurs with:

- Kidney disease
  - Renal vascular disease
  - Pyelonephritis
  - Glomerulonephritis
  - Renal failure
  - Renal injury
  - Renal tumor
- Adrenal disorder
  - Cushing's disease
  - Pheochromocytoma (tumor of adrenal medulla)
  - Hyperaldosteronism
- Coarctation of the aorta
- Central nervous system disorders
  - Brain tumor
  - Head injury
- Medication side effect
  - Pressor agents (epinephrine, isoproterenol, ephedrine)
  - Corticosteroids
  - Oral contraceptives
  - Amphetamines
- Volume overload

Bibliography

Abraham SJ, Clifford L, Najjar MF: Height and weight of adults 18–74 years of age in the United States. Advancedata 3:1–8, 1976.

Bahr RT Sr, Gress L: Blood pressure readings and selected parameter relationships on an elderly ambulatory population. J Gerontol Nurs 8:159–163, 1982.

Baker NC, Cerone SB, Gaze N, Knapp TR: The effect of type of thermometer and length of time inserted on oral temperature measurements of afebrile subjects. Nurs Res 33:109–111, 1984.

Barr GD, Allen CM, Shinefield HR: Height and weight of 7,500 children of three skin colors. Am J Dis Child 124:866–872, 1972.

Battaglia FC, Lubchenco LO: A practical classification of newborn infants by weight and gestational age. J Pediatr 71(2):159–163, 1967.

Blainey CG: Site selection in taking body temperature. Am J of Nurs 74:1859–1861, 1974.

Blumenthal S, Epps RR, Heavenrich R, et al: National Heart, Lung and Blood Institute's Report of the task force on blood pressure control in children. Pediatrics 59(5)(Suppl.):797–820, 1977.

Britton CV: Blood pressure measurement and hypertension in children. Pediatr Nurs 7:13–17, 1981.

Brues AM: People and Races. New York, Macmillan, 1977.

Burch GG, DePasquale NP: Primer of Clinical Measurement of Blood Pressure. St. Louis, MO, CV Mosby, 1962.

Dubowitz LM, Dubowitz V, Goldberg C: Clinical assessment of gestational age in the newborn infant. J Pediatr 77(1):1–10, 1970.

Eoff MJ: Temperature measurement in infants. Nurs Res 23:457–460, 1974.

Eoff MJ, Joyce B: Temperature measurements in children. Am J Nurs 81:1010–1011, 1981.

Erickson R: Oral temperature differences in relation to thermometer and technique. Nurs Res 29:157–164, 1980.

Frohlich ED, Grim C, Labarthe DR, et al: Recommendations for human blood pressure determination by sphygmomanometers. Report of a Special Task Force appointed by the Steering Committee, American Heart Association. Circulation 77:501A–514A, 1988.

Gelfant B: Hypertension protocol. Nurse Pract. 8:25–34, 1983.
Hahn WK, Brooks JA, Hite R: Blood pressure norms for healthy young adults: Relation to sex, age and reported parental hypertension. Res Nurs Health 12:53–56, 1989.
Hait HI, Lemeshow S, Rosenman KD: A longitudinal study of blood pressure in a national survey of children. Am J Public Health 72:1285–1287, 1982.
Henneman EA, Henneman PL: Intricacies of blood pressure measurement: Reexamining the rituals. Heart Lung 18:263–273, 1989.
Hill MN, Cunningham SL: The latest words for high BP. AJN 89(4):504–510, 1989.
Hulse FS: The breakdown of isolates and hybrid vigor among the Italian Swiss. Proceedings of the 12th International Congress on Genetics 2:177, 1968.
Hunt JC, Frolich ED, Moser M, et al: Devices used for self-measurement of blood pressure. Arch Intern Med 145:2231–2234, 1985.
Jarvis CM: Vital Signs — A Preview of Problems. Assessing Vital Functions Accurately. 2nd ed. Springhouse, PA, Springhouse, 1983.
Joint National Committee on Detection, Evaluation, and Treatment of High Blood Pressure: The 1984 Report. U.S. Department of Health and Human Services, NIH Publication No. 84-1088, June 1984.
Jones ML: Accuracy of pulse rates counted for fifteen, thirty and sixty seconds. Milit Med, 135(12):1127–1136, 1970.
Kirkendall WM, Burton AC, Epstein FH, Fries ED: Committee of the American Heart Association: Recommendations for human blood pressure determination by sphygmomanometers. Circulation 36:980–988, 1967.
Lubchenco LO, Hansman C, Boyd E: Intrauterine growth in length and head circumference as estimated from live births at gestational ages from 26 to 42 weeks. Pediatrics 37(3):403–408, 1966.
Lubchenco LO, Hansman C, Dressler M, Boyd E: Intrauterine growth as estimated from liveborn birth-weight data at 24 to 42 weeks of gestation. Pediatrics 32:793–800, 1963.
McCarron, K: Fever, The cardinal vital sign. CCQ 9(1):15–18, 1986.
Moss AJ: Indirect methods of blood pressure measurement. Pediatr Clin North Am 25:3–14, 1978.
Nichols GA: Taking adult temperatures — rectal measurements. Am J Nurs 72:1092–1093, 1972.
Nichols GA, and Kucha D: Oral measurements. Am J Nurs 72:1091–1093, 1972.
Overfield T: Biologic Variation in Health and Illness: Race, Age and Sex Differences. Menlo Park, CA, Addison Wesley, 1985.
Robson JR, Larkin FH, Bursick JH, Peri KP: Growth standards for infants and children: A cross-sectional study. Pediatrics 56:1014–1020, 1975.
Task Force on Blood Pressure Control in Children: Report of Second Task Force on Blood Pressure Control in Children. Pediatrics 79:1–15, 1987.
Whaley LF, Wong DL: Nursing Care of Infants and Children. 4th ed. St. Louis, CV Mosby, 1990.

CHAPTER

9 Assessing the Skin, Hair, and Nails

STRUCTURE AND FUNCTION

Think of the skin as the body's largest organ system — it covers 20 square feet of surface area in the average adult. The skin is the sentry that guards the body from environmental stresses (e.g., trauma, pathogens, dirt) and adapts it to other environmental influences (e.g., heat, cold).

SKIN

The skin has two layers — the outer highly-differentiated *epidermis* and the inner supportive *dermis* (Fig. 9 – 1). Beneath these layers is a third layer, the *subcutaneous* layer of adipose tissue.

Epidermis. The *epidermis* is thin but tough. It forms a rugged protective barrier. It is stratified into several zones. The inner *stratum germinativum,* or basal cell layer, forms new skin cells. Their major ingredient is the tough, fibrous protein *keratin.* The melanocytes interspersed along this layer produce the pigment melanin, which gives brown tones to the skin and hair. All people have the same number of melanocytes — the amount of melanin they produce varies with genetic, hormonal, and environmental influences.

From the basal layer, the new cells migrate up and flatten into the *stratum corneum.* This outer horny cell layer consists of dead keratinized cells that are interwoven and closely packed. The cells are constantly being shed, or desquamated, and are replaced with new cells from below. The epidermis is completely replaced every 4 weeks. In fact, each person sheds about 1 pound of skin each year.

The epidermis is uniformly thin except on the surfaces that are exposed to friction, such as the palms and the soles. On these surfaces, skin is thicker because of abrasion and weight-bearing. The epidermis is avascular; it is nourished by blood vessels in the dermis below.

Skin color is derived mainly from the brown pigment melanin. Color also comes from the yellow-orange tones of the pigment carotene and from the red-purple tones in the underlying vascular bed. All people have skin of varying shades of brown, yellow, and red; the relative proportion of these shades affects the prevailing color. Skin color is further modified by the thickness of the skin and by the presence of edema.

Dermis. The *dermis* is the inner supportive layer consisting mostly of connective tissue, or *collagen.* This is the tough, fibrous protein that enables the skin to resist tearing. The dermis also has resilient elastic tissue that allows the skin to stretch with body movements. The nerves, sensory receptors, blood vessels, and lymphatics lay in the dermis. Also, appendages from the epidermis, such as the hair follicles, sebaceous glands, and sweat glands, are embedded in the dermis.

Subcutaneous Layer. The *subcutaneous layer* is adipose tissue, which is made up of lobules of fat cells. The subcutaneous tissue stores fat for energy, provides insulation for temperature control, and aids in protection by its soft cushioning effect.

EPIDERMAL APPENDAGES

These structures are formed by a tubular invagination of the epidermis down into the underlying dermis.

Hair. Hair is *vestigial* for humans; it no longer is needed for protection from cold or trauma. However, hair is highly significant in most cultures for its cosmetic and psychological meaning (see Cultural Considerations).

The hair shaft is the visible projecting part, and the root is below the surface embedded in the follicle. At the root, the bulb matrix is the expanded area where new cells are produced at a high rate. Hair growth is cyclical with active and resting phases. Each follicle functions independently so that while some hairs are resting, others are growing. Around the hair follicle are the muscular *arrector pili,* which contract and elevate the hair so that it resembles "goose flesh" when the skin is exposed to cold or in emotional states.

People have two types of hair. Fine, faint *vellus* hair

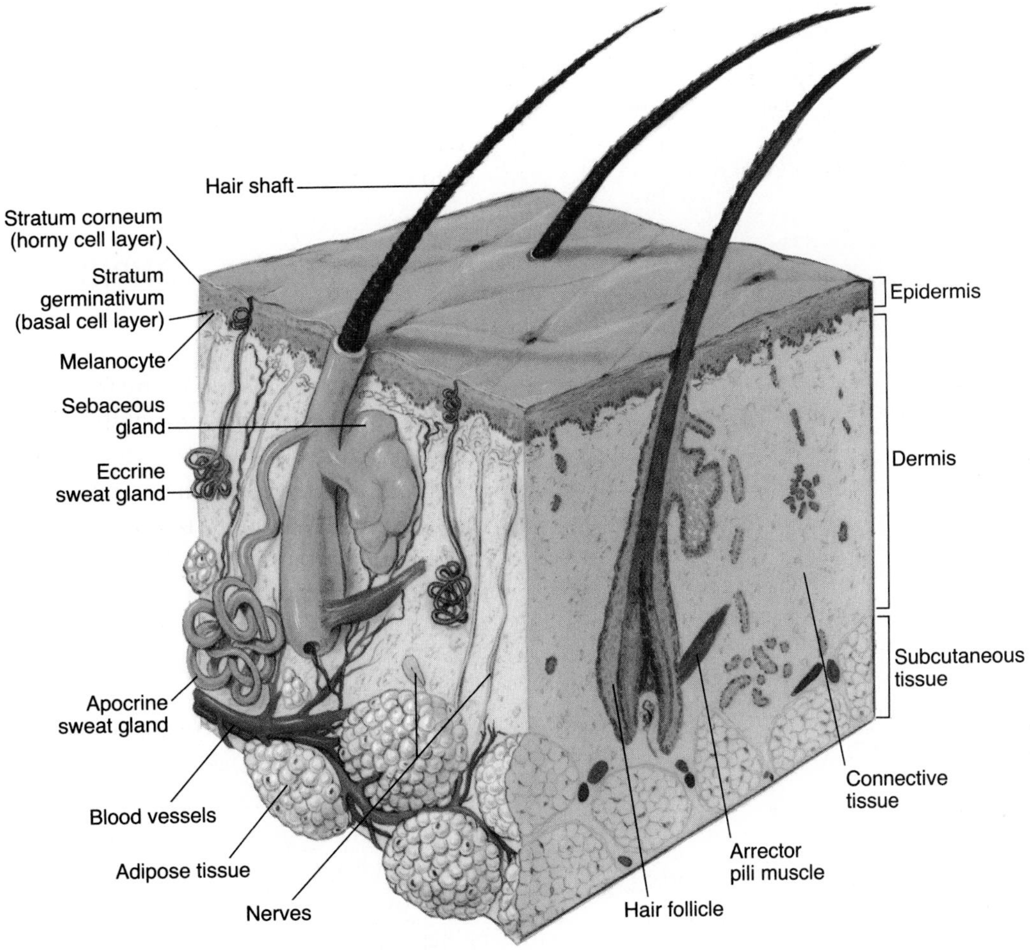

► **Figure 9 – 1**

covers most of the body (except the palms and soles, the dorsa of the distal parts of the fingers, the umbilicus, the glans penis, and inside the labia). *Terminal hair* is the darker thicker hair that grows on the scalp and eyebrows and, after puberty, the axillae, pubic area, and the face and chest in the male.

Sebaceous Glands. These glands produce a protective lipid substance, sebum, which is secreted through the hair follicles. Sebum oils and lubricates the skin and hair and forms an emulsion with water that retards water loss from the skin. (Dry skin results from loss of water, not directly from loss of oil.) Sebaceous glands are everywhere except on the palms and soles. They are most abundant in the scalp, forehead, face, and chin.

Sweat Glands. There are two types. The *eccrine* glands are coiled tubules that open directly onto the skin surface and produce a dilute saline solution called sweat. The evaporation of sweat reduces body temperature. Eccrine glands are widely distributed through the body and are mature in the 2-month-old infant.

The *apocrine* glands produce a thick milky secretion and open into the hair follicles. They are located mainly in the axillae, anogenital area, nipples, and navel and are vestigial in humans. They become active during puberty, and secretion occurs with emotional and sexual stimulation. Bacterial flora residing on the skin surface reacts with apocrine sweat to produce characteristic musky body odor. Their functioning decreases in the aging adult.

Nails. The nails are hard plates of keratin on the dorsal edges of the fingers and toes (Fig. 9 – 2). The nail plate is clear with fine longitudinal ridges that become prominent in aging. Nails take their pink color from the underlying nail bed of highly vascular epithelial cells. The

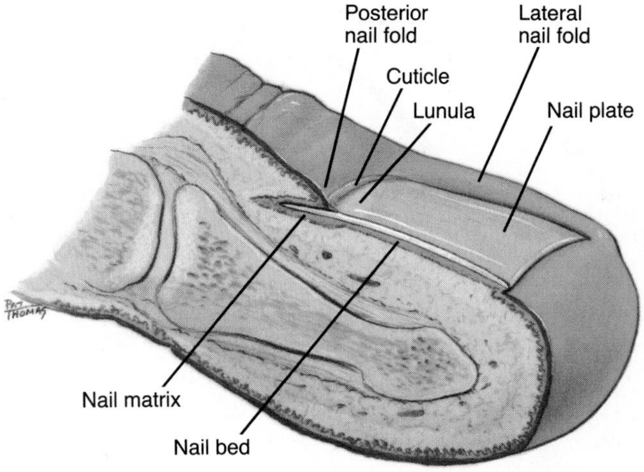

▶ **Figure 9–2**

lunula is the white opaque semilunar area at the proximal end of the nail. It lies over the nail matrix where new keratinized cells are formed. The nail folds overlap the posterior and lateral borders.

FUNCTION

The skin is a waterproof, almost indestructible covering that has protective and adaptive properties:

- Protection: Minimizes injury from physical, chemical, thermal, and light wave sources.
- Prevents penetration: A barrier that stops invasion of microorganisms and loss of water and electrolytes from within the body.
- Perception: A vast sensory surface holding the neurosensory end-organs for touch, pain, temperature, and pressure.
- Temperature regulation: Allows heat dissipation through sweat glands and heat storage through subcutaneous insulation.
- Identification: People identify one another by unique combinations of facial characteristics, hair, skin color, and even fingerprints. Self-image is often enhanced or deterred by the way society's standards of beauty measure up to each person's perceived characteristics.
- Communication: Emotions are expressed in the sign language of the face and in the body posture. Vascular mechanisms also signal emotional states such as blushing or blanching.
- Wound repair: Cell replacement of surface wounds.
- Absorption and excretion: Limited excretion of some metabolic wastes, by-products of cellular decomposition such as minerals, sugars, amino acids, cholesterol, uric acid, and urea.
- Production of vitamin D: The skin is the surface on which ultraviolet light converts certain compounds into vitamin D.

DEVELOPMENTAL CONSIDERATIONS

Infants and Children

The hair follicles develop in the fetus at 3 months' gestation; by mid-gestation most of the skin is covered with *lanugo,* the fine downy hair of the newborn. In the first few months after birth, this is replaced by fine vellus hair. Terminal hair on the scalp, if present at birth, tends to be soft and suffer a patchy loss, especially at the temples and occiput. Also present at birth is *vernix caseosa,* the thick cheesy substance made up of sebum and shed epithelial cells.

The newborn's skin is similar in structure to the adult's, but many of its functions are not fully developed. The newborn's skin is thin, smooth, and elastic and is relatively more permeable than that of the adult so the infant is at greater risk for fluid loss. Sebum, which holds water in the skin, is present for the first few weeks of life, producing milia and cradle cap in some babies. Then sebaceous glands decrease in size and production and do not resume functioning until puberty. Temperature regulation is ineffective. Eccrine sweat glands do not secrete in response to heat until the first few months of life and then only minimally throughout childhood. The skin cannot protect much against cold either because it cannot contract and shiver and because the subcutaneous layer is inefficient. Also, the pigment system is inefficient at birth.

As the child grows, the epidermis thickens, toughens, and darkens and the skin becomes better lubricated. Hair growth accelerates. At puberty, secretion from apocrine sweat glands increases in response to heat and emotional stimuli, producing body odor. Sebaceous glands become more active—the skin looks oily, and acne develops. Subcutaneous fat deposits increase, especially in females.

Secondary sex characteristics that appear during adolescence are evident in the integument. In the female, the diameter of the areola enlarges and darkens and breast tissue develops. Coarse pubic hair develops in males and females, then axillary hair, and then coarse facial hair in males.

The Pregnant Female

The change in hormone levels results in increased pigment in the areolae and nipples, vulva, and sometimes in the midline of the abdomen (linea nigra) or in the face (chloasma). Hyperestrogenemia probably also causes the common vascular spiders and palmar erythema. There is increased fragility of connective tissue, resulting in *striae gravidarum,* which may develop in the skin of the abdomen, breasts, or thighs. Metabolism is increased in pregnancy; as a way to dissipate heat, the peripheral vasculature dilates and the sweat and sebaceous glands increase secretion. Fat deposits are laid down, particularly in the buttocks and hips, as maternal reserves for the nursing baby.

The Aging Adult

The skin is a mirror reflecting aging changes that proceed in all our organ systems; it is just the one organ we can view directly. The aging process carries a slow atrophy of skin structures. The aging skin loses its elasticity, it folds and sags. By the seventh to eighth decade, it looks parchment thin, lax, dry, and wrinkled.

The epidermis's outer layer, *stratum corneum,* thins and flattens. This allows chemicals easier access into the body. Wrinkling occurs because the underlying dermis thins and flattens. There is a loss of elastin, collagen, and subcutaneous fat and reduced muscle tone. The loss of collagen increases the risk for shearing, tearing injuries.

Sweat glands and sebaceous glands decrease in number and function, leaving dry skin. Decreased response of the sweat glands to thermoregulatory demand also puts the aging person at greater risk for heat stroke. The vascularity of the skin diminishes, while the vascular fragility increases; a minor trauma may produce discolored areas, or *senile purpura.*

The skin areas that have been chronically exposed to sunlight have greatly accentuated aging changes. Fine wrinkling, decreased elasticity, speckled and uneven coloring, more pigment changes, and a yellowed leathery texture occur. Chronic sun damage is even more prominent in pale or light-skinned persons.

An accumulation of factors place the aging person at risk for skin disease and breakdown: the thinning of the skin, the decrease in vascularity and nutrients, the loss of protective cushioning of the subcutaneous layer, a lifetime of environmental trauma to skin, the social changes of aging (e.g., less nutrition, financial resources), the increasingly sedentary lifestyle, and the chance of immobility. When skin breakdown does occur, cell replacement is slower and wound healing is delayed.

In the aging hair matrix, the number of functioning melanocytes decreases so the hair looks gray or white and feels thin and fine. A person's genetic script determines the onset of graying and the number of gray hairs. Hair distribution changes. Males may have a symmetric W-shaped balding in the frontal areas. Some testosterone is present in both males and females; as it decreases with age, axillary and pubic hair decrease. As the female's estrogen also decreases, testosterone is unopposed and the female may develop some bristly facial hairs. Nails grow more slowly. Their surface is lusterless and is characterized by longitudinal ridges due to local trauma at the nail matrix.

Because the aging changes in the skin and hair can be viewed directly, they carry profound psychologic impact. For many people, self-esteem is linked to a youthful appearance. This view is compounded by media advertising in Western society. Although sagging and wrinkling skin and graying and thinning hair are a normal process of aging, they prompt a loss of self-esteem for many adults.

TRANSCULTURAL CONSIDERATIONS

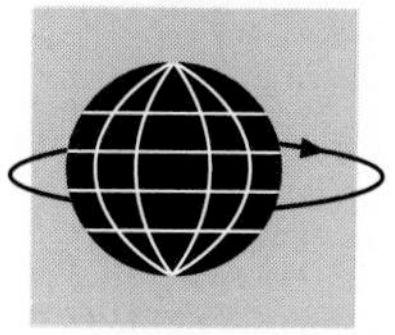

Awareness of normal biocultural differences and the ability to recognize the unique clinical manifestations of disease is especially important for darkly pigmented people. As described earlier, melanin is responsible for the various colors and tones of skin observed among people from culturally diverse backgrounds. Melanin protects the skin against harmful ultraviolet rays, a genetic advantage accounting for the lower incidence of skin cancer among darkly pigmented black and Native American people. Areas of the skin affected by hormones and, in some cases, differing for culturally diverse people, are the sexual skin areas, such as the nipples, areola, scrotum, and labia majora. In general, these areas are darker than other parts of the skin in both adults and children, especially among black and Asian people.

The apocrine and eccrine sweat glands are important for fluid balance and for thermoregulation. When apocrine gland secretions are contaminated by normal skin flora, odor results. Most Asians and Native Americans have a mild body odor or none at all, whereas whites and blacks tend to have strong body odor.

Eskimos have made an interesting environmental adaptation whereby they sweat less than whites on their trunks and extremities but more on their faces (Schaefer, 1974). This adaptation allows for temperature regulation without causing perspiration and dampness of their clothes, which would decrease their ability to insulate against severe cold weather and would pose a serious threat to their survival.

The amount of chloride excreted by sweat glands varies widely, and blacks have lower salt concentrations in their sweat than whites do. A study of Ashkenazi Jews (Jews of European descent) and Sephardic Jews (Jews of Northern African and Middle Eastern descent) revealed that those of European origins had a lower percentage of sweat chlorides (Levin, 1966).

Perhaps one of the most obvious and widely variable racial differences occurs with the hair. The hair of black people varies widely in texture. It is very fragile and ranges from long and straight to short, spiralled, thick, and kinky. The hair and scalp have a natural tendency to be dry and require daily combing, gentle brushing, and the application of oil. In comparison, people of Asian backgrounds generally have straight, silky hair.

Hair condition is significant in diagnosing and treating certain disease states. For example, hair texture becomes dry, brittle, and lusterless with inadequate nutrition. The hair of black children with severe malnutrition, e.g., marasmus, frequently changes not only in texture but in color. The child's hair often becomes less kinky and assumes a copper-red color.

SUBJECTIVE DATA

Previous history of skin disease (allergies, hives, psoriasis, eczema)

Change in pigmentation

Change in mole (size or color)

Excessive dryness or moisture

Pruritus

Excessive bruising

Rash or lesion

Medications

Hair loss

Change in nails

Environmental or occupational hazards

Self-care behaviors

EXAMINER ASKS:	RATIONALE:
1. Do you have any **previous skin disease** or problem? How was this treated? Is there any family history of allergies or allergic skin problems?	Significant familial predisposition: allergies, hay fever, psoriasis, atopic dermatitis (eczema), acne.
Do you have any known allergies to drugs, plants, animals?	Identify offending allergen.
Do you have any birthmarks, tattoos?	Use of nonsterile equipment to apply tattoos increases risk of hepatitis.
2. Have you noted any **change in skin color** or **pigmentation?**	Localized change: Vitiligo—loss of pigmentation; Hyperpigmentation—increase in color
Was it a generalized color change (all over), or localized?	Generalized change suggests systemic illness: pallor, jaundice, cyanosis.

EXAMINER ASKS:	RATIONALE:
3. Have you noticed any **change in a mole:** color, shape, sudden appearance of tenderness, bleeding, itching? Any "sores" that do not heal?	Signs suggest neoplasm in pigmented nevus. Person may be unaware of change in nevus on back or buttock that he or she cannot see.
4. Have you noticed any change in the feel of your skin? temperature, **moisture,** texture?	Seborrhea — oily
Any excess **dryness?** Is this seasonal or constant?	Xerosis — dry
5. Do you have any skin itching? Is this mild (prickling, tingling) or intense (intolerable)? Does it awaken you from sleep?	**Pruritus** is the most common of skin symptoms. Note index of severity.
Where is the itching? When did it start?	Presence or absence of pruritus may be significant for diagnosis. Scratching may cause excoriation of primary lesion.
Do you have any other skin pain or soreness? Where?	
6. Have you noticed any excess **bruising?** Where on the body?	Multiple cuts and bruises, bruises in various stages of healing, bruises above knees and elbows, and illogical explanation — consider the possibility of abuse. Frequent falls may be due to dizziness of neurologic or cardiovascular origin. Also, frequent minor trauma may be a side effect of alcoholism or other drug abuse.
7. Do you have any skin **rash or lesion?**	Rashes are a common cause of seeking health care. A careful history is important; it may be an accurate predictor of the type of lesion you will see in the examination and its cause.
Onset. When did you first notice it?	
Location. Where did it start?	Identify the primary site — it may give clue to cause.
Where did it spread?	Migration pattern, evolution.
Character or quality. Describe the color.	
Is it raised or flat? Any crust, odor? Does it feel tender, warm?	
Duration. How long have you had it? Describe the frequency and course.	
Setting. Anyone at home or work with a similar rash? Have you been camping, have a new pet, tried a new food, drug? Does the rash seem to come with stress?	Identify new or relevant exposure.
Alleviating and aggravating factors. What home care have you tried? Bath, lotions, heat? Do they help, or make it worse?	Myriad of over-the-counter remedies available. Many people have tried them and only seek professional help when they do not see improvement.
Associated symptoms. Any itching, fever?	

EXAMINER ASKS:	RATIONALE:
What do you think rash/lesion means?	Assess person's perception of cause. May need to deal with fear of cancer, tick-borne illnesses, and so forth.
Coping strategies. How has rash/lesion affected your self-care, hygiene, ability to function at work/home/socially?	Assess effectiveness of coping strategies. Chronic skin diseases may increase risk of loss of self-esteem, social isolation, and anxiety.
Any new or increased stress in your life?	Stress can exacerbate chronic skin illness.
8. What **medications** do you take? Prescription and over-the-counter? Recent change?	Drugs may produce skin eruption: aspirin, antibiotics, barbiturates, some laxatives, and tonics. Drugs may increase sunlight sensitivity and give burn response: sulfonamides, thiazide diuretics, oral hypoglycemic agents, and tetracycline.
How long on medication?	Even after a long time on medication, a person may develop sensitivity.
9. Have you noticed any recent **hair loss?** Was it a gradual or sudden onset? Was it symmetric? Is it associated with fever, illness, increased stress?	Alopecia
Have you noticed any unusual hair growth?	Hirsutism
Any recent change in texture, appearance?	
10. Have you noticed any **change in nails:** shape, color, brittleness? Do you tend to bite or chew nails?	
11. Now I would like to ask you about **environmental** and **occupational hazards.** Are there any hazard-related problems with your occupation, e.g., dyes, toxic chemicals, radiation? How about hobbies? Do you perform any household or furniture repair work?	Majority of skin neoplasms result from occupational or environmental agents. Some people at risk include coal workers; sun exposure to farmers, sailors, outdoor workers; also creosote workers, roofers.
How much sun exposure do you get from outdoor work, leisure activities, sunbathing?	Unprotected sun exposure accelerates aging and produces lesions. At more risk: light-skinned people over 40 and those regularly in sun.
Have you recently been bitten by insect: bee, tick, mosquito?	Identify contactants that produce lesions or contact dermatitis.
Any recent exposure to plants, animals in yard work, camping?	For people with chronic recurrent urticaria (hives), tell them to keep diary of meals and environment to identify precipitating factors.

EXAMINER ASKS:	RATIONALE:

12. What do you do to care for your skin, hair, nails? What cosmetics, soaps, chemicals do you use?

Assess **self-care** and influence on self-concept—may be important with this society's media stress on high norms of beauty. Many over-the-counter remedies are costly and exacerbate skin problems.

If you have allergies, how do you control your environment to minimize exposure?

ADDITIONAL QUESTIONS FOR INFANTS AND CHILDREN

Does the child have any birthmarks?

Was there any change in skin color as a newborn? Any jaundice? Which day after birth? Any cyanosis? What were the circumstances?

Have you noted any rash or sores? What seems to bring it on? Have you introduced a new food or formula? When? Does your child eat chocolate, cow's milk, eggs?

Generalized rash—consider allergic reaction to new food.

Irritability and general fussiness may indicate the presence of pruritus.

A careful history is important for any lesion that may indicate child abuse or neglect: cigarette burns; excessive bruising, especially above knees or elbows; linear whip marks. With abuse, the history often will not coincide with the physical appearance of lesion.

Does the child have any diaper rash? How do you care for this? How do you wash diapers? Do you use rubber pants? How do you clean skin?

Occlusive diapers or infrequent changing may cause rash. Infant may be allergic to certain detergent or to disposable wipes.

Has the child had any exposure to contagious skin conditions: scabies, impetigo, lice? Or to communicable diseases: measles, chicken pox, scarlet fever? Or to toxic plants: poison ivy?

Are the child's vaccinations up to date?

Does the child have any habits or habitual movements, e.g., nail-biting, twisting hair, rubbing head on mattress?

ADDITIONAL QUESTIONS FOR THE AGING ADULT

What changes have you noticed in your skin in the last few years?

Assess impact of aging on self-concept. For some, normal aging changes may cause distress.

Note that many changes attributed to aging are due to chronic sun damage. Aging people are at greater risk of sun damage.

Any delay in wound healing?

EXAMINER ASKS:	RATIONALE:
Have you noticed any skin itching?	Pruritus is very common with aging. Consider side effect of medicine or systemic disease (e.g., liver or kidney disease, cancer, lymphoma), but senile pruritus is usually due to dry skin (xerosis). Exacerbated by too frequent bathing or use of soap. Scratching with dirty jagged fingernails produces excoriations.
Do you have any other skin pain?	Some diseases produce more intense sensations of pain, itching in aging people, e.g., herpes zoster (shingles). Other diseases may reduce pain sensation in extremities, e.g., diabetes. Also, some aging people tolerate chronic pain as "part of growing old," and hesitate to "complain."
Have you noticed any change in feet, toenails? Any bunions? Is it possible to wear shoes?	Some aging people cannot reach down to their feet to give self-care.
Do you experience frequent falls?	Multiple bruises, trauma from falls.
Do you have a history of diabetes, peripheral vascular disease?	
What do you do to care for your skin?	The application of bland lotions is important to retain moisture in aging skin. But dermatitis may ensue from certain cosmetics, creams, ointments, and dyes applied to achieve a youthful appearance. Aging skin has a delayed inflammatory response when exposed to irritants. If the person is not alerted by warning signs (e.g., pruritus, redness), exposure may continue and dermatitis may ensue.

OBJECTIVE DATA

METHOD OF EXAMINATION

Equipment Needed

Strong direct lighting (natural daylight is ideal to evaluate skin characteristics but is usually not available in the clinical area)
Small centimeter ruler
Penlight

Needed for special procedures:
Wood's light (filtered ultraviolet light)
Magnifying glass, for minute lesions
Materials for laboratory tests: potassium hydroxide (KOH), glass slide

Preparation

Try to control external variables that may influence skin color and confuse your findings, both in light-skinned and in dark-skinned persons (Table 9–1).

Learn to consciously attend to skin characteristics. The danger is one of omission. You grow so accustomed to seeing the skin that you are likely to ignore it as you assess the organ systems underneath. Yet the skin holds information about the body's circulation, nutritional status, and signs of systemic diseases as well as topical data on the integument itself.

The Complete Physical Examination. Although it is presented alone in this chapter, skin assessment is integrated throughout the complete examination; it is not a separate step. At the beginning of the examination, assessing the person's hands and fingernails is a nonthreatening way to accustom him or her to your touch. Most people are used to having relative strangers shake their hand or touch their arm. As you move through the examination scrutinize the outer skin surface first before you concentrate on the underlying

Table 9–1 ► External Variables Influencing Skin Color

VARIABLE	CAUSES	OUTCOME
Emotions		
Fear, anger	Peripheral vasoconstriction	False pallor
Embarrassment	Flushing in face and neck	False erythema
Environment		
Hot room	Vasodilatation	False erythema
Chilly or air-conditioned room, mist tents	Vasoconstriction	False pallor, coolness
Cigarette smoking	Vasoconstriction	False pallor
Physical		
Prolonged elevation	Decreased arterial perfusion	Pallor, coolness
Dependent position	Venous pooling	Redness, warmth, distended veins
Immobilization, prolonged inactivity	Slowed circulation	Pallor, coolness, nail beds pale, prolonged capillary filling time

(Data from Roach L.: Dark skins: Recognizing and interpreting color changes. Crit Care Update 5–15, 1977.)

structures. Separate intertriginous areas (areas with skin folds) such as under large breasts, obese abdomen, and the groin and inspect them thoroughly. These areas are dark, warm, and moist and provide the perfect conditions for irritation or infection. Last, always remove the person's socks and inspect the feet, toenails, and the area between the toes.

The Regional Examination. At times, an individual seeks health care because of a skin change and your assessment will be focused on the skin alone. Ask the person to remove his or her clothing and assess the skin as one entity. Stand back at first to get an overall impression; this helps reveal distribution patterns. Then inspect lesions carefully. With a skin rash, check all areas of the body because there are some locations the person cannot see. You cannot rely on the history alone that the rash is limited to one location. Inspect mucous membranes, too, because some disorders have characteristic lesions here.

The skills used are inspection and palpation because some skin changes have accompanying signs that can be felt.

NORMAL RANGE OF FINDINGS	ABNORMAL FINDINGS

SKIN

Inspect and palpate

Color

General Pigmentation

1. Observe the skin tone. Normally, it is consistent with genetic background and varies from pinkish tan to ruddy dark tan, or from light to dark brown, and may have yellow or olive overtones. Dark-skinned people normally have areas of lighter pigmentation on the palms, nail beds, and lips. An acquired condition is *vitiligo*, the complete absence of melanin pigment in patchy areas of white or light skin on the face, neck, hands, feet, body folds, and around orifices (Fig. 9–3). Otherwise, the depigmented skin is normal. Vitiligo can occur in all races, although dark-skinned people seem more severely affected and potentially suffer a greater threat to their body image.

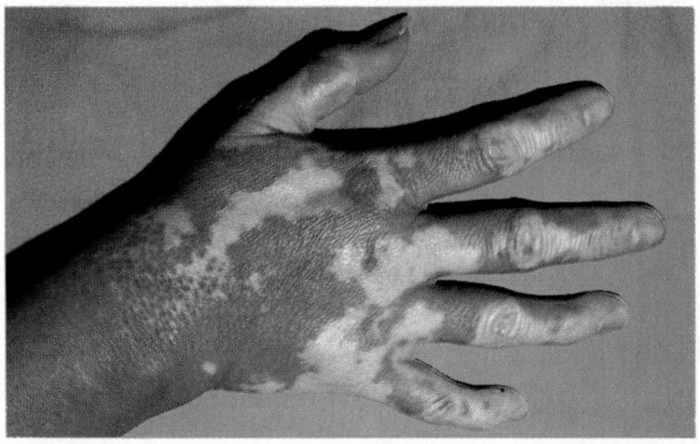

Vitiligo

▶ Figure 9–3

NORMAL RANGE OF FINDINGS

General pigmentation is darker in sun-exposed areas. Common (benign) pigmented areas also occur (Fig. 9–4a):

Freckles (ephelides)—small, flat macules of brown melanin pigment

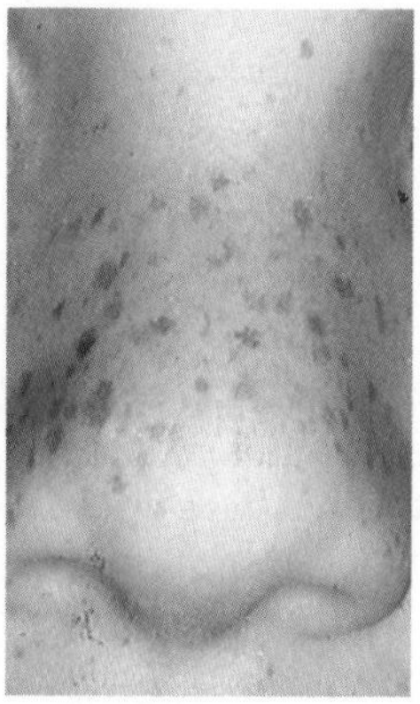

Freckles

► Figure 9–4a

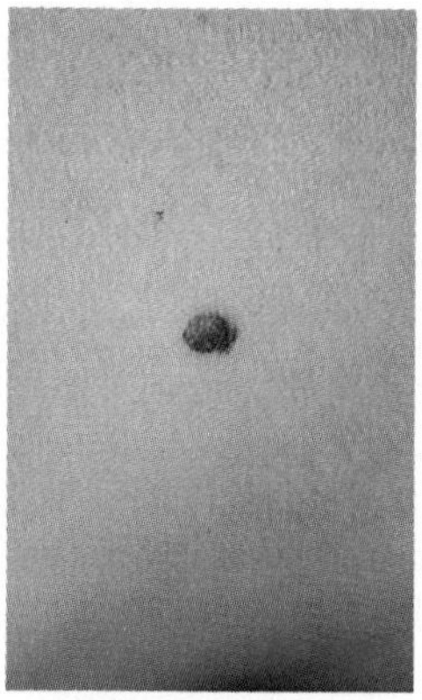

Junctional nevus

► Figure 9–4b

Moles (pigmented nevi)—a proliferation of melanocytes, tan to brown color, flat or raised. The junctional nevus (Fig. 9–4b) is macular only. The compound nevus (Fig. 9–4c) is macular and papular. The intradermal nevus (Fig. 9–4d) has nevus cells in only the dermis.

Birthmarks—may be tan to brown color

Advise anyone with moles or birthmarks to perform periodic skin self-examinations. Watch for danger signs listed here. Ask a family member to check any areas the person cannot see (e.g., the back).

ABNORMAL FINDINGS

Danger signs: Note the following abnormal characteristics in pigmented lesions and refer to the proper health care specialist:

1. sudden enlargement
2. change in color
3. an irregular border with notching or a butterfly shape, or a previously flat mole becoming elevated
4. variegated color, i.e., an irregular range of blue, red, white, mixed with brown or black
5. clumping of pigment instead of an even color tone
6. change in surface features (scaling, flaking, oozing)
7. change in sensation (itching, tenderness)
8. change in surrounding skin (redness, swelling)
9. ulceration or bleeding in mole (late sign)

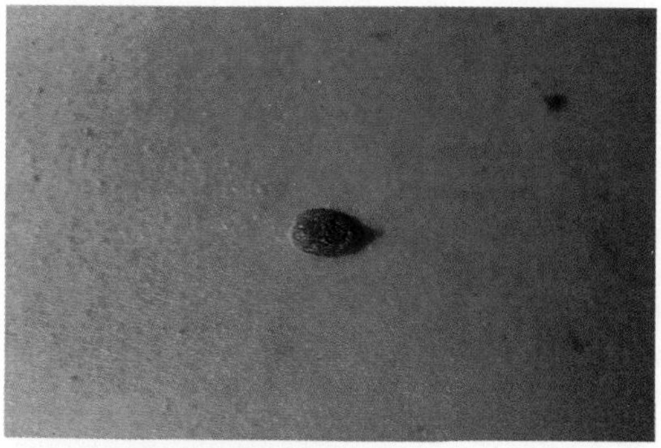

Compound nevus

► Figure 9–4c

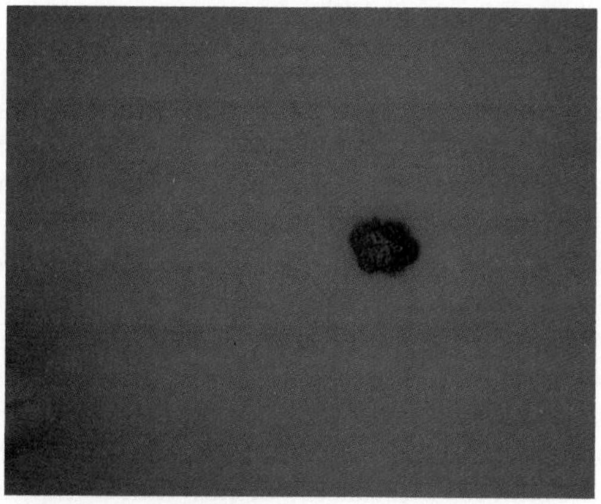

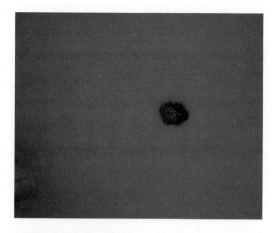

Intradermal nevus

► Figure 9–4d

NORMAL RANGE OF FINDINGS	ABNORMAL FINDINGS

Widespread Color Change

Note any color change over the entire body skin, such as pallor (white), erythema (red), cyanosis (blue), and jaundice (yellow). Note whether the color change is transient and expected or if it is due to pathology. In dark-skinned people, the amount of normal pigment may mask color changes. Lips and nail beds show some color change, but they vary with the person's skin color and may not always be accurate signs. The more reliable sites are those with the least pigmentation, such as under the tongue, the buccal mucosa, the palpebral conjunctiva, and the sclera. See Table 9 – 2 for specific clues to assessment.

Pallor. When the red-pink tones from the oxygenated hemoglobin in the blood are absent, the skin takes on the color of connective tissue (collagen), which is mostly white. Pallor is common in acute high stress states such as anxiety or fear, due to the powerful peripheral vasoconstriction from sympathetic nervous system stimulation. The skin also looks pale with vasoconstriction from exposure to cold and cigarette smoking and in the presence of edema.

Abnormal: Ashen gray color, marked pallor, due to anemia, shock, arterial insufficiency (see Table 9 – 2).

Pallor in dark-skinned people may be observed by the absence of the underlying red tones that normally give brown or black skin its luster. The brown-skinned individual demonstrates pallor with a more yellowish-brown color, and the black-skinned person will appear ashen or gray. Generalized pallor can be observed in the mucous membranes, lips, and nail beds. The palpebra, conjunctiva, and nail beds are preferred sites for assessing the pallor of anemia. When inspecting the conjunctiva, lower the lid sufficiently to visualize the conjunctiva near the outer canthus as well as the inner canthus. The coloration is often lighter near the inner canthus.

Abnormal: The pallor of impending shock is accompanied by other subtle manifestations, such as increasing pulse rate, oliguria, apprehension, and restlessness. Anemias, particularly chronic iron deficiency anemia, may become manifest by "spoon" nails, which have a concave shape. A lemon yellow tint of the face and slightly yellow sclera accompany pernicious anemia, which is also indicated by neurologic deficits and a red, painful tongue. Fatigue, exertional dyspnea, rapid pulse, dizziness, and impaired mental function accompany most severe anemias.

Erythema. This is an intense redness of the skin due to excess blood (hyperemia) in the dilated superficial capillaries. This is a sign that is to be expected with fever, local inflammation, or with emotional reactions, e.g., blushing in vascular flush areas (cheeks, neck, and upper chest).

Abnormal: Polycythemia, venous stasis, carbon monoxide poisoning, extravascular presence of red blood cells (petechiae, ecchymosis, hematoma) (See Tables 9 – 2 and 9 – 7).

When erythema is associated with fever or localized inflammation, it is characterized by increased skin temperature. The degree of redness is determined by the quantity of blood present in the capillaries, whereas the warmth of the skin is related to the rate of blood flow through the blood vessels. When assessing inflammation in dark-skinned persons, it is often necessary to palpate the skin for increased warmth, taut or tightly pulled surfaces that may be indicative of edema, and hardening of deep tissues or blood vessels.

Cyanosis. This is a bluish mottled color that signifies decreased perfusion; the tissues are not adequately perfused with oxygenated blood. Be aware that cyanosis can be a nonspecific sign. A person who is anemic

Abnormal: Hypoxemia

NORMAL RANGE OF FINDINGS	ABNORMAL FINDINGS
could have hypoxemia without ever looking blue because not enough hemoglobin is present (either oxygenated or reduced) to color the skin. On the other hand, a person with polycythemia (an increase in the number of red blood cells) looks ruddy-blue at all times and may not necessarily be hypoxemic. This person just is unable to fully oxygenate the massive numbers of red blood cells. Lastly, do not confuse cyanosis with the common and normal bluish tone on the lips of dark-skinned persons of Mediterranean origin. Cyanosis is difficult to observe in darkly pigmented persons (see Table 9–2). Given that most conditions causing cyanosis also cause decreased oxygenation of the brain, other clinical signs, such as changes in level of consciousness and signs of respiratory distress, will be evident.	
Jaundice. Jaundice is exhibited by a yellow color, indicating rising amounts of bilirubin in the blood. Jaundice is first noted in the junction of the hard and soft palate in the mouth, and in the sclera. But do not confuse scleral jaundice with the normal yellow subconjunctival fatty deposits that are common in the outer sclera of dark-skinned persons. The scleral yellow of jaundice extends up to the edge of the iris. As levels of serum bilirubin rise, jaundice is evident in the skin over the rest of the body. This is best assessed in direct natural daylight. Common calluses on palms and soles often look yellow—do not interpret these as jaundice. Except for physiologic jaundice in the newborn (p. 245), jaundice does not occur normally.	Liver inflammation Hemolytic disease Light or clay-colored stools and dark golden urine often accompany jaundice in both light- and dark-skinned people.
Temperature	
Note the temperature of your own hands. Then use the backs (dorsa) of your hands to palpate the person and check bilaterally. The skin should be warm, and the temperature should be equal bilaterally; warmth suggests normal circulatory status. Hands and feet may be slightly cooler in a cool environment.	
Hypothermia. Generalized coolness may be induced, such as in hypothermia used for surgery or high fever. Localized coolness is expected with an immobilized extremity, as when a limb is in a cast or with an IV infusion.	General hypothermia accompanies central circulatory disturbance, such as in shock. Localized hypothermia occurs in peripheral arterial insufficiency and Raynaud's disease.
Hyperthermia. Generalized hyperthermia occurs with an increased metabolic rate, such as in fever, or after heavy exercise. A localized area feels hyperthermic with trauma, infection, or sunburn.	Hyperthyroidism
Moisture	
Perspiration appears normally on the face, hands, axilla, and skin folds in response to activity, a warm environment, or anxiety. *Diaphoresis,* or profuse perspiration, accompanies an increased metabolic rate, such as occurs in heavy activity or fever. Dehydration is evident in the oral mucous membranes. They look dry, and the lips looks parched and cracked. Be aware that dark skin may normally look dry and flaky, but this does not necessarily indicate systemic dehydration.	Diaphoresis occurs with thyrotoxicosis and with stimulation of the nervous system with anxiety or pain With extreme dryness the skin is fissured, resembling cracks in a dry lake bed.

NORMAL RANGE OF FINDINGS	ABNORMAL FINDINGS

Texture

Normal skin feels smooth and firm, with an even surface.

Hyperthyroidism—the skin feels smoother and softer, like velvet. Hypothyroidism—the skin feels rough, dry, and flaky.

Thickness

The epidermis is uniformly thin over most of the body, although thickened callus areas are normal on palms and soles. A callus is a circumscribed overgrowth of epidermis and is an adaptation to excessive pressure. On the palms and soles, calluses develop from the friction of work and weight-bearing.

Very thin, shiny skin (atrophic) occurs with arterial insufficiency.

Edema

Edema is fluid accumulating in the intercellular spaces and is not present normally. Edema is most evident in dependent parts of the body (feet, ankles, and sacral areas), where the skin looks puffy and tight. Edema makes the hair follicles more prominent, so you note a pig-skin or orange-peel look.

Unilateral edema—consider a local or peripheral cause.

Bilateral edema or edema that is generalized over the whole body (anasarca)—consider a central problem such as congestive heart failure, kidney failure.

To check for edema, imprint your thumbs firmly against the ankle malleolus or the tibia. If your pressure leaves a dent in the skin, "pitting" edema is present. Its presence is graded on a 4-point scale; from 1+ for mild edema, to 4+ for deep pitting edema. This scale is somewhat subjective; outcomes vary among examiners.

Edema masks normal skin color as well as obscures pathologic conditions such as jaundice or cyanosis because the fluid lies between the surface and the pigmented and vascular layers. It makes dark skin look lighter.

Mobility and Turgor

Pinch up a large fold of skin on the anterior chest under the clavicle (Fig. 9–5). Mobility is the skin's ease of rising, and turgor is its ability to return to place promptly when released. This reflects the elasticity of the skin.

Mobility is decreased when edema is present.

Poor turgor is evident in severe dehydration or extreme weight loss; the pinched skin recedes slowly or "tents" and stands by itself.

Scleroderma, literally "hard skin," is a connective tissue disorder associated with decreased mobility.

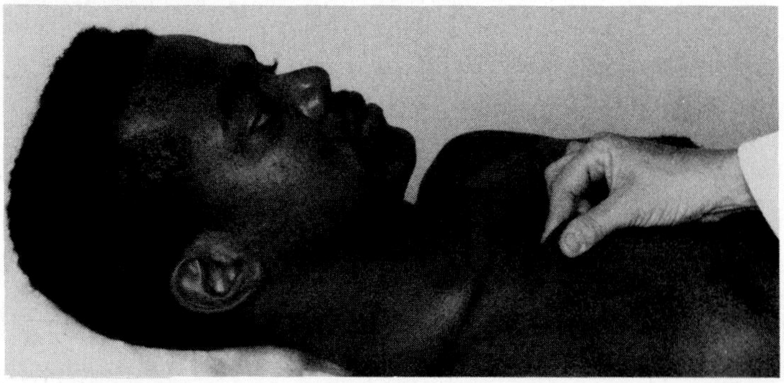

► **Figure 9–5**

NORMAL RANGE OF FINDINGS	ABNORMAL FINDINGS

Hygiene

Skin should be clean and free of body odor.

Vascularity or Bruising

Cherry (senile) angiomas are small, punctate, slightly raised bright red dots that commonly appear on the trunk in all adults over 30 (Fig. 9–6). They normally increase in size and number with aging.

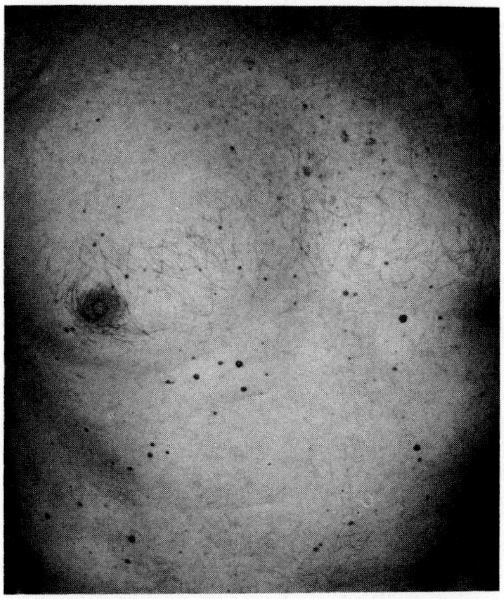

► Figure 9–6

Any bruising should be consistent with the expected trauma of life. There are normally no venous dilatation or varicosities.

Multiple bruises at different stages of healing and excessive bruises above knees or elbows should raise concern about physical abuse.

Document the presence of any tattoos (a permanent skin design from indelible pigment) on the person's chart. Advise the person that the use of tattoo needles and tattoo parlor equipment of doubtful sterility increases the risk of hepatitis.

Needle marks or tracks from IV injection of street drugs may be visible on the antecubital fossae or forearms, or on any available vein.

Lesions

Note:

1. Color
2. Elevation: flat, raised, or pedunculated
3. Pattern or shape: The grouping or distinctness of each lesion, for example, annular, grouped, confluent, linear. The pattern may be characteristic of a certain disease.
4. Size, in centimeters: Use a ruler to measure. Avoid descriptions such as "quarter size," or "pea size."
5. Location and distribution on body. Is it generalized or localized to area of a specific irritant; around jewelry, watchband, around eyes?
6. Any exudate. Note its color or odor.

See Table 9–3.

NORMAL RANGE OF FINDINGS	ABNORMAL FINDINGS

Lesions are traumatic or pathologic changes in previously normal structures. When a lesion develops on previously unaltered skin, it is primary. However, when a lesion changes over time or changes due to a factor such as scratching or infection, it is secondary. Study Tables 9–4 and 9–5 for the characteristics of primary and secondary skin lesions. The terms used (macule, papule, and so forth) are helpful to describe any lesion you encounter.

Palpate lesions. Roll a nodule between the thumb and index finger to assess depth. Gently scrape a scale to see if it comes off. Note the nature of its base or if it bleeds when the scale comes off. Note the surrounding skin temperature. However, the erythema associated with rashes is not always accompanied by noticeable increases in skin temperature.

Does the lesion blanch with pressure or stretch? Red macules from dilated blood vessels *will* blanch momentarily, whereas those from extravasated blood (petechiae) do not. Blanching also helps identify a macular rash in dark-skinned people. Stretching the area of skin between your thumb and index finger decreases (blanches) the normal underlying red tones, thus providing more contrast and brightening the macules.

Use a penlight for closer inspection of the lesion. Use a Wood's light, an ultraviolet light filtered through a special glass, to detect fluorescing lesions. With the room darkened, shine the Wood's light on the area.

Lesions with blue-green fluorescence indicate fungal infection, e.g., tinea capitis (scalp ringworm).

Potassium Hydroxide (KOH) Preparation. Microscopic examination of skin scrapings helps diagnose superficial fungal infections. Use a sharp sterile blade and lightly scrape the lesion, especially in a vesicular area, if present. Place on a clean slide. Add 1 drop of 10 to 20 percent potassium hydroxide (KOH) to dissolve nonfungal skin debris and send to the lab.

HAIR

Inspect and palpate

Color

Hair color comes from melanin production and may vary from pale blonde to total black. Graying begins as early as the third decade of life due to reduced melanin production in the follicles. Genetic factors affect the age of onset of graying.

Texture

Scalp hair may be fine or thick and may look straight, curly, or kinky. It should look shiny, although this characteristic may be lost with the use of some beauty products such as dyes, rinses, or permanents.

Note dull, coarse, or brittle scalp hair.

Gray, scaly, well-defined areas with broken hairs accompany tinea capitis, a ringworm infection found in children (see Table 9–10).

Distribution

Fine vellus hair coats the body, whereas coarser terminal hairs grow at the eyebrows, eyelashes, and scalp. During puberty, distribution conforms to normal male and female patterns. At first, coarse curly hairs develop in the pubic area, then in the axillae, and last in the facial area in boys. In the genital area, the female pattern is an inverted triangle, the male pattern is

Genital hair absent or with abnormal configuration suggests endocrine abnormalities.

NORMAL RANGE OF FINDINGS | **ABNORMAL FINDINGS**

an upright triangle with pubic hair extending up to the umbilicus. In Asians, body hair may be diminished.

Hirsutism—excess body hair. In females, this forms a male pattern of hair distribution on the face and chest and indicates the presence of endocrine abnormalities.

Lesions

Separate the hair into sections and lift it, observing the scalp. The area should be clean and free of any lesions or pest inhabitants. Many people normally have seborrhea (dandruff), which is indicated by loose white flakes.

Head or pubic lice. Distinguish dandruff from nits (eggs) of lice, which are oval, adherent to hair shaft, and cause intense itching.

NAILS

Inspect and palpate

Shape and Contour

The nail surface is normally slightly curved or flat, and the posterior and lateral nail folds are smooth and rounded. Nail edges are smooth, rounded, and clean, suggesting adequate self-care.

Spoon nails (see Table 9–11). Jagged nails, bitten to the quick, or traumatized nail folds from chronic nervous picking suggest nervous habits.

Chronically dirty nails suggest poor self-care or some occupations in which it is impossible to keep them clean.

View the index finger at its profile and note the angle of the nail base; it should be about 160 degrees (Fig. 9–7). The nail base is firm to palpation. Curved nails are a variation of normal with a convex profile. They may look like clubbed nails, but notice that the angle between nail base and nail is normal, i.e., 160 degrees or less.

Clubbing of nails occurs with congenital chronic cyanotic heart disease and with emphysema and chronic bronchitis.

In early clubbing, the angle straightens out to 180 degrees and the nail base feels spongy to palpation.

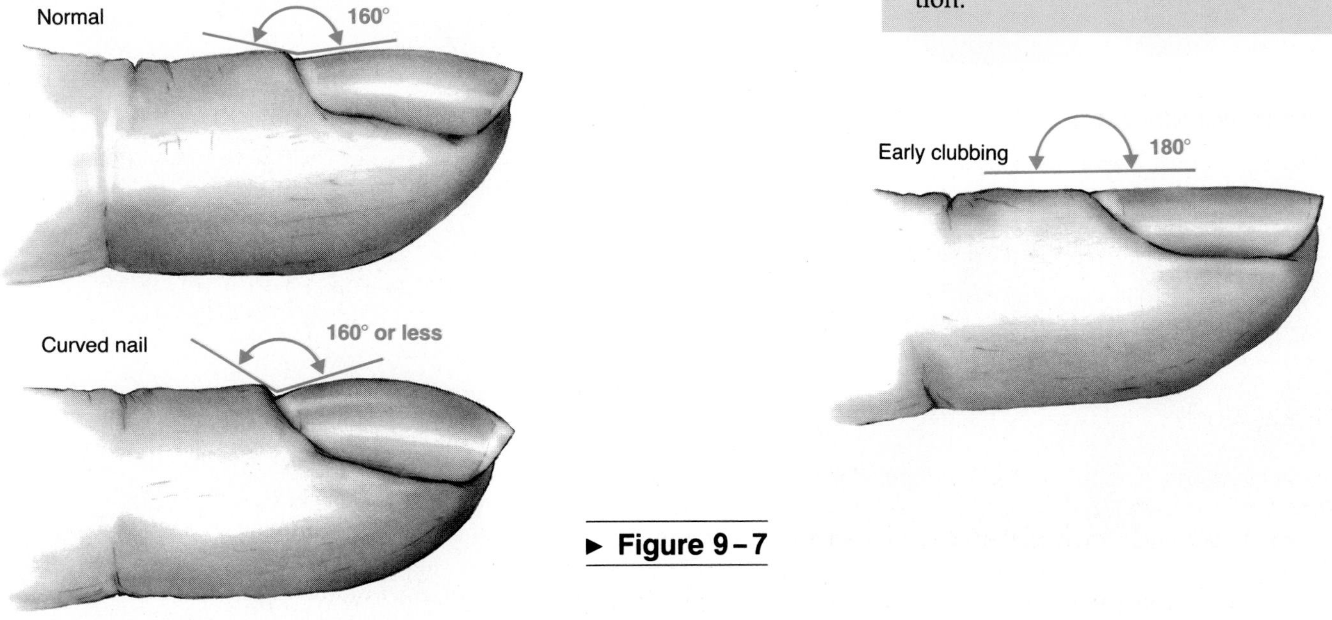

► Figure 9–7

NORMAL RANGE OF FINDINGS	ABNORMAL FINDINGS

Consistency

The surface is smooth and regular, not brittle or splitting.

Pits, transverse grooves, or lines may indicate a nutrient deficiency or may accompany acute illness in which nail growth is disturbed.

Nail thickness is uniform.

Nails are thickened and ridged with arterial insufficiency.

The nail is firmly adherent to the nail bed and the nail base is firm to palpation.

A spongy nail base accompanies clubbing.

Color

The translucent nail plate is a window to the even, pink nail bed underneath.

Cyanosis or marked pallor.

Dark-skinned people may have brown-black pigmented areas or linear bands or streaks along the nail edge (Fig. 9–8). All people normally may have white hairline linear markings from trauma or picking at the cuticle (Fig. 9–9). Note any abnormal marking in the nail beds.

Brown linear streaks are abnormal in light-skinned people and may indicate melanoma.

Splinter hemorrhages, transverse ridges or Beau's lines (see Table 9–11).

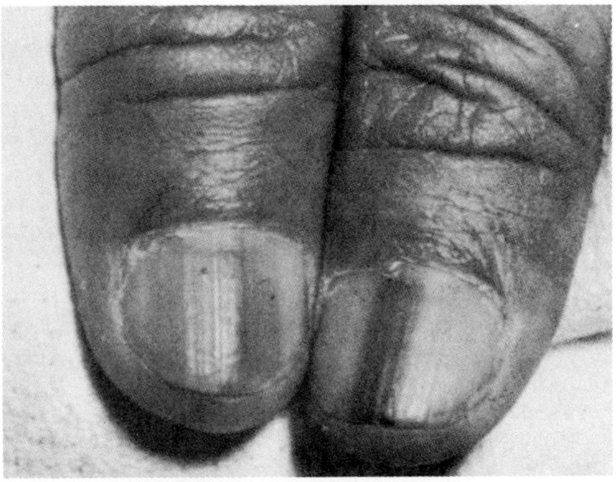

Linear pigmentation ► **Figure 9–8**

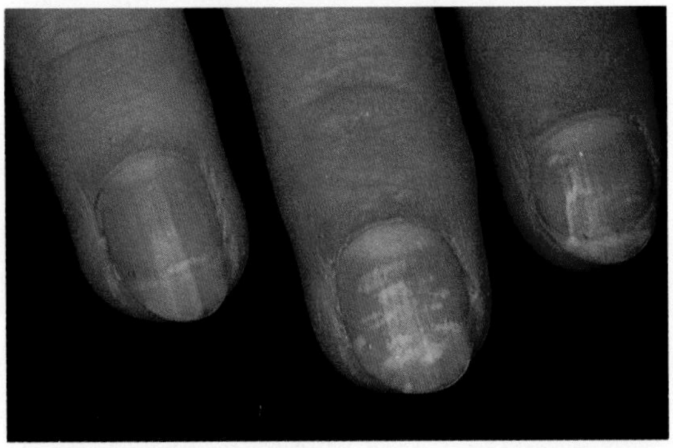

Leukonychia striata ► **Figure 9–9**

NORMAL RANGE OF FINDINGS

Depress the nail edge to blanch and then release, noting the return of color. Normally, color return is instant, or at least within a few seconds in a cold environment. This indicates the status of the peripheral circulation. A sluggish color return takes longer than 1 or 2 seconds.

Inspect the toenails. Separate the toes and note the smooth skin in between.

ABNORMAL FINDINGS

Cyanotic nail beds or sluggish color return, consider cardiovascular or respiratory dysfunction.

DEVELOPMENTAL CONSIDERATIONS

Use the same examination as described in the previous sections for the adult. Common variations follow.

Infants

Skin Color — General Pigmentation. Black newborns initially have lighter toned skin than their parents due to a pigment function that is not yet in full production. Their full melanotic color is evident in the nail beds and scrotal folds. The *Mongolian spot* is a common variation of hyperpigmentation in black, Native American, Latin, and Asian newborns (Fig. 9 – 10).

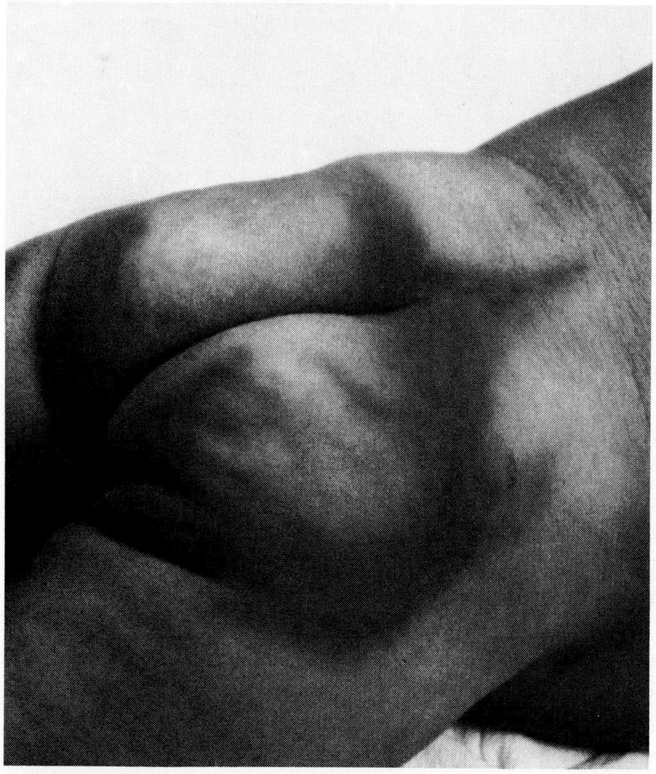

Mongolian spot

► Figure 9 – 10

NORMAL RANGE OF FINDINGS

It is a blue-black to purple macular area at the sacrum or buttocks, but sometimes it occurs on the abdomen, thighs, shoulders, or arms. It is due to deep dermal melanocytes. It gradually fades during the first year. By adulthood these spots are lighter but are frequently still visible. Mongolian spots are present in 90 percent of blacks, 80 percent of Asians and Native Americans, and 9 percent of whites. If you are unfamiliar with Mongolian spots, be careful not to confuse them with bruises. Recognition of this normal variation is particularly important when dealing with children who might be erroneously identified as victims of child abuse.

The *café au lait spot* is a large round or oval patch of light brown pigmentation (hence, the name "coffee with cream"), which is usually present at birth (Fig. 9–11). Most of these patches are normal, but occasionally they may be associated with neurofibromatosis.

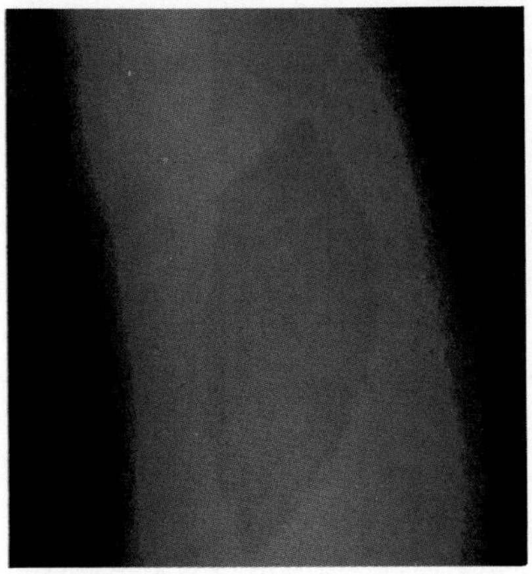

Café au lait spot

► Figure 9–11

Skin Color Change. Some erythematous states are common variations in the neonate. The newborn's skin has a beefy red flush for the first 24 hours due to vasomotor instability, then the color fades to its normal color. Another finding, the *Harlequin color change,* occurs when the baby is in a side-lying position. The lower half of the body turns red and the upper half blanches with a distinct demarcation line down the midline. The cause is unknown, and its occurrence is transient. Finally, *erythema toxicum* is a common rash that appears in the first 3 to 4 days of life. It consists of tiny, punctate, red macules and papules on the cheeks, trunk, chest, back, and buttocks (Fig. 9–12). The cause is unknown; no treatment is needed.

A newborn may have *acrocyanosis,* a bluish color around the lips, hands and fingernails, and feet and toenails. This may last for a few hours and disappear with warming. *Cutis marmorata* is a transient mottling in the trunk and extremities in response to cooler room temperatures (Fig. 9–13). It forms a reticulated red or blue pattern over the skin.

ABNORMAL FINDINGS

Persistent genalized cyanosis indicates distress, possibly cyanotic congenital heart disease.

Persistent or pronounced cutis marmorata occurs with Down syndrome or prematurity.

NORMAL RANGE OF FINDINGS

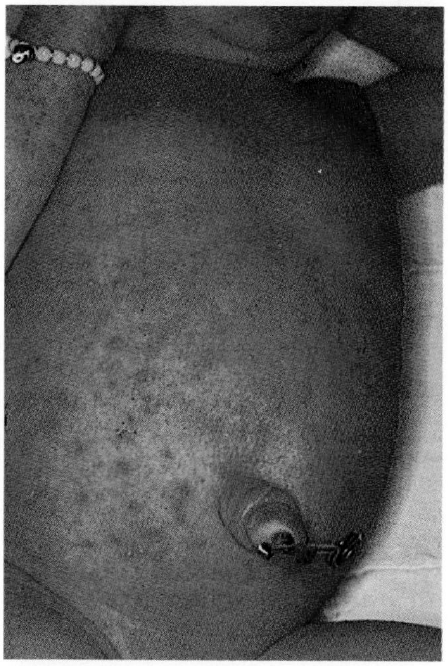

Erythema toxicum

► **Figure 9-12**

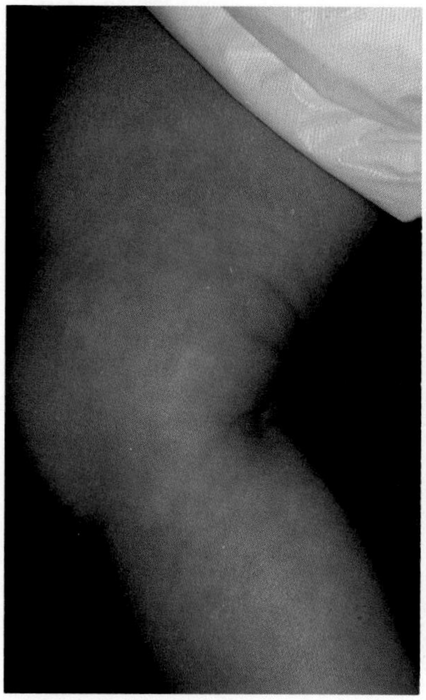

Cutis marmorata

► **Figure 9-13**

Physiologic jaundice is a common variation in about half of all newborns. A yellowing of the skin, sclera, and mucous membranes develops after the third or fourth day of life due to the increased numbers of red blood cells that hemolyze following birth. The hemoglobin in the red blood cells is metabolized by the liver and spleen; its pigment is converted into bilirubin.

Carotenemia also produces a yellow-orange color in light-skinned persons but no yellowing in the sclera or mucous membranes. It comes from ingesting large amounts of foods containing carotene, a vitamin A precursor. Carotene-rich foods are popular as prepared infant foods, and the absorption of carotene is enhanced by mashing, pureeing, and cooking. The color is best seen on the palms and soles, the forehead, tip of the nose and nasolabial folds, the chin, behind the ears, and over the knuckles; it fades to normal color within 2 to 6 weeks of withdrawing carotene-rich foods from the diet.

Moisture. The vernix caseosa is the moist, white, cheese-like substance that covers part of the skin in all newborns. Perspiration is present after 1 month of age.

ABNORMAL FINDINGS

Jaundice on the first day of life may indicate hemolytic disease. Jaundice after 2 weeks of age may indicate biliary tract obstruction.

In children, excessive sweating may accompany hypoglycemia, heart disease, or hyperthyroidism.

NORMAL RANGE OF FINDINGS

Texture. A common variation occurring in the infant is *milia* (Fig. 9 – 14). Milia are tiny white papules on the cheeks, forehead, across the nose and chin due to sebum that occludes the opening of the follicles. Tell parents not to squeeze the lesion; milia resolve spontaneously within a few weeks.

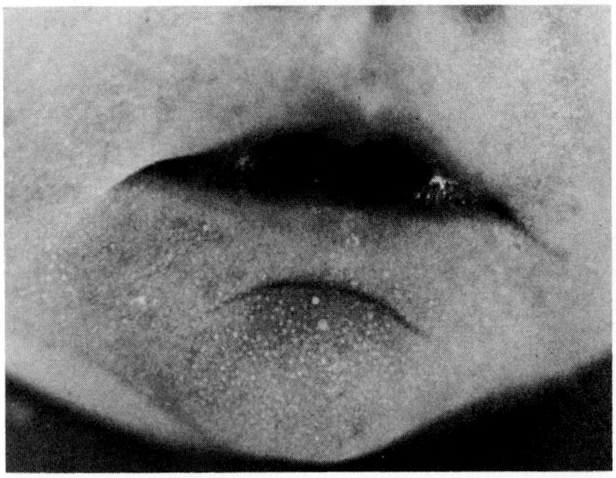

► **Figure 9 – 14**

Dermatoglyphics are the unique patterns of handprints and footprints.

Thickness. In the neonate, the epidermis is normally thin but you will also note well-defined areas of subcutaneous fat. The baby's skin dimples over joints, but there is no break in the skin. Check for any defect or break in the skin especially over the length of the spine.

Mobility and Turgor. Test mobility and turgor over the abdomen in an infant.

Vascularity or Bruising. Some vascular markings are common birthmarks in the newborn. A *storkbite* (salmon patch) is a flat, irregularly shaped red or pink patch found on the forehead, eyelid, or upper lip, but most commonly at the back of the neck (nuchal area) (Fig. 9 – 15). It is present at birth and usually fades during the first year.

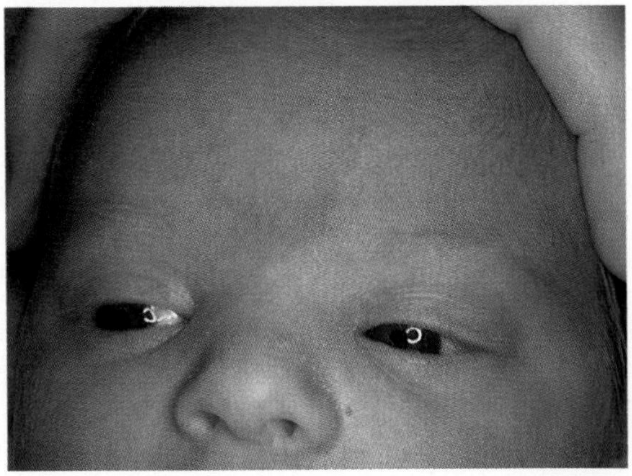

► **Figure 9 – 15**

ABNORMAL FINDINGS

A single palmar crease, called a *simian crease,* is a single transverse fold at the base of the fingers in children with Down syndrome.

Lack of subcutaneous fat occurs in prematurity and malnutrition.

A red sacrococcygeal dimple occurs with a pilonidal cyst or sinus (see Table 23 – 1).

Poor turgor, or "tenting," indicates dehydration or malnutrition.

Port-wine stain, strawberry mark (immature hemangioma), cavernous hemangioma (see Table 9 – 6). Bruising may suggest abuse (see Table 9 – 7).

NORMAL RANGE OF FINDINGS

Hair. A newborn's skin is covered with fine downy lanugo. Scalp hair may be lost in the few weeks following birth, especially at the temples and occiput. It grows back slowly.

Nails. A newborn's nail beds may be blue (cyanotic) for the first few hours of life; then they turn pink.

Adolescents

The increase in sebaceous gland activity creates increased oiliness and acne (Fig. 9–16). Acne is the most common skin problem of adolescence. Almost all teens have some acne, even if it is the milder form of open comedones (blackheads) and closed comedones (whiteheads). Severe acne includes papules, pustules, and nodules. Acne lesions usually appear on the face and sometimes on the chest, back, and shoulders. Acne may appear in children as early as 7 to 8 years of age, then the lesions increase in number and severity, and peak at 14 to 16 years in girls and 16 to 19 years in boys.

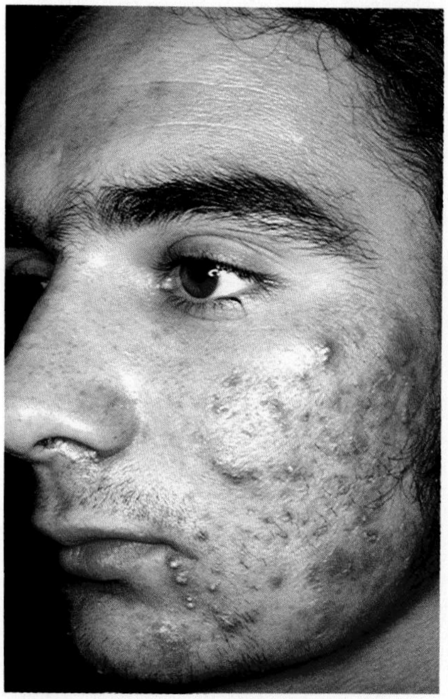

► **Figure 9–16**

The Pregnant Female

Striae are jagged linear "stretch marks" of silver to pink color that appear during the second trimester on the abdomen, breasts, and sometimes, thighs. They occur in one-half of all pregnancies. They fade after delivery but do not disappear. Another skin change on the abdomen is the *linea nigra,* a brownish black line down the midline. *Chloasma* is an irregular brown patch of hyperpigmentation on the face. It may occur with pregnancy or in women taking oral contraceptive pills. Chloasma disappears after delivery or stopping the pills. *Vascular spiders* occur in two-thirds of pregnancies in white women and less often in blacks. These lesions have tiny red centers with radiating branches and occur on the face, neck, upper chest, and arms.

ABNORMAL FINDINGS

Scaly crusted scalp occurs with seborrheic dermatitis (cradle cap) (see Table 9–10).

NORMAL RANGE OF FINDINGS | **ABNORMAL FINDINGS**

The Aging Adult

Skin Color and Pigmentation. The lesions discussed in the following sections are common variations of hyperpigmentation:

Senile Lentigines. These lesions are commonly called liver spots and are small, flat, brown macules (Fig. 9–17). These circumscribed areas are clusters of melanocytes that appear following extensive sun exposure. They appear on the forearms and dorsa of the hands. They are not malignant and require no treatment.

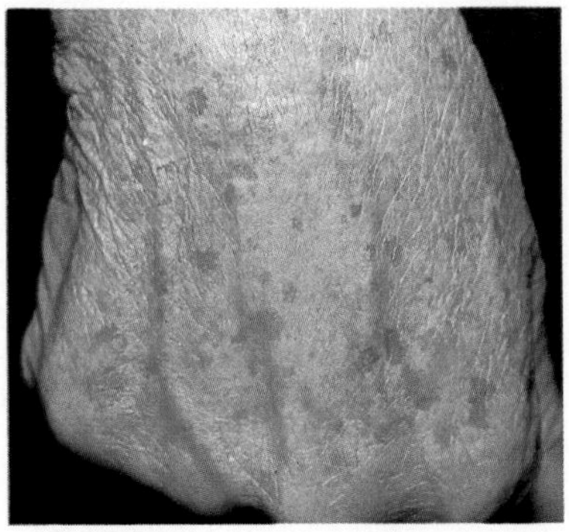

Lentigines ▶ **Figure 9–17**

Keratoses. These lesions are raised, thickened areas of pigmentation which look crusted, scaly, and warty. One type, *seborrheic keratoses,* look dark, greasy, and "stuck on" (Fig. 9–18). They develop mostly on the trunk, but also on the face and hands, and on unexposed as well as on sun-exposed areas. They do not become cancerous.

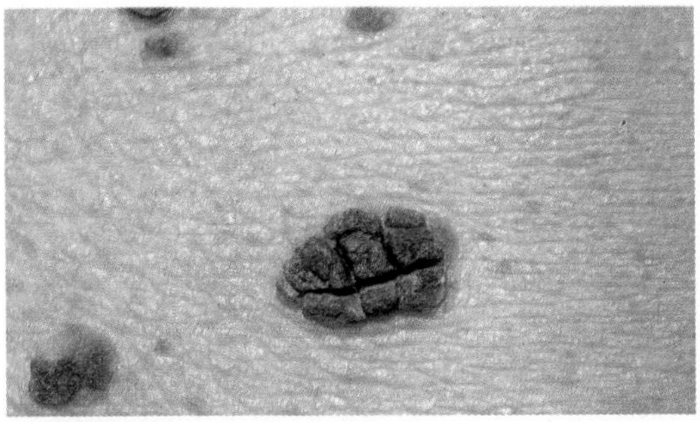

Seborrheic keratosis ▶ **Figure 9–18**

Another type, *actinic (senile or solar) keratoses,* are less common (Fig. 19–19). These lesions are red-tan scaly plaques that increase over the years to become raised and roughened. They may have a silvery white scale adherent to the plaque. They occur on sun-exposed surfaces and are

NORMAL RANGE OF FINDINGS | ABNORMAL FINDINGS

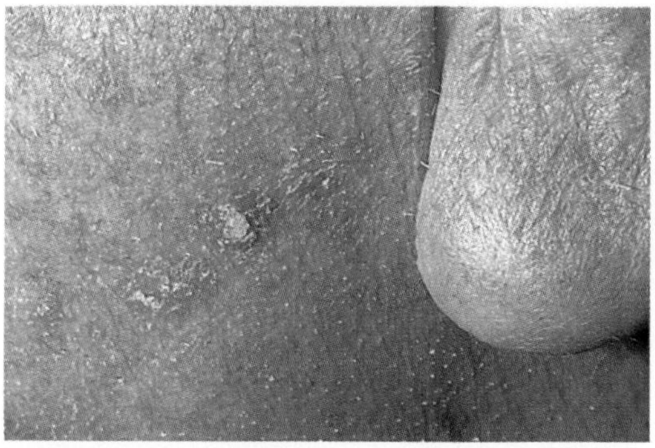

Actinic keratosis ► **Figure 9–19**

directly related to sun exposure. They are premalignant and may develop into squamous cell carcinoma.

Moisture. Dry skin (xerosis) is common in the aging person because of a decline in the size, number, and output of the sweat glands and sebaceous glands. The skin itches and looks flaky and loose.

Texture. Common variations occurring in the aging adult are *acrochordons,* or "skin tags," which are overgrowths of normal skin that form a stalk and are polyp-like (Fig. 9–20). They occur frequently on eyelids, cheeks and neck, and axillae and trunk.

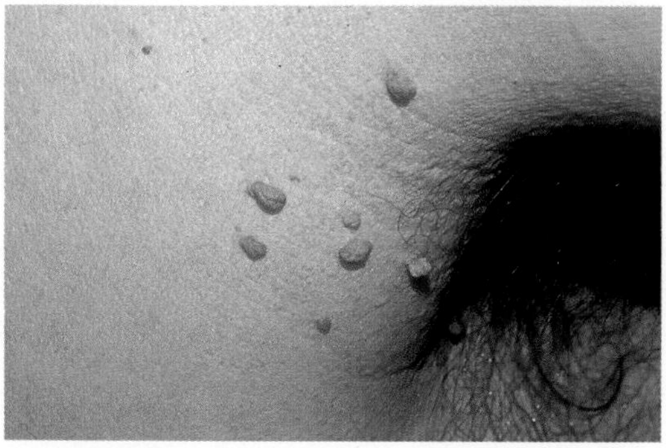

Skin tags ► **Figure 9–20**

Sebaceous hyperplasia are raised yellow papules with a central depression. They are more common in men, occurring over the forehead, nose, or cheeks. They have a pebbly look.

Thickness. With aging, the skin looks as thin as parchment and the subcutaneous fat diminishes. Thinner skin is evident over the dorsa of the hands, forearms, lower legs, dorsa of feet, and over bony prominences. The skin may feel thicker over the abdomen and chest.

NORMAL RANGE OF FINDINGS	ABNORMAL FINDINGS

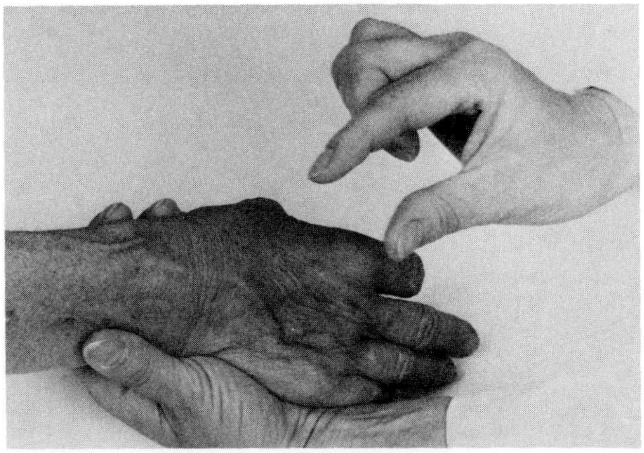

► Figure 9-21

Mobility and Turgor. The turgor is decreased (less elasticity) and the skin recedes slowly or "tents" and stands by itself (Fig. 9-21).

Hair. With aging, the hair growth decreases, and the amount decreases in the axillae and pubic areas. After menopause, white women may develop bristly hairs on the chin or upper lip resulting from unopposed androgens. In men, coarse terminal hairs develop in the ears, nose, and eyebrows, although the beard is unchanged. Male-pattern balding, or alopecia, is a genetic trait. It is usually a gradual receding of the anterior hairline in a symmetric W shape. In men and women, scalp hair gradually turns gray because of the decrease in melanocyte function.

Nails. With aging, the nail growth rate decreases and local injuries in the nail matrix may produce longitudinal ridges. The surface may be brittle or peeling and sometimes yellowed. Toenails also are thickened and may grow misshapen, almost grotesque. The thickening may be a process of aging, or it may be due to chronic peripheral vascular disease.

Fungal infections are common in aging, with thickened crumbling toenails and erythematous scaling on contiguous skin surfaces.

☑ SUMMARY CHECKLIST

1 ► Inspect the skin for:
- Color
- General pigmentation
- Areas of hypopigmentation or hyperpigmentation
- Abnormal color changes

2 ► Palpate the skin for:
- Temperature
- Moisture
- Texture
- Thickness
- Edema
- Mobility and turgor
- Hygiene
- Vascularity or bruising

3 ► Note any lesions:
- Color
- Shape and configuration
- Size
- Location and distribution on body

4 ► Inspect and palpate the hair for:
- Texture
- Distribution
- Any scalp lesions

5 ► Inspect and palpate the nails for:
- Shape and contour
- Consistency
- Color

SAMPLE RECORDING

Subjective

► No history of skin disease; no present change in pigmentation or in nevi; no pruritus, bruising, rash, or lesions. On no medications. No work-related skin hazards. Uses sun block cream when outdoors.

Objective

► Skin: Color tan-pink, warm to touch, turgor good, no lesions
Hair: Normal distribution and texture
Nails: No clubbing or deformities, nail beds pink with prompt capillary refill

SAMPLE CLINICAL PROBLEM 1*

Ethan E. is a 3-year-old white male present with his mother, who seeks health care because of Ethan's fever, fatigue, and rash of 3 days' duration.

Subjective

► 2 weeks prior to arrival (PTA)—Ethan was playing with child who was subsequently diagnosed as having varicella.
3 days PTA—Mother reports fever 100° to 101° and fatigue, irritability. That evening noted "tiny blisters" on chest and back.
1 day PTA—Blisters on chest changed to white with scab on top. New eruption of blisters on shoulders, thighs, face. Intense itching and scratching.

Objective

► Temp 38.0°C (100.4°F), P 110, R 24
Generalized vesiculopustular rash covering face, trunk, upper arms, and thighs. Small vesicles on face, pustules and red-honey–colored crusts on trunk.

Assessment

► Varicella
Impaired skin integrity R/T infection and scratching

* Please note that space does not allow a detailed plan for each sample clinical problem in this text. Please consult the appropriate text for current treatment plans.

SAMPLE CLINICAL PROBLEM 2

Myra G. is a 79-year-old widowed, retired college professor, in good health up until recent hospitalization following a fall.

Problem List 1 Fractured right hip—hip pinning 11/24

11/27

Subjective

- Aching pain in left hip (nonoperative side)

Objective

- Erosion 2 × 2 cm with surrounding erythema covering L ischium. Erosion is moist, no active bleeding. Area very warm and tender to touch.

Assessment

- Pressure sore, L hip
  Impaired skin integrity R/T immobility and pressure
  Pain, acute

NURSING DIAGNOSES COMMONLY ASSOCIATED WITH SKIN, HAIR, AND NAIL DISORDERS

Diagnosis	Related Factors (Etiology)	Defining Characteristics (Symptoms and Signs)
Impaired skin integrity	Altered Nutritional state Oxygen transport Sensation Autoimmune dysfunction Decreased circulation Edema Effects of aging, medication Infection Skeletal prominence Excretions/secretions Allergy (drugs, foods) Chemical substances on skin Immobility Insect/animal bites Pressure	Blisters Bruising Callus Chafing Cyanosis Disruption of skin surface skin layers Dryness Erythema Induration Lesions Necrosis Pallor Pruritus

Diagnosis	Related Factors (Etiology)	Defining Characteristics (Symptoms and Signs)
Impaired skin integrity (*continued*)	Radiation Restraint Stress Surgery	
Self-care deficit: bathing/hygiene	Effects of Aging Trauma Surgery Chronic illness Muscular weakness Fatigue Pain Immobility Presence of external devices—IV lines, casts, traction Visual impairment Stiffness Depression Knowledge deficit Lack of motivation Perceptual or cognitive impairment Confusion Grieving	Dirt or stains on body Requests help in bathing Body odor Halitosis Inability to wash body or body parts
Fluid volume deficit	Loss of body fluids or electrolytes Diaphoresis Diarrhea Increased insensible water loss Nausea and/or vomiting Excessive drainage through artificial orifices or lumens, wounds or drainage tubes Diuretic therapy Exposure to extreme heat Excessive use of alcohol, enemas, or laxatives	Concentrated urine, blood Decreased Blood pressure Skin turgor Urine output Dry skin Dry mucous membranes Increased Body temperature Pulse rate Thirst Sudden weight loss

ABNORMAL CONDITIONS

Table 9-2 ▶ Color Changes in Light and Dark Skin

	APPEARANCE	
ETIOLOGY	**Light Skin**	**Dark Skin**
PALLOR		
Anemia—decreased Hct Shock—decreased perfusion, vasoconstriction	Generalized pallor	Brown skin appears yellow-brown, dull; black skin appears ashen gray, dull. Skin loses its healthy glow. Check areas with least pigmentation, such as conjunctivae, mucous membranes
Local arterial insufficiency	Marked localized pallor, e.g., lower extremities, especially when elevated	Ashen gray, dull; cool to palpation
Albinism—total absence of pigment melanin throughout the integument	Whitish pink	Tan, cream, white
Vitiligo—patchy depigmentation from destruction of melanocytes	Patchy milky white spots, often symmetric bilaterally	Same
CYANOSIS		
Increased amount of unoxygenated hemoglobin: Central—chronic heart and lung disease cause arterial desaturation	Dusky blue	Dark but dull, lifeless. Only severe cyanosis is apparent in skin. Check conjunctiva, oral mucosa, nail beds
Peripheral—exposure to cold, anxiety	Nail beds dusky	
ERYTHEMA		
Hyperemia—increased blood flow through engorged arterioles, such as in inflammation, fever, alcohol intake, blushing	Red, bright pink	Purplish tinge, but difficult to see. Palpate for increased warmth with inflammation, taut skin, and hardening of deep tissues

Table 9-2 ▸ Color Changes in Light and Dark Skin *Continued*

	APPEARANCE	
ETIOLOGY	**Light Skin**	**Dark Skin**
Polycythemia—increased RBCs, capillary stasis	Ruddy blue in face, oral mucosa, conjunctiva, hands and feet	Well concealed by pigment. Check for redness in lips.
Carbon monoxide poisoning	Bright cherry red in face and upper torso	Cherry red color in nail beds, lips, and oral mucosa
Venous stasis—decreased blood flow from area, engorged venules	Dusky rubor of dependent extremities. A prelude to necrosis with pressure sore	Easily masked; use palpation for warmth or edema
JAUNDICE		
Increased serum bilirubin, over 2 to 3 mg/100 ml due to liver inflammation or hemolytic disease such as after severe burns, some infections	Yellow in sclera, hard palate, mucous membranes, then over skin	Check sclera for yellow near limbus. Do not mistake normal yellowish fatty deposits in the periphery under the eyelids for jaundice. Jaundice best noted in junction of hard and soft palate; also palms
Carotenemia—increased serum carotene from ingestion of large amounts of carotene-rich foods	Yellow orange in forehead, palms and soles, nasolabial folds, but no yellowing in sclera or mucous membranes	Yellow orange tinge in palms and soles
Uremia—renal failure causes retained urochrome pigments in the blood	Orange-green or gray overlying pallor of anemia. May also have ecchymoses and purpura	Easily masked; rely on laboratory and clinical findings
BROWN-TAN		
Addison's disease—cortisol deficiency stimulates increased melanin production	Bronzed appearance, an "eternal tan," most apparent around nipples, perineum, genitalia, and pressure points (inner thighs, buttocks, elbow, axillae)	Easily masked, rely on lab and clinical findings
Café au lait spots—due to increased melanin pigment in basal cell layer	Tan to light brown, irregularly shaped, oval patch with well-defined borders	

Table 9–3 ▶ Common Shapes and Configurations of Lesions

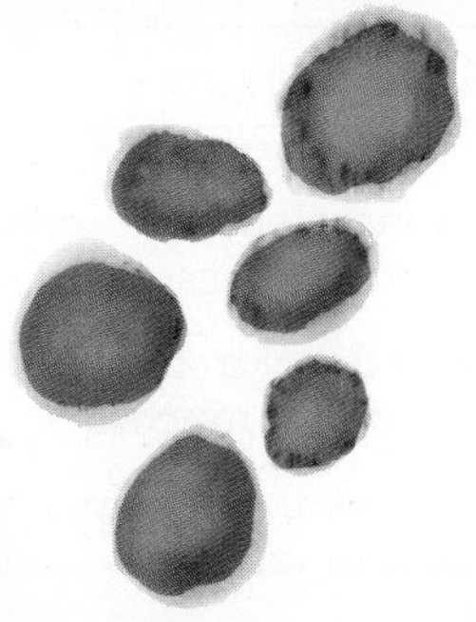

ANNULAR, or circular, begins in center and spreads to periphery, e.g., ringworm, tinea versicolor, pityriasis rosea

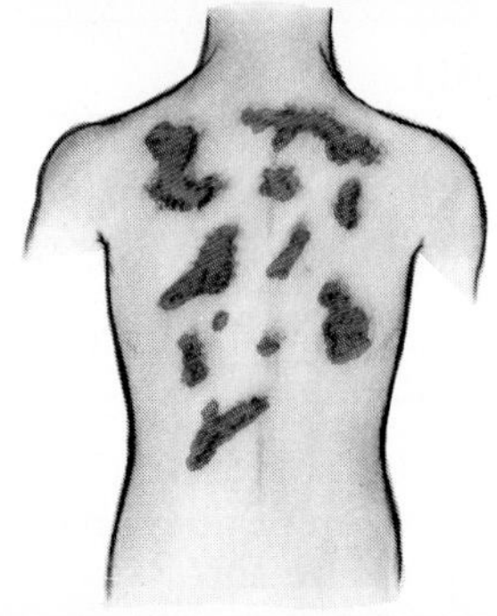

CONFLUENT, lesions run together, e.g., urticaria

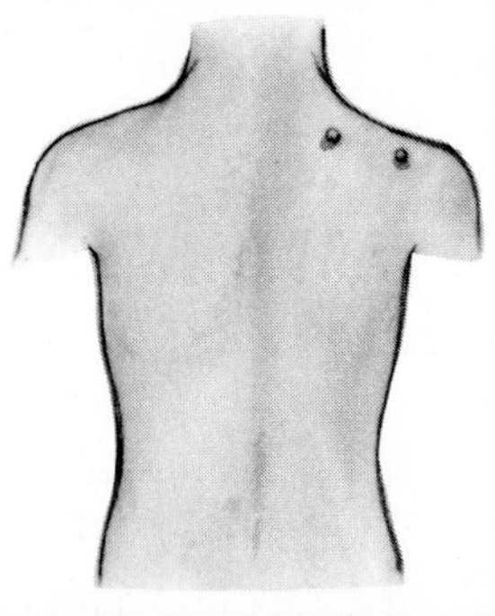

DISCRETE, distinct, individual lesions which remain separate

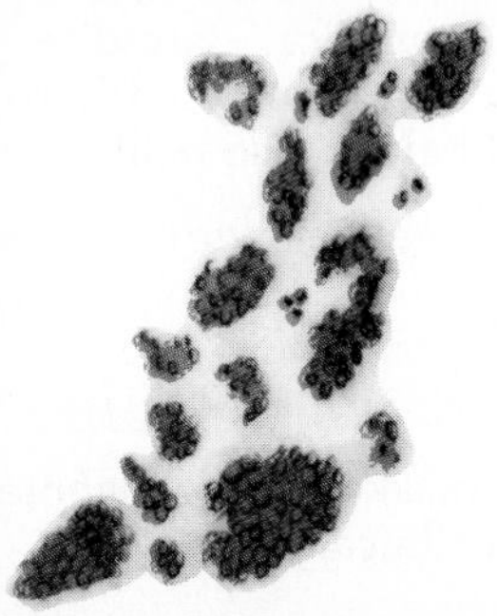

GROUPED, clusters of lesions, e.g., vesicles of contact dermatitis

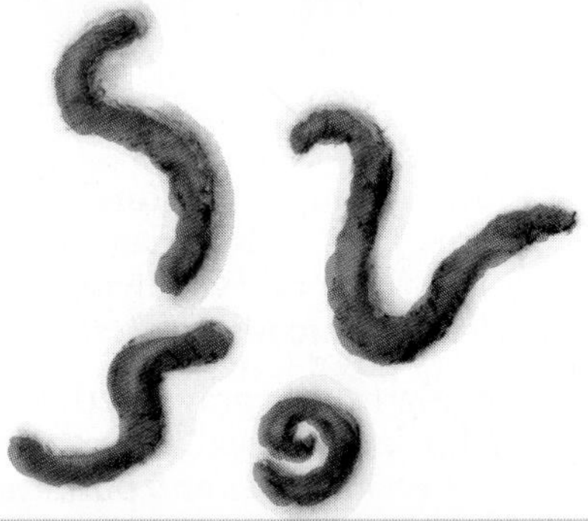

GYRATE, twisted, coiled spiral, snakelike

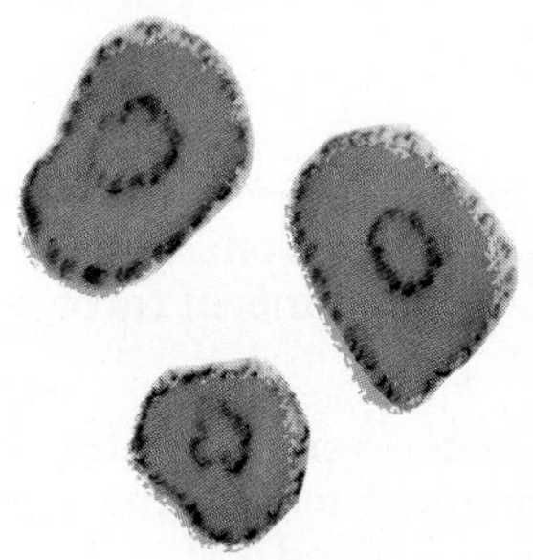

IRIS, or target, resembles iris of eye, concentric rings of lesions

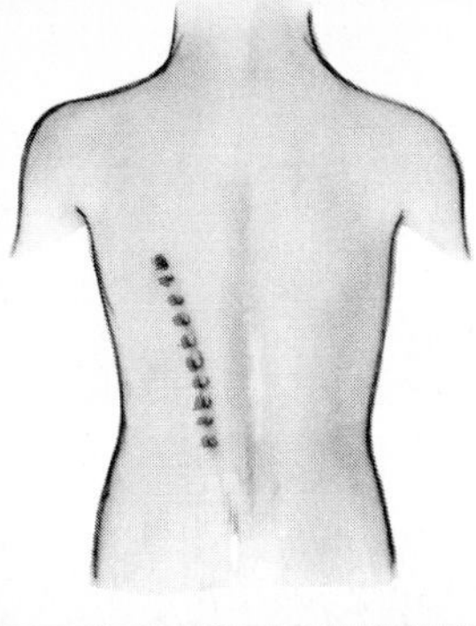

LINEAR, a scratch, streak, line, or stripe

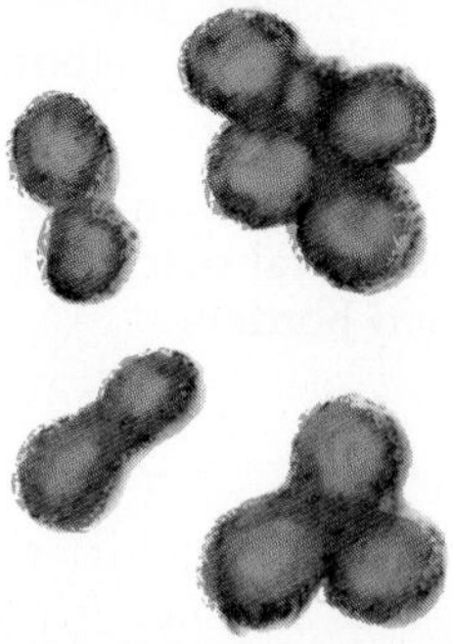

POLYCYCLIC, annular lesions grow together

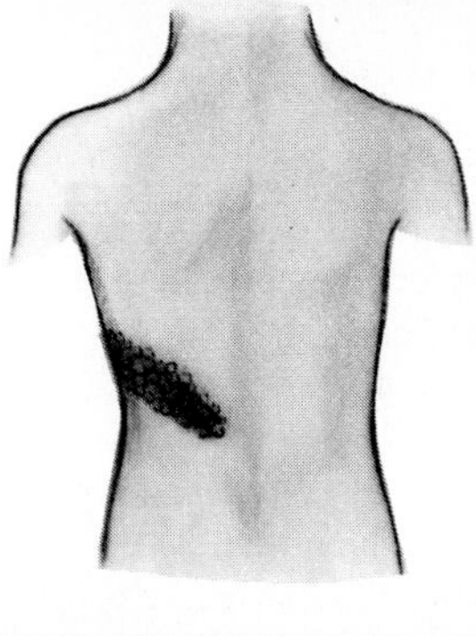

ZOSTERIFORM, linear arrangement along a nerve route, e.g., herpes zoster

Table 9-4 ▸ Primary Skin Lesions*

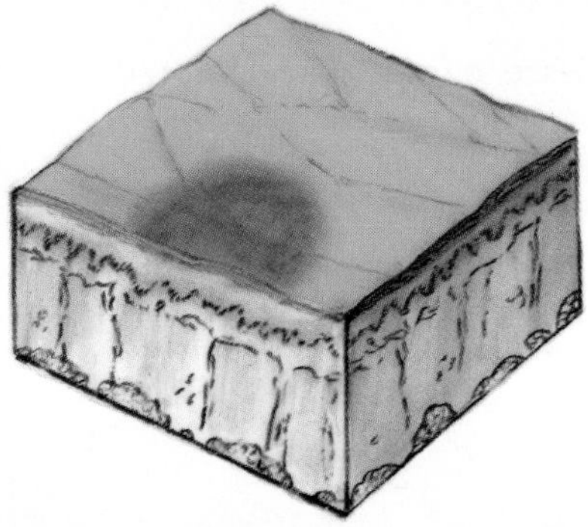

MACULE

Solely a color change, flat and circumscribed, less than 1 cm. Examples: freckles, flat nevi, hypopigmentation, petechiae, measles, scarlet fever

PATCH (not illustrated)

Macules larger than 1 cm. Examples: mongolian spot, vitiligo, café au lait spot, chloasma, measles rash

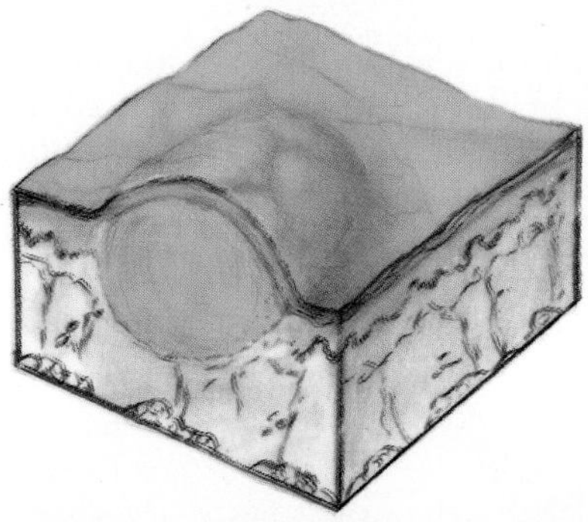

PAPULE

Something you can feel, i.e., solid, elevated, circumscribed, less than 1 cm diameter, due to superficial thickening in the epidermis. Examples: elevated nevus (mole), lichen planus, molluscum, wart (verruca)

PLAQUE (not illustrated)

Papules coalesce to form surface elevation wider than 1 cm. A plateau-like, disc-shaped lesion. Examples: psoriasis, lichen planus

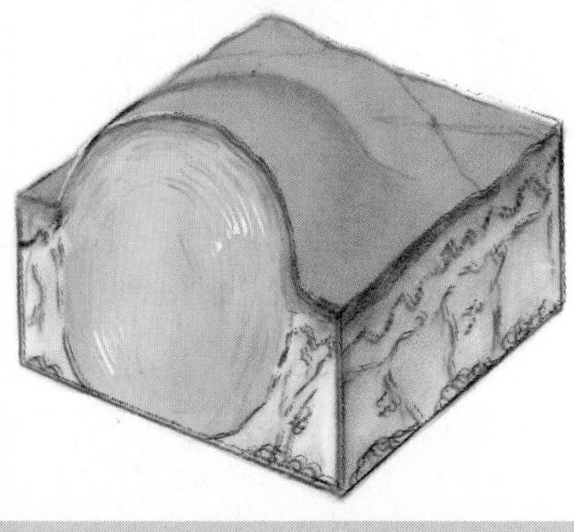

NODULE

Solid, elevated, hard or soft, larger than 1 cm. May extend deeper into dermis than papule. Examples: xanthoma, fibroma, intradermal nevi

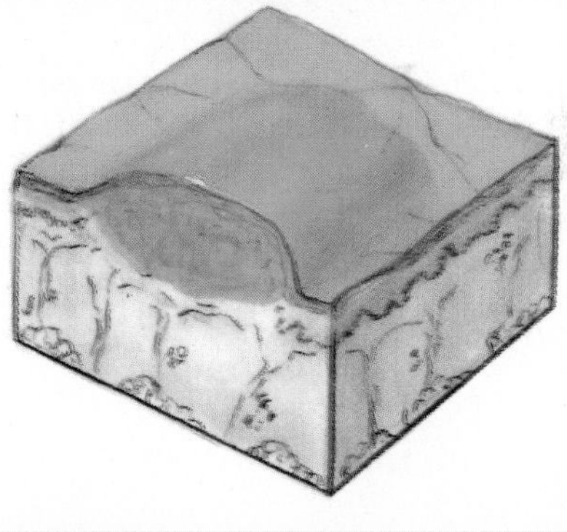

WHEAL

Superficial, raised, transient, and erythematous; slightly irregular shape due to edema (fluid held diffusely in the tissues). Examples: mosquito bite, allergic reaction, dermographism

Table continued on following page

Table 9-4 ▶ Primary Skin Lesions* *Continued*

TUMOR

Larger than a few centimeters in diameter, firm or soft, deeper into dermis; may be benign or malignant, although "tumor" implies "cancer" to most people. Examples: lipoma, hemangioma

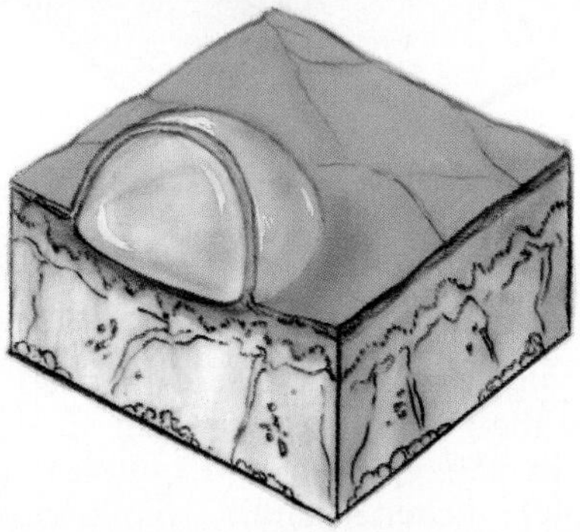

URTICARIA (HIVES)

Wheals coalesce to form extensive reaction, intensely pruritic.

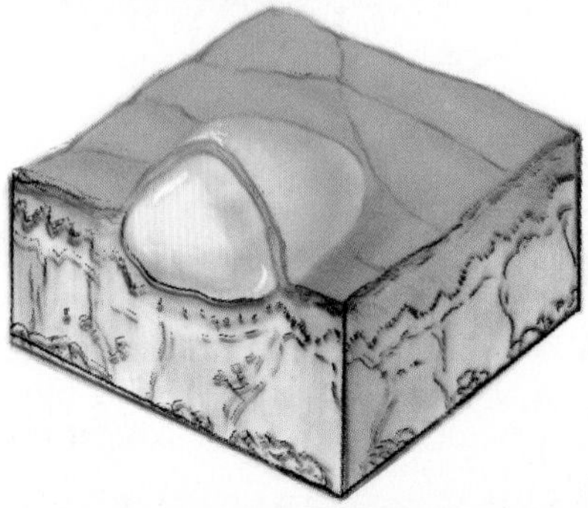

VESICLE

Elevated cavity containing free fluid, up to 1 cm. Clear serum flows if wall is ruptured. Examples: herpes simplex, early varicella (chicken pox), herpes zoster (shingles), contact dermatitis

BULLA

Larger than 1 cm diameter; usually single-chambered (unilocular); superficial in epidermis; it is thin walled, so it ruptures easily. Examples: friction blister, pemphigus, burns, contact dermatitis

PUSTULE

Turbid fluid (pus) in the cavity. Circumscribed and elevated. Examples: impetigo, acne

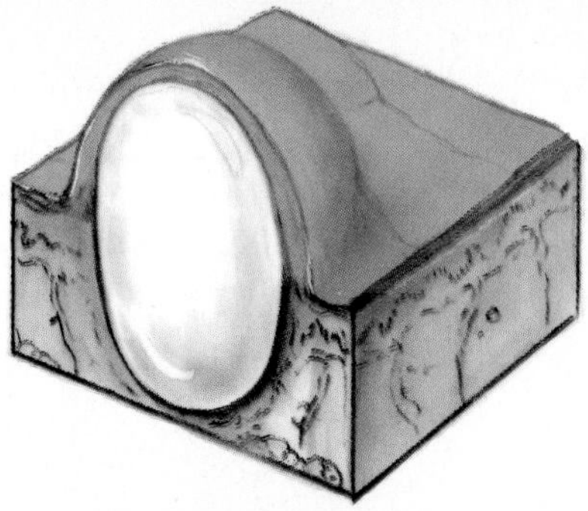

CYST

Encapsulated, fluid-filled cavity in dermis or subcutaneous layer, tensely elevating skin. Examples: sebaceous cyst, wen

* The immediate result of a specific causative factor; primary lesions develop on previously unaltered skin.

Table 9-5 ▸ Secondary Skin Lesions*

DEBRIS ON SKIN SURFACE

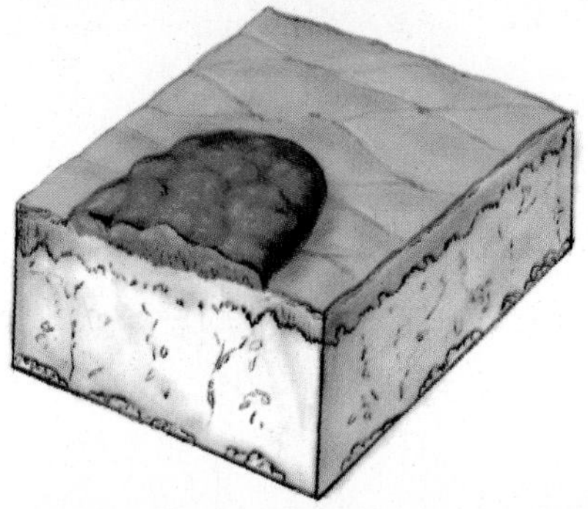

Crust

The thickened, dried-out exudate left when vesicles/ pustules burst or dry up. Color can be red-brown, honey, or yellow, depending on the fluid's ingredients (blood, serum, pus). Example: impetigo (dry, honey colored), weeping eczematous dermatitis, scab following abrasion

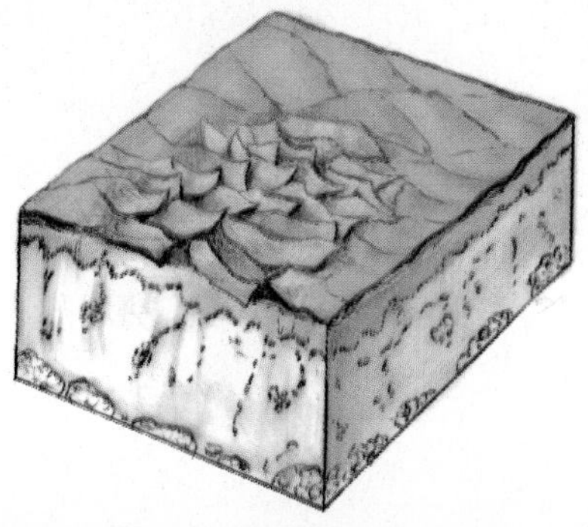

Scale

Compact, desiccated flakes of skin, dry or greasy, silvery or white, from shedding of dead excess keratin cells. Examples: following scarlet fever or drug reaction (laminated sheets), psoriasis (silver, mica-like), seborrheic dermatitis (yellow, greasy), eczema, ichthyosis (large, adherent, laminated), dry skin

BREAK IN CONTINUITY OF SURFACE

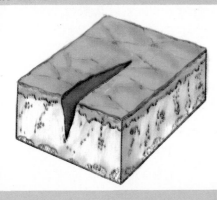

Fissure

Linear crack with abrupt edges, extends into dermis, dry or moist. Examples: Cheilosis—at corners of mouth due to excess moisture; athlete's foot

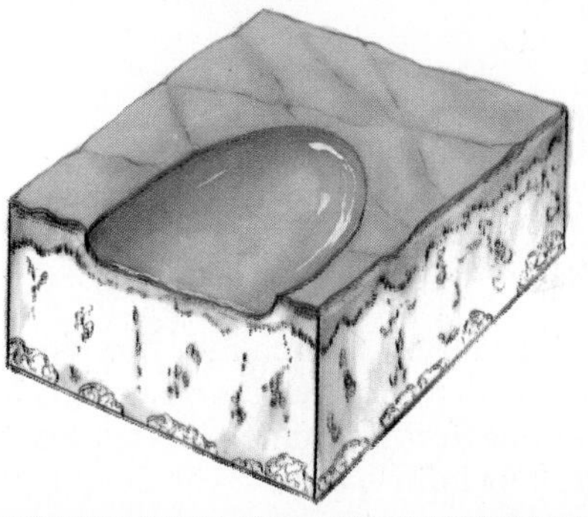

Erosion

Scooped out but shallow depression. Superficial; epidermis lost; moist but no bleeding; heals without scar because erosion does not extend into dermis

Table continued on following page

Table 9–5 ▸ Secondary Skin Lesions* *Continued*

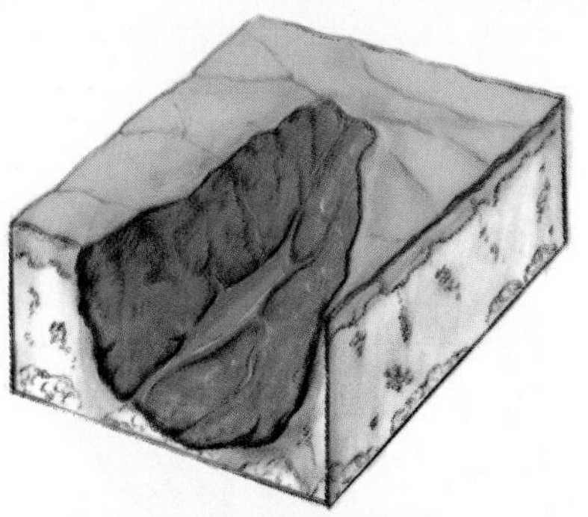

Ulcer

Deeper depression extending into dermis, irregular shape; may bleed; leaves scar when heals. Examples: stasis ulcer, pressure sore, chancre

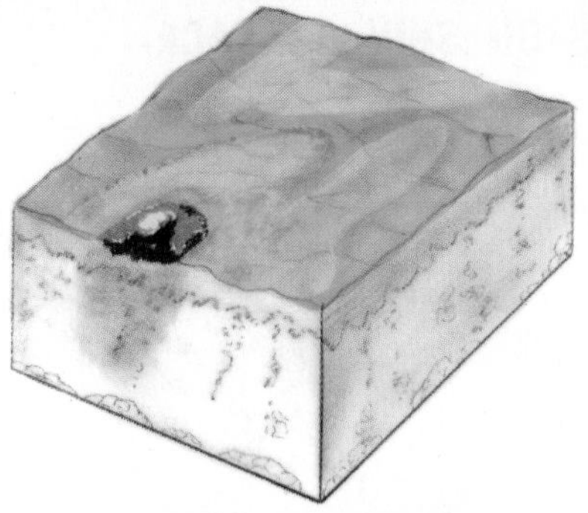

Excoriation

Self-inflicted abrasion; superficial; sometimes crusted; scratches from intense itching. Examples: insect bites, scabies, dermatitis, varicella

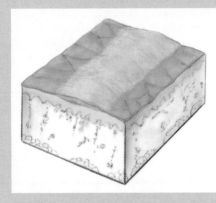

Scar

After a skin lesion is repaired, normal tissue is lost and replaced with connective tissue (collagen). This is a permanent fibrotic change. Examples: healed area of surgery or injury, acne

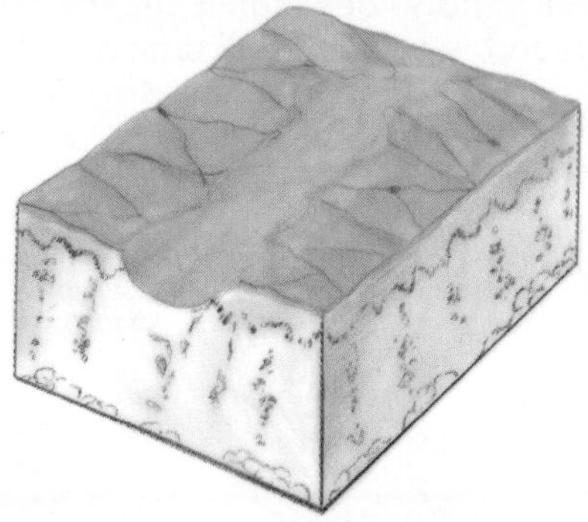

Atrophic Scar

Resulting skin level depressed with loss of tissue; a thinning of the epidermis. Example: striae

Table 9-5 ► Secondary Skin Lesions* *Continued*

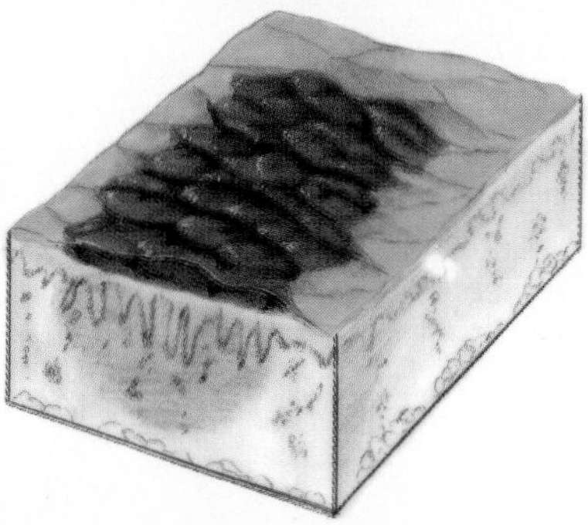

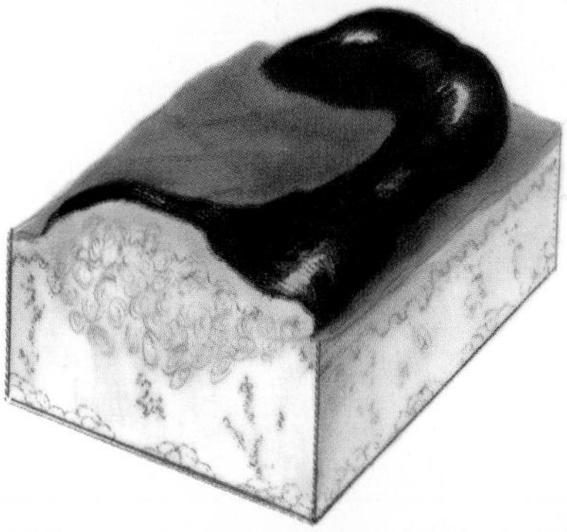

Lichenification

Prolonged intense scratching eventually thickens the skin and produces tightly packed sets of papules; looks like surface of moss (or lichen).

Keloid

A hypertrophic scar. The resulting skin level is elevated by excess scar tissue, which is invasive beyond the site of original injury. May increase long after healing occurs. Looks smooth, rubbery, "clawlike," and has a higher incidence among blacks.

---

* Resulting from a change in a primary lesion due to the passage of time; an evolutionary change.
Note: Combinations of primary and secondary lesions may coexist in the same person. Such combined designations may be termed papulosquamous, maculopapular, vesiculopustular, or papulovesicular.

Table 9-6 ► Vascular Nevi—Hemangiomas

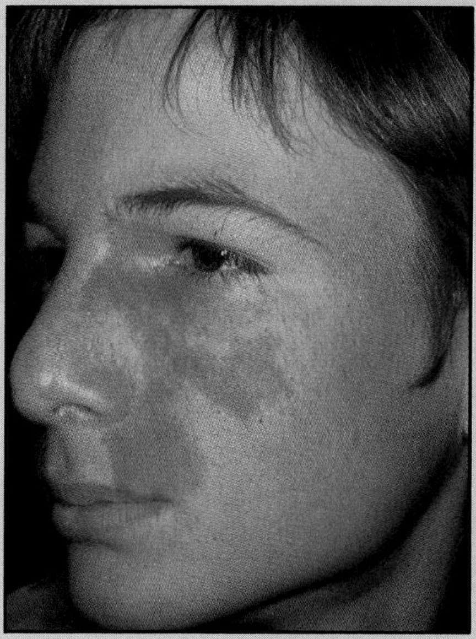

Port-Wine Stain (Nevus Flammeus)

A large, flat macular patch covering the scalp or face, frequently along the distribution of cranial nerve V. The color is dark red, bluish, or purplish and intensifies with crying, exertion, or exposure to heat or cold. The marking consists of mature capillaries. It is present at birth and usually does not fade. It may be associated with neurologic disease.

Table continued on following page

Table 9-6 ► Vascular Nevi—Hemangiomas *Continued*

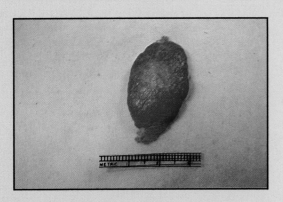

Strawberry Mark (Immature Hemangioma)

A raised bright red area with well-defined borders about 2 to 3 cm in diameter. It does not blanch with pressure. It consists of immature capillaries, is present at birth or develops in the first few months, and usually disappears by age 5 to 7. Requires no treatment, although it may be of concern to parents.

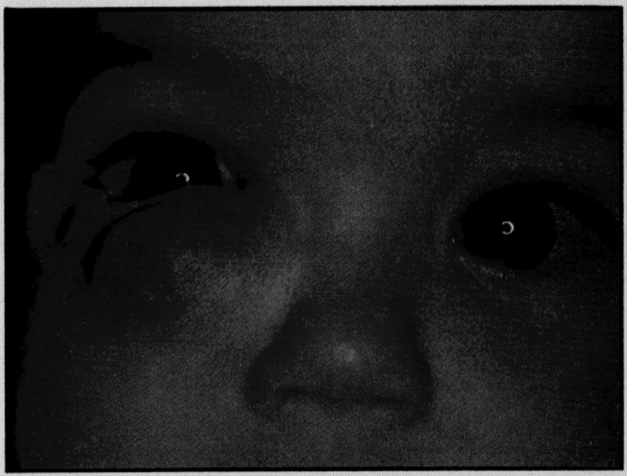

Cavernous Hemangioma (Mature)

A reddish-blue, irregularly shaped, solid and spongy mass of blood vessels. It may be present at birth, may enlarge during the first 10 to 15 months, and will not involute spontaneously.

Table 9-7 ► Vascular Lesions

TELANGIECTASES

Due to vascular dilatation; permanently enlarged and dilated blood vessels that are visible on the skin surface. Examples are

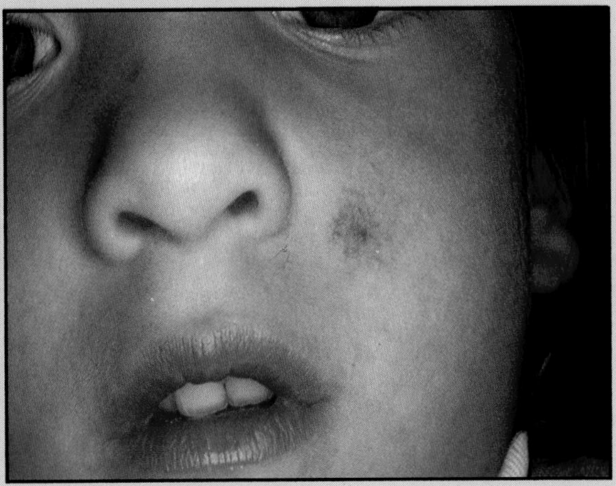

Spider Angioma

A fiery red, star-shaped marking with a solid circular center. Capillary radiations extend from the central arterial body. With pressure, note a central pulsating body and blanching of extending legs. Develops on face, neck, or chest; may be associated with pregnancy, liver disease, or estrogen therapy, or may be normal.

Venous Star (not illustrated)

A blue dilatation of blood vessels in a star-shaped, linear, or flaring pattern. Does not blanch. Suggests an increased pressure in superficial veins. Located on the legs near varicose veins and also on the chest.

Table 9-7 ▸ Vascular Lesions *Continued*

PURPURIC LESIONS

Due to blood flowing out of breaks in the vessels. Red blood cells and blood pigments are deposited in the tissues (extravascular). Difficult to see in dark-skinned people.

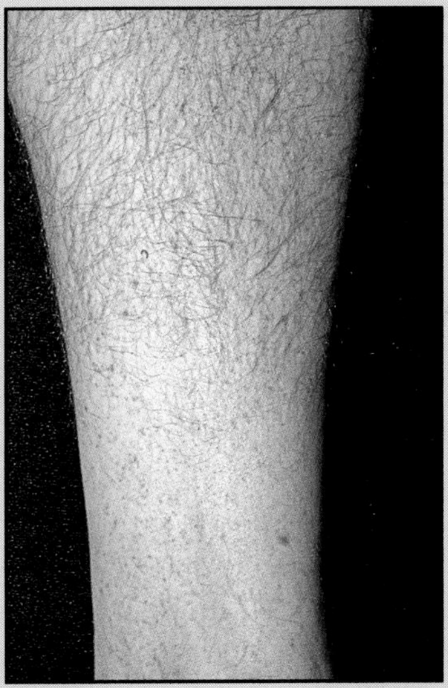

Petechiae

Tiny punctate hemorrhages, <2 mm, round and discrete, dark red, purple, or brown in color. Due to bleeding from superficial capillaries; will not blanch. May indicate abnormal clotting factors. In dark-skinned people petechiae are best visualized in the areas of lighter melanization, such as the abdomen, buttocks, and volar surface of the forearm. When the skin is black or very dark brown, petechiae cannot be seen in the skin. Most of the diseases that cause bleeding and microembolism formation, such as thrombocytopenia, subacute bacterial endocarditis, and other septicemias, are characterized by the presence of petechiae in the mucous membranes as well as on the skin. Thus, you should inspect for petechiae in the mouth, particularly the buccal mucosa, and in the conjunctiva.

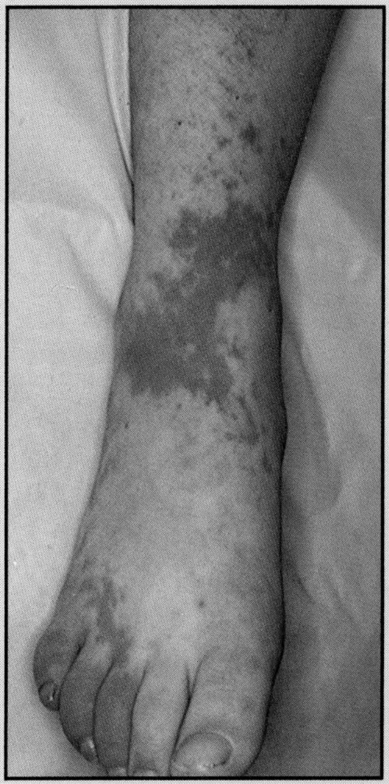

Purpura

Confluent and extensive patch of petechiae and ecchymoses, flat macular hemorrhage. Seen in generalized disorders such as thrombocytopenia and scurvy.

Table continued on following page

Table 9-7 ► Vascular Lesions *Continued*

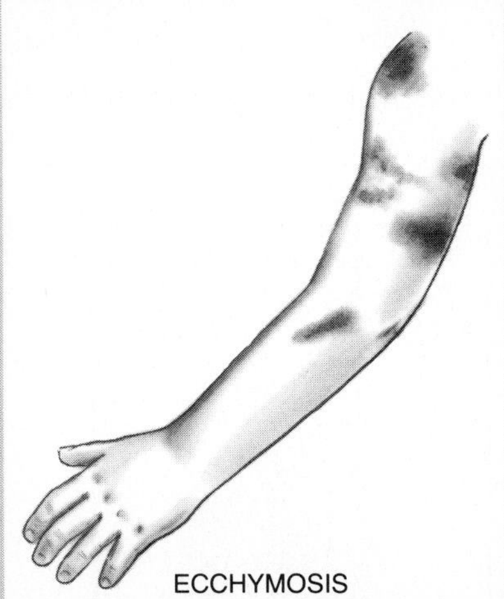

ECCHYMOSIS

Ecchymosis (Bruise)

A larger patch of capillary bleeding into tissues. Color in light-skinned person is first blue-purple, then green-brown, then yellow. Bruise in dark-skinned person is deep dark purple. Pressure on a bruise will *not* cause it to blanch. A bruise usually occurs from trauma; also from bleeding disorders and liver dysfunction.

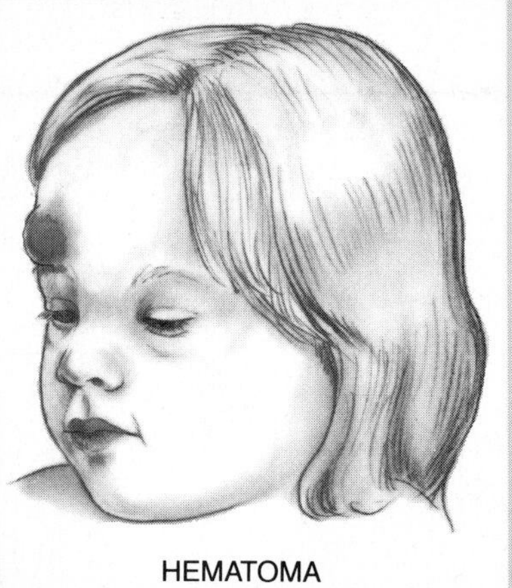

HEMATOMA

Hematoma

A bruise you can feel, elevates the skin and is seen as swelling.

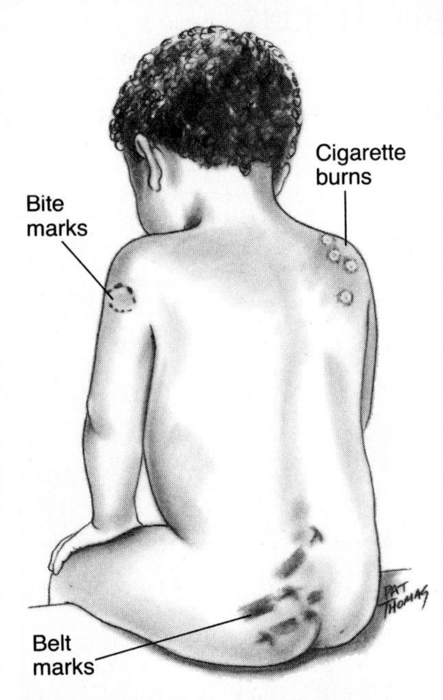

PATTERN INJURIES

Pattern Injury

Pattern injury is a bruise or wound whose shape suggests the instrument or weapon that caused it, e.g., belt buckle, broomstick, burning cigarette, pinch marks, bite marks, or scalding hot liquid. These physical signs suggest child abuse, together with a history that does not match the severity or type of injury, and indicates impaired or dysfunctional parent/child relationship.

Table 9-8 ▸ Common Skin Lesions in Children

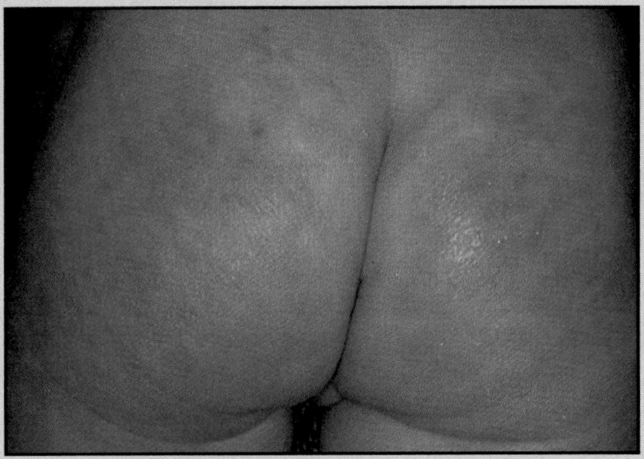

DIAPER DERMATITIS

Red moist maculopapular patch with poorly defined borders in diaper area, extending along inguinal and gluteal folds. History of infrequent diaper changes or occlusive coverings. Inflammatory disease due to skin irritation from ammonia, heat, moisture, occlusive diapers.

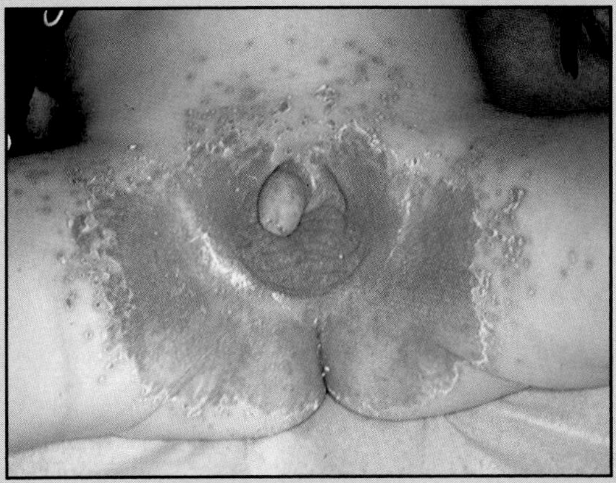

INTERTRIGO (CANDIDIASIS)

Scalding red, moist patches with sharply demarcated borders, some loose scales. Usually in genital area extending along inguinal and gluteal folds. Infectious disease aggravated by urine, feces, heat, moisture.

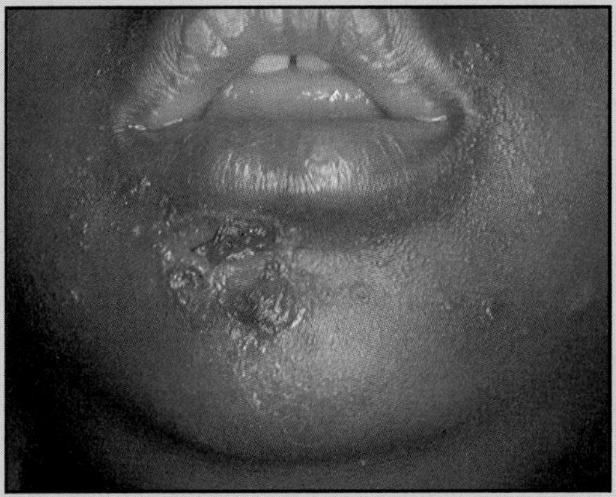

IMPETIGO

Moist, thin-roofed vesicles with thin erythematous base. Rupture to form thick honey-colored crusts. Contagious bacterial infection of skin; most common in infants and children.

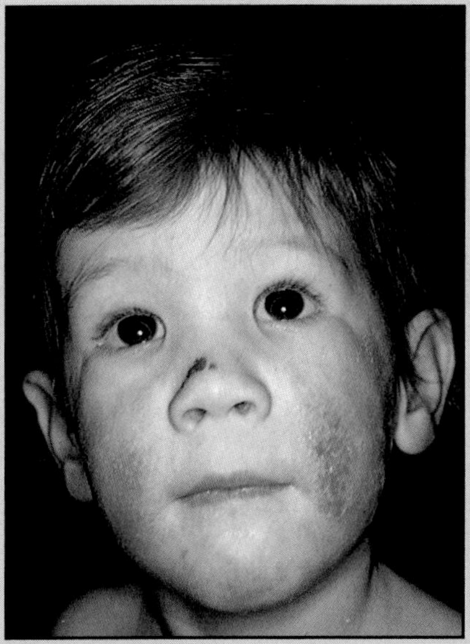

ATOPIC DERMATITIS (ECZEMA)

Erythematous papules and vesicles, with weeping, oozing, and crusts. Lesions usually on scalp, forehead, cheeks, forearms and wrists, elbows, backs of knees. Paroxysmal and severe pruritus. Family history of allergies.

Table continued on following page

Table 9-8 ▶ Common Skin Lesions in Children *Continued*

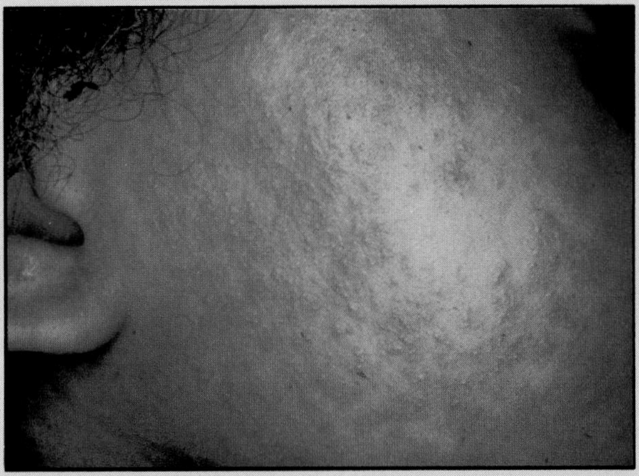

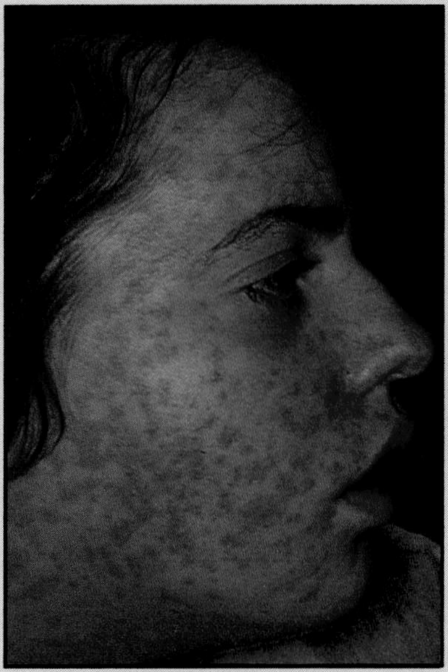

MEASLES (RUBEOLA)

Red-purple maculopapular blotchy rash in dark skin (on left) and in light skin (on right), appears on third or fourth day of illness. Rash appears first behind ears and spreads over face, then over neck, trunk, arms and legs; looks "coppery" and does not blanch. Also characterized by Koplik's spots in mouth—bluish white, red-based elevations of 1 to 3 mm.

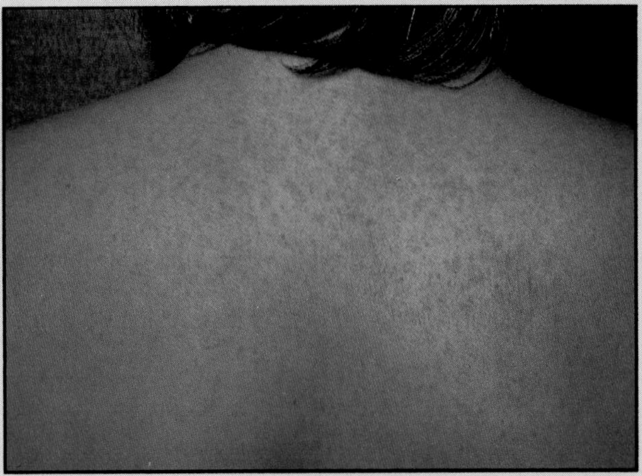

GERMAN MEASLES (RUBELLA)

Pink papular rash (similar to measles but paler) first appears on face, then spreads. Distinguished from measles by presence of neck lymphadenopathy and absence of Koplik's spots.

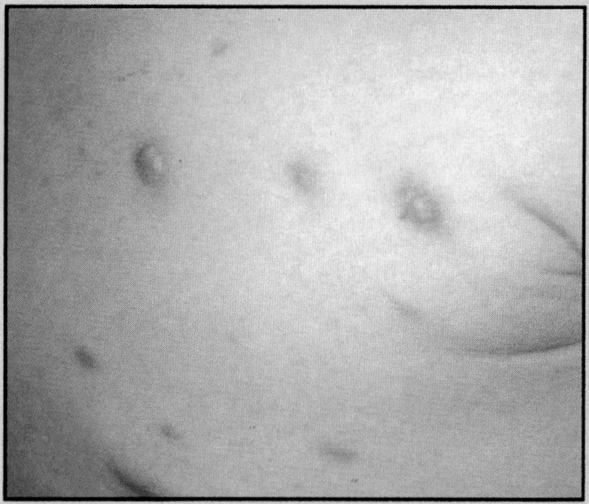

CHICKEN POX (VARICELLA)

Small tight vesicles first appear on trunk, then spread to face, arms and legs (not palms or soles). Vesicles erupt in succeeding crops over several days, then become pustules, and then crusts. Intensely pruritic.

Table 9-9 ▶ Common Skin Lesions

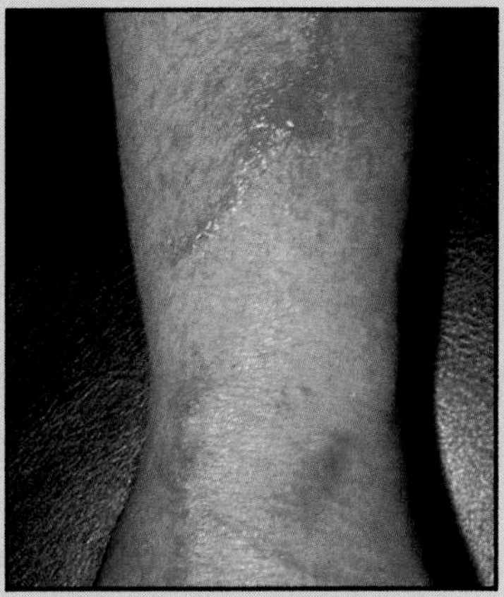

PRIMARY CONTACT DERMATITIS

Local inflammatory reaction to an irritant in the environment or an allergy. Characteristic location of lesions often give clue. Often erythema shows first, followed by swelling, wheals, or urticaria, or maculopapular vesicles, scales. Often accompanied by intense pruritus. Example here: poison ivy

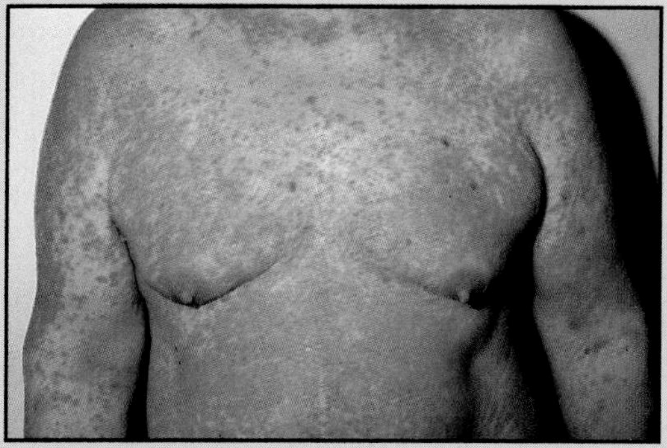

ALLERGIC DRUG REACTION

Erythematous and symmetric rash, usually generalized. Some drugs produce urticarial rash, or vesicles and bullae. History of drug ingestion.

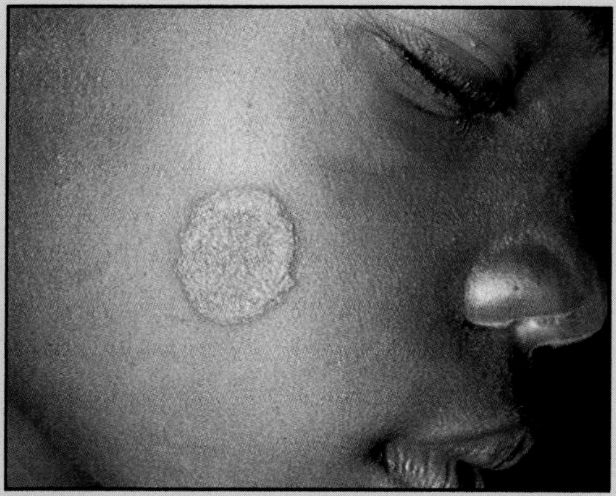

TINEA CORPORIS (RINGWORM OF THE BODY)

Scales—hyperpigmented in whites, depigmented in dark-skinned persons—on chest, abdomen, back of arms, forming multiple circular lesions with clear centers.

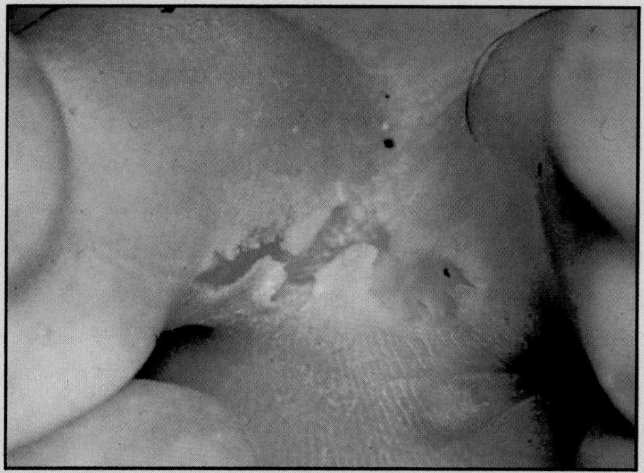

TINEA PEDIS (RINGWORM OF THE FOOT)

"Athlete's foot," a fungal infection, first appears as small vesicles between toes, sides of feet, soles. Then grows scaly and hard. Found in chronically warm moist feet: children after gymnasium activities, athletes, aging adults who cannot dry their feet well.

Table continued on following page

Table 9-9 ► Common Skin Lesions *Continued*

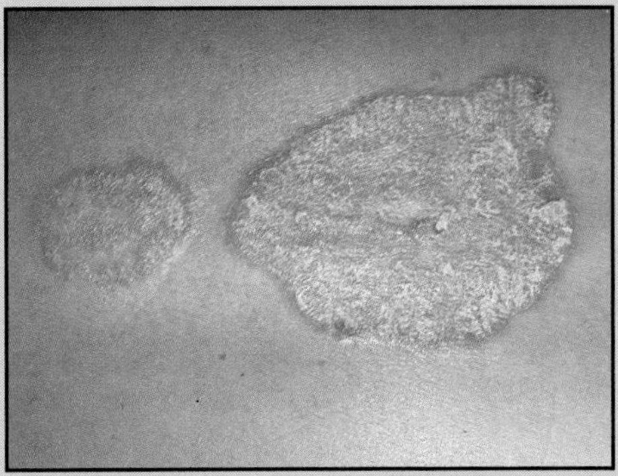

PSORIASIS

Scaly erythematous patch, with silvery scales on top. Usually on scalp, outside of elbows and knees, low back, and anogenital area.

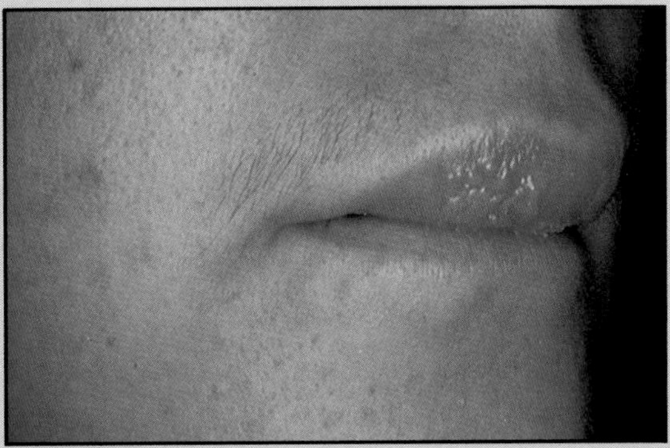

HERPES SIMPLEX (COLD SORES)

Prodrome of skin tingling and sensitivity. Then erupts with tight vesicles, then pustules, then crust. Common location is upper lip, also in genitalia.

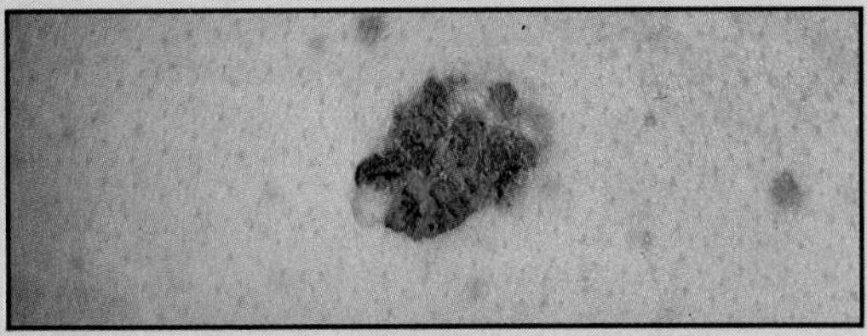

MALIGNANT MELANOMA

Half of these lesions arise from pre-existing nevi. Usually brown, can be tan, black, pink-red, purple, or mixed pigmentation. Often irregular or notched borders. May have scaling, flaking, oozing texture.

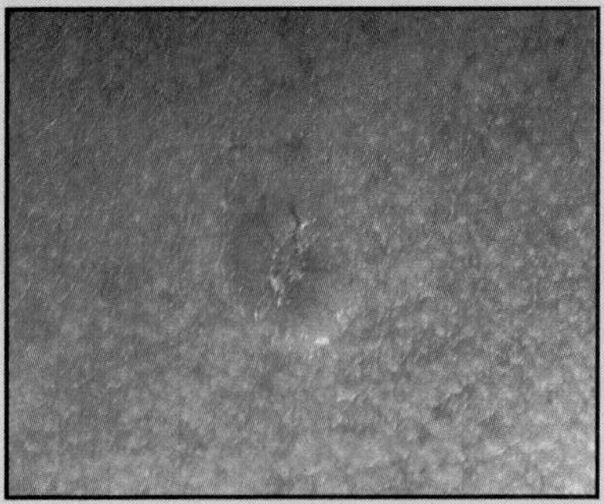

BASAL CELL CARCINOMA

Usually starts as a skin-colored papule (may be deeply pigmented) with a translucent top and overlying telangiectasia. Then develops rounded pearly borders with central red ulcer, or looks like large open pore with central yellowing. Most common form of skin cancer; slow but inexorable growth.

SQUAMOUS CELL CARCINOMA
(not illustrated)

Erythematous scaly patch with sharp margins, 1 cm or more. Develops central ulcer and surrounding erythema. Usually on hands or head, areas exposed to solar radiation. Less common than basal cell carcinoma but grows rapidly.

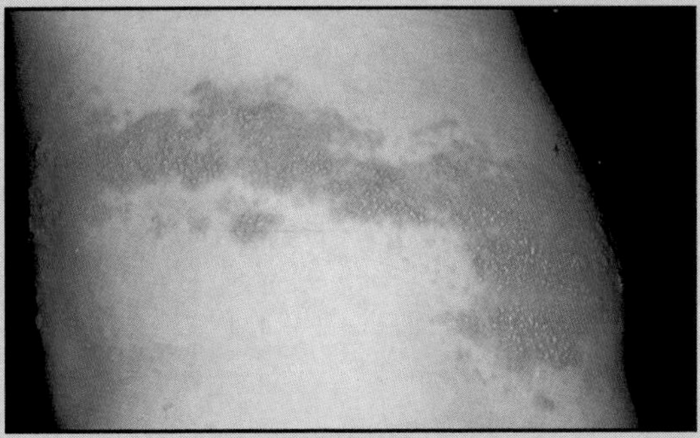

HERPES ZOSTER (SHINGLES)

Small grouped vesicles along route of cutaneous sensory nerve, then pustules, then crusts. Virus of chicken pox is dormant, then erupts. Acute appearance, practically always unilateral. Commonly on trunk, can be anywhere. If on ophthalmic branch of cranial nerve V, it poses risk to eye. Pain is often severe in aging adults.

Table 9–10 ▸ Abnormal Conditions of Hair

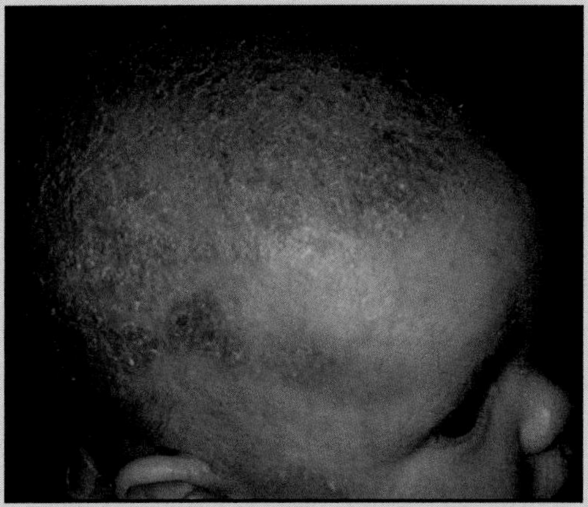

SEBORRHEIC DERMATITIS (CRADLE CAP)

Thick, yellow, greasy, adherent scales on scalp and forehead; very common in early infancy. Resembles eczema lesions except cradle cap is distinguished by absence of pruritus, "greasy" yellow-pink lesions, and negative family history of allergy.

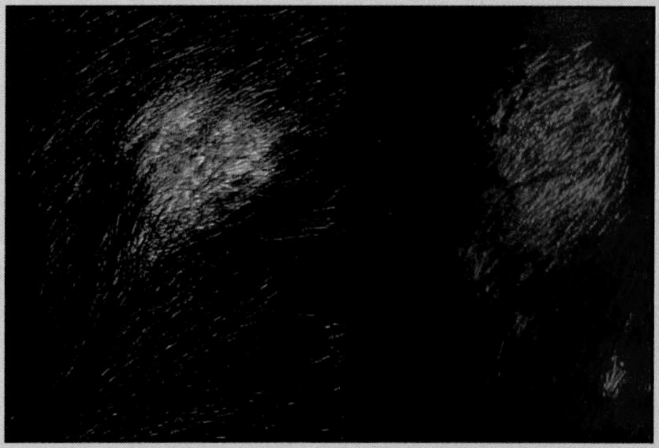

TINEA CAPITIS (SCALP RINGWORM)

Rounded patchy hair loss on scalp, leaving broken off hairs, pustules, and scales on skin. Due to fungal infection; lesions fluoresce under Wood's light. Usually seen in children and farmers; highly contagious.

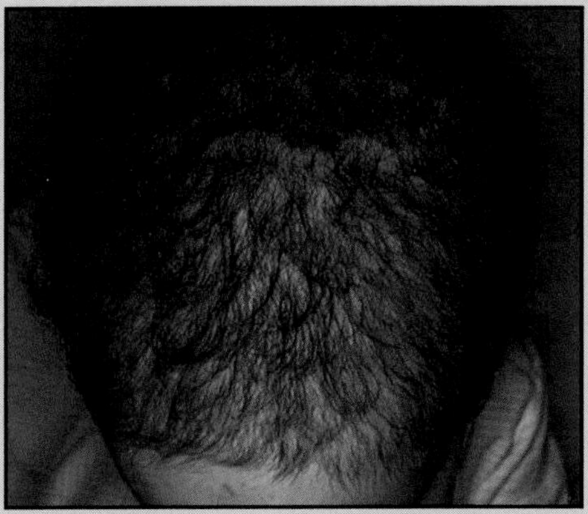

TOXIC ALOPECIA

Patchy, asymmetric balding that accompanies severe illness or use of chemotherapy where growing hairs are lost and resting hairs are spared. Regrowth occurs after illness or discontinuation of toxin.

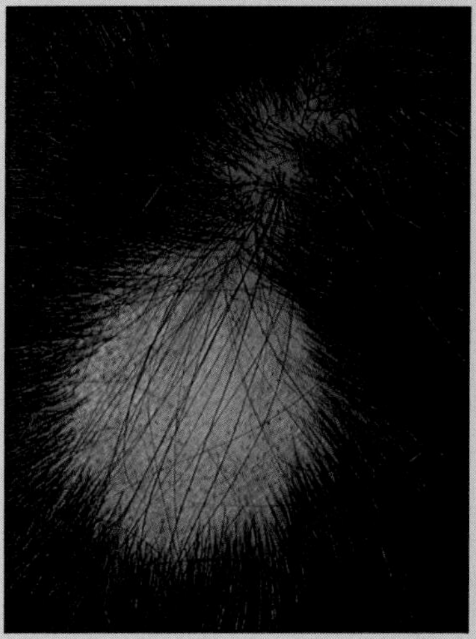

ALOPECIA AREATA

Sudden appearance of a sharply circumscribed, round or oval balding patch, usually with smooth, soft, hairless skin underneath. Unknown cause; when limited to a few patches, person usually has complete regrowth.

Table continued on following page

Table 9-10 ► Abnormal Conditions of Hair *Continued*

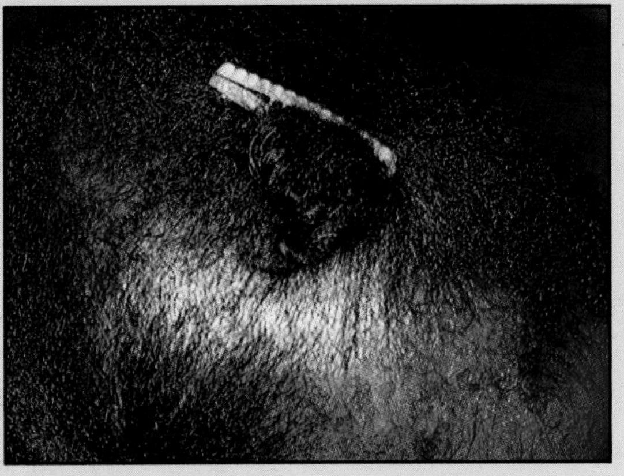

TRAUMATIC ALOPECIA: TRACTION ALOPECIA

Linear or oval patch of hair loss along hair line, a part, or scattered distribution; due to trauma from hair rollers, tight braiding, tight pony tail, barrettes.

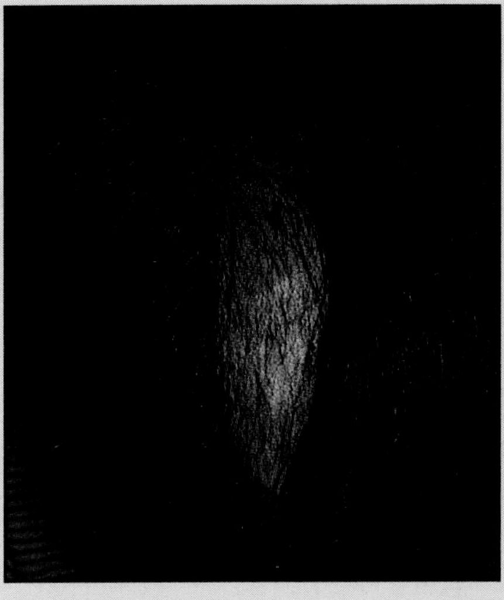

TRICHOTILLOMANIA

Self-induced hair loss usually due to habit. Forms irregularly shaped patch, with broken off, stublike hairs of varying lengths; person is never completely bald. Occurs as child rubs or twirls area absently while falling asleep, reading, or watching television.

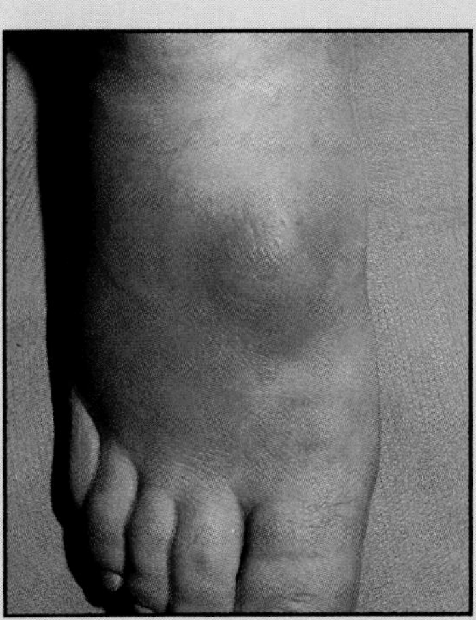

FURUNCLE AND ABSCESS

Red, swollen, hard, tender, pus-filled lesion due to acute localized bacterial (usually staphylococcal) infection; usually on back of neck, buttocks, occasionally on wrists or ankles. Furuncles are due to infected hair follicles, whereas abscesses are due to traumatic introduction of bacteria into the skin. Abscesses are usually larger and deeper than furuncles.

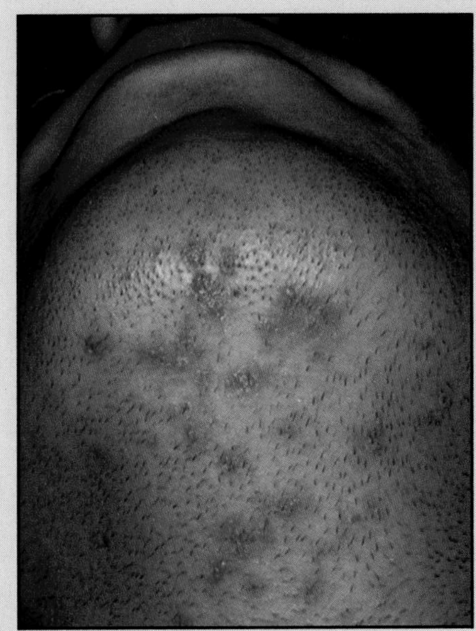

FOLLICULITIS

Superficial infection of hair follicles. Multiple pustules, "whiteheads," with hair visible at center and erythematous base. Usually on arms, legs, face, and buttocks.

Table 9-10 ► Abnormal Conditions of Hair *Continued*

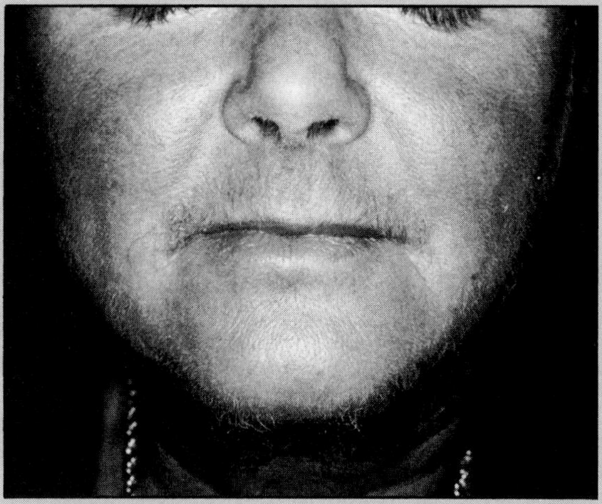

HIRSUTISM

Excess body hair in females forming a male sexual pattern (upper lip, face, chest, abdomen, arms, legs), due to endocrine or metabolic dysfunction, or occasionally idiopathic.

Table 9-11 ► Abnormal Conditions of the Nails

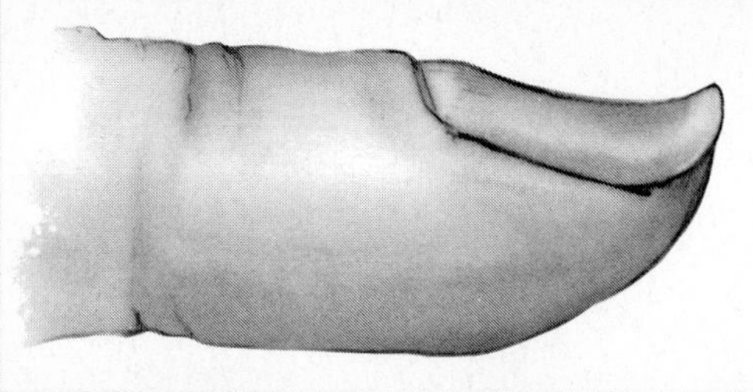

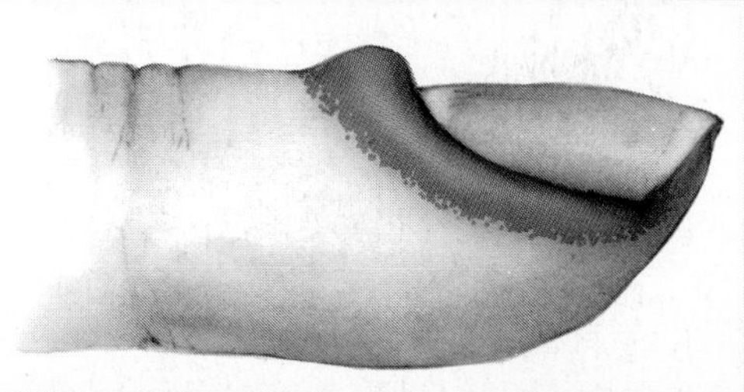

KOILONYCHIA (SPOON NAILS)

Thin depressed nails with lateral edges tilted up, forming a concave profile. May be congenital or a hereditary trait, occasionally due to hypochromic anemia.

PARONYCHIA

Red, swollen, tender inflammation of the nail folds.

Table continued on following page

Table 9-11 ▶ Abnormal Conditions of the Nails *Continued*

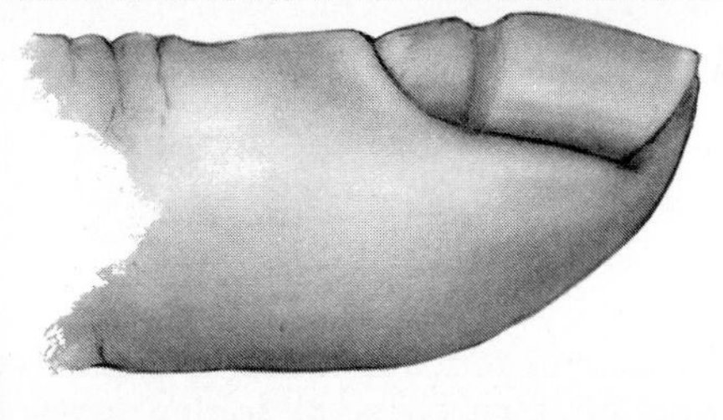

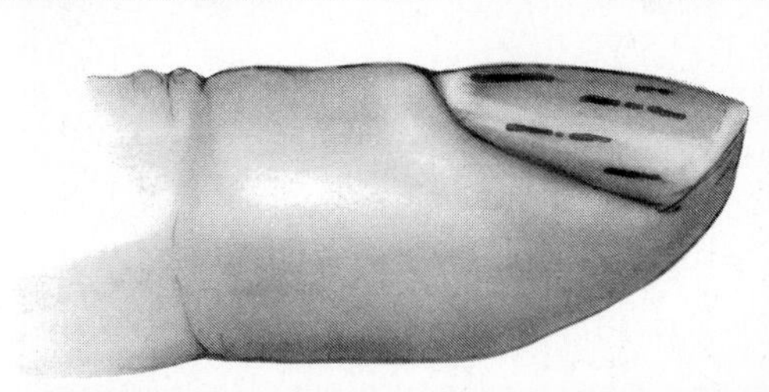

BEAU'S LINE

Transverse furrow or groove. A depression across the nail that extends down to the nail bed. Occurs with any trauma that temporarily impairs nail formation, such as acute illness, toxic reaction, or local trauma. Dent appears first at the cuticle and moves forward as nail grows.

SPLINTER HEMORRHAGES

Red-brown streaks, embolic lesions, occur with subacute bacterial endocarditis; also may be a nonspecific sign.

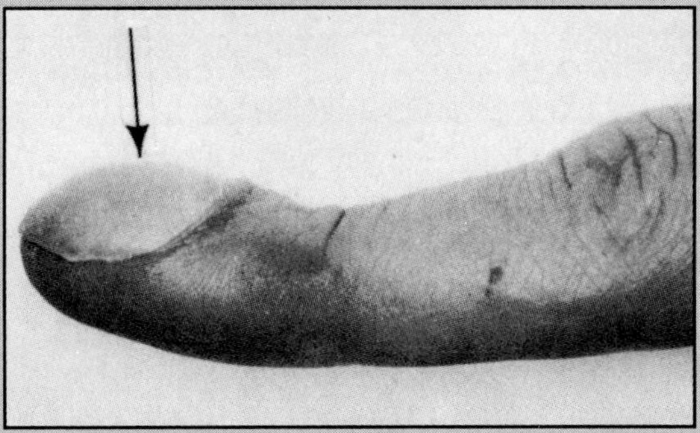

LATE CLUBBING

Proximal edge of nail elevates, angle is greater than 180 degrees. Distal phalanx looks rounder and wider. Seen with chronic obstructive pulmonary disease and congenital heart disease with cyanosis. Occurs first in thumb and index finger.

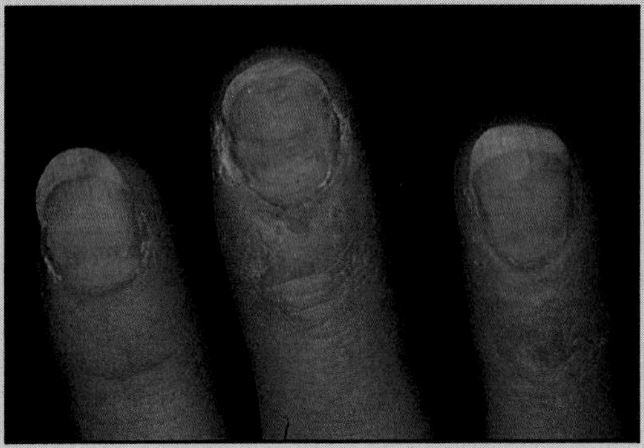

HABIT—TIC DYSTROPHY

Depression down middle of nail or multiple horizontal ridges, due to continuous picking of cuticle by another finger of same hand, which causes injury to nail base and nail matrix.

Table 9-11 ▶ Abnormal Conditions of the Nails *Continued*

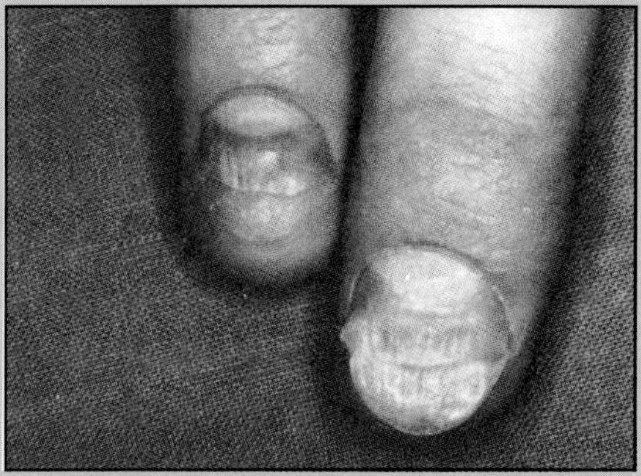

ONYCHOLYSIS

Loosening of the nail plate, usually beginning at the distal edge and progressing proximally.

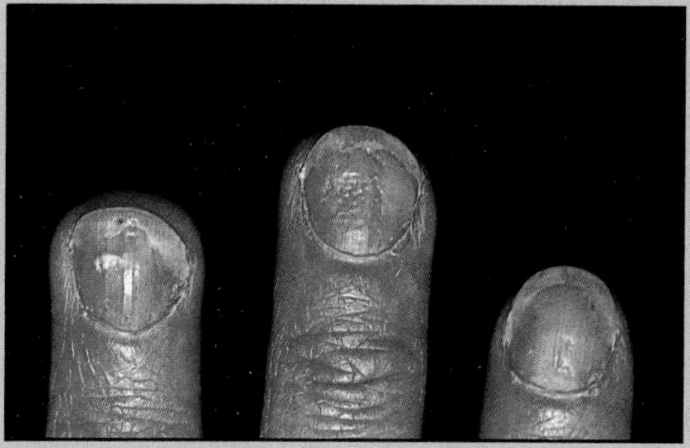

PITTING

Pitting, crumbling of the nails with distal detachment often occurs with psoriasis.

Bibliography

Berliner H: Aging skin: Part I. Am J Nurs 86:1138–1141, 1986.

Berliner H: Aging skin: Part II. Am J Nurs 86:1259–1261, 1986.

Boodley CA, Jaquis JL: Measles, mumps, rubella and chicken pox in the adult population. Nurse Pract 14:12–22, 1989.

Cohen S: Skin rashes in infants and children. Am J Nurs 78:1041–1072, 1978.

DeNicola P, Morsiani M: Nail Diseases in Internal Medicine. Springfield, IL, Charles C Thomas, 1974.

De Villez RL: Externally and internally caused skin problems of aging. Geriatrics 38:71–73, 77–78, 1983.

Domonkos AN, Arnold HL, Odom RB: Andrews' Diseases of the Skin. 7th ed. Philadelphia, WB Saunders, 1982.

Fenske N, et al: Common problems of aging skin. Patient care. 23(7):225–228, 1989.

Fleming J: Common dermatologic conditions in children. MCN 6:346–354, 1981.

Fraser MC, McGuire DB: Skin cancer's early warning signs. Am J Nurs 84:1232–1236, 1984.

Habif TP: Clinical Dermatology. St. Louis, CV Mosby, 1985.

Hurwitz S: Clinical Pediatric Dermatology. Philadelphia, WB Saunders, 1981.

Levin S: Effect of age, ethnic background and disease on sweat chloride. Isr J Med Sci 2(3):333–337, 1966.

Lookingbill DP: Yield from a complete skin examination — findings in 1157 new dermatology patients. J Am Acad Dermatol 18(1):31–37, 1988.

Lookingbill DP, Marks JG: Principles of Dermatology. Philadelphia, WB Saunders, 1986.

McKenna DF: Lyme disease: A review for primary health care providers. Nurse Pract 14:18–29, 1989.

Mittleman RE, Mittleman HS, Wetli CV: What child abuse really looks like. Am J Nurs 87:1185–1188, 1987.

Neilley LK, Ellis RA: Nailing down a diagnosis. Nurse Pract 9:26–34, 1984.

Pillsbury D, Heaton C: A Manual of Dermatology. Philadelphia, WB Saunders, 1980.

Polednak A: Connective tissue responses in negroes in relation to disease. Am J Physical Anthropol 41:49–55, 1974.

Roach L: Dark skins: Recognizing and interpreting color changes. Crit Care Update 5–15, 1977.

Robinson JK: Skin problems of aging. Geriatrics 38:57, 1983.

Rosen T, Martin S: Atlas of Black Dermatology. Boston, Little, Brown & Co, 1981.

Sauer GC: Manual of Skin Diseases. 5th ed. Philadelphia, JB Lippincott, 1985.

Schaefer O: Regional sweating in Eskimos compared with Caucasians. Can J Physiol Pharmacol 52(5):960–965, 1974.

Shelley WB, Shelley ED: The ten major problems of aging skin. Geriatrics 37:107, 1982.

Solomon L. Adolescent Dermatology. Philadelphia, WB Saunders, 1978.

CHAPTER

10 Assessing the Head and Neck, Including Regional Lymphatics

STRUCTURE AND FUNCTION

THE HEAD

The skull is a rigid bony box that protects the brain and special sense organs, and it includes the bones of the cranium and the face (Fig. 10–1). Note the location of these cranial bones: frontal, parietal, occipital, and temporal. Use these names to describe any of your findings in the corresponding areas.

The seven cranial bones unite at immovable joints called the *sutures.* The bones are not firmly joined at birth; the sutures gradually ossify during early childhood. The coronal suture crowns the head from ear to ear at the union of the frontal and parietal bones. The sagittal suture separates the head lengthwise between the two parietal bones. The lambdoid suture separates the parietal bones crosswise from the occipital bone.

The 14 facial bones also articulate at sutures (note the nasal bone, zygomatic bone, and maxilla), except for the mandible (the lower jaw). It moves up, down, and sideways from the temporomandibular joint, which is anterior to each ear.

The cranium is supported by the cervical vertebrae: C1, the "atlas"; C2, the "axis"; and down to C7. The C7 vertebra has a long spinous process that is palpable when the head is flexed. Feel this useful landmark, the *vertebra prominens,* on your own neck.

The bones of the fetal skull are separated by sutures and by *fontanels,* the spaces where the sutures intersect (Fig. 10–2). These membrane-covered "soft spots" allow for growth of the brain during the first year. They gradually ossify; the triangular shaped posterior fontanel is closed by 1 to 2 months, and the diamond shaped anterior fontanel closes between 9 months and 2 years.

The human face has myriad appearances and a large array of facial expressions, each reflecting the person's mood. The expressions are formed by the facial muscles, which are mediated by cranial nerve VII, the facial nerve

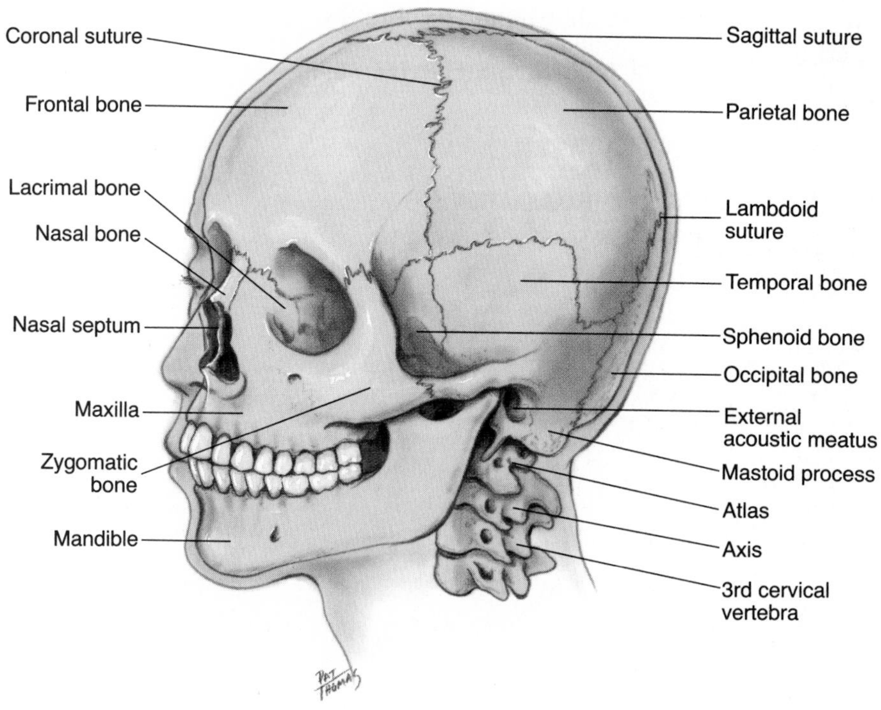

▶ **Figure 10–1**

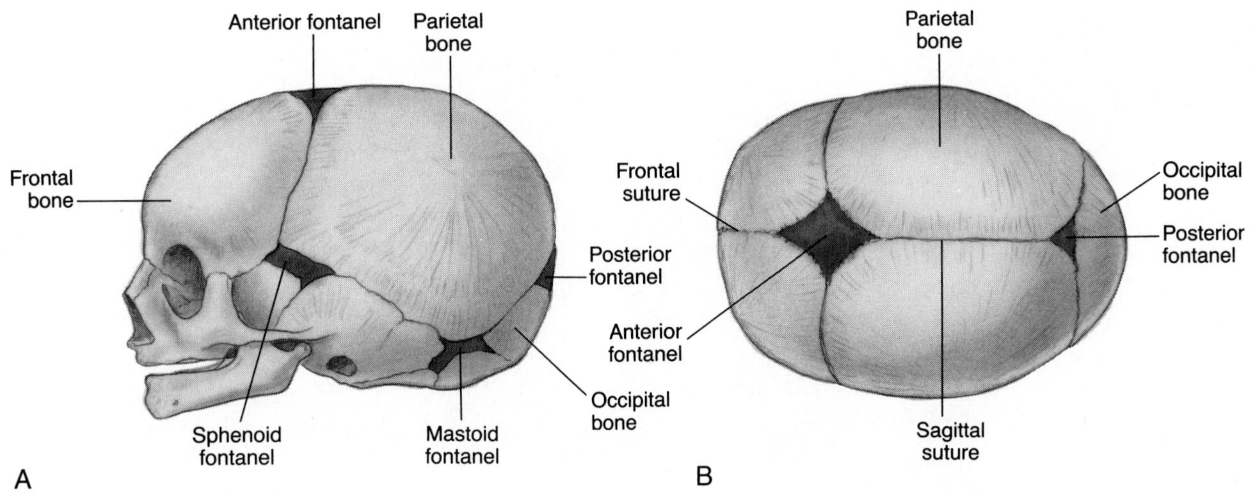

► **Figure 10–2**

(Fig. 10–3). Facial muscle function is symmetric bilaterally, except for an occasional quirk or wry expression.

Facial structures also are symmetric; the eyebrows, eyes, ears, nose and mouth appear about the same on both sides. The palpebral fissures, the openings between the eyelids, are equal bilaterally. Also, the nasolabial folds, the crease extending from the nose to each corner of the mouth, should look symmetric. Facial sensations of pain or touch are mediated by cranial nerve V, the trigeminal nerve. (Testing for sensory function is described in Chapter 20, Assessing the Neurologic System).

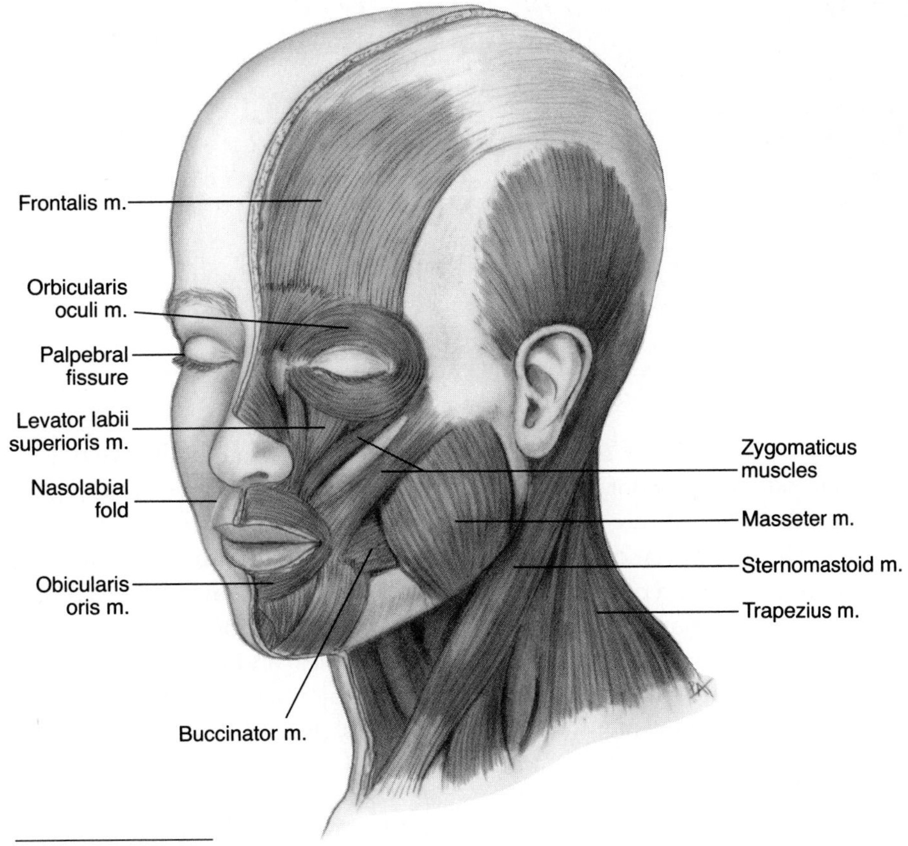

► **Figure 10–3**

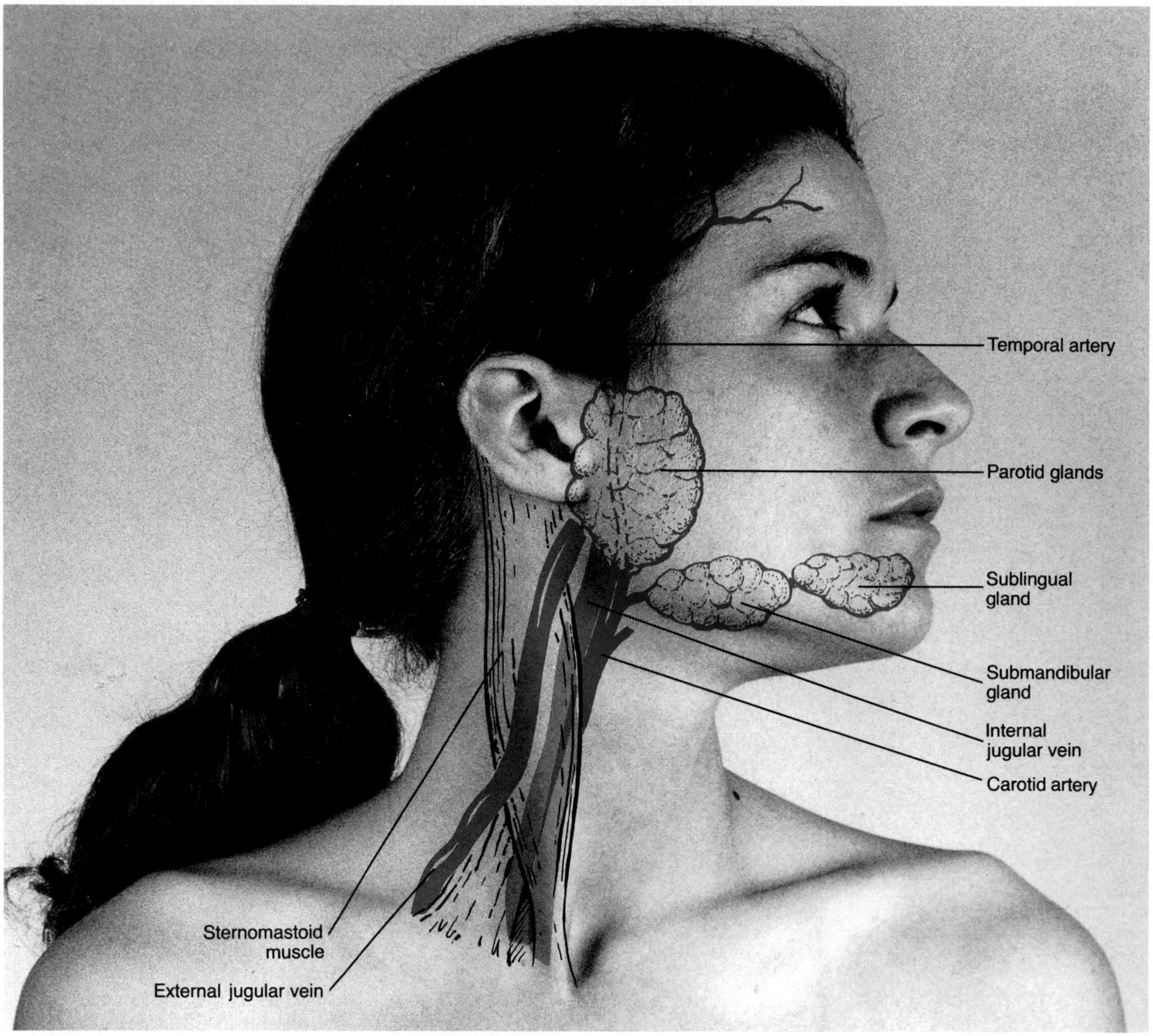

► **Figure 10–4**

The temporal artery lies superior to the temporalis muscle, and its pulsation is palpable anterior to the ear (Fig. 10–4). Two pairs of salivary glands are accessible to examination on the face. The *parotid* glands are in the cheeks over the mandible, anterior to and below the ear. They are the largest of the salivary glands but are not normally palpable. The *submandibular* glands are beneath the mandible at the angle of the jaw. A third pair, the *sublingual* glands, lie in the floor of the mouth. (Salivary gland function follows in Chapter 13.)

THE NECK

The neck contains many structures lying in close proximity. Blood vessels course through the neck. The carotid artery and internal jugular vein lie beneath the sternomastoid muscle. The external jugular vein runs diagonally across the sternomastoid muscle. (Assessment of the neck vessels is discussed in Chapter 16.) The neck also is an area of passage between the head and thorax containing parts of the respiratory and digestive systems, nerves, and lymphatics.

The major neck muscles are the *sternomastoid* and the *trapezius* (Fig. 10–5); they are innervated by cranial nerve XI, the spinal accessory. The sternomastoid muscle arises from the sternum and the medial part of the clavicle and extends diagonally across the neck to the mastoid process behind the ear. It accomplishes head rotation and head flexion. The two trapezius muscles form a trapezoid shape on the upper back. Each arises

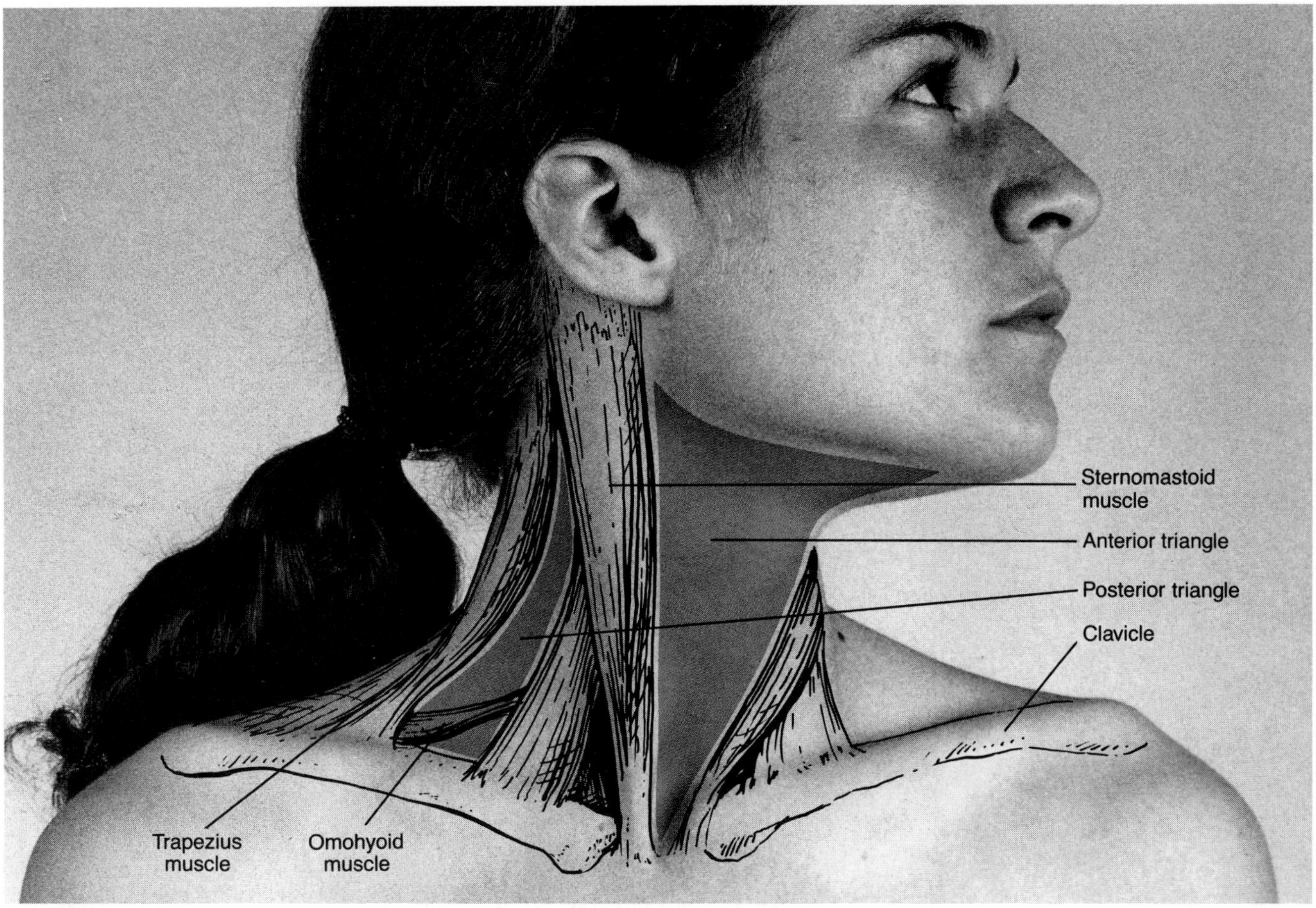

► **Figure 10–5**

from the occipital bone and the vertebrae and extends to the scapula and clavicle. The trapezius muscles move the shoulders and extend and turn the head.

The sternomastoid muscle divides each side of the neck into two triangles. In front of the sternomastoid, the *anterior triangle* extends to the mandible above, and the midline of the body medially. Behind the sternomastoid muscle, the trapezius muscle is to the other side of the *posterior triangle,* and the clavicle is below. These triangles are helpful guidelines when describing findings in the neck.

The *thyroid gland* straddles the trachea in the middle of the neck (Fig. 10–6). This highly vascular endocrine gland secretes thyroxine (T_4) and triiodothyronine (T_3), hormones that stimulate the rate of cellular metabolism. The gland has two lobes, both conical in shape, each curving posteriorly between the trachea and the sternomastoid muscle. The lobes are connected in the middle by a thin isthmus lying over the second and third tracheal rings. (Sometimes there is a third lobe, the pyramidal lobe. It is cone shaped, usually on the left, and extends up toward the hyoid bone from the isthmus or from the neighboring lobe.)

Just above the thyroid isthmus, within about 1 cm, is the cricoid cartilage or upper tracheal ring. The thyroid cartilage is above that, with a small palpable notch in its upper edge. This is the prominent "Adam's apple" in males. And the highest is the hyoid bone, palpated high in the neck at the level of the floor of the mouth.

LYMPHATICS

The head and neck have a rich supply of *lymph nodes* (Fig. 10–7). Although sources differ as to their nomenclature, one commonly used system is given here. Note that their labels correspond to adjacent structures.

Preauricular, in front of the ear.
Posterior auricular (mastoid), superficial to the mastoid process.
Occipital, at the base of the skull.
Submental, midline, behind the tip of the mandible.
Submaxillary (submandibular), half way between the angle and the tip of the mandible.

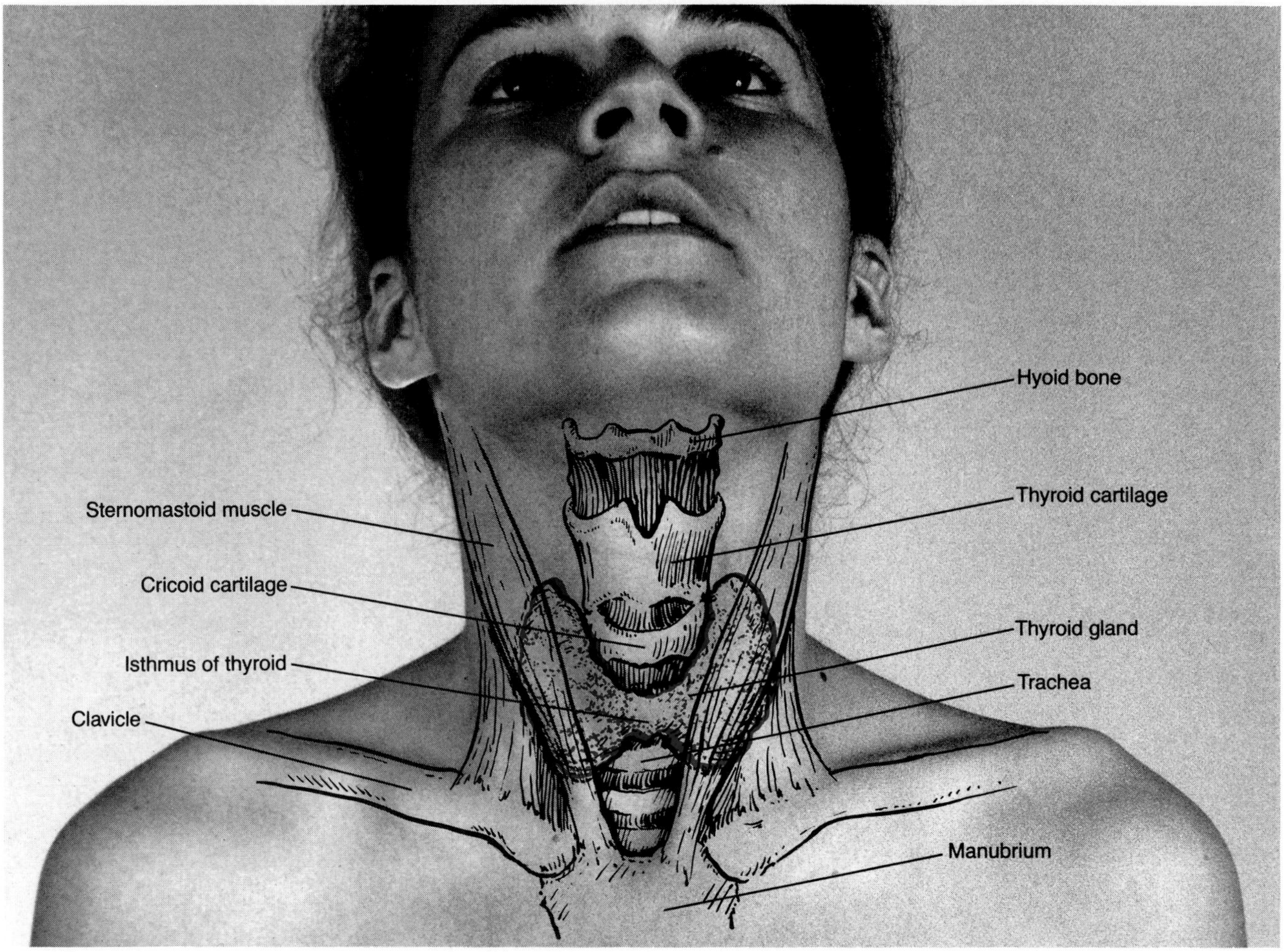

► **Figure 10-6**

Jugulodigastric, under the angle of the mandible.
Superficial cervical, overlying the sternomastoid muscle.
Deep cervical, deep under the sternomastoid muscle.
Posterior cervical, in the posterior triangle along the edge of the trapezius muscle.
Supraclavicular, just above and behind the clavicle, at the sternomastoid muscle.

You also should be familiar with the direction of the drainage patterns of the lymph nodes (Fig. 10-8). When nodes are abnormal, check the area they drain for the source of the problem. Explore the area proximal (upstream) to the location of the abnormal node.

The lymphatic system is an extensive vessel system, which is separate from the cardiovascular system and phylogenetically older. The lymphatics are a major part of the immune system, whose job it is to detect and eliminate foreign substances from the body. The vessels allow the flow of clear, watery fluid (lymph) from the tissue spaces into the circulation. Lymph nodes are set at intervals along the lymph vessels like beads on a string. The nodes are small oval clusters of lymphatic tissue. They filter the lymph and engulf pathogens, preventing potentially harmful substances from entering the circulation. Nodes are located throughout the body, but are accessible to examination only in four areas: head and neck, arms, axillae, and inguinal region. The greatest supply is in the head and neck.

DEVELOPMENTAL CONSIDERATIONS

Note the relative proportions of the head and trunk at different ages (Fig. 10-9). At birth, the head is one-fourth the total length; whereas in the adult, the head is one-eighth of the overall length.

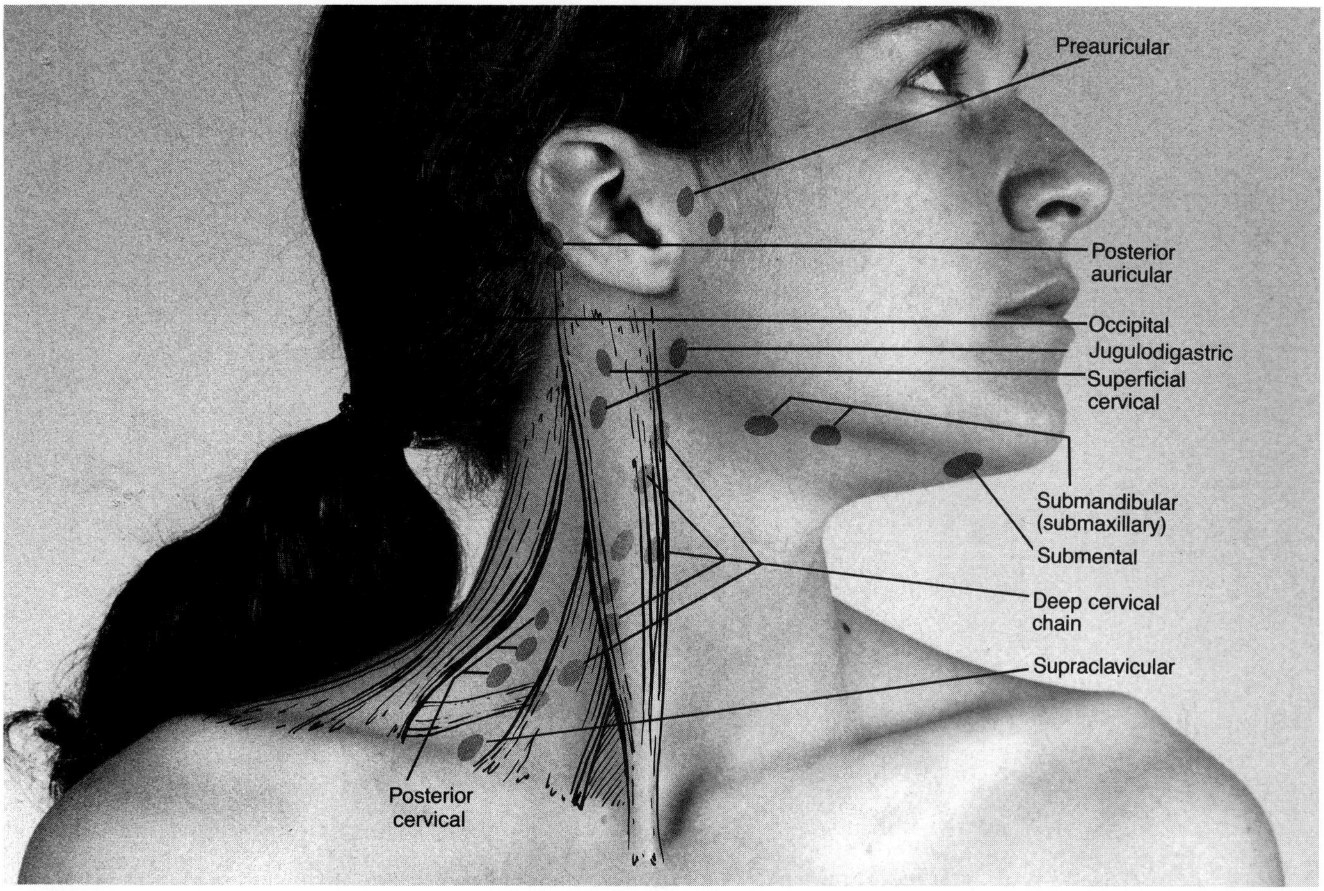

► **Figure 10-7 Lymph nodes of the head and neck**

Infants and Children

During the fetal period, head growth predominates. Head size is greater than chest circumference at birth. The head size grows during childhood, reaching 90 percent its final size when the child is age 6. But during infancy, trunk growth predominates so head size changes in proportion to body height. Facial bones grow at varying rates, especially nasal and jaw bones. In the toddler, the mandible and maxilla are small and the nasal bridge is low, so that the whole face seems small compared with the skull.

Lymphoid tissue is well developed at birth and grows to adult size when the child is age 6. The child's lymphatic tissue continues to grow rapidly until age 10 or 11, actually exceeding its adult size before puberty. Then the lymphatic tissue slowly atrophies.

The appearance of acne in adolescence was discussed in the previous chapter. Facial hair also appears on boys at this time—first on the upper lip, then on cheeks and lower lip, last on the chin. There is a noticeable enlargement of the thyroid cartilage and with it the voice deepens.

The Pregnant Female

The thyroid gland enlarges slightly during pregnancy owing to hyperplasia of the tissue and increased vascularity.

The Aging Adult

The facial bones and orbits appear more prominent, and the facial skin sags owing to decreased elasticity, decreased subcutaneous fat, and decreased moisture in the skin. The lower face may look smaller if teeth have been lost.

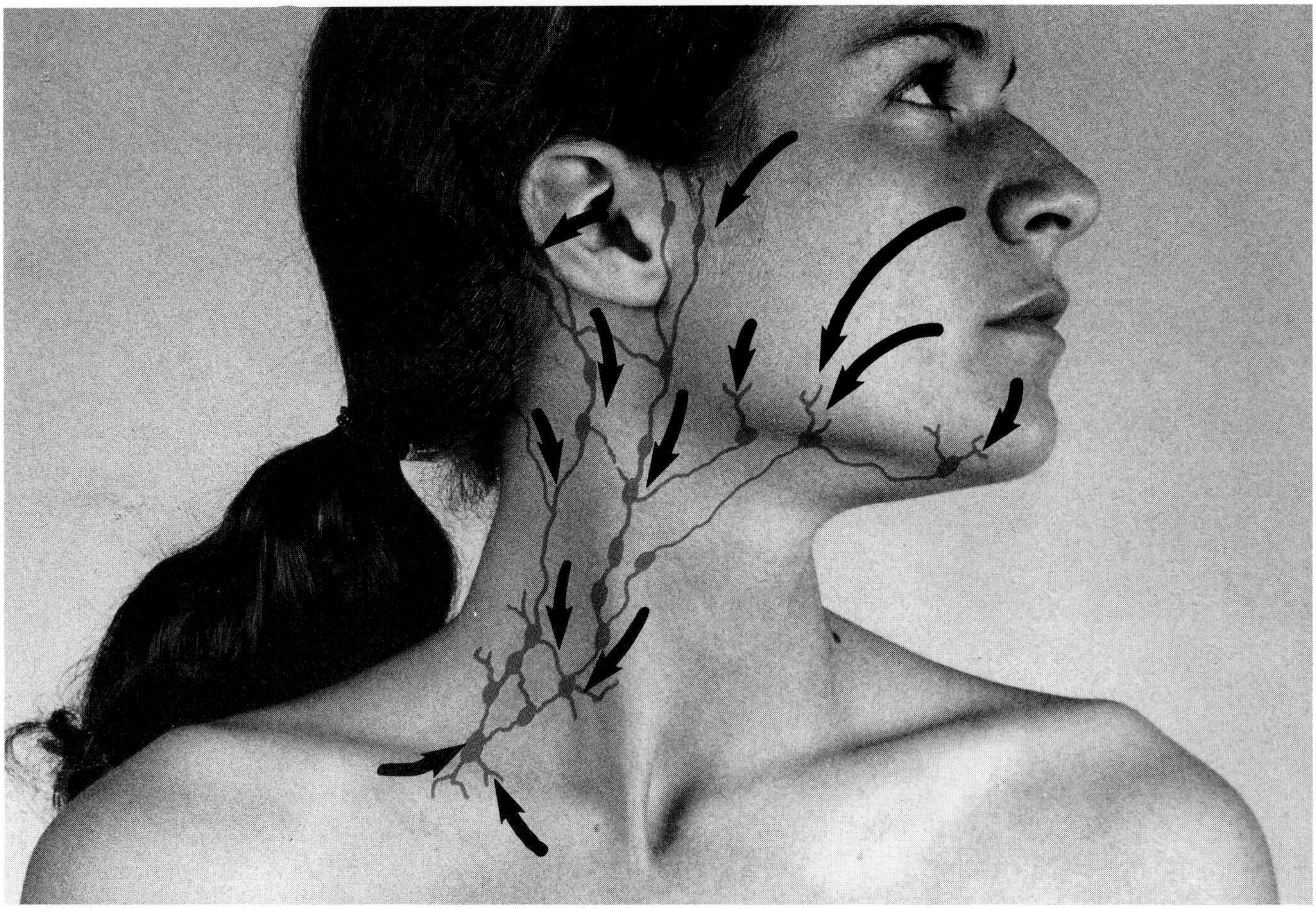

► **Figure 10–8 Lymphatic drainage patterns**

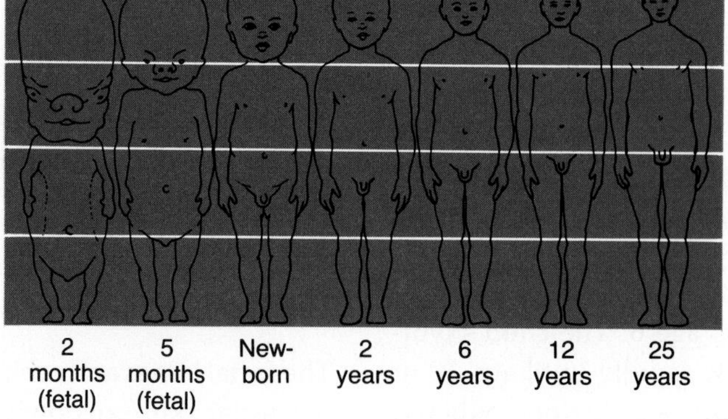

► **Figure 10–9**

SUBJECTIVE DATA

Headache
Head injury
Dizziness
Neck pain
Limitation of motion
Lumps or swelling

EXAMINER ASKS:	RATIONALE:
1. Do you have any *unusually frequent* or *unusually severe* **headaches**? Onset. When did *this kind* of headache start? Was it gradual, over hours, or a day? Or, suddenly, over minutes, or less than 1 hour?	This is a more meaningful question than, "Do you ever have headaches?," because most people have had at least one headache. Since many conditions have a headache as a symptom, a detailed history is important.
Location. Where do you feel it? Is it frontal, temporal, behind your eyes, like a band around the head, in the sinus area, or in the occipital area?	Tension headaches tend to be occipital or frontal or with bandlike tightness; migraines (vascular) tend to be supraorbital, retro-orbital, or frontotemporal; cluster headaches (vascular) produce pain around the eye, temple, forehead, and cheek.
Is pain localized on one side, or all over?	Unilateral or bilateral, e.g., with cluster headaches pain is always unilateral and always on the same side of the head.
Character. What does the headache feel like? Is it throbbing (pounding, shooting), or aching (viselike, constant pressure, dull)?	Character is typically viselike with tension headache, throbbing with migraine or temporal arteritis.
Is it mild, moderate, or severe?	Quantity is often severe with migraine, or excruciating with cluster headache.
Course and Duration. What time of day do the headaches occur? In the morning, in the evening? Do they awaken you from sleep? How long do they last? Do they last hours, days? Have you noted any daily headaches, or several within a time period?	Migraines occur about two per month, each lasting 1 to 3 days; 1 to 2 cluster headaches occur per day, each lasting 1/2 to 2 hours

EXAMINER ASKS:	RATIONALE:
	for 1 or 2 months, then complete remission may last for months or years.
Precipitating Factors. What do you think brings it on, for example, activity or exercise, work environment, emotional upset, anxiety, alcohol? (Also note signs of depression.)	Alcohol ingestion and daytime napping typically precipitate cluster headaches; whereas alcohol, letdown after stress, menstruation, and eating chocolate or cheese precipitate migraines.
Associated Factors. Is there any relation to other symptoms? For example, any nausea and vomiting? (Note which came first, headache or nausea.) Have you noted any vision changes, pain with bright lights, neck pain or stiffness, fever, weakness, moodiness, stomach problems?	Nausea, vomiting, and visual disturbances are associated with migraines; eye reddening and tearing, eyelid drooping, rhinorrhea, and nasal congestion are associated with cluster headaches; anxiety and stress are associated with tension headaches; nuchal rigidity and fever are associated with the headache of meningitis or encephalitis.
Do you have any other illness?	Hypertension, fever, hypothyroidism, and vasculitis produce headaches.
Do you take any medications?	Oral contraceptives, bronchodilators, alcohol, nitrates, and carbon monoxide produce headaches.
What makes it worse? Does movement aggravate the headache? Or, do coughing, straining, exercise aggravate it?	
Pattern. Is there any family history of headache? What is the frequency of your headaches? Once a week? Are your headaches occurring closer together? Are they getting worse? Or, are they getting better? Do you have any symptoms during the time between attacks? (For females) When do they occur in relation to your menstrual periods?	Migraines are associated with family history of migraine.
Effort to Treat. What seems to help: for example, going to sleep, medications, positions, rubbing the area?	With migraines, people lie down to feel better, whereas with cluster headaches they need to move to feel better, even to pace the floor.
Coping Strategies. How have these headaches affected your self-care, or your ability to function at work, home, and socially?	
2. Have you had any **head injury** or blow to your head?	
Onset. When was this? Please describe exactly what happened. How about the setting? Were there any hazardous conditions? Were you wearing a helmet or hard hat? How about yourself just before injury? Were you dizzy, lightheaded, had a blackout, had a seizure?	

EXAMINER ASKS:	RATIONALE:
Did you lose consciousness and then fall? (Note which came first.) Were you knocked unconscious? Or did you lose consciousness a few minutes later?	Loss of consciousness before a fall may have a cardiovascular cause, e.g., heart block.
Do you have any history of illness, e.g., heart trouble, diabetes, epilepsy?	
Location. Exactly where did you hit your head?	
Duration. How long were you unconscious?	
Did you have any symptoms afterward—headache, vomiting, projectile vomiting?	
Have you noted any change in level of consciousness; are you dazed or sleepy?	A change in the level of consciousness is of prime importance in evaluating a neurologic deficit.
Associated Symptoms. Have you noted any pain in the head or the neck, vision change, discharge from ear or nose—is it bloody or watery? Are you able to move all extremities? Do you have any tremors, staggered walk, numbness and tingling?	
Pattern. Have the symptoms become worse, better, unchanged since injury?	
Effort to Treat. Were you seen in the emergency department, or hospitalized?	
Have you taken any medications?	
3. Have you experienced any **dizziness**?	
(Determine exactly what the person means by dizziness.) Was it a feeling of lightheadedness or of falling? Or, was it a spinning sensation?	Dizziness is a lightheaded, swimming sensation or a feeling of falling. Vertigo is true rotational spinning owing to neurologic dysfunction (labyrinthine-vestibular apparatus, vestibular nuclei in brain stem). When vertigo is objective, the perception is that the room spins. When vertigo is subjective, the perception is that the person spins.
Onset. Was the dizziness abrupt or gradual? Did it occur after a change in position, such as sudden standing?	
Associated Factors. Have you noted any nausea and vomiting, pallor, immobility, decreased hearing acuity, or tinnitus along with the dizziness?	
4. Do you have any **neck pain**?	
Onset. Did the pain start with injury, automobile accident, after lifting, from a fall? Or, with fever? Or, did it have a gradual onset?	Acute onset of stiffness along with headache and fever occurs with meningeal inflammation.
Location. Does pain radiate? To the shoulders, arms?	

EXAMINER ASKS:	RATIONALE:
Associated Symptoms. Have you noted any **limitations to range of motion**, numbness or tingling in shoulders, arms, or hands?	
Precipitating Factors. What movements cause pain? Does neck movement aggravate it or alleviate it? Do you need to lift or bend at work or home?	
Does stress seem to bring it on?	Pain creates a vicious circle. Tension increases pain and disability, which produces more anxiety.
Coping Strategies. Are you able to do your work, to sleep?	
5. Do you have any **lumps or swelling** in the neck?	
Do you have any recent infection? Do you have any tenderness?	Tenderness usually indicates acute infection.
For a lump that persists, how long have you had it? Has it changed in size?	A persistent lump should arouse suspicion of malignancy.
Do you have any history of prior irradiation of head, neck, upper chest?	Increased risk for salivary and thyroid tumors.
Do you have any difficulty swallowing?	Dysphagia.
	For persons over 40 years, suspect any neck lump as malignant until it is proved otherwise.
Do you smoke? For how long? How many packs a day? Do you chew tobacco?	Smoking and chewing tobacco increases risk of oral and respiratory cancer.
How much alcohol do you drink a day? Are you exposed to any industrial toxins?	Smoking and large alcohol consumption together increase the risk of cancer.
Were you ever told you had a thyroid problem? Was it over-functioning or under-functioning? How was it treated? Surgery or irradiation? Any medication?	
6. Have you ever had surgery of the head or neck? For what condition? When did the surgery occur?	Surgery for head and neck cancer often is disfiguring and increases risk of body image disturbance.
How do you feel about results?	

ADDITIONAL QUESTIONS FOR INFANTS AND CHILDREN

Did the mother use alcohol or street drugs during pregnancy? How often was it used? How much was used per episode?	Alcohol increases the risk of fetal alcohol syndrome. Cocaine use causes neurologic, developmental, and emotional problems.
Was delivery vaginal or by cesarean section? Any difficulty? Use of forceps?	Forceps may increase the risk of caput succedaneum, cephalhematoma, and Bell's palsy.

EXAMINER ASKS:	RATIONALE:
What were you told about the baby's growth? Was it on schedule? Did the head seem to grow and fontanels close on schedule? Is the neck growing along with the body? At what age (in months) did the baby achieve head control? Have you noticed that the head shape of the baby is different from that of siblings or other children?	

ADDITIONAL QUESTIONS FOR THE AGING ADULT

If dizziness is a problem, how does this affect your daily activities? Are you able to drive safely, maneuver about the house safely?	Assess self-care. Assess potential for injury.
If neck pain is a problem, how does this affect your daily activities? Are you able to drive, perform at work, do housework, sleep, look down when using stairs?	Assess self-care. Assess potential for injury.

OBJECTIVE DATA

METHOD OF EXAMINATION

NORMAL RANGE OF FINDINGS	ABNORMAL FINDINGS
Preparation	
Remove any wig or hairpiece.	
THE HEAD	
Inspect and palpate the skull	
Note the general size and shape. *Normocephalic* is the term that denotes a round symmetric skull that is appropriately related to body size. Be aware that "normal" includes a wide range of sizes.	Deformities include microcephaly, abnormally small head; macrocephaly, abnormally large head, e.g., hydrocephaly; and acromegaly, Paget's disease, see Table 10–1.
To assess shape, place your fingers in the person's hair and palpate the scalp. The skull normally feels symmetrical and smooth. The cranial bones that have normal protrusions are the forehead, the lateral edge of each parietal bone, the occipital bone, and the mastoid process behind each ear. There is no tenderness to palpation.	Note lumps, depressions, or abnormal protrusions.
Palpate the temporal artery above the zygomatic (cheek) bone between the eye and top of the ear.	The artery looks more tortuous and feels hardened and tender with

NORMAL RANGE OF FINDINGS	ABNORMAL FINDINGS

The temporomandibular joint is just below the temporal artery and anterior to the tragus. Palpate the joint as the person opens the mouth, and note normally smooth movement with no limitation or tenderness.

Crepitation, limited range of motion, or tenderness.

Inspect the face

Inspect the face, noting the facial expression and its appropriateness to behavior or reported mood. Anxiety is common in the hospitalized or ill person.

Hostility or embarrassment.
Tense, rigid muscles may indicate anxiety or pain; a flat affect may indicate depression; excessive smiling may be inappropriate.

Although the shape of facial structures may vary somewhat among races, they always should be symmetric. Note symmetry of eyebrows, palpebral fissures, nasolabial folds, and sides of the mouth. Note any abnormal facial structures (coarse facial features, exophthalmos, changes in skin color or pigmentation), or any abnormal swelling. Also note any involuntary movements (tics) in the facial muscles. Normally there are none.

Marked asymmetry with central brain lesion (e.g., cerebrovascular accident) or with peripheral cranial nerve VII damage (Bell's palsy). See Table 10–5.
Edema in the face is noted first around the eyes (periorbital) and the cheeks where the subcutaneous tissue is relatively loose.
Note grinding of jaws, tics, fasciculations, or excessive blinking. (See Table 20–6).

THE NECK

Inspect and palpate the neck

Symmetry

Head position is centered in the midline, and the accessory neck muscles should be symmetric. The head should be held erect and still.

Head tilt occurs with muscle spasm.
Rigid head and neck occur with arthritis.

Range of Motion

Note any limitation of movement during active motion. Ask the person to touch the chin to the chest, turn the head to the right and left, try to touch each ear to the shoulder (without elevating shoulders), and to extend the head backward. When the neck is supple, motion is smooth and controlled.

Note pain at any particular movement.
Note ratchety movement or limitation of movement that may be due to cervical arthritis or inflammation of neck muscles. With arthritis, the neck is rigid and the person turns at the shoulders rather than the neck.

Test muscle strength and the status of cranial nerve XI by trying to resist the person's movements with your hands as the person shrugs the shoulders and turns the head to each side.

As the person moves the head, note enlargement of the salivary glands and lymph glands. Normally there is no enlargement. Note a swollen parotid gland when the head is extended; look for swelling below the angle of the jaw. Also, note thyroid gland enlargement. This may be

See Table 10–2.

NORMAL RANGE OF FINDINGS

unilateral, or it may be diffuse and look like a doughnut lying across the lower neck. Normally there is no enlargement.

Also note any obvious pulsations. The carotid artery runs medial to the sternomastoid muscle, and it creates a brisk localized pulsation just below the angle of the jaw. Normally, there are no other pulsations while the person is in the sitting position (see Chapter 16, Assessing the Heart and Neck Vessels).

Lymph Nodes

Using a gentle circular motion of your fingerpads, palpate the lymph nodes (Fig. 10–10). (Normally, the salivary glands are not palpable, but the parotid may become swollen with the onset of mumps. When symptoms warrant, check for parotid tenderness by palpating in a line from the outer corner of the eye to the lobule of the ear.) Beginning with the preauricular lymph nodes in front of the ear, palpate the 10 groups of lymph nodes in a routine order. There are many nodes closely packed, so you must be systematic and thorough in your examination. Once you establish your sequence, do not vary or you may miss some small nodes.

Use gentle pressure because strong pressure could push the nodes into the neck muscles. It is usually most efficient to palpate with both hands,

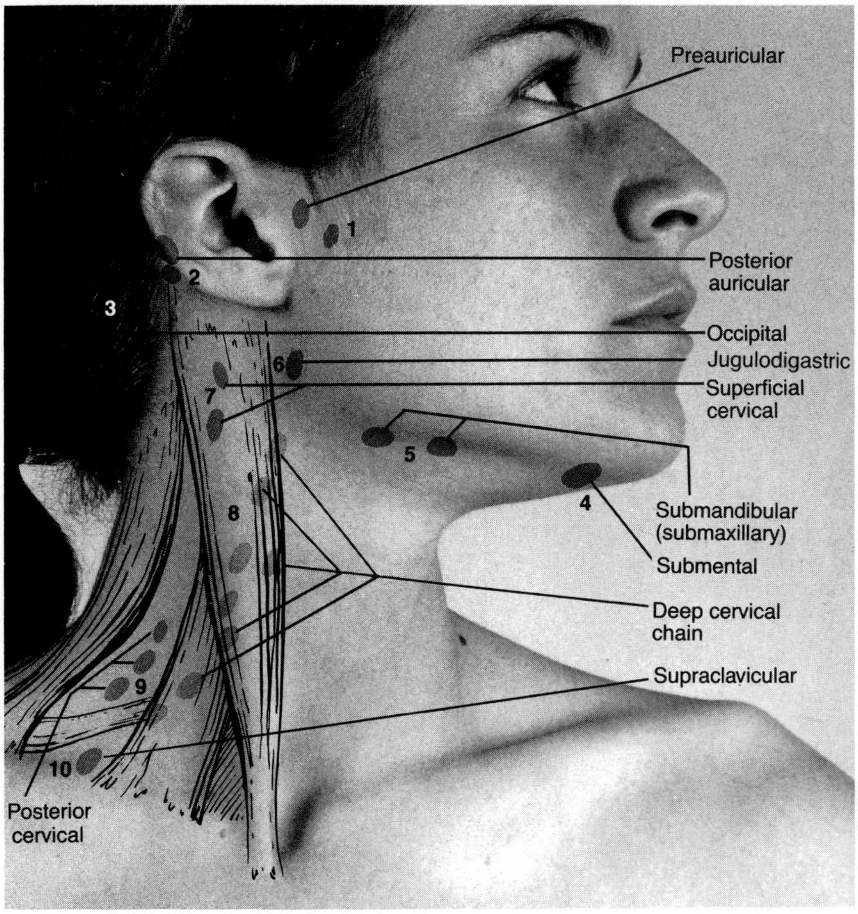

► Figure 10–10

ABNORMAL FINDINGS

NORMAL RANGE OF FINDINGS	ABNORMAL FINDINGS

comparing the two sides symmetrically. However, the submental gland is easier to explore with one hand. When you palpate with one hand, use your other hand to position the person's head. For the deep cervical chain, tip the person's head toward the side being examined to relax the ipsilateral muscle (Fig. 10–11). Then you can press your fingers under the

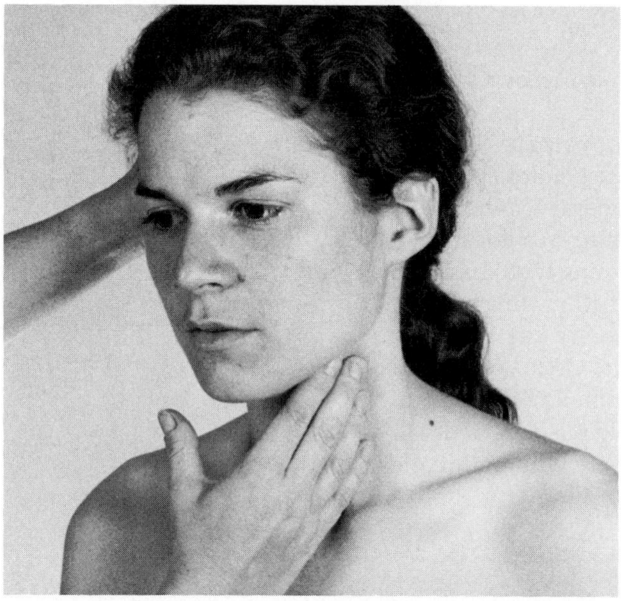

► **Figure 10–11**

muscle. Search for the supraclavicular node by having the person hunch the shoulders and elbows forward (Fig. 10–12); this relaxes the skin. The inferior belly of the omohyoid muscle crosses the posterior triangle here; do not mistake it for a lymph node.

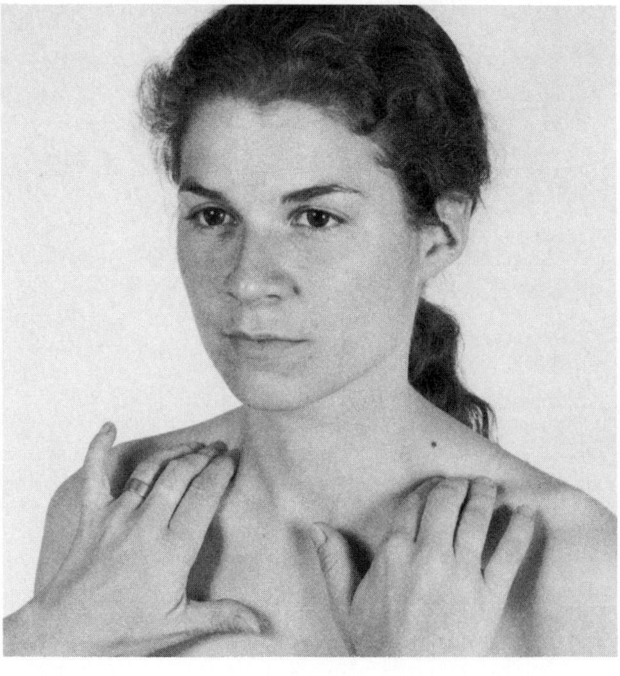

► **Figure 10–12**

NORMAL RANGE OF FINDINGS

If any nodes are palpable, note their location, size, shape, delimitation (discrete or matted together), mobility, consistency, and tenderness. Cervical nodes often are palpable in healthy persons, although this palpability decreases with age. Normal nodes feel movable, discrete, soft, and nontender.

If nodes are enlarged or tender, check the area they drain for the source of the problem. Look *proximal* (upstream) to the location of the node. For example, those in the upper cervical or submandibular area often relate to inflammation or a neoplasm in the head and neck. Follow up on or refer your findings. An enlarged lymph node, particularly when you cannot find the source of the problem, deserves prompt attention.

Trachea

Normally, the trachea is midline; palpate for any tracheal shift. Place your index finger on the trachea in the sternal notch, and slip it off to each side. The space should be symmetric on both sides. Note any deviation from the midline.

Thyroid Gland

The thyroid gland is difficult to palpate; arrange your setting to maximize your likelihood of success. Position a standing lamp to shine tangentially across the neck to highlight any possible swelling. Supply the person with a glass of water, and first inspect the neck as the person takes a sip and swallows. Thyroid tissue moves up with a swallow.

ABNORMAL FINDINGS

Lymphadenopathy — enlargement of the lymph nodes due to infection, allergy or neoplasm.

The following criteria are common clues but are not definitive in all circumstances.

- Acute infection—nodes are bilateral, enlarged, warm, tender, and firm but freely moveable.
- Chronic inflammation, e.g., in tuberculosis the nodes are clumped.
- Cancerous nodes are hard, unilateral, nontender and fixed.
- Nodes with asymptomatic human immunodeficiency virus (HIV) infection are firm but not hard, and are nontender and mobile.
- An enlarged supraclavicular node may indicate a neoplasm in the thorax or abdomen.

Conditions of tracheal shift:

- The trachea is pushed to the unaffected side with an aortic aneurysm, a tumor, unilateral thyroid lobe enlargement, and pneumothorax.
- The trachea is pulled toward the affected side with large atelectasis, pleural adhesions, or fibrosis.
- Tracheal tug is a rhythmic downward pull that is synchronous with systole and that occurs with aortic arch aneurysm.

Look for diffuse enlargement or a nodular lump.

NORMAL RANGE OF FINDINGS	ABNORMAL FINDINGS

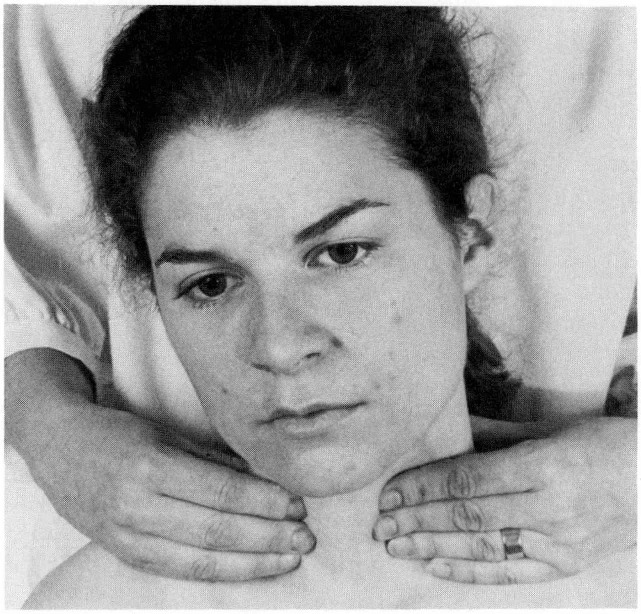

► Figure 10–13

To palpate, move behind the person (Figs. 10–13 and 10–14). Ask the person to sit up very straight, then to bend the head slightly forward and to the right. This will relax the neck muscles. Use the fingers of your left hand to push the trachea slightly to the right.

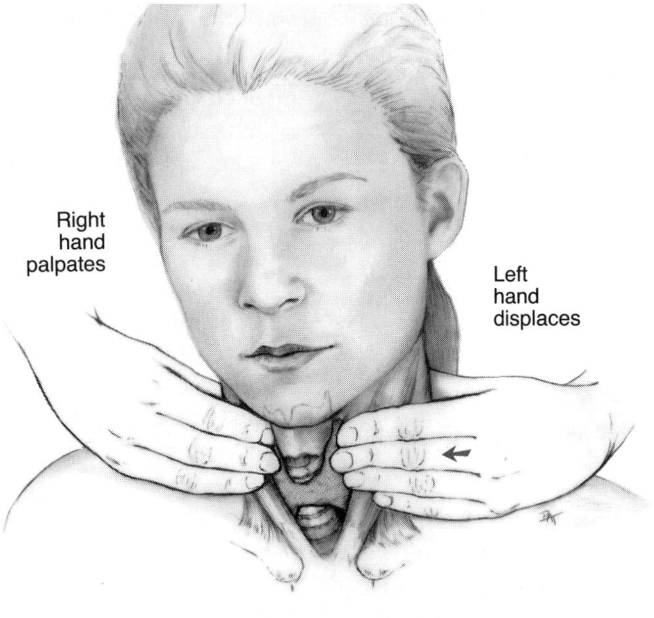

► Figure 10–14

Then curve your right fingers between the trachea and the sternomastoid muscle, retracting it slightly, and ask the person to take a sip of water. The thyroid moves up under your fingers with the trachea and larynx as the person swallows. Reverse the procedure for the left side.

Usually you cannot palpate the normal adult thyroid. If the person has a long thin neck, you sometimes will feel the isthmus over the tracheal rings. The lateral lobes usually are not palpable; check them for enlarge-

Abnormalities include enlarged lobes that are easily palpated before swallowing, or are tender to

NORMAL RANGE OF FINDINGS

ment, consistency, symmetry, and the presence of nodules.

Anterior Approach. This is an alternate method of palpating the thyroid, but it is more awkward to perform, especially for a beginning examiner. Stand facing the person. Ask him or her to tip the head forward and to the right. Use your right thumb to displace the trachea slightly to the person's right. Hook your left thumb and fingers around the sternomastoid muscle. Feel for lobe enlargement as the person swallows (Figs. 10–15 and 10–16).

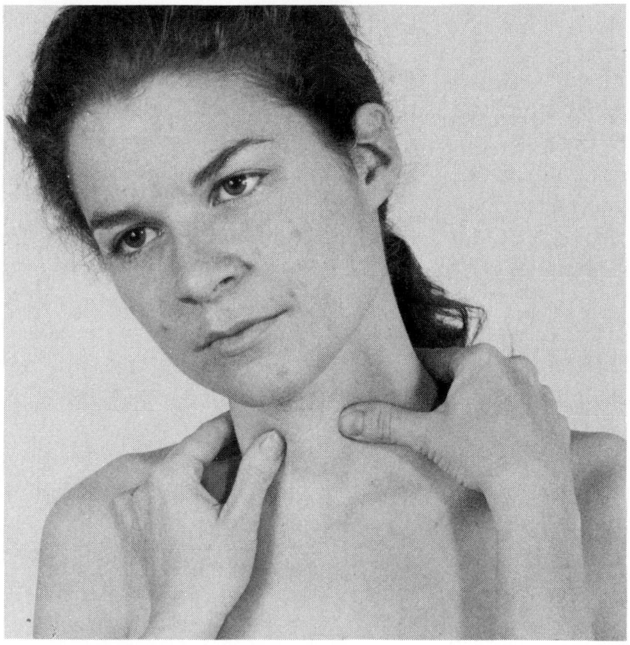

► **Figure 10–15**

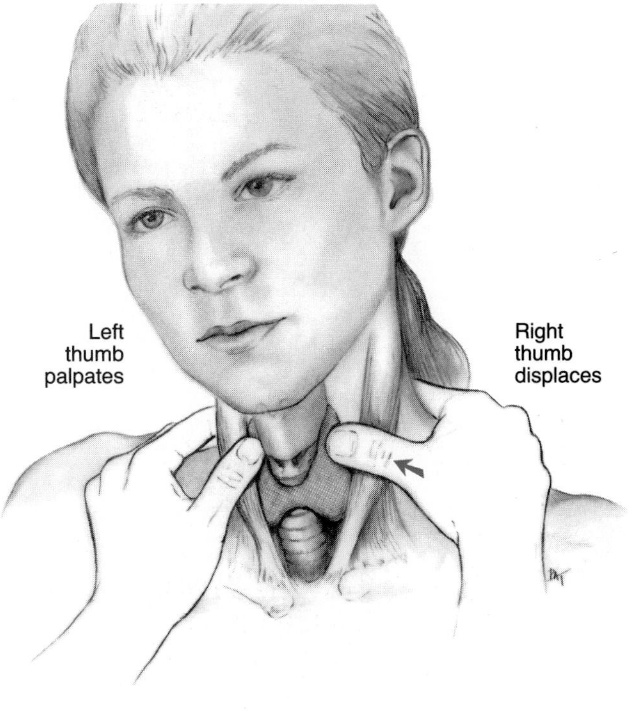

► **Figure 10–16**

ABNORMAL FINDINGS

palpation, or the presence of nodules or lumps. See Table 10–2.

NORMAL RANGE OF FINDINGS	ABNORMAL FINDINGS

Auscultate the thyroid

If the thyroid gland is enlarged, auscultate it for the presence of a *bruit.* This is a soft, pulsatile, whooshing, blowing sound heard best with the bell of the stethoscope. The bruit is not present normally.

A bruit occurs with accelerated or turbulent blood flow, indicating hyperplasia of the thyroid, e.g., hyperthyroidism.

DEVELOPMENTAL CONSIDERATIONS

Infants and Children

Skull

An infant's head size is measured with measuring tape at each visit up to age 2. You may have the parent hold the child to ensure a still position. Circle the tape around the head at the frontal and occipital bones; the widest span is correct. Plot the measurement on standardized growth charts. Compare the infant's head size with that expected for age. A series of measurements is more valuable than a single figure to show the *rate* of head growth. (Measurement of head circumference is presented in detail in Chapter 8.)

Microcephalic—head circumference below norms for age. Macrocephalic—an enlarged head for age, or rapidly increasing in size. This may be due to hydrocephalus (increased cerebrospinal fluid).

The newborn's head measures about 32 to 38 cm (average around 34 cm), and is 2 cm larger than chest circumference. At age 2, both measurements are the same. During childhood, the chest circumference grows to exceed head circumference by 5 to 7 cm.

Note an abnormal increase in head size or failure to grow.

Observe the infant's head from all angles, not just the front. The contour should be symmetric. There is some racial variation in normal head shapes; Nordic children tend to have long heads and Asian children have broad heads.

Frontal bulges or "bossing" occur with prematurity, rickets, or congenital syphilis.

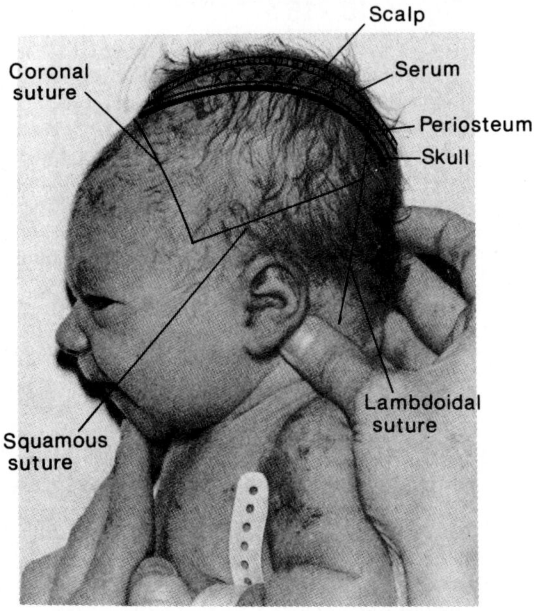

► **Figure 10-17 Caput succedaneum**

NORMAL RANGE OF FINDINGS	ABNORMAL FINDINGS

Two common variations in the newborn cause the shape of the skull to look markedly asymmetric: A *caput succedaneum* is edematous swelling and ecchymosis of the presenting part of the head due to birth trauma (Fig. 10–17). It feels soft, and it may extend across suture lines. It gradually resolves during the first few days of life and needs no treatment.

A *cephalhematoma* is a subperiosteal hemorrhage, which is also a result of birth trauma (Fig. 10–18). It is soft, fluctuant, and well defined over one cranial bone. It appears several hours after birth and gradually increases in size. There is no discoloration, but it looks bizarre, so parents need reassurance that it will be reabsorbed during the first few weeks of life without treatment. Rarely, a large hematoma may persist to 3 months.

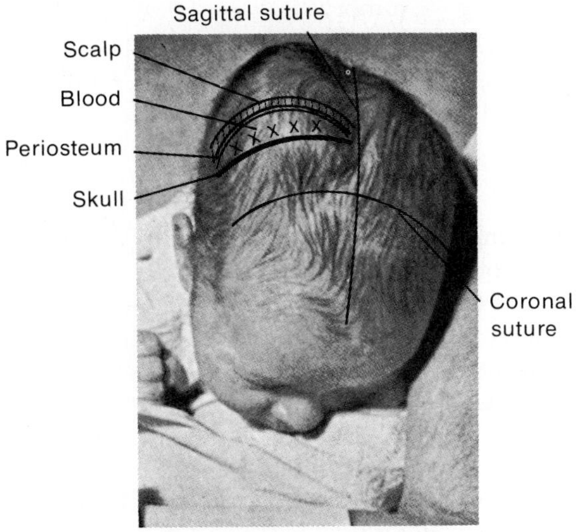

► Figure 10–18 Cephalhematoma

As you palpate the newborn's head, the suture lines feel like ridges. By 5 to 6 months, they are smooth and not palpable.

Abnormal findings: Sutures palpable when the child is older than 6 months.

A newborn's head may feel asymmetric and the involved ridges more prominent due to *molding* of the cranial bones during engagement and passage through the birth canal. Molding is overriding of the cranial bones; usually, the parietal bone overrides the frontal or occipital bone. Reassure parents that this lasts only a few days or a week. Babies delivered by cesarean section are noted for their evenly round heads. Also, some asymmetry may occur if an infant continually sleeps in one position; this is a flattening of the dependent cranial bone, usually the occiput.

Abnormal findings: Marked asymmetry, as in *craniosynostosis,* a severe deformity due to premature closure of the sutures, is abnormal. See Table 10–1.

Flattening also occurs with rickets or mental retardation.

Gently palpate the skull and fontanels while the infant is calm and somewhat in a sitting position (crying, lying down, or vomiting may cause the anterior fontanel to look full and bulging). The skull should feel smooth and fused except at the fontanels. The fontanels feel firm, slightly concave, and well defined against the edges of the cranial bones. You may see slight arterial pulsations in the anterior fontanel.

Abnormal findings: A true tense or bulging fontanel occurs with acute increased intracranial pressure.

Depressed and sunken fontanels occur with dehydration or malnutrition.

Marked pulsations occur with increased intracranial pressure.

NORMAL RANGE OF FINDINGS	ABNORMAL FINDINGS
The posterior fontanel may not be palpable at birth. If it is, it measures 1 cm and closes by 1 to 2 months. The anterior fontanel may be small at birth, and enlarge to 2.5 cm by 2.5 cm. A large diameter of 4 to 5 cm occasionally may be normal under 6 months. And, a small fontanel usually is normal. The anterior fontanel closes between 9 months and 2 years. Early closure may be insignificant if head growth proceeds normally.	Delayed closure or larger than normal fontanels occur with hydrocephalus, Down syndrome, hypothyroidism, or rickets. A small fontanel is a sign of microcephaly, as is early closure.
Note the infant's head posture and head control. The infant can turn the head side to side by 2 weeks and shows the tonic neck reflex when supine and the head is turned to one side (extension of same arm and leg, flexion of opposite arm and leg). The tonic neck reflex disappears between 3 and 4 months, and then the head is maintained in the midline. Head control is achieved by 4 months, when the baby can hold the head erect and steady when pulled to a vertical position. (See Chapter 19, Assessing the Musculoskeletal System, and Chapter 20, Assessing the Neurologic System, for further details.)	Tonic neck reflex lasting longer than 5 months indicates brain damage. In children, head tilt occurs with habit spasm, poor vision, and brain tumor. Head lag after 4 months is significant; it may indicate mental or motor retardation.

Face

Check facial features for symmetry, appearance, and presence of swelling. Note symmetry of wrinkling when the infant cries or smiles, e.g., both sides of the lips rise and both sides of forehead wrinkle. Children love to comply when you ask them to "make a face." Normally, no swelling is evident. Parotid gland enlargement is seen best when the child sits and looks up at the ceiling; the swelling appears below the angle of the jaw.	Unilateral immobility indicates nerve damage (central or peripheral), e.g., note angle of mouth droop on paralyzed side. Some facies are characteristic of congenital abnormalities or of chronic allergy. See Tables 10–3 and 10–4.

Neck

An infant's neck looks short; it lengthens during the first 3 to 4 years. You can see the neck better by supporting the infant's shoulders and tilting the head back a little. This positioning also enhances palpation of the trachea, which is buried deep in the neck. Feel for the row of cartilaginous rings in the midline or just slightly to the right of midline.	A short neck or webbing (loose fanlike folds) may indicate a congenital abnormality, such as Down or Turner syndrome, or it may occur alone.
Assess muscle development with gentle passive range of motion. Cradle the infant's head with your hands, and turn it side to side and test forward flexion, extension, and rotation. Note any resistance to movement, especially flexion. Ask a child to actively move through the range of motion, as you would an adult.	Head tilt and limited range of motion occur with torticollis (wryneck), or due to sternomastoid muscle injury during birth, or a congenital defect. Resistance to flexion (nuchal rigidity) and pain on flexion indicate meningeal irritation or meningitis.
During infancy, cervical lymph nodes are not palpable normally. But a child's lymph nodes are—they feel more prominent than an adult's until after puberty when lymphoid tissue begins to atrophy. Palpable nodes less than 3 mm are normal. They may be up to 1 cm in size in the cervical and inguinal areas but are discrete, move easily, and are nontender. Children have a higher incidence of infection, so you will expect a greater incidence of inflammatory adenopathy. There should be no other mass in the neck.	Cervical nodes larger than 1 cm are considered enlarged. Thyroglossal duct cyst—cystic lump high up in midline, freely movable, and rises up when swallowing. Supraclavicular nodes enlarge with Hodgkin's disease.

NORMAL RANGE OF FINDINGS

The thyroid gland is difficult to palpate in an infant due to the short thick neck, unless it is enlarged. The child's thyroid may be palpable normally.

Special Procedures

Palpation. *Craniotabes* is a softening of the skull's outer layer. With a newborn, pressure along the suture of the parietal and occipital bones above the ear produces a snapping sensation due to the pliable skull bone. It is like indenting a ping pong ball and feeling it snap back. Do not attempt this unless craniotabes is suspected because of other abnormal findings, and even then avoid excessive pressure. Craniotabes may be normal, especially with premature infants.

Percussion. With an infant, you may directly percuss with your plexor finger against the head surface. This yields a resonant or "cracked pot" sound, which is normal before closure of the fontanels.

Auscultation. Bruits are common in the skull in children under 4 or 5 years of age or in children with anemia. They are systolic or continuous and are heard over the temporal area.

Transillumination. Use this procedure if you suspect an abnormal head size or an intracranial lesion. In a completely darkened room, hold a rubber-collared flashlight firmly against the infant's skull. You need a tight fit against the head. Explore all regions of the head: frontal, both sides, occiput (Fig. 10–19). A small ring of light around the flashlight is normal (less than 2 cm in the frontal area, less than 1 cm in the occipital area). But you should not see a larger halo around the rubber collar.

ABNORMAL FINDINGS

Craniotabes may occur with rickets, hydrocephaly, or congenital syphilis.

The sound occurs with hydrocephalus due to separation of cranial sutures (Macewen's sign).

After 5 years of age, bruits indicate increased intracranial pressure, aneurysm, or arteriovenous shunt.

Presence of a halo of light through the skull indicates a loss or thinning of cerebral cortex. If the cortex is absent, the entire cranium lights up (Fig. 10–20).

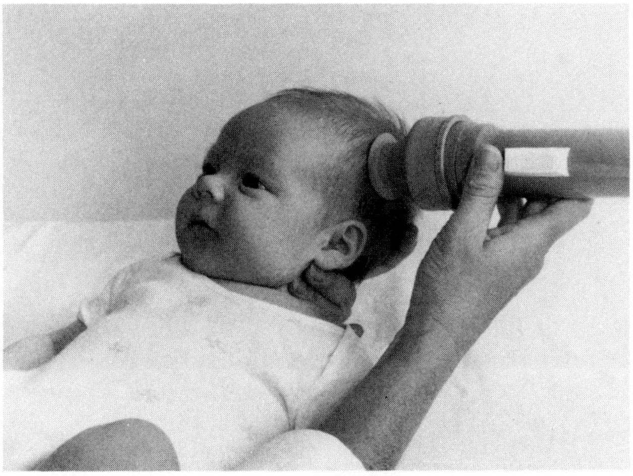

► **Figure 10–19**

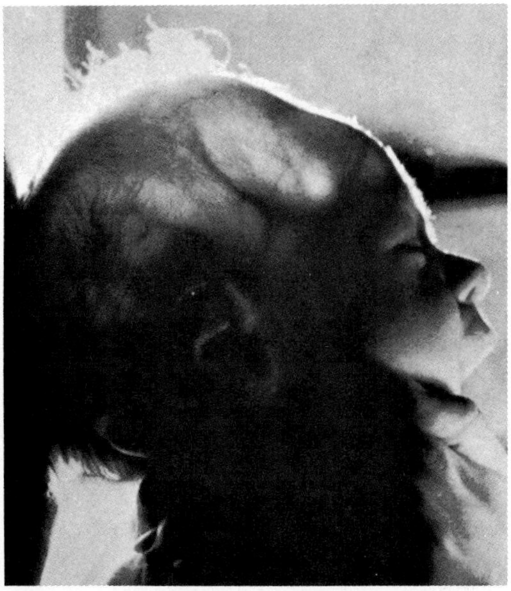

► **Figure 10–20 Hydranencephaly**

NORMAL RANGE OF FINDINGS	ABNORMAL FINDINGS

The Pregnant Female

During the second trimester, chloasma may show on the face. This is a blotchy hyperpigmented area over the cheeks and forehead that fades after delivery. The thyroid gland may be palpable normally during pregnancy.

The Aging Adult

The temporal arteries may look twisted and prominent. In some aging adults, a mild rhythmic tremor of the head may be normal. *Senile tremors* are benign and include head nodding (as if saying yes or no) and tongue protrusion. If some teeth have been lost, the lower face looks unusually small, with the mouth sunken in.

The neck may show an increased cervical concave curve when the head and jaw are extended forward to compensate for kyphosis of the spine. During the examination, direct the aging person to perform range of motion slowly; he or she may experience dizziness with side movements. An aging person may have prolapse of the submandibular glands, which could be mistaken for a tumor. But drooping submandibular glands will feel soft and be present bilaterally.

☑ SUMMARY CHECKLIST

1 ► Inspect and palpate the skull:
General size and contour
Note any deformities, lumps, tenderness
Palpate temporal artery, temporomandibular joint

2 ► Inspect the face:
Facial expression
Symmetry of movement (cranial nerve VII)
Any involuntary movements, edema, lesions

3 ► Inspect and palpate the neck:
Active range of motion
Enlargement of salivary glands, lymph nodes, thyroid gland
Position of the trachea

4 ► Auscultate the thyroid (if enlarged) for bruit

SAMPLE RECORDING

Subjective

- Denies any unusually frequent or severe headache, no history of head injury, dizziness or syncope, no neck pain, limitation of motion, lumps or swelling.

Objective

- Head. Normocephalic, no lumps, no lesions, no tenderness
  Face. Symmetric, no weakness, no involuntary movements
  Neck. Supple with full ROM, no pain
  Symmetric, no lymphadenopathy or masses, trachea midline, thyroid not palpable
  No bruits

SAMPLE CLINICAL PROBLEM

- Problem list

1 ▶ Chronic hypertension

2 ▶ Benign prostatic hypertrophy — Surgery, transurethral resection of prostate, March 3

Subjective

- Frank V. is a 57-year-old insurance executive who is in his 4th postop day following TUR of the prostate. His postop course has been unremarkable until today when he complained of dizziness, a lightheaded feeling that occurred on standing and cleared on sitting. No previous episodes of dizziness. Denies palpitations, nausea, or vomiting. States urine pink tinged as it was yesterday with no red blood. No pain meds today. On 2nd day of same antihypertensive medication he took before surgery.

Objective

- BP 142/88 RA Sitting, 108/58 RA Standing. Pulse 84 sitting and standing, regular rhythm, no skipped beats. Temp 37° C. Color tannish-pink, no pallor, skin warm and dry. Neuro: alert and oriented X 3. Speech clear and fluent. Moving all extremities, no weakness. No nystagmus, no ataxia, past pointing normal. Romberg's sign negative (normal). Intake/Output in balance. Urine faint pink tinged, no clots.
  Lab: Hct 45, serum chemistries normal.

Assessment

- Orthostatic hypotension
- Potential for injury R/T orthostatic hypotension.

NURSING DIAGNOSES COMMONLY ASSOCIATED WITH HEAD AND NECK DISORDERS

Diagnosis	Related Factors (Etiology)	Defining Characteristics (Symptoms and Signs)
Body image disturbance	Effects of loss of body part(s) Effects of loss of body function	Verbal or nonverbal response to actual or perceived change in structure and/or function Verbalization of Fear of rejection or of reaction by others Negative feelings about body Not looking at and/or touching body part Preoccupation with loss or change Refusal to verify actual change or loss Hiding or overexposing body part Change in social involvement Depersonalization of part or loss by use of impersonal pronouns
Impaired swallowing	Neuromuscular impairment Decreased/absent gag reflex Facial paralysis Decreased strength or excursion of muscles of mastication Mechanical obstruction Edema Tracheostomy tube Tumor Limited awareness Excessive/inadequate salivation Fatigue Reddened, irritated oropharyngeal cavity	Observed evidence of difficulty swallowing Evidence of aspiration Reported pain on swallowing Dehydration Weight loss

ABNORMAL FINDINGS

Table 10-1 ▶ Abnormalities in Head Size and Contour

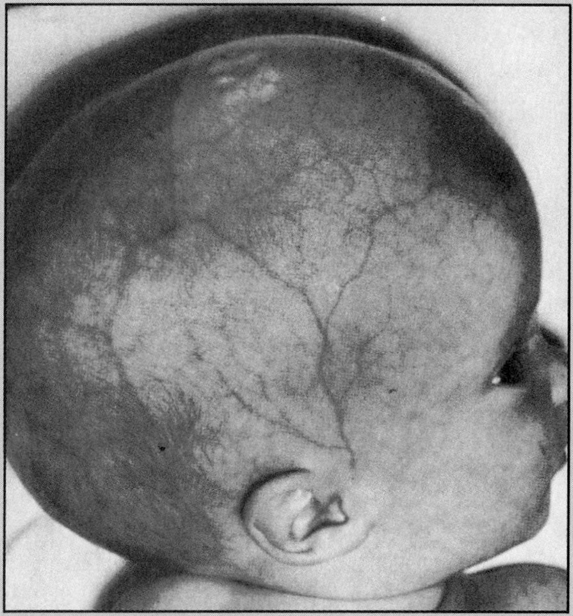

HYDROCEPHALUS

Obstruction of drainage of cerebrospinal fluid results in excessive accumulation, increasing intracranial pressure, and enlargement of the head. The face looks small compared with the enlarged cranium. The increasing pressure also produces dilated scalp veins, frontal bossing, and downcast or "setting sun" eyes (sclera visible above iris). The cranial bones thin, sutures separate, and percussion yields a "cracked pot" sound (Macewen's sign).

PAGET'S DISEASE OF BONE (OSTEITIS DEFORMANS) (not illustrated)

A localized bone disease of unknown etiology that softens, thickens, and deforms bone. It affects 3 percent of adults over age 40, and 10 percent over age 80 and occurs more often in males. The disease is characterized by bowed long bones, sudden fractures, and enlarging skull bones, which form an acorn shaped cranium. Enlarging skull bones press on cranial nerves, causing symptoms of headache, vertigo, tinnitus, and progressive deafness.

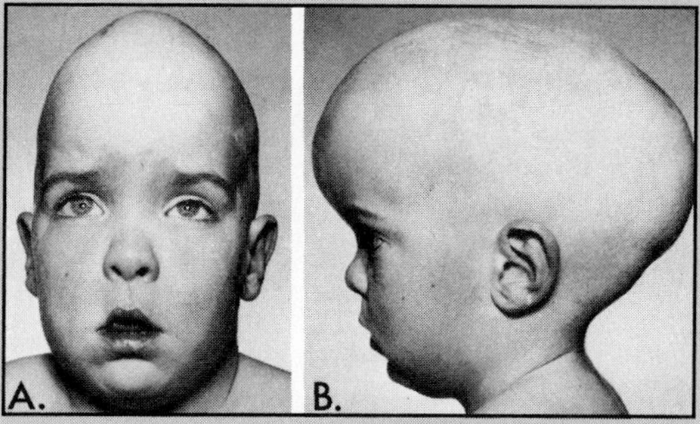

CRANIOSYNOSTOSIS

Premature closure of one or more sutures while brain growth continues. Skull growth stops at right angles to closed suture. Deformity depends on involved sutures; closure of the sagittal suture results in a long narrow head, and closure of the coronal suture involves the head, the face, and the orbits. Also note exophthalmos and drooping eyelids.

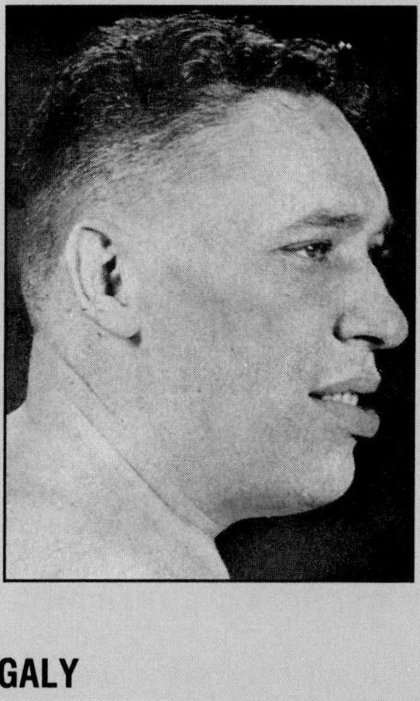

ACROMEGALY

Excessive secretion of growth hormone creates an enlarged skull and thickened cranial bones. Note the elongated head, massive face, prominent nose and lower jaw, heavy eyebrow ridge, and coarse facial features.

Table 10-2 ▸ Swellings on the Head or Neck

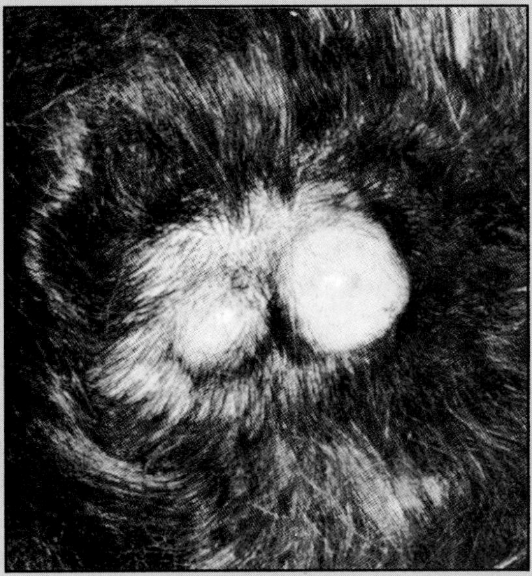

PILAR CYST (SEBACEOUS CYST, WEN)

Smooth, firm, fluctuant swelling on the scalp. Tense pressure of the contents causes overlying skin to be shiny and taut. It is a benign growth.

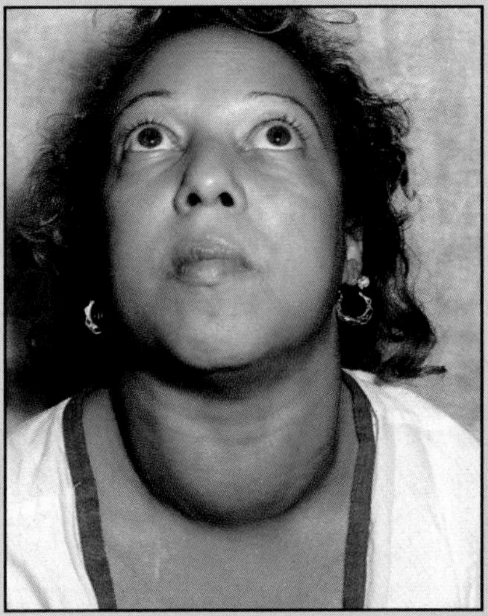

THYROID—DIFFUSE ENLARGEMENT

The isthmus and the lobes are palpable. This occurs with endemic goiter, Hashimoto's thyroiditis, and hyperthyroidism.

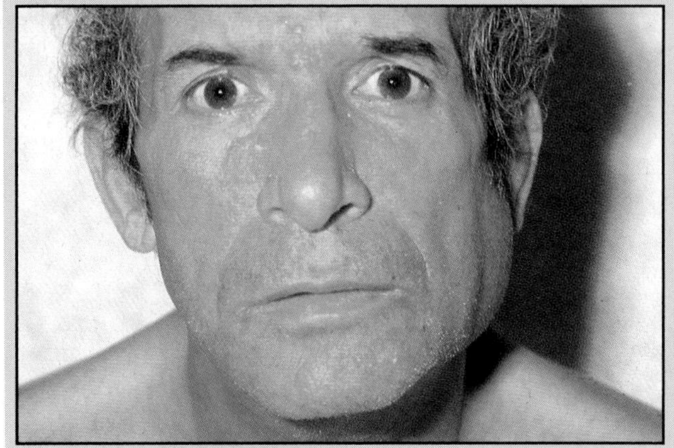

PAROTID GLAND ENLARGEMENT

Rapid painful inflammation occurs with mumps. Parotid swelling also occurs with abscess or tumor. Note swelling anterior to lower ear lobe.

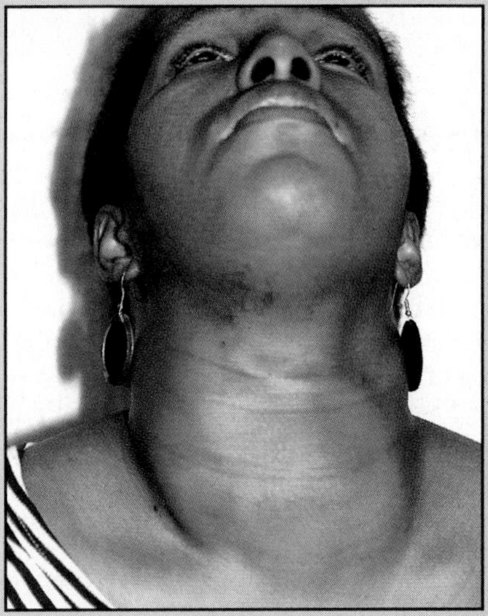

THYROID—MULTIPLE NODULES

Multiple nodules usually indicate inflammation or a multinodular goiter rather than a neoplasm. However, suspect any rapidly enlarging or firm nodule.

Table 10-2 ▸ Swellings on the Head or Neck *Continued*

THYROID — SINGLE NODULE (not illustrated)

Most solitary nodules are benign, although a solitary nodule poses a greater risk of malignancy than do multiple nodules, and poses a greater risk in a young person. Suspect any painless, rapidly growing nodule, especially the appearance of a single nodule in a young person. Cancerous nodules tend to be hard and are fixed to surrounding structures.

TORTICOLLIS →

Congenital shortening or spasm of one sternomastoid muscle, resulting in limited range of motion. You may feel a firm mass in mid-muscle on the involved side. This requires treatment or the muscle becomes fibrotic and permanently shortened with permanent limitation of range of motion and asymmetry of head and face.

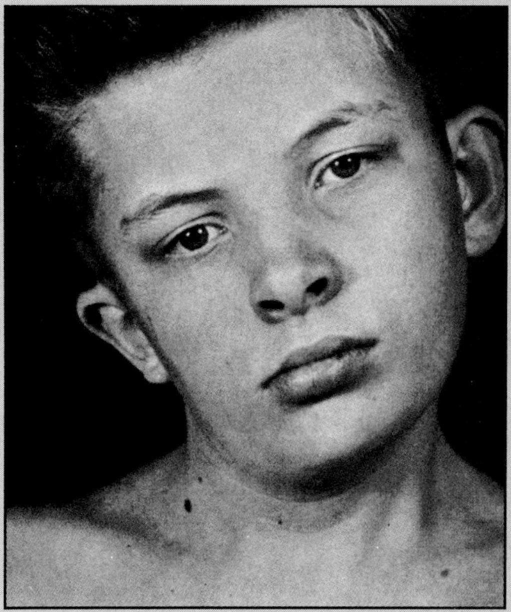

Table 10-3 ▸ Pediatric Facial Abnormalities

CRANIAL NERVE VII PARALYSIS (CARDIOFACIAL SYNDROME) (not illustrated)

Asymmetric crying facies is a congenital defect involving partial paralysis of cranial nerve VII. One side of the face is affected; the lower lip does not depress with crying, although the infant is able to smile and suck. It is *not* caused by forceps injury. It often is accompanied by cardiac defects, so a thorough examination is indicated.

DOWN SYNDROME →

Chromosomal aberration (trisomy-21). Head and face characteristics may include slanted eyes with inner epicanthal folds, flat nasal bridge, small broad flat nose, protruding thick tongue, ear dysplasia, and short broad neck with webbing.

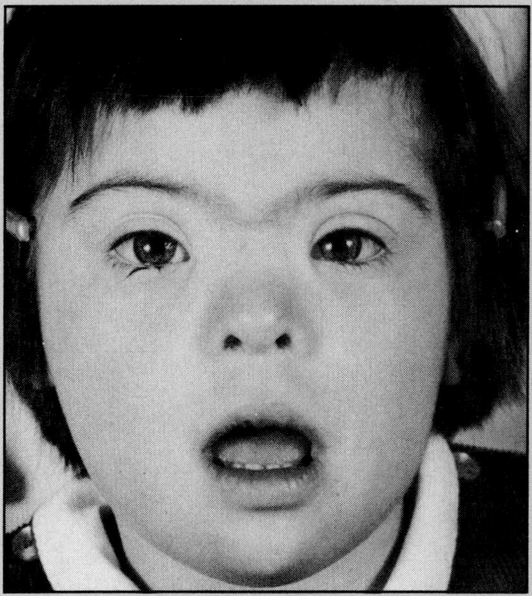

Table continued on following page

Table 10-3 ▸ Pediatric Facial Abnormalities *Continued*

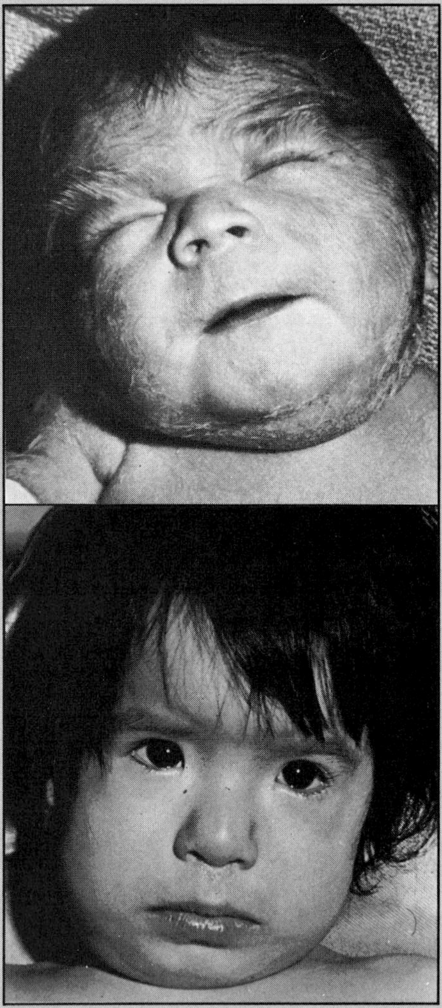

FETAL ALCOHOL SYNDROME

A pregnant woman who abuses alcohol is at great risk of producing a baby with a wide range of growth and developmental abnormalities. Facial malformations may be recognizable at birth. Characteristic facies include narrow palpebral fissures, epicanthal folds, and midfacial hypoplasia. Photo on top, at birth; photo on bottom, at one year.

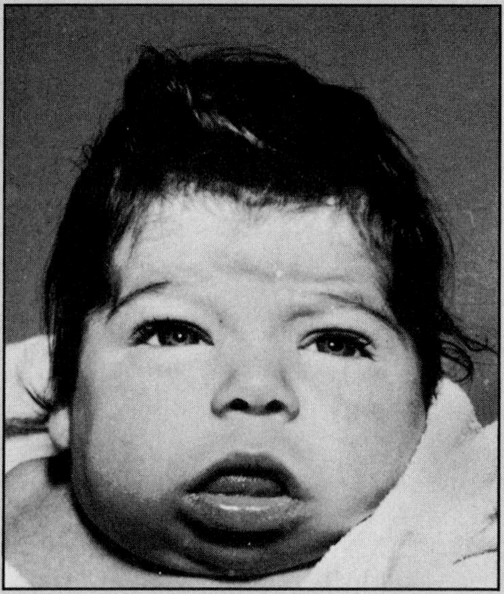

CRETINISM — CONGENITAL HYPOTHYROIDISM

Thyroid deficiency at an early age produces impaired growth and neurologic deficit. Characteristic facies include low hairline, hirsute forehead, swollen eyelids, narrow palpebral fissures, widely spaced eyes, depressed nasal bridge, puffy face, thick tongue protruding through an open mouth, and a dull expression. Head size is normal, but the anterior and posterior fontanels are wide open.

Table 10-4 ► Facial Features with Chronic Allergies

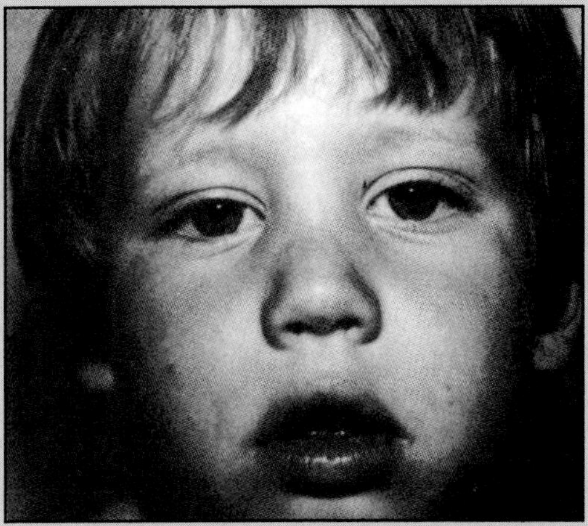

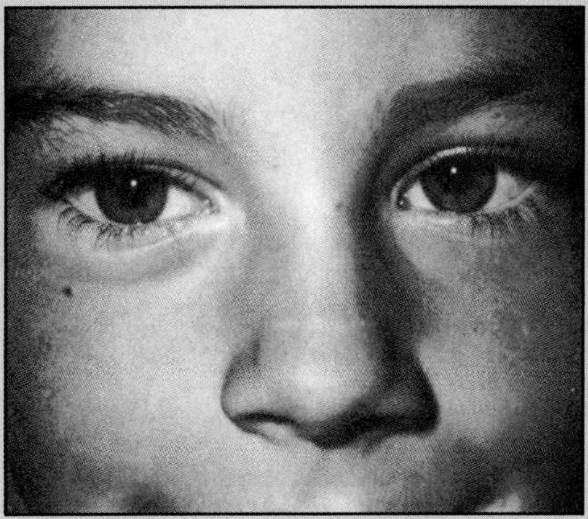

ATOPIC (ALLERGIC) FACIES

Children with chronic allergies such as atopic dermatitis often develop characteristic facial features. These include blue shadows below the eyes ("allergic shiners"), a double or single crease on the lower eyelids (Morgan's lines), central facial pallor, and open-mouth breathing (allergic gaping).

ALLERGIC SALUTE

This transverse line on the nose is also a feature of chronic allergies. It is formed when the child chronically uses the hand to push the nose up and back to relieve itching and to free swollen turbinates, which allows air passage.

Table 10-5 ► Abnormal Facial Appearances with Chronic Illnesses

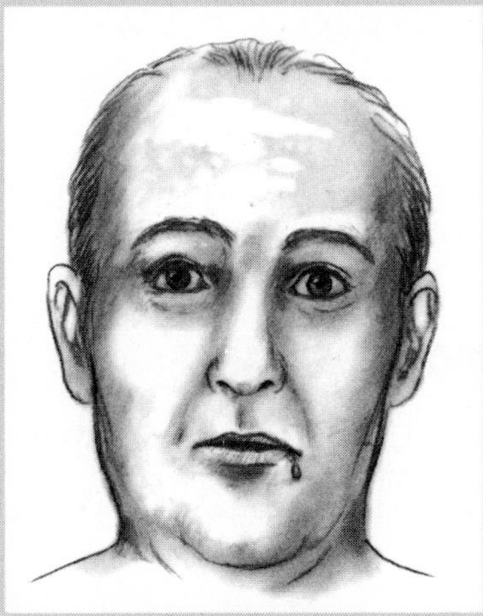

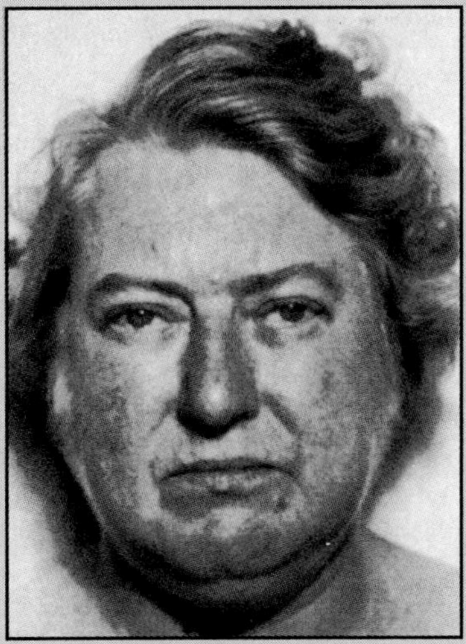

PARKINSON'S SYNDROME

A deficiency of the neurotransmitter dopamine and degeneration of the basal ganglia in the brain. The immobility of features produces a face that is flat and expressionless, "masklike," with elevated eyebrows, staring gaze, oily skin, and drooling.

CUSHING'S SYNDROME

With excessive secretion of adrenocorticotropic hormone (ACTH) and chronic steroid use, the person develops a plethoric, rounded, "moonlike" face, prominent jowls, red cheeks, and hirsutism on the upper lip, lower cheeks, and chin.

Table continued on following page

Table 10-5 ► Abnormal Facial Appearances with Chronic Illnesses *Continued*

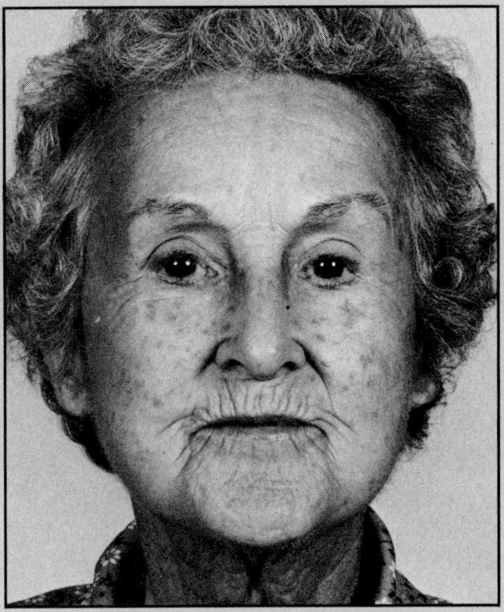

SCLERODERMA

"Hard skin," a collagen disease with proliferation of connective tissue. Characteristic facies: skin atrophy, with marked tightening and thinning; person may not be able to close the lips over the teeth.

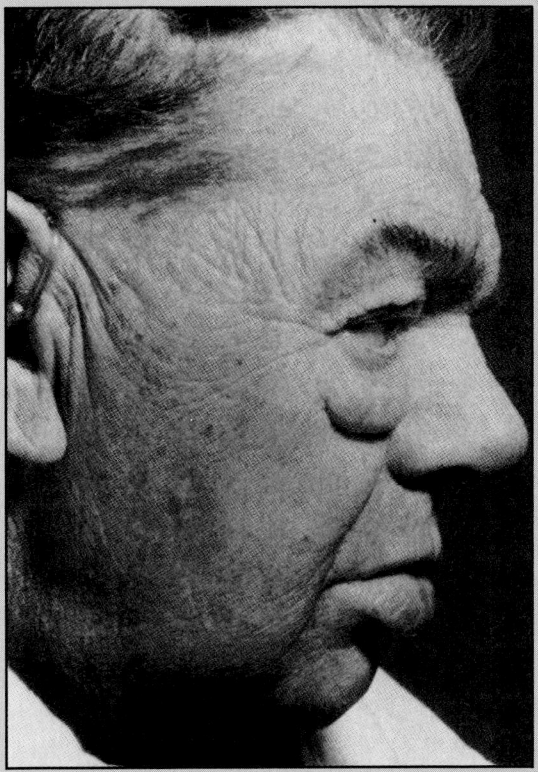

MYXEDEMA (HYPOTHYROIDISM)

A deficiency of thyroid hormone, when severe, causes a nonpitting edema or myxedema. Note puffy edematous face especially around eyes (periorbital edema), coarse facial features, dry skin, and dry coarse hair and eyebrows.

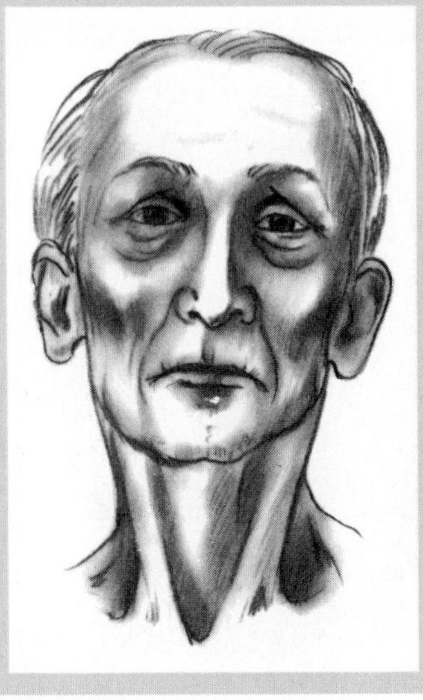

CACHECTIC APPEARANCE

Accompanies chronic wasting diseases such as cancer, dehydration, and starvation. Features include sunken eyes, hollow cheeks, and exhausted defeated expression.

Table 10-5 ► Abnormal Facial Appearances with Chronic Illnesses *Continued*

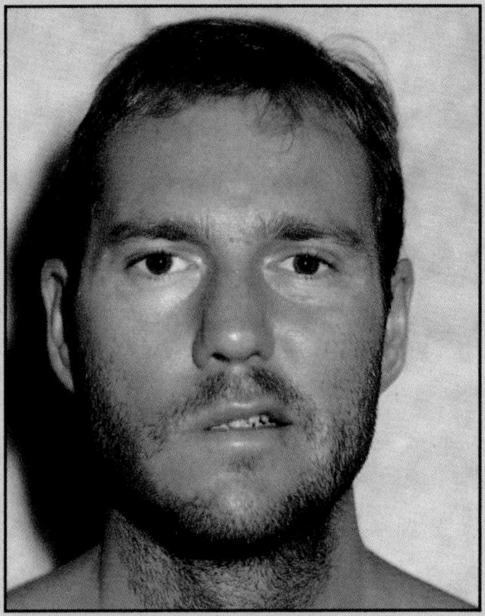

BELL'S PALSY

A lower motor neuron lesion (peripheral), producing cranial nerve VII paralysis, which is almost always unilateral. It has a rapid onset, and its cause is unknown, but perhaps is viral. Note complete paralysis of one-half of the face; person cannot raise eyebrow, close eye, whistle, or show teeth.

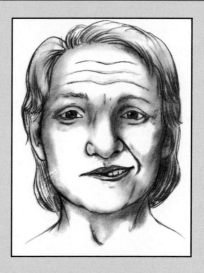

CEREBROVASCULAR ACCIDENT

An upper motor neuron lesion (central). Note paralysis of lower facial muscles, but upper half of face is not affected owing to the intact nerve from the unaffected hemisphere. The person is still able to wrinkle the forehead and to close the eyes.

Bibliography

Abrams DI, Foon KA, Gold JW: Lymphadenopathy: A diagnostic plan. Patient Care 22(8):94–112, 1988.

Baker KH, Feldman JE: Cancers of the head and neck. Cancer Nurs 10:293–299, 1987.

Bierman CW, Pearlman DS: Allergic Diseases from Infancy to Adulthood. 2nd ed. Philadelphia, WB Saunders, 1988.

Braun BL, Amundson LR: Quantitative assessment of head and shoulder posture. Arch Phys Med Rehabil 70:322–329, 1989.

Burrow GN, Oppenheimer JH, Volpe R: Thyroid Function and Disease. Philadelphia, WB Saunders, 1989.

Crumley R: Diagnosis and treatment of idiopathic facial paralysis. Prim Care 9:429–437, 1982.

Gabai IJ, Spierings ELH: Diagnosis and management of cluster headaches. Nurse Pract 15(10):32–36, 1990.

Gambert SR, Brensinger, JF: Assessing thyroid function in the elderly. Nurse Pract 8:38–43, 1983.

Ingbar SH: The thyroid gland. *In* Wilson JD and Foster DW (Eds): Williams Textbook of Endocrinology, 7th ed. Philadelphia, WB Saunders, 1985, pp 742–743.

Linet OI, Metzler, C: Incidence of palpable cervical nodes in adults. Postgrad Med 62:210–213, 1977.

Mechner F: Patient assessment: Examination of the head and neck. Am J Nurs 75:PI 1–24, May 1975.

Nellhaus G: Head circumference from birth to eighteen years. Pediatrics 41:106–133, 1968.

Sapar JR: Headache disorders: Current concepts and treatment strategies. Littleton, MA, PSG Publishing, 1982.

Southwick HW. Head and neck cancer: Early detection. Cancer 47(Suppl):1188–1192, 1981.

Wollenberg SP: Primary care diagnosis and management of Bell's palsy. Nurse Pract 14(12):14–18, 1989.

Yeomans AC: Assessment and management of hypothyroidism. Nurse Pract 15(11):8–16, 1990.

CHAPTER

11 Assessing the Eyes and Visual Status

STRUCTURE AND FUNCTION

EXTERNAL ANATOMY

The eye is the sensory organ of vision. Because this sense is so important to humans, the eye is well protected by the bony orbital cavity surrounded with a cushion of fat. The *eyelids* are like two moveable shades that further protect the eye from injury, strong light, and dust. The eyelashes curve outward from the lid margins, filtering out dust and dirt.

The *palpebral fissure* is the open space between the eyelids (Fig. 11–1). When closed, the lid margins approximate completely. When open, the upper lid covers part of the iris. The lower lid margin is just at the *limbus*, the border between the cornea and sclera. The *canthus* is the corner of the eye, the angle where the lids meet. At the inner canthus, the *caruncle* is a small fleshy mass containing sebaceous glands.

Within the upper lid, *tarsal plates* are strips of connective tissue that give it shape (Fig. 11–2). The tarsal plates contain the *meibomian glands*, modified sebaceous glands that secrete an oily lubricating material onto the lids.

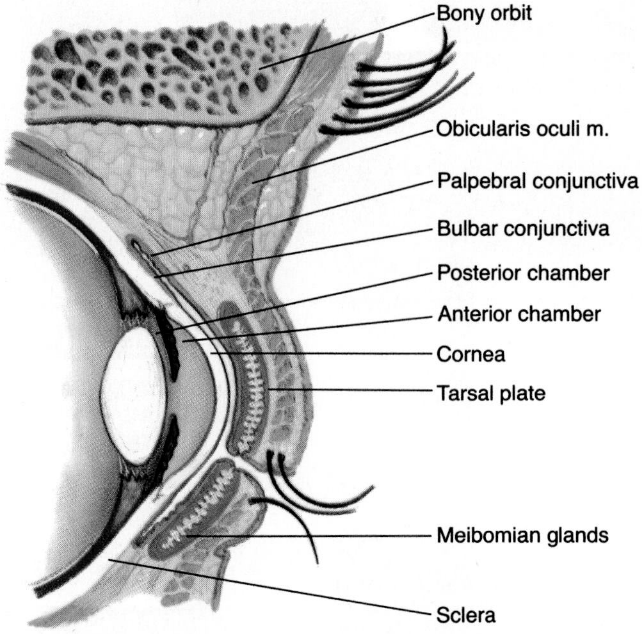

► **Figure 11–2**

The exposed part of the eye has a transparent protective covering, the *conjunctiva*. The conjunctiva is a thin mucous membrane shaped like an envelope between the eyelids and the eyeball. The *palpebral* conjunctiva lines the lids and is clear, with many small blood vessels. It forms a deep recess and then folds back over the eye.

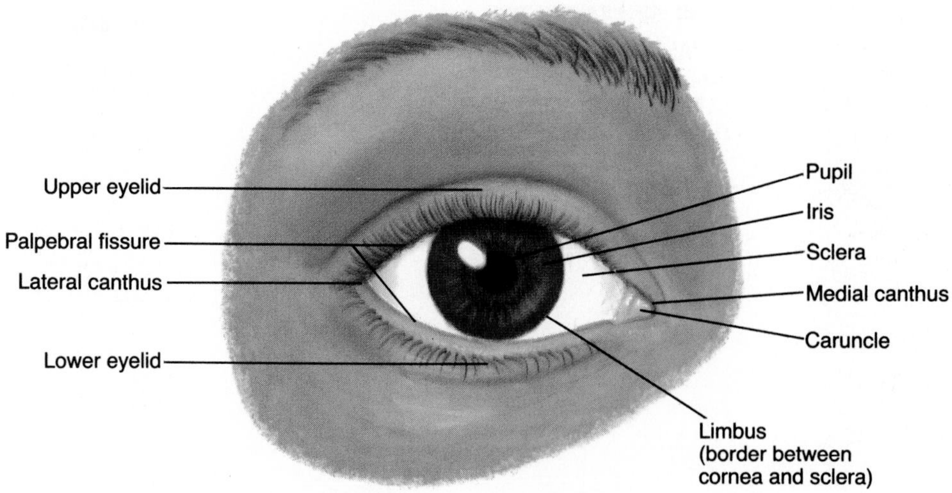

► **Figure 11–1**

The *bulbar* conjunctiva overlays the eyeball, with the white sclera showing through. At the limbus, the conjunctiva merges with the cornea. The cornea covers and protects the iris and pupil.

The *lacrimal apparatus* provides constant irrigation to keep the conjunctiva and cornea moist and lubricated (Fig. 11–3). The lacrimal gland, in the upper outer corner over the eye, secretes tears. The tears wash across the eye and are drawn up evenly as the lid blinks. The tears drain into the *puncta,* visible on the upper and lower lids at the inner canthus. The tears then drain into the nasolacrimal sac, through the nasolacrimal duct, and empty into the inferior meatus inside the nose.

Extraocular Muscles. Six muscles attach the eyeball to its orbit (Fig. 11–4). These extraocular muscles give the

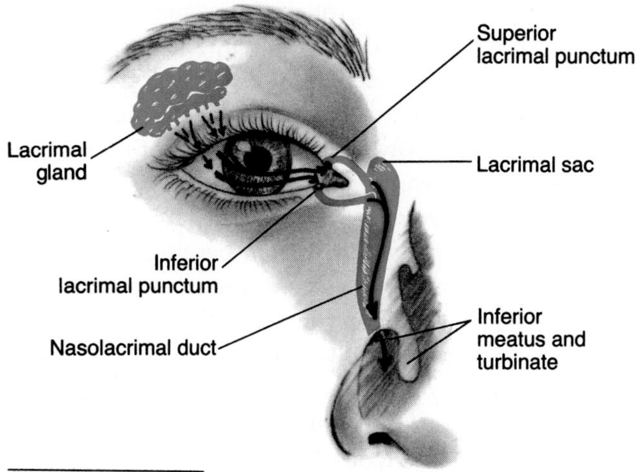

► **Figure 11–3**

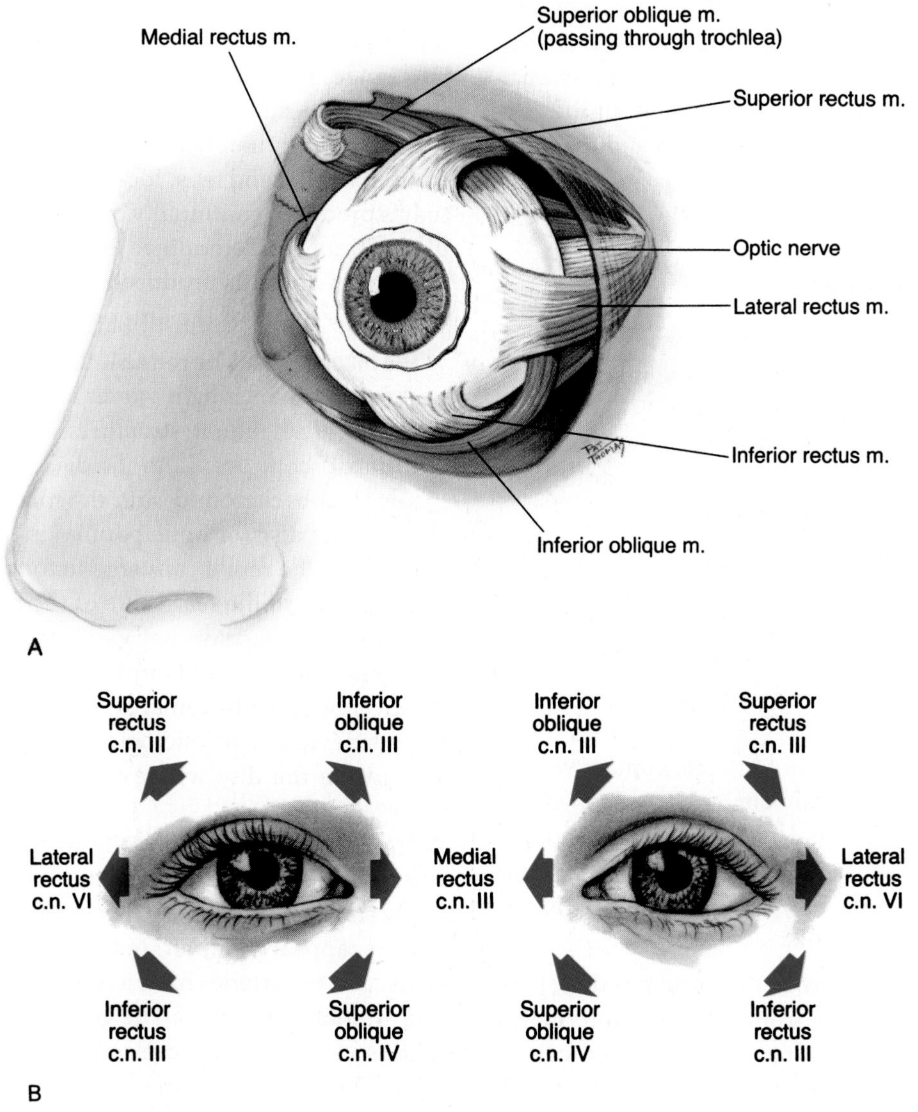

► **Figure 11–4 Muscle attachments *(A)* and direction of movement *(B)***

eye both straight and rotary movement. The four straight, or *rectus,* muscles are the superior, inferior, lateral, and medial rectus muscles. The two slanting, or *oblique,* muscles are the superior and inferior muscles.

Each muscle is coordinated, or yoked, with one in the other eye. This ensures that when the two eyes move, their axes always remain parallel (called *conjugate movement*). Parallel axes are important because the human brain must see only one image. Although some animals can perceive two different pictures through each eye, human beings have a binocular, single-image visual system. This occurs because our eyes move as a pair. For example, the two yoked muscles that allow looking to the far right are the right lateral rectus and the left medial rectus.

Movement of the extraocular muscles is stimulated by three cranial nerves. Cranial nerve VI, the abducens nerve, innervates the lateral rectus muscle (which abducts the eye); cranial nerve IV, the trochlear nerve, innervates the superior oblique muscle; and cranial nerve III, the oculomotor nerve, innervates all the rest — the superior, inferior and medial rectus and the inferior oblique muscles.

INTERNAL ANATOMY

The eye is a sphere composed of three concentric coats: (1) the outer fibrous *sclera,* (2) the middle vascular *choroid,* and (3) the inner nervous *retina* (Fig. 11–5). Inside the retina is the transparent vitreous body. The only parts accessible to examination are the sclera anteriorly and the retina through the ophthalmoscope.

The Outer Layer. The sclera is a tough, protective, white covering. It is continuous anteriorly with the smooth, transparent cornea, which covers the iris and pupil. The cornea is part of the refracting media of the eye, bending incoming light rays so they will be focused on the inner retina.

The cornea is very sensitive to touch; contact with a wisp of cotton stimulates a blink in both eyes, called the *corneal reflex.* The trigeminal nerve (cranial nerve V) carries the afferent sensation into the brain, and the facial nerve (cranial nerve VII) carries the efferent message that stimulates the blink.

The Middle Layer. The vascular choroid has dark pigmentation to prevent light from reflecting internally. Anteriorly, the choroid is continuous with the ciliary body and the iris. The muscles of the ciliary body control the thickness of the lens. The iris functions as a diaphragm, varying the opening at its center, the pupil. This controls the amount of light admitted into the retina. The muscle fibers of the iris contract the pupil in bright light and to accommodate for near vision, and dilate the pupil when the light is dim and for far vision. The color of the iris varies from person to person.

The pupil is round and regular. Its size is determined by a balance between the parasympathetic and sympathetic chains of the autonomic nervous system. Stimulation of the parasympathetic branch, through cranial nerve III, causes constriction of the pupil. Stimulation of the sympathetic branch dilates the pupil and elevates the eyelid. As mentioned earlier, the pupil size also reacts to the amount of ambient light and to accommodation, or focusing an object on the retina.

The lens is a biconvex disc located just posterior to the pupil. The transparent lens serves as a refracting medium, keeping a viewed object in continual focus on the retina. Its thickness is controlled by the ciliary body; the lens bulges for focusing on near objects, and flattens for far away objects.

The anterior chamber is posterior to the cornea and in front of the iris and lens. It contains the aqueous humor that is produced continually by the ciliary body. Intraocular pressure is determined by a balance between the amount of aqueous produced and resistance to its outflow at the angle of the anterior chamber.

The Inner Layer. The retina is the visual receptive layer of the eye in which light waves are changed into nerve impulses. The retinal structures viewed through the ophthalmoscope are the optic disc, the retinal vessels, the general background, and the macula (Fig. 11–6).

The optic disc (or optic papilla) is the area in which fibers from the retina converge to form the optic nerve. Located toward the nasal side of the retina, it has these characteristics: a color that varies from creamy yellow-orange to pink; a round or oval shape; margins that are distinct and sharply demarcated, especially on the temporal side; and a physiologic cup, the smaller circular area inside the disc where the blood vessels exit and enter.

The retinal vessels normally include a paired artery and vein extending to each quadrant, growing progressively smaller in caliber as they reach the periphery. The arteries appear brighter red and narrower than the veins, and the arteries have a thin sliver of light on them (the arterial light reflex). The general background of the fundus varies in color, depending on the person's skin color. The macula is located on the temporal side of the fundus. It contains the fovea centralis at its center, the

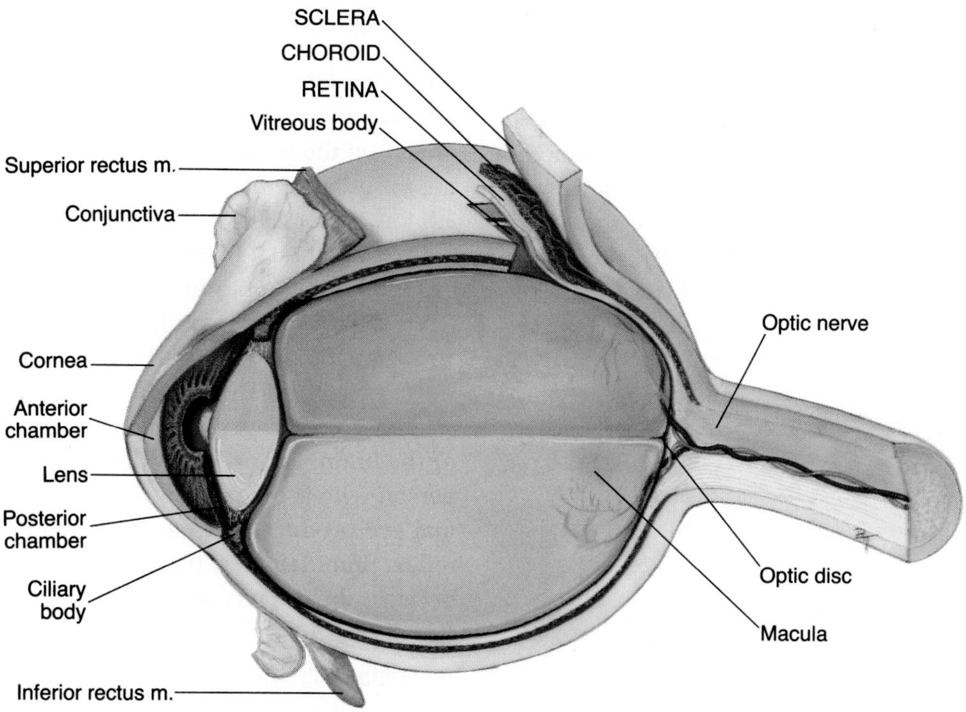

► **Figure 11-5**

area of sharpest and keenest vision. The macula looks slightly darker than the rest of the fundus.

VISUAL PATHWAYS AND VISUAL FIELDS

Objects reflect light. The light rays are refracted through the transparent media (cornea, aqueous humor, lens, and vitreous body), and strike the retina. The retina transforms the light stimulus into nerve impulses that are conducted through the optic nerve and the optic tract to the visual cortex of the occipital lobe.

The image formed on the retina is upside down and reversed from its actual appearance in the outside world (Fig. 11-7). That is, an object in the upper temporal visual field of the right eye reflects its image onto the

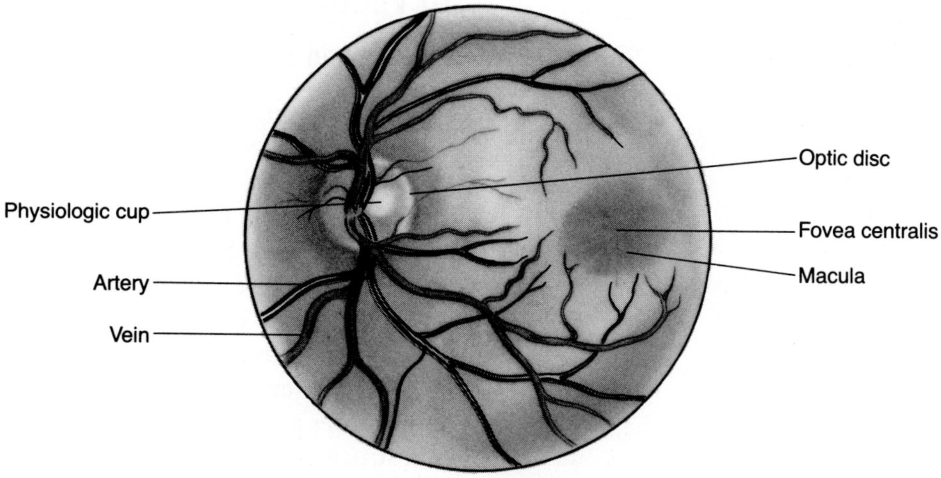

► **Figure 11-6**

lower nasal area of the retina. All retinal fibers collect to form the optic nerve but they maintain this same spatial arrangement, with nasal fibers running medially and temporal fibers running laterally.

At the optic chiasm, nasal fibers (from both temporal visual fields) cross over. The left optic tract now has fibers from the left half of each retina, and the right optic tract contains fibers only from the right. Thus the right side of the brain looks at the left side of the world.

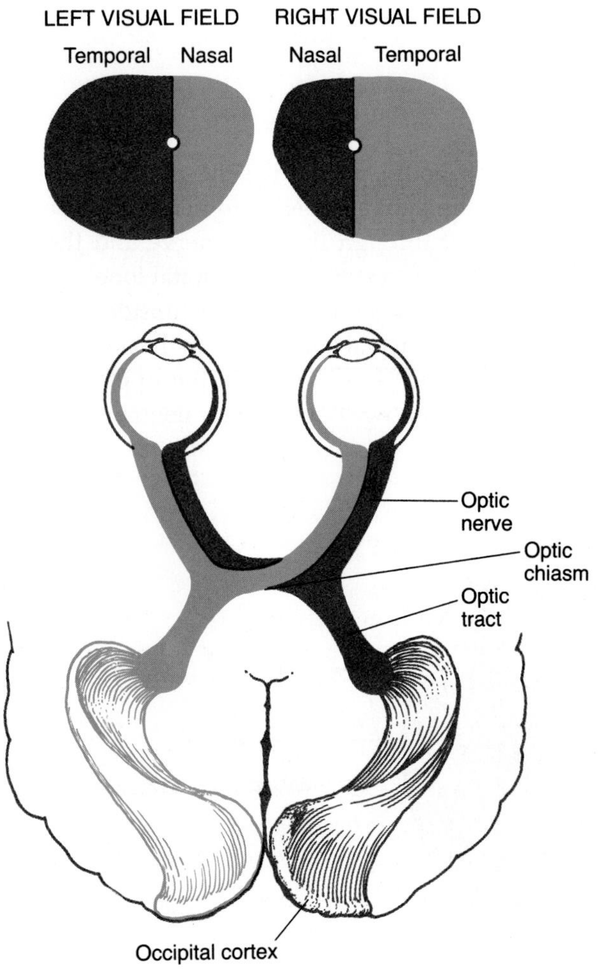

▶ **Figure 11-7**

VISUAL REFLEXES

Pupillary Light Reflex. The pupillary light reflex is the normal constriction of the pupils when bright light shines on the retina (Fig. 11-8). It is a subcortical reflex arc (i.e., there is no conscious control over it); the afferent link is cranial nerve II, the optic nerve, and the efferent path is cranial III, the oculomotor nerve. When one eye is exposed to bright light, a *direct light reflex* occurs (constriction of that pupil), as well as a *consensual light reflex* (simultaneous constriction of the other pupil). This happens because the optic nerve carries the sensory afferent message in and then synapses with both sides of the brain. For example, consider the light reflex in a person who is blind in one eye. Stimulation of the normal eye produces both a direct and a consensual light reflex. Stimulation of the blind eye causes no response because the sensory afferent in cranial nerve II is destroyed.

Fixation. This is a reflex direction of the eye toward an object attracting a person's attention. The image is fixed in the center of the visual field, the fovea centralis. Although this is a cortical reflex, it takes a strong conscious effort to avoid fixation.

Accommodation. This is adaptation of the eye for near vision. It is accomplished by increasing the curvature of the lens through movement of the ciliary muscles. Although the lens cannot be observed directly, the components of accommodation that can be observed are convergence of the axes of the eyeballs and pupillary constriction.

DEVELOPMENTAL CONSIDERATIONS

Infants and Children

At birth, eye function is limited but will mature fully during the early years (Table 11-1). Peripheral vision is intact in the newborn. The macula, the area of keenest vision, is absent at birth but is developing by 4 months and is mature by 8 months. Eye movements may be poorly coordinated at birth. By 3 to 4 months of age, the infant establishes binocularity and can fixate on a single image with both eyes simultaneously. Most neonates (80 percent) are born farsighted; this gradually decreases after age 7 to 8.

In structure, the eyeball reaches adult size by 8 years. At birth, the iris shows little pigment and the pupils are small. The lens is nearly spherical at birth, growing flat-

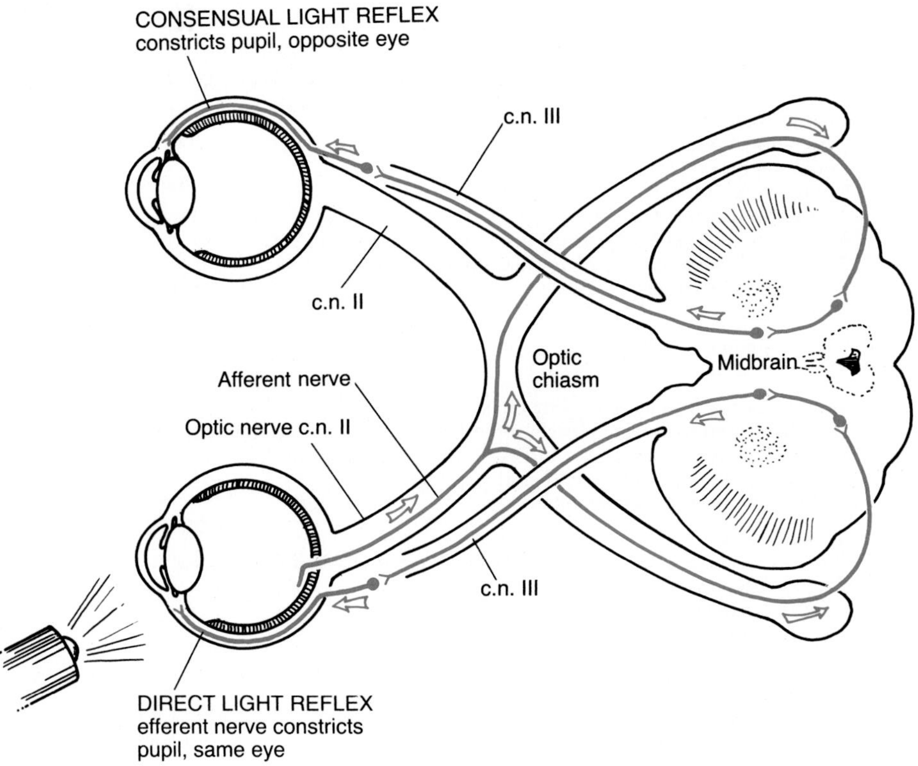

▶ **Figure 11-8**

ter throughout life. Its consistency changes from that of soft plastic at birth to rigid glass in old age.

The Aging Adult

Changes in eye structure contribute greatly to the distinct facial changes of the aging person. The skin loses its elasticity, causing wrinkling and drooping; fat tissues and muscles atrophy; and the external eye structures appear as on p. 340. Lacrimal glands involute, causing decreased tear production and a feeling of dryness and burning.

On the globe itself, the cornea may show an infiltration of degenerative lipid material around the limbus (see discussion of *arcus senilus,* p. 341). Pupil size decreases. The lens loses elasticity, becoming hard and glasslike. This glasslike quality decreases its ability to change shape in order to accommodate for near vision, and this condition is termed *presbyopia.* Almost all people experience presbyopia beginning around age 42 to 46 years (Vaughan, 1989). By age 70 years, the normally transparent fibers of the lens begin to thicken and yellow. This is nuclear sclerosis, or the beginning of a senile cataract.

Inside the globe, floaters appear in the vitreous due to deposits or exudates. Retinal structures are described on p. 342.

Visual acuity may diminish gradually after age 50 years, and even more so after age 70 years. Yet, central visual acuity remains good for most aging people, up to 85 percent of those to age 90 years (Rossman, 1986). Near vision is commonly affected owing to the decreased power of accommodation in the lens (presbyopia). As early as the fourth decade, a person may have blurred vision and difficulty reading. Also, the aging person needs more light to see because of a decreased adaptation to darkness, and this condition may affect the function of night driving.

In the aging population, the most common causes of decreased visual functioning are:

1. Cataract formation, or lens opacity. Some cataract formation should be expected by age 70. Studies indicate that everyone eventually develops cataracts if they live long enough (Rossman, 1986).

Table 11-1 ▶ Chronology of Visual Function

BIRTH	Moderate photophobia—usually keeps eyes closed Eyes blink in response to light Pupils miotic, do react to light Corneal reflex present Tear glands do not function In 75 percent of newborns, visual acuity approximates 20/300 Transitory fixation, usually monocular but binocular at times Pupils start to enlarge Tearing begins
2 TO 4 WEEKS	Some attending to bright light Some attending to near objects in line of vision with some following to midline
6 TO 12 WEEKS	Short binocular fixation to moving object 8 weeks—Alert to moving objects, although convergence and following are jerky 12 weeks—Follows with head and eye through 180 degrees Fascinated with light objects and bright colors Tear glands function with emotion
4 TO 5 MONTHS	Inspects hands One-inch test cubes stimulate immediate fixation if within 2 feet of eyes Central vision maturing. Acuity 20/200 Recognition of strangers yields shy response Fundus looks pale owing to absent pigmentation Macula area maturing, with fovea now distinguishable
5 TO 7 MONTHS	Color preference for bright reds and yellows Accommodation-convergence reflexes start to organize Hand-eye coordination developing Maintains voluntary fixation of stationary object Binocular fixation is well established Ultimate color of iris now apparent
9 TO 11 MONTHS	Depth perception beginning at 9 months Approaches small objects with extended index finger Hand preference begins Extends head to gaze upward
12 MONTHS	Pupils enlarged to midposition Central acuity close to 20/100 Fusion present but easily interrupted Amblyopia may develop with any loss of binocularity Discriminates geometric forms Stares intently at facial expressions
12 TO 18 MONTHS	Keen interest in pictures Can identify forms, associate simple visual experiences Able to crayon linear marks on paper
18 MONTHS	Convergence is well established Interpretation of spatial intervals immature, runs into objects
2 YEARS	Central acuity approaches 20/40 Fascinated with minute objects, which demands maturing of convergence and accommodation
3 YEARS	Central acuity close to 20/30 Convergence is now smoother Attention span fair—fixation with small pictures or toys approaches 50 seconds
4 YEARS	Acuity nearly 20/20 Lacrimal glands fully developed Reading readiness is present
5 YEARS	True depth perception is present Now only moderate risk for amblyopia Color recognition is well established
6 YEARS	Central acuity fully established Gross attention span extends to 20 minutes Detailed attention span lasts about 2 minutes Differentiates color shading

Adapted from Johnson TR, Moore WM, Jeffries JE (eds): Children Are Different: Developmental Physiology. 2nd ed. Columbus OH: Ross Laboratories, 1978, pp. 48–50. Reprinted with permission of Ross Laboratories, Columbus, OH 43216, from Children Are Different: Developmental Physiology, © 1978 Ross Laboratories.

2. Glaucoma, or increased ocular pressure. The incidence increases from age 45 to 60, then levels off. Chronic, open-angle glaucoma is the most common type and involves a gradual loss of peripheral vision. With acute, narrow-angle glaucoma, a person experiences sudden clouding of vision, sudden eye pain, and halos around lights. This condition requires emergency treatment to avoid permanent vision loss.
3. Macular degeneration. Loss of central vision, the area of clearest vision, affects 30 percent of those older than 65, and the percentage increases gradually with succeeding decades (Rossman, 1986). With this, the person is unable to read fine print, sew, or do fine work, and may have difficulty distinguishing faces. Depending on how much the lifestyle is oriented around activities requiring close work, loss of central vision may cause great distress. Peripheral vision is not affected, so the person can manage self-care and will not become completely disabled.

TRANSCULTURAL CONSIDERATIONS

Racial differences are evident in the palpebral fissures. Persons of Asian origins are often identified by their characteristic eyes, whereas the presence of narrowed palpebral fissures in non-Asian individuals may be diagnostic of a serious congenital anomaly, *Down syndrome.*

There is culturally based variability in the color of the iris and in retinal pigmentation, with darker irides having darker retinas behind them (Hoffman, 1975). Individuals with light retinas generally have better night vision but can suffer pain in an environment that has too much light. One needs to be sensitive to the illumination of rooms and to the discomfort that bright lights might cause (Overfield, 1985).

SUBJECTIVE DATA

Vision difficulty (decreased acuity, blurring, blind spots)

Pain

Strabismus, diplopia

Redness, swelling

Watering, discharge

Past history of ocular problems

Glaucoma

Does the person wear glasses or contact lenses

Self-care behaviors

EXAMINER ASKS:	RATIONALE:
1. Do you have any **difficulty seeing?** Has this come on suddenly, or did it progress slowly? Is this problem in one eye or both? Do you have any blurring? Does it occur in both eyes or just one? Is it constant, or does it come and go? Do objects appear out of focus, or does it feel like a clouding over objects? Does it feel like "grayness" of vision?	
Do spots move in front of your eyes, called "floaters" or "flashes"? How many? One or many? Does this occur in one or both eyes?	Floaters are common sensation with myopia or after middle age owing to condensed vitreous fibers. Usually, they are not significant.
Have you ever noticed a halo/rainbows around objects? Or rings around lights?	Halos around lights occur with acute narrow-angle glaucoma.

EXAMINER ASKS:	RATIONALE:
Do you have any blind spots? Does it move as you shift your gaze? Have you noted any loss of peripheral vision?	*Scotoma* is a blind spot in the visual field surrounded by an area of normal or decreased vision. This occurs with glaucoma and with optic nerve and visual pathway disorders.
Any night blindness?	Night blindness occurs with optic atrophy, glaucoma, or vitamin A deficiency.
2. Do you have any **eye pain?** Please describe. Did this come on suddenly?	Note: Consider *sudden onset* of eye symptoms or vision change (pain, floaters, blind spot, loss of peripheral vision) as a possible emergency. Refer immediately.
What is the quality of the pain? Would you say, burning or itching?	Quality may be valuable diagnostic indicator.
Or, sharp, stabbing pain or pain with bright light? Is it a foreign body sensation? Or, deep, aching? Or, headache in brow area?	*Photophobia* is the inability to tolerate light. (Note: some common eye diseases cause no pain, e.g., refractive errors, cataract, glaucoma.)
3. Do you have a history of crossed eyes? Now or in the past? Does this occur with eye fatigue?	**Strabismus** is a deviation in the anteroposterior axis of the eye.
Do you ever see double? Is this constant, or does it come and go? Does this occur in one eye or when both are open?	**Diplopia** is the perception of two images of a single object.
4. Do you have any **redness** or **swelling** in the eyes? Any infections? Now or in the past? When do these occur? Do they recur in a particular time of year? Are they seasonal?	
5. Do you have any **watering,** or excessive tearing?	Lacrimation (tearing) and epiphora (excessive tearing) are due to irritants or obstruction in drainage of tears.
Do you have any **discharge?** Any matter in the eyes? Is it hard to open your eyes in the morning? What color is the discharge?	Purulent discharge is thick and yellow colored. Crusts form at night.
How do you remove matter from eyes?	Assess hygiene practices and knowledge of cross-contamination.
6. Is there any **past history** of injury or surgery to eye? Or, any history of allergies?	Allergens may cause irritation of conjunctiva or cornea, e.g., make-up, contact lens solution.
7. Have you ever been tested for **glaucoma?** What were the results? Is there any family history of glaucoma?	Glaucoma is an eye disease characterized by increased intraocular pressure.
8. Do you wear **glasses** or **contact lenses?** How do they work for you? Are you able to function as you would like all day? When was the last time your prescription was checked? Was it changed? If you wear contact lenses, are there any problems such as pain, photophobia, watering, or swelling?	
How do you care for contacts? How long do you wear them? How do you clean them? Do you remove them for certain activities?	Assess self-care behaviors.

EXAMINER ASKS:	RATIONALE:

9. Have you ever had your vision tested? Who tested it?
Have you ever been tested for color vision?
Are there any environmental conditions at home or at work that may affect your eyes? For example, flying sparks, metal bits, smoke, dust, chemical fumes? If so, do you wear goggles to protect your eyes?

Self care behaviors for eyes and vision.

Ocular diseases or injuries may be work related, e.g., an auto mechanic with a foreign body from metal working.

10. What medications are you taking? Is that systemic or topical? Do you take any medication specifically for the eyes?

Some medications have ocular side effects, e.g., prednisone may cause cataracts or increased intraocular pressure.

11. If you have experienced a vision loss, how do you cope? Do you have books with large print, books on audio tape, Braille?
Do you maintain living environment the same?
Do you sometimes fear complete loss of vision?

A constant spatial layout eases navigation through the home.

ADDITIONAL QUESTIONS FOR INFANTS AND CHILDREN

Were there any vaginal infections in the mother at time of delivery?

Certain forms of vaginitis (gonorrhea, genital herpes) have ocular sequelae for the newborn.

Considering age of child, which developmental milestones of vision have you (parent) noted?

Studies indicate the parent is most often the one to detect vision problems.

Does the child have routine vision testing at school?
Are you (parent) aware of safety measures to protect child's eye from trauma? Do you inspect toys? Have you taught the child safe care of sharp objects, and how to carry and how to use them?

ADDITIONAL QUESTIONS FOR THE AGING ADULT

Have you noticed any visual difficulty with climbing stairs or driving?

Any loss of depth perception.

When was the last time you were tested for glaucoma? Have you noted any aching pain around eyes? Any loss of peripheral vision?
If you have glaucoma, how do you manage your eyedrops?

Assess compliance; it may be a problem if symptoms are absent. Assess ability to administer eyedrops.

Do you have any problem with night vision?
Is there a history of cataracts? Have you noted any loss or progressive blurring of vision?
Do your eyes ever feel dry? burning? What do you do for this?

Decreased tear production may occur with aging.

OBJECTIVE DATA

Equipment Needed

Snellen eye chart
Handheld visual screener
Opaque card or occluder
Penlight
Applicator stick
Ophthalmoscope

PREPARATION

Position the person sitting up with the head at your eye level.

METHOD OF EXAMINATION

NORMAL RANGE OF FINDINGS	ABNORMAL FINDINGS

CENTRAL VISUAL ACUITY

Test visual acuity

Snellen Eye Chart. The Snellen alphabet chart is the most commonly used and accurate measure of visual acuity. It has lines of letters arranged in decreasing size.

Place the Snellen chart in a well-lit spot at eye level. Position the person on a mark exactly 20 feet from the chart. Hand the person an opaque card with which to shield one eye at a time during the test; inadvertent peeking may result when shielding the eye with the person's own fingers (Fig. 11–9). If the person wears glasses or contact lenses, leave them on. Remove only reading glasses because they will blur distance vision. Ask the person to read through the chart to the smallest line of letters possible. Encourage the person to try the next smallest line also. (Note: use a Snellen "E" chart for people who cannot read letters. See p. 336).

Abnormal findings: Hesitancy, squinting, leaning forward, misreading letters.

Record the result using the numeric fraction at the end of the last successful line read. Indicate whether or not the person missed any letters or if corrective lenses were worn, e.g., "O.D.* 20/30 −1, with glasses."

Normal visual acuity is 20/20. Contrary to some people's impression, the numeric fraction is *not* a percentage of normal vision. Instead, the top number (numerator) indicates the distance the person is standing from the chart, while the denominator gives the distance at which a normal eye

Abnormal findings: The larger the denominator, the poorer the vision. If vision is poorer than 20/30, refer the person to an ophthalmologist or optometrist. Impaired vision may be

* O.D., oculus dexter, or right eye.

NORMAL RANGE OF FINDINGS

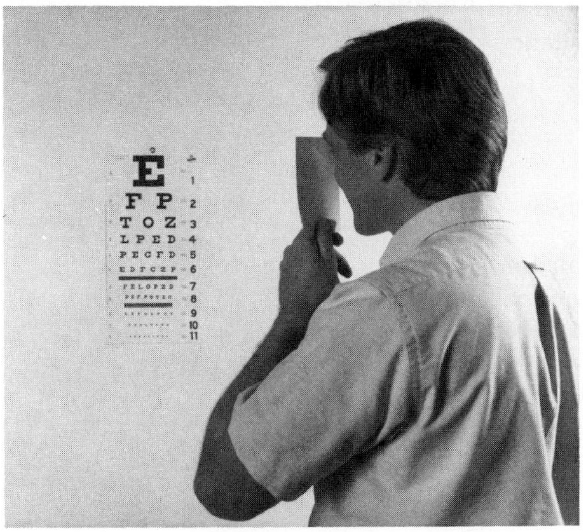

► **Figure 11-9**

could have read that particular line. Thus "20/20" means, "You can read at 20 feet what the normal eye could have read at 20 feet."

If the person is unable to see even the largest letters, shorten the distance to the chart until it is seen and record that distance, e.g., "10/200." If there is even less visual acuity, assess if the person can count your fingers when they are spread in front of the eyes or distinguish light perception using your penlight.

Near Vision. For people over 40 years of age or for those who report increasing difficulty reading, test near vision using a handheld vision screener with various sizes of print (e.g., a Jaeger card) (Fig. 11-10). Hold the card in good light about 35 cm (14 inches) from the eye—this distance

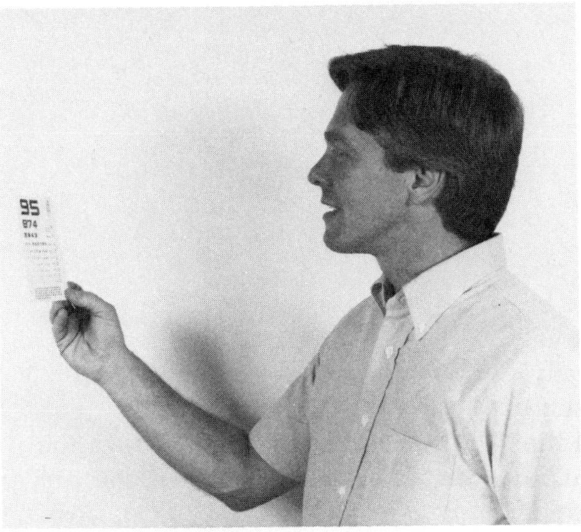

► **Figure 11-10**

ABNORMAL FINDINGS

due to refractive error, opacity in the media (cornea, lens, vitreous), or disorder in the retina or optic pathway.

Presbyopia, the decrease in power of accommodation with aging, is suggested when the card is moved farther away.

NORMAL RANGE OF FINDINGS | **ABNORMAL FINDINGS**

equals the print size on the 20 foot chart. Test each eye separately, with glasses on. A normal result is "14/14" in each eye, read without hesitancy and without moving the card closer or farther away.

VISUAL FIELDS

Test visual fields

Confrontation Test. This is a gross measure of peripheral vision. It compares the person's peripheral vision with your own, assuming yours is normal (Fig. 11–11). Position yourself at eye level with the person, about 2 feet away. Direct the person to cover one eye with an opaque card, and with the other eye to look straight at you. Hold a pencil or your finger midline between you and the other person, and slowly advance it in from the periphery in several directions.

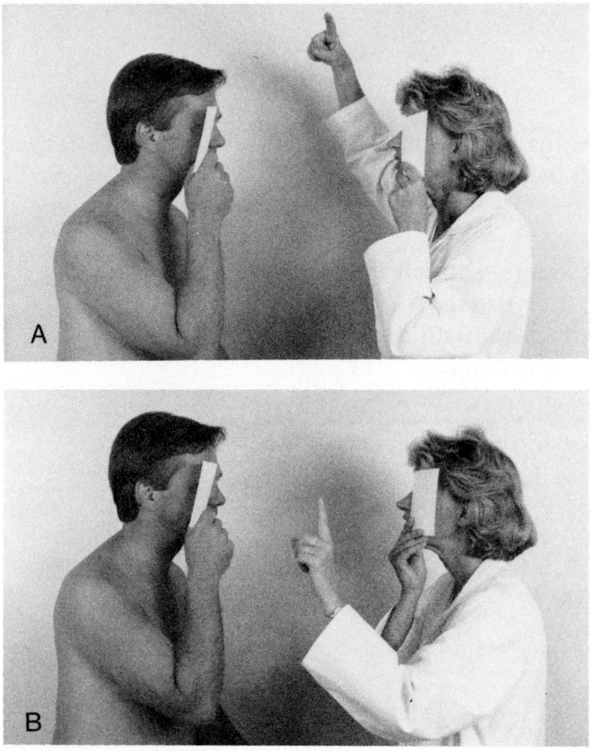

► **Figure 11–11**

Ask the person to say "Now" as the object is first seen; this should be just as you see the object also. (This works with all but the temporal visual field, with which you would need a 6-foot arm to avoid being seen initially! With the temporal direction, start the object somewhat behind the person.) Estimate the angle between the anteroposterior axis of the eye and the peripheral axis where the object is first seen. Normal results are about 50 degrees upward, 90 degrees temporal, 70 degrees down, and 60 degrees nasal (Fig. 11–12).

If the person is unable to see the object as examiner does, the test suggests peripheral field loss. Refer the person for more precise testing using a tangent screen (see Table 11–2).

NORMAL RANGE OF FINDINGS	ABNORMAL FINDINGS

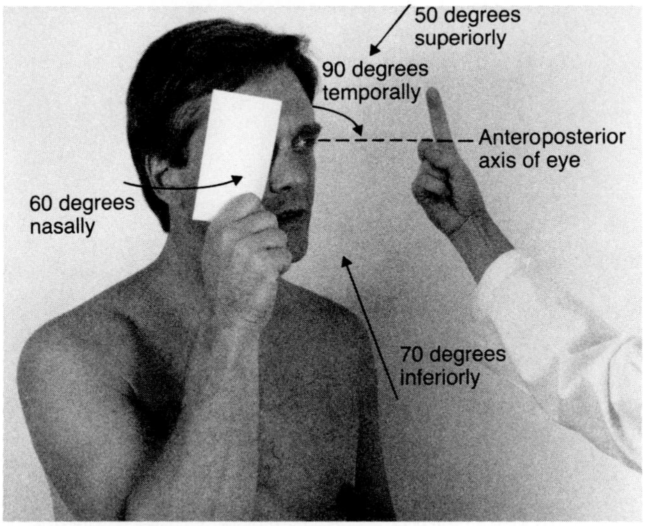

Range of peripheral vision

► **Figure 11-12**

EXTRAOCULAR MUSCLE FUNCTION

Inspect extraocular muscle function

Corneal Light Reflex (The Hirschberg Test). Assess the parallel alignment of the eye axes by shining a light toward the person's eyes. Direct the person to stare straight ahead as you hold the light about 30 cm (12 inches) away. Note the reflection of the light on the corneas; it should be in exactly the same spot on each eye. See Figure 11-28 for symmetry of the corneal light reflex.

Asymmetry of the light reflex indicates deviation in alignment due to eye muscle weakness or paralysis. If noted, perform the cover test.

Cover Test. This test detects small degrees of deviated alignment by interrupting the fusion reflex that normally keeps the two eyes parallel. Ask the person to stare straight ahead at your nose even though the gaze may be interrupted. With an opaque card, cover one eye. As it is covered, note the uncovered eye. A normal response is a steady fixed gaze (Fig. 11-13*A*).

If the eye jumps to fixate on the designated point, it was out of alignment before.

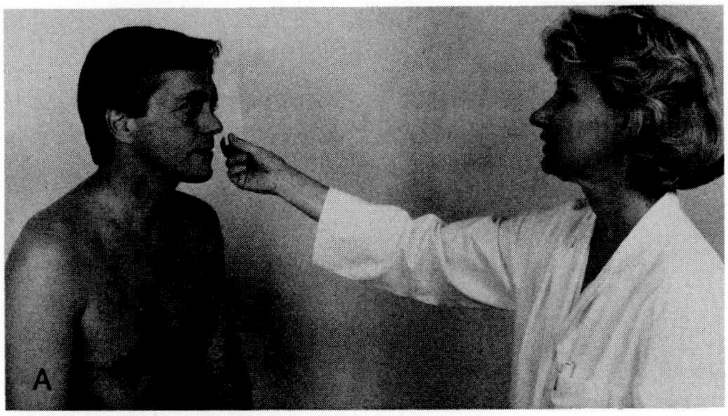

► **Figure 11-13*A***

NORMAL RANGE OF FINDINGS	ABNORMAL FINDINGS

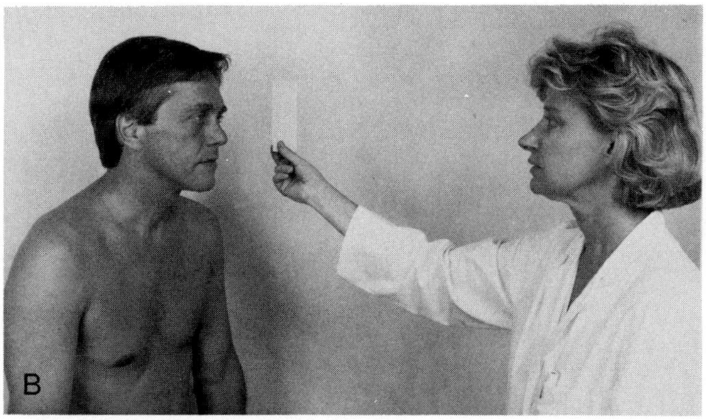

► Figure 11–13*B*

Meanwhile, the macular image has been suppressed on the covered eye. If muscle weakness exists, the covered eye will drift into a relaxed position. Now uncover the eye and observe it for movement. It should stare straight ahead (Fig. 11–13*B*). If it jumps to re-establish fixation, eye muscle weakness exists. Repeat with the other eye.

A *phoria* is a mild weakness noted only when fusion is blocked. *Tropia* is more severe, a constant malalignment of the eyes (see Table 11–3).

Diagnostic Positions Test. Leading the eyes through the six cardinal positions of gaze will elicit any muscle weakness during movement (Fig. 11–14). Ask the person to hold the head steady and to follow the movement of your finger, pen, or penlight only with the eyes. Hold the object back about 12 inches so the person can focus on it comfortably, and move it to each of the six positions, hold it momentarily, then back to center. Progress clockwise. A normal response is parallel tracking of the object with both eyes.

Eye movement is not parallel. Failure to follow in a certain direction indicates weakness of an extraocular muscle (EOM) or dysfunction of cranial nerve innervating it.

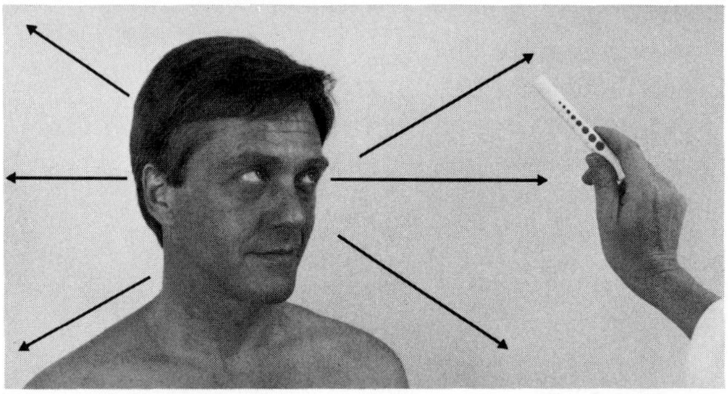

► Figure 11–14

In addition to parallel movement, note any *nystagmus,* a fine oscillating movement best seen around the iris. Mild nystagmus at extreme lateral gaze is normal; nystagmus at any other position is not. Finally, note that the upper eyelid continues to overlap the superior part of the iris, even during downward movement. You should not see a white rim of sclera between the lid and the iris. If noted, this is termed "lid lag."

Nystagmus.

Lid lag occurs with hyperthyroidism.

NORMAL RANGE OF FINDINGS	ABNORMAL FINDINGS

EXTERNAL OCULAR STRUCTURES

Inspect external eye structures

Begin with the most external points, and logically work your way inward.

General. Already you will have noted the person's ability to move around the room, with vision functioning well enough to avoid obstacles, and respond to your directions. Also note the facial expression; a relaxed expression accompanies adequate vision.

Groping with hands.

Squinting or craning forward.

Eyebrows. Normally the eyebrows are present bilaterally, move symmetrically as the facial expression changes, and have no scaling or lesions.

Absent lateral third of hair with hypothyroidism.
Unequal or absent movement with nerve damage.
Scaling with seborrhea.

Eyelids and Lashes. The upper lids normally overlap the superior part of the iris, and approximate completely with the lower lids when closed. The skin is intact without redness, swelling, discharge, or lesions.

Lid lag with hyperthyroidism.
Incomplete closure creates risk for corneal damage.

The palpebral fisures are horizontal in non-Asians, whereas Asians normally have an upward slant.

Ptosis, drooping of upper lid.
Periorbital edema, lesions (see Tables 11–4 and 11–5).

Note that the eyelashes are evenly distributed along the lid margins, and curve outward.

Ectropion and entropion (see Table 11–4).

Eyeballs. The eyeballs are aligned normally in their sockets with no protrusion or sunken appearance. Blacks normally may have a slight protrusion of the eyeball beyond the supraorbital ridge.

Exophthalmos, protruding eyes and enophthalmos, sunken eyes (see Table 11–4).

Conjunctiva and Sclera. Ask the person to look up. Using your thumbs, slide the lower lids down along the bony orbital rim. Take care not to push against the eyeball. Inspect the exposed area (Fig. 11–15). The eyeball

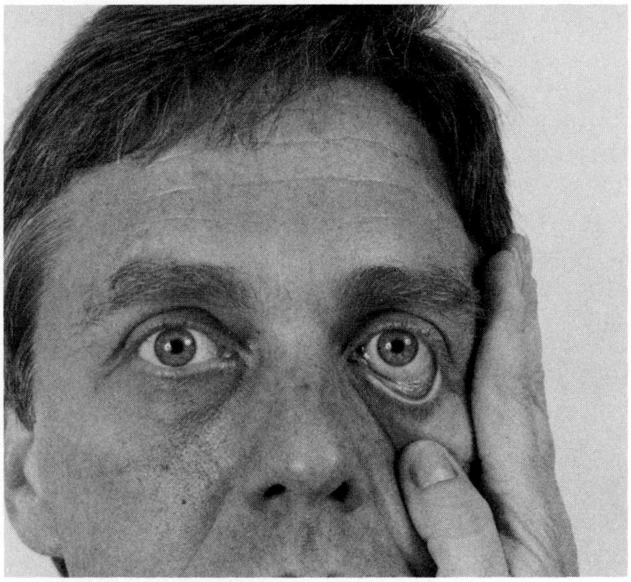

▶ **Figure 11–15**

NORMAL RANGE OF FINDINGS	ABNORMAL FINDINGS
looks moist and glossy. Numerous small blood vessels normally show through the transparent conjunctiva. Otherwise, the conjunctivae are clear and show the normal color of the structure below—pink over the lower lids, and white over the sclera. Note any color change, swelling, or lesions.	General reddening (injected) (see Table 11–6). Cyanosis of the lower lids. Pallor near the outer canthus of the lower lid may indicate anemia (the inner canthus normally contains less pigment).
Blacks occasionally have a gray-blue or "muddy" color to the sclera. Also in dark-skinned people, you normally may see small brown macules (like freckles) on the sclera, which should not be confused with foreign bodies or petechiae. Lastly, blacks may have yellowish fatty deposits beneath the lids away from the cornea. Do not confuse these yellow spots with the overall scleral yellowing that accompanies jaundice.	*Scleral icterus* is a yellowing of the sclera extending up to the cornea, indicating jaundice. Tenderness, foreign body, discharge, or lesions.

Eversion of the Upper Lid. This maneuver is not part of the normal examination, but it is useful when you must inspect the conjunctiva of the upper lid, as with eye pain or suspicion of a foreign body. Most people are apprehensive of any eye manipulation. Enhance their cooperation by using a calm and gentle, yet deliberate, approach.

1. Ask the person to look down. This relaxes the eyelid, whereas closing it would tense the orbicularis muscle.
2. Slide the upper lid up along the bony orbit to lift up the eyelashes.
3. Grasp the lashes between your thumb and forefinger and gently pull down and outward.
4. With your other hand, place the tip of an applicator stick on the upper lid above the level of the internal tarsal plates (Fig. 11–16).

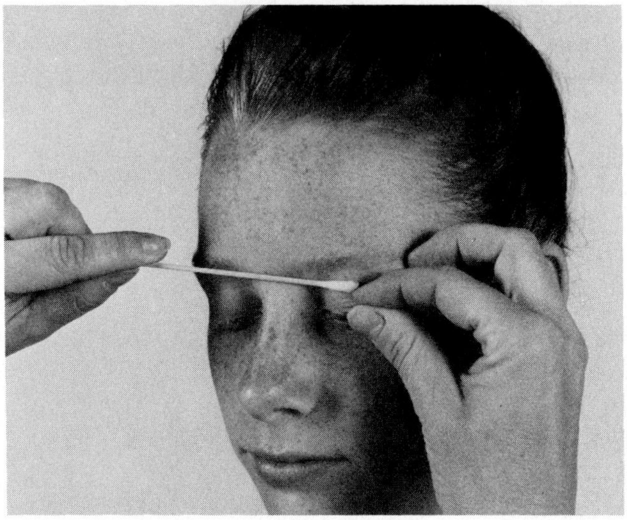

► **Figure 11–16**

5. Gently push down with the stick as you lift the lashes up. This flips the lid inside out. Take special care not to push in on the eyeball.
6. Secure the everted position by holding the lashes against the bony orbital rim (Fig. 11–17).

NORMAL RANGE OF FINDINGS | **ABNORMAL FINDINGS**

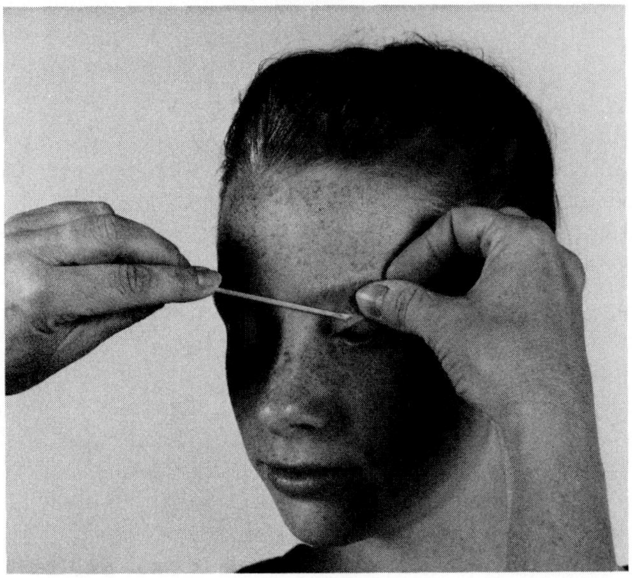

► **Figure 11–17**

7. Inspect for any color change, swelling, lesion, or foreign body.
8. To return to normal position, gently pull the lashes outward as the person looks up.

Lacrimal Apparatus. Ask the person to look down. With your thumbs, slide the outer part of the upper lid up along the bony orbit. Inspect for any redness or swelling.

Swelling of the lacrimal gland may show as a visible bulge in the outer part of the upper lid.

Normally, the puncta drain the tears into the lacrimal sac. Presence of excessive tearing may indicate blockage of the nasolacrimal duct. Check this by pressing the index finger against the sac, just inside the lower orbital rim, not against the side of the nose (Fig. 11–18). Pressure will slightly evert the lower lid, but there should be no other response to pressure.

Puncta red, swollen, tender to pressure.

Watch for any regurgitation out of the puncta, which confirms duct blockage.

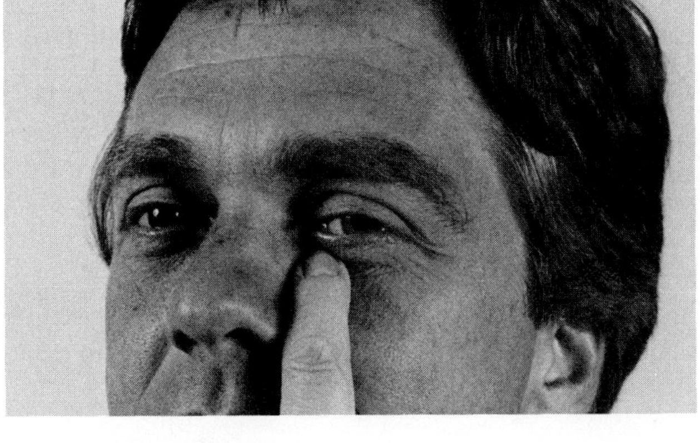

► **Figure 11–18**

NORMAL RANGE OF FINDINGS	ABNORMAL FINDINGS

ANTERIOR EYEBALL STRUCTURES

Inspect anterior eyeball structures

Cornea and Lens. Shine a light from the side across the cornea, and check for smoothness and clarity. This oblique view highlights any abnormal irregularities in the corneal surface. There should be no opacities (cloudiness) in the cornea, anterior chamber, or in the lens behind the pupil. Do not confuse an *arcus senilis* with an opacity. This is a normal finding in aging persons and is illustrated on p. 341.

Abnormal: A corneal abrasion causes irregular ridges in reflected light, producing a shattered look to light rays (see Table 11–7).

Iris and Pupils. The iris normally appears flat, with a round regular shape and even coloration. Normally the pupils appear round, regular, and of equal size in both eyes. In the adult, resting size is from 3 to 5 mm. A small number of people (5 percent) normally have pupils of two different sizes, termed *anisocoria.*

Abnormal: Irregular shape.

Although they may be normal, all unequally sized pupils call for a consideration of central nervous system injury.

To test the **pupillary light reflex,** darken the room and ask the person to gaze into the distance. (This dilates the pupils.) Advance a light in from the side* and note the response. Normally you will see (1) constriction of the same sided pupil (a *direct light reflex*) and (2) simultaneous constriction of the other pupil (a *consensual light reflex*).

Abnormal: Dilated pupils.
Dilated and fixed pupils.
Constricted pupils.
Unequal or no response to light (see Table 11–9).

In the acute care setting, gauge the pupil size in millimeters, both before and after the light reflex. Recording the pupil size in millimeters is more accurate when many nurses and physicians care for the same person, or when small changes may be significant signs of increasing intracranial pressure. Normally, the resting size is 3, 4, or 5 mm, and decreases equally in response to light. A normal response is designated by

$$R\,\frac{3}{1} = \frac{3}{1}\,L.$$

This indicates that both pupils measure 3 mm in the resting state and both constrict to 1 mm in response to light. A graduated scale printed on a handheld vision screener or taped onto a tongue blade facilitates your measurement (see Fig. 20–56).

Test for **accommodation** by asking the person to focus on a distant object (Fig. 11–19). This process dilates the pupils. Then have the person shift the gaze to a near object, such as your finger held about 7 to 8 cm (3 in) from the nose. A normal response includes (1) pupillary constriction and (2) convergence of the axes of the eyes.

Abnormal: Absence of constriction or convergence.
Asymmetric response.

Record the normal response to all these maneuvers as PERRLA, or *P*upils *E*qual, *R*ound, *R*eact to *L*ight and *A*ccommodation.

---

* Always advance the light in from the *side* to test the light reflex. If you advance from the front, the pupils will constrict to accommodate for near vision. Thus you do not know what the pure response to the light would have been.

NORMAL RANGE OF FINDINGS | ABNORMAL FINDINGS

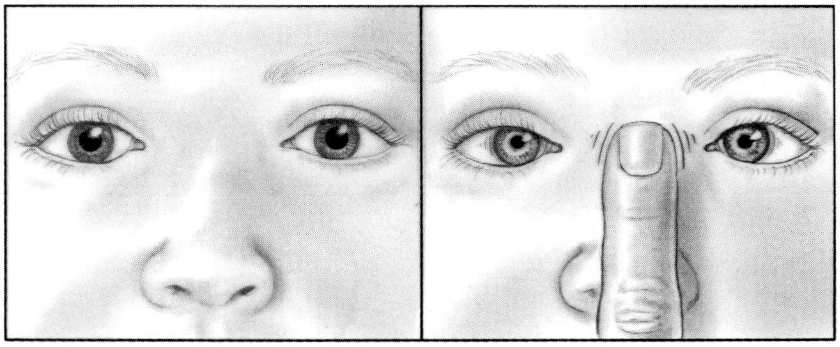

▶ **Figure 11-19**

THE OCULAR FUNDUS

Inspect the ocular fundus

The ophthalmoscope enlarges your view of the eye so that you can inspect the media (anterior chamber, lens, vitreous) and the ocular fundus (the internal surface of the retina). It accomplishes this by directing a beam of light through the pupil to illuminate the inner structures. Thus using the ophthalmoscope is like peering through a keyhole (the pupil) into an interesting room beyond.

The ophthalmoscope should function as an appendage of your own eye. This takes some practice. Practice holding the instrument and focusing at objects around the room before you approach a "real" person. Hold the ophthalmoscope right up to your eye, braced firmly against the cheek and brow. Extend your index finger onto the lens selector dial so that you can refocus as needed during the procedure without taking your head away from the ophthalmoscope to look. Now, look about the room, moving your head and the instrument together, as one unit. Keep both your eyes open; just view the field through the ophthalmoscope.

Recall that the ophthalmoscope contains a set of lenses that control the focus (Fig. 11-20). The unit of strength of each lens is the *diopter*. The black numbers indicate a positive diopter; they focus on objects nearer in space to the ophthalmoscope. The red numbers show a negative diopter and are for focusing on objects farther away.

To examine a person, darken the room to help dilate the pupils. (Dilating eyedrops are not needed during a screening examination. When indicated, they dilate the pupils for a wider look at the fundus background and macular area. Eyedrops are used only when glaucoma can be completely ruled out, because dilating the pupils in the presence of glaucoma

NORMAL RANGE OF FINDINGS | **ABNORMAL FINDINGS**

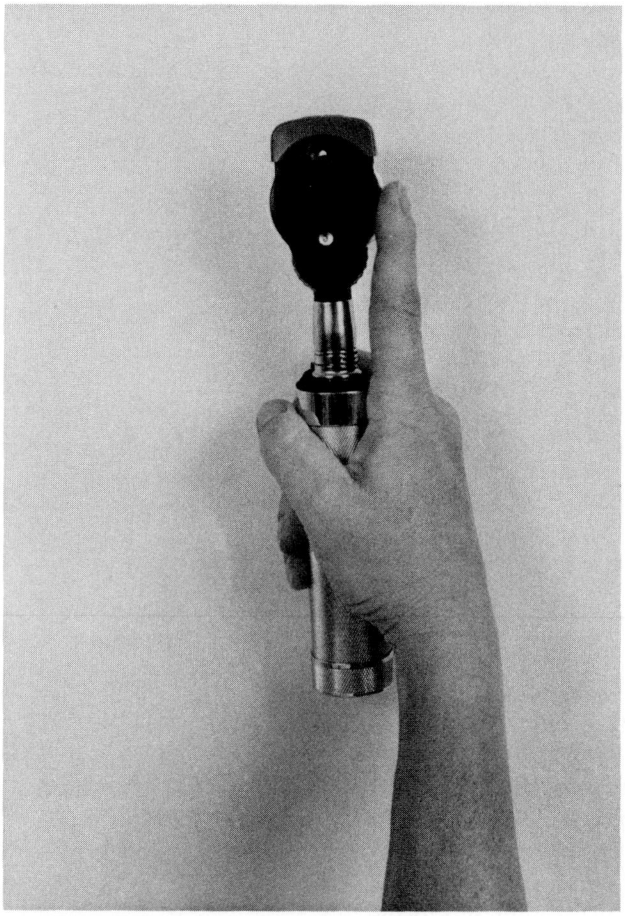

► **Figure 11-20**

can precipitate an acute episode.) Remove eyeglasses from yourself or the other person; they obstruct close movement and you can compensate for their correction by using the diopter setting. Contact lenses may be left in; they pose no problem as long as they are clean.

Select the large round aperture with the white light for the routine examination. If the pupils are small, use the smaller white light. (Although the instrument has other shape and colored apertures, these are rarely used in a screening examination.) The light must have maximum brightness; replace old or dim batteries.

Tell the person, "Please keep looking at that light switch (or mark) on the wall across the room, even though my head will get in the way." Staring at a distant fixed object helps to dilate the pupils and to hold the retinal structures still.

Match sides with the person. That is, hold the ophthalmoscope in your *right* hand up to your *right* eye to view the person's *right* eye. You must do this to avoid bumping noses during the procedure. Place your free hand on the person's shoulder or forehead (Fig. 11-21*A*). This helps

NORMAL RANGE OF FINDINGS | **ABNORMAL FINDINGS**

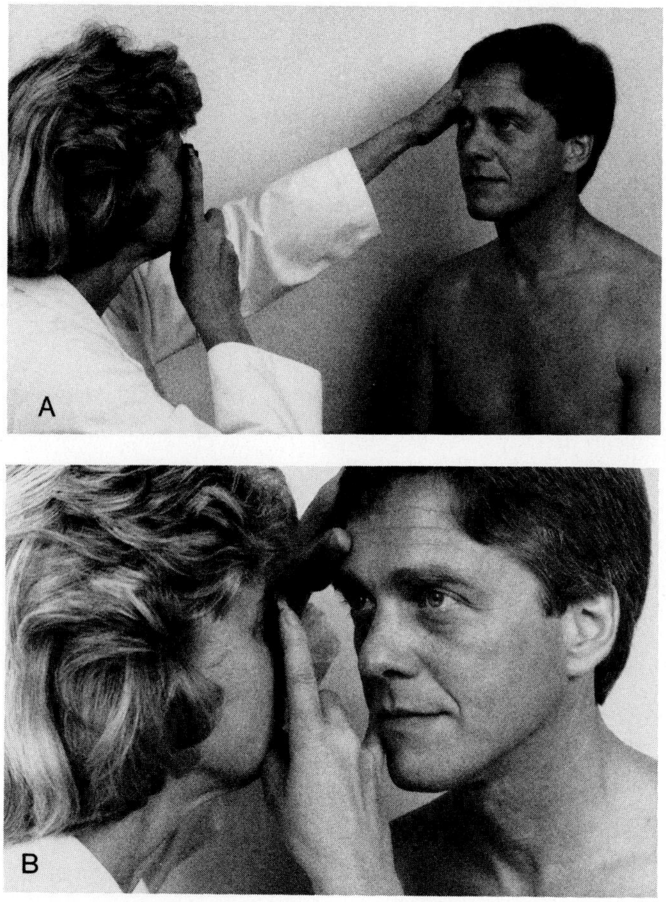

► **Figure 11-21**

orient you in space, because once you have the ophthalmoscope in position, you only have a very narrow range of vision.

Begin about 25 cm (10 inches) away from the person at an angle about 15 degrees lateral to the person's line of vision. Note the red glow filling the person's pupil. This is the *red reflex,* caused by the reflection of your ophthalmoscope light off the inner retina. Keep sight of the red reflex, and steadily move closer to the eye. If you lose the red reflex, the light has wandered off the pupil and onto the iris or sclera. Adjust your angle to find it again.

As you advance, adjust the lens to +6 and note any opacities in the media. These appear as dark shadows or black dots interrupting the red reflex. Normally, there are none.

Progress toward the person until your foreheads almost touch (Fig. 11-21*B*). Adjust the diopter setting to bring the ocular fundus into sharp focus. If you and the person have normal vision, this should be at 0. Moving the diopters compensates for nearsightedness or farsightedness. Use the red lenses for nearsighted eyes and the black for farsighted eyes (Fig. 11-22).

NORMAL RANGE OF FINDINGS	ABNORMAL FINDINGS

NORMAL EYE

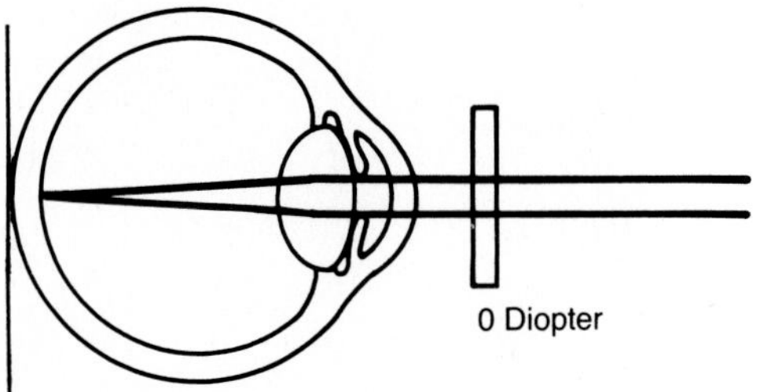

The person's eye and your eye are normal. The 0 diopter (clear glass) will focus sharply on the retina

MYOPIA (nearsighted)

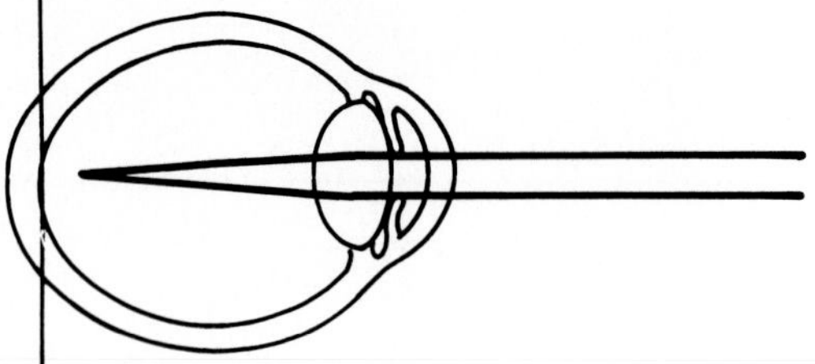

In myopia, the globe is longer than normal and light rays focus in *front* of the retina

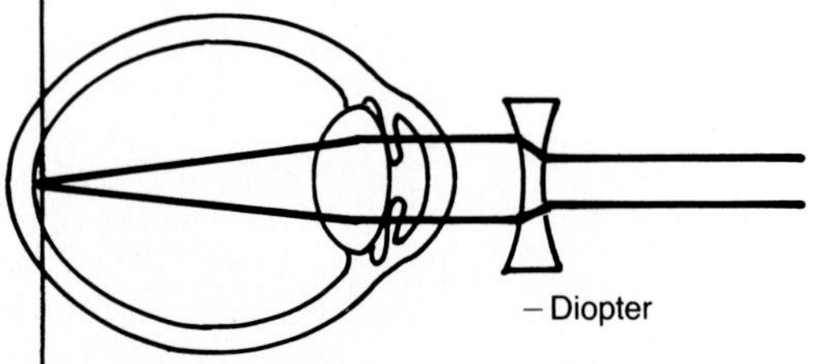

Compensate for myopia in yourself or the client by using a negative diopter (red or concave lens). This corrects the focal point onto the retina

HYPEROPIA (farsighted)

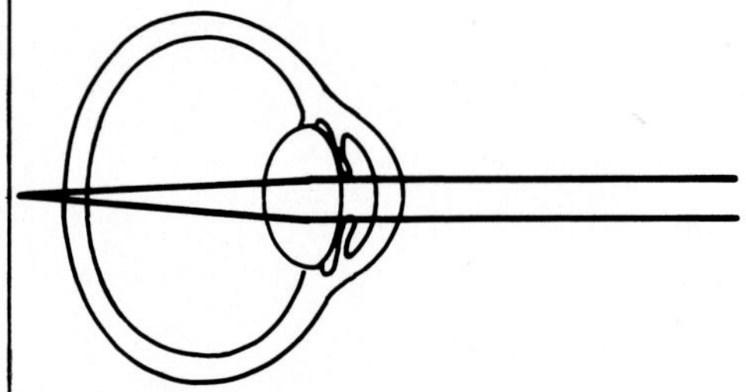

In hyperopia, the globe is shorter than normal. Light rays would focus behind the retina (if they could pass through)

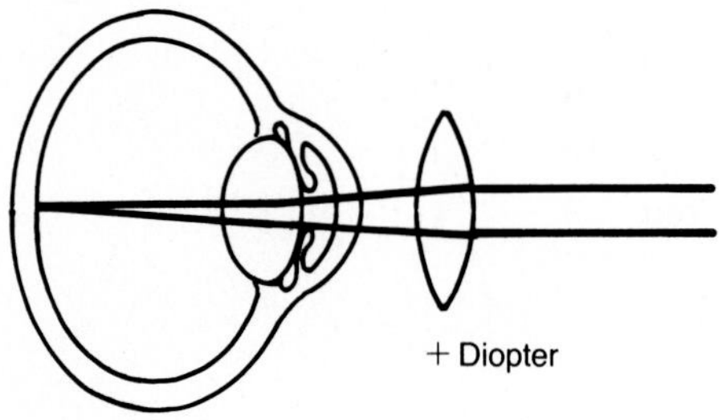

Compensate for hyperopia by using a positive diopter (black or convex lens). This bends the light rays so the focal point is on the retina

► **Figure 11–22**

NORMAL RANGE OF FINDINGS

ABNORMAL FINDINGS

Moving in on the 15-degree lateral line should bring your view just to the optic disc. If the disc is not in sight, track a blood vessel as it grows larger and it will lead you to the disc. Systematically inspect the structures in the ocular fundus: (1) optic disc, (2) retinal vessels, (3) general background, and (4) macula (Fig. 11–23). (Note the illustration here shows a large area of the fundus. Your actual view through the ophthalmoscope is much smaller, slightly larger than 1 disc diameter.)

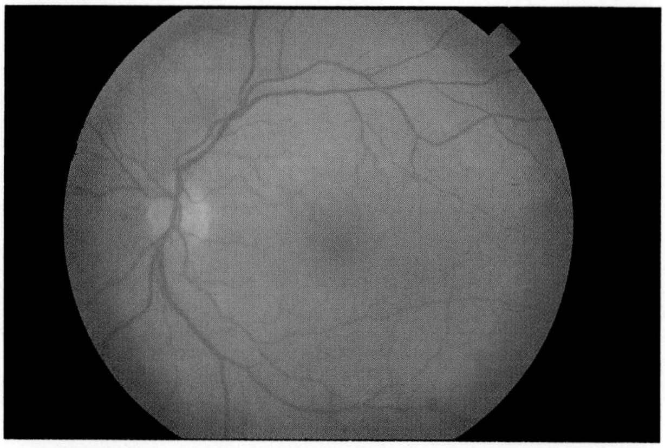

▸ **Figure 11–23 Normal ocular fundus**

Optic Disc. The most prominent landmark is the optic disc, located on the nasal side of the retina. Explore these characteristics:

	Normal	Abnormal
1. Color	Creamy yellow-orange to pink.	Pallor. Hyperemia.
2. Shape	Round or oval.	Irregular.
3. Margins	Distinct and sharply demarcated, though the nasal edge may be slightly fuzzy.	Blurred margins.
4. Cup disc ratio	Distinctness varies. When visible, physiologic cup is a brighter yellow-white than rest of the disc. Its width is not more than one-half the disc diameter.	Cup extending to the disc border (see Table 11–11).

Two normal variations may occur around the disc margins. A *scleral crescent* is a gray-white new moon shape (Fig. 11–24). It occurs when pigment

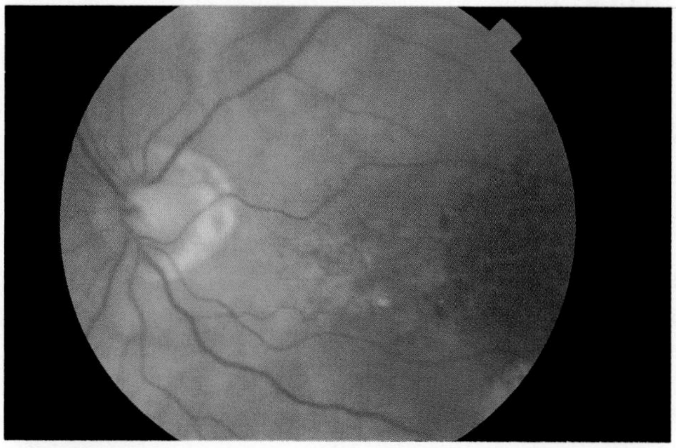

▸ **Figure 11–24 Scleral crescent and drusen**

NORMAL RANGE OF FINDINGS	ABNORMAL FINDINGS

is absent in the choroid layer and you are looking directly at the sclera. A *pigment crescent* is black, and is due to accumulation of pigment in the choroid.

The diameter of the disc, or DD, is a standard of measure for other fundus structures (Fig. 11–25). To describe a finding, note its clock-face position as well as its relationship to the disc in size and distance, e.g., ". . . at 5:00, 3 DD from the disc."

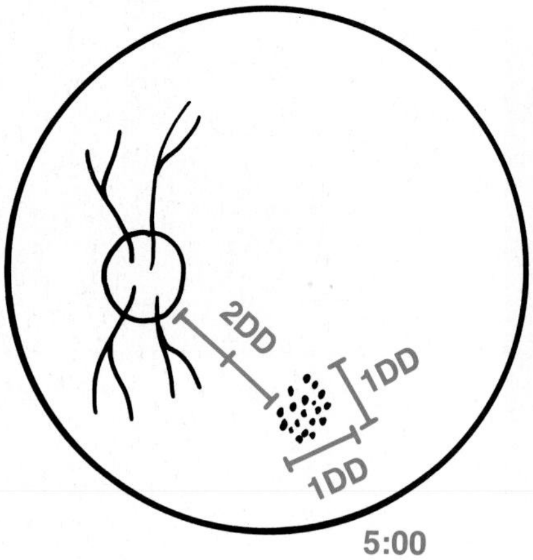

► **Figure 11–25**

Retinal Vessels. This is the only place in the body where you can view blood vessels directly. Many systemic diseases that affect the vascular system show signs in the retinal vessels. Follow a paired artery and vein out to the periphery in the four quadrants (see Fig. 11–23), noting these points:

	Normal	Abnormal
1. Number	A paired artery and vein pass to each quadrant. Vessels look straighter at the nasal side.	Absence of major vessels.
2. Color	Arteries are brighter red than veins. Also, they have the arterial light reflex, with a thin stripe of light down middle.	
3. A:V ratio	The ratio comparing the artery-to-vein width is 2:3 or 4:5.	Arteries too constricted. Veins dilated.
4. Caliber	Arteries and veins show a regular decrease in caliber as they extend to periphery.	Focal constriction. Neovascularization.
5. A-V (arteriovenous) crossing	An artery and vein may cross paths. This is not significant if within 2 DD of disc and if no sign of interruption in blood flow. There should be no indenting or displacing of vessel.	Crossings more than 2 DD away. Nicking or pinching of underlying vessel. Vessel engorged peripheral to crossing.
6. Tortuosity	Mild vessel twisting when present in both eyes is usually congenital and not significant.	Extreme tortuosity or markedly asymmetric in two eyes.
7. Pulsations	Present in veins near disc as their drainage meets the intermittent pressure of arterial systole. (Often hard to see.)	Absent pulsations (see Table 11–12).

NORMAL RANGE OF FINDINGS

General Background of the Fundus. The color normally varies from light red to dark brown-red, generally corresponding with the person's skin color. Your view of the fundus should be clear; there should be no lesions obstructing the retinal structures.

Macula. The macula is 1 DD in size and located 2 DD temporal to the disc. Inspect this area last in the funduscopic examination. A bright light on this area of central vision causes some watering and discomfort and pupillary constriction. Note that the normal color of the area is somewhat darker than the rest of the fundus but even and homogenous. Clumped pigment may occur with aging.

Within the macula, you may note the foveal light reflex. This is a tiny white glistening dot reflecting your ophthalmoscope light.

ABNORMAL FINDINGS

Abnormal lesions: hemorrhages, exudates, microaneurysms (see Table 11–13).

Clumped pigment occurs with trauma or retinal detachment.

Hemorrhage or exudate in the macula occurs with senile macular degeneration.

DEVELOPMENTAL CONSIDERATIONS

Infants and Children

The eye examination is often deferred at birth because of transient edema of the lids from birth trauma or from the instillation of silver nitrate for prophylaxis. The eyes should be examined within a few days, and at every well child visit thereafter.

Visual Acuity

The child's age determines the screening measures used. With a newborn, test visual reflexes and attending behaviors. Test *light perception* using the blink reflex; the neonate blinks in response to bright light (Fig. 11–26). Also the pupillary light reflex shows that the pupils constrict in response to

Absent blinking.

Absent pupillary light reflex, especially after 3 weeks, indicates blindness.

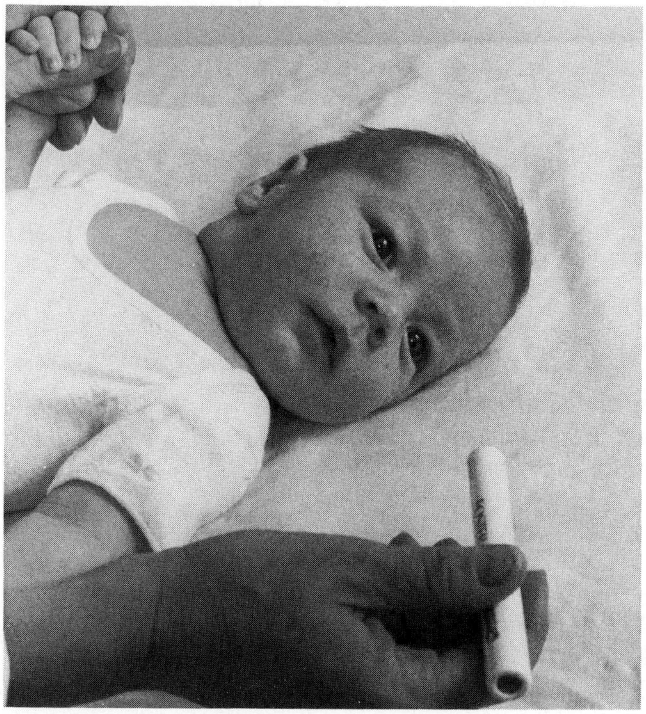

► **Figure 11–26**

NORMAL RANGE OF FINDINGS

light. These reflexes indicate that the lower portion of the visual apparatus is intact. But you cannot infer that the infant can *see;* that requires later observation to show that the brain has received images and can interpret them (Whaley and Wong, 1990).

As you introduce an object to the infant's line of vision, note these attending behaviors:

Birth to 2 weeks — Refusal to reopen eyes after exposure to bright light; increasing alertness to object; infant may fixate on an object.

By 2 to 4 weeks — Infant can fixate on an object.

By 1 month — Infant can fixate and follow a light or bright toy.

By 3 to 4 months — Infant can fixate, follow, and reach for the toy.

By 6 to 10 months — Infant can fixate and follow the toy in all directions.

The Allen test (picture cards) screens children from 2 1/2 years to 2 years and 11 months of age, and even is reliable with cooperative toddlers as young as 2 years of age. The test contains seven cards of familiar objects (birthday cake, teddy bear, tree, house, car, telephone, and horse and rider). First, show the pictures up close to the child to make sure the child can identify them. Then, present each picture at a distance of 15 feet. Results are normal if the child can name three out of seven cards within three to five trials.

Use the Snellen E chart for the preschooler from 3 to 6 years of age. The chart shows the capital letter E in varying sizes pointing in different directions. The child points his or her fingers in the direction the "table legs" are pointing on each designated E. By age 7 to 8 years of age when the child is familiar with reading letters, begin to use the standard Snellen alphabet chart. Normally, a child achieves 20/20 acuity by 6 to 7 years of age.

Visual Fields

Assess peripheral vision with the confrontation test in children older than age 3 years when the preschooler is able to stay in position. As with the adult, the child should see the moving object at the same time your normal eyes do. Often a young child forgets to say "now" or "stop" as the moving object is seen. Rather, note the instant the child's eyes deviate or head shifts position to gaze at the moving object. Match this nearly automatic response with your own sighting.

Color Vision

Color blindness is an inherited recessive X-linked trait affecting about 8 percent of white males and 4 percent of black males. It is rare in females

ABNORMAL FINDINGS

The National Society for Prevention of Blindness states these criteria for referral:

1. Age 3 — vision 20/50 or less in either eye.
2. Age 4 and over — 20/40 or less in either eye.
3. Difference between two eyes is one line or more.
4. Child shows other signs of vision impairment, regardless of acuity.

Screen two separate times before referral.

NORMAL RANGE OF FINDINGS

(0.4 percent). "Color deficient" is a more accurate term, because the condition is relative and not disabling. Often, it is just a social inconvenience, although it may affect the person's ability to discern traffic lights, or it may affect school performance in which color is a learning tool.

Test only boys for color vision once between the ages of 4 and 8. Use Ishihara's test, a series of polychromatic cards. Each card has a pattern of dots printed against a background of many colored dots. Ask the child to identify each pattern. A boy with normal color vision can see each pattern. A color blind person cannot see the letter against the field color.

Extraocular Muscle Function

Testing for strabismus (squint, crossed eye) is an important screening measure to perform during early childhood. Untreated strabismus can lead to permanent visual damage. Strabismus causes disconjugate vision because one eye deviates off the fixation point. To avoid diplopia or unclear images, the brain begins to suppress data from the weak eye (a suppression scotoma). Then, visual acuity in this otherwise normal eye begins to deteriorate from disuse. The resulting loss of vision due to disuse is *amblyopia ex anopsia.* Early recognition and treatment are essential to restore binocular vision. Diagnosis after age 6 years has a poor prognosis. Test malalignment by the corneal light reflex and the cover test.

Check the *corneal light reflex* by shining a light toward the child's eyes. The light should be reflected at exactly the same spot in the two corneas. Some asymmetry (where one light falls off center) under age 6 months is normal.

Perform the cover test on all children as described on p. 323. Some examiners omit the opaque card and place their hand on the child's head. The examiner's thumb extends down and blocks vision over the eye without actually touching the eye. One can use a familiar character puppet to attract the child's attention. The normal results are the same as those listed in the adult section.

Function of the extraocular muscles during movement can be assessed during the early weeks by following a brightly colored toy. An older infant can sit on the parent's lap as you move the toy in all directions. After age 2 years, direct the child's gaze through the 6 cardinal positions of gaze. You may stabilize the child's chin with your hand to avoid moving the entire head.

External Eye Structures

Inspect the ocular structures as described in the earlier section. A neonate usually holds the eyes tightly shut. Do not attempt to pry them open; that just increases contraction of the orbicularis oculi muscle. Hold the newborn supine and gently lower the head; the eyes will open. Also the eyes will open when you hold the infant at arm's length and slowly turn the infant in one direction (Fig. 11–27). In addition to inspecting the ocular structures, this also tests the vestibular function reflex. That is, the baby's eyes will look in the same direction as the body is being turned. When the turning stops, the eyes will shift to the opposite direction after a few quick beats of nystagmus. Also termed "doll's eyes," this reflex disappears by 2 months of age.

ABNORMAL FINDINGS

Asymmetry in the corneal light reflex after 6 months is abnormal and must be referred.

NORMAL RANGE OF FINDINGS

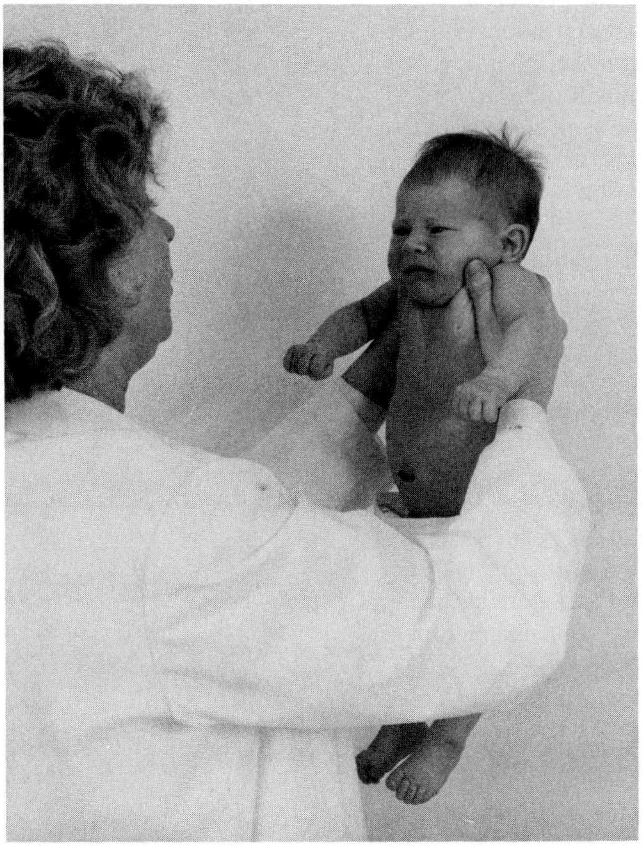

► **Figure 11-27**

Eyelids and Lashes. Normally, the upper lids overlie the superior part of the iris. In newborns, the *setting-sun sign* is common. The eyes appear to deviate down and you see a white rim of sclera over the iris. It may show as you rapidly change the neonate from a sitting to a supine position.

Many infants have an *epicanthal fold,* an excess skin fold extending over the inner corner of the eye, partly or totally overlapping the inner canthus. It occurs frequently in Asian children and in 20 percent of whites. In non-Asians it disappears as the child grows, usually by age 10 years. While they are present, epicanthal folds give a false appearance of malalignment, termed *pseudostrabismus* (Fig. 11-28). Yet the corneal light reflex is normal.

Asian infants normally have an upward slant of the palpebral fissures. Entropion, a turning inward of the eyelid, is found normally in some Asian children. If the lashes do not abrade the corneas, it is not significant.

ABNORMAL FINDINGS

The setting-sun sign also occurs with hydrocephalus as the globes protrude.

Blank sunken eyes accompany malnutrition, dehydration, and a severe illness.

Mongolian slant—An upward lateral slope together with epicanthal folds and hypertelorism (large spacing between the eyes) occurs with Down syndrome.

NORMAL RANGE OF FINDINGS | **ABNORMAL FINDINGS**

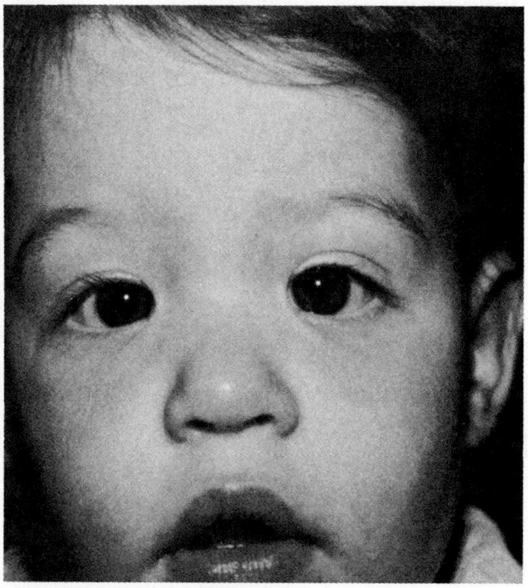

Pseudostrabismus

▶ **Figure 11-28**

Conjunctiva and Sclera. A newborn may have a transient chemical conjunctivitis due to the instillation of silver nitrate. This appears within 1 hour and lasts not more than 24 hours after birth. The sclera should be white and clear, although it may have a blue tint due to thinness at birth. The lacrimal glands are not functional at birth.

Ophthalmia neonatorum (conjunctivitis of the newborn) is a purulent discharge due to chemical irritant, bacterial, or viral agent acquired from the birth canal.

Iris and Pupils. The iris normally is a deep blue, blue, or slate gray in light-skinned newborns, and brown in the dark-skinned infants. By 6 to 9 months, the permanent color is differentiated. You may note Brushfield's spots, or white specks around the edge of the iris. This may be normal in the newborn but suggests Down syndrome.

Absence of iris color occurs with albinism.

A searching nystagmus is common just after birth. The pupils are small but constrict to light.

Constant nystagmus, prolonged setting-sun sign, marked strabismus, and slow lateral movements suggest vision loss.

The Ocular Fundus

The amount of data gathered during the funduscopic examination depends on the child's ability to hold the eyes still and on your ability to glean as much data as possible in a brief period of time.

A complete funduscopic examination is difficult to perform on an infant, but at least check the red reflex when the infant fixates at the bright light for a few seconds. Note any interruption.

An interruption in the red reflex indicates an opacity in the cornea or lens. An absent red reflex occurs with congenital cataracts or retinal disorders.

Perform a funduscopic examination on an infant between 2 and 6 months of age. Position the infant (up to 18 months) lying on the table.

NORMAL RANGE OF FINDINGS

The fundus appears pale, and the vessels are not fully developed. There is no foveal light reflection because the macula area will not be mature until 1 year.

Inspect the fundus of the young child and school-aged child as described in the adult section. Allow the child to handle the equipment. Explain why you are darkening the room and that you will leave a small light on. Assure the child that the procedure will not hurt. Direct the young child to look at an appealing picture, perhaps Mickey Mouse or an animal, during the examination.

The Aging Adult

Visual Acuity

Perform the same examination as described in the adult section. Central acuity may decrease, particularly after age 70. Peripheral vision may be diminished.

Ocular Structures

The eyebrows may show a loss of the outer one-third to one-half of hair due to a decrease in hair follicles. The remaining brow hair is coarse (Fig. 11–29). Owing to atrophy of elastic tissues, the skin around the eyes may show wrinkles or crow's feet. The upper lid may be so elongated as to rest on the lashes, resulting in a pseudoptosis.

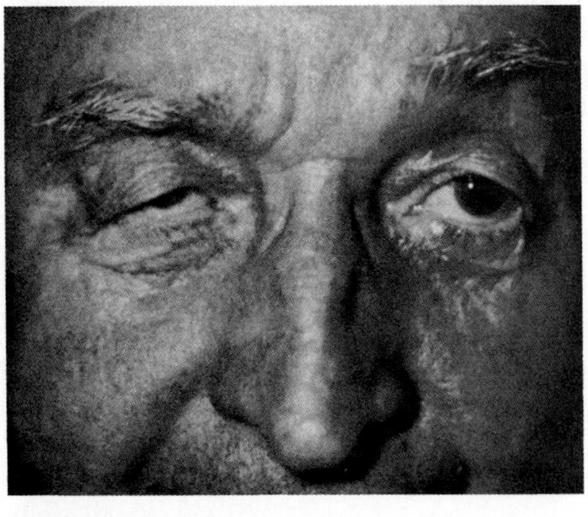

► **Figure 11–29**

The eyes may appear sunken owing to atrophy of the orbital fat. Also, the orbital fat may herniate, causing bulging at the lower lids and inner third of the upper lids.

Atrophy of the levator palpebrae muscle causes a partial ptosis. In contrast with the baggy lids described above, ptosis is an actual drooping.

ABNORMAL FINDINGS

Papilledema is rare in the infant because the fontanels and open sutures will absorb any increased intracranial pressure if it occurs.

NORMAL RANGE OF FINDINGS

Atrophy of elastic and fibrous tissues may cause the lower lid to drop away from the globe, or *ectropion.* This compromises the globe structures, because the tears cannot drain into the out-turned puncta. Alternately, *entropion,* or a turning inward of the lower lid, may irritate the eye from friction of lashes.

The lacrimal apparatus may decrease tear production, causing the eyes to look dry and lusterless and the person to report a burning sensation. *Pingueculae* commonly show on the sclera (Fig. 11–30). These yellowish elevated nodules are due to a thickening of the bulbar conjunctiva from prolonged exposure to sun, wind, and dust. Pingueculae appear at the 3 and 9 o'clock positions, first on the nasal side, then on the temporal side.

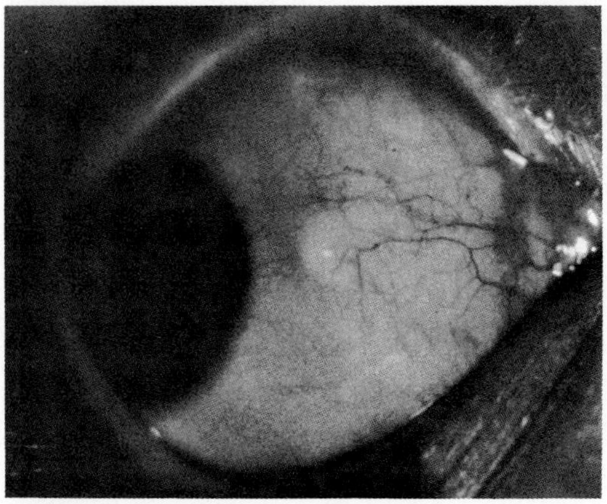

▶ Figure 11–30 Pinguecula

The cornea may look cloudy with age. An *arcus senilis* commonly is seen around the cornea (Fig. 11–31). This is a gray-white arc or circle around the limbus and is due to deposition of lipid material. As more lipid accumulates, the cornea may look thickened and raised, but the arcus has no effect on vision.

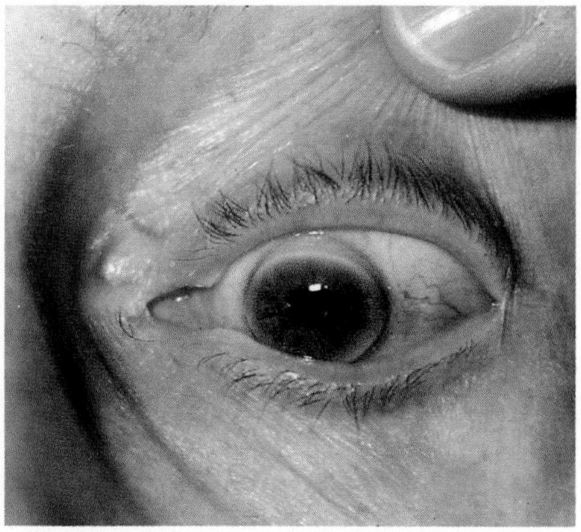

▶ Figure 11–31 Arcus senilis

ABNORMAL FINDINGS

See ectropion and entropion (Table 11–4).

NORMAL RANGE OF FINDINGS	ABNORMAL FINDINGS

Xanthelasma are soft, raised yellow plaques occurring on the lids at the inner canthus (Fig. 11–32). They commonly occur around the fifth decade of life and more frequently in women. They occur with both high and normal blood levels of cholesterol and have no pathologic significance.

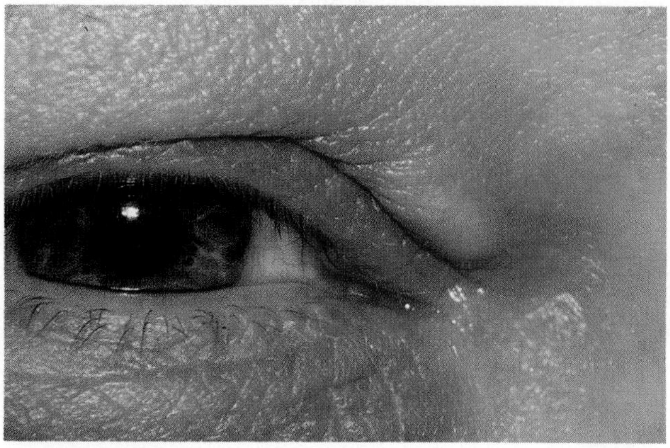

Xanthelasma

▶ Figure 11–32

Pupils are small in old age, and the pupillary light reflex may be slowed. The lens loses transparency, and looks opaque.

The Ocular Fundus

Retinal structures generally have less shine. The blood vessels look paler, narrower, and attenuated. Arterioles appear paler and straighter, with a narrower light reflex. More arteriovenous (AV) crossing defects occur.

A normal development on the retinal surface are *drusen,* or benign degenerative hyaline deposits (see Fig. 11–24). They are small round yellow dots that are scattered haphazardly on the retina. Although they do not occur in a pattern, they are usually symmetrically placed in the two eyes. They have no effect on vision.

Drusen are easily confused with the abnormal finding, *hard exudates* (see Table 11–13).

☑ SUMMARY CHECKLIST

1 ▶ Test visual acuity
   Snellen eye chart
   Near vision (those older than 40 years or those having difficulty reading)

2 ▶ Test visual fields—confrontation test

3 ▶ Inspect extraocular muscle (EOM) function
   Corneal light reflex (Hirschberg test)
   Cover test
   Diagnostic positions test

4 ▶ Inspect external eye structures
   General
   Eyebrows
   Eyelids and lashes
   Eyeball alignment
   Conjunctiva and sclera
   Lacrimal apparatus

5 ▶ Inspect anterior eyeball structures
   Cornea and lens
   Iris and pupil
      Pupillary light reflex
      Accommodation

6 ▶ Inspect the ocular fundus
   Optic disc (color, shape, margins, cup-disc ratio)
   Retinal vessels (number, color, artery/vein [A/V] ratio, caliber, arteriovenous crossings, tortuosity, pulsations)
   General background (color, integrity)
   Macula

SAMPLE RECORDING

Subjective

▶ Vision reported good with no recent change. No eye pain, no inflammation, no discharge, no lesions. Wears no corrective lenses, vision last tested 1 year PTA, test for glaucoma at that time was normal.

Objective

▶ Snellen chart—O.D. 20/20, O.S. 20/20 $^{-}1$. Fields normal by confrontation. EOMs intact. Brows and lashes present. No ptosis. Conjunctiva clear. Sclera white. No lesions. PERRLA. Fundi: Red reflex present bilaterally. Discs flat with sharp margins. Vessels present in all quadrants without crossing defects. Retinal background has even color with no hemorrhages or exudates. Macula has even color.

SAMPLE CLINICAL PROBLEM 1

Emma K. is a 34-year-old white, married homemaker, brought to the Emergency Department by police following a reported domestic quarrel.

Subjective

- States husband struck her about the face and eyes with his fists about 1 hour PTA. "I ruined the dinner again. I can't do anything right." Pain in left cheek and both eyes felt immediately and continues. Alarmed at "bright red blood on eyeball." No bleeding from eye area or cheek. Vision intact just after trauma. Now reports difficulty opening lids.

Objective

- Sitting quietly and hunched over, hands over eyes. Voice tired and flat. L cheek swollen and discolored, no laceration. Lids edematous and discolored both eyes. No skin laceration. L lid swollen almost shut. L eye—round 1-mm bright red patch over lateral aspect of globe. No active bleeding out of eye, iris intact, anterior chamber clear. R eye—conjunctiva clear, sclera white, cornea and iris intact, anterior chamber clear. PERRLA, Pupils $\frac{4}{1} = \frac{4}{1}$. Vision $\frac{14}{14}$ both eyes by Jaeger card.

Assessment

- Ecchymoses L cheek and both eyes
  Subconjunctival hemorrhage L eye
  Self-esteem disturbance R/T effects of domestic violence

SAMPLE CLINICAL PROBLEM 2

Sam T. is a 63-year-old white postal carrier admitted to the Medical Center for surgery for suspected brain tumor. Following postanesthesia recovery, Sam T. is admitted to the Neuro ICU, awake, lethargic with slowed but correct verbal responses, oriented ×3, moving all four extremities, vital signs stable, Pupils $\frac{4}{2} = \frac{4}{2}$ with sluggish response. Assessments are made q 15 minutes.

Subjective

- No response now to verbal stimuli.

Objective

- Semi-comatose — no response to verbal stimuli, does withdraw R arm and leg purposefully to painful stimuli. No movement L arm or leg. Pupils R $\frac{5}{5} \neq$ L $\frac{4}{2}$. Vitals remain stable as noted on graphic sheet.

Assessment

- Unilateral dilated and fixed R pupil
  Clouding of consciousness
  Focal motor deficit — no movement L side
  Altered tissue perfusion: cerebral R/T interruption of flow

SAMPLE CLINICAL PROBLEM 3

Trung Q. is a 4-year-old male born in southeast Asia, who arrived in this country 1 month PTA. Lives with parents, 2 siblings. Speaks only native language, here with uncle to act as interpreter.

Subjective

- Seeks care because RN in church sponsoring family noted "crossed eyes." Uncle states vision seemed normal to parents. Plays with toys and manipulates small objects without difficulty. Identifies objects in picture books, does not read.

Objective

- With uncle interpreting directions for test to Trung, vision by Snellen E chart — O.D. 20/30, O.S. 20/50 $^{-}$1. Fields seem intact by confrontation — jerks head to gaze at object entering field.
  EOMs — asymmetric corneal light reflex with outward deviation L eye. Cover test — as R eye covered, L eye jerks to fixate, R eye steady when uncovered. As L eye covered, R eye holds steady gaze, L eye jerks to fixate as uncovered. Diagnostic positions — able to gaze in 6 positions, although L eye obviously malaligned at extreme medial gaze.
  Eye structures — Brows and lashes present and normal bilaterally. Upward palpebral slant, epicanthal folds bilaterally — consistent with racial heritage. Conjunctiva clear, sclera white, iris intact, PERRLA. Fundi: discs flat with sharp margins. Observed vessels normal. Unable to see in all 4 quadrants, unable to see macular area.

Assessment

- L exotropia
  Abnormal vision in L eye
  Sensory/perceptual alteration: visual R/T effects of neurologic impairment

SAMPLE CLINICAL PROBLEM 4

Vera K. is an 87-year-old black homemaker, living independently, who is admitted to hospital for observation and adjustment of digitalis medication. Cardiac status has been stable during hospital stay.

Subjective

- Reports desire to monitor own medication at home but fears problems owing to blurred vision. First noted distant vision blurred 5 years ago but near vision seemed to improve at that time, "I started to read better without my glasses!" Since then, blurring at distant vision has increased, near vision now blurred also. Able to navigate home environment without difficulty. Fixes simple meals with cold foods. Receives hot meal from "Meals on Wheels" at lunch. Enjoys television, though somewhat blurred. Unable to write letters, sew, or read paper, which she regrets.

Objective

- Vision by Jaeger card O.D. 20/200. O.S. 20/400 −1 with glasses on. Fields intact by confrontation. EOMs intact. Brow hair absent lateral third. Upper lids have folds of redundant skin but lids do not droop. Lower lids and lashes intact. Xanthelasma present both inner canthi. Conjunctiva clear, sclera white, iris intact, L pupil looks cloudy, PERRLA, pupils $\frac{3}{2} = \frac{3}{2}$. Fundi: Red reflex has central dark spot both eyes. Discs flat, with sharp margins. Observed vessels normal. Unable to see in all 4 quadrants or macular area owing to small pupils.

Assessment

- Central opacity, both eyes
  Central visual acuity deficit, both eyes
  Diversional activity deficit R/T poor vision

NURSING DIAGNOSES COMMONLY ASSOCIATED WITH THE EYES AND VISUAL DISORDERS

Diagnosis	Related Factors (Etiology)	Defining Characteristics (Symptoms and Signs)
Sensory/perceptual alteration: visual	Restriction of head/neck motion Effects of Aging Stress Neurologic impairment Failure to use protective eye devices Improper use of contact lens Difficulty in adjusting to corrective lens Persistent visual stimulation	Headache Blurring Spots Double vision Excessive tearing Inflammation Lack of blink or corneal reflex Squinting Holding objects too close or at a distance for viewing Colliding with objects Abnormal results of vision testing
Diversional activity deficit	Effects of chronic illness Physical limitations Poor vision Social isolation Decreased economic resources Confined to bedrest Preoccupation with job	Restlessness Napping during day Apathy or hostility Complaints of boredom Verbalizes desire for activity Inability to participate in usual activities or hobbies because of physical limitations Depression Preoccupation with self Weight loss or gain
Impaired home maintenance management	Impaired mental status Effects of chronic debilitating disease (loss of vision) Inadequate support system Substance abuse Depression Lack of knowledge Lack of motivation Decreased financial resources	Offensive odors Presence of rodents or vermin Accumulation of dirt, food, dirty laundry, or hygienic wastes Reports by patient or family of difficulty maintaining home in comfortable fashion Inappropriate room temperature Lack of necessary equipment

Table 11-2 ► Visual Field Loss

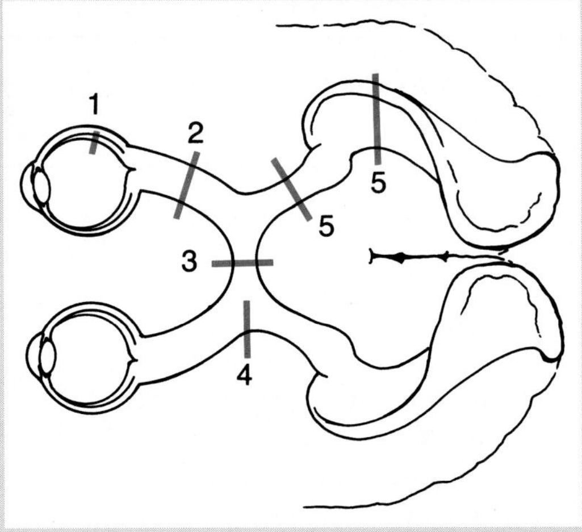

1. Retinal damage
   - Macula—central blind area, e.g. diabetes.

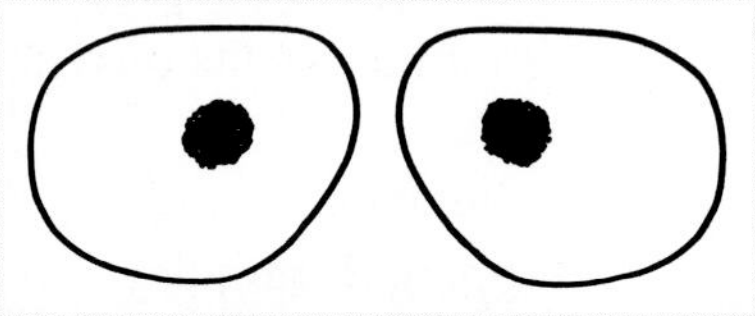

   - Localized damage—blind spot (scotoma) corresponding to particular area.

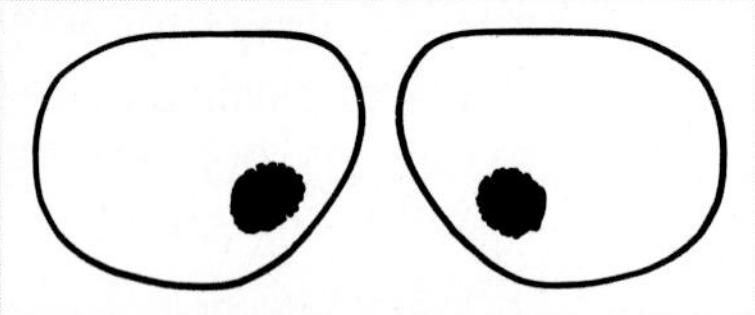

   - Increasing intraocular pressure—decrease in peripheral vision, e.g., glaucoma. Starts with paracentral scotoma in early stage.

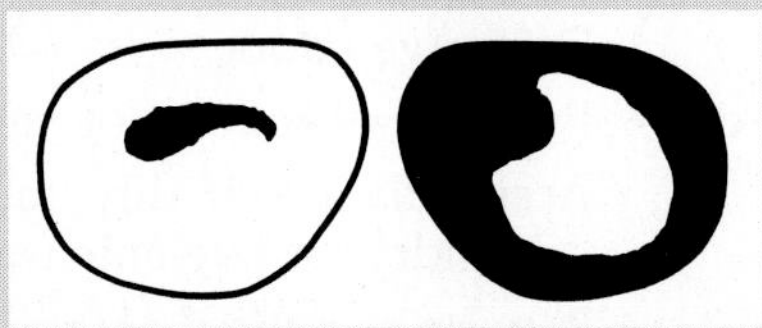

   - Retinal detachment. Person has shadow or diminished vision in one quadrant or one half visual field.

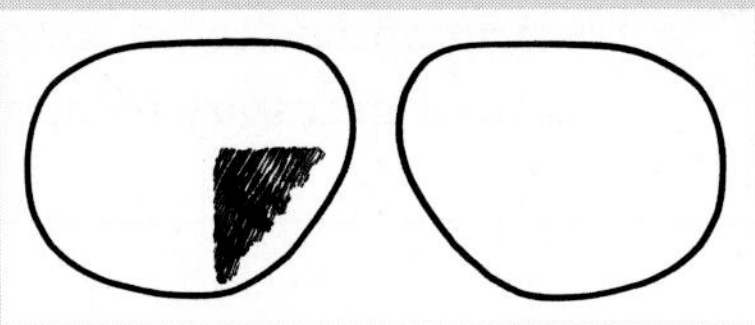

2. Lesion in globe or optic nerve.
   Injury here yields one blind eye, or unilateral blindness.

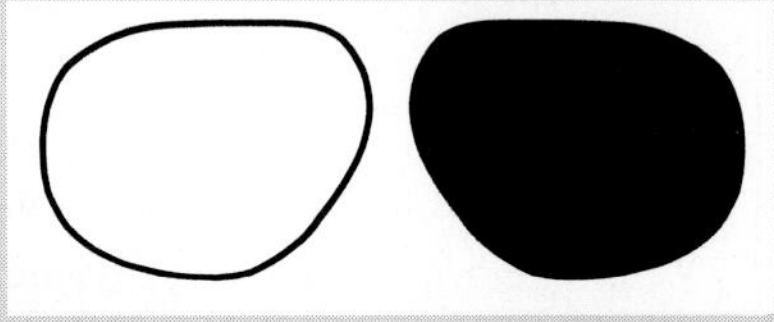

3. Lesion at optic chiasm (e.g., pituitary tumor)—Injury to crossing fibers only yields a loss of nasal part of each retina and a loss of both temporal visual fields.
   Bitemporal (heteronymous) hemianopsia.

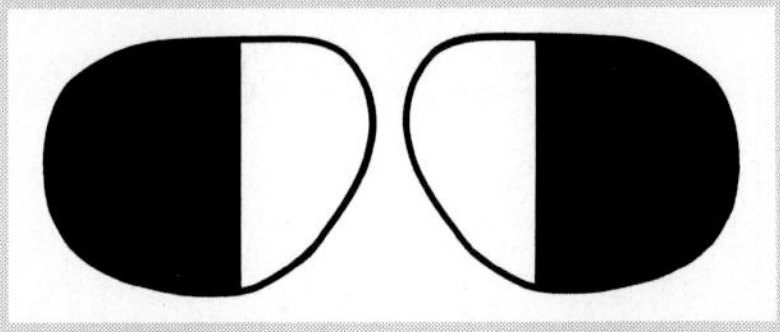

4. Lesion of outer uncrossed fibers at optic chiasm, e.g., aneurysm of left internal carotid artery exerts pressure on uncrossed fibers. Injury yields left nasal hemianopsia.

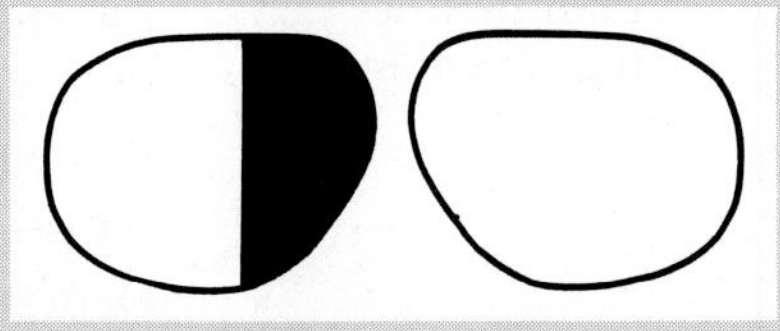

5. Lesion R optic tract or R optic radiation.
   Visual field loss in R nasal and L temporal fields.
   Loss of same half visual field in both eyes is homonymous hemianopsia.

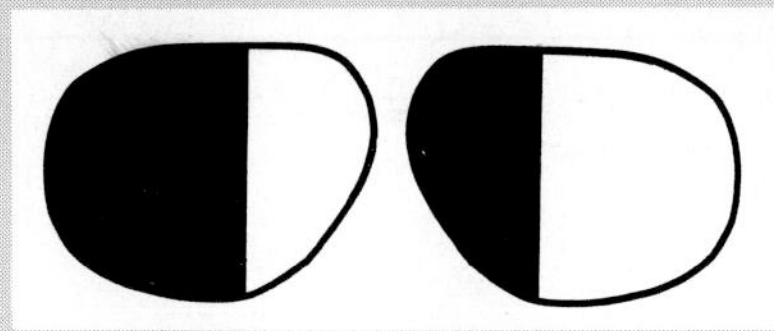

Table 11-3 ▶ Extraocular Muscle Dysfunction

CORNEAL LIGHT REFLEX

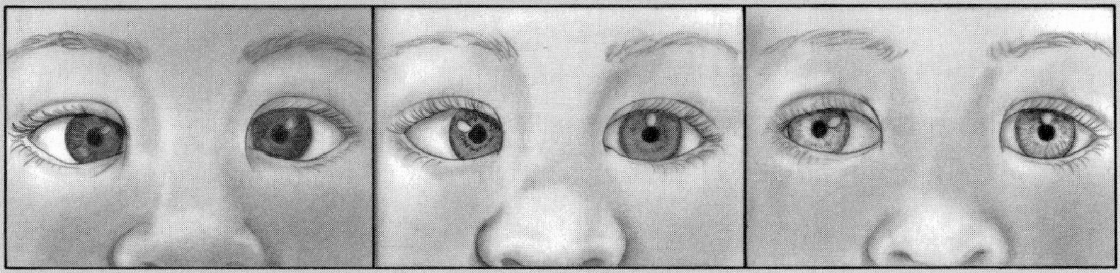

A Pseudostrabismis B R Esotropia C R Exotropia

Symmetric Corneal Light Reflex

A. *Pseudostrabismus* has the appearance of strabismus due to epicanthic fold, but is normal for a young child.

Asymmetric Corneal Light Reflex

Strabismus is true disparity of the eye axes. This constant malalignment is also termed tropia and is likely to cause amblyopia.

B. Esotropia—inward turn of the eye.

C. Exotropia—outward turn of the eye.

COVER TEST

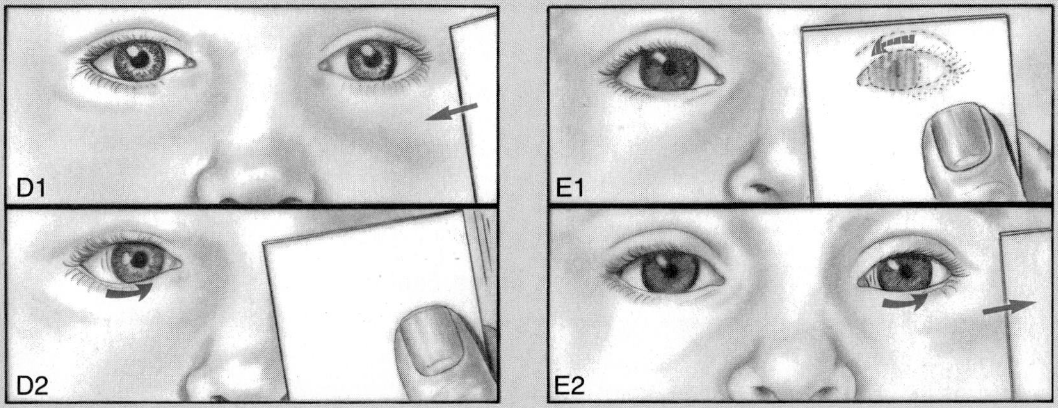

D Right, uncovered eye is weaker E Left, covered eye is weaker

D. Uncovered eye—if it jumps to fixate on designated point, it was out of alignment before (i.e., when you cover the stronger eye, the weaker eye now tries to fixate).

E. Covered eye—If this is the weaker eye, once macular image is suppressed it will drift to relaxed position.

As eye is uncovered—if it jumps to reestablish fixation, weakness exists.

Phoria—mild weakness, apparent only with the cover test and less likely to cause amblyopia than a tropia but still possible.

Esophoria—nasal (inward) drift.

Exophoria—temporal (outward) drift.

Table continued on following page

Table 11-3 ▸ Extraocular Muscle Dysfunction *Continued*

DIAGNOSTIC POSITIONS TEST

(Paralysis apparent during movement through 6 cardinal positions of gaze.)

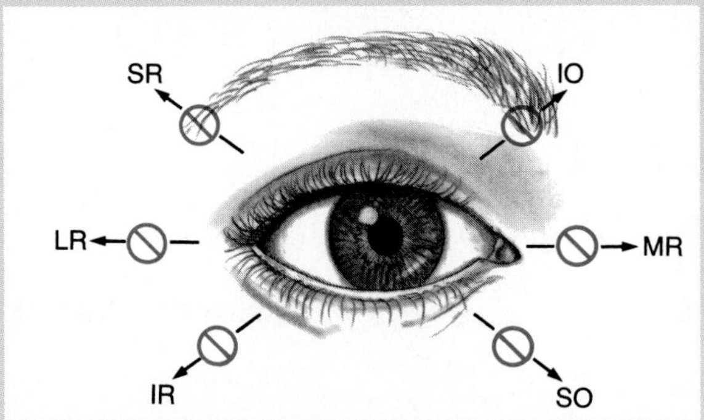

If eye will not turn:	Paralysis in:	or Cranial Nerve
Straight nasal	medial rectus	III
Up and nasal	inferior oblique	III
Up and temporal	superior rectus	III
Straight temporal	lateral rectus	VI
Down and temporal	inferior rectus	III
Down and nasal	superior oblique	IV

Table 11-4 ▸ Abnormalities in the Eyelids

ENOPHTHALMOS (SUNKEN EYES) (not illustrated)

Enophthalmos occurs with chronic wasting illnesses. See Cachexia in Table 10-5.

EXOPHTHALMOS (PROTRUDING EYES) ⟶

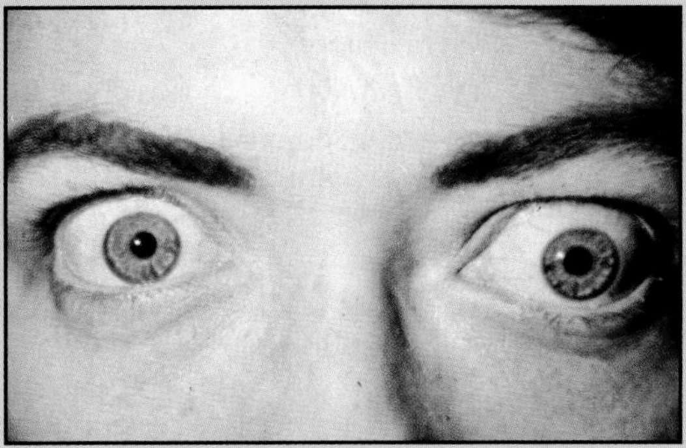

Exophthalmos is a forward displacement associated with thyroid disease. Note "lid lag," the upper lid rests well above the limbus and white sclera is visible. This is evident when you direct the person's gaze from up to down.

Table 11-4 ▶ Abnormalities in the Eyelids *Continued*

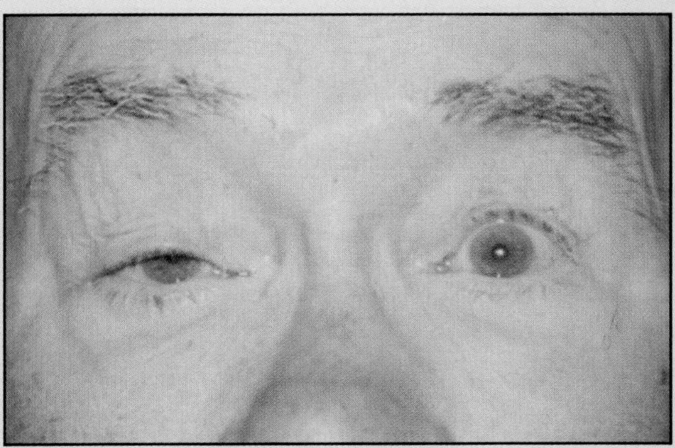

PTOSIS (DROOPING UPPER LID)

Ptosis occurs from neuromuscular weakness (e.g., myasthenia gravis), oculomotor cranial nerve III damage, or sympathetic nerve damage (e.g., Horner's syndrome). It is a positional defect that gives the person a sleepy appearance.

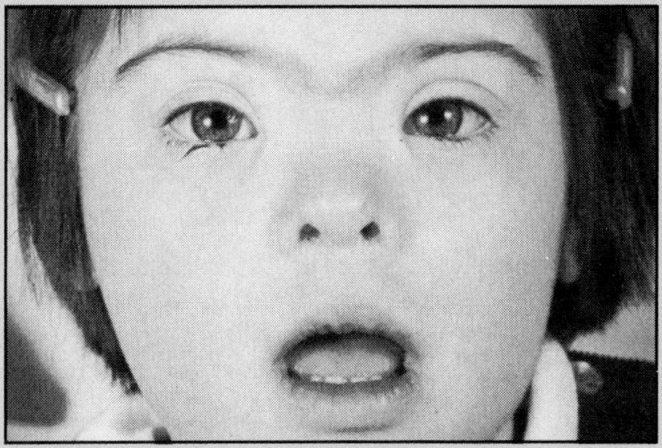

UPWARD PALPEBRAL SLANT

Although normal in many children, when combined with epicanthal folds and hypertelorism (large spacing between the eyes), indicates Down syndrome.

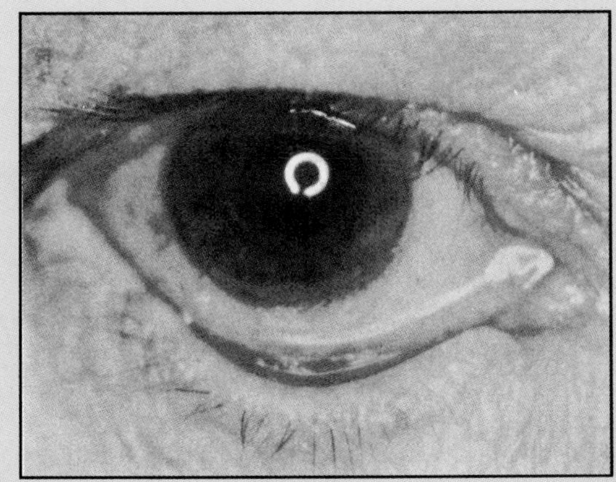

ECTROPION

The lower lid is loose and rolling out, does not approximate to eyeball. Puncta cannot siphon tears effectively so excess tearing results. Exposed palpebral conjunctiva increases risk for inflammation.

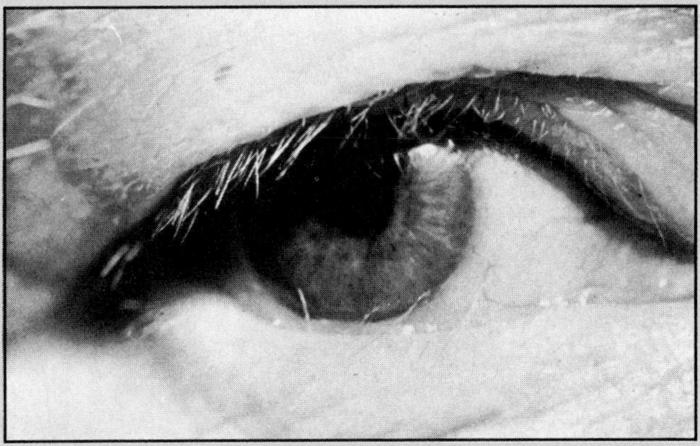

ENTROPION

The lower lid rolls in owing to spasm of lids or scar tissue contracting. Lashes may irritate cornea.

Table continued on following page

Table 11-4 ▶ Abnormalities in the Eyelids *Continued*

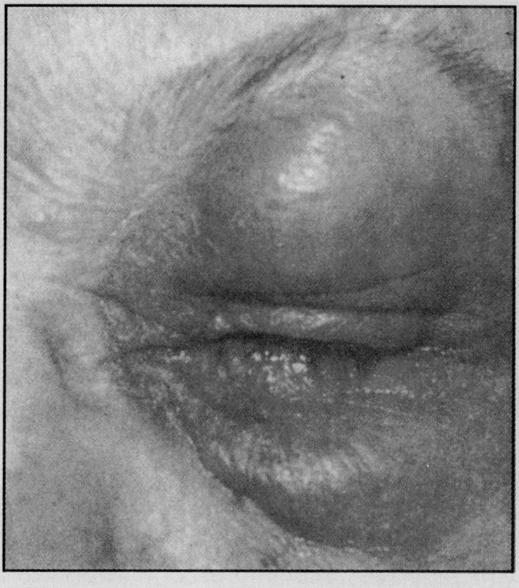

PERIORBITAL EDEMA

Lids are swollen and puffy. Lid tissues are loosely connected so excess fluid is easily apparent. This occurs with local infections, crying, and systemic conditions such as congestive heart failure, renal failure, allergy, hypothyroidism (myxedema).

Table 11-5 ▶ Lesions on Eyelids

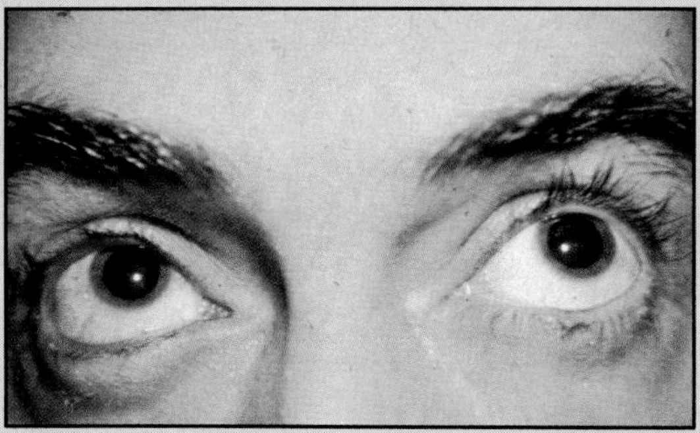

BLEPHARITIS (INFLAMMATION OF THE EYELIDS)

Red scaly crusted lid margins occur with staphylococcal infection or seborrheic dermatitis of the lid edge.

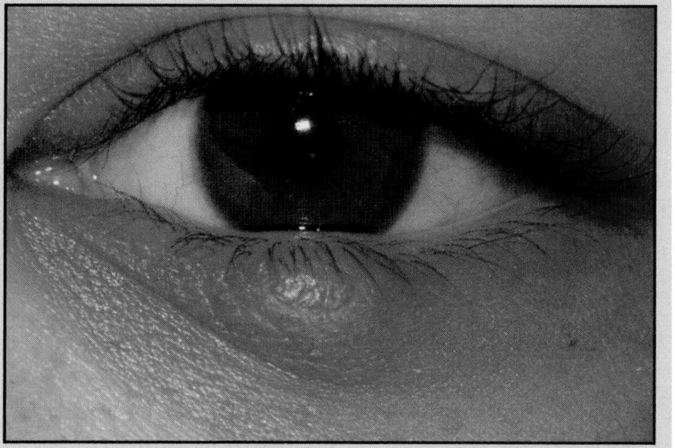

CHALAZION

A beady nodule protruding on the lid, chalazion is an infection or retention cyst of a meibomian gland. It is a nontender, firm, discrete swelling with freely moveable skin overlying the nodule. If it becomes inflamed, it points inside and not on lid margin (in contrast with sty).

Table 11-5 ▶ Lesions on Eyelids *Continued*

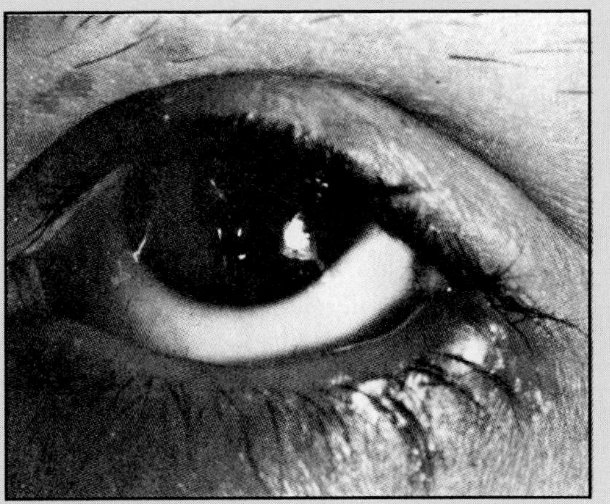

HORDEOLUM (STY)

Hordeolum is a localized staphylococcal infection of the hair follicles at the lid margin. It is painful, red, and swollen; it resembles a pustule at the lid margin.

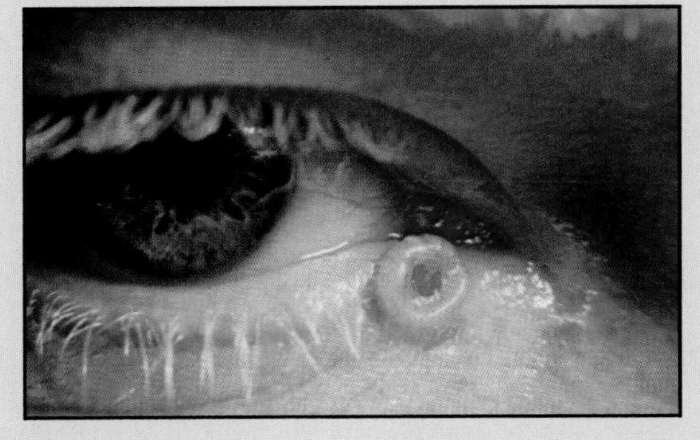

BASAL CELL CARCINOMA

Carcinoma is rare, but it occurs most often on the lower lid. It looks like a papule with an ulcerated center. Note the rolled out pearly edges.

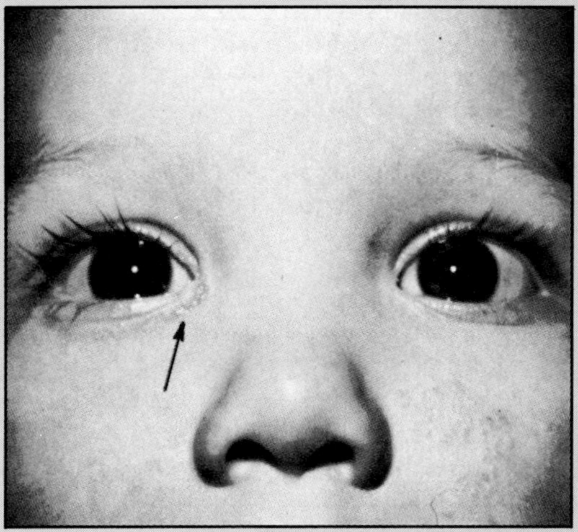

DACROCYSTITIS (INFLAMMATION OF THE LACRIMAL SAC)

Dacrocystitis is infection and blockage of sac and duct. Pain, warmth, redness, and swelling occur below the inner canthus toward nose. Tearing is present. Pressure on sac yields purulent discharge from puncta.

DACROADENITIS (INFLAMMATION OF THE LACRIMAL GLAND) (not illustrated)

Dacroadenitis is an infection of the lacrimal gland. Pain, swelling, and redness occur in outer third of upper lid. It occurs with mumps, measles, and infectious mononucleosis, or from trauma.

Table 11-6 ▶ Vascular Disorders of the External Eye

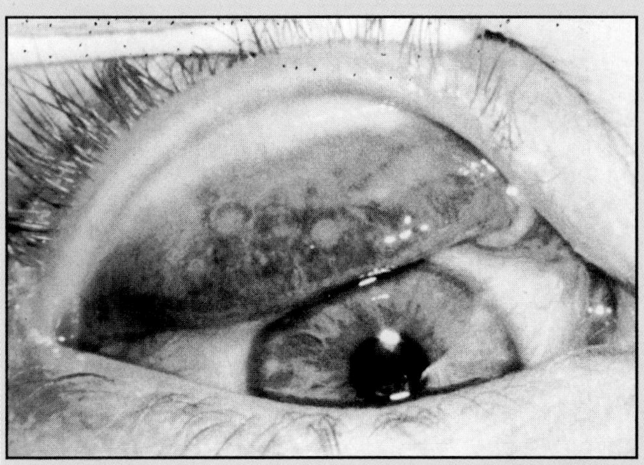

CONJUNCTIVITIS

Infection of the conjunctiva has red beefy-looking vessels at periphery but looks clearer around iris. This is a common disorder due to bacterial or viral infection, allergy, or chemical irritation. Purulent discharge accompanies bacterial infection. Often, the person has a history of an upper respiratory infection (URI).

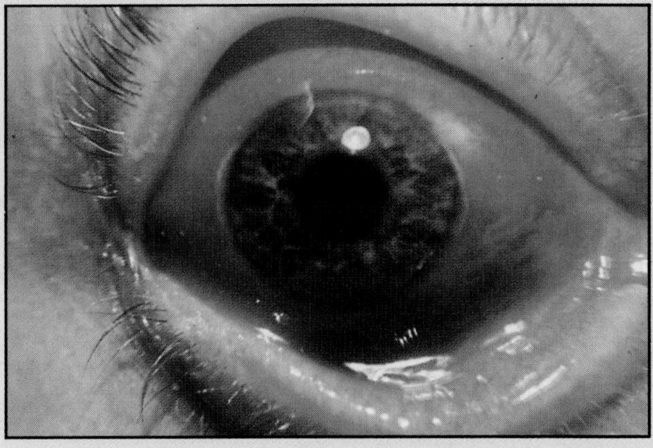

SUBCONJUNCTIVAL HEMORRHAGE

A red patch on the sclera, subconjunctival hemorrhage looks alarming but is usually not serious. The red patch has sharp edges like a spot of paint, although here it is extensive. It occurs from increased intraocular pressure from coughing, physical activity, trauma, or spontaneous bleeding.

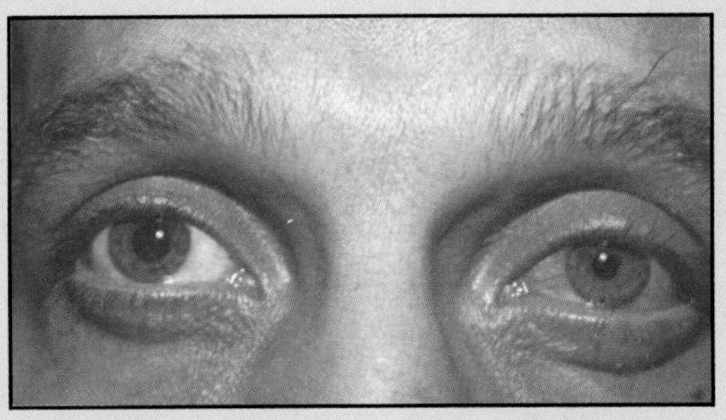

IRITIS (CIRCUMCORNEAL REDNESS)

Deep dull red halo around the iris and cornea. Note red is around iris, in contrast with conjunctivitis, in which redness is more prominent at the periphery. Pupil shape may be irregular from swelling of iris. Person also has marked photophobia, constricted pupil, blurred vision, and throbbing pain. Warrants immediate referral.

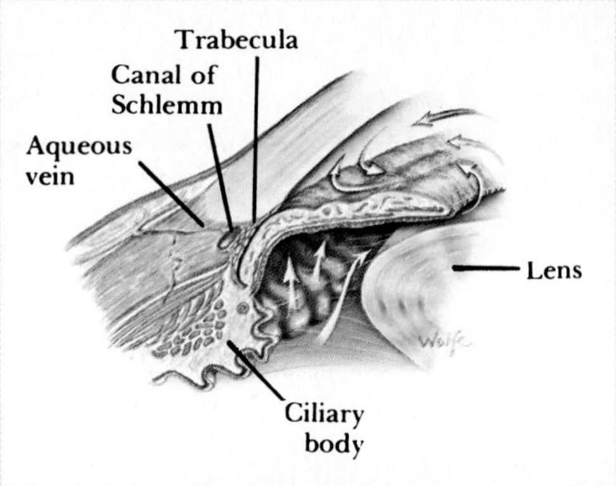

ACUTE GLAUCOMA

This is circumcorneal redness with a dilated pupil. Acute glaucoma has redness radiating around iris. Pupil is oval, dilated, cornea looks "steamy." Anterior chamber is shallow. Occurs with sudden increase in intraocular pressure due to blocked outflow from anterior chamber. This is an emergency situation.

Table 11-7 ▶ Abnormalities on the Cornea

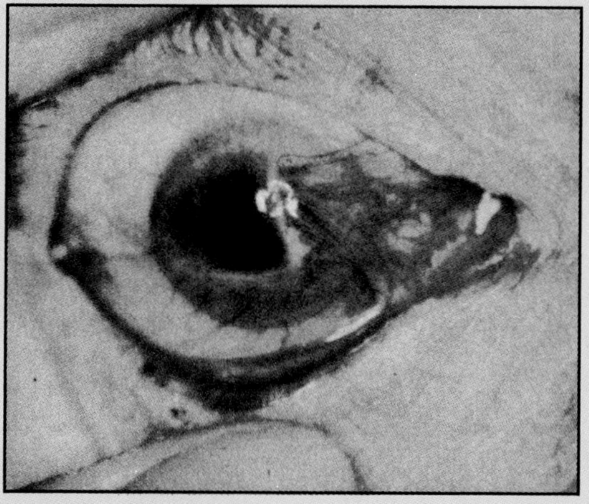

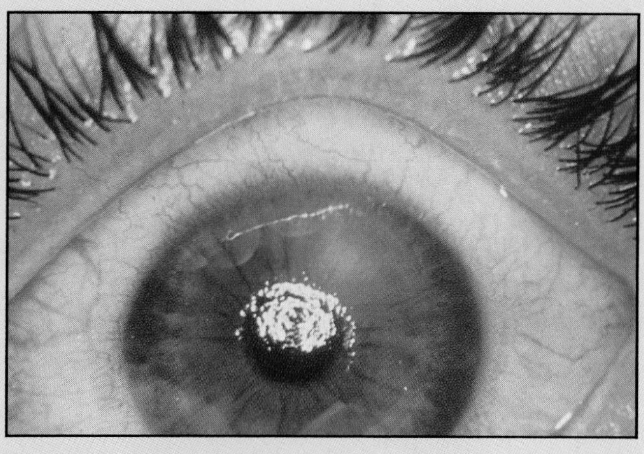

PTERYGIUM

A triangular opaque wing of bulbar conjunctiva grows toward the center of the cornea. It usually invades from nasal side, and it may obstruct vision as it covers pupil. Occurs usually from chronic exposure to hot, dry, sandy climate.

CORNEAL ABRASION

Irregular ridges are usually visible only when fluorescein stain reveals yellow-green branching. Top layer of corneal epithelium removed. A common disorder from scratches or poorly fitting or overworn contact lenses. Because the area is rich in nerve endings, the person feels intense pain, a foreign-body sensation, and lacrimation, redness, and photophobia.

Table 11-8 ▶ Abnormalities in the Anterior Chamber

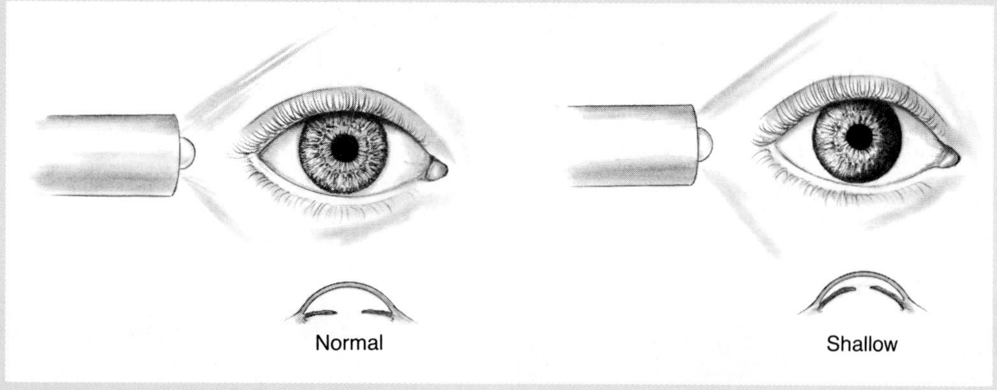

NORMAL ANTERIOR CHAMBER (FOR CONTRAST)

A light directed across the eye from the temporal side illuminates the entire iris evenly because the normal iris is flat and creates no shadow.

SHALLOW ANTERIOR CHAMBER

The iris is pushed anteriorly because of increased intraocular pressure. Because direct light is received from the temporal side, only the temporal part of iris is illuminated; the nasal side is shadowed. This may be a sign of acute angle-closure glaucoma.

Table continued on following page

Table 11–8 ▶ Abnormalities in the Anterior Chamber *Continued*

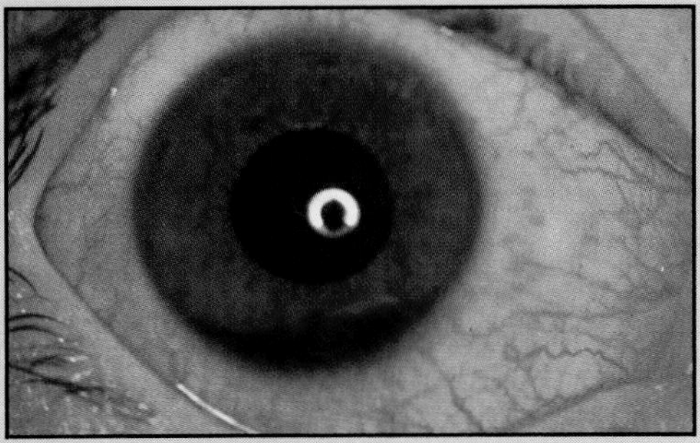

HYPHEMA

Blood in anterior chamber is a serious result of trauma or spontaneous hemorrhage. Suspect scleral rupture or major intraocular trauma. Note that gravity settles blood.

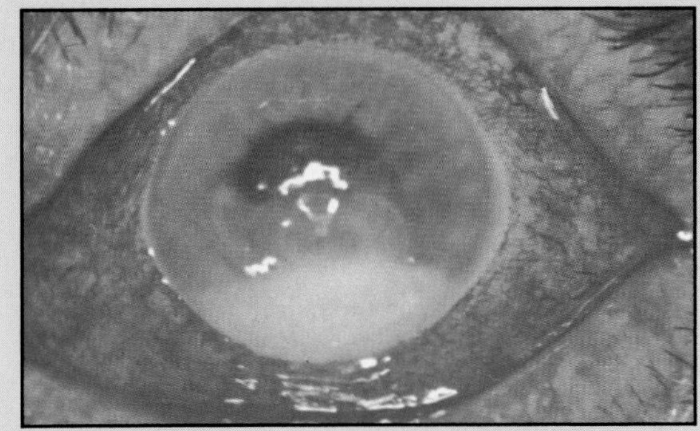

HYPOPYON

Purulent matter in anterior chamber occurs with inflammation in the anterior chamber.

Table 11–9 ▶ Abnormalities in the Pupil

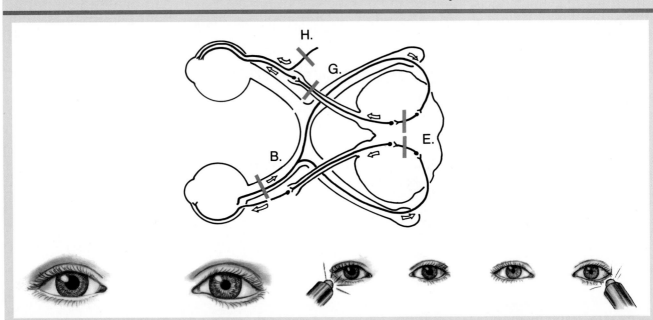

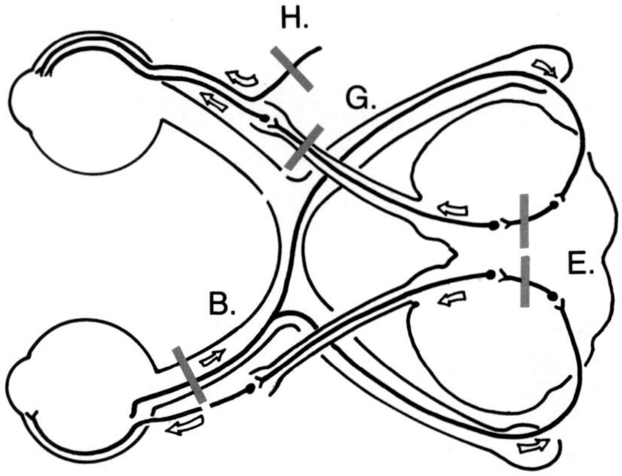

A. UNEQUAL PUPIL SIZE—ANISOCORIA

Although this exists normally in 5 percent of the population, consider central nervous system disease.

B. MONOCULAR BLINDNESS

When light is directed to the blind eye, there is no response in either eye. When light is directed to normal eye, both pupils constrict (direct and consensual response to light) as long as the oculomotor nerve is intact.

Table 11-9 ▶ Abnormalities in the Pupil *Continued*

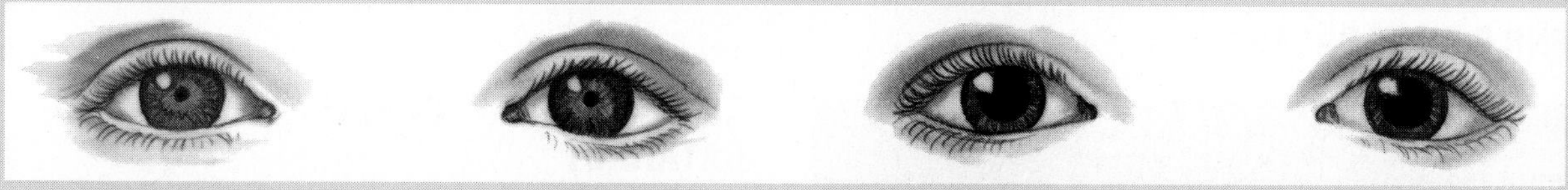

C. CONSTRICTED AND FIXED PUPILS—MIOSIS

Miosis occurs with the use of pilocarpine drops for glaucoma treatment, the use of narcotics, with iritis, and with brain damage of pons.

D. DILATED AND FIXED PUPILS—MYDRIASIS

Enlarged pupils occur with stimulation of the sympathetic nervous system, reaction of sympathomimetic drugs, use of dilating drops, acute glaucoma, past or recent trauma. Also, they herald central nervous system injury, circulatory arrest, or deep anesthesia.

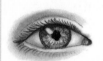

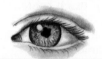

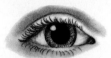

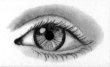

E. ARGYLL ROBERTSON PUPIL

No reaction to light, pupil does constrict with accommodation. Small and irregular bilaterally. Argyll Robertson pupil occurs with central nervous system syphilis, brain tumor, meningitis, and chronic alcoholism.

F. TONIC PUPIL (ADIE'S PUPIL)

Sluggish reaction to light and accommodation. Tonic pupil is usually unilateral, a large regular pupil that does react, but sluggishly after long latent time. No pathologic significance.

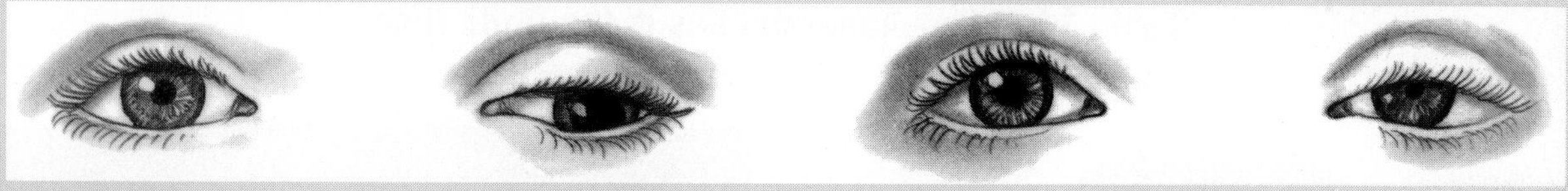

G. CRANIAL NERVE III DAMAGE

Unilateral dilated pupil with no reaction to light or accommodation, occurs with oculomotor nerve damage. May also have ptosis with eye deviating down and laterally.

H. HORNER'S SYNDROME

Unilateral, small, regular pupil does react to light and accommodation. Occurs with Horner's syndrome, a lesion of the sympathetic nerve. Also, note ptosis and absence of sweat (anhidrosis) on same side.

Table 11-10 ► Opacities in the Lens

SENILE CATARACTS

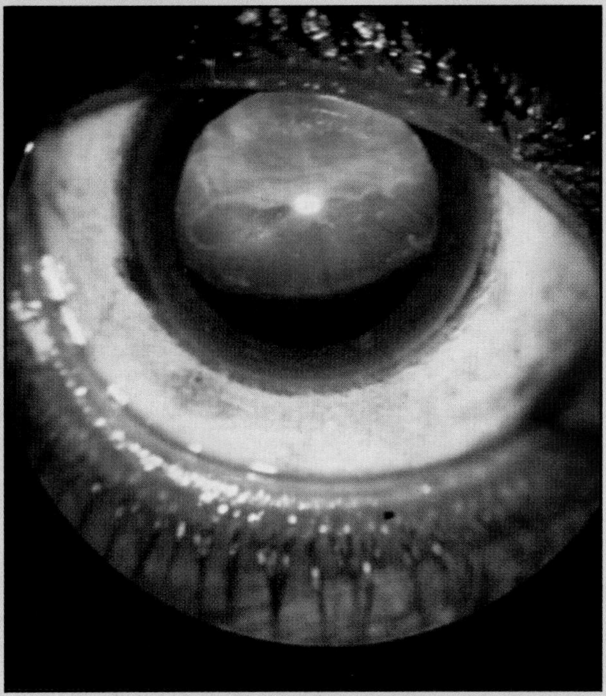

CENTRAL GRAY OPACITY—NUCLEAR CATARACT

Nuclear cataract shows as an opaque gray surrounded by black background as it forms in lens nucleus. Through the ophthalmoscope, it looks like a black center against the red reflex. It begins after age 40 and develops slowly.

STAR-SHAPED OPACITY—CORTICAL CATARACT (not illustrated)

Cortical cataract shows as peripheral gray wedges with black center. Through ophthalmoscope, black spokes are evident against the red reflex. This forms in outer cortex of lens, progressing faster than nuclear cataract.

Table 11-11 ► Abnormalities in the Optic Disc

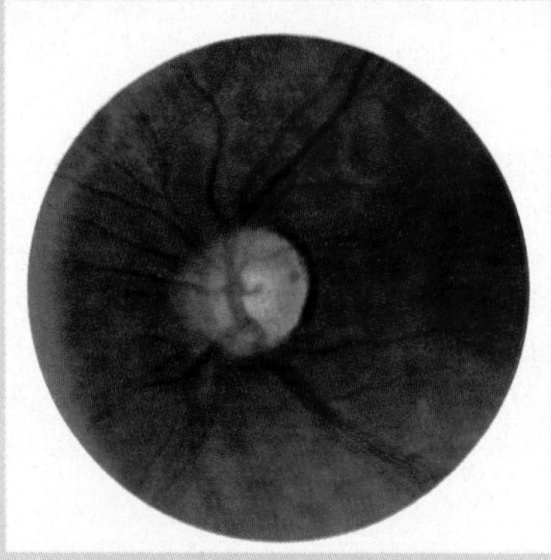

OPTIC ATROPHY (DISC PALLOR)

Optic atrophy is a chalky whiteness of the disc due to partial or complete death of the optic nerve.

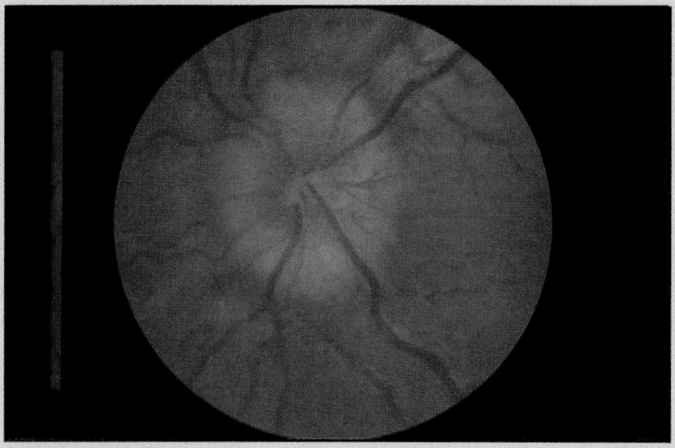

PAPILLEDEMA (CHOKED DISC)

Increased intracranial pressure causes venous stasis in the globe, showing redness, congestion, and elevation of the disc, blurred margins, hemorrhages, and absent venous pulsations. This is a serious sign of intracranial pressure.

Table 11-11 ▶ Abnormalities in the Optic Disc *Continued*

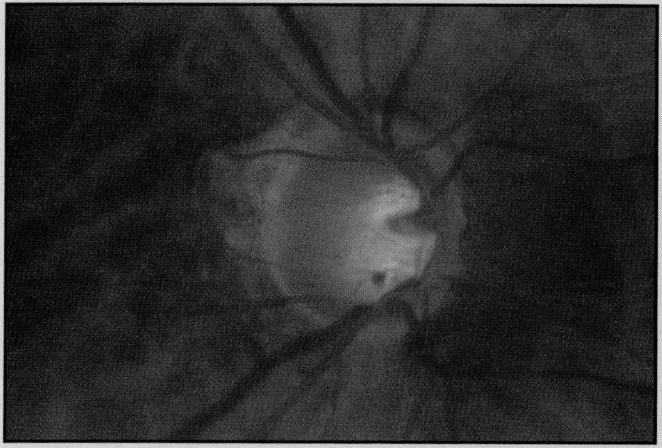

EXCESSIVE CUP-DISC RATIO

With glaucoma, the increased intraocular pressure decreases blood supply to retinal structures. The physiologic cup enlarges to more than 1/2 of the disc diameter, vessels appear to plunge over edge of cup, and the vessels are displaced nasally.

Table 11-12 ▶ Abnormalities in the Retinal Vessels

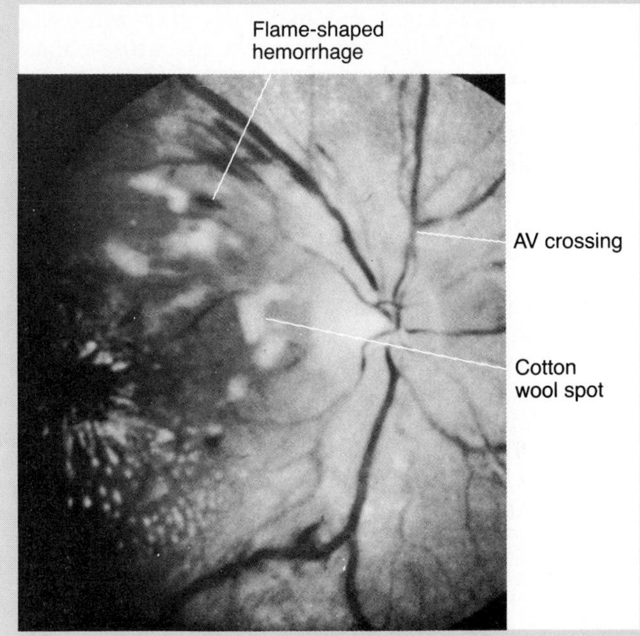

ARTERIOVENOUS CROSSING

Arteriovenous crossing with interruption of blood flow. When vein is occluded, it dilates distal to crossing.

VESSEL NICKING

Nicking is a localized narrowing in vein caused by arteriole crossing. It is seen with hypertension and arteriosclerosis.

NARROWED ARTERIES

This is a generalized decrease in diameter. The light reflex also narrows. It occurs with severe hypertension, occlusion of central retinal artery, and with retinitis pigmentosa.

SILVERWIRE ARTERIES

With hypertension, the arteriole wall thickens and becomes opaque so that no blood is seen inside it.

COPPERWIRE ARTERIES

The light reflex widens, showing a metallic copper color. This is seen with hypertension.

Table 11-13 ► Abnormalities in the General Background

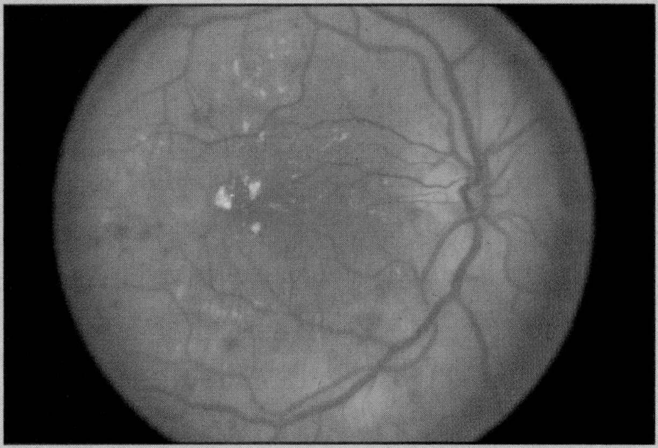

MICROANEURYSMS

Microaneurysms are round punctate red dots that are localized dilatations of a small vessel. Their edges are smooth and discrete. The vessel itself is too small to view with the ophthalmoscope, only the isolated red dots are seen. This occurs with diabetes.

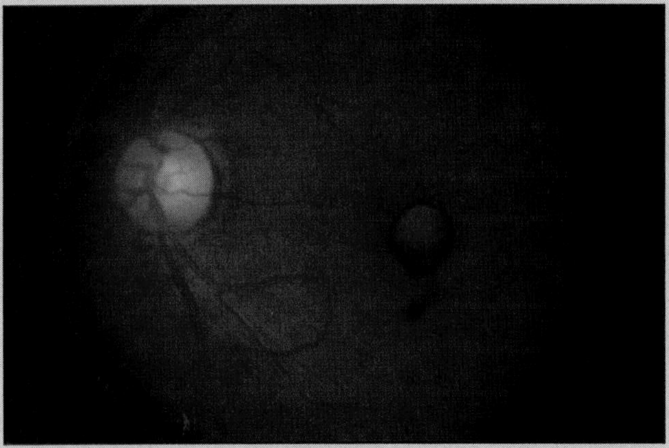

PRERETINAL HEMORRHAGE

Preretinal hemorrhage is a solid dark area due to blood accumulating in a pocket between the retina and vitreous body. Note the top has horizontal fluid level from gravity and that it conceals the retinal vessels behind.

DOT-SHAPED HEMORRHAGES

Deep intraretinal hemorrhages look splattered on. These occur with diabetes. They may be distinguished from microaneurysms by the blurred irregular edges.

FLAME-SHAPED HEMORRHAGES

Flame-shaped hemorrhages are superficial retinal hemorrhages that look linear and spindle shaped. They occur with hypertension (see Figure in Table 11-12).

SOFT EXUDATES

"Cotton wool" areas look like fluffy gray-white cumulus clouds. They are arteriolar microinfarctions that envelop and obscure the vessels. They occur with diabetes, hypertension, subacute bacterial endocarditis (SBE), lupus, and papilledema of any cause (see Table 11-12).

HARD EXUDATES

These are numerous small yellow-white spots, having distinct edges and a smooth, solid-looking surface. They often form a circular pattern, clustered around a venous microinfarction. They also may form a linear or star pattern. (This is in contrast with the normal Drusen, which have a scattered haphazard location (see in Figure with microaneurysms on this page).

Bibliography

Arsham GM, Colenbrander A, Spivey BE: Basic instruction in ophthalmoscopy. Iowa City, IA, University of Iowa, Department of Ophthalmology, 1971.

Boyd-Monk H: Examining the external eye. Part 1. Nursing 80 10(5):58–63, 1980.

Boyd-Monk H: Examining the external eye. Part 2. Nursing 80 10(6):58–63, 1980.

Hiles DA: Strabismus. Am J Nurs 74:1082–1089, 1974.

Hoffman MJ: Retinal pigmentation, visual acuity and brightness levels. Am J Phys Anthropology 43(3):417–424, 1975.

Johnson JH, Cryan M: Homonymous hemianopsia—assessment and nursing management. Am J Nurs 79:2131–2135, 1979.

Jones, M., Tippett T: Assessment of the red eye. Nurse Pract 5:10–15, 1980.

Meltzer DW: Ophthalmic Aspects. *In* Steinberg FU (Ed.): Care of the Geriatric Patient. St. Louis, CV Mosby, 1983, pp. 450–461.

Newell FW: Ophthalmology: Principles and Concepts (6th ed.) St. Louis, CV Mosby, 1986.

Norman S: The pupil check. Am J Nurs 82:588–591, April 1982.

Overfield T: Biologic Variation in Health and Illness: Race, Age, and Sex Differences. Menlo Park, CA, Addison-Wesley, 1985.

Patient Assessment: Examination of the eye. Am J Nurs—Part 1. 74:P11–24, 1974. Patient assessment—Part 2. 75:P11–24, 1975.

Rossman I (Ed): Clinical Geriatrics. 3rd ed. Philadelphia, J.B. Lippincott, 1986.

Scheie HG, Albert DM: Textbook of Ophthalmology. 9th ed. Philadelphia, W.B. Saunders, 1977.

Tumulty G, Resler: Eye trauma. Am J Nurs 84:740–744, June 1984.

Vaughan D, Asbury T: General Ophthalmology. 12th ed. East Norwalk, CT, Appleton & Lange, 1989.

Whaley LF, Wong DL: Nursing Care of Infants and Children. 4th ed. St. Louis, CV Mosby, 1990.

CHAPTER

12 Assessing the Ears and Hearing Status

STRUCTURE AND FUNCTION

The ear is the sensory organ for hearing and maintaining equilibrium. The ear has three parts: the external, middle, and inner ear. The external ear is called the *auricle,* or *pinna,* and consists of movable cartilage and skin (Fig. 12–1). Note the landmarks of the auricle and use these terms to describe your findings. The mastoid process, the bony prominence behind the lobule, is not part of the ear but is an important landmark.

EXTERNAL EAR

The external ear funnels sound into its opening, the *external auditory canal* (Fig. 12–2). The canal is a cul-de-sac 2.5 to 3 cm long in the adult and terminates at the tympanic membrane. It is lined with glands that secrete cerumen, a yellow waxy material that lubricates and protects the ear. Two types of earwax exist among races. It looks wet, sticky and honey colored in whites and blacks, and it looks dry and flaky in Asians and Native Americans (see section on Transcultural Considerations).

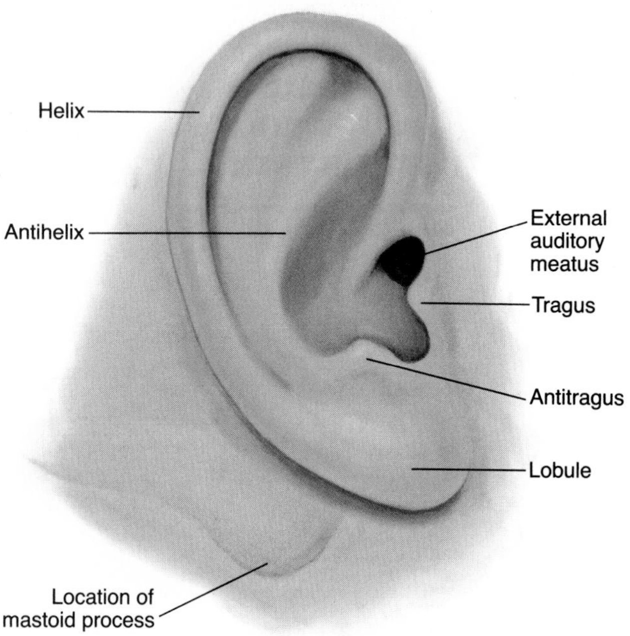

▶ **Figure 12–1**

The outer one-third of the canal is cartilage; the inner two-thirds consists of bone covered by thin sensitive skin. The canal has a slight S-curve in the adult. The outer one-third curves up and toward the back of the head, whereas the inner two-thirds angles down and forward toward the nose.

The *tympanic membrane* separates the external and middle ear and is tilted obliquely to the ear canal. It is a translucent membrane with a pearly gray color and a prominent cone of light in the anteroinferior quadrant, which is the reflection of the otoscope light (Fig. 12–3). The drum is slightly concave, pulled in at its center by one of the middle ear ossicles, the *malleus.* The parts of the malleus show through the translucent drum; these are the *umbo,* the *manubrium* (handle), and the *short process.* The small, slack, superior section of the tympanic membrane is called the *pars flaccida.* The remainder of the drum, which is more taut, is the *pars tensa.* The *annulus* is the outer fibrous rim of the drum.

MIDDLE EAR

The middle ear is a tiny air-filled cavity inside the temporal bone (Fig. 12–2). It contains tiny ear bones or auditory ossicles: the *malleus, incus,* and *stapes.* There are several openings into the middle ear. Its opening to the outer ear is covered by the eardrum or tympanic membrane. The openings to the inner ear are the oval window at the end of the stapes and the round window. Another opening is the *eustachian tube,* which connects the middle ear with the nasopharynx and allows passage of air.

The middle ear has three functions: (1) It conducts sound vibrations from the outer ear to the central hearing apparatus in the inner ear; (2) it protects the inner ear by reducing the amplitude of loud sounds; and (3) its eustachian tube allows equalization of air pressure on each side of the tympanic membrane so that the membrane does not rupture.

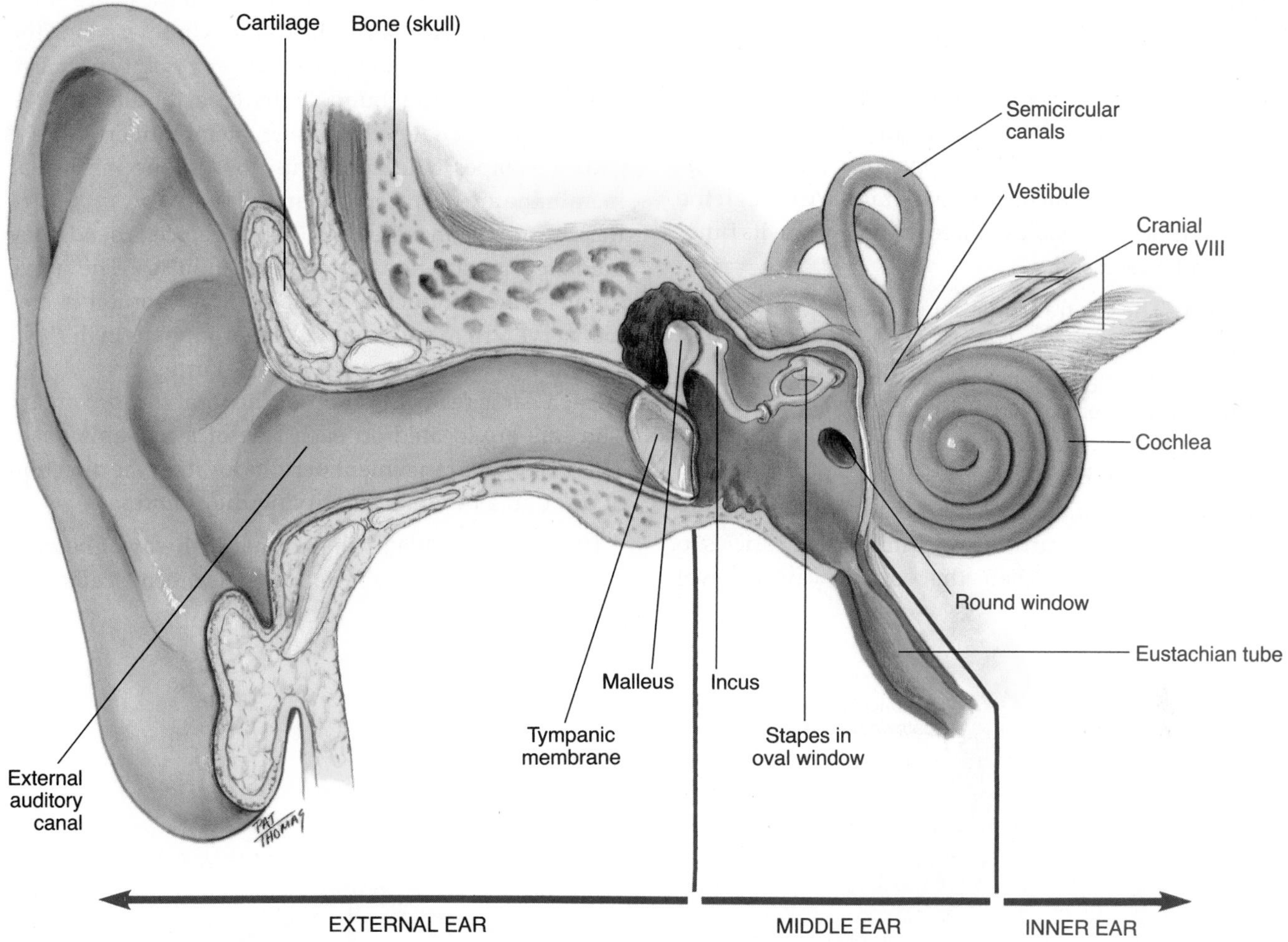

► **Figure 12-2**

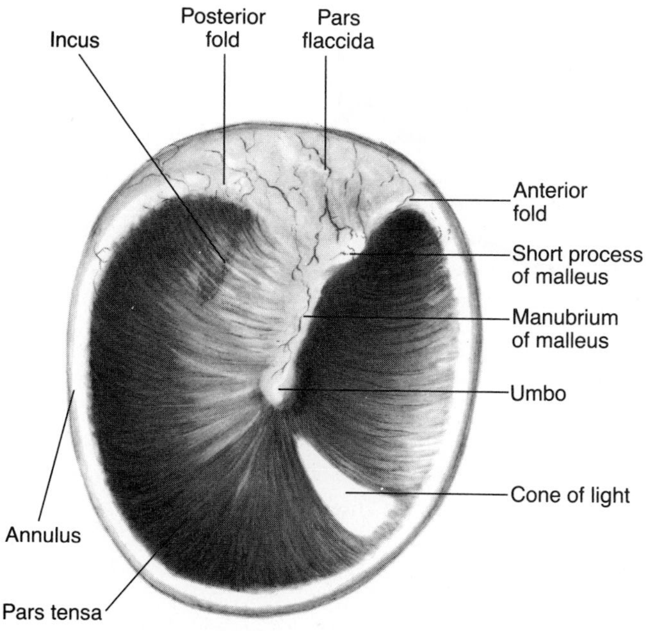

► **Figure 12-3**

INNER EAR

The inner ear contains the *bony labyrinth,* which holds the sensory organs for equilibrium and hearing. Within the bony labyrinth, the *vestibule* and the *semicircular canals* comprise the vestibular apparatus, and the *cochlea* contains the central hearing apparatus. Although the inner ear is not accessible to direct examination, its functions can be assessed.

Hearing. The ear transmits sound and converts its vibrations into nerve impulses. For example, you hear an alarm bell ringing in the hall. Its sound waves travel instantly to your ears (Fig. 12–4). The *amplitude* is how loud the alarm is; its *frequency* is the pitch (in this case, high) or the number of cycles per second. The sound waves produce vibrations on your tympanic membrane. These vibrations are carried by the middle ear ossicles to your oval window. Then the sound waves travel through your cochlea, which is coiled like a snail's shell, and are dissipated against the round window. Along the way, the *basilar membrane* vibrates at a point specific to the frequency of the sound. In this case, the alarm's high frequency stimulates the basilar membrane at its base near the stapes. The numerous fibers along the basilar membrane are the receptor hair cells of the *organ of Corti,* the sensory organ of hearing. As the hair cells bend, they mediate the vibrations into nerve impulses. The nerve impulses are conducted by the auditory portion of cranial nerve VIII to your brain. All this happens in the split second it takes you to react to the alarm.

Each ear is really one-half of the total sensory organ. The ears are located on each side of a movable head. This *binaural* arrangement permits locating the direction of a sound as well as identifying the sound.

Pathways of Hearing. The normal pathway of hearing is air conduction described above; it is the most efficient.

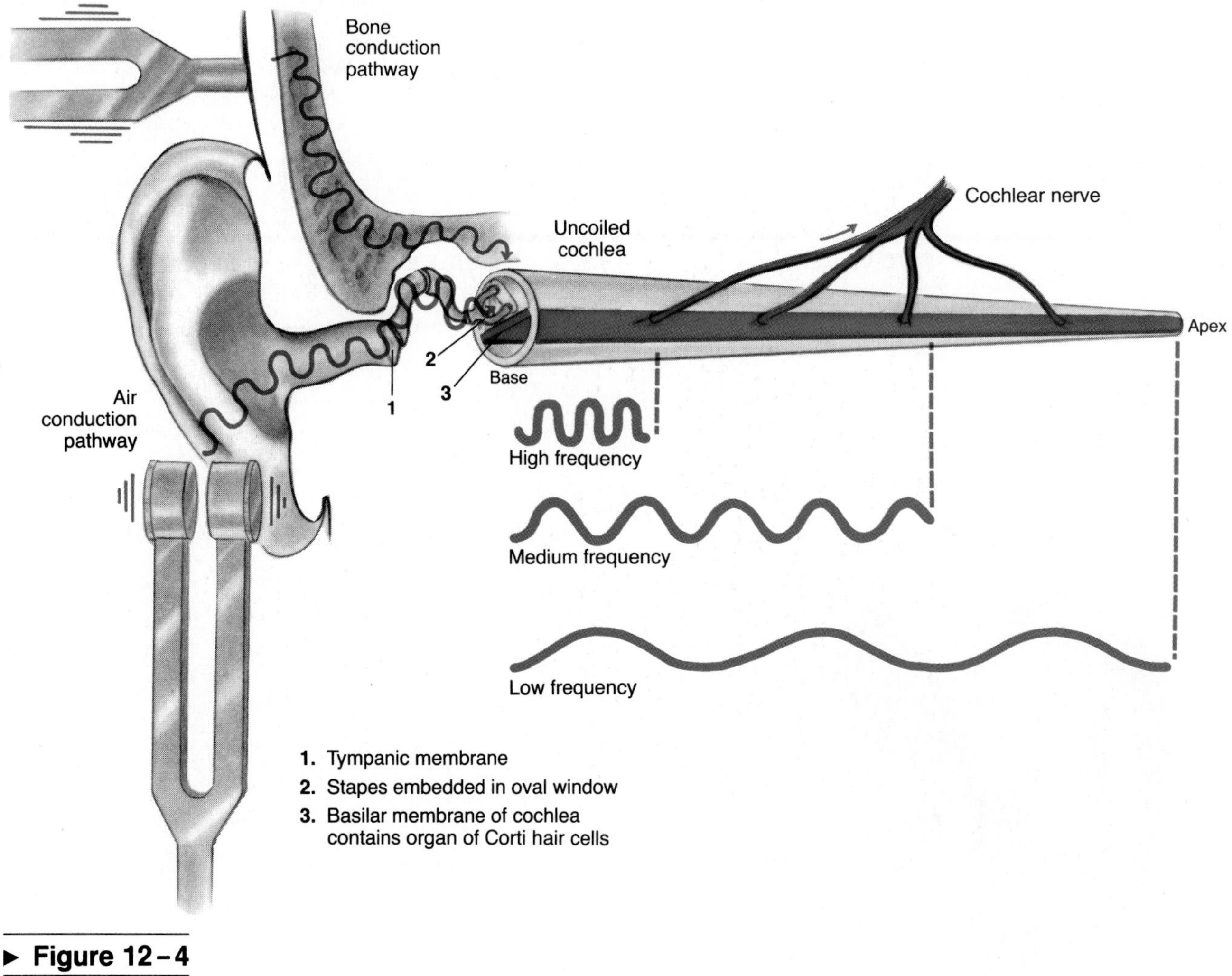

► **Figure 12–4**

An alternate route of hearing is by bone conduction. Here, the bones of the skull vibrate. These vibrations are transmitted directly to the inner ear and to cranial nerve VIII.

Hearing Loss. Anything that obstructs the transmission of sound impairs hearing. A *conductive* hearing loss involves dysfunction of the external or middle ear. It is a partial loss because the person is able to hear if the sound amplitude is increased enough to reach normal nerve elements in the inner ear. Conductive hearing loss may be caused by impacted cerumen, foreign bodies, a perforated tympanic membrane, pus or serum in the middle ear, and otosclerosis (a decrease in mobility of the ossicles).

Sensorineural (or perceptive) loss signifies pathology of the inner ear, cranial nerve VIII, or the auditory areas of the cerebral cortex. A simple increase in amplitude may not enable the person to understand words. Sensorineural hearing loss may be caused by *presbycusis,* a gradual nerve degeneration that occurs with aging, and ototoxic drugs, which affect the hair cells in the cochlea.

A *mixed* loss is a combination of conductive and sensorineural types in the same ear.

Equilibrium. The labyrinth in the inner ear constantly feeds information to your brain about your body's position in space. It works like a plumb line to determine verticality or depth. The ear's plumb lines register the angle of your head in relation to gravity. If the labyrinth ever becomes inflamed, it feeds the wrong information to the brain, creating a staggering gait and a strong, whirling sensation called vertigo.

DEVELOPMENTAL CONSIDERATIONS

Infants and Children

The inner ear starts to develop early in the fourth week of gestation. If maternal rubella infection occurs during the first trimester, it can damage the organ of Corti and impair hearing. The infant's eustachian tube is relatively shorter, relatively wider, and its position is more horizontal than the adult's, so it is easier for pathogens from the nasopharynx to migrate through to the middle ear (Fig. 12–5). The lumen is surrounded by lymphoid tissue, which increases during childhood; thus, the lumen is easily occluded. These factors place the infant at greater risk for middle ear infections than the adult.

The infant's and the young child's external auditory canal is shorter and has an opposite slope than the adult's (see Fig. 12–17).

The Adult

Otosclerosis is a common cause of conductive hearing loss in young adults between the ages of 20 and 40. It is a gradual hardening that causes the foot plate of the stapes to become fixed in the oval window, impeding the transmission of sound and causing progressive deafness.

The Aging Adult

In the aging person, cilia lining the ear canal become coarse and stiff. This condition may cause decreased

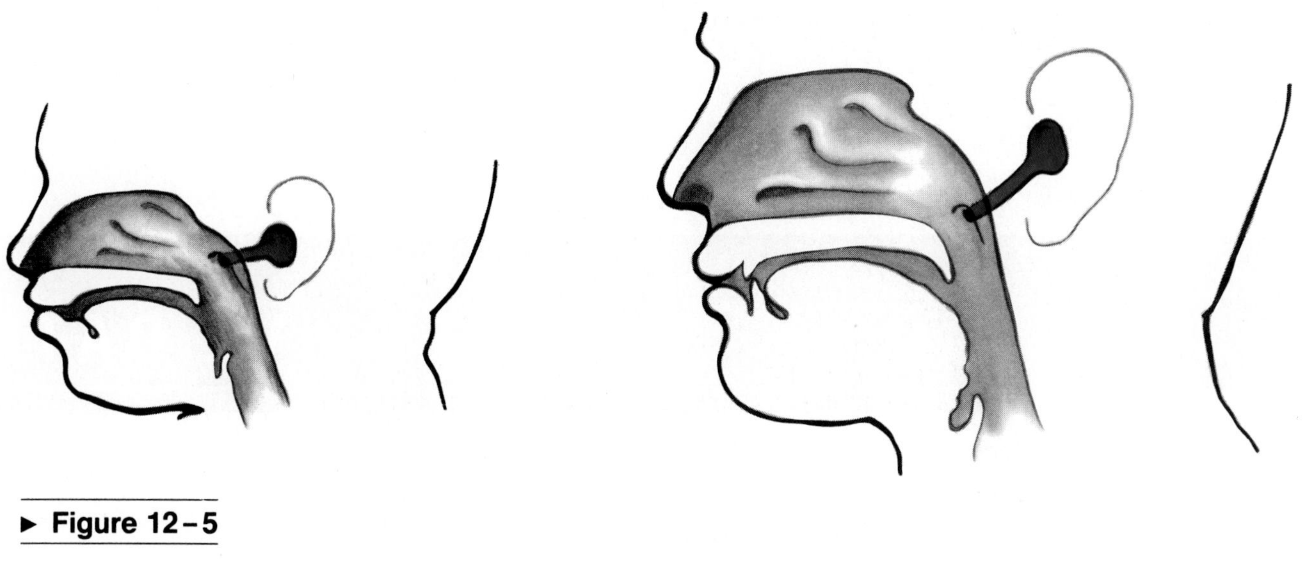

► **Figure 12–5**

hearing since it impedes sound waves traveling toward the tympanic membrane. It also causes cerumen to accumulate and oxidize, which greatly reduces hearing. The cerumen itself is drier because of atrophy of the apocrine glands. Also, an older person with a life history of frequent ear infections may have noticeable scarring on the drum.

A person living in a noise-polluted area (e.g., near an airport or a busy highway) has a greater risk of hearing loss. But *presbycusis* is a type of hearing loss that occurs with aging, even in people living in a quiet environment. It is a gradual sensorineural loss caused by nerve degeneration in the inner ear or auditory nerve. Its onset usually occurs in the fifth decade, and then it slowly progresses. The person first notices a high-frequency tone loss; it is harder to hear consonants (high-pitched components of speech) than vowels. This makes words sound garbled. The ability to localize sound is impaired also. This communication dysfunction is accentuated when background noise is present (e.g., with music, with dishes clattering, or in a large noisy party).

Lastly, the "auditory reaction time" increases after age 70 (Rossman, 1986). That is, it takes longer for the older adult to process sensory input and to respond to it.

TRANSCULTURAL CONSIDERATIONS

Middle ear infection (otitis media) occurs because of obstruction of the eustachian tube and/or passage of nasopharyngeal secretions into the middle ear. Otitis media is one of the most common illnesses in children. An epidemiologic study of over 2500 children revealed that 71 percent had at least one episode of acute otitis media by age 3 years (Teele, 1980). The incidence and severity are increased in Native Americans and Alaskan and Canadian Eskimos (Bluestone and Klein, 1988). American black children have less incidence of otitis media than American white children (Bluestone and Klein, 1988).

The incidence of otitis media also is increased in premature infants, in those with Down syndrome, and in babies fed by bottle in a supine position. In the supine position, the effects of gravity and sucking tend to draw the nasopharyngeal contents directly into the middle ear. The parent should be urged to hold the baby partly upright against the arm while feeding. Do not prop the bottle or let the baby take a bottle to bed. Encouraging breast-feeding helps prevent this problem.

The most important side effect of acute otitis media is the persistence of fluid in the middle ear after treatment. One study found the persistence of middle ear effusion to be frequent in all children, although it is more likely in children under 2 years of age and in white children (Shurin et al, 1979). This can impair hearing, placing the child at risk for cognitive development.

Cerumen is genetically determined and comes in two major types: (1) dry cerumen, which is gray, flaky, and frequently forms a thin mass in the ear canal and (2) wet cerumen, which is honey to dark brown and moist. Asians and Native Americans have an 84 percent frequency of dry cerumen whereas blacks have a 99 percent and whites have a 97 percent frequency of wet cerumen (Overfield, 1985). The clinical significance of this occurs when examining or irrigating the ears. The presence and composition of cerumen are not related to poor hygiene, and caution should be exercised to avoid mistaking the flaky dry cerumen for eczematous lesions.

SUBJECTIVE DATA

Earaches	Environmental noise
Infections	Tinnitus
Discharge	Vertigo
Hearing loss	Self-care behaviors

EXAMINER ASKS:	RATIONALE:
1. Do you have any **earache** or other pain in ears? Location—Does it feel close to the surface or deep in the head? Does it hurt when you push on the ear? Character—Is the pain dull, aching or sharp, stabbing? Is it constant or does it come and go? Is it affected by changing position of head?	Pain may be directly due to ear disease or may be referred pain from a problem in teeth or oropharynx.
Do you have accompanying cold symptoms or sore throat? Are there any problems with sinuses or teeth?	Virus/bacteria from upper respiratory infection (URI) may migrate up eustachian tube to involve middle ear.
Have you ever been hit on the ear or on the side of the head, or had any sport injury? Have you had any trauma from a foreign body?	Trauma may rupture the tympanic membrane.
What have you tried to relieve pain?	Assess effect of coping strategies.
2. Have you had any ear **infections?** As an adult, or in childhood? How frequent were they? How were they treated?	A history of chronic ear problems alerts you to possibility of sequelae.
3. Is there any **discharge** from your ears?	Discharge suggests infection; it may come from canal or may indicate a perforated eardrum. For example:
Does it look like pus, or bloody?	*External otitis*—purulent, sanguinous, or watery discharge. *Acute otitis media with perforation*—purulent discharge.
Any odor to the discharge?	*Cholesteatoma*—dirty yellow/gray discharge, foul odor.
Is there any relation between the discharge and the ear pain?	Typically with perforation—ear pain occurs first, stops with a popping sensation, then drainage occurs.
4. **Hearing loss**	
Have you ever had any trouble hearing? Onset—Did the loss come on slowly or all at once?	Presbycusis has a gradual onset over years, whereas a loss due to trauma is often sudden. Any sudden loss in one or both ears *not* associated with upper respiratory infection warrants referral.
Character—Has all your hearing decreased, or just on hearing certain sounds?	
In what situations do you notice the loss: conversations, using the telephone, listening to TV, at a party?	Loss may be apparent when there is competition from background noise, e.g., at a party.
Do people seem to shout at you?	*Recruitment*—There is a marked loss when sound is at low intensity, but sound actually may become painful when repeated in a loud voice.
Is there any family history of hearing loss?	
Effort to treat—Have you tried any hearing aid or other device? Do you do anything to help hearing?	
Coping strategies—How does the loss affect your daily life? Is there any job problem? Do you feel some social isolation? Do you find less pleasure at leisure activities? How do your family, friends react?	

EXAMINER ASKS:	RATIONALE:
Note to examiner — During history, note these clues from normal conversation, which indicate possible hearing loss. 1. Person lip reading or watching your face and lips closely rather than your eyes. 2. Frowning or straining forward to hear. 3. Posturing of head to catch sounds with better ear. 4. Misunderstands your questions, or frequently asks you to repeat. 5. Acts irritable or shows startle reflex when you raise your voice. (Recruitment) 6. Person's speech sounds garbled, possibly vowel sounds distorted. 7. Inappropriately loud voice. 8. Flat monotonous tone of voice.	
5. **Environmental noise.** Are you around any loud noises at home or on the job? For example, do you live in a noise polluted area, near an airport, or busy traffic area? Are you near other noises such as heavy machinery, loud persistent music, gun shots while hunting?	
Are you around environmental noise now or have you been at any time in the past?	Old trauma to hearing initially goes unnoticed, yet results in further decibel loss in later years.
Coping strategies — Do you take any steps to protect your ears, such as headphones or ear plugs?	
6. **Tinnitus.** Have you ever felt ringing, crackling, or buzzing in your ears? When did this occur?	The sound of tinnitus originates within the person. Tinnitus accompanies some hearing loss or ear disorders.
Does this sound seem louder at night?	Tinnitus seems louder when there is no competition from environmental noise.
Are you taking any medications?	Consider medications with possible ototoxic sequelae: aspirin, streptomycin, gentamicin, kanamycin, neomycin, ethacrynic acid (Edecrin), furosemide (Lasix), indomethacin (Indocin), quinine, vancomycin.
7. Have you ever felt **vertigo,** that is, the room spinning around or yourself spinning? Vertigo is a true twirling motion.	True rotational spinning with dysfunction of labyrinth. Objective vertigo — feels like room spins. Subjective vertigo — feels like person spins.
Ever felt dizzy, like you are not quite steady, like falling or losing your balance? Giddy, lightheaded?	Distinguish true vertigo from dizziness or lightheadedness.
8. **Self care.** How do you clean your ears?	Assess potential trauma from invasive instruments. Cleaning with cotton tipped applicators can impact cerumen, causing hearing loss.
When was the last time you had your hearing checked? If a hearing loss was noted, did you obtain a hearing aid? How long have you had it? Do you wear it? How does it work? Do you have any trouble with upkeep, cleaning, changing batteries?	Prescribe frequency of hearing assessment according to person's age and/or risk factors.

EXAMINER ASKS: | **RATIONALE:**

ADDITIONAL QUESTIONS FOR INFANTS AND CHILDREN

Ear infections. At what age was the child's first episode? How many ear infections in the last 6 months? How many total? How were these treated?

Has the child had any surgery, such as insertion of ear tubes or removal of tonsils?

Are the infections increasing in frequency, in severity, or staying the same?

Does the child seem to be hearing well?

Have you noticed that the infant startles with loud noise? Did the infant babble around 6 months? Does he or she talk; at what age did talking start? Was the speech intelligible?

Ever had the child's hearing tested? If there was a hearing loss, did it follow any diseases in the child, or in mother during pregnancy?

(Note: It is important to catch any problem early, because a child with hearing loss is at risk for delayed speech and social development and learning deficit.)

If two or more episodes occurred in the first year, the child is "otitis-prone" and will have twice as many subsequent episodes as the child with one episode or no episodes during the first year (Howie, 1975).

Children at risk for hearing deficit include those exposed to maternal rubella and maternal ototoxic drugs in utero, premature infants, low birth weight infants, and infants with congenital liver or kidney disease.

In children, the incidence of meningitis, measles, mumps, otitis media, and any illness with persistent high fever may increase risk of hearing deficit.

3. Does the child tend to put objects in the ears? Is the older child or adolescent active in contact sports?

These children are at increased risk for trauma.

ADDITIONAL QUESTIONS FOR THE AGING ADULT

Vertigo. Offer same general questions as listed above, but note that unsteadiness is very common in aging people.

OBJECTIVE DATA

Equipment Needed

Otoscope with bright light (fresh batteries give off white, not yellow, light)
Pneumatic bulb attachment, sometimes used with infant or young child
Tuning forks in 512, 1024 Hz

Preparation

Position the adult sitting up straight with his or her head at your eye level. Occasionally the ear canal is partially filled with cerumen, which obstructs your view of the tympanic membrane. You may use a cerumen spoon to curette out the wax only if you are proficient and comfortable with this instrument. If the eardrum is intact, a preferred method of cleaning the canal is to soften the cerumen with a warmed solution of mineral oil and hydrogen peroxide. Then the canal is irrigated with warm water using a bulb syringe or a low-pulsatile dental irrigator (Water-Pik). (Do not irrigate if the history or the examination suggests perforation.)

METHOD OF EXAMINATION

NORMAL RANGE OF FINDINGS	ABNORMAL FINDINGS
THE EXTERNAL EAR	
Inspect and palpate the external ear.	
Size and Shape	
The ears are of equal size bilaterally with no swelling or thickening. Ears of unusual size and shape may be a normal familial trait with no clinical significance.	*Microtia*—ears smaller than 4 cm vertically *Macrotia*—ears larger than 10 cm vertically Edema (See Table 12–1, Abnormalities of the External Ear)
Skin Condition	
The skin color is consistent with the person's facial skin color. The skin is intact, with no lumps or lesions. On some people you may note *Darwin's tubercle,* a small painless nodule at the helix. This is a congenital variation and is not significant (see Table 12–2).	Reddened, excessively warm skin indicates inflammation. Crusts and scaling occur with otitis externa and with eczema, contact dermatitis, and seborrhea. Enlarged tender lymph nodes in the region indicate inflammation of the pinna or mastoid process. Red-blue discoloration indicates frostbite. Tophi, sebaceous cyst, chondrodermatitis, keloid, carcinoma (see Table 12–2).
Tenderness	
Move the pinna, and push on the tragus. They should feel firm, and movement should produce no pain. Palpating the mastoid process should be painless.	Pain with movement occurs with otitis externa and furuncle. Pain at the mastoid process may indicate mastoiditis or lymphadenitis of the posterior auricular node.

NORMAL RANGE OF FINDINGS

The External Auditory Meatus

Note the size of the opening to direct your choice of speculum for the otoscope. There should be no swelling, redness, or discharge.

Some cerumen is usually present. The color varies from gray-yellow to light brown and black, and the texture varies from moist and waxy to dry and desiccated. A large amount of cerumen obscures visualization of the canal and drum.

THE OTOSCOPIC EXAMINATION

Inspect, using the otoscope.

As you inspect the external ear, note the size of the auditory meatus. Then, choose the largest speculum that will fit comfortably in the ear canal and attach it to the otoscope. Tilt the person's head slightly away from you toward the opposite shoulder. This method brings the obliquely sloping eardrum into better view.

Pull the pinna up and back on an adult or older child; this helps straighten the S-shape of the canal (Fig. 12–6). (Pull the pinna down on an infant and child under 3 years of age) (see Fig. 12–17.) Hold the pinna gently but firmly. Do not release traction on the ear until you have finished the examination and the otoscope is removed.

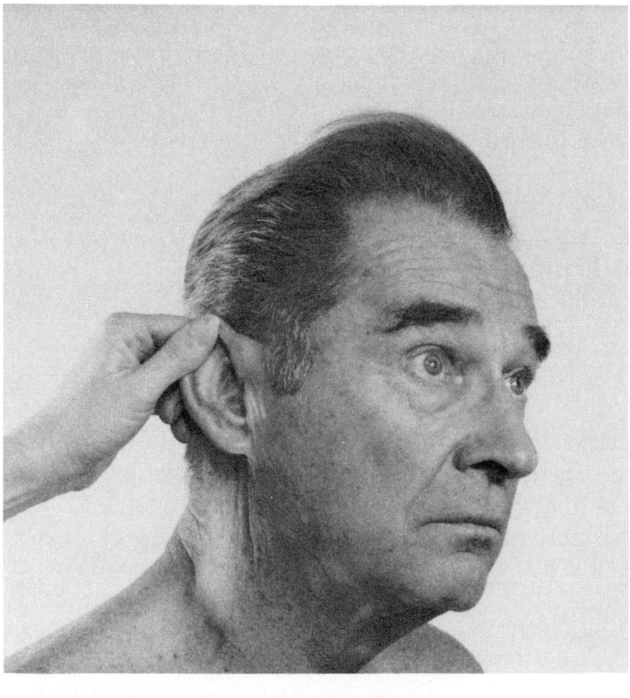

► **Figure 12–6**

ABNORMAL FINDINGS

Atresia — absence or closure of the ear canal.

A sticky yellow discharge accompanies otitis externa, or it may indicate otitis media if the drum has ruptured.

Impacted cerumen is a common cause of conductive hearing loss.

NORMAL RANGE OF FINDINGS | **ABNORMAL FINDINGS**

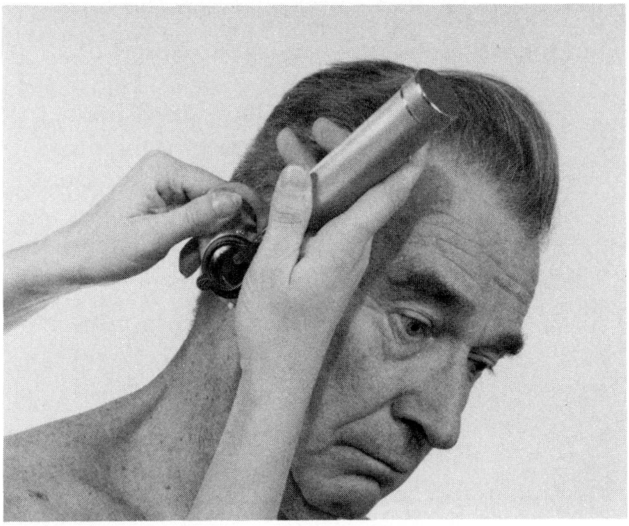

► **Figure 12–7**

Hold the otoscope "upside down" along your fingers, and have the dorsa (back) of your hand along the person's cheek braced to steady the otoscope (Fig. 12–7). This position feels awkward to you only at first. It soon will feel natural and you will find it useful to prevent forceful insertion. Also your stabilizing hand acts as a protecting lever if the person suddenly moves the head.

Insert the speculum slowly and carefully along the axis of the canal. Watch the insertion; then put your eye up to the otoscope. Avoid touching the inner "bony" section of the canal wall, which is covered by a thin epithelial layer and is sensitive to pain. Sometimes you cannot see anything but canal wall. If so, try to reposition the person's head, apply more traction on the pinna, and re-angle the otoscope to look forward toward the person's nose.

Once it is in place, you may need to rotate the otoscope slightly to visualize all of the drum; do this gently. Lastly, perform the otoscopic examination before you test hearing; ear canals with impacted cerumen give the erroneous impression of pathologic hearing loss.

The External Canal

Note any redness and swelling, lesions, foreign bodies, or discharge. If any discharge is present, note the color and odor. (Also, clean discharge from the speculum before examining the other ear to avoid contamination with possibly infectious material.) For a person with a hearing aid, note any irritation on the canal wall from poorly fitting earmolds.

Redness and swelling occur with otitis externa; canal may be completely closed with swelling.

Purulent otorrhea suggests otitis externa, or otitis media may be indicated if the drum has ruptured.

Frank blood or clear watery drainage (cerebrospinal fluid leak) following trauma suggests basal

NORMAL RANGE OF FINDINGS	ABNORMAL FINDINGS

skull fracture and warrants immediate referral. Cerebrospinal fluid feels oily and produces a positive glucose finding on Testape.

Foreign body, exostosis, polyp, furuncle (see Table 12–3, Abnormalities in the Ear Canal).

The Tympanic Membrane

Color and Characteristics

Systematically explore its landmarks (Fig. 12–8). The normal eardrum is shiny and translucent, with a pearl-gray color. The cone-shaped light reflex is prominent in the anteroinferior quadrant (at 5 o'clock in the right drum and 7 o'clock in the left drum). This is the reflection of your otoscope light. Sections of the malleus are visible through the translucent drum: the umbo, manubrium, and short process. (Infrequently, you also may see the incus behind the drum; it shows as a whitish haze in the upper posterior area.) At the periphery, the annulus looks whiter and denser.

Yellow-amber color of the drum occurs with serous otitis media.

Red color occurs with acute otitis media.

Absent or distorted landmarks.

Air/fluid level or air bubbles behind drum indicate serous otitis media (see Table 12–4 and Table 12–5).

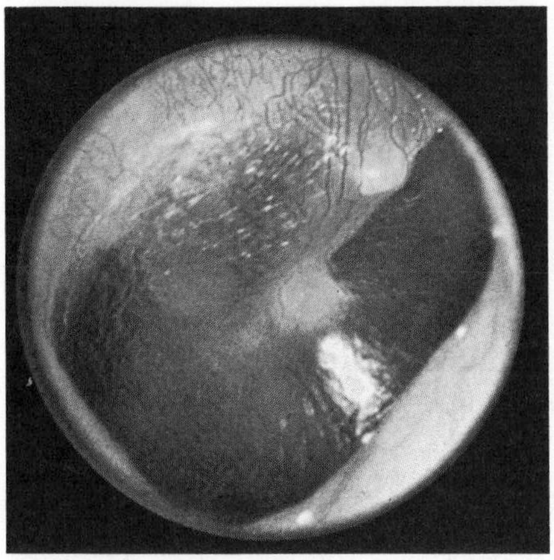

Normal tympanic membrane, right

► Figure 12–8

Position

The eardrum is flat, slightly pulled in at the center, and flutters when the person performs the Valsalva maneuver or holds the nose and swallows (insufflation). You may elicit these maneuvers to assess drum mobility. Avoid them with an aging person because they may disrupt equilibrium. Also avoid middle ear insufflation in a person with upper respiratory infection because it could propel infectious matter into the middle ear.

Retracted drum due to vacuum in middle ear.

Bulging drum from increased pressure.

Drum does not move (see Table 12–5).

NORMAL RANGE OF FINDINGS	ABNORMAL FINDINGS

Integrity of Membrane

The normal tympanic membrane is intact. Some adults may show scarring, or a dense white patch on the drum, as a sequela of repeated ear infections.

Perforation shows as a dark oval area or as a larger opening on the drum.

Vesicles on drum (see Table 12–5).

HEARING ACUITY

Test hearing acuity.

Your screening for a hearing deficit begins during the history; how well does the person hear conversational speech? An audiometer gives a precise quantitative measure of hearing by assessing the person's ability to hear sounds of varying frequency. Since this equipment usually is not available in the clinical setting, you may use alternate screening measures. These are "crude" tests. They are nonquantitative; they are useful to document the *presence* of hearing loss but do not measure the degree of loss. Refer any abnormal findings for more accurate measures with pure tone audiometry.

Voice Test

Test one ear at a time while masking hearing in the other ear to prevent sound transmission around the head. This is done by placing one finger on the tragus and rapidly pushing it in and out of the auditory meatus. Shield your lips so the person cannot compensate for a hearing loss (consciously or unconsciously) by lip reading or using the "good" ear. With your head 30 to 60 cm (1–2 ft) from the person's ear, exhale and whisper slowly some two-syllable words, such as Tuesday, armchair, baseball, and fourteen. Normally, the person repeats each word correctly after you say it.

The person is unable to hear whispered words. A whisper is a high-frequency sound and is used to detect high-tone loss.

Tuning Fork Tests

Tuning fork tests measure hearing by air conduction (AC) or by bone conduction (BC) in which the sound vibrates through the cranial bones to the inner ear. The AC route through the ear canal and middle ear is usually the more sensitive route. To activate the tuning fork, hold it by the stem and strike the tines softly on the back of your hand (Fig. 12–9). A hard strike makes the tone too loud, and it takes a long time to fade out.

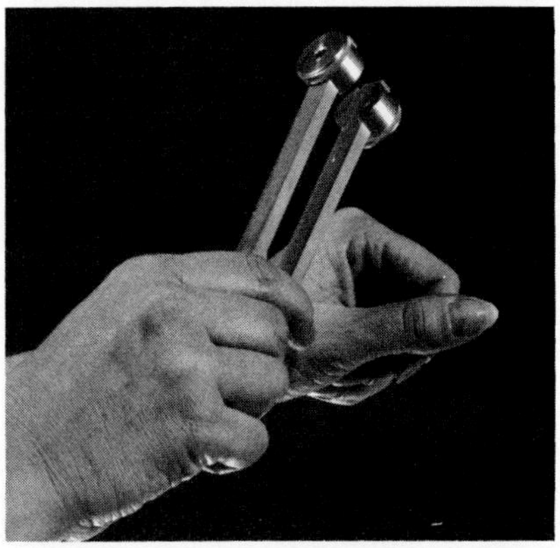

▸ **Figure 12–9**

NORMAL RANGE OF FINDINGS

ABNORMAL FINDINGS

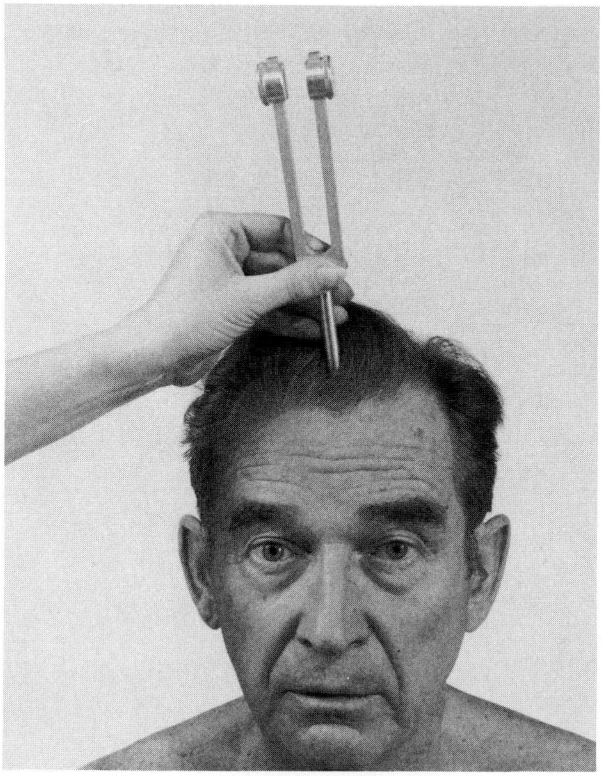

► Figure 12–10

Weber test

The *Weber test* is valuable when a person reports hearing better with one ear than the other. Place a vibrating tuning fork in the midline of the person's skull, and ask if the tone sounds the same in both ears or better in one (Fig. 12–10). The person should hear the tone by bone conduction through the skull, and it should sound equally loud in both ears.

Sound lateralizes to one ear (see Table 12–6).

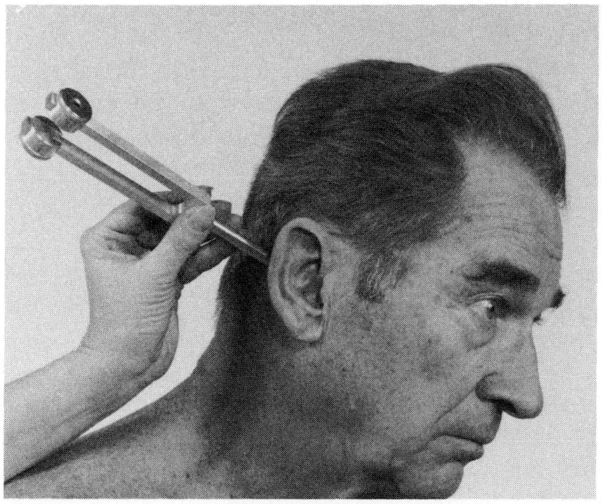

► Figure 12–11

The *Rinne test* compares AC and BC sound (Fig. 12–11). Place the stem of the vibrating tuning fork on the person's mastoid process, and ask him or her to signal when the sound goes away. Quickly invert the fork so

NORMAL RANGE OF FINDINGS	ABNORMAL FINDINGS

the vibrating end is near the ear canal; the person should still hear a sound (Fig. 12-12). Normally, the sound is heard twice as long by AC (next to ear canal) as by BC (through the mastoid process). A normal response is a positive Rinne test, or "AC > BC." Repeat with the other ear.

Ratio of AC to BC is altered with hearing loss (see Table 12-6).

Sound is heard longer by bone conduction.

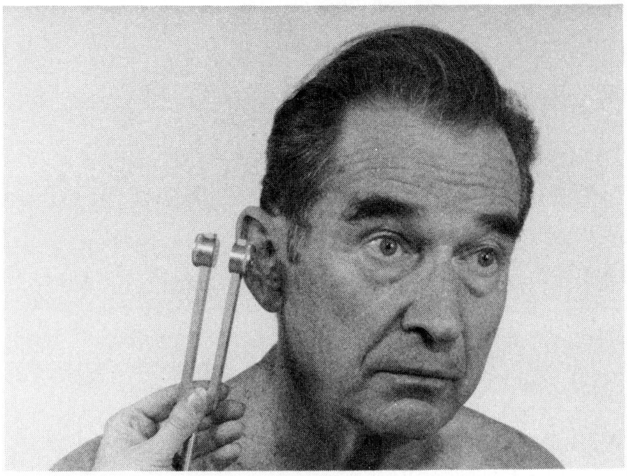

▶ **Figure 12-12**

THE VESTIBULAR APPARATUS

Assess the vestibular apparatus.

The *Romberg test* assesses the ability of the vestibular apparatus in the inner ear to help maintain standing balance. Ask the person to stand with feet together and arms to the side, then to close the eyes. Wait about 20 seconds. The person's position should be steady, even with the visual orienting information blocked. You must stand close to the person, in case he or she sways and loses balance. A mild swaying may occur; this is normal. This test is not done in the screening examination of children. The Romberg test also assesses intactness of the cerebellum and proprioception and is discussed in Chapter 20, Assessing the Neurologic System (see Fig. 20-17).

The person loses balance and falls. The person needs to have feet apart for a wider base of support.

DEVELOPMENTAL CONSIDERATIONS

Infants and Young Children

Examination of the external ear is similar to that described for the adult, with the addition of examination of position and alignment on head. Note the ear position. The top of the pinna should match an imaginary line extending from the corner of the eye to the occiput. Also, the ear should be positioned within 10 degrees of vertical (Fig. 12-13).

Low-set ears or deviation in alignment may indicate mental retardation or a genitourinary malformation.

NORMAL RANGE OF FINDINGS | ABNORMAL FINDINGS

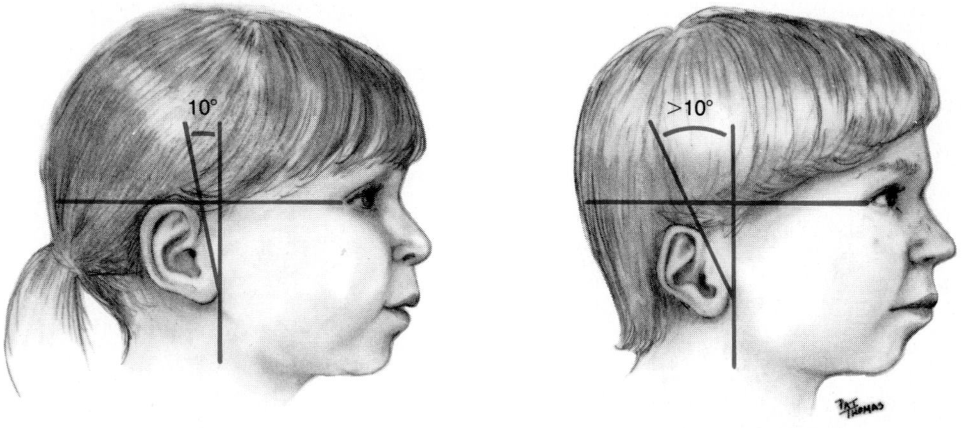

Normal alignment

Low set ears and deviation in alignment

► Figure 12–13

Otoscopic Examination. In addition to its place in the complete examination, eardrum assessment is mandatory for any infant or child requiring care for illness or fever. For the infant or young child, the timing of the otoscopic examination is best toward the end of the complete examination. Many young children protest vigorously during this procedure no matter how well you prepare, and it is difficult to reestablish cooperation afterward. Save the otoscopic examination until last. Then the parent can hold and comfort the child.

To help prepare the child, let the child hold your funny-looking "flashlight." You may wish to have the child look in the parent's ear as you hold the otoscope (Fig. 12–14).

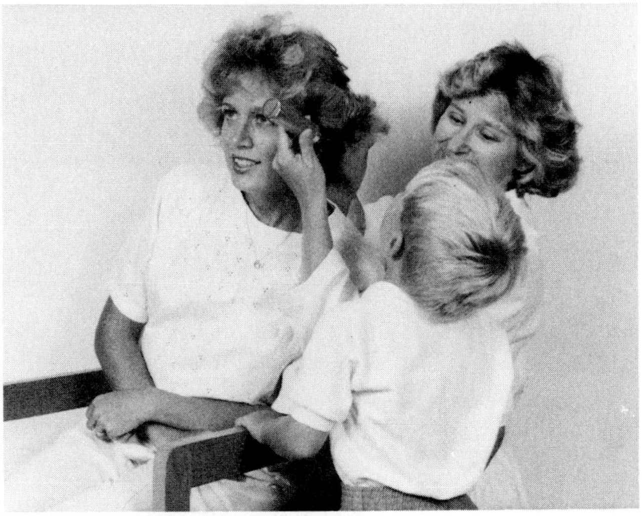

► Figure 12–14

NORMAL RANGE OF FINDINGS	ABNORMAL FINDINGS

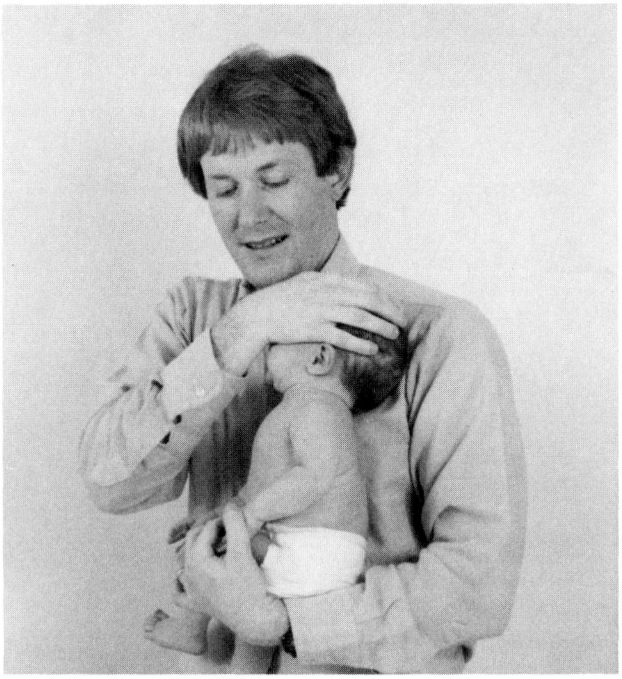

► **Figure 12–15**

Positioning is important. You need a clear view of the canal, and you must protect the eardrum from injury in case of sudden head movement. Enlist the aid of a cooperative parent. Prop an infant upright against the parent's chest or shoulder, with the parent's arm around the upper part of the head (Fig. 12–15). A toddler can be held in the parent's lap or may lie on the examining table with the child's arms secured (Fig. 12–16). In each case, the child's head is stabilized to avoid movement against the otoscope.

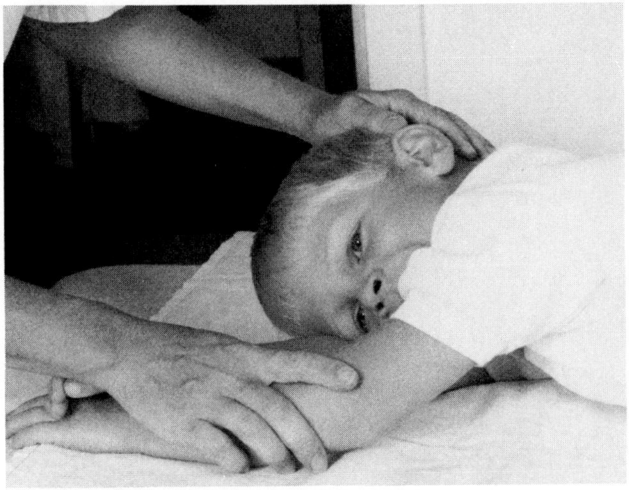

► **Figure 12–16**

NORMAL RANGE OF FINDINGS	ABNORMAL FINDINGS

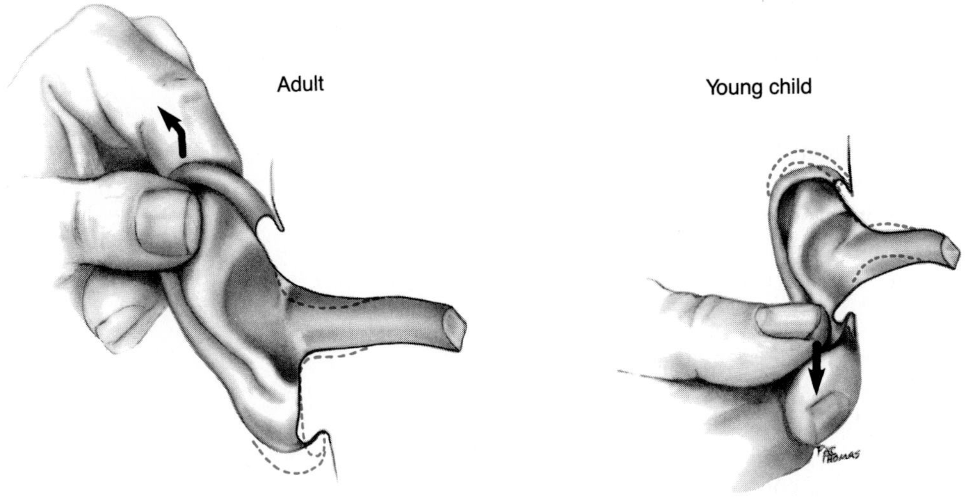

Adult — pull pinna up and back   Infant — pull pinna straight down

► Figure 12–17

Remember to pull the pinna straight down on an infant or child under 3 years old. This method will match the slope of the ear canal (Fig. 12–17).

At birth, the patency of the ear canal is determined but the otoscopic examination is not performed because the canal is filled with amniotic fluid and vernix caseosa. After a few days, the tympanic membrane is examined. During the first few days, the tympanic membrane often looks thickened and opaque. It may look "injected" and have a mild redness due to increased vascularity. The drum also looks injected in infants after crying. The position of the eardrum is more horizontal in the neonate, making it more difficult to see completely and harder to differentiate from the canal wall. By 1 month of age, the drum is in the oblique (more vertical) position of the older child and examination is a bit easier.

When examining an infant or young child, a pneumatic bulb attachment enables you to direct a light puff of air toward the drum to assess vibrability (Fig. 12–18). Choose the largest speculum that will fit in the ear

An abnormal response is no movement. Drum hypomobility indicates effusion or a high vacuum in the middle ear. For the newborn's first 6 weeks, drum immobility is the best indicator of middle ear infection.

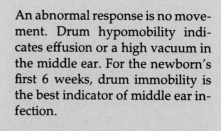

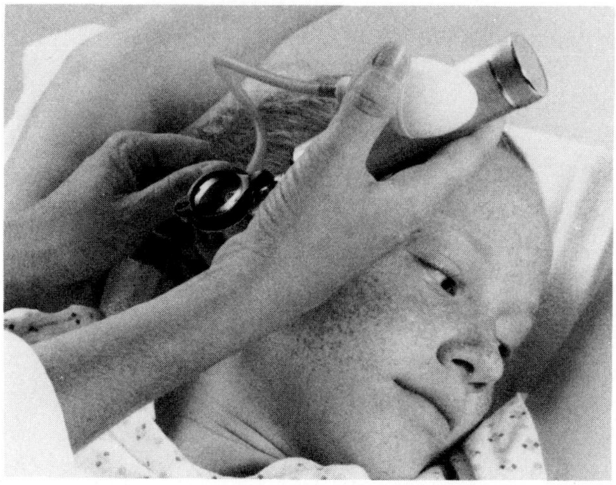

► Figure 12–18

NORMAL RANGE OF FINDINGS | **ABNORMAL FINDINGS**

canal without causing pain, for a secure seal. A rubber tip on the end of the speculum gives a better seal. Give a small pump to the bulb (positive pressure), then release the bulb (negative pressure). Normally the tympanic membrane moves inward with a slight puff and outward with a slight release.

Normally, the tympanic membrane is intact. In a child being treated for chronic otitis media, you may note the presence of a myringotomy tube in the central part of the drum. This is inserted surgically to equalize pressure and drain secretions. Finally, although the condition is not normal, it is not uncommon to note a foreign body in a child's canal, such as a small stone or a bead.

Abnormal findings: See Table 12–5. Foreign body (see Table 12–3).

Test Hearing Acuity. Use the developmental milestones, mentioned in this section, to assess hearing in an infant. Also, attend to the parents' concern over the infant's inability to hear; their assessment is usually well founded.

The room should be silent and the baby contented. Make a loud sudden noise (hand clap or squeeze toy) out of the baby's peripheral range of vision of about 30 cm (12 in). You may need to repeat a few times, but you should note these responses:

Newborn — startle (Moro) reflex, acoustic blink reflex

3 to 4 months — acoustic blink reflex, infant stops movement and appears to "listen," halts sucking, quiets if crying, cries if quiet

Abnormal findings: Absence of alerting behavior may indicate congenital deafness.

6 to 8 months — infant turns head to localize sound, responds to own name

Abnormal findings: Failure to localize sound

Preschool and school age child — child must be screened with audiometry

Abnormal findings: No intelligible speech by 2 years of age.

Note that a young child may be unaware of a hearing loss because the child does not know how one "ought" to hear. Note these behavioral manifestations of hearing loss:

1. The child is inattentive in casual conversation
2. The child reacts more to movement and facial expression than to sound
3. The child's facial expression is strained or puzzled
4. The child frequently asks to have statements repeated
5. The child confuses words that sound alike
6. The child has an accompanying speech problem; speech is monotonous or garbled, mispronounces or omits sounds
7. The child appears shy and withdrawn and "lives in a world of his own"
8. The child frequently complains of earaches
9. The child hears better at times when the environment is more conducive to hearing

The Aging Adult

An aging person may have pendulous earlobes with linear wrinkling because of loss of elasticity of the pinna. Coarse, wiry hairs may be present at the opening of the ear canal. During otoscopy, the drum normally may be whiter in color and more opaque, duller than in the younger adult. It also may look thickened. A high-tone frequency hearing loss is apparent for those affected with presbycusis, the hearing loss that occurs with aging.

NORMAL RANGE OF FINDINGS	ABNORMAL FINDINGS
This condition is revealed in difficulty hearing whispered words in the voice test, and difficulty hearing consonants during conversational speech.	

☑ SUMMARY CHECKLIST

1 ▶ Inspect external ear
   A. Size and shape of auricle
   B. Position and alignment on head
   C. Note skin condition—color, lumps, lesions
   D. Check movement of auricle and tragus for tenderness
   E. Evaluate external auditory meatus. Note size, swelling, redness, discharge, cerumen, lesions, foreign bodies

2 ▶ Otoscopic examination
   A. External canal
      1. Cerumen, discharge, foreign bodies, lesions
      2. Redness or swelling of canal wall
   B. Inspect tympanic membrane
      1. Color and characteristics
      2. Note position (flat, bulging, retracted)
      3. Integrity of membrane

3 ▶ Test hearing acuity
   A. Note behavioral response to conversational speech
   B. Voice test
   C. Tuning fork tests—Weber and Rinne

SAMPLE RECORDING

Subjective:

▶ States hearing is good, no earaches, infections, discharge, hearing loss, tinnitus, or vertigo.

Objective:

▶ No masses, lesions, tenderness, discharge. Both TM pearly gray c̄ light reflex & landmarks intact, no perforations. Whispered words heard bilaterally. Weber midline s̄ lateralization. Rinne AC > BC and = bilaterally.

SAMPLE CLINICAL PROBLEM 1

Todd R. is a 15-year-old high school student who comes to the Health Center to seek care for "cough off and on all winter and earache since last night."

Progress Notes

Subjective

- 6 weeks PTA—Non-productive cough throughout day, no fever, no nasal congestion, no chest soreness. Todd's father gave him OTC decongestant, which helped, but cough continued off/on since. Does not smoke.
  1 day PTA—Intermittent cough continues, nasal congestion c̄ thick white mucus. Also earache R ear, treated self with heating pad, pain unrelieved. Pain is moderate, not deep and throbbing. Says R ear feels full, "hollow headed," voices sound muffled and far away, switches telephone to L ear to talk. No sore throat, no fever, no chest congestion or soreness.

Objective

- T 37° C oral, P 76, B/P 106/72
  L ear, canal, TM normal. R ear and canal normal, R TM retracted, with multiple air bubbles, drum color is yellow/amber. No sinus tenderness.
  Nose—turbinates injected and swollen, mucopurulent discharge.
  Throat—not injected, tonsils 1+.
  Neck—1 R ant. cervical node enlarged, firm, moveable, tender. All others normal.
  Chest—clear to auscultation, resonant to percussion throughout.
  Hearing—Weber lateralizes to R.

Assessment

- Serous otitis media, R ear, with mild URI
  Transient conductive hearing loss
  Sensory/perceptual alteration (auditory) R/T excessive fluid in middle ear
  Pain R/T middle ear pressure

SAMPLE CLINICAL PROBLEM 2

Emma S., 78 years old, has a medical diagnosis of angina pectoris, which has responded to nitroglycerin prn and periods of rest between activity. She has been independent in her own home, is coping well with activity restrictions through help from neighbors and family. Now hospitalized for evaluation of acute chest pain episode; M.I. has been ruled out, pain diagnosed as anginal, to be released to own home with a beta-blocking medication and nitroglycerin prn.

Just before this hospitalization Mrs. S. received a hearing aid following evaluation by audiologist at Senior Center. Mrs. S. was born in Germany, immigrated to U.S. at age 5, considers English her primary language.

Complete Problem List

Problem No.	Title	Date Entered
1	Angina pectoris	5/20/
2	Hearing loss	6/3/

Progress Notes

Subjective

- Since this hospitalization, feels "irritable and nervous." Relates this to worry about heart and also, "I get so mixed up in here, this room is so strange, and I just can't hear the nurses. They talk like cavemen, 'oo-i-ee-uou.'" Tried using her new hearing aid but no relief, "It just kept screeching in my ear, and it made the monitor beep so loud it drove me crazy." States no tinnitus, no vertigo.

Objective

- Pinna with elongated lobes, but no tenderness to palpation, no discharge, no masses or lesions. Both canals clear of cerumen. Both TM appear gray-white, slightly opaque and dull, though all landmarks visible, ō perforation.
  Hearing—Unable to hear whispered voice bilaterally. Weber midline though unable to hear 1024 Hz fork, used 512 Hz. Rinne positive, AC > BC, but time reduced overall.

Assessment

- Knowledge deficit R/T lack of teaching on hearing aid
  Sensory/perceptual alteration (auditory) R/T effects of aging
  Anxiety R/T change in cardiovascular health status and inability to communicate effectively

NURSING DIAGNOSES COMMONLY ASSOCIATED WITH THE EARS AND HEARING DISORDERS

Diagnosis	Related Factors (Etiology)	Defining Characteristics (Symptoms and Signs)
Sensory/perceptual alteration: auditory	Effects of aging Neurologic impairment Effects of certain antibiotics Excessive earwax, fluid, or foreign body in ear Social isolation Stress Failure to use protective ear devices Continuous exposure to excessive noise Psychoses	Tinnitus Abnormal hearing test Lack of startle reflex Failure to respond to verbal stimuli Cupping of ears Inattentiveness Withdrawal Daydreaming Auditory hallucinations Inappropriate responses Delayed speech or language development

ABNORMAL FINDINGS

Table 12-1 ▸ Abnormalities of the External Ear

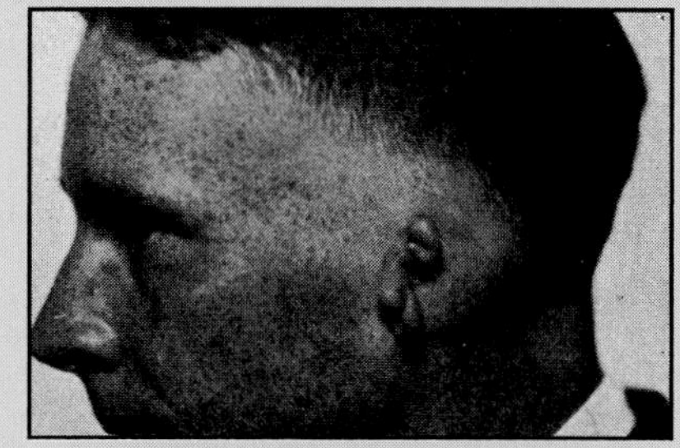

CONGENITAL MICROTIA AND ATRESIA

Small rudimentary auricle appears as a vertical curved ridge. Also note atresia (absence or closure) of ear canal, with hearing loss.

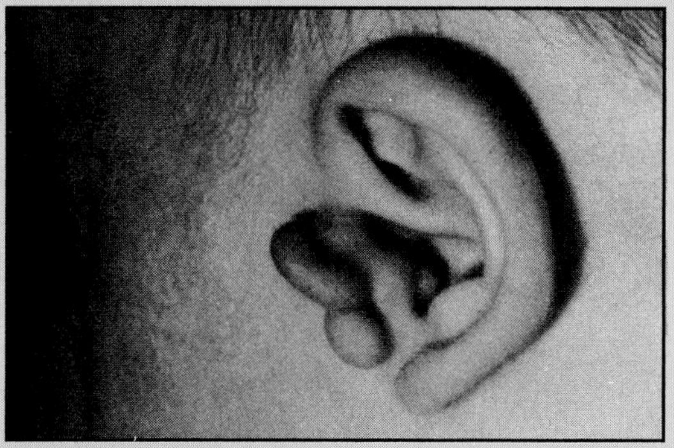

ACCESSORY AURICLE

Auricular appendages are a common finding and usually appear as skin tags. Usually they are unilateral and single but are multiple here. They occur most often in the preauricular area, in front of the tragus.

Table 12-1 ▸ Abnormalities of the External Ear *Continued*

FROSTBITE (not illustrated)

Reddish blue discoloration and swelling of auricle following exposure to extreme cold. Vesicles or bullae may develop, and the person feels pain and tenderness.

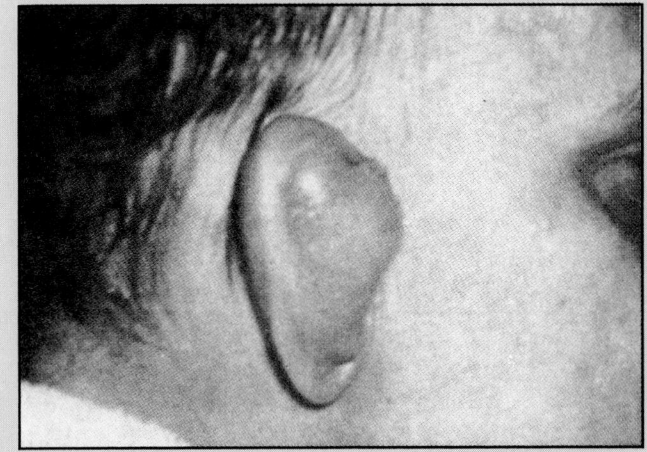

CAULIFLOWER EAR

Thickened gnarled auricle results from repeated trauma, as in chronic hemorrhage or chronic perichondritis (infection around cartilage).

CEREBROSPINAL FLUID OTORRHEA (not illustrated)

Skull fracture of temporal bone causes cerebrospinal fluid to leak from ear canal and pool in concha when the person is supine. Cerebrospinal fluid feels oily and gives a positive glucose reaction on Testape.

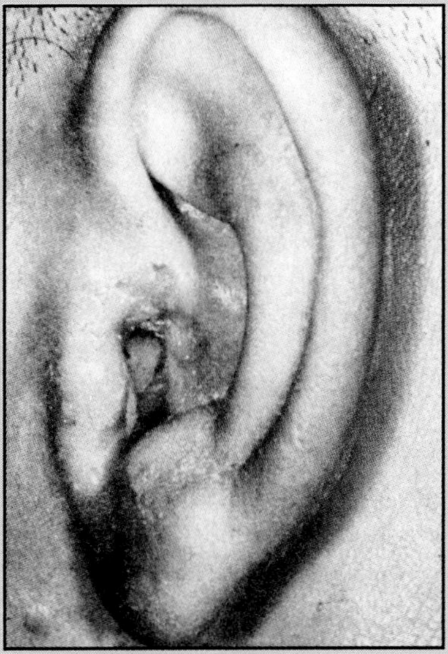

OTITIS EXTERNA

An infection of the outer ear, with severe painful movement of the pinna and tragus, redness and swelling of pinna and canal, scanty purulent discharge, scaling, itching, fever, and enlarged tender regional lymph nodes. Hearing is normal or slightly diminished. More common in hot humid weather; also called swimmer's ear. Canal becomes waterlogged and swells; skin folds are set up for infection.

Table 12-2 ▸ Lumps and Lesions on the External Ear

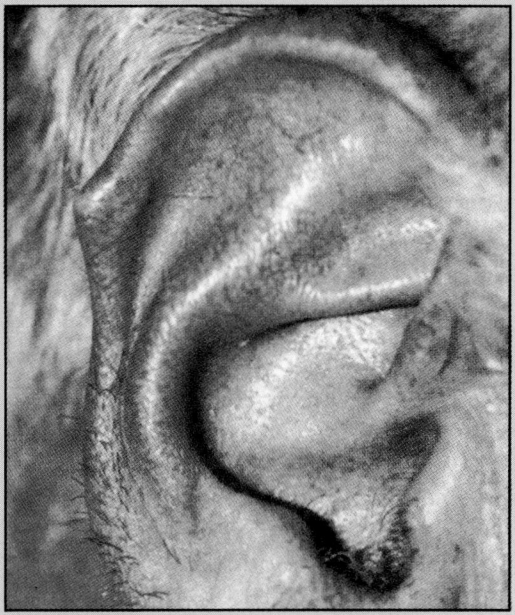

DARWIN'S TUBERCLE

Small painless nodule at the helix. It is a congenital variation and is not significant. Do not mistake it for a tophus.

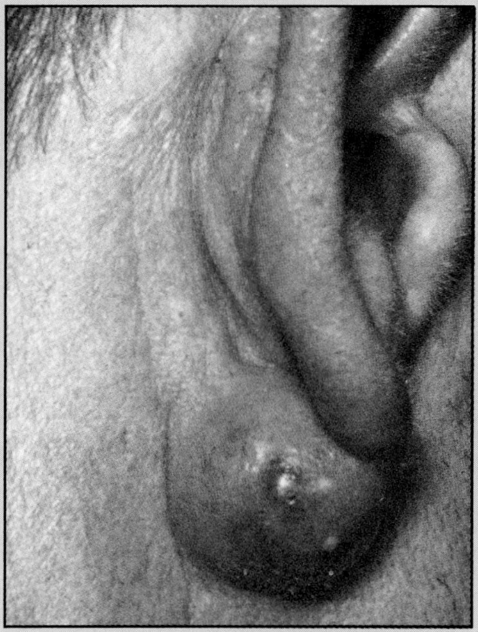

SEBACEOUS CYST

More common behind lobule, in the postauricular fold. A small nodule with central black punctum indicates blocked sebaceous gland. It is painful if it becomes infected. Often are multiple.

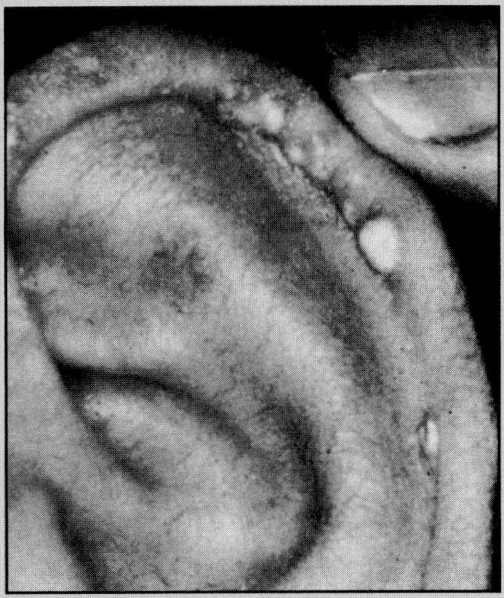

TOPHI

Small, whitish-yellow, hard, nontender nodules in or near helix or antihelix. Contain greasy chalky material of uric acid crystals and are a sign of gout.

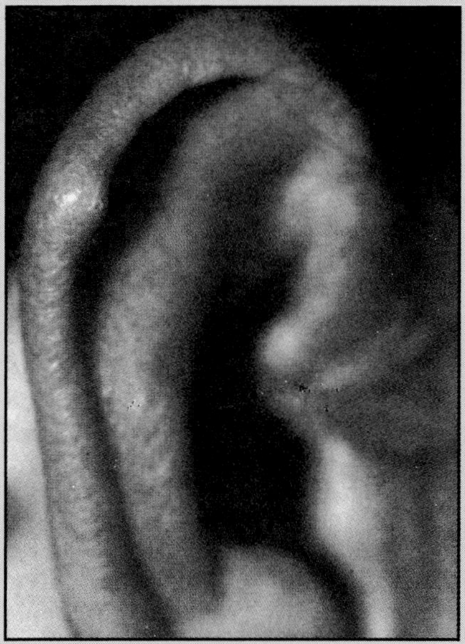

CHONDRODERMATITIS

Painful nodules on the rim of the helix. They are small, indurated, and very painful. Their cause is unknown.

Table 12-2 ▸ Lumps and Lesions on the External Ear *Continued*

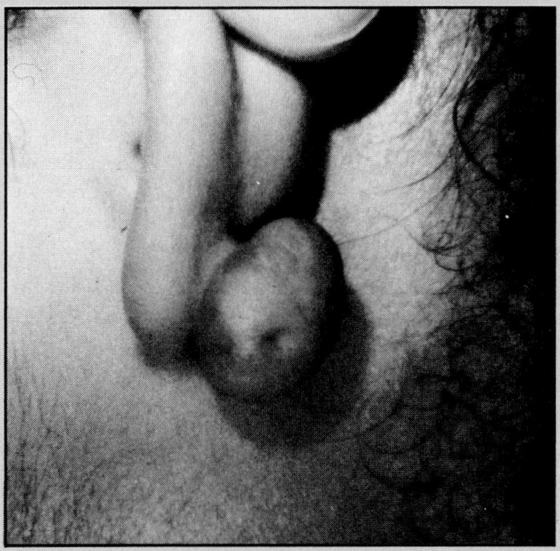

KELOID

Overgrowth of scar tissue, which invades original site of trauma. It is more common in dark-skinned people, although it also occurs in whites. In the ear, it is most common at lobule at the site of a pierced earring.

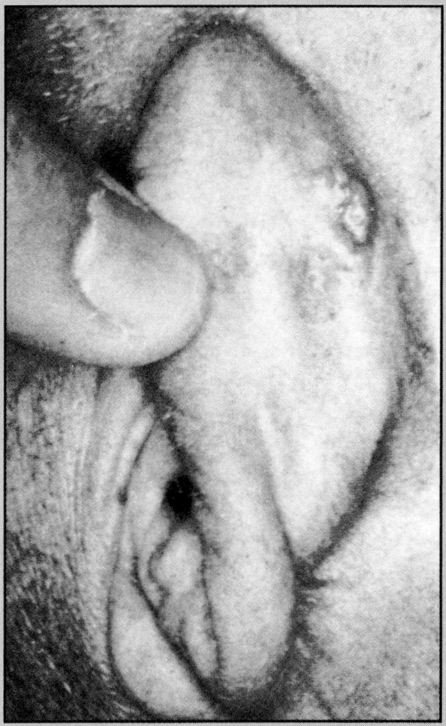

CARCINOMA

Ulcerated crusted nodule with indurated base that fails to heal. Bleeds intermittently. Must refer for biopsy. May occur also in ear canal and show chronic discharge that is either serosanguineous or bloody. There is pain and swelling of the canal.

Table 12-3 ▸ Abnormalities in the Ear Canal

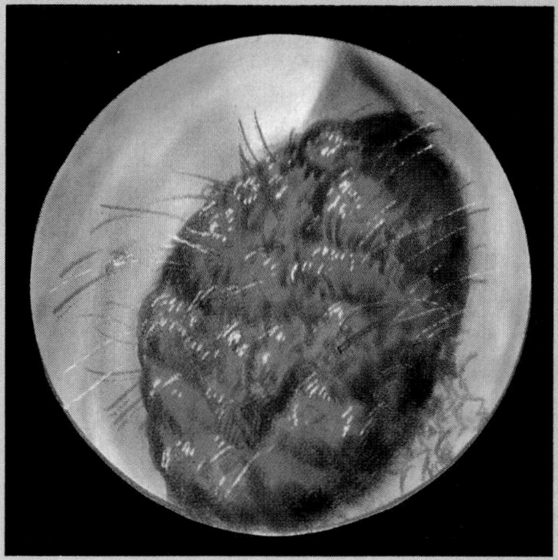

EXCESSIVE CERUMEN

Excessive cerumen is produced or is impacted owing to narrow tortuous canal or cleaning method. May show as round ball partially obscuring drum or totally occluding canal. With total occlusion, person experiences ear fullness and impaired hearing.

Table continued on following page

Table 12–3 ► Abnormalities in the Ear Canal *Continued*

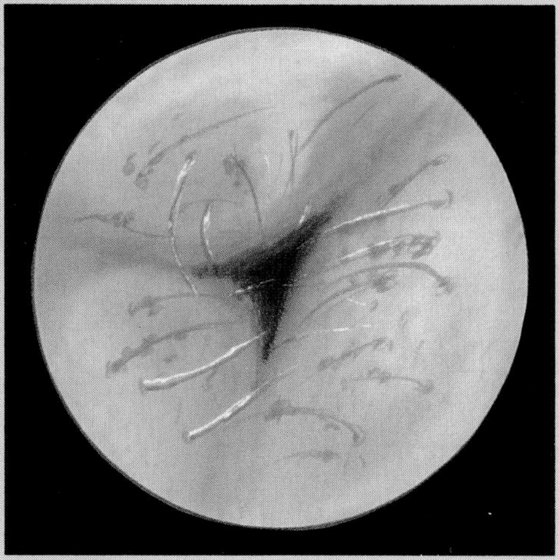

OTITIS EXTERNA

Severe swelling of canal; inflammation; tenderness. Here canal lumen is narrowed to one-quarter normal size.

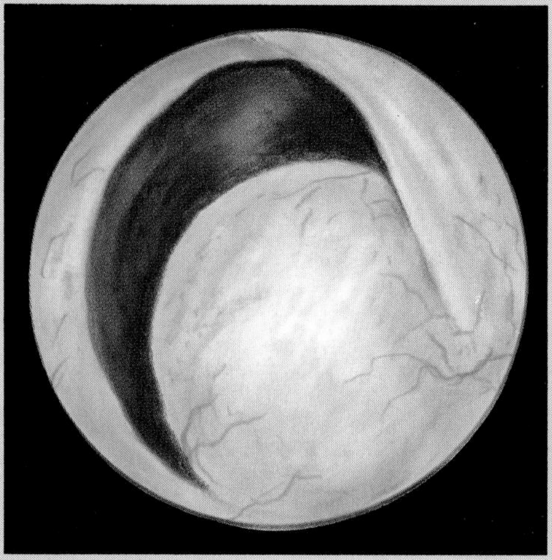

OSTEOMA

Single, stony hard, rounded nodule that obscures the drum; nontender; overlying skin appears normal. Attached to inner third, the bony part, of canal. Benign but refer for removal.

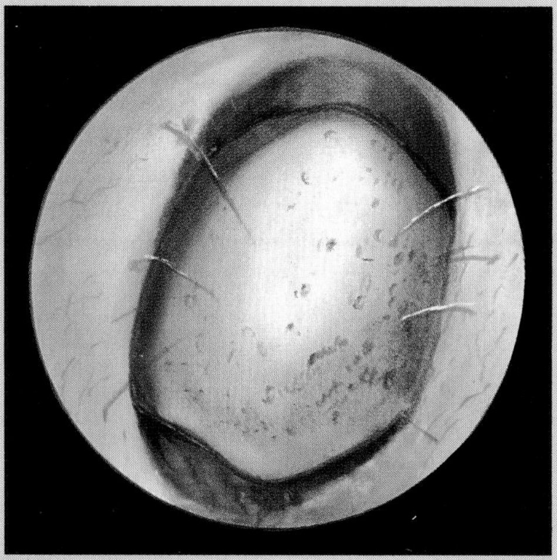

FOREIGN BODY

Here, a stone completely occludes the canal. It is usually seen in children. Common objects are beans, corn, jewelry beads, small stones, sponge rubber. Cotton is most common in adults and is impacted from cotton-tipped applicators.

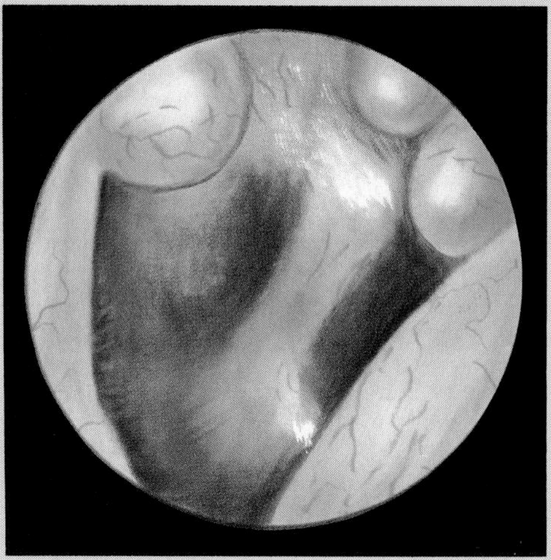

EXOSTOSIS

More common than osteoma. Small, bony hard, rounded nodules of hypertrophic bone, covered with normal epithelium. They arise near the drum but usually do not obstruct the view of the drum. They are usually multiple and bilateral. They may occur more frequently in cold water swimmers (Adams, 1989). The condition needs no treatment, athough it may cause accumulation of cerumen, which blocks the canal.

Table 12-3 ► Abnormalities in the Ear Canal *Continued*

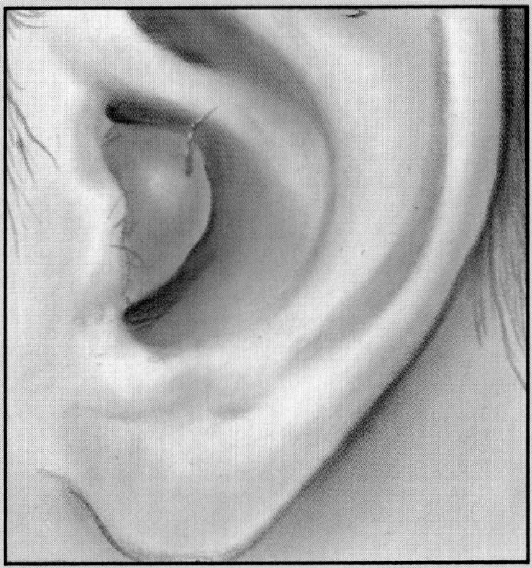

FURUNCLE

Exquisitely painful, reddened, infected hair follicle. Here, it occurs on the tragus but also may be on cartilaginous part of ear canal. Regional lymphadenopathy often accompanies a furuncle.

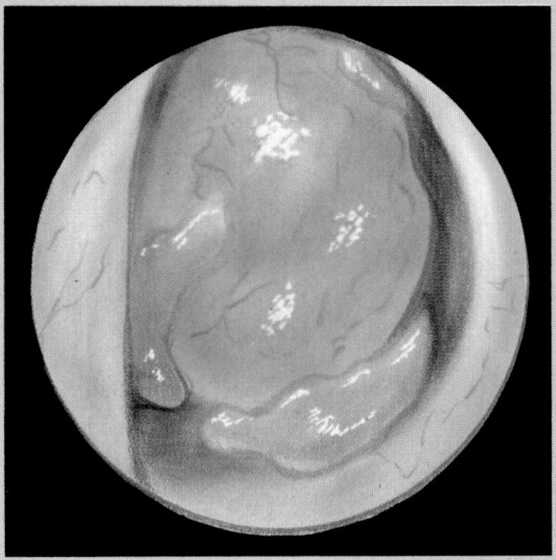

POLYP

Arises in canal from granulomatous or mucosal tissue; redder than surrounding skin and bleeds easily; bathed in foul purulent discharge; indicates chronic ear disease. Benign but refer for excision.

Table 12-4 ► Abnormal Findings Seen on Otoscopy

APPEARANCE OF EARDRUM	INDICATES	SUGGESTED CONDITION
Yellow-amber color	Serum or pus	Serous otitis media or chronic otitis media
Prominent landmarks	Retraction of drum	Negative pressure in middle ear from an obstructed eustachian tube
Air/fluid level or air bubbles	Serous fluid	Serous otitis media
Absent or distorted light reflex	Bulging of eardrum	Acute otitis media
Bright red color	Infection in middle ear	Acute purulent otitis media
Blue or dark red color	Blood behind drum	Trauma, skull fracture
Dark oval areas	Perforation	Drum rupture
White dense areas	Scarring	Sequelae of infections
Diminished or absent landmarks	Thickened drum	Chronic otitis media
Black or white dots on drum or canal	Colony of growth	Fungal infection

Reprinted by permission of Elsevier Science Publishing Co., Inc., from Sherman JL, Fields, SK: Guide to Patient Evaluation. 3rd ed, p. 122. Copyright 1978 by Medical Examination Publishing Company, Inc.

Table 12-5 ► Abnormalities of the Tympanic Membrane

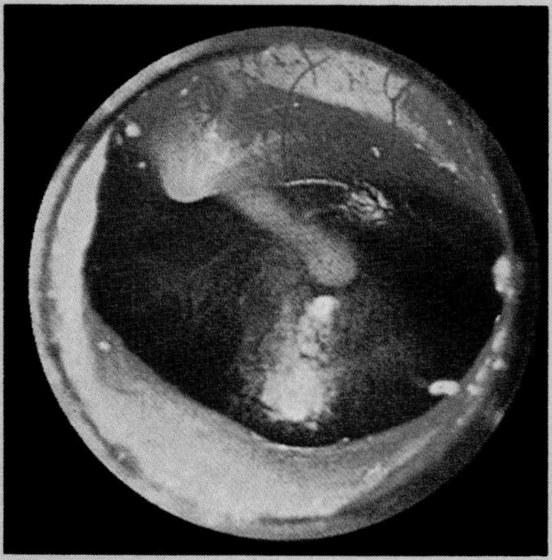

RETRACTED DRUM

Landmarks look more prominent and well defined. Malleus handle looks shorter and more horizontal than normal. Short process is very prominent. Light reflex is absent or distorted. The drum is dull and lusterless and does not move. These signs indicate negative pressure and middle ear vacuum due to obstructed eustachian tube and serous otitis media.

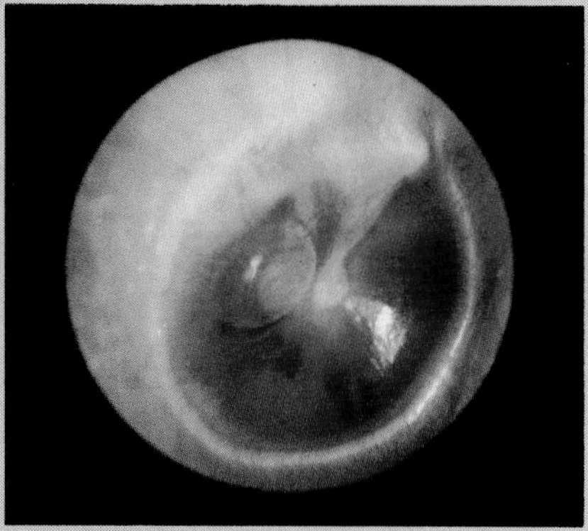

SEROUS OTITIS MEDIA

An amber-yellow drum suggests serum in middle ear that transudates to relieve negative pressure from the blocked eustachian tube. You may note an air/fluid level with fine black dividing line, or air bubbles visible behind drum. Symptoms are feeling of fullness, transient hearing loss, popping sound with swallowing. Also called: secretory otitis media, middle ear effusion, glue ear.

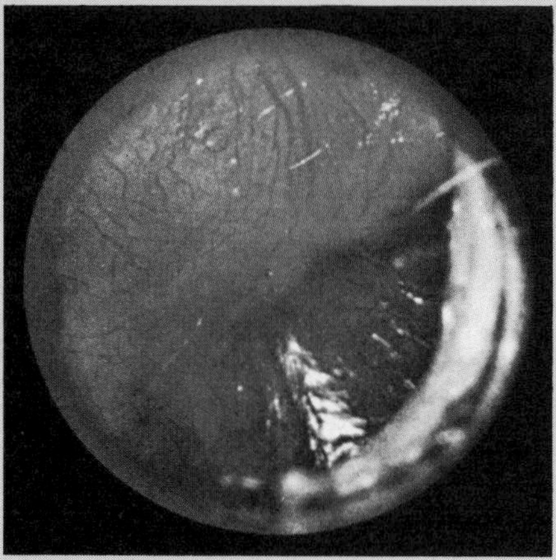

Early stage

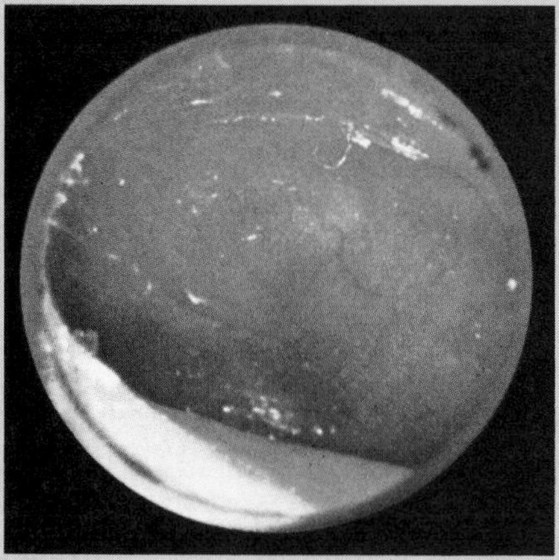

Later stage

ACUTE PURULENT OTITIS MEDIA

This results when the middle ear fluid is infected. An absent light reflex due to increasing middle ear pressure is an early sign. Redness and bulging are first noted in superior part of drum (pars flaccida), along with earache and fever. Then fiery red bulging of entire drum occurs; deep throbbing pain; fever; transient hearing loss. Pneumatic otoscopy reveals drum hypomobility.

Table 12-5 ► Abnormalities of the Tympanic Membrane *Continued*

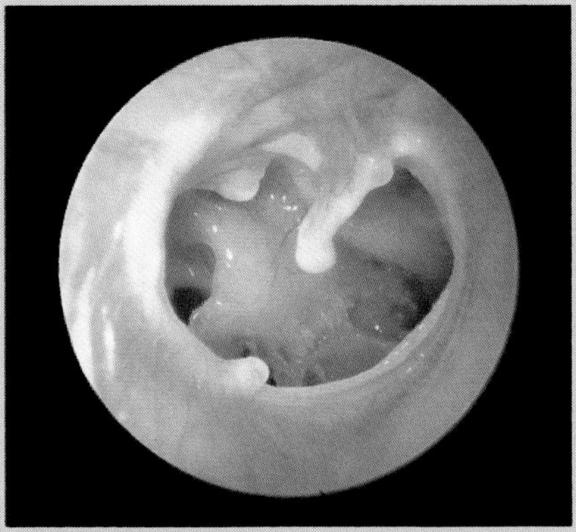

PERFORATION

If the acute otitis media is not treated, the drum may rupture from increased pressure. Perforations also occur from trauma (e.g., a slap on the ear). Usually, the perforation appears as a round or oval darkened area on the drum, but in this photo the perforation is very large. *Central* perforations occur in the pars tensa. *Marginal* perforations occur at the annulus. Marginal perforations are called attic perforations when they occur in superior part of the drum, the pars flaccida.

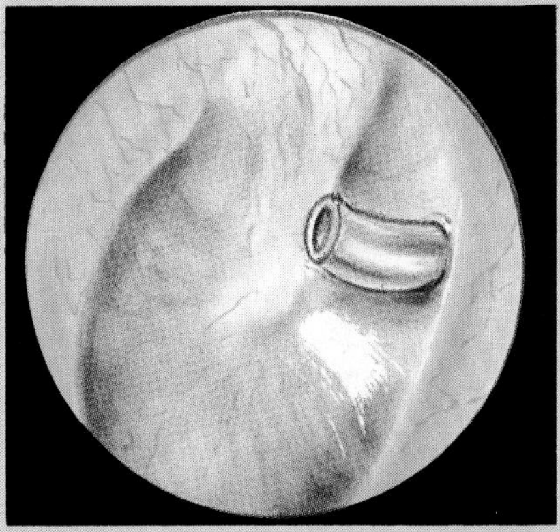

INSERTION OF TYMPANOSTOMY TUBES

Polyethylene tubes are inserted surgically into the eardrum to relieve middle ear pressure and promote drainage of chronic or recurrent middle ear infections. Tubes extrude spontaneously in 6 months to 1 year.

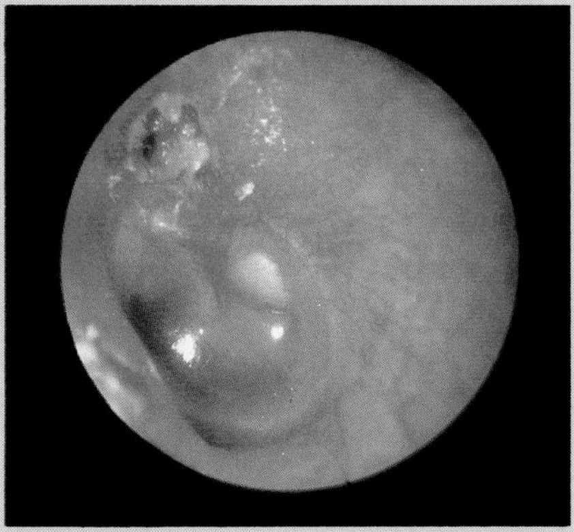

CHOLESTEATOMA

A malignant overgrowth of epidermal tissue may result over the years following a marginal perforation. It has a pearly white cheesy appearance. Growth of cholesteatoma can erode bone and produce hearing loss.

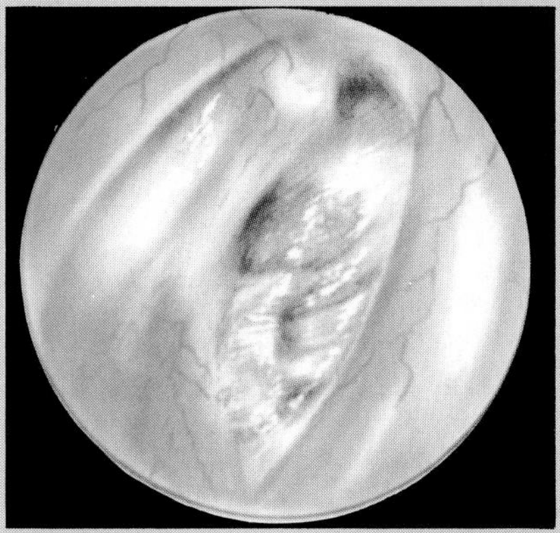

SCARRED DRUM

Dense white patches are sequelae of repeated ear infections. They do not necessarily affect hearing.

Table continued on following page

Table 12-5 ▶ Abnormalities of the Tympanic Membrane *Continued*

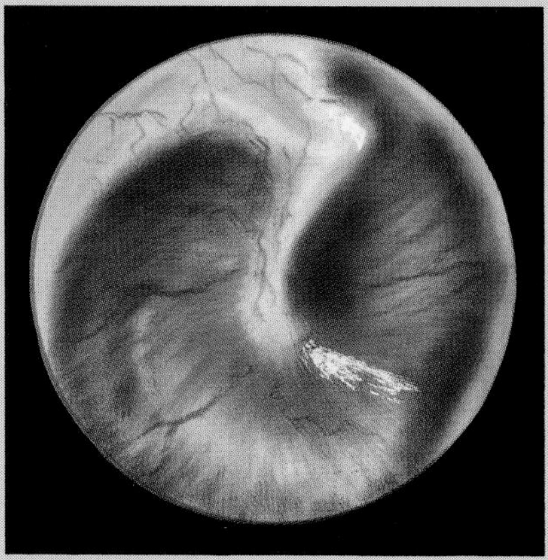

BLUE DRUM (HEMOTYMPANUM)

This indicates blood in the middle ear, as in trauma resulting in skull fracture.

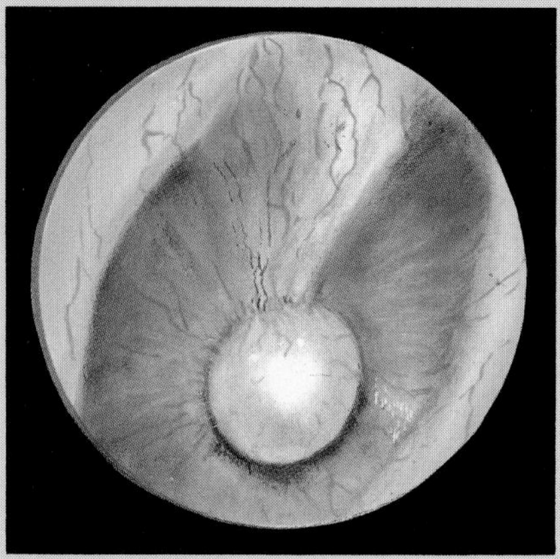

BULLOUS MYRINGITIS

Small vesicles on the drum; accompany mycoplasma pneumonia and virus infections.

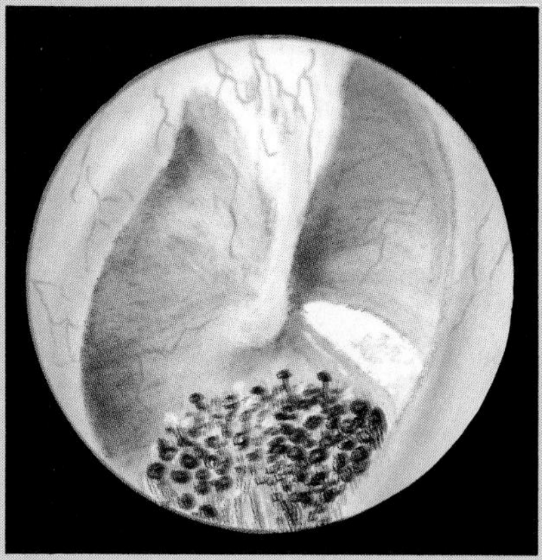

FUNGAL INFECTION (OTOMYCOSIS)

Colony of black or white dots on drum or canal wall suggests a yeast or fungal infection.

Table 12-6 ▶ Tuning Fork Tests

WEBER TEST	RINNE TEST
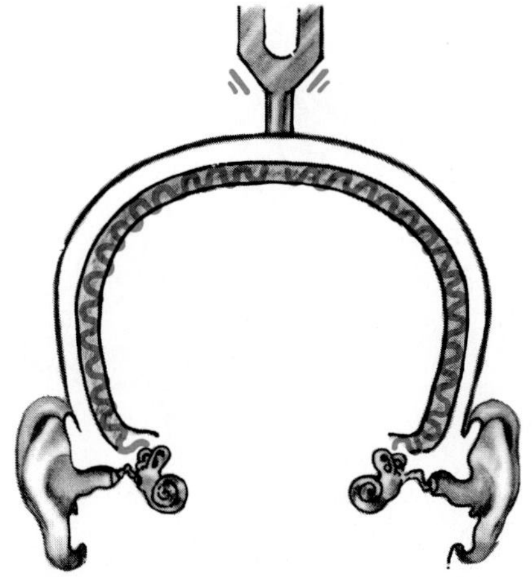	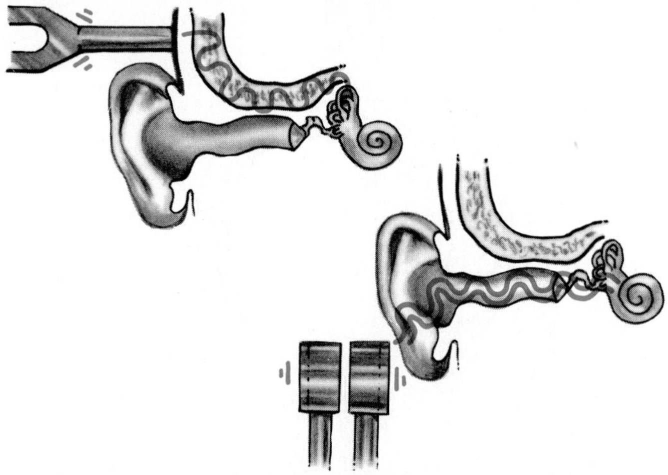
Normal—sound should be equally loud in both ears; sound does not lateralize.	Normal—sound is heard twice as long by air conduction as by bone conduction; a "positive" Rinne, or AC > BC.
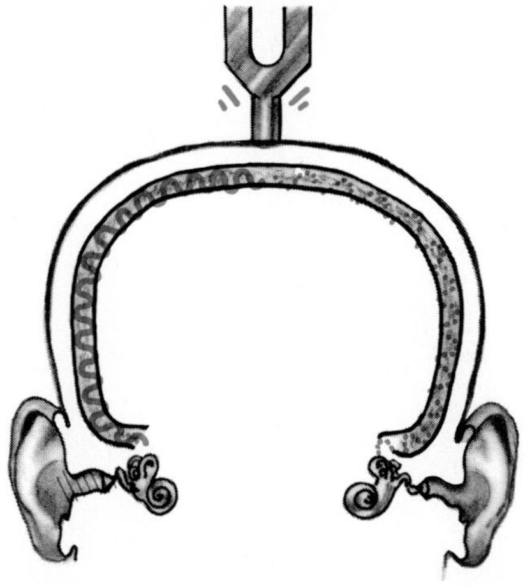	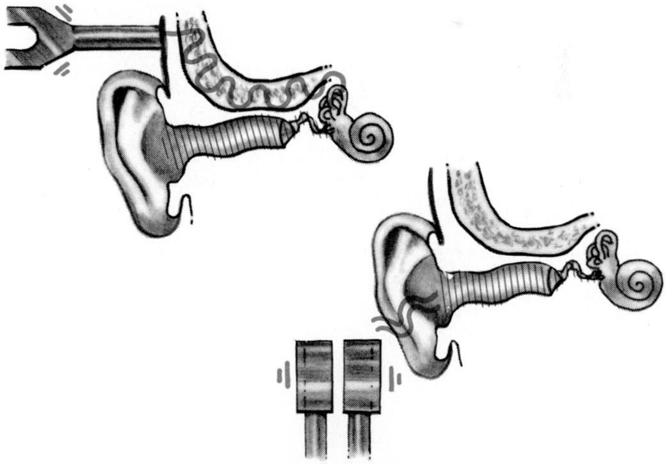
Conductive loss—sound lateralizes to "poorer" ear owing to background room noise, which masks hearing in normal ear. "Poorer" ear (the one with conductive loss) is not distracted by background noise, thus has a better chance to hear bone-conducted sound. Examples: transient conductive loss with serous or purulent otitis media.	Conductive loss—person hears as long by bone conduction (AC = BC) or even longer (AC < BC), a "negative" finding on the Rinne test.

Table continued on following page

Table 12-6 ► Tuning Fork Tests *Continued*

WEBER TEST

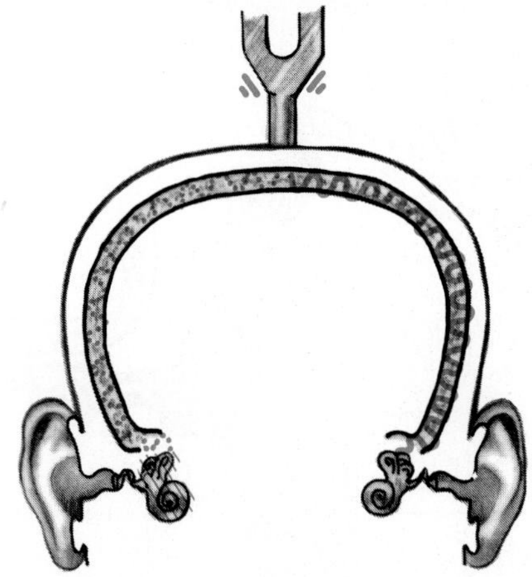

Sensorineural loss — sound lateralizes to "better" ear or unaffected ear. Poor ear (the one with nerve loss) is unable to perceive the sound.

RINNE TEST

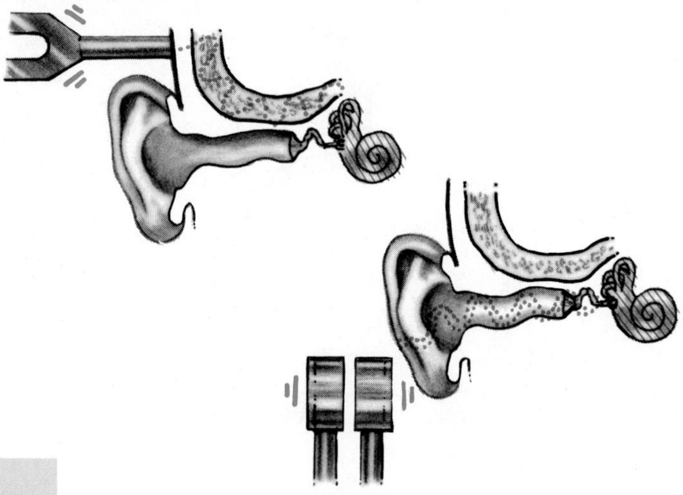

Sensorineural loss — normal ratio of AC > BC is intact, but is reduced overall. That is, person hears poorly both ways.

Bibliography

Adams GL, Boies LR, Hilger PA: Boies Fundamentals of Otolaryngology. 6th ed. Philadelphia, W.B. Saunders, 1989.

Alberti PW, Ginsberg IA, Goode RL: Managing adult hearing loss. Patient Care 22(3):54–76, 1988.

Anderson RG: Otologic manifestations of aging. Otolaryngol Clin North Am 15:353–370, 1982.

Becker W, Buckingham RA, Holinger PH, et al: Atlas of Ear, Nose and Throat Diseases. 2nd ed. Philadelphia, W.B. Saunders, 1984.

Bluestone CD, Klein, JO: Otitis Media in Infants and Children. Philadelphia, WB Saunders, 1988.

Bluestone CD, Shurin PA: Middle ear disease in children—pathogenesis, diagnosis, and management. Pediatr Clin North Am 21:379–400, 1974.

Cotton RT, Farrer SM, Grundfast KM, Stool SE: Detecting childhood hearing loss. Patient Care 23(5):55–70, 1989.

DeWeese D, Saunders W: Textbook of Otolaryngology. St. Louis, C.V. Mosby, 1982.

Facione N: Otitis media: An overview of acute and chronic disease. Nurse Pract 15(10):11–22, 1990.

Hamill B: Comparing two methods of preschool and kindergarten hearing screening. Journal of School Health 58(3):95–97, 1988.

Harkess C: Clearing the occluded auditory canal. Pediatr Nurse 8:23–25, 1982.

Howie VM, Ploussard JH, Sloyer J: The "otitis-prone" condition. Am J Dis Child 129:676–678, 1975.

Kass JR, Meebe ME: Serious otitis media. Nurse Pract 4:25–28, 1979.

Miller J: The body in question. New York, Random House, 1978.

Overfield T: Biologic Variation in Health and Illness: Race Age, and Sex Differences. Menlo Park, CA, Addison-Wesley Publishing, 1985.

Rambur BA: Sudden hearing loss. Nurse Pract 14:8–19, 1989.

Rossman I: Clinical Geriatrics. 3rd ed. Philadelphia, J.B. Lippincott, 1986.

Rowe DS: Acute suppurative otitis media. Pediatrics 56:285–294, 1975.

Shurin PA, et al: Persistence of middle-ear effusion after acute otitis media in children. N Engl J Med 300:1121–1123, 1979.

Teele DW, Klein JO, Rosner BA: Epidemiology of otitis media in children. Ann Otol Rhinol Laryngol 89 (Suppl 68):5–6, 1980.

CHAPTER

13 Assessing the Nose, Mouth, and Throat

STRUCTURE AND FUNCTION

NOSE

The nose is the first segment of the respiratory system. It warms, moistens, and filters the inhaled air, and it is the sensory organ for smell. The external nose is shaped like a triangle with one side attached to the face (Fig. 13–1). On its leading edge, the superior part is the *bridge* and the free corner is the *tip*. The oval openings at the base of the triangle are the *nares;* just inside, each naris widens into the *vestibule.* The *collumella* divides the two nares and is continuous inside with the nasal septum. The *ala* is the lateral outside wing of the nose on either side. The upper third of the external nose is made up of bone; the rest is cartilage.

Inside, the *nasal cavity* is much larger than the external nose would indicate (Fig. 13–2). It extends back over the roof of the mouth. The anterior edge of the cavity is lined with numerous coarse nasal hairs, or vibrissae. The rest of the cavity is lined with a blanket of ciliated mucous membrane. The nasal hairs filter the coarsest matter from inhaled air, whereas the mucous blanket filters out dust and bacteria. Nasal mucosa appears redder than oral mucosa because of the rich blood supply present to warm the inhaled air.

The nasal cavity is divided medially by the *septum* into two slitlike air passages. The anterior part of the septum holds a rich vascular network, *Kiesselbach's plexus,* the most common site of nosebleeds. In many people, the nasal septum is not absolutely straight and may deviate toward one passage.

The lateral walls of each nasal cavity contain three parallel bony projections — the superior, middle and inferior *turbinates.* They increase the surface area so that more blood vessels and mucous membrane are available to warm, humidify, and filter the inhaled air. Underlying each turbinate is a cleft, the *meatus,* which is named for the turbinate above. The sinuses drain into the middle meatus, and tears from the nasolacrimal duct drain into the inferior meatus.

The olfactory receptors (hair cells) lie at the roof of the nasal cavity and in the upper one-third of the septum. These receptors for smell merge into the olfactory nerve, cranial nerve I, which transmits to the temporal lobe of the brain. Although it is not necessary for human survival, the sense of smell adds to nutrition by enhancing the pleasure and taste of food.

The *paranasal sinuses* are air-filled pockets within the cranium (Fig. 13–3). They communicate with the nasal

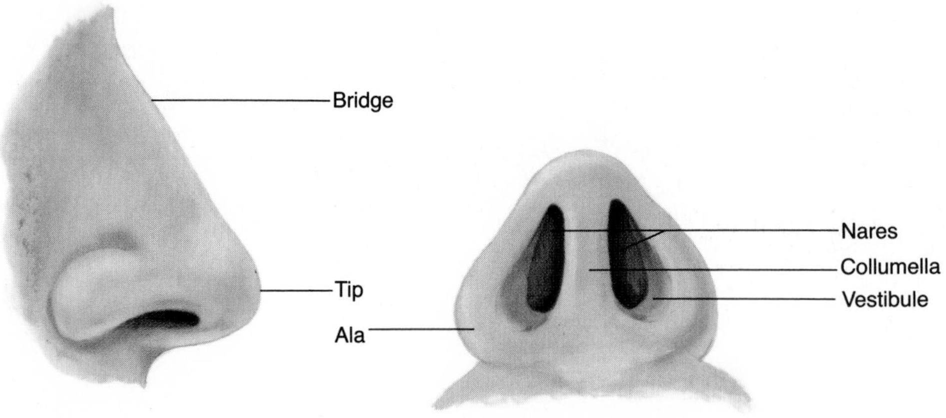

► **Figure 13–1**

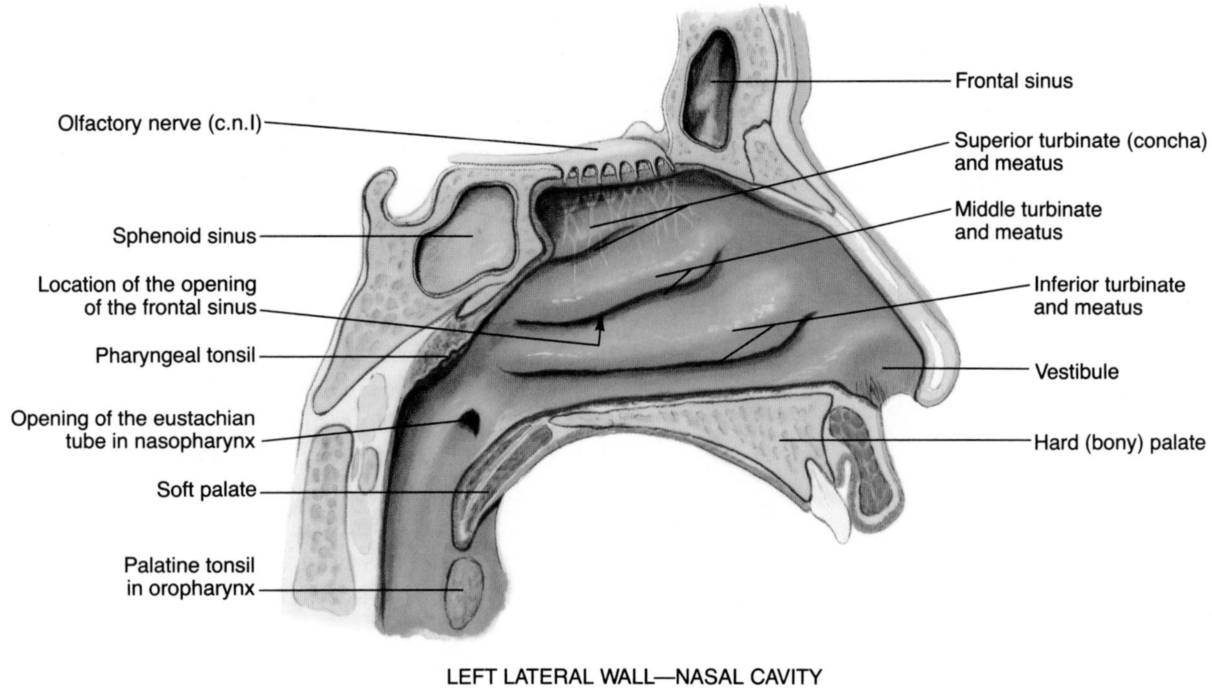

► **Figure 13-2**

cavity and are lined with the same type of ciliated mucous membrane. They lighten the weight of the skull bones, serve as resonators for sound production, and provide mucus, which drains into the nasal cavity. The sinus openings are narrow and easily occluded, which may cause inflammation or sinusitis.

Two pairs of sinuses are accessible to examination: the *frontal* sinuses in the frontal bone above and medial to

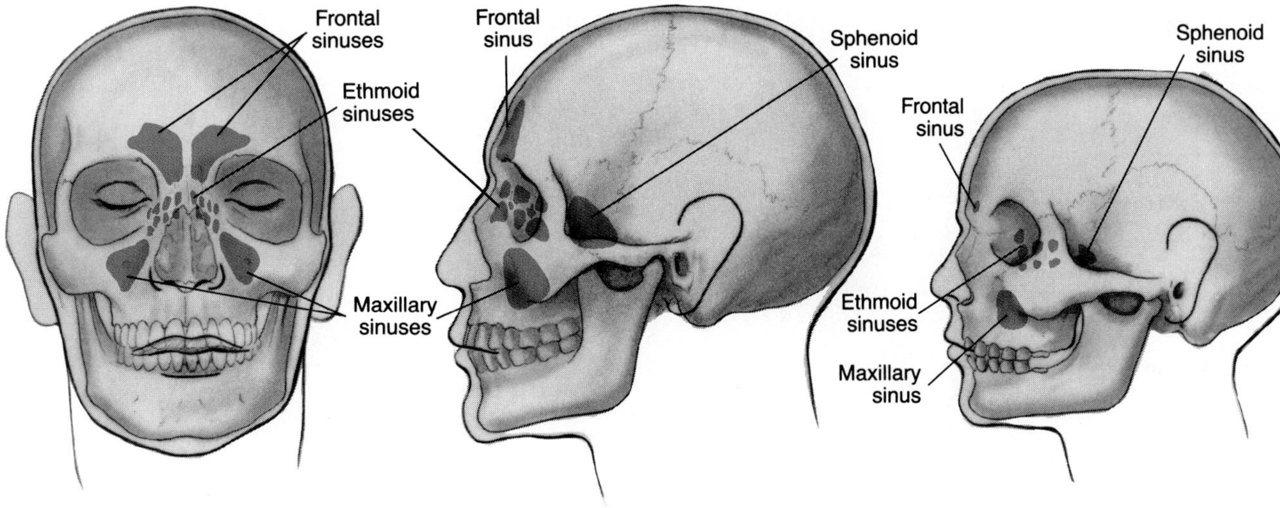

► **Figure 13-3**

the orbits, and the *maxillary* sinuses in the maxilla (cheekbone) along the side walls of the nasal cavity. The other two sets are smaller and deeper: the *ethmoid* sinuses between the orbits, and the *sphenoid* sinuses deep within the skull in the sphenoid bone.

Only the maxillary and ethmoid sinuses are present at birth. The maxillary sinuses reach full size after all permanent teeth have erupted. The ethmoid sinuses grow rapidly between 6 and 8 years and after puberty. The frontal sinuses are absent at birth, are fairly well developed between 7 and 8 years, and reach full size after puberty. The sphenoid sinuses are minute at birth and develop after puberty.

MOUTH

The mouth is the first segment of the digestive system and an airway for the respiratory system. The *oral cavity* is a short passage bordered by the lips, palate, cheeks, and tongue. It contains the teeth and gums, tongue, and salivary glands (Fig. 13–4).

The lips are the anterior border of the oral cavity—the transition zone from the outer skin to the inner mucous membrane lining the oral cavity. The arching roof of the mouth is the palate; it is divided into two parts. The anterior *hard palate* is made up of bone and is a whitish color. Posterior to this is the *soft palate,* an arch of muscle that is pinker in color and mobile. The *uvula* is the free projection hanging down from the middle of the soft palate. The cheeks are the side walls of the oral cavity.

The floor of the mouth consists of the horseshoe-shaped mandible bone, the tongue, and underlying muscles. The *tongue* is a mass of striated muscle arranged in a crosswise pattern so that it can change shape and position. The papillae are the rough, bumpy elevations on its dorsal surface. Note the larger vallate papillae in an inverted V shape across the posterior base of the tongue, and do not confuse them with abnormal growths. Underneath, the ventral surface of the tongue is smooth and shiny and has prominent veins. The *frenulum* is a midline fold of tissue that connects the tongue to the floor of the mouth.

The tongue's ability to change shape and position enhances its functions in mastication, swallowing, cleansing the teeth, and in the formation of speech. The tongue also functions in taste sensation. Microscopic taste buds are in the papillae at the back and along the sides of the tongue and on the soft palate.

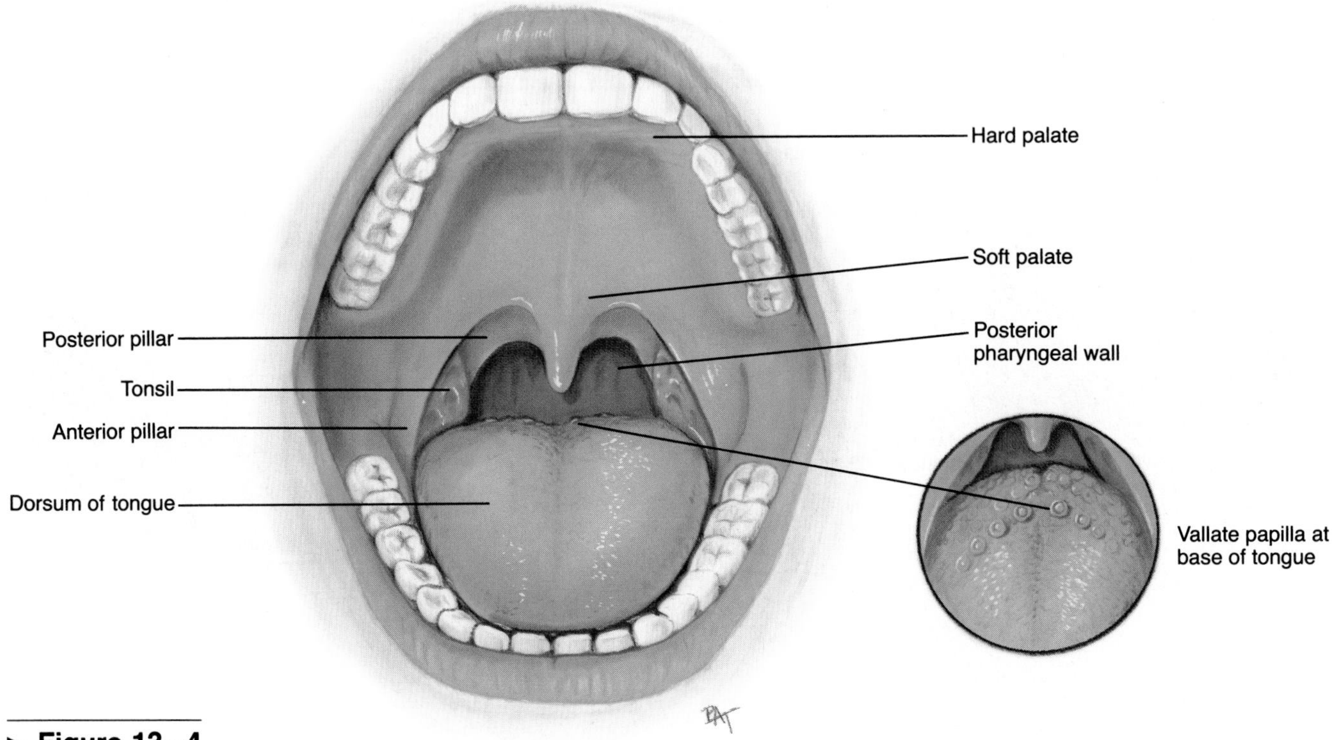

▸ Figure 13–4

The mouth contains three pairs of salivary glands (Fig. 13–5). The largest, the *parotid* gland, lies within the cheeks in front of the ear extending from the zygomatic arch down to the angle of the jaw. Its duct, Stensen's duct, runs forward to open on the buccal mucosa opposite the second molar. The *submandibular* gland is the size of a walnut. It lies beneath the mandible at the angle of the jaw. Wharton's duct runs up and forward to the floor of the mouth and opens at either side of the frenulum. The smallest, the almond shaped *sublingual* gland, lies within the floor of the mouth under the tongue. It has many small openings along the sublingual fold under the tongue.

The glands secrete saliva, the clear fluid that moistens and lubricates the food bolus, starts digestion, and cleans and protects the mucosa.

There are 32 *permanent* teeth, 16 in each arch in the adult. Each tooth has three parts: the crown, the neck, and the root. The gums (gingivae) collar the teeth. They are thick fibrous tissues covered with mucous membrane. The gums are different from the rest of the oral mucosa by their pale pink color and stippled surface.

THROAT

The throat, or pharynx, is the area behind the mouth and nose. The *oropharynx* is separated from the mouth by a fold of tissue on each side, the anterior tonsillar pillar. Behind the folds are the *tonsils,* each a mass of lymphoid tissue. The tonsils are the same color as the surrounding mucous membrane, though they look more granular and their surface shows deep crypts. Tonsillar tissue enlarges during childhood until puberty, then involutes. The posterior pharyngeal wall is seen behind these structures. Some small blood vessels may show on it.

The *nasopharynx* is continuous with the oropharynx, although it is above the oropharynx and behind the nasal cavity. The pharyngeal tonsils (adenoids) and the eustachian tube openings are located here (see Fig. 13–2).

The oral cavity and throat have a rich lymphatic network. Review the lymph nodes and their drainage patterns in Chapter 10, and keep this in mind when evaluating the mouth.

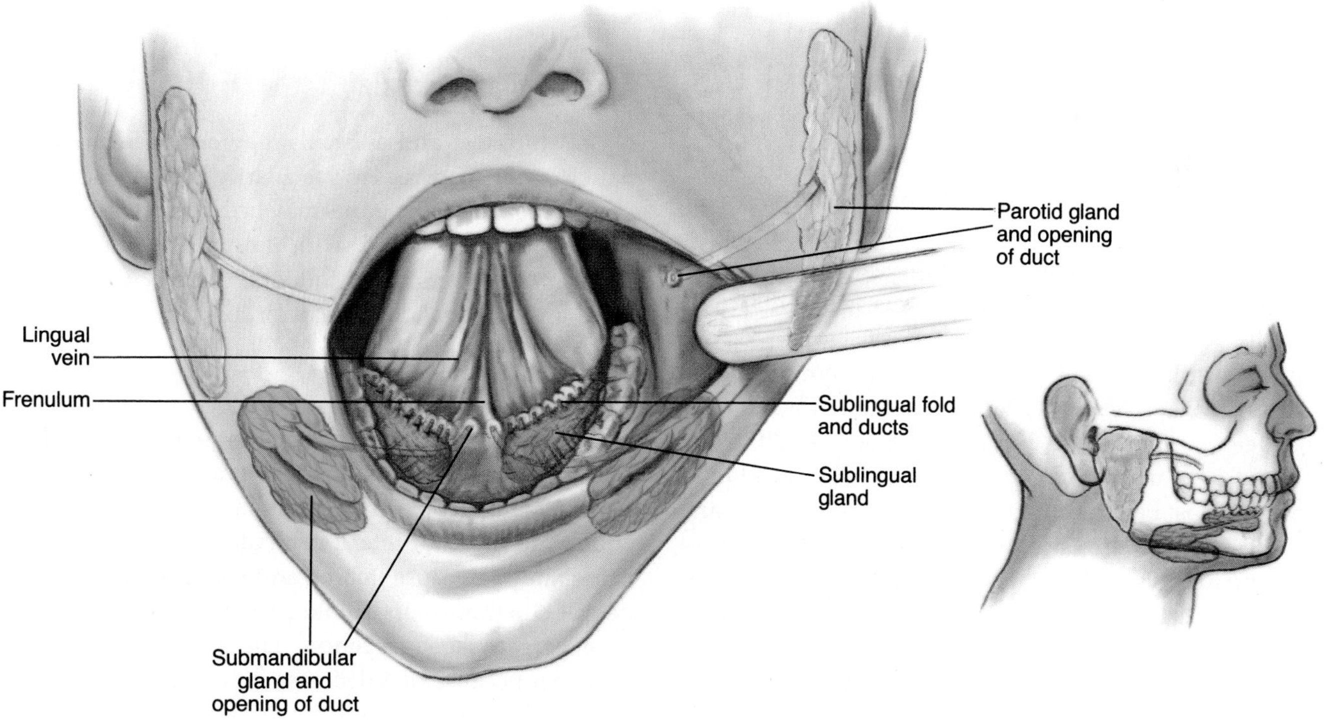

► **Figure 13–5**

UPPER DECIDUOUS

	Erupt (months)	Shed (years)
Central incisor	6 to 8	6 to 7
Lateral incisor	8 to 11	8 to 9
Canine (cuspid)	16 to 20	11 to 12
First molar	10 to 16	10 to 11
Second molar	20 to 30	10 to 12

UPPER PERMANENT

	Erupt (years)
Central incisor	7 to 8
Lateral incisor	8 to 9
Canine (cuspid)	11 to 12
First premolar	10 to 11
Second premolar	10 to 12
First molar	6 to 7
Second molar	12 to 13
Third molar	17 to 25

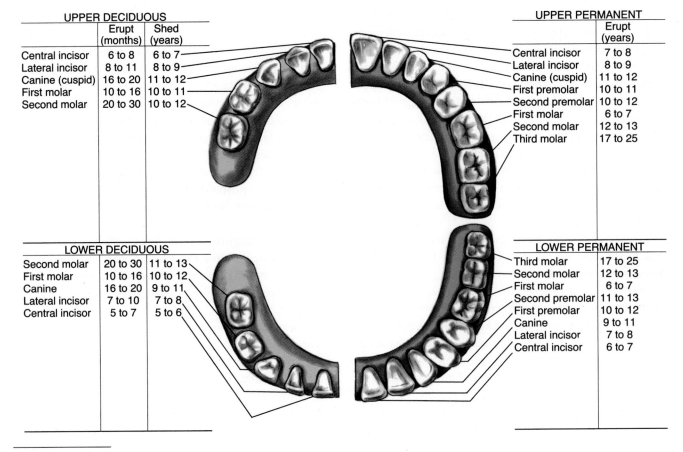

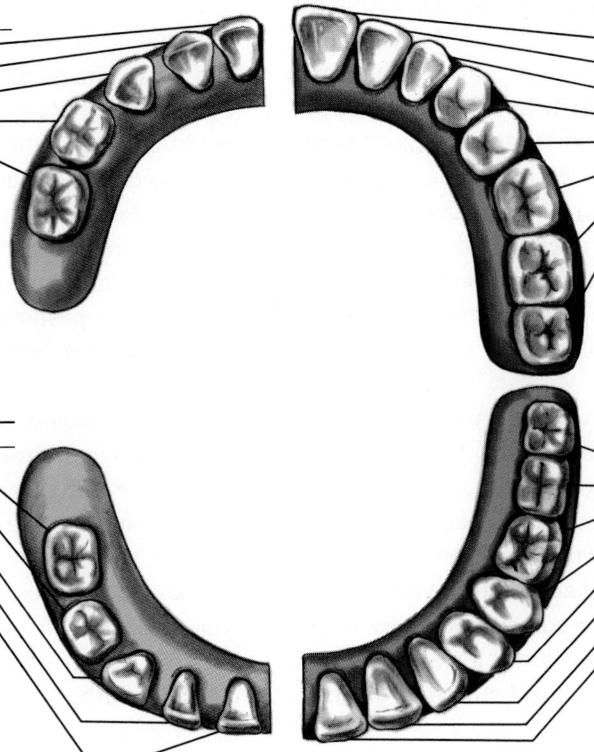

LOWER DECIDUOUS

Second molar	20 to 30	11 to 13
First molar	10 to 16	10 to 12
Canine	16 to 20	9 to 11
Lateral incisor	7 to 10	7 to 8
Central incisor	5 to 7	5 to 6

LOWER PERMANENT

Third molar	17 to 25
Second molar	12 to 13
First molar	6 to 7
Second premolar	11 to 13
First premolar	10 to 12
Canine	9 to 11
Lateral incisor	7 to 8
Central incisor	6 to 7

► **Figure 13-6**

DEVELOPMENTAL CONSIDERATIONS

Infants and Children

In the infant, salivation starts at 3 months. The baby will drool periodically for a few months before learning to swallow the saliva. This drooling does not herald the eruption of the first tooth, although many parents think it does.

The teeth, both sets, begin development in utero. There are 20 *deciduous,* or temporary teeth. These erupt between 6 months and 24 months of age. All 20 teeth should appear by 2 1/2 years of age. The deciduous teeth are lost beginning age 6 through age 12. They are replaced by the permanent teeth, starting with the central incisors (Fig. 13-6). The permanent teeth appear earlier in girls than in boys, and they erupt earlier in black children than in white children.

The nose develops during adolescence, along with other secondary sex characteristics. This growth starts at age 12 or 13, reaching full growth at age 16 in females and age 18 in males.

The Pregnant Female

Nasal stuffiness and epistaxis may occur during pregnancy owing to increased vascularity in the upper respiratory tract. Also, the gums may be hyperemic and softened, and may bleed with normal toothbrushing. Contrary to superstitious folklore, there is no sign that pregnancy causes tooth decay or loss.

The Aging Adult

A gradual loss of subcutaneous fat starts during later middle adult years, making the nose appear more prominent in some people. The nasal hairs grow coarser and stiffer and may not filter the air as well. The hairs protrude and may cause itching and sneezing. Many older people clip these hairs, thinking them unsightly, but this practice can cause infection. The sense of smell may diminish because of a decrease in the number of olfactory nerve fibers. Research studies find a decrease in the sensation of smell in the sixth and seventh decades, but especially during the eighth decade (Rossman, 1986).

In the oral cavity, the soft tissues atrophy and the epithelium thins, especially in the cheek and tongue. This results in loss of taste buds, with about an 80 percent reduction in taste functioning (Rossman, 1986). Atrophic tissues ulcerate easily, which places the older person at risk for infections such as oral moniliasis. There is also an increased risk of malignant oral lesions.

Many dental changes occur with aging. The tooth surface is abraded. The gums begin to recede and the teeth begin to erode at the gum line. A smooth V-shaped cavity forms around the neck of the tooth, exposing the nerve and making the tooth hypersensitive. Some tooth loss may occur owing to bone resorption (osteoporosis), which decreases the inner tooth structure and its outer support. Natural tooth loss is exacerbated by years of inadequate dental care, decay, and poor oral hygiene.

If tooth loss occurs, the remaining teeth drift, causing *malocclusion.* The stress of chewing with maloccluding teeth causes further problems: (1) There is excessive bone resorption with further tooth loss. (2) there is muscle imbalance resulting from a mandible and maxilla now out of alignment. This produces muscle spasms, tenderness of muscles of mastication, and chronic headaches. (3) The temporomandibular joint is stressed, leading to osteoarthritis, pain, and inability to fully open the mouth (Carotenuto, 1980).

A diminished sense of taste and smell decreases the aging person's interest in food and may contribute to malnutrition. There may be decreased saliva production. Saliva acts as a solvent for food flavors and helps move food around the mouth. Decreased saliva also reduces the mouth's self-cleaning property. The major cause of decreased saliva flow is not the aging process itself, but use of medications (Ofstehage, 1986). Over 250 medications may cause the mouth to be dry.

The absence of some teeth and trouble with mastication encourage the older person to eat soft foods (usually high in carbohydrates) and to decrease meat and fresh vegetable intake. This produces a risk of nutritional deficit for protein, vitamins, and minerals.

TRANSCULTURAL CONSIDERATIONS

Bifid uvula, a condition in which the uvula is split either completely or partially, occurs in 18 percent of some Native American groups and 10 percent of Asians. The occurrence in whites and blacks is rare (Schaumann et al, 1970).

Cleft lip and *cleft palate* are most common in Asians and Native Americans and least common in blacks (Emanuel, 1972; Overfield, 1985). *Torus palatinus,* a bony ridge running the middle of the hard palate, is more common in Native Americans (55 percent) and in Eskimos and Asians (up to 77 percent) (Jarvis and Gorlin, 1972).

Leukoedema, a grayish-white benign lesion occurring on the buccal mucosa, is present in 68 to 90 percent of blacks but only 43 percent of whites (Martin and Crump, 1972). Oral hyperpigmentation also varies according to race (Waserman, 1974). Usually absent at birth, hyperpigmentation increases with age. By age 50 years, 10 percent of whites and 50 to 90 percent of blacks will show oral hyperpigmentation, a condition that is believed to be caused by a lifetime of accumulation of postinflammatory oral changes (Overfield, 1985).

Because teeth are often used as indicators of developmental, hygienic, and nutritional adequacy, biocultural differences are important. Although it is rare for a white baby to be born with teeth (1 in 3000), the incidence rises to 1 in 11 among Tlingit Indians and to 1 or 2 in 100 among Canadian Eskimo infants (Jarvis and Gorman, 1972). Although congenital teeth are usually not problematic, extraction is necessary for some breast-fed infants.

The size of teeth varies widely, with the teeth of whites being the smallest, followed by blacks, then Asians and Native Americans. The largest teeth are found among Eskimos and Australian Aborigines (Overfield, 1985). Larger teeth cause some groups to have prognathic, or protruding, jaws, a condition that is seen more frequently in blacks and Asians. The condition is normal and does not reflect an orthodontic problem.

Agenesis (absence) of teeth varies by race, with absence of the third molar occurring in 18 to 35 percent of Asians, 9 to 25 percent of whites, and 1 to 11 percent of blacks (Brothwell et al, 1963). Throughout life, whites have more tooth decay than blacks. Complete tooth loss occurs more often in whites than in blacks despite the higher incidence of periodontal disease in blacks. Approximately one third of whites 45 years or older have lost all their teeth, compared with 25 percent of blacks in the same age group (Kelly et al, 1967).

The differences in tooth decay between blacks and whites can be explained by the fact that blacks have harder and denser tooth enamel that makes their teeth less susceptible to the organisms that cause caries.

SUBJECTIVE DATA

Nose

- Discharge
- Frequent colds (upper respiratory infections)
- Sinus pain
- Trauma
- Epistaxis
- Allergies
- Altered smell

Mouth and Throat

- Sores or lesions
- Sore throat
- Bleeding gums
- Toothache
- Hoarseness
- Dysphagia
- Altered taste
- Smoking, alcohol consumption
- Self-care behaviors
  - Dental care pattern
  - Dentures or appliances

EXAMINER ASKS:	RATIONALE:
NOSE	
1. Do you have any **nasal discharge,** or runny nose? Is this continuous?	Rhinorrhea
Character: Is the discharge watery, purulent, mucoid, bloody? Is it from one side or both?	Unilateral or bilateral.
2. Do you have any unusually **frequent or severe colds (upper respiratory infections)?** How often do these occur?	Most people have occasional colds. Asking a more precise question yields meaningful data.
3. Do you have any **sinus pain** or sinusitis? How is this treated? Do you have chronic postnasal drip?	
4. Have you ever had any **trauma** or a blow to the nose?	
Can you breathe through your nose? Are both sides obstructed or just the right, or left?	Nares obstructed.
5. Do you have any nosebleeds? How often do these occur? How much bleeding is there—a teaspoonful or does it pour out? What is the color of the blood—red or brown? Are there clots? Does it come from one nostril or both? Does it seem to be aggravated by nose picking or scratching? How do you treat the nosebleeds? Are they difficult to stop?	**Epistaxis.**
6. Do you have any **allergies,** or hay fever? To what are you allergic? How was this determined? What type of environment makes it worse? Do you use inhalers, nasal spray, nose drops? How often? Which type? How long have you used this?	"Seasonal" rhinitis if due to pollen; "perennial" if allergen is dust. Misuse of over-the-counter nasal medications irritates the mucosa and causes rebound swelling, a common problem.
7. Have you experienced any **change in sense of smell?**	

EXAMINER ASKS:	RATIONALE:

MOUTH AND THROAT

1. Have you noticed any **sores or lesions** in the mouth, tongue, or gums? How long have you had it?
Is the sore constant, or does it come and go? Does it seem to be associated with stress, season change, food?
How have you treated the sore? Have you applied any local medication?

2. How about **sore throats?** How frequently do you get them? Do you have a sore throat now? When did it start?
Is it associated with: cough, fever, fatigue, decreased appetite, headache, postnasal drip, or hoarseness?
Is it worse when arising? What is the humidity level in the room where you sleep? Do you experience any dust or smoke inhaled at work?
Do you usually get a throat culture for the sore throats? Were any documented as streptococcal?
How have you treated this sore throat: medication, gargling? How effective are these? Have your tonsils or adenoids been taken out?

3. Have you noted any **bleeding gums?** How long have you had this?

4. Do you have any **toothache?** Do your teeth seem sensitive to hot, cold? Have you lost any teeth?

5. Do you have any **hoarseness,** voice change? For how long?
Does it feel like having to clear your throat? Or, like a "lump in your throat?"
Do you use your voice a lot at work, recreation?
Does the hoarseness seem associated with a cold, sore throat?

A disorder of the larynx due to many causes, e.g., overuse of the voice, upper respiratory infection, chronic inflammation, lesions, or a neoplasm.

6. Do you have any difficulty swallowing? How long have you had it?
Does it feel like food gets stopped at a certain point?
Is there any pain with this?

Dysphagia

7. Do you have any **change in sense of taste?**

8. Do you smoke? Pipe or cigarettes? Smokeless tobacco? How many packs per day? For how many years?
When was your last alcoholic drink? How much alcohol did you drink that time? How much alcohol do you usually drink?

Chronic use of tobacco in any form and heavy alcohol consumption increase risk of oral cancers.

9. **Self-care behaviors.** Tell me about your daily dental care. Do you use a toothbrush and floss regularly?

Assess self-care behaviors for oral hygiene.

When was your last dental examination? Do dental problems affect which foods you eat? Are there any foods you are unable to eat?

Periodic dental screening is necessary to note caries.

Do you have a dental appliance: braces, bridge, headgear?
Do you wear dentures? How long have you had this set? How do they fit? Are they tight or wobbly? Do you wear dentures all the time?
Have you noticed any sores or irritation on the palate, or gums? Do you have any problems with talking—do the dentures whistle or drop? Can you chew all foods with them? How do you clean them?

Lesions may arise from ill-fitting dentures. Or the presence of dentures may mask the eruption of new lesion.

EXAMINER ASKS:	RATIONALE:

ADDITIONAL QUESTIONS FOR INFANTS AND CHILDREN

Does the child have any mouth infections or sores, such as thrush or canker sores? How frequently do these occur?	
Does the child have frequent sore throat, or tonsillitis? How often? How are these treated? Have they ever been documented as streptococcal infections?	
Have you noticed the child grinding his or her teeth? Does this happen at night?	Bruxism—occurs in sleep, usually from nervous tension.
Does the child tend to put objects up his or her nose? Have you noted unilateral nose drainage?	Foreign body.
Did the child's teeth erupt about on time?	Many delayed teeth may impair nutrition. Eruption is delayed with Down syndrome, cretinism, rickets.
Do the teeth seem straight to you?	Malocclusion.
Is the child using a bottle? How often during the day? Does the child go to sleep with a bottle at night?	Constant use of a bottle during day or when going to sleep places infant at risk for caries and middle ear infections.
Have you noticed any thumbsucking after the child's secondary teeth came in?	Prolonged thumbsucking (after age 6 to 7) may affect occlusion.
Self-care behaviors. How are the child's dental habits? Does he or she use a toothbrush regularly? How often does the child see a dentist?	Evaluate child's self-care. Early self-care has best compliance.
Do you use fluoridated water or fluoride supplement?	

ADDITIONAL QUESTIONS FOR THE AGING ADULT

Do you have any dryness in the mouth? Are you taking any medications? (Note prescribed and over-the-counter medications.)	Xerostomia (dry mouth) is a side effect of many drugs used by older people: antidepressants, anticholinergics, antispasmodics, antihypertensives, antipsychotics, bronchodilators.
Have you had any loss of teeth? Can you chew all types of food?	Note a decrease in eating meat, fresh vegetables, and cleansing foods such as apples.
Are you able to care for your own teeth or dentures?	Ability to perform self-care may be decreased by physical disability (arthritis), vision loss, confusion, or depression.
Have you noticed a change in your sense of taste or smell?	Some people add condiments to enhance food when taste begins to wane. Note salt and sugar additives, especially. Also, diminished smell may decrease the person's ability to detect food spoilage, natural gas leaks, or smoke from a fire (Blair, 1990).

OBJECTIVE DATA

Equipment Needed

Otoscope with short, wide-tipped nasal speculum attachment or nasal speculum and penlight
Tongue blade
Cotton gauze pad (4 × 4 inches)
Gloves
Occasionally: Long-stem light attachment for otoscope

Preparation

Position the person sitting up straight with his or her head at your eye level. If the person wears dentures, offer a paper towel and ask the person to remove them.

METHOD OF EXAMINATION

NORMAL RANGE OF FINDINGS	ABNORMAL FINDINGS

THE NOSE

Inspect and palpate the nose.

Healthy nasal function requires patent airways and intact mucous membrane lining.

External Nose

Normally, the nose is symmetric, in the midline, and in proportion to other facial features (Fig. 13–7). Inspect for any deformity, asymmetry, inflam-

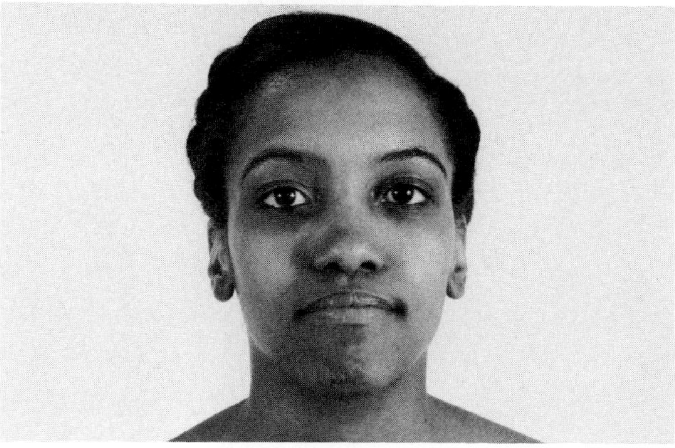

► **Figure 13–7**

NORMAL RANGE OF FINDINGS	ABNORMAL FINDINGS

mation, or skin lesions. If an injury is reported or suspected, palpate gently for any pain or break in contour.

Test the patency of the nostrils by pushing each nasal wing shut with your finger while asking the person to sniff inward through the other naris. This reveals any obstruction, which later is explored using the nasal speculum. The sense of smell, mediated by cranial nerve I, is usually not tested in a routine examination. The procedure for assessing smell is presented with cranial nerve testing in Chapter 20.

Absence of sniff indicates obstruction.

Nasal Cavity

There are two possible techniques to explore the nasal cavity. You may use a nasal speculum to open the vestibule and a penlight to illuminate the cavity (Fig. 13–8). Hold the speculum in your left palm with its blades pointing away from you. Insert the closed blades 1 cm into the vestibule (Fig. 13–9). Keep the blades vertical to avoid any pressure on the sensitive

► Figure 13–9

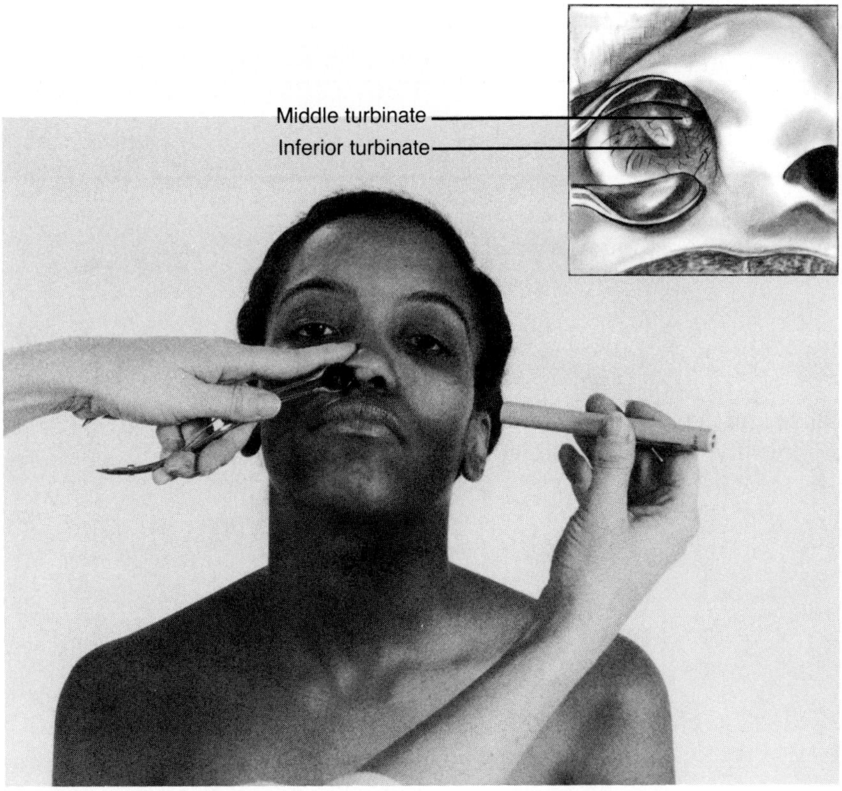

► Figure 13–8

NORMAL RANGE OF FINDINGS

nasal septum. Keep your index finger on the nasal wing to stabilize the instrument. Use your free hand to hold the penlight and to change position of the person's head.

An alternate technique is to attach the short wide-tipped speculum to the otoscope head and insert this combined apparatus into the nasal vestibule, again avoiding pressure on the nasal septum (Fig. 13–10). Gently lift up the tip of the nose with your finger before inserting.

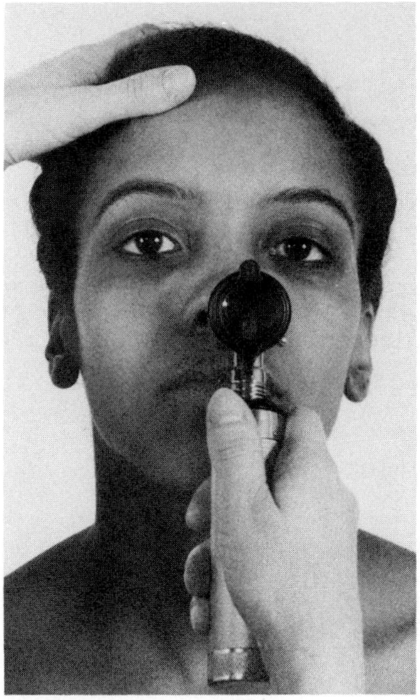

▸ **Figure 13–10**

View each nasal cavity with the person's head erect, then with the head tilted back. Inspect the nasal mucosa, noting its normal red color and smooth moist surface (see Fig. 13–9). Note any swelling, discharge, bleeding, or foreign body.

ABNORMAL FINDINGS

Rhinitis—nasal mucosa is swollen and bright red with an upper respiratory infection.

Discharge is common with rhinitis and sinusitis, varying from watery and copious to thick, purulent, and green-yellow.

With chronic allergy, mucosa looks swollen, boggy, pale, and gray.

NORMAL RANGE OF FINDINGS	ABNORMAL FINDINGS

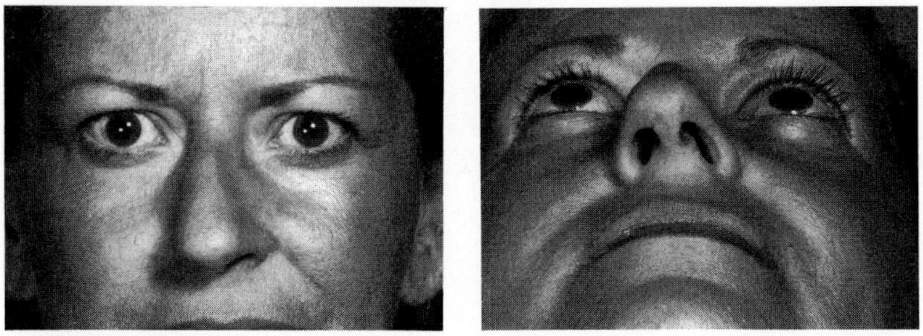

▶ Figure 13-11

Observe the nasal septum for deviation (Fig. 13-11). A deviated septum is common and is not significant unless air flow is obstructed. (If present in a hospitalized patient, document the deviated septum in the event the person needs nasal suctioning or a nasogastric tube.) Also note any perforation or bleeding in the septum.

A deviated septum looks like a hump or shelf in one nasal cavity. Perforation is seen as a spot of light from penlight shining in other naris.

Epistaxis commonly comes from anterior septum (see Table 13-1).

Inspect the turbinates, the bony ridges curving down from the lateral walls. The superior turbinate will not be in your view, but the middle and inferior turbinates appear the same light red color as the nasal mucosa. Note any swelling but do not try to push the speculum past it. Turbinates are quite vascular and tender if touched.

Note any polyps, which are benign growths that accompany chronic allergy, and distinguish them from the normal turbinates.

Polyps are smooth, pale gray in color, avascular, mobile, and nontender (see Table 13-1).

THE SINUS AREAS

Palpate the sinus areas.

Using your thumbs, press over the frontal sinuses below the eyebrows (Fig. 13-12) and over the maxillary sinuses below the cheekbones (Fig.

Sinus areas are tender to palpation in persons with chronic allergies and acute infection (sinusitis).

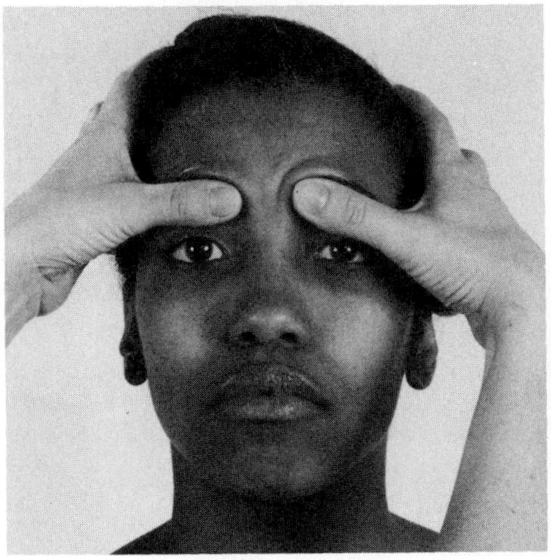

▶ Figure 13-12

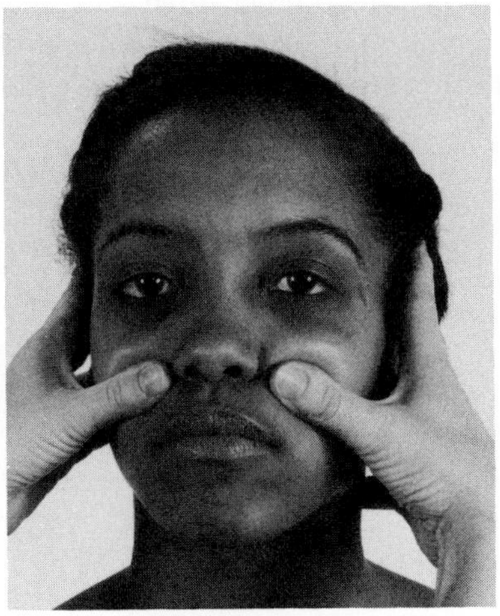

▶ Figure 13-13

NORMAL RANGE OF FINDINGS

13–13). Take care not to press directly on the eyeballs. The person should feel firm pressure but no pain.

Transillumination

You may use this technique when you suspect sinus inflammation, although it is of limited usefulness. Darken the examining room. Affix a strong narrow light to the end of the otoscope, and hold it under the superior orbital ridge against the location of the frontal sinus area (Fig. 13–14). Cover with your hand. A diffuse red glow is a normal response (Fig. 13–15). It comes from the light shining through the air in the healthy sinus. An inflamed sinus filled with fluid does not transilluminate.

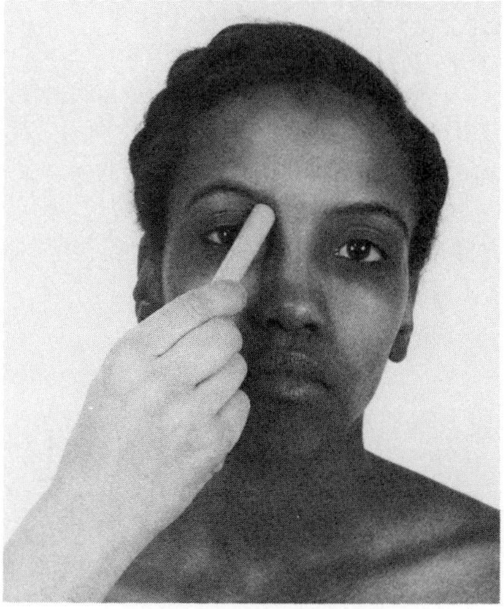

► **Figure 13–14**

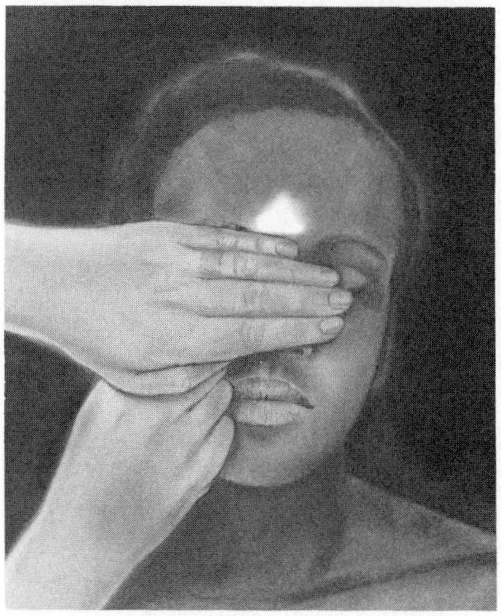

► **Figure 13–15**

ABNORMAL FINDINGS

NORMAL RANGE OF FINDINGS | **ABNORMAL FINDINGS**

You may use the same technique with the maxillary sinuses, providing the person has no upper denture that would impede the light (Fig. 13–16). Place the light into the mouth and ask the person to close the lips around it. Shine the light on one side of the hard palate, then the other. Note a dull glow under the eyes as the light transmits through the sinuses (Fig. 13–17). Healthy sinuses contain air and may light up symmetrically. But be aware that asymmetry is not a reliable sign of sinus inflammation because many healthy sinuses normally will not transilluminate. Clean the light before and after use.

A significant finding is one sinus illuminated and the other clouded. If one has fluid, it looks darker than the healthy one.

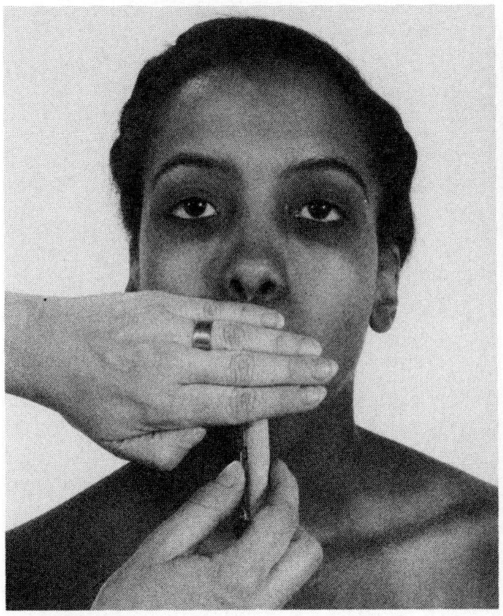

► Figure 13–16

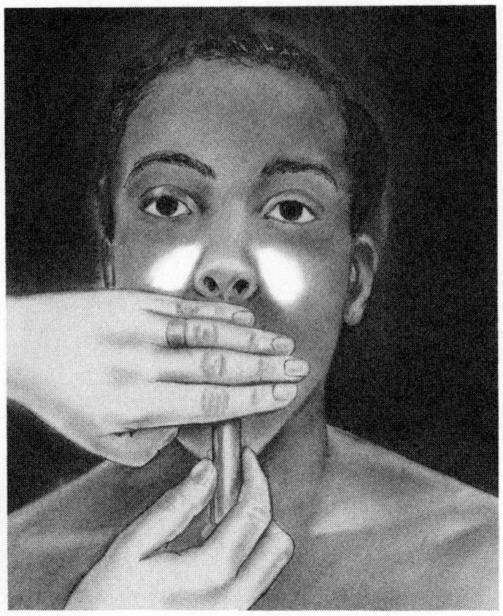

► Figure 13–17

THE MOUTH

Inspect the mouth.

Begin with anterior structures and move posteriorly. Use a tongue blade to retract structures and a bright light for optimal visualization.

Lips

Inspect the lips for color, moisture, cracking, or lesions. Retract the lips and note their inner surface as well (Fig. 13–18). Black persons normally may have bluish lips.

In light-skinned people: circumoral pallor occurs with shock and anemia; cyanosis with hypoxemia and chilling; cherry red lips with carbon monoxide poisoning, acidosis from aspirin poisoning, or ketoacidosis.

Cheilosis—cracking at the corners.

Herpes simplex, other lesions (see Table 13–2).

NORMAL RANGE OF FINDINGS | **ABNORMAL FINDINGS**

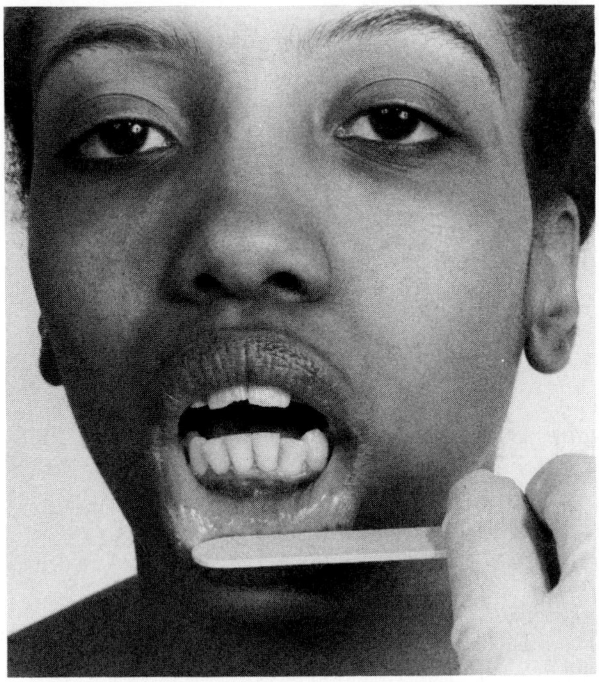

► Figure 13-18

Teeth and Gums

The condition of the teeth is an index of the person's general health. Your examination should not replace the regular dental examination, but you should note any diseased, absent, loose, or abnormally positioned teeth. The teeth normally look white, straight and evenly spaced, and clean and free of debris or decay.

Discolored teeth: appear brown with excessive fluoride use; yellow with tobacco use.

Compare the number of teeth with the number expected for the person's age. Ask the person to bite as if chewing something and note alignment of upper and lower jaw. Normal occlusion in the back is the upper teeth resting directly on the lowers; in the front, the upper incisors slightly override the lower incisors.

Grinding down of tooth surface.

Plaque—soft debris.

Caries—decay.

Malocclusion (poor biting relationship), e.g., protrusion of upper or lower incisors (see Table 13-3).

Normally, the gums look pink or coral with a stippled (dotted) surface. The gum margins at the teeth are tight and well defined. Check for swelling; retraction of gingival margins; and spongy, bleeding, or discolored gums. Black people normally may have a dark melanotic line along the gingival margin.

Gingival hypertrophy (see Table 13-3), crevices between teeth and gums, pockets of debris.

Gums bleed with slight pressure.

Dark line on gingival margins occurs with lead and bismuth poisoning.

Tongue

Check the tongue for color, surface characteristics, and moisture. The color is pink and even. The dorsal surface is normally roughened from the papillae. A thin white coating may be present. Ask the person to touch the

Beefy red swollen tongue. Smooth glossy areas (see Table 13-5).

Enlarged tongue occurs with

NORMAL RANGE OF FINDINGS

tongue to the roof of the mouth. Its ventral surface looks smooth, glistening, and shows veins. Saliva is present.

Inspect carefully the entire U-shaped area under the tongue. Oral malignancies are most likely to develop here. Note any white patches, nodules, or ulcerations. If lesions are present, or with any person over 50 or with a positive history of smoking or alcohol use, put on a glove* and palpate the area. Place your other hand under the jaw to stabilize the tissue and "capture" any abnormality (Fig. 13–19). Notice any induration.

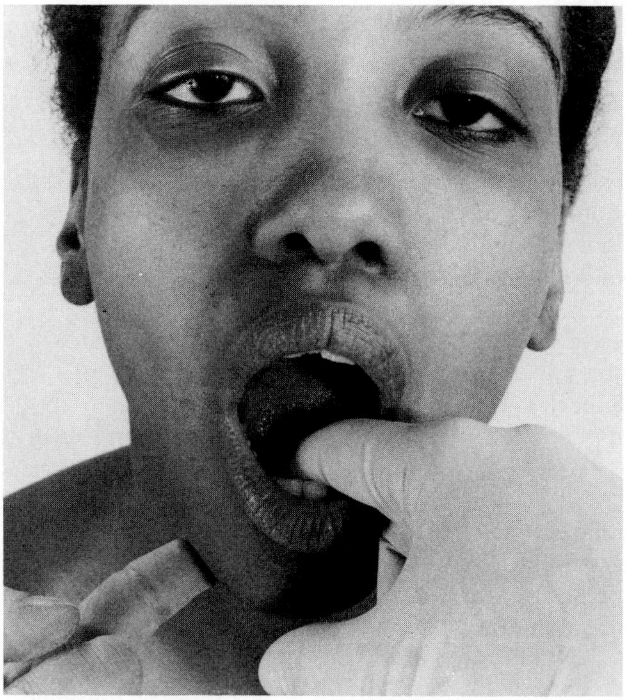

▶ **Figure 13–19**

Hold the tongue using a cotton gauze pad for traction, and swing the tongue out and to each side (Fig. 13–20). Inspect for any white patches or lesions—normally there are none. If any occur, palpate these lesions for induration.

* Always wear gloves to examine mucous membranes. This follows universal precautions to prevent the spread of possible communicable disease.

ABNORMAL FINDINGS

mental retardation, hypothyroidism, acromegaly.

A small tongue accompanies malnutrition.

Dry mouth occurs with dehydration, fever; tongue has deep vertical fissures.

Saliva is decreased while the person is taking anticholinergic and other medication.

Excess saliva and drooling occur with gingivostomatitis and neurologic dysfunction.

Any lesion or ulcer persisting for more than 2 weeks must be investigated.

An indurated area may be a mass or lymphadenopathy, and it must be investigated.

NORMAL RANGE OF FINDINGS	ABNORMAL FINDINGS

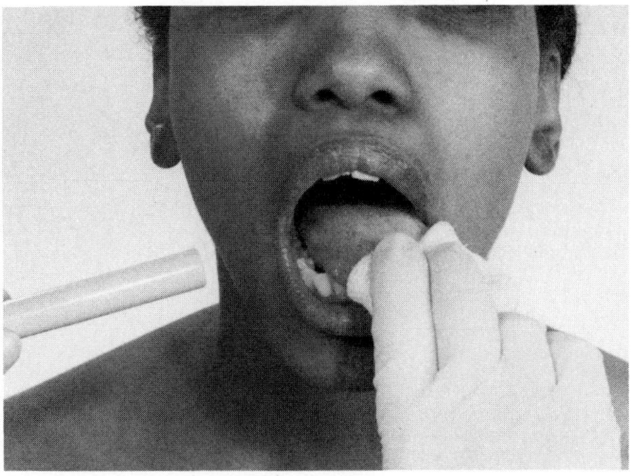

► Figure 13-20

Buccal Mucosa

Hold the cheek open with a wooden tongue blade, and check the buccal mucosa for color, nodules, or lesions. It looks pink, smooth, and moist, although patchy hyperpigmentation is common and normal in dark-skinned people.

Dappled brown patches present with Addison's disease (chronic adrenal insufficiency).

An expected finding is Stensen's duct, the opening of the parotid salivary gland. It looks like a small dimple opposite the upper second molar. You also may see a raised occlusion line on the buccal mucosa parallel with the level the teeth meet due to the teeth closing against the cheek.

Orifice of Stensen's duct looks red with mumps.

Koplik's spots—a prodromal sign of measles.

Leukoplakia (see Table 13-4).

A larger patch also may be present along the buccal mucosa. This is *leukoedema,* a benign grayish opaque area, more common in blacks and East Indians. When it is mild, the patch disappears as you stretch the cheeks. The severity of the condition increases with age, looking grayish white and thickened. The cause of the condition is unknown. Do not mistake leukoedema for oral infections such as candidiasis (thrush).

Fordyce granules are small, isolated white or yellow papules on the mucosa of cheek, tongue, and lips (Fig. 13-21). These little sebaceous cysts are painless and not significant.

The chalky white raised patch of *leukoplakia* is abnormal (see Table 13-4).

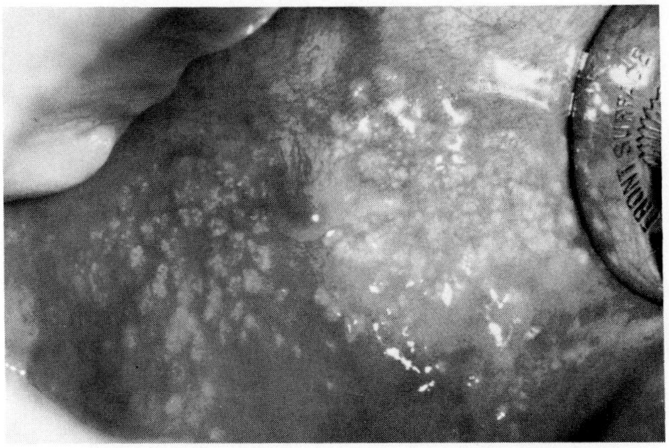

► Figure 13-21

NORMAL RANGE OF FINDINGS | ABNORMAL FINDINGS

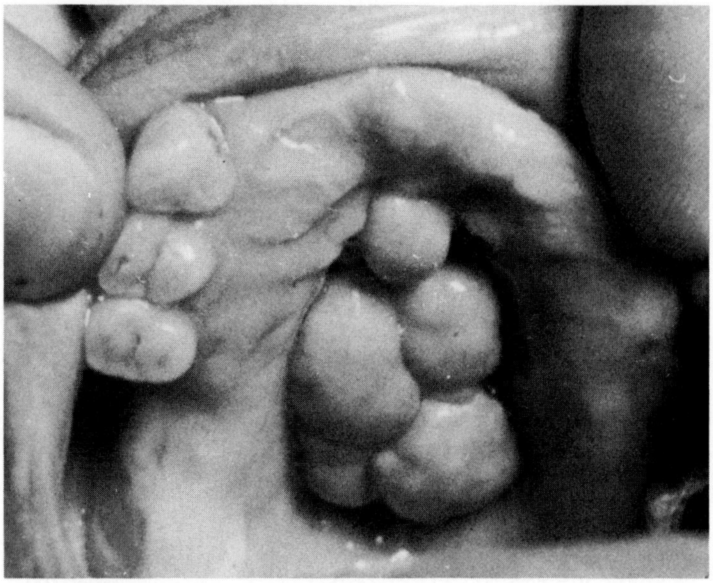

▶ Figure 13-22

Palate

Shine your light up to the roof of the mouth. The more anterior hard palate is white with irregular transverse rugae. The posterior soft palate is pinker, smooth, and upwardly movable. A normal variation is a nodular bony ridge down the middle of the hard palate, a *torus palatinus* (Fig. 13-22). This benign growth arises after puberty and is present in 25 percent of females and 15 percent of males (Adams et al, 1989). It is a more common finding in Native Americans, Eskimos, and Asians.

The hard palate appears yellow with jaundice. In blacks with jaundice, it may look yellow, muddy yellow, or green-brown.

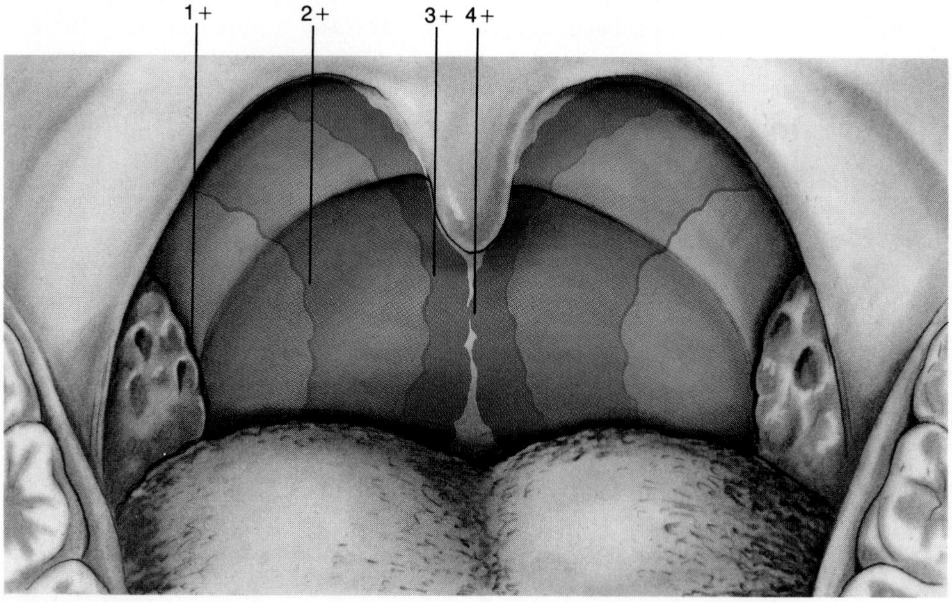

▶ Figure 13-23

NORMAL RANGE OF FINDINGS	ABNORMAL FINDINGS

Observe the uvula; it normally looks like a fleshy pendant hanging in the midline (Fig. 13–23). Ask the person to say "ahhh" and note the soft palate and uvula rise in the midline. This tests one function of cranial nerve X, the vagus nerve.

A *bifid* uvula looks like it is split in two; more common in Native Americans (see Table 13–6).

Any deviation to the side or absent movement indicates nerve damage, which also occurs with poliomyelitis and diphtheria.

THE THROAT

Inspect the throat.

Using your light, observe the oval, rough-surfaced *tonsils* behind the anterior tonsilar pillar (Fig. 13–23). Their color is the same pink as the oral mucosa, and their surface is peppered with indentations, or crypts. In some people, the crypts collect small plugs of whitish cellular debris. This does not indicate infection. However, there should be no exudate on the tonsils. Tonsils are graded in size as:

1+—visible;

2+—halfway between tonsillar pillars and uvula;

3+—touching the uvula;

4+—touching each other.

With an acute infection, tonsils are bright red, swollen, and may have exudate or large white spots. A white membrane covering the tonsils may accompany infectious mononucleosis, leukemia and diphtheria.

You may normally see 1+ or 2+ tonsils in healthy people, especially in children, because lymphoid tissue is proportionately enlarged until puberty.

Tonsils are enlarged to 2+, 3+, or 4+, with an acute infection.

Enlarge your view of the posterior pharyngeal wall by depressing the tongue with a tongue blade. Push down halfway back on the tongue; if you push on its tip, the tongue will hump up in back. Press slightly off center to avoid eliciting the gag reflex. (Some people can depress their own tongue so the tongue blade is not needed.) Scan the posterior wall for color, exudate, or lesions. When finished, discard the tongue blade.

Although usually it is not done in the screening examination, touching the posterior wall with the tongue blade elicits the gag reflex. This tests cranial nerves IX and X, the glossopharyngeal and vagus. Test cranial nerve XII, the hypoglossal nerve, by asking the person to stick out the tongue. It should protrude in the midline. Children enjoy this request. Note any tremor, loss of movement, or deviation to the side.

With damage to cranial nerve XII, the tongue deviates *toward* the paralyzed side.

A fine tremor of the tongue occurs with hyperthyroidism; a coarse tremor with cerebral palsy and alcoholism.

Ankyloglossia, "tongue-tie," limits protrusion and causes speech defects (see Table 13–5). Also a neoplasm may restrict protrusion.

During the examination, notice any breath odor, *halitosis.* This is common and usually is due to a local cause, such as poor oral hygiene, consumption of odoriferous foods, alcohol consumption, heavy smoking, or dental infection. Occasionally, it may indicate a systemic disease.

Diabetic ketoacidosis has a sweet fruity breath odor; this acetone smell also occurs in children with malnutrition or dehydration. Others are an ammonia breath

NORMAL RANGE OF FINDINGS | **ABNORMAL FINDINGS**

odor with uremia; a musty odor with liver disease; a foul, fetid odor with dental or respiratory infections; alcohol odor with alcohol ingestion or chemicals; a mouse-like smell of the breath with diphtheria.

DEVELOPMENTAL CONSIDERATIONS

Infants and Children

Preparation

Since the oral examination is intrusive for the infant or young child, the timing is best toward the end of the complete examination, along with the ear examination. But if any crying episodes occur earlier, seize the opportunity to examine the mouth and oropharynx.

As with the ear examination, let the parent help position the child. Place the infant supine on the examining table, with the arms restrained by the parent (Fig. 13–24). The older infant and toddler may be held on the parent's lap with one of the parent's hands holding the arms down and the other hand restraining the child's head against the parent's chest. Though not often needed, the parent's leg can reach over and capture the child's legs between the parent's own (Fig. 13–25).

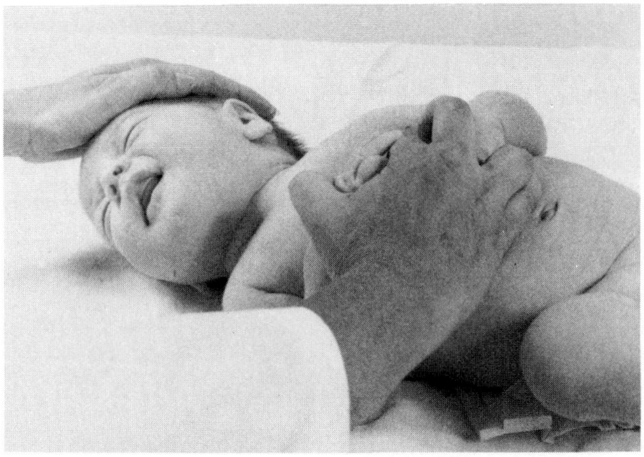

► **Figure 13–24**

Use a game to help prepare the young child. Encourage the preschool child to use a tongue blade to look into a puppet's mouth. Or place a mirror so that the child can look into the mouth while you do. The school-age child is usually cooperative and loves to show off missing or new teeth (Fig. 13–26).

NORMAL RANGE OF FINDINGS

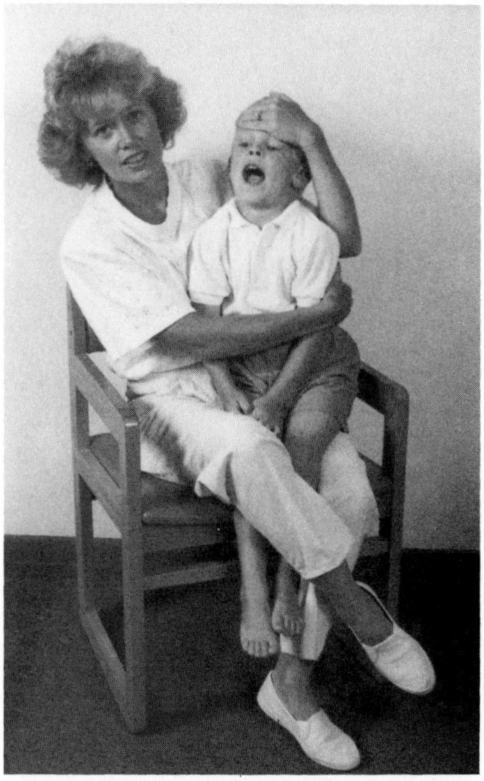

► Figure 13-25

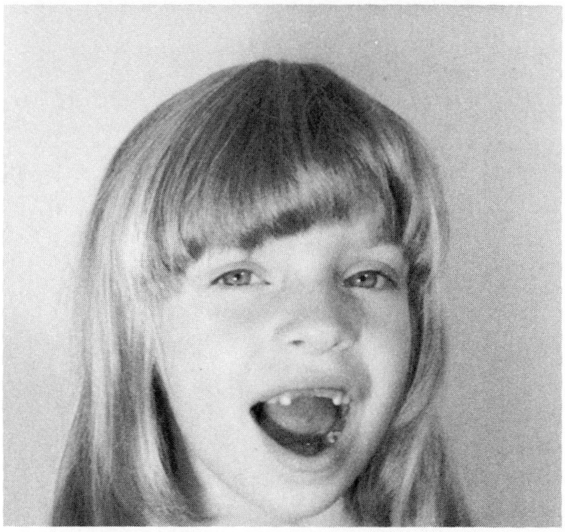

► Figure 13-26

Be discriminating in your use of the tongue blade. It may be necessary for a full view of oral structures, but it produces a strong gag reflex in the infant. You may avoid the tongue blade completely with a cooperative preschooler and school-aged child. Try asking the young child to open the mouth "as big as a lion" and to move the tongue in different directions. To enlarge your view of the oropharynx, ask the child to stick out the tongue and "pant like a dog."

ABNORMAL FINDINGS

NORMAL RANGE OF FINDINGS	ABNORMAL FINDINGS

At some point, you will encounter an uncooperative young child who clenches the teeth and refuses to open the mouth. If all your other efforts have failed, slide the tongue blade along the buccal mucosa and turn it between the back teeth. Push down to depress the tongue. This stimulates the gag reflex and the child opens the mouth wide for a few seconds. You will have a *brief* look at the throat.

Nose

The newborn may have milia across the nose. The nasal bridge may be flat in black and Asian children. There should be no nasal flaring or narrowing with breathing.

Nasal flaring in the infant indicates respiratory distress.

A transverse ridge across the nose occurs in a child with chronic allergy from wiping the nose upward with palm (see Table 10–4). Nasal narrowing on inhalation is seen with chronic nasal obstruction and mouth-breathing.

It is essential to determine the patency of the nares in the immediate newborn period because most newborns are obligate nose-breathers. Nares blocked with amniotic fluid are suctioned gently with a bulb syringe. If obstruction is suspected, a small lumen (5 to 10 Fr) catheter is passed down each naris to confirm patency.

Inability to pass catheter through nasal cavity indicates choanal atresia, which needs immediate intervention (see Table 13–1).

Avoid the nasal speculum when examining the infant and young child. Instead, gently push up the tip of the nose with your thumb while using your other hand to shine the light into the naris. With a toddler, be alert for the possible foreign body lodged in the nasal cavity (see Table 13–1). Only in children older than 8 years do you need to palpate the child's sinus areas. In younger children, sinus areas are too small for palpation.

Mouth and Throat

A normal finding in infants is the sucking tubercle, a small pad in the middle of the upper lip from friction of breast- or bottle-feeding. Note the number of teeth, and whether or not it is appropriate for the child's age. Also note pattern of eruption, position, condition, and hygiene. Use this guide for children under 2 years; the child's age in months minus the number 6 should equal the expected number of deciduous teeth. Normally, all 20 deciduous teeth are in by 2 1/2 years. Saliva is present after 3 months of age, and shows in excess with teething children.

No teeth by age 1 year.

Discolored teeth: appear yellow or yellow-brown with infants taking tetracycline or whose mothers took the drug during the last trimester; appear green or black with excessive iron ingestion, although this reverses when the iron is stopped.

Malocclusion: upper or lower dental arches are out of alignment.

NORMAL RANGE OF FINDINGS

Mobility should allow the tongue to extend at least as far as the alveolar ridge.

Note any bruising or laceration on the buccal mucosa or gums of infant or young child.

On the palate, *Epstein's pearls* are a normal finding in newborns and infants (Fig. 13–27). They are small, yellow-white, glistening, pearly papules along the median raphe of the hard palate and on the gums where they look like teeth. They are small retention cysts and disappear in the first few weeks.

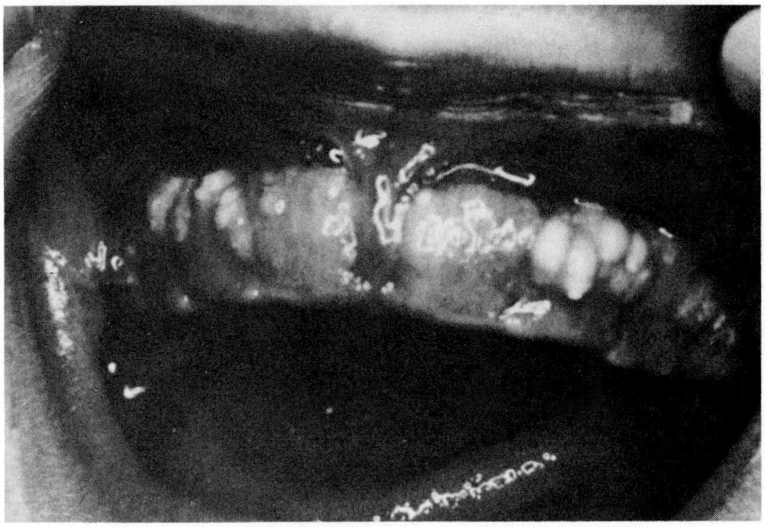

Epstein's pearls

▸ Figure 13–27

Bednar aphthae are traumatic areas or ulcers on the posterior hard palate on either side of the midline. They result from abrasions while sucking.

The tonsils are not visible in the newborn. They gradually enlarge during childhood, remaining proportionately larger until puberty. Tonsils appear still larger if the infant is crying or gagging. Normally, the newborn can produce a strong, lusty cry.

Insert your finger into the baby's mouth and palpate the hard and soft palate as the baby sucks. The sucking reflex can be elicited in infants up to 12 months.

ABNORMAL FINDINGS

A short lingual frenulum can impair speech development (see Table 13–5).

Trauma may indicate child abuse due to forced feeding of bottle or spoon.

A high-arched palate is usually normal in the newborn, but a very narrow or high arch also occurs with Turner's syndrome, Ehlers-Danlos syndrome, Marfan's syndrome, Treacher Collins syndrome, or develops in the mouth-breather in chronic allergies.

NORMAL RANGE OF FINDINGS	ABNORMAL FINDINGS

The Pregnant Female

Gum hypertrophy (surface looks smooth and stippling disappears) may occur normally at puberty or during pregnancy (pregnancy gingivitis).

The Aging Adult

The nose may appear more prominent on the face due to a loss of subcutaneous fat. In the edentulous person, the mouth and lips fold in, giving a "purse-string" appearance. The teeth may look slightly yellowed though the color is uniform. Yellowing results from the dentin visible through worn enamel. The surface of the incisors may show vertical cracks from a lifetime of exposure to extreme temperatures. The teeth may look longer as the gum margins recede.

The surfaces look worn down or abraded. Old dental work deteriorates, especially at the gum margins. The teeth loosen with bone resorption and may move with palpation.

The tongue looks smoother owing to papillary atrophy. The aging adult's buccal mucosa is thinned and may look shinier, as though it was "varnished."

☑ SUMMARY CHECKLIST

NOSE

1 ▶ Inspect external nose for symmetry, any deformity, or lesions.

2 ▶ Palpation—Test patency of each nostril.

3 ▶ Inspect using nasal speculum.
- A. Color and integrity of nasal mucosa.
- B. Septum—note any deviation, perforation, or bleeding.
- C. Turbinates—note color, any exudate, swelling, or polyps.

4 ▶ Palpate the sinus areas—note any tenderness.

MOUTH AND THROAT

1 ▶ Inspect using penlight.
- A. Lips, teeth and gums, tongue, buccal mucosa. Note color; if structures are intact, any lesions.
- B. Palate and uvula—note integrity and mobility as person phonates.
- C. Grade tonsils.
- D. Pharyngeal wall—note color, any exudate, or lesions.

2 ▶ Palpation
- A. When indicated in adults, bimanual palpation of mouth.
- B. With the neonate, palpate for integrity of palate and to assess sucking reflex.

SAMPLE RECORDING

Subjective

▶ **Nose.** No history of discharge, sinus problems, obstruction, epistaxis, or allergy. Colds 1–2/yr, mild. Fractured nose during high school sports, treated by M.D.

Mouth and Throat. No pain, bleeding gums, dysphagia, or hoarseness. Occasional sore throat with colds. Tonsillectomy, age 8. Smokes cigarettes 1 PPD × 9 years. Alcohol—1–2 drinks socially, about 2×/month. Visits dentist annually, dental hygenist 2×/year, flosses daily. No dental appliance.

Objective

▶ **Nose.** No deformity. Nares patent. Mucosa pink, no septal deviation or perforation.

Mouth. Can clench teeth. Mucosa and gingivae pink, no masses or lesions. Teeth in good repair. Tongue protrudes in midline, no tremor.

Throat. Mucosa pink, no lesions. Uvula rises in midline on phonation. Tonsils out. Gag reflex present.

SAMPLE CLINICAL PROBLEM 1

Brad D., a 34-year-old electrician, seeks care for "sore throat for 2 days."

Progress Notes

Subjective

▶ 2 days PTA—sudden onset of sore throat, swollen glands, fever 101°F, occasional shaking chills, extreme fatigue.
Today—symptoms remain. Cough productive of yellow sputum. Treated self with ASA for minimal relief. Unable to eat last 2 days because "throat on fire." Taking adequate fluids, on bedrest. Not aware of exposure to other sick persons. Does not smoke.

Objective

▶ Ears. TMs normal with landmarks intact.
Nose. No discharge. Mucosa pink, no swelling.

Mouth. Mucosa and gingivae pink, no lesions.
Throat. Tonsils 3+. Pharyngeal wall bright red with yellow-white exudate, exudate also on tonsils.
Neck. Enlarged anterior cervical nodes bilaterally, painful to palpation.
Chest. Resonant to percussion throughout. Breath sounds normal anterior and posterior. No adventitious sounds.

Assessment

► Pharyngitis
Pain R/T inflammation
Altered nutrition: less than body requirements R/T dysphagia

SAMPLE CLINICAL PROBLEM 2

Calvin W., a 53-year-old white businessman, is in the hospital awaiting coronary bypass surgery for coronary artery disease. As part of a pre-op teaching plan for coughing and deep breathing, a respiratory assessment is performed.

Problem List

No.	Title	Date Entered
1	CAD	7/4/
2	Chronic allergy to dust, or animal hair	7/4/

Progress Notes

Subjective

► States understanding of reason for admission to hospital, and extent of coronary artery disease. Unaware of details of surgical procedure and post-op care. Interested, "I do better when I know what I'm dealing with." History of exertional angina after walking one short block or climbing one flight of stairs, treats self with nitroglycerin. Does not smoke. Chronic watery nasal discharge, "comes and goes, but present most of time."

Objective

- Nose. Only R naris patent. Mucosa gray and boggy bilaterally. L naris has mobile, gray, nontender mass, obstructing view of turbinates and rest of nasal cavity.
  Mouth and Throat. Mucosa pink, no lesions. Uvula midline, rises on phonation. Tonsils absent. No lumps or lesions on palpation.
  Chest. Thorax symmetric, AP $<$ transverse diameter, respirations 18/min effortless. Resonant to percussion. Breath sounds normal. No adventitious sounds.

Assessment

- L nasal mass, appears as polyp
  Knowledge deficit for surgery and expected post op course R/T lack of exposure

SAMPLE CLINICAL PROBLEM 3

Esther V. is a 61-year-old professor who has been admitted to the hospital for chemotherapy for carcinoma of the breast. This is her 5th hospital day. An oral assessment is performed when she complains of "soreness and a white coating" in the mouth.

Subjective

- Felt soreness on tongue and cheeks during night. Now pain persists, and E.V. can see a "white coating" on tongue and cheeks. "I'm worried. Is this more cancer?"

Objective

- E.V. generally appears restless and overly aware.
  Oral mucosa pink. Large white cheesy patches covering most of dorsal surface of tongue and buccal mucosa. Will scrape off with tongue blade, revealing red eroded area beneath. Bleeds with slight contact. Posterior pharyngeal wall pink, no lesions. Patches are soft to palpation. No palpable lymph nodes.

Assessment

- Oral lesion, appears as candidiasis
  Altered oral mucous membrane R/T effects of chemotherapy
  Pain R/T infectious process
  Anxiety R/T threat to health status

NURSING DIAGNOSES COMMONLY ASSOCIATED WITH NOSE, MOUTH, THROAT DISORDERS

Diagnosis	Related Factors (Etiology)	Defining Characteristics (Symptoms and Signs)
Altered oral mucous membrane	Dehydration Effects of chemotherapy medication radiation to head/neck diabetes mellitus oral cancer Immunosuppression Inadequate oral hygiene Infection Lack of knowledge Mouth-breathing Malnutrition/vitamin deficiency NPO for >24 hours Chemical trauma acidic foods alcohol drugs noxious agents tobacco Mechanical trauma braces broken teeth endotracheal tube fractured mandible ill-fitting dentures nasogastric tube Vomiting	Atrophy of gums Coated tongue Dry mouth (xerostomia) Edema of mucosa Halitosis Hemorrhagic gingivitis Hyperemia Lack of or decreased salivation Leukoplakia Oral lesions pain or discomfort plaque redness ulcers vesicles Purulent drainage Stomatitis
Impaired swallowing	Effects of cleft lip/palate cerebrovascular accident cranial nerve damage (V, VII, IX, X) neuromuscular disorder (e.g., cerebral palsy, muscular dystrophy, Guillain-Barré syndrome, myasthenia gravis, poliomyelitis), oral/pharyngeal cancer	Coughing/choking Dehydration Evidence of aspiration Regurgitation of fluids/solids through mouth or nose Reported pain on swallowing Stasis of food in oral cavity Weight loss

Diagnosis	Related Factors (Etiology)	Defining Characteristics (Symptoms and Signs)

	Excessive/inadequate salivation
	Fatigue
	Limited awareness
	Mechanical obstruction
	  edema
	  tracheostomy tube
	  tumor
	Neuromuscular impairment
	  decreased/absent gag reflex
	  decreased strength of muscles of mastication
	  perceptual impairment
	  facial paralysis
	Reddened irritated oropharynx	

Pain	Effects of surgery or trauma
	Experiences during diagnostic tests
	Infectious process
	Inflammation
	Muscle spasm
	Immobility
	Obstructive processes
	Overactivity
	Pressure points
		Reports of pain
		Anxiety
		Clutching of painful area
		Crying or moaning
		Distraction behavior
		Focused on self
		Immobilization
		Painful response to palpation
		Facial mask of pain
		Changes in posture or gait
		Withdrawal reflex
		Changes in muscle tone—listless to rigid
		Autonomic responses
		  Increased blood pressure, pulse, respirations
		  Diaphoresis
		  Dilated pupils
		Social withdrawal
		Impaired thought process
		Altered time perception
		Feelings of guilt, despair, or helplessness

Sensory/perceptual alteration: olfactory	Effects of aging Foreign body in nares Inflammation of nasal mucosa Neurologic impairment Obstruction in nares	Decreased sensitivity to smells Decreased appetite

Diagnosis	Related Factors (Etiology)	Defining Characteristics (Symptoms and Signs)
gustatory	Effects of aging Effects of trauma to tongue Inflammation of nasal mucosa Neurologic impairment Side effects of specific medications	Decreased sensitivity to tastes Decreased appetite Increased seasoning of foods

ABNORMAL FINDINGS

Table 13-1 ► Abnormalities of the Nose

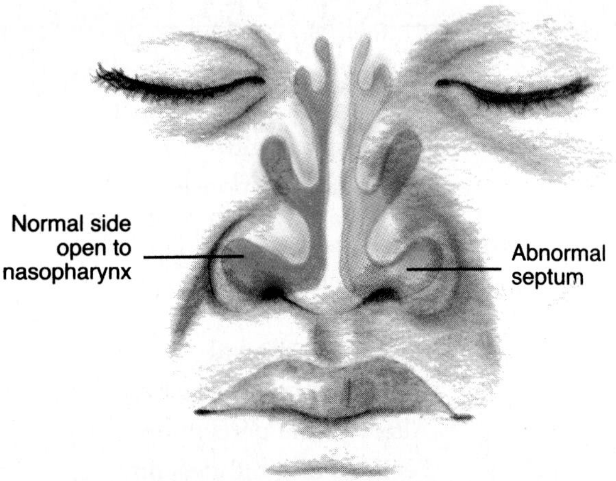

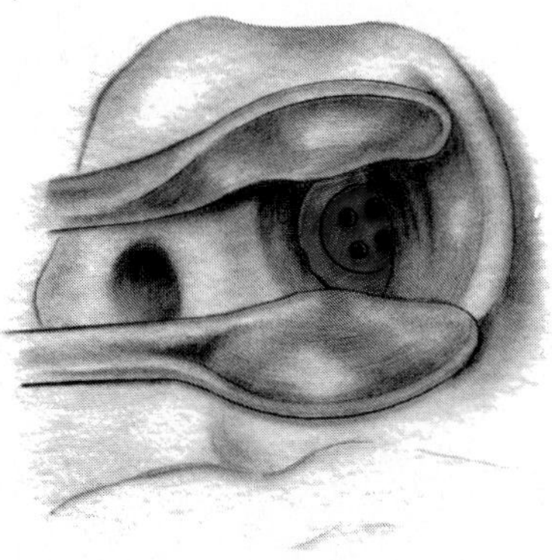

CHOANAL ATRESIA

A bony or membranous septum between the nasal cavity and the pharynx. When the condition is bilateral, it requires the immediate insertion of an oral airway to prevent asphyxia because most newborns are obligate nose-breathers. When the condition is unilateral, the infant may be asymptomatic until the onset of his or her first respiratory infection.

FOREIGN BODY

Children particularly are apt to put an object up the nose, producing unilateral purulent drainage and foul odor.

Table 13–1 ► Abnormalities of the Nose *Continued*

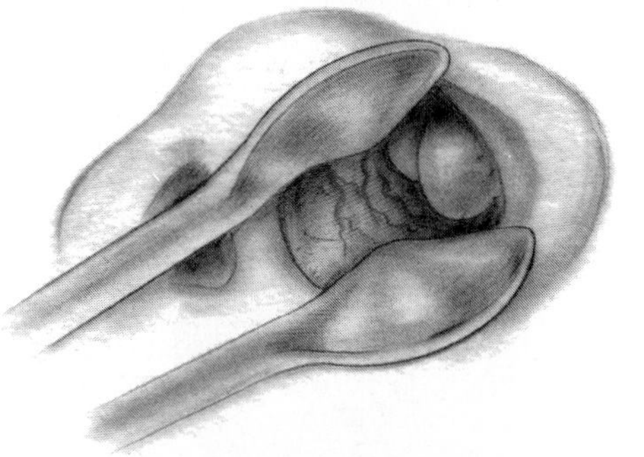

EPISTAXIS

The most common site of a nosebleed is Kiesselbach's plexus in the anterior septum. It may be spontaneous from a local cause or a sign of underlying illness. Causes include nose-picking, forceful coughing or sneezing, fracture, foreign body, rhinitis, following heavy exertion, or with hypertension or a coagulation disorder. Bleeding from the anterior septum is easily controlled and rarely severe. A posterior hemorrhage is less common (<10 percent) but is more profuse, harder to manage, and more serious.

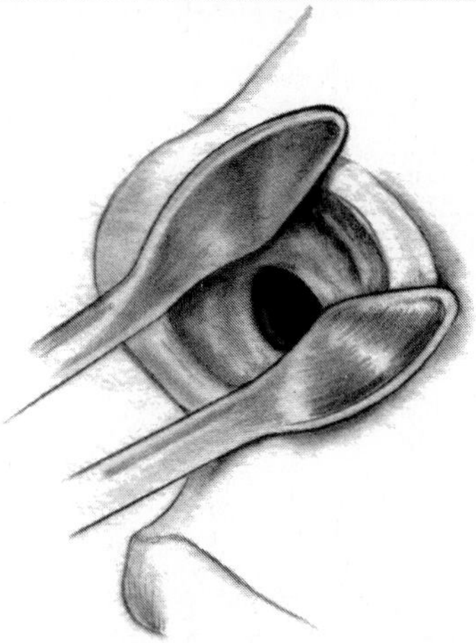

PERFORATED SEPTUM

A hole in the septum, usually the cartilaginous part, may be caused by chronic infection, trauma from continual picking of crusts, sniffing cocaine, or from nasal surgery. It is seen as a spot of light when the penlight is directed into the other naris.

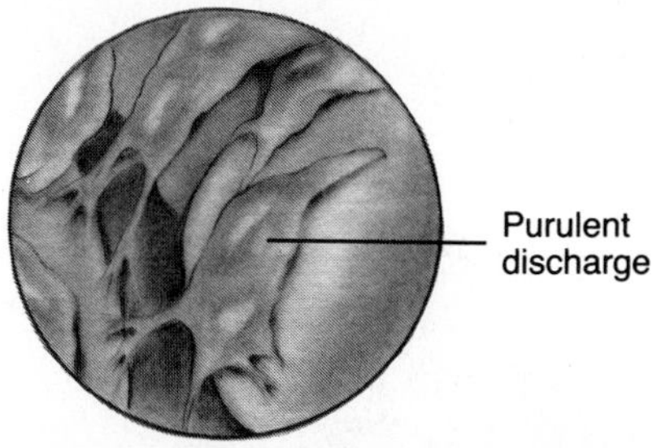

ACUTE RHINITIS

The first sign is a watery discharge, rhinorrhea, which becomes purulent. This is accompanied by sneezing and swollen mucosa, which causes nasal obstruction.

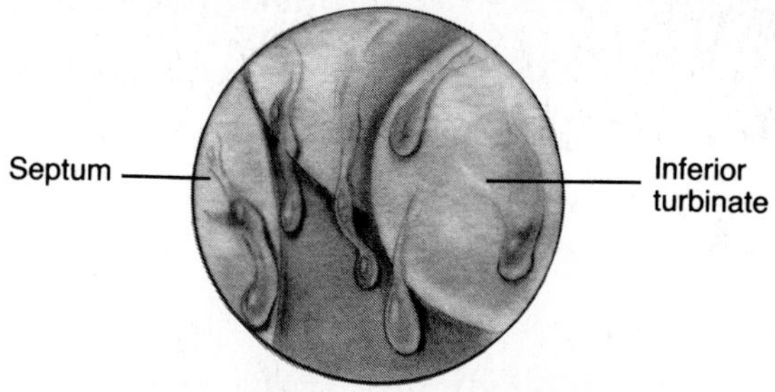

ALLERGIC RHINITIS

Rhinorrhea, itching of nose and eyes, lacrimation, and sneezing are present. Note serous edema and swelling of turbinates to fill the air space. Turbinates are usually pale (though may appear violet) and their surface looks smooth and glistening. May be seasonal or perennial, depending on allergen.

Table continued on following page

Table 13-1 ▶ Abnormalities of the Nose *Continued*

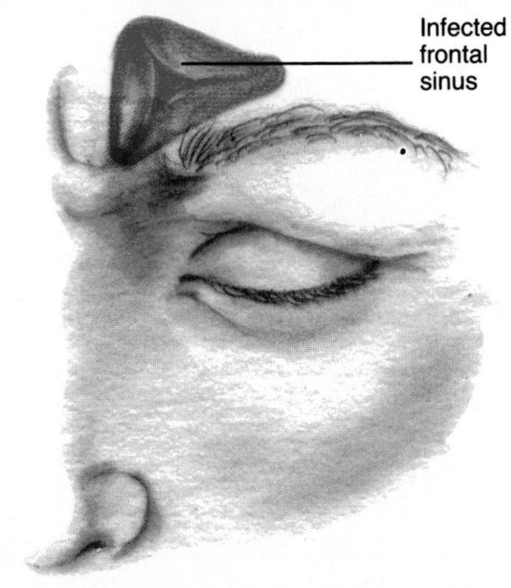

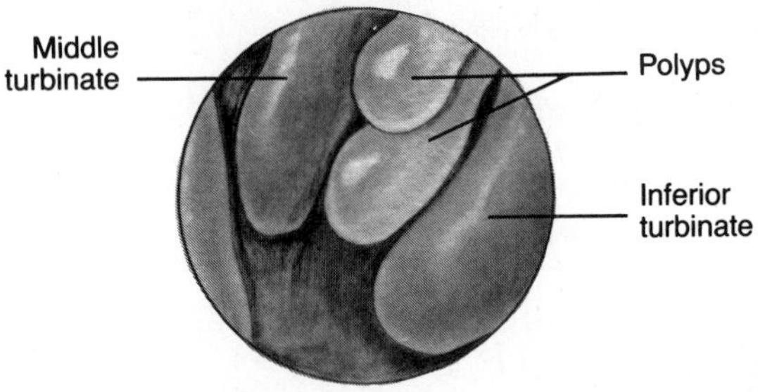

SINUSITIS

Facial pain following upper respiratory infection; signs include red swollen nasal mucosa, swollen turbinates, and purulent discharge. Person also experiences fever, chills, malaise. With maxillary sinusitis, there is dull throbbing pain in cheeks and teeth on the same side and pain with palpation. With frontal sinusitis, pain is above the supraorbital ridge.

POLYPS

Smooth, pale gray nodules, which are overgrowths of mucosa, most commonly caused by chronic allergic rhinitis. May be stalked. A common site is protruding from the middle meatus. Often multiple, they are mobile and nontender in contrast to turbinates. They may obstruct air passageways as they get larger.

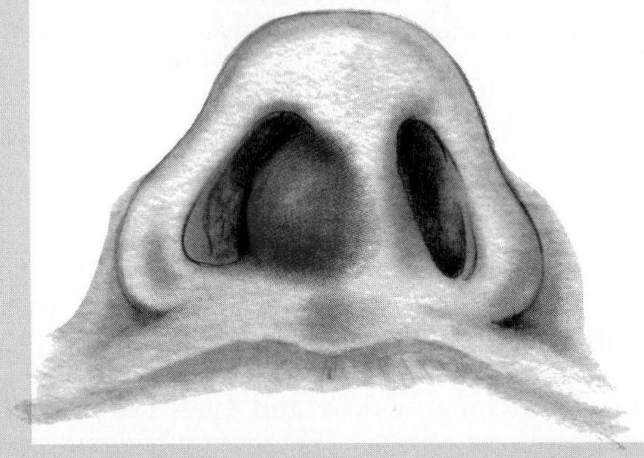

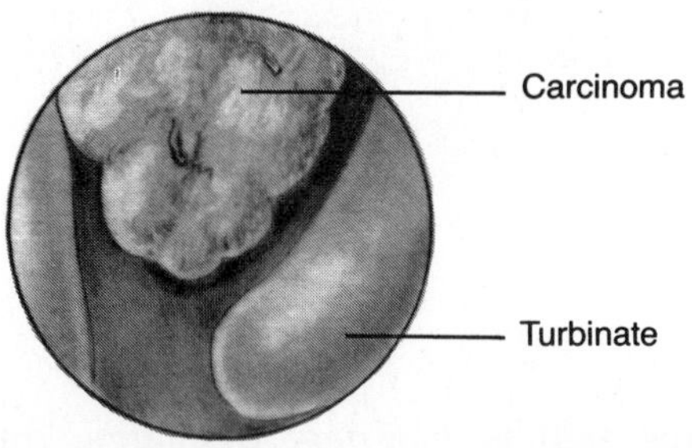

FURUNCLE

A small boil located in the skin or mucous membrane; appears red and swollen; and is quite painful. Avoid any manipulation or trauma that may spread the infection.

CARCINOMA

This appears gray-white and nontender. It may produce slow bloody unilateral discharge, in contrast to the profuse bleeding that accompanies epistaxis. It is not a common lesion.

Table 13-2 ▶ Abnormalities of the Lips

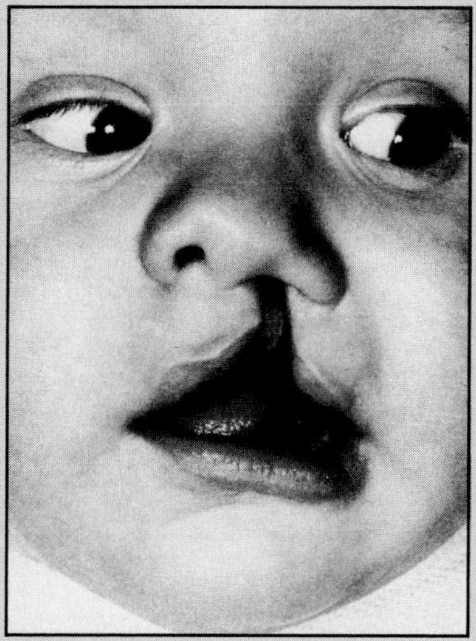

CLEFT LIP

Maxillofacial clefts are among the more common types of congenital anomalies. The incidence of cleft lip, with or without cleft palate, is about 1/1000 white births. The incidence is higher in Asians at 1.7/1000 births, and it is lower in blacks at 1/2500 births (Adams et al, 1989). Early treatment preserves the functions of speech and language formation and deglutition (swallowing).

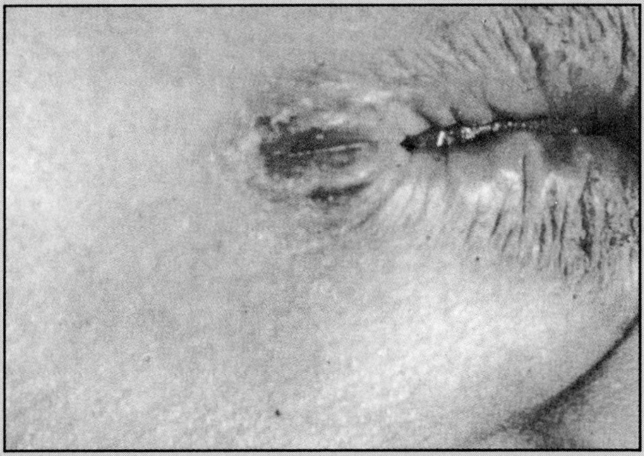

CHEILOSIS (ANGULAR STOMATITIS, PERLECHE)

Painful fissures at the corners of the mouth occur with excess salivation and monilial infection. It is often seen in edentulous persons and in those with poorly fitting dentures causing folding in of corners of mouth. It also occurs from riboflavin deficiency (rare).

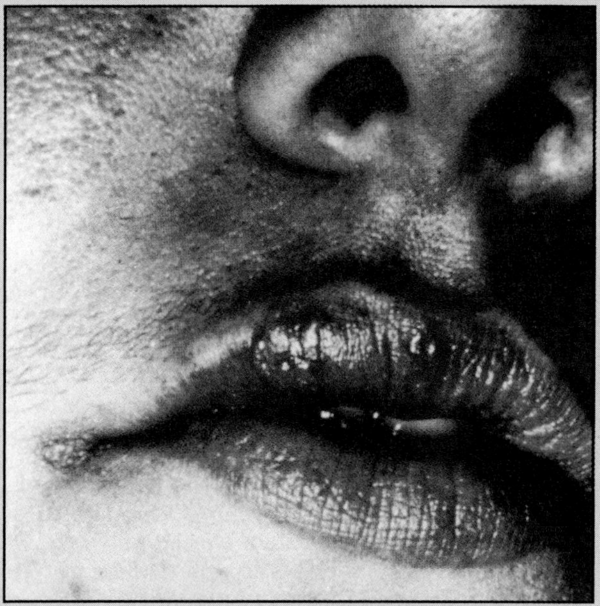

HERPES SIMPLEX I

The cold sores are groups of clear vesicles with a surrounding erythematous base. These evolve into pustules or crusts and heal in 4 to 10 days. The most likely site is the lip-skin junction; infection often recurs in same site. It may be precipitated by sunlight, fever, colds, allergy. It is a very common lesion, affecting 50 percent of adults.

CARCINOMA (not illustrated)

The initial lesion is round and indurated, then it becomes crusted and ulcerated with an elevated border. The vast majority occur between the outer and middle thirds of lip. Any lesion that is still unhealed after 2 weeks should be referred.

RETENTION "CYST" (MUCOCELE) (not illustrated)

A round, well-defined nodule that may be very small or up to 1 or 2 cm. It is a pocket of mucus that forms when a duct of a minor salivary gland ruptures. The benign lesion also may occur on the buccal mucosa, floor of the mouth, or under the tip of the tongue.

Table 13-3 ► Abnormalities of the Teeth and Gums

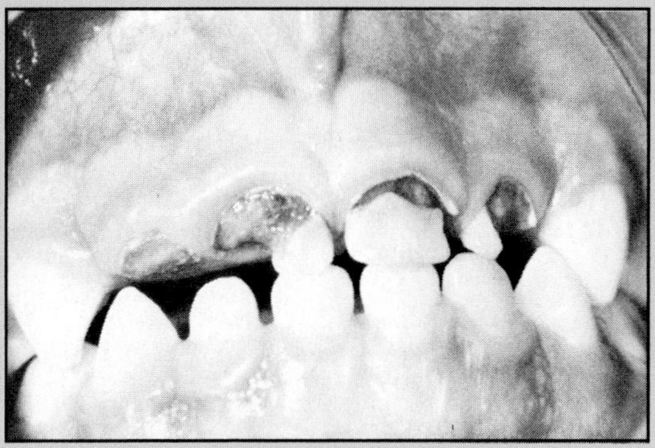

BABY BOTTLE CARIES

Destruction of upper deciduous teeth may occur in older infants and toddlers who take a bottle of milk, juice, or sweetened drink to bed. Liquid pools around the upper front teeth. Mouth bacteria act on carbohydrates in the liquid, especially sucrose, forming metabolic acids. Acids break down tooth enamel and destroy its protein.

DENTAL CARIES

Progressive destruction of tooth. Decay initially looks chalky white. Later, it may turn brown or black and form a cavity. Early decay is apparent only on x-ray study. Susceptible sites are tooth surfaces where food debris, bacterial plaque, and saliva collect.

MALOCCLUSION (not illustrated)

Upper or lower dental arches are out of alignment and incisors protrude owing to developmental problem of mandible or maxilla or incompatibility between jaw size and tooth size. The condition increases risk of facial deformity, negative body image, chewing problems, or speech dysfluency.

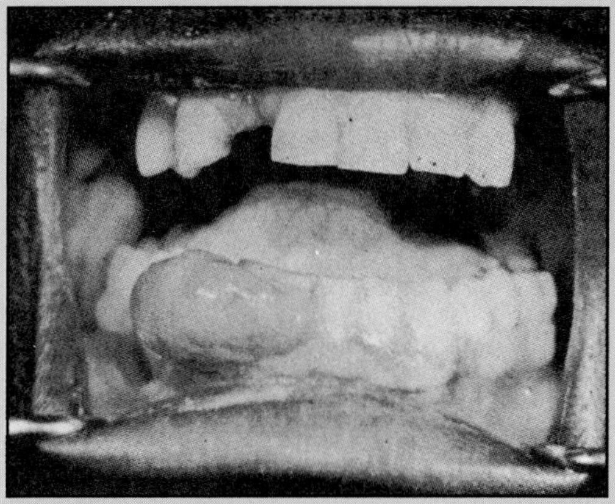

EPULIS

A nontender, fibrous nodule of the gum, seen emerging between the teeth.

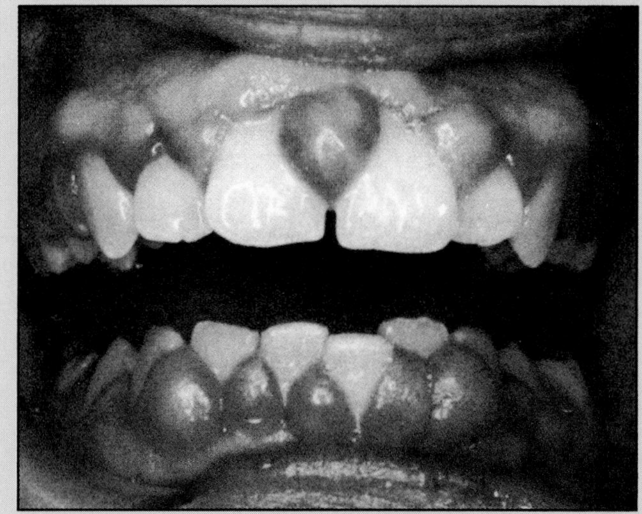

GINGIVAL HYPERPLASIA

Painless enlargement of gums, sometimes overreaching the teeth. This occurs with puberty, pregnancy, leukemia, and with long therapeutic use of phenytoin (Dilantin).

Table 13-3 ▸ Abnormalities of the Teeth and Gums *Continued*

GINGIVITIS

Gum margins are red, swollen, and bleed easily. Note bulbous gingivae between the teeth. Inflammation is usually due to poor dental hygiene or vitamin C deficiency. The condition may occur in pregnancy and puberty because of changing hormonal balance.

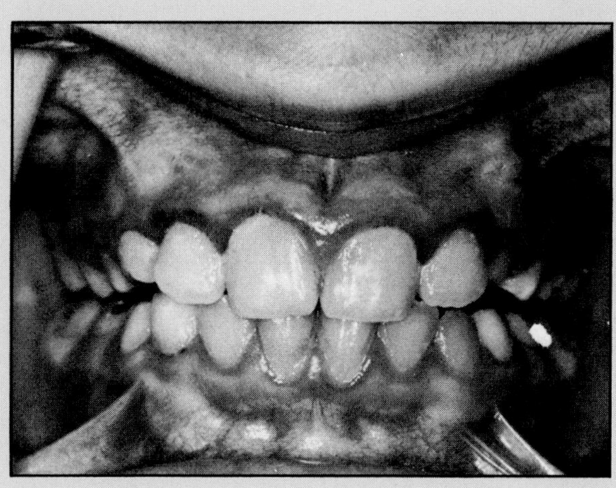

Table 13-4 ▸ Abnormalities on the Buccal Mucosa

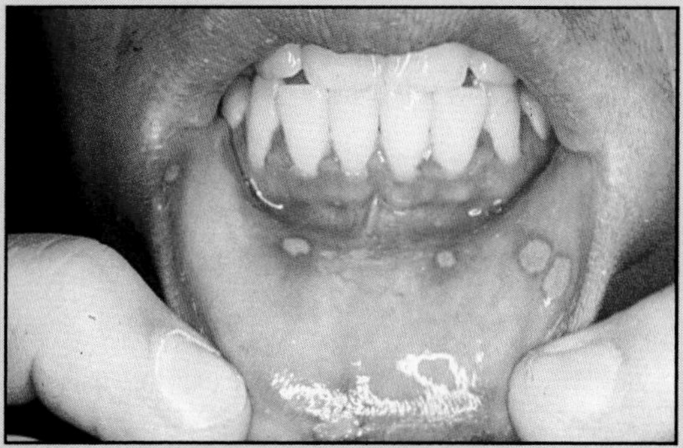

APHTHOUS ULCERS

A "canker sore" is a vesicle at first, then a small round ulcer with white base surrounded by a red halo. It is quite painful and lasts for 1 to 2 weeks. The cause is unknown, although it is associated with stress, fatigue, and food allergy. It is common, affecting 20 percent of the population.

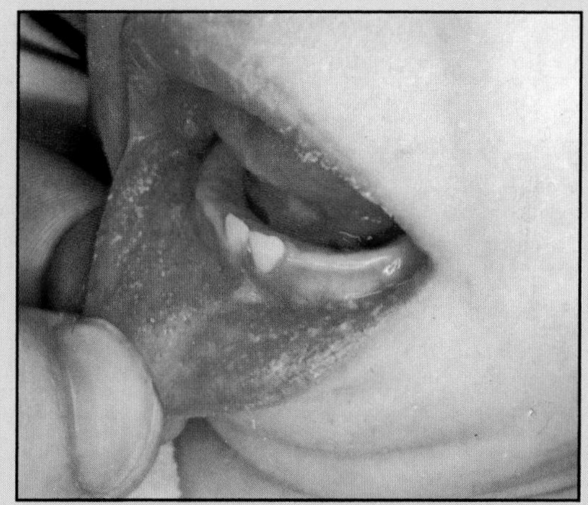

KOPLIK'S SPOTS

Small blue-white spots with irregular red halo scattered over mucosa opposite the molars. An early sign, and pathognomonic of measles.

Table continued on following page

Table 13-4 ▶ Abnormalities on the Buccal Mucosa *Continued*

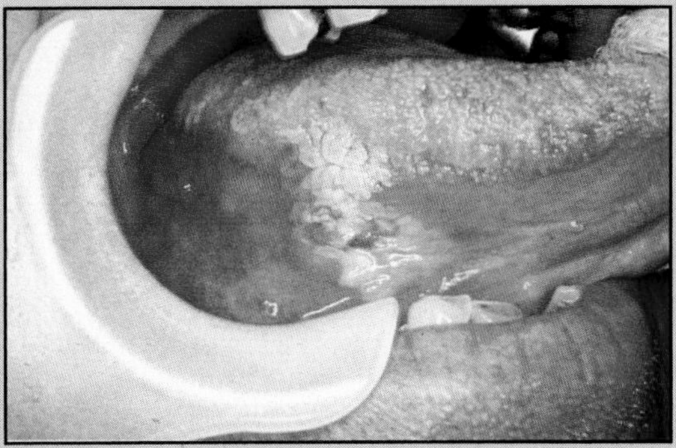

LEUKOPLAKIA

Chalky white, thick, raised patch with well-defined borders. The lesion is firmly attached and does not scrape off. It may occur on the lateral edges of tongue. It is due to chronic irritation, and occurs more frequently with heavy smoking and heavy alcohol use. Lesions are precancerous, and the person should be referred. (Here, the lesion is associated with squamous carcinoma.)

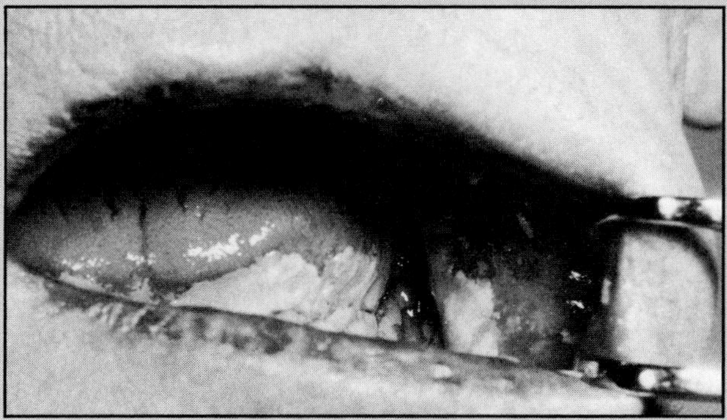

CANDIDIASIS OR MONILIAL INFECTION

A white, cheesy, curdlike patch on the buccal mucosa and tongue. It scrapes off, leaving raw, red surface that bleeds easily. Termed "thrush" in the newborn. It also occurs after the use of antibiotics, corticosteroids, and in immunosuppressed persons.

Table 13-5 ▶ Abnormalities of the Tongue

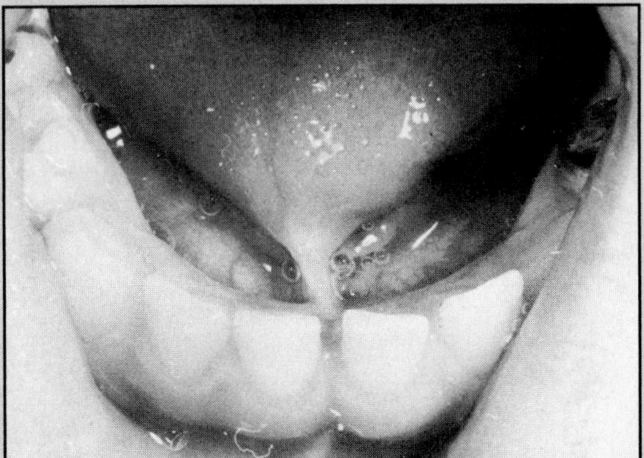

ANKYLOGLOSSIA

(Tongue-tie) A short lingual frenulum, here fixing the tongue tip to the floor of the mouth and gums. This limits mobility and will affect speech (pronunciation of a, d, n) if the tongue tip cannot be elevated to the alveolar ridge. A congenital defect.

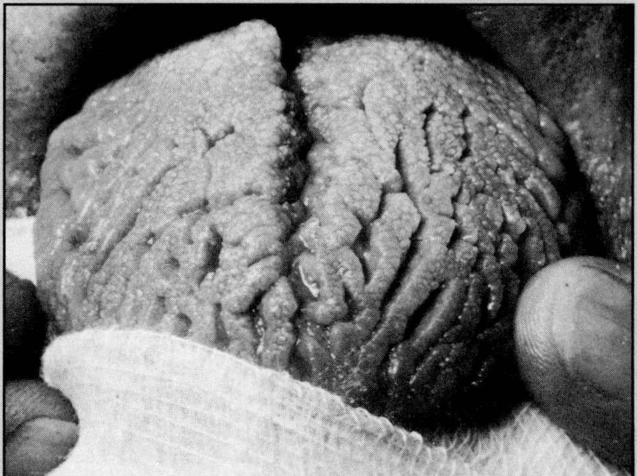

FISSURED OR SCROTAL TONGUE

Deep furrows divide the papillae into small irregular rows. The condition is congenital and is not significant. The incidence increases with age. (Vertical, or longitudinal, fissures also occur with dehydration because of reduced volume of the tongue.)

Table 13-5 ► Abnormalities of the Tongue *Continued*

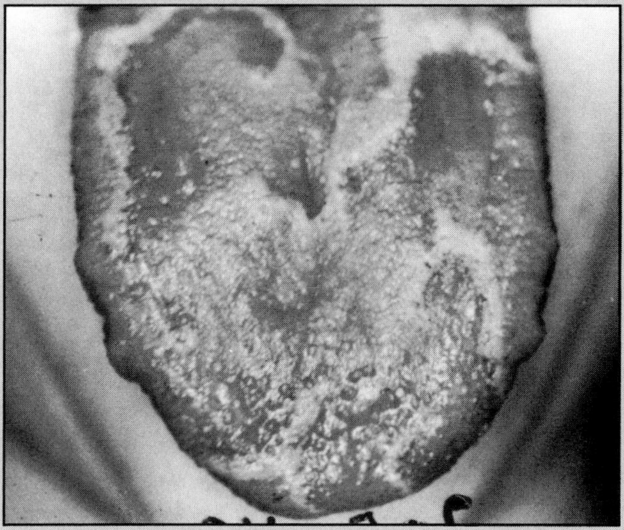

GEOGRAPHIC TONGUE (MIGRATORY GLOSSITIS)

Pattern of normal coating interspersed with bright red, shiny, circular bald areas, having raised pearly borders. Pattern resembles a map, and changes in a few days. Not significant, and its cause is not known.

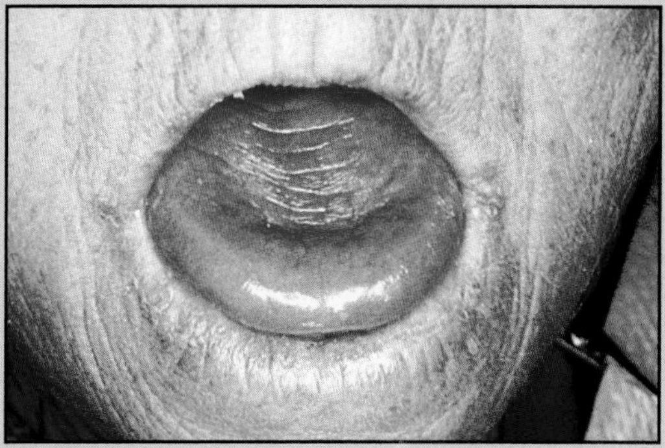

SMOOTH GLOSSY (ATROPHIC GLOSSITIS)

The surface is slick and shiny; the mucosa thins and looks red from decreased papillae. Accompanied by dryness of tongue and burning. Occurs with B_{12} deficiency (pernicious anemia), folic acid deficiency, and iron deficiency anemia. Here, also note angular cheilosis.

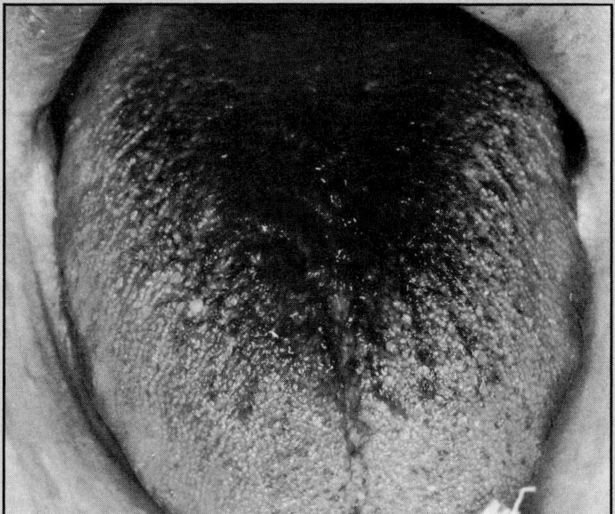

BLACK HAIRY TONGUE

This is not really hair but the elongation of filiform papillae and painless overgrowth of mycelial threads of fungus infection on the tongue. It occurs following use of antibiotics, which inhibit normal bacteria and allow proliferation of fungus.

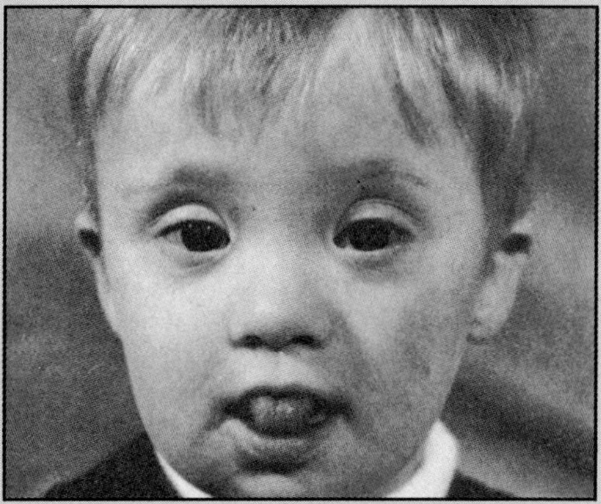

ENLARGED TONGUE (MACROGLOSSIA)

The tongue is enlarged and may protrude from mouth. The condition is not painful but may impair speech development. Here, it occurs with Down syndrome; it also occurs with cretinism, myxedema, acromegaly. Also a transient swelling occurs with local infections.

Table continued on following page

Table 13–5 ▸ Abnormalities of the Tongue *Continued*

CARCINOMA

An ulcer with rolled edges; indurated. Occurs particularly at sides, base, and under the tongue. When it is in the floor of mouth, it may cause painful movement or limited movement of tongue. There is risk of early metastasis due to rich lymphatic drainage. Heavy smoking and heavy alcohol use place persons at greater risk.

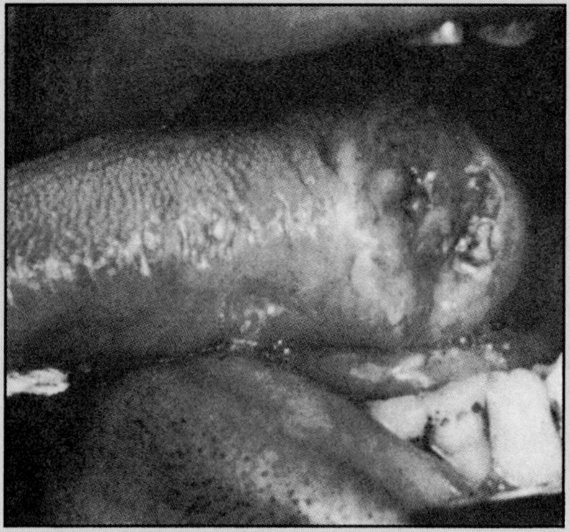

Table 13–6 ▸ Abnormalities of the Oropharynx

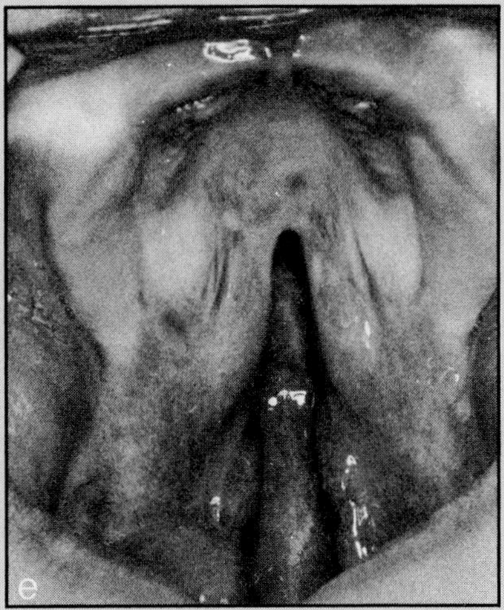

CLEFT PALATE

A congenital defect, the failure of fusion of the maxillary processes. There is wide variation in extent of cleft formation, from upper lip only, palate only, uvula only, to cleft of the nostril and the hard and soft palates.

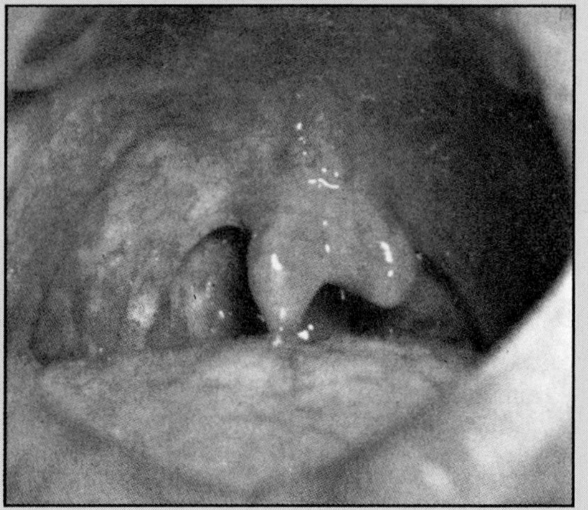

BIFID UVULA

The uvula looks partly severed. May indicate a submucous cleft palate, which feels like a notch at the junction of the hard and soft palates. The submucous cleft palate may affect speech development because it prevents necessary air trapping. The incidence of bifid uvula varies among racial groups: It is common in Native Americans, uncommon in whites, and rare in blacks.

Table 13-6 ▸ Abnormalities of the Oropharynx *Continued*

ACUTE TONSILLITIS AND PHARYNGITIS

Bright red throat, swollen tonsils, white or yellow exudate on tonsils and pharynx, swollen uvula, and enlarged tender cervical and tonsillar nodes. Accompanied by severe sore throat, high fever of sudden onset. (Caution: Cannot discriminate bacterial from viral infection on clinical data alone; need a throat culture.)

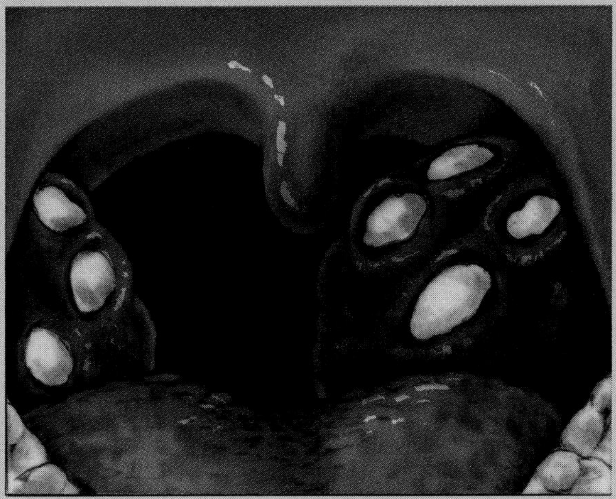

Bibliography

Adams GL, Boies LR, Hilger PA: Boies Fundamentals of Otolaryngology. 6th ed. Philadelphia, W.B. Saunders, 1989.

Becker W, Buckingham RA, Holinger PH et al: Atlas of Ear, Nose and Throat Diseases. Philadelphia, W.B. Saunders, 1984.

Blair KA: Aging: Physiological aspects and clinical implications. Nurse Pract 15(2):14–28, 1990.

Brothwell DR, Carbonell VM, Goose DH: Congenital absence of teeth in human populations. *In* Brothwell DR (Ed): Dental Anthropology. New York, Pergamon Press, 1963, pp 179–189.

Burgraf V, Donlon, B: Assessing the elderly—system by system. Part 1. Am J Nurs 85(9):974–984, 1985.

Carotenuto R, Bullock J: Physical Assessment of the Gerontologic Client. Philadelphia, FA Davis, 1980.

Cornelius, J: Screening for head and neck cancers. Nurse Pract 4:15–19, 1979.

DeWeese DD, Saunders WH: Textbook of Otolaryngology. 6th ed. St. Louis, C.V. Mosby, 1982.

DiIorio C, Price ME: Swallowing: An assessment guide. Am J Nurs 90(7):38–46, 1990.

Emanuel I: The incidence of congenital malformations in a Chinese population: The Taipei collaborative study. Teratology 5(2):159–170, 1972.

Jarvis A, Gorlin R: Minor orofacial abnormalities in an Eskimo population. Oral Surg 33:417–426, 1972.

Kelly J, VanKirk L, Garst C: Total teeth loss in adults. Vital Health Stat 11(27):1–23, 1967.

Martin J, Crump E: Leukoedema of the buccal mucosa in Negro children and youth. Oral Surg 34:49–58, 1972.

Ofstehage JC, Magilvy K: Oral health and aging. Geriatr Nurs 7(5):238–241, 1986.

Overfield T: Biologic Variation in Health and Illness: Race, Age, and Sex Differences. Menlo Park, CA, Addison-Wesley Publishing, 1985.

Rossman I: Clinical Geriatrics. 3rd ed. Philadelphia, J.B. Lippincott, 1986.

Schaumann BF, Peagler FD, Gorlin RJ: Minor orofacial anomalies among a Negro population. Oral Surg 29(4):566–575, 1970.

Wasserman HP: Ethnic Pigmentation: Historical, Physiological and Chemical Aspects. New York, American Elsevier, 1974.

Williams RA: Textbook of black-related diseases. New York, McGraw-Hill, 1975.

CHAPTER

14 Breasts and Regional Lymphatics

STRUCTURE AND FUNCTION

The breasts, or mammary glands, are present in both sexes, although in the male they are rudimentary throughout life. The female breasts are accessory reproductive organs whose function is to produce milk for nourishing the newborn.

SURFACE ANATOMY

The breasts lie anterior to the pectoralis major and serratus anterior muscles (Fig. 14–1). The breasts are located between the second and sixth ribs, extending from the side of the sternum to the midaxillary line. The superior lateral corner of breast tissue, called the axillary *tail of Spence*, projects up and laterally into the axilla.

The *nipple* is just below the center of the breast. It is rough, round, and usually protuberant; its surface looks wrinkled and indented with tiny milk duct openings. The *areola* surrounds the nipple for a 1- to 2-cm radius. In the areola are small elevated sebaceous glands, called Montgomery's glands. These secrete a protective lipid

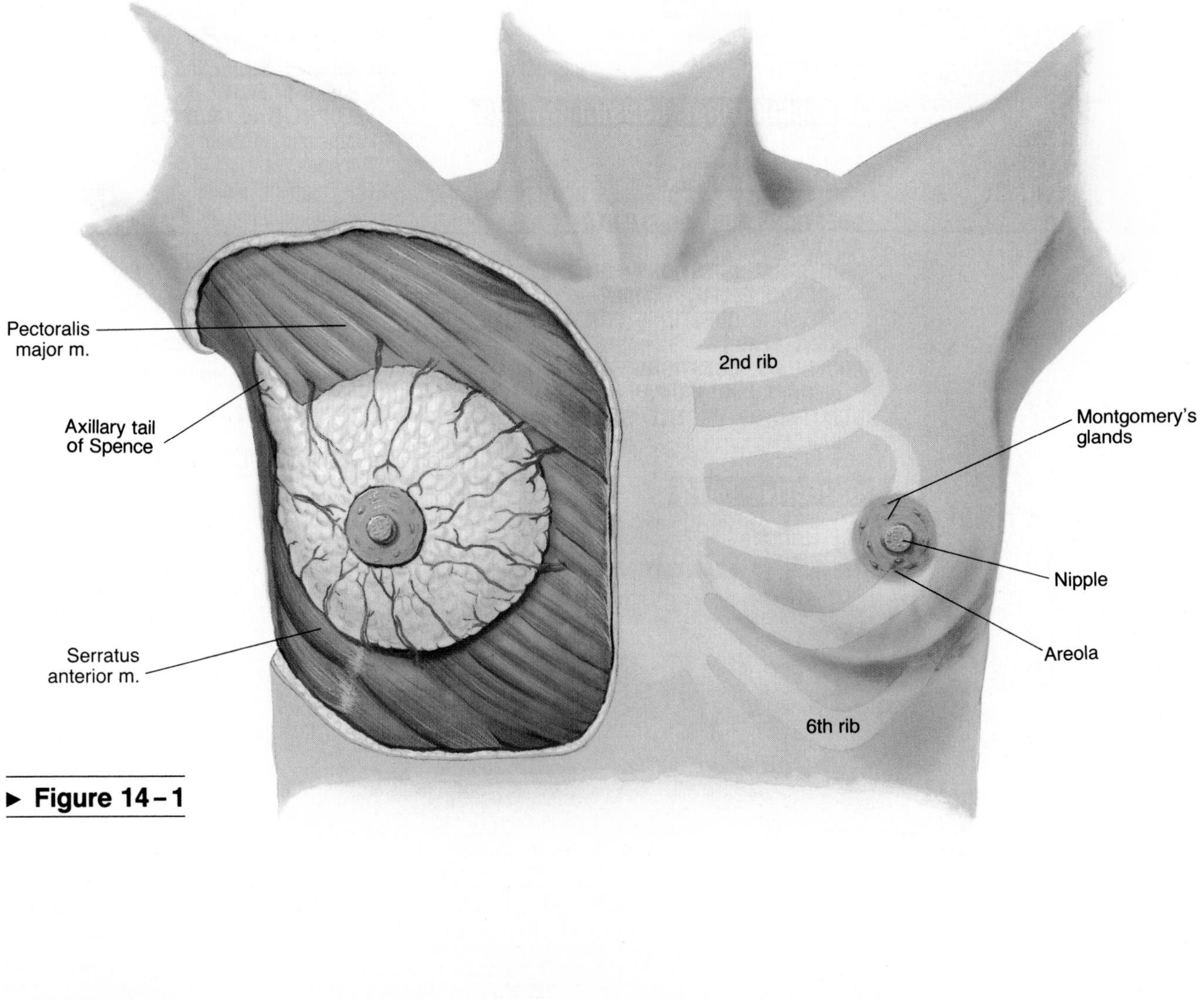

► **Figure 14–1**

material during lactation. The areola also has smooth muscle fibers that cause nipple erection when stimulated. Both the nipple and areola are more darkly pigmented than the rest of the breast surface; the color varies from pink to brown depending on the person's skin color and parity.

INTERNAL ANATOMY

The breast is composed of (1) glandular tissue, (2) fibrous tissue including the suspensory ligaments, and (3) adipose tissue (Fig. 14–2). First, the glandular tissue contains 15 to 20 lobes radiating from the nipple, and these are composed of lobules. Within each lobule are clusters of alveoli that produce milk. Each lobe empties into a lactiferous duct. The 15 to 20 lactiferous ducts form a collecting duct system converging toward the nipple. There, the ducts form ampullae, or lactiferous sinuses, behind the nipple, which are reservoirs for storing milk.

Second, the suspensory ligaments, or *Cooper's ligaments,* are fibrous bands extending vertically from the surface to attach on chest wall muscles. These support the breast tissue. They become contracted in cancer of the breast, producing pits or dimples in the overlying skin.

Finally, the lobes are embedded in adipose tissue. These layers of subcutaneous and retromammary fat actually provide most of the bulk of the breast. The relative proportion of glandular, fibrous, and fatty tissue varies depending on age, cycle, pregnancy, lactation, and general nutritional state.

The breast may be divided into four quadrants by imaginary horizontal and vertical lines intersecting at the nipple (Fig. 14–3). This makes a convenient map to describe clinical findings. In the upper outer quadrant, note the axillary *tail of Spence,* the cone-shaped breast tissue that projects up into the axilla, close to the pectoral group of axillary lymph nodes. The upper outer quadrant is the site of most breast tumors.

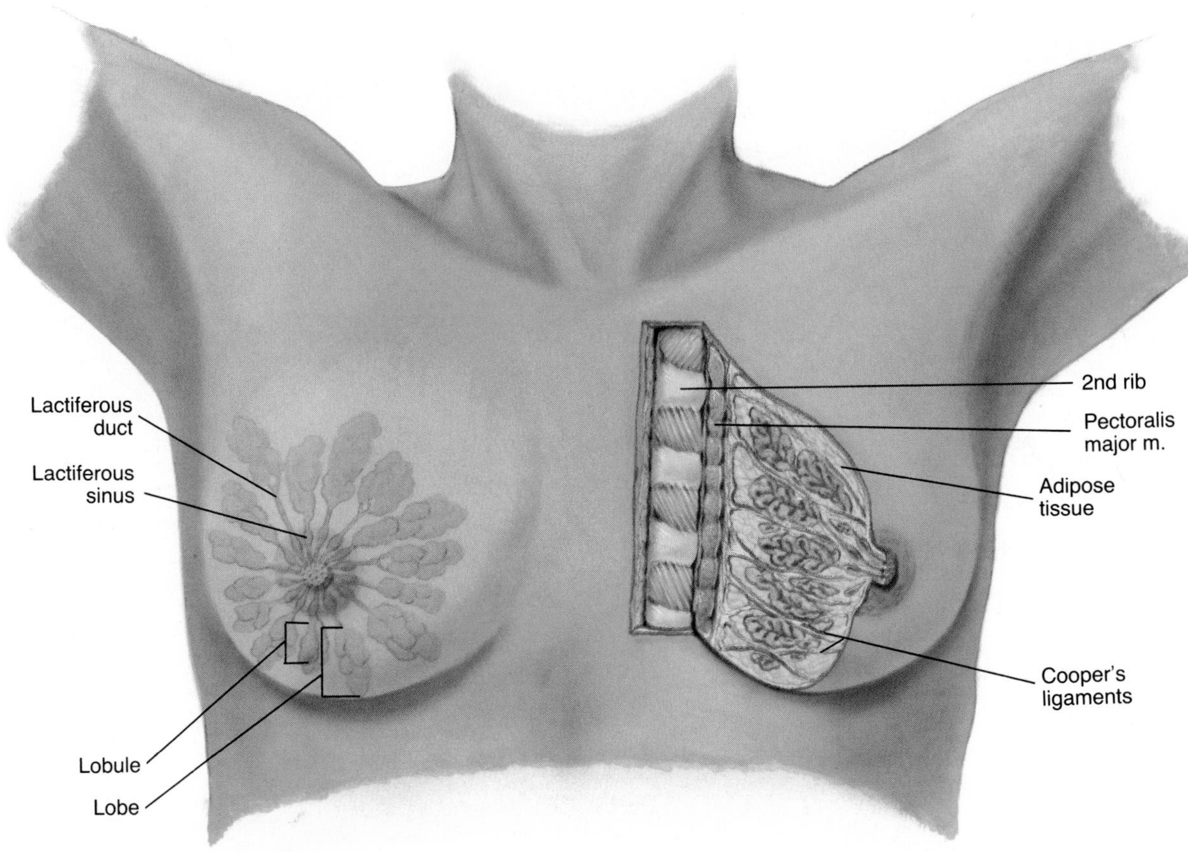

► Figure 14–2

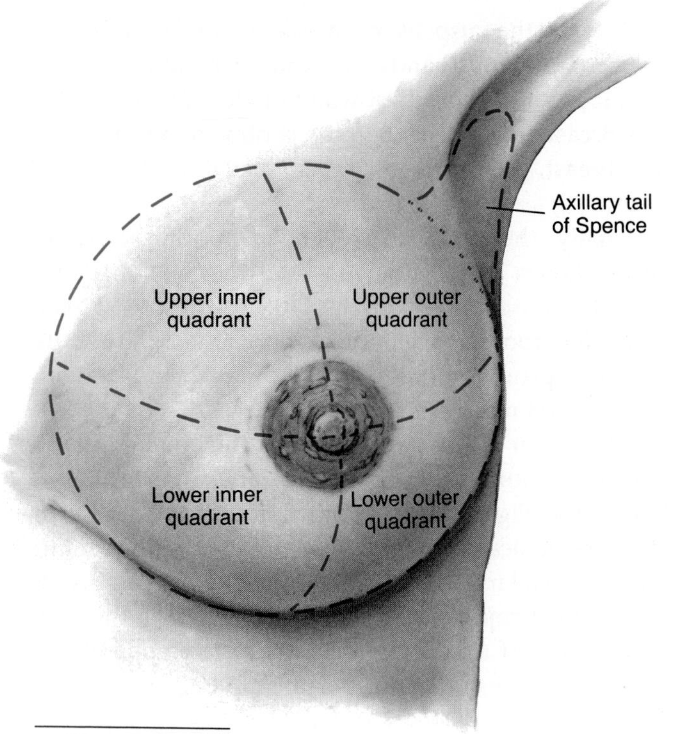

► **Figure 14–3**

The breast has extensive lymphatic drainage. Most of the lymph, more than 75 percent, drains into the ipsilateral axillary nodes. There are four groups of axillary nodes (Fig. 14–4):

1. Central axillary nodes — high up in the middle of the axilla, over the ribs and serratus anterior muscle. These receive lymph from:
2. Pectoral (anterior) — along the lateral edge of the pectoralis major muscle, just inside the anterior axillary fold.
3. Subscapular (posterior) — along the lateral edge of the scapula, deep in the posterior axillary fold.
4. Lateral — along the humerus, inside the upper arm.

From the central axillary nodes, drainage flows up to the infraclavicular and supraclavicular nodes.

A smaller amount of lymphatic drainage does not take these channels but flows directly up to the infraclavicular group, deep into the chest, or into the abdomen, or directly across to the opposite breast.

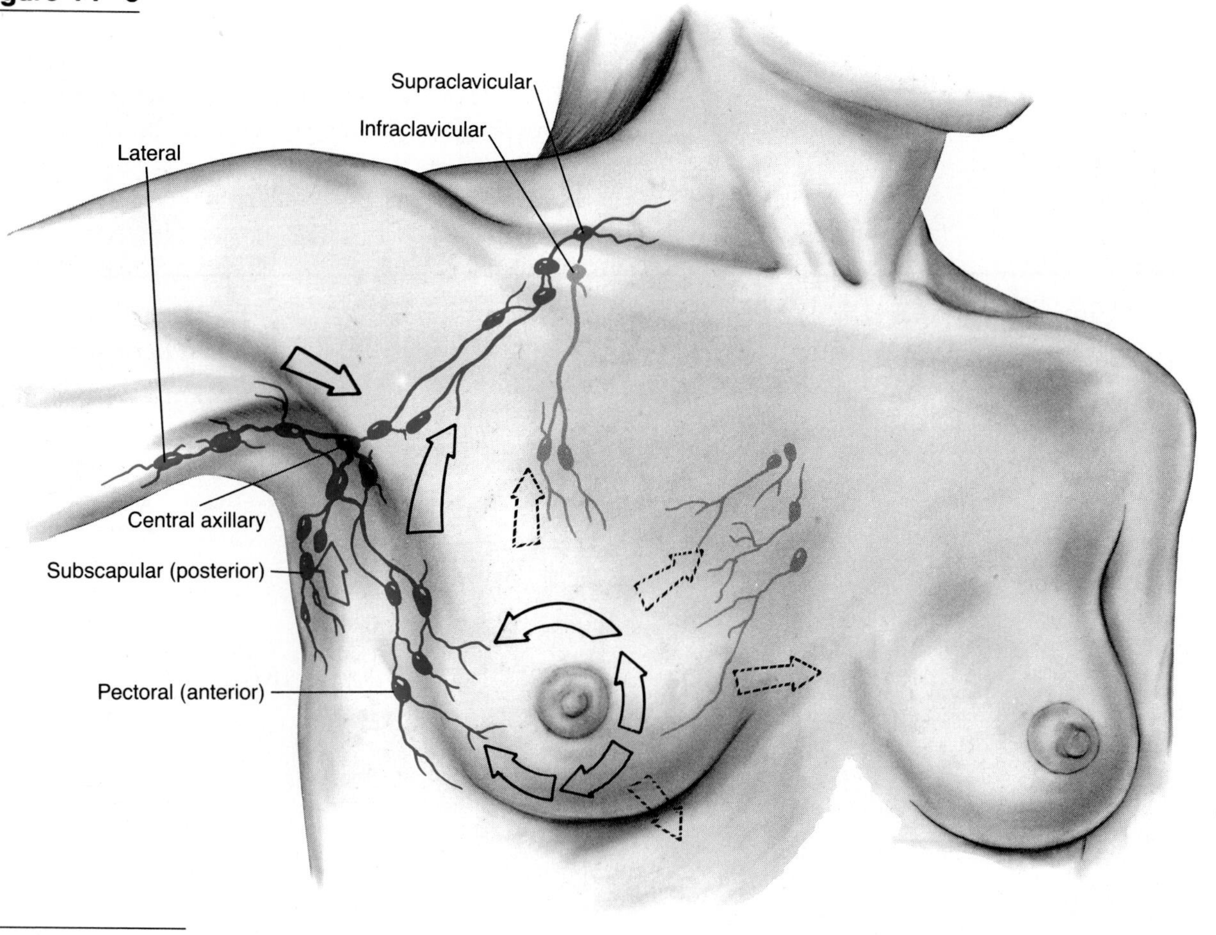

► **Figure 14–4**

Arrows indicate direction of lymph flow

DEVELOPMENTAL CONSIDERATIONS

During embryonic life, there are mammary ridges, or "milk lines," which curve down from the axilla to the groin (Fig. 14–5). The breast develops along the ridge, and the rest of the ridge usually atrophies. Occasionally a *supernumerary nipple or breast* persists and is visible somewhere along the track of the mammary ridge (see Fig. 14–8).

At birth, the only breast structures present are the lactiferous ducts within the nipple. No alveoli have developed. There is little change until puberty.

The Adolescent

At puberty, the estrogen hormones stimulate breast changes (Table 14–1). The breasts enlarge, mostly due to extensive fat deposition. The duct system also grows and branches, and masses of small, solid cells develop at the duct endings. These are potential alveoli.

Average breast development begins between 10 and 11 years of age, although the normal range is between 8 and 13 years. Occasionally, one breast may grow faster than the other, producing a temporary asymmetry. This may cause some distress; reassurance is necessary. Tenderness is common also. Although the age of onset varies widely, the five stages of breast development follow this pattern described by Tanner's sexual maturity rating or SMR (Tanner, 1962).

Full development from stage 2 to stage 5 takes an average of 3 years, although the range is 1.5 to 6 years. During this time, pubic hair develops, and axillary hair appears 2 years after the onset of pubic hair. The beginning of breast development precedes menarche by about 2 years. Menarche occurs in breast development stage 3 or 4, usually just after the peak of the adolescent growth spurt, which occurs around age 12. Note the relationship of these events (Fig. 14–6).

This knowledge aids in assessing the development of adolescent girls and increasing their knowledge about their own development. Be aware that Tanner's figures are derived from studies of white British females and may not necessarily generalize to other racial groups. Tanner's results did agree closely with the U.S. Health Examination Survey, finding close correlation of Tanner stages for breast and pubic hair development. One significant difference was that black girls were shown to develop secondary sex characteristics earlier than white

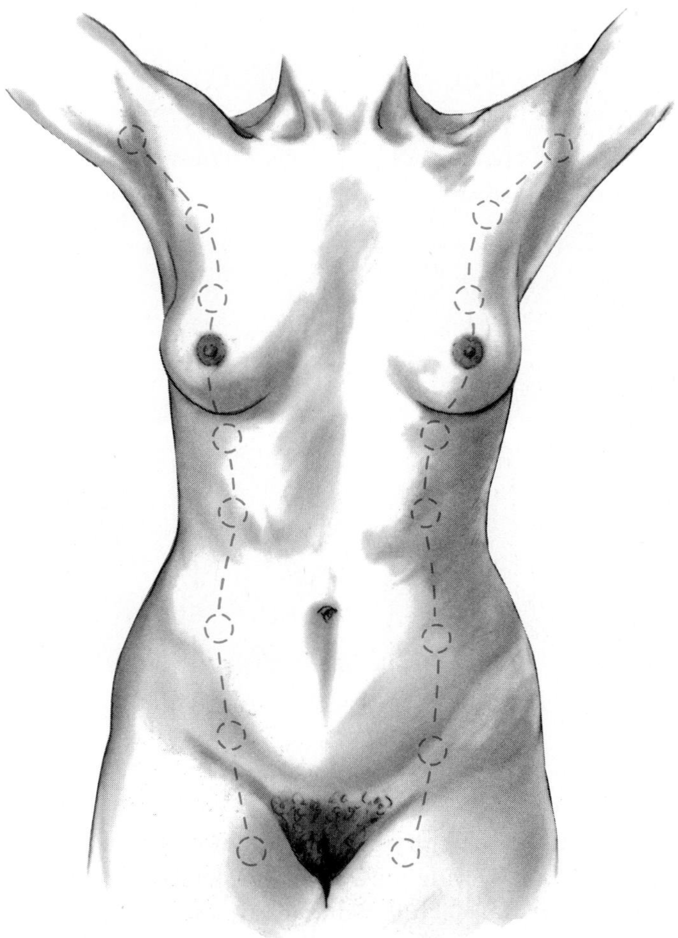

► **Figure 14–5**

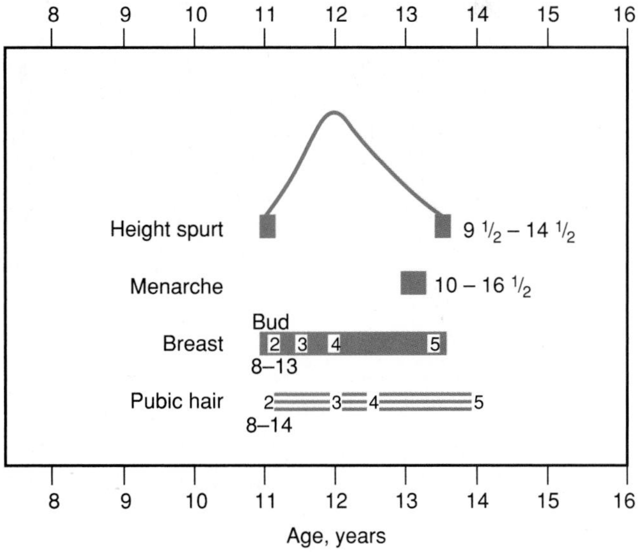

► **Figure 14–6**

Table 14–1 ► Sexual Maturity Rating in Girls

Stage	
1	Preadolescent. Only a small elevated nipple.
2	Breast bud stage. A small mound of breast and nipple develops. The areola widens.
3	The breast and areola enlarge. The nipple is flush with the breast surface.
4	The areola and nipple form a secondary mound over the breast.
5	Mature breast; only the nipple protrudes, the areola is flush with the breast contour. (The areola may continue as a secondary mound in some normal women.)

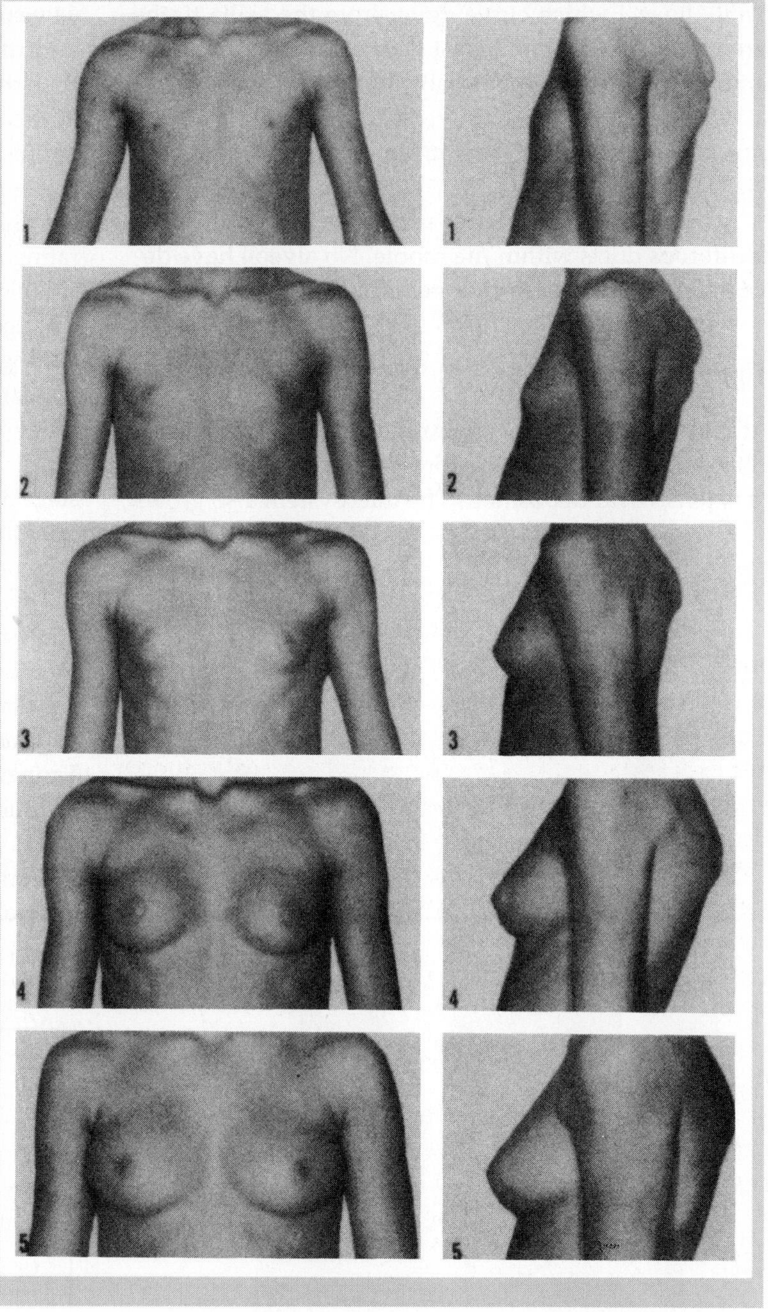

girls of the same age (Harlan, 1977). Other differences are that axillary hair appears earlier in black females, and Asian women normally have fine sparse pubic hair.

Breasts of the nonpregnant woman change with the ebb and flow of hormones during the monthly menstrual cycle. Nodularity increases from midcycle up to menstruation. During the 3 to 4 days before menstruation, the breasts feel full, tight, heavy, and occasionally sore. The breast volume is smallest on days 4 to 7 of the menstrual cycle.

The Pregnant Female

During pregnancy, breast changes start during the second month and are an early sign of pregnancy for most women. Pregnancy stimulates the expansion of the ductal system and supporting fatty tissue as well as development of the true secretory alveoli. Thus the breasts enlarge and feel more nodular. The nipples are larger, darker, and more erectile. The areolae become larger and grow a darker brown as pregnancy progresses. (The brown color fades after lactation, but the areolae never return to the original color.) A venous pattern is prominent over the skin surface. After the fourth month, *colostrum* may be expressed. This thick yellow fluid is the precursor of milk, containing the same amount of protein and lactose but practically no fat. Milk production (lactation) begins 1 to 3 days postpartum.

The Aging Female

After menopause, the glandular tissue atrophies and is replaced with connective tissue. The fat envelope atrophies also, beginning in the middle years and becoming marked in the eighth and ninth decades. These changes decrease breast size and elasticity so the breasts droop and sag, looking flattened and flabby. Drooping is accentuated by the kyphosis in some older women.

The decreased breast size makes inner structures more prominent. A breast lump may have been present for years but is suddenly palpable. Around the nipple the lactiferous ducts are more palpable and feel firm and stringy because of fibrosis and calcification. Breast shrinkage and fibrosis may cause nipple retraction. Although the nipple usually can be everted and there is no associated breast lump, this arouses suspicion of cancer and must be distinguished (Rossman, 1986). The axillary hair decreases.

THE MALE BREAST

The male breast is a rudimentary structure consisting of a thin disc of undeveloped tissue underlying the nipple. The areola is well developed, although the nipple is relatively very small. During adolescence, it is common for the breast tissue to temporarily enlarge, producing *gynecomastia.* This condition is usually unilateral and temporary. Reassurance is necessary for the adolescent male, whose attention is riveted on his body image. Gynecomastia may reappear in the aging male, and may be due to testosterone deficiency.

TRANSCULTURAL CONSIDERATIONS

The superficial veins of the chest form a network over the entire chest, called the mammary venous plexus. It flows in either a transverse or a longitudinal pattern. In the transverse pattern, the veins radiate laterally and toward the axillae. In the longitudinal pattern, the veins radiate downward and laterally like a fan. These two patterns occur with different frequencies in the two populations that have been studied. The transverse pattern is more common. White women have the recessive longitudinal pattern 6 to 10 percent of the time, whereas this pattern occurs 30 percent of the time in Navajos. An alteration of either pattern is produced by breast tumor (Spuhler, 1950).

Racial differences in sexual maturity already have been mentioned.

The incidence of breast cancer varies with different cultural groups. In the search for an environmental influence to account for this difference, researchers suspect a diet rich in fat. The high incidence of breast cancer rates in the United States, Britain and the Netherlands correlates with a high amount of fat in the diet of those nations. In Japan, Peru, Singapore, and Romania, where people eat a lean diet, the incidence of breast cancer is one-sixth to one-half that in the United States (American Cancer Society, 1991). However, migratory studies show that when Japanese move to the United States, their previously low incidence rises as they adapt to a western diet (Secretary's Task Force on Black & Minority Health, 1986).

SUBJECTIVE DATA

Breast

- Pain
- Lump
- Discharge
- Rash
- Swelling
- Trauma
- History of breast disease
- Surgery
- Perform breast self-examination
- Last mammogram

Axilla

- Tenderness
- Lump or swelling
- Rash

In Western culture, the female breasts signify more than their primary purpose of lactation. Women are surrounded by messages that feminine norms of beauty and desirability are enhanced by and dependent on the size of the breasts and their appearance. More recently, women leaders have tried to refocus this attitude, stressing women's self-worth as individual human beings, not as stereotyped sexual objects. The intense cultural emphasis is gradually changing, yet the breasts still are crucial to a woman's self-concept and her perception of her femininity. Matters pertaining to the breast affect a woman's body image and generate deep emotional responses.

This emotionality may take strong forms that you observe as you discuss the woman's history. One woman may be acutely embarrassed talking about the breasts, as evidenced by lack of eye contact, minimal response, nervous gestures, or inappropriate humor. Another woman may talk wryly and disparagingly about the size or development of her breasts. A young adolescent is acutely aware of her own development in relation to her peers. Or, a woman who has found a breast lump may come to you with fear, high anxiety, and even panic. Although a high percentage of breast lumps are benign, many women initially assume the worst possible outcome — cancer, disfigurement, and death. While you are collecting the subjective data, tune in to cues for these behaviors that call for a straightforward and reasoned attitude.

EXAMINER ASKS:	RATIONALE:
1. Do you have any **pain** or tenderness in the breasts? When did you first notice it? Where is the pain? Does it seem localized or all over? Characteristics: Is the painful spot sore to touch? Do you feel a burning or pulling sensation?	Contrary to common belief, pain can be a symptom of cancer. One study of women with breast cancer found 13 percent reporting pain as their initial symptom, the second most common after a lump. It was a "vague pain," "a pulling, burning, a funny feeling" (Bullough, 1980).

EXAMINER ASKS:	RATIONALE:
Is the pain cyclic? What relation does the pain have to your menstrual period?	Cyclic pain is common with normal breasts, use of oral contraceptives, and with fibrocystic disease.
Is the pain brought on by strenuous activity, especially involving one arm; a change in activity; manipulation during sex; part of underwire bra; exercise?	Is pain spontaneous or related to specific cause?
2. Have you ever noticed a **lump or thickening** in the breast? Where in the breast? When did you first notice it? Has it changed at all since then? Does the lump have any relation to your menstrual period? Have you noticed any change in the overlying skin: redness, warmth, dimpling, swelling?	The presence of any lump must be carefully explored. A lump that has been present for many years and exhibiting no change may not be serious but still should be explored. Approach any recent change or new lump with suspicion.
3. Do you have any **discharge** from the nipple? When did you first notice this? Characteristics: What color is the discharge? What is the consistency—thick or runny? Is there an odor?	Note use of medications that may cause clear nipple discharge, such as oral contraceptives, phenothiazines, diuretics, digitalis, and steroids. Also, tricyclic tranquilizers, reserpine, and methyldopa. Bloody or blood-tinged discharge always is significant. Any discharge in the presence of a lump is significant.
4. Have you noted any **rash** on the breast? When did you first notice this? Where did it start? On the nipple, areola, or surrounding skin?	Paget's disease starts with a small crust on the nipple apex, then spreads to areola. Eczema or other dermatitis rarely starts at nipple unless it is due to breast-feeding. It usually starts on the areola or surrounding skin and then spreads to the nipple.
5. Have you noted any **swelling** in the breasts? Is this in one spot or all over? Does the swelling seem to be related to your menstrual period, pregnancy, or breast-feeding? Have you noticed any change in bra size?	
6. Have you had any **trauma** or injury to the breasts? Did it result in any swelling, lump, or break in skin?	A lump from an injury is due to local hematoma or edema and should resolve shortly. Or, trauma may cause a woman to feel the breast and find a lump that really was there before.
7. Do you have any **history of breast disease** yourself? What type? How was this diagnosed? When did this occur? How is it being treated?	A history of breast cancer increases the risk of recurrent cancer (see Breast Cancer Risk Factors). The presence of fibrocystic disease makes it more difficult to examine the breasts; the general lumpiness of the breast conceals a new lump.

EXAMINER ASKS:	RATIONALE:

Has there been any breast cancer in your family? Who? Sister, mother, maternal grandmother, maternal aunts?
At what age did this relative have breast cancer?

The finding of breast cancer occurring before menopause in certain family members increases risk for this woman (see Breast Cancer Risk Factors).

8. Have you ever had **surgery** on the breasts? Was this a biopsy? Mastectomy? Mammoplasty—augmentation or reduction?

9. Self-care behaviors.

Have you ever been taught **breast self-examination?**

(If so:) How often do you perform it? What helps you remember?

That is an excellent way to be in charge of your own health. I would like you to show me your technique after we do your examination.

(If not:) This will be an excellent way that you can take charge of your own health. You can make breast self-examination a very routine health habit, just like brushing your teeth. I will teach you the technique after we do your examination.

Have you ever had **mammography,** a screening x-ray examination of the breasts? When was the last x-ray?

The monthly practice of breast self-examination is an excellent routine health habit. Most lumps are not cancerous but need to be examined by a professional. Mammography (x-ray examination using low-level radiation) can reveal cancers too small to be detected by the woman or by the most experienced examiner. The American Cancer Society recommends a baseline mammogram for all women between the ages of 35 and 39. Asymptomatic women between the ages of 40 and 49 should have a mammogram every 1 to 2 years; for asymptomatic women over 50 years of age, a mammogram should be performed every year. Also, the Society recommends a professional physical examination of the breast every 3 years for women 20 to 40 years of age, and every year for those older than 40 years of age (American Cancer Society, 1991).

AXILLA

1. Have you noticed any **tenderness** or **lump** in the underarm area? Where? When did you first notice this?

Breast tissue extends up into the axilla. Also, the axilla contains numerous lymph nodes.

2. Do you have an axillary **rash?** Please describe it. Does it seem to be a reaction to deodorant?

ADDITIONAL QUESTIONS FOR THE PREADOLESCENT FEMALE

Have you noticed your breasts changing?
How long has this been happening?
Many girls notice other changes in their bodies, too, that come with growing up. What have you noticed?

Developing breasts are the most obvious sign of puberty. This is the focus of attention for most girls, especially in comparison to their

EXAMINER ASKS:	RATIONALE:
What do you think about all this?	peers. Assess each adolescent's perception of her own development, and provide teaching and reassurance as indicated.

ADDITIONAL QUESTIONS FOR THE PREGNANT FEMALE

Have you noticed any enlargement or fullness in the breasts? Is there any tenderness or tingling? Are the veins more prominent on the skin surface? Do the nipples seem more erect?	Breast changes are expected and normal during pregnancy. Assess the woman's knowledge and provide reassurance.
Do you have a history of inverted nipples? Have you noticed darkening of nipple and areola?	Inverted nipples may need special care in preparation for breastfeeding.
Are you able to express thick, yellowish fluid from breasts? (This is a late sign of pregnancy.)	Colostrum.

ADDITIONAL QUESTIONS FOR THE MENOPAUSAL WOMAN

Have you noticed any change in the breast contour, size, or firmness? (Note: Change may not be as apparent to the obese woman, or to the woman whose earlier pregnancies already have produced breast changes.)	Decreased estrogen level causes decreased firmness. Rapid decrease in estrogen level causes actual shrinkage.

RISK FACTOR PROFILE FOR BREAST CANCER

Breast cancer is the second major cause of death from cancer in women. One out of 9 women will acquire breast cancer at some point in her lifetime (American Cancer Society, 1991). Although incidence rates continue to increase, early detection and improved treatment have increased survival rates. The 5-year survival rate for localized breast cancer has increased from 78 percent in the 1940s to 91 percent today. If the cancer is not invasive, the survival rate is close to 100 percent. If the cancer has spread regionally, the survival rate is 69 percent; if the cancer has distant metastases, the survival rate is 18 percent (American Cancer Society, 1991). Early treatment of breast cancer greatly increases survival, and breast self-examination promotes early case finding. A Gallup Organization poll revealed that although most women questioned were aware of breast self-examination (95 percent), few practiced it (25 percent). Reasons for this lack included fear and anxiety, and lack of knowledge and confidence in the technique (Public Awareness of Cancer Detection Tests, 1975). One study concurred that women are more likely to practice frequent breast self-examination if they have been shown how to do it and are confident in their ability to detect a lump (Bennett, 1983). As a health professional, you can be instrumental in increasing the practice of breast self-examination by teaching all women the skill and bolstering their confidence in their tech-

EXAMINER ASKS:	RATIONALE:

Table 14-2 ▶ Breast Cancer Risk Factors

Documented hereditary cancer syndrome
Family history of breast cancer in first-degree relatives
Nulliparity or first childbirth after age 30
Early menarche and late menopause
Proliferative breast lesion (especially with atypical cells)
High-dose radiation exposure to the chest area
Hormone replacement therapy (in women at increased risk)*
High-fat diet
Obesity (especially postmenopause)

**Documented with total accumulated doses of more than 1500 mg.*
(Adapted from Counseling Women with Respect to Lifestyles, Life Events, and Breast Cancer Risks. AAOHN Journal 37:158–165, 1989.)

nique. (See section on teaching breast self-examination, p. 461.) Although all women need to learn breast self-examination, the above-mentioned historical data will highlight those at higher risk (Table 14–2).

OBJECTIVE DATA

Equipment Needed:

Small pillow

Ruler marked in centimeters

Pamphlet or teaching aid for breast self-examination

Preparation

The woman is sitting up, disrobed to the waist, facing the examiner. An alternative draping method is to use a short gown, open at the back, and lift it up to the woman's shoulders during inspection. During palpation when the woman is supine, cover one breast with the gown while examining the other. Be aware that many women are embarrassed to have their breasts examined; use a sensitive but matter-of-fact approach.

Following your examination, be prepared to teach the woman breast self-examination.

METHOD OF EXAMINATION

NORMAL RANGE OF FINDINGS	ABNORMAL FINDINGS

THE BREASTS

Inspect the Breasts.

General Appearance

Note symmetry of size and shape (Fig. 14–7). It is common to have a slight asymmetry in size; often the left breast is slightly larger than the right.

A sudden increase in the size of one breast signifies inflammation or new growth.

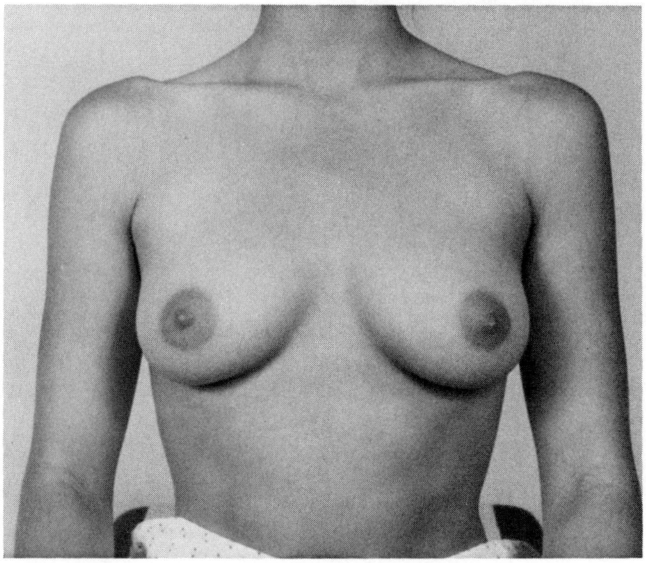

► **Figure 14–7**

Skin

The skin normally is smooth and of even color. Note any localized areas of redness, bulging, or dimpling. Also, note any skin lesions or focal vascular pattern. A fine blue vascular network is visible normally during pregnancy. Pale linear striae, or stretch marks, often follow pregnancy.

Normally there is no edema. Edema exaggerates the hair follicles, giving a "pig skin" or "orange peel" look (also called *peau d'orange*).

Hyperpigmentation.

Redness and heat with inflammation.

Unilateral dilated superficial veins in a nonpregnant woman. See Table 14–3.

Lymphatic Drainage Areas

Observe the axillary and supraclavicular regions. Note any bulging, discoloration, or edema.

NORMAL RANGE OF FINDINGS | **ABNORMAL FINDINGS**

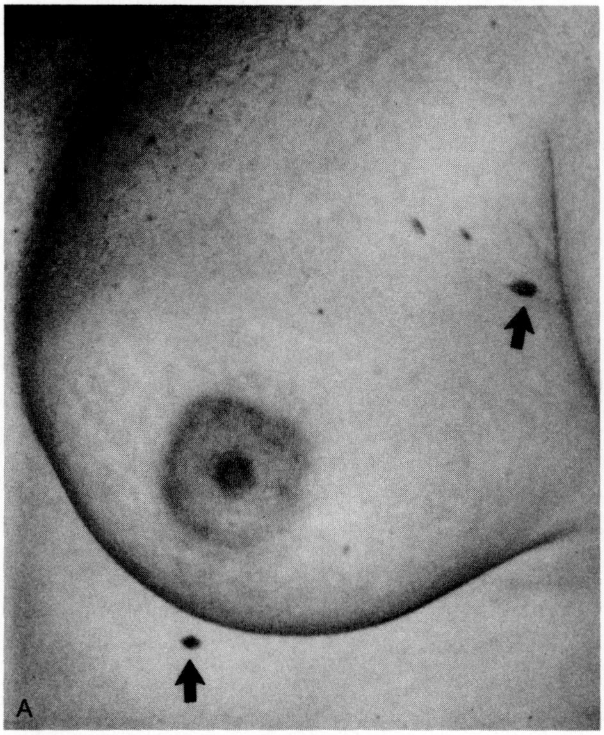

Supernumerary nipples

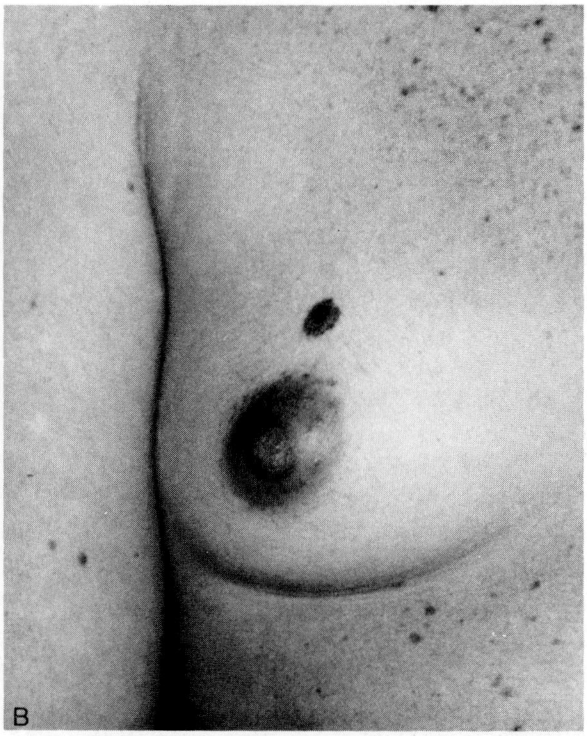

Supernumerary nipple and areolar complex

▶ Figure 14–8

Nipple

The nipples should be symmetrically placed on the same plane on the two breasts. Nipples usually protrude, although some are flat and some are inverted. They tend to stay in their original condition. Distinguish a recently retracted nipple from one that has been inverted for many years or since puberty. Normal nipple inversion may be unilateral or bilateral and usually can be pulled out (i.e., it is not fixed).

Deviation in pointing (see Table 14–3).

Recent nipple retraction signifies acquired disease (see Table 14–3).

Note any dry scaling, any fissure or ulceration, and bleeding or other discharge.

Any discharge must be explored, especially in the presence of a breast mass.

A normal variation in about 1 percent of men and women is a *supernumerary nipple* (Fig. 14–8). An extra nipple along the embryonic "milk line" on the thorax or abdomen is a congenital finding. Usually, it is 5 to 6 cm below the breast near the midline and has no associated glandular tissue. It looks like a mole, although a close look reveals a tiny nipple and areola. It is not significant; merely distinguish it from a mole.

Rarely, glandular tissue, a supernumerary breast, or polymastia, is present.

Maneuvers to Screen for Retraction

Direct the woman to change position while you check the breasts for skin retraction signs. First ask her to lift the arms slowly over the head. Both breasts should move up symmetrically (Fig. 14–9).

Retraction signs are due to fibrosis in the breast tissue, usually caused by growing neoplasms. The fibro-

NORMAL RANGE OF FINDINGS

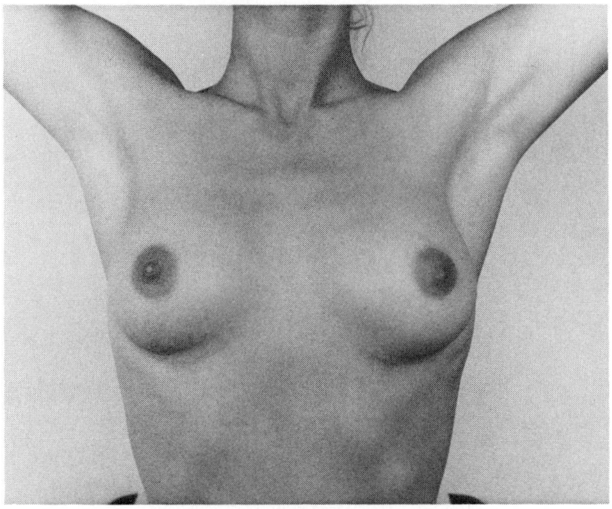

► Figure 14-9

Next ask her to push her hands onto her hips (Fig. 14-10) and to push her two palms together (Fig. 14-11). These maneuvers contract the pectoralis major muscle. There will be a slight lifting of both breasts.

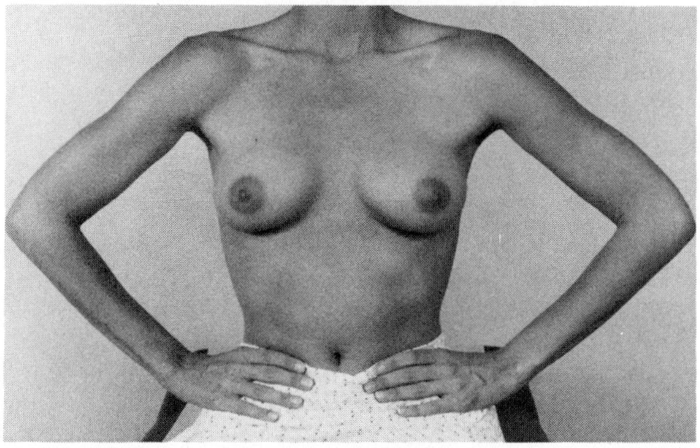

► Figure 14-10

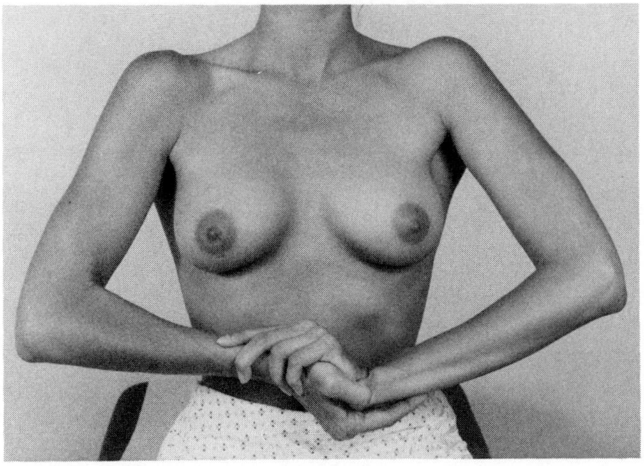

► Figure 14-11

ABNORMAL FINDINGS

sis shortens with time, causing contrasting signs with the normally loose breast tissue.

Note a lag in movement of one breast.

Note a dimpling or a pucker, which indicates skin retraction (see Table 14-3).

NORMAL RANGE OF FINDINGS	ABNORMAL FINDINGS

Ask the woman with large pendulous breasts to lean forward while you support her forearms. Note the symmetric free-forward movement of both breasts (Fig. 14–12).

Note fixation to chest wall or skin retraction (see Table 14–3).

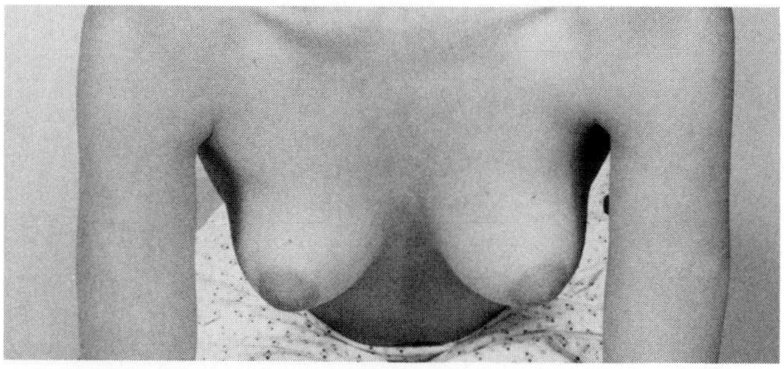

► **Figure 14–12**

THE AXILLAE

Inspect and palpate the axillae

Examine the axillae while the woman is sitting. Inspect the skin, noting any rash or infection. Lift the woman's arm and support it yourself, so that her muscles are loose and relaxed. Use your right hand to palpate the left axilla (Fig. 14–13). Reach your fingers high into the axilla. Move them firmly down in four directions: down the chest wall in a line from the middle of the axilla, the anterior border of the axilla, the posterior border, and along the inner aspect of the upper arm. Move the woman's arm through range-of-motion to increase the surface area you can reach.

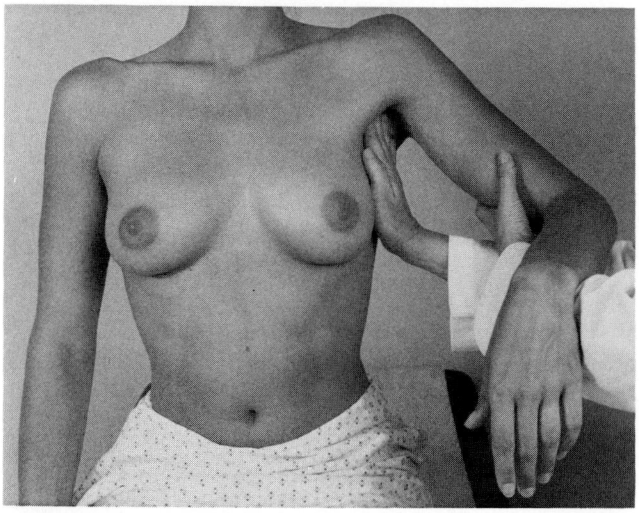

► **Figure 14–13**

NORMAL RANGE OF FINDINGS | **ABNORMAL FINDINGS**

Usually nodes are not palpable, although you may feel a small, soft, nontender node in the central group. Expect some tenderness when palpating high in the axilla. Note any enlarged and tender lymph nodes.

Nodes enlarge with any local infection of the breast, arm, or hand, and with breast cancer metastases.

BREAST PALPATION

Help the woman to a supine position. Tuck a small pad under the side to be palpated and raise her arm over her head. These maneuvers will flatten the breast tissue and displace it medially. Any significant lumps will then feel more distinct (Fig. 14–14).

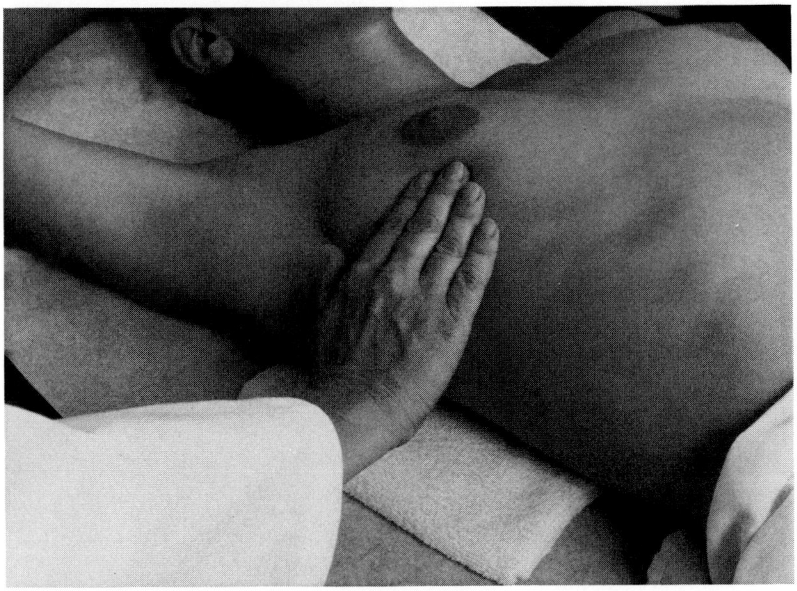

▸ **Figure 14–14**

Use the pads of your first three fingers and make a gentle rotary motion on the breast. Choose one of two patterns for palpation. (1) You may start at the nipple and palpate out to the periphery as if following spokes on a wheel (Fig. 14–15). (2) Or, start at the nipple and palpate in concentric circles, increasing out to the periphery (Fig. 14–16). With either pattern, move in a clockwise direction taking care to examine every square inch of the breast. Also, take care to palpate the tail of Spence extending from the upper outer quadrant into the axilla. It does not matter which method of palpation you use, but be consistent and thorough.

Heat, redness, and swelling in nonlactating and nonpostpartum breasts indicate inflammation.

In nulliparous women, normal breast tissue feels firm, smooth, and elastic. After pregnancy, the tissue feels softer and looser. Premenstrual engorgement is normal owing to increasing progesterone. This consists of a slight enlargement, a tenderness to palpation, and a generalized nodularity; the lobes feel prominent and their margins more distinct.

NORMAL RANGE OF FINDINGS

ABNORMAL FINDINGS

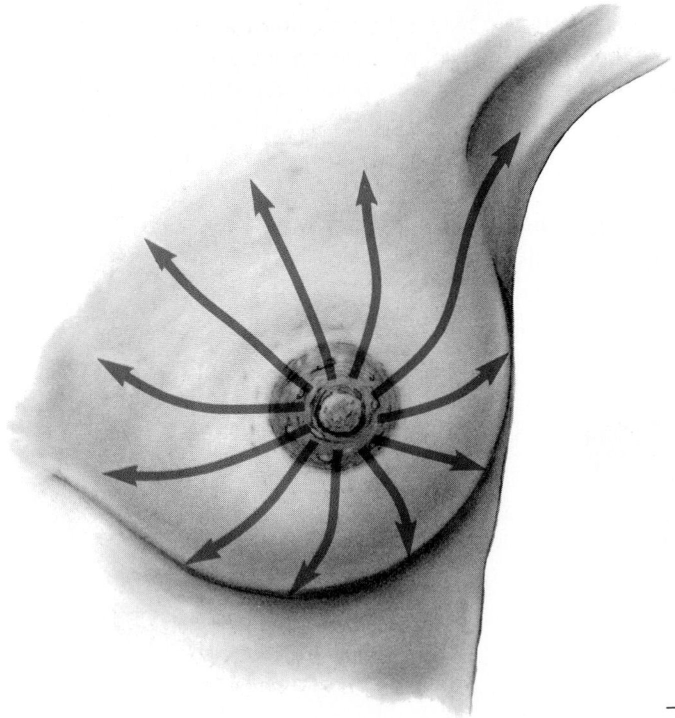

Spokes-on-a-wheel pattern of palpation

► **Figure 14–15**

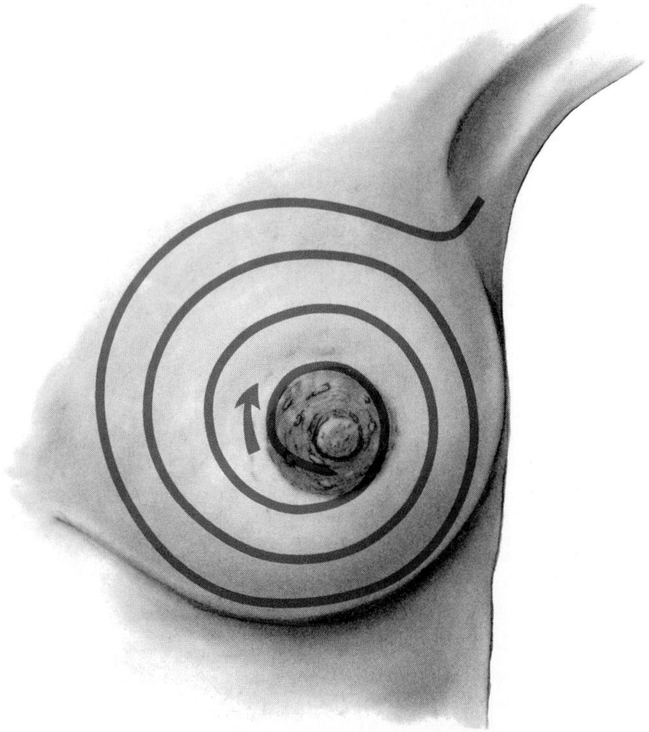

Concentric circles pattern of palpation

► **Figure 14–16**

Also, normally you may feel a firm transverse ridge of compressed tissue in the lower quadrants. This is the *inframammary ridge,* and it is especially noticeable in large breasts. Do not confuse it with an abnormal lump.

NORMAL RANGE OF FINDINGS

After palpating over the four breast quadrants, palpate the nipple (Fig. 14–17). Note any induration or subareolar mass. Use your thumb and forefinger to apply gentle pressure or a stripping action to the nipple. If any discharge appears, note its color and consistency.

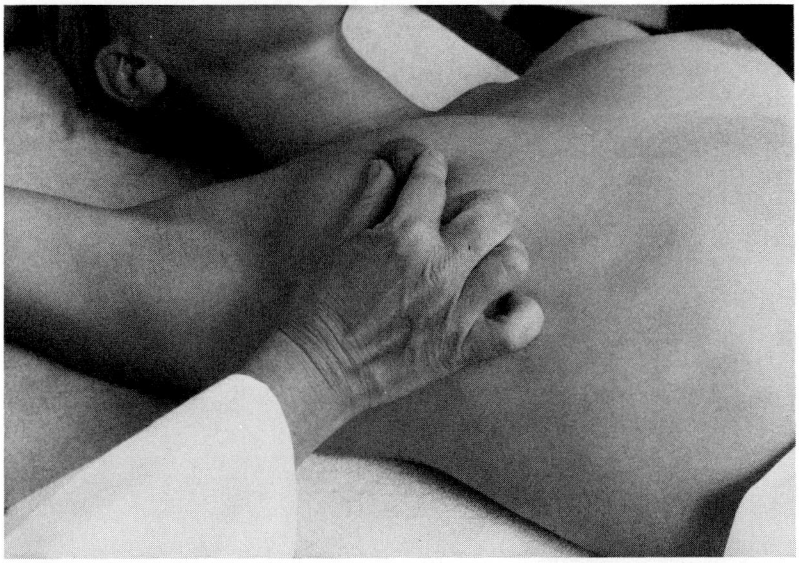

▶ **Figure 14–17**

For the woman with large pendulous breasts, you may palpate using a bimanual technique (Fig. 14–18). The woman is in a sitting position, leaning forward. Support the inferior part of the breast with one hand. Use your other hand to palpate the breast tissue against your supporting hand.

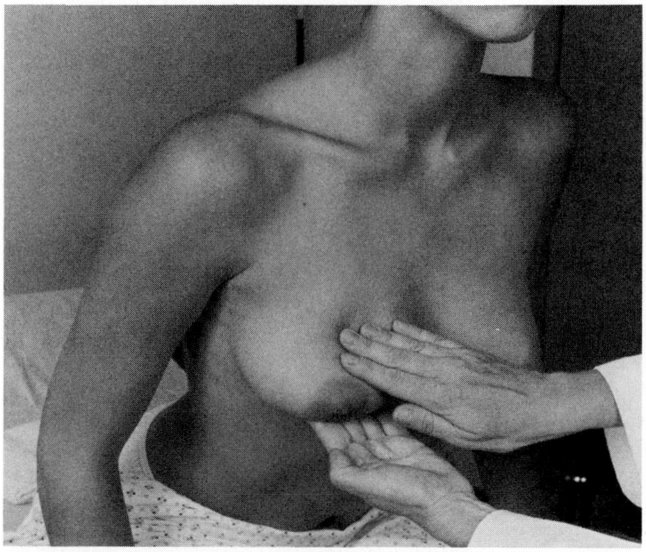

▶ **Figure 14–18**

ABNORMAL FINDINGS

Except in pregnancy and lactation, discharge is abnormal.

NORMAL RANGE OF FINDINGS

If the woman mentions a breast lump she has discovered herself, examine the unaffected breast first to learn a baseline of normal consistency for this individual. If you do feel a lump or mass, note these characteristics:

1. Location—Using the breast as a clock face, describe the distance in centimeters from the nipple, e.g. "2:00, 3 cm from the nipple." Or, diagram the breast in the woman's record and mark in the location of the lump.
2. Size—Judge in centimeters in three dimensions: width × length × thickness (Fig. 14–19).
3. Shape—State if the lump is oval, round, lobulated, or indistinct.
4. Consistency—State if the lump is soft, firm or hard.
5. Moveable—Is the lump freely moveable, or is it fixed when you try to slide it over the chest wall?
6. Distinctness—Is the lump solitary or multiple?
7. Nipple—Is it displaced or retracted?
8. Note the skin over the lump—Is it erythematous, dimpled or retracted?
9. Tenderness—Is the lump tender to palpation?
10. Lymphadenopathy—Are any regional lymph nodes palpable?

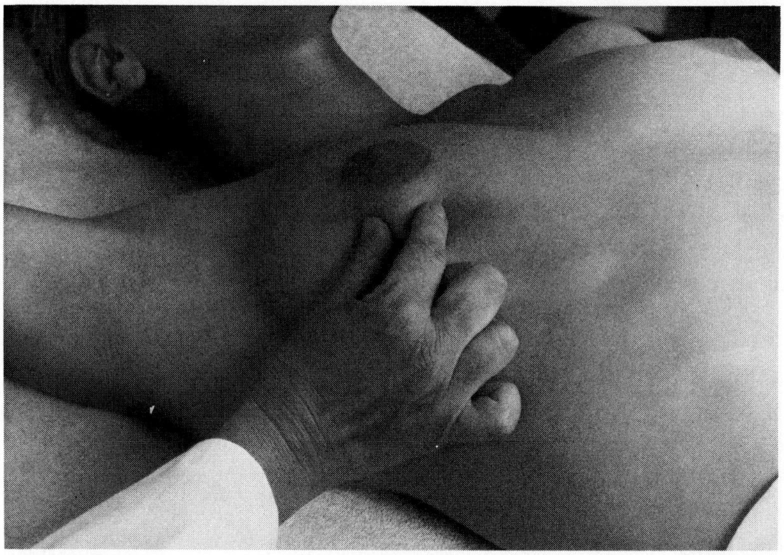

► **Figure 14–19**

The *friction-free examination* incorporates hot, soapy lather applied to the breasts before palpation. The soap acts as a lubricant and greatly enhances the breast features. Talcum powder also can be used. Some high-risk breast clinics advocate this technique as a valuable tool for detection of lumps because the details are so clearly defined. The heat also enhances detection of any nipple secretions. Following the examination the breasts are cleaned with a hot wet towel.

ABNORMAL FINDINGS

See Tables 14–4 and 14–5 for description of common breast lumps using these characteristics.

NORMAL RANGE OF FINDINGS | ABNORMAL FINDINGS

THE BREAST SELF-EXAMINATION

Finish your own assessment first; then teach the self-examination. You need to focus your skill and concentration on the examination, and you may be diverted by teaching at the same time. The same is true for the woman. She waits to hear your examination of her is normal. Once reassured, she can relax about the findings and concentrate on your teaching.

Help each woman establish a regular schedule of self-care. The best time to conduct breast self-examination is right after the menstrual period, or the fourth through seventh day of the menstrual cycle, when the breasts are the smallest and least congested. Advise the pregnant or menopausal woman who is not having menstrual periods to select a familiar date to examine her breasts each month, for example her birthdate or the day the rent is due.

Stress that a regular monthly self-examination will familiarize her with her own breasts and their normal variation. This is a positive step that will reassure her of her healthy state. Emphasize the absence of lumps (not the presence of them). However, do encourage her to report any deviation promptly.

While teaching, focus on the positive aspects of breast self-examination. Avoid citing frightening mortality statistics about breast cancer. This may generate excessive fear and denial that actually obstructs a woman's self-care action. Rather, be selective in your choice of factual material:

The majority of women will never get breast cancer.

The great majority of breast lumps are benign.

Early detection of breast cancer is important; if the cancer is not invasive, the survival rate is close to 100 percent.

Emphasize self-care through knowledge of risk factors, regular performance of breast self-examination to increase confidence in detecting abnormalities, and early referral for any suspicious findings.

Describe the correct technique and rationale, and the expected findings to note as the woman inspects her own breasts. Teach the woman to do this in front of a mirror while she is disrobed to the waist. At home, she can start palpation in the shower where soap and water assist palpation. Then, palpation should be performed while lying supine. Encourage the woman to palpate her own breasts while you are there to monitor her technique. Use the return demonstration to assess her technique and understanding of the procedure.

Many examiners use a simulated breast model so that the woman can palpate a "lump." Pamphlets also are helpful reinforcers; just be sure they conform to the method you teach, e.g., circular approach versus radiating line approach to palpation. Give the woman two pamphlets to take home and encourage her to give one to a relative or friend. This may promote discussion, which is reinforcing.

THE MALE BREAST

Your examination of the male breast can be much more abbreviated, but do not omit it. Inspect the chest wall noting the skin surface and any lumps

NORMAL RANGE OF FINDINGS

or swelling. Palpate the nipple area for any lump or tissue enlargement. It should feel even with no nodules.

The normal male breast has a flat disc of undeveloped breast tissue beneath the nipple. *Gynecomastia* is an enlargement of this breast tissue, making it clinically distinguishable from the other tissues in the chest wall (Fig. 14–20). It feels like a smooth, firm, moveable disc. This occurs normally during puberty. It usually affects only one breast and is temporary.

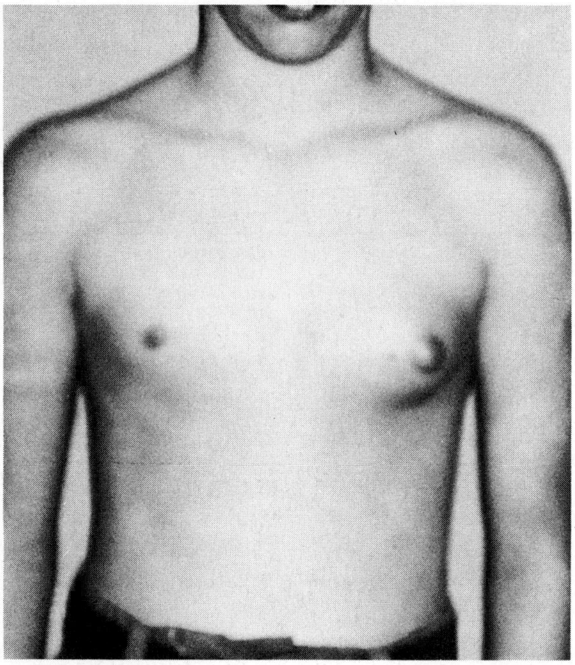

Gynecomastia

▶ **Figure 14–20**

The adolescent male is acutely aware of his body image. Reassure him that this change is normal, common, and temporary.

An obese male has an increase of fatty, not glandular, tissue.

DEVELOPMENTAL CONSIDERATIONS

Infants and Children

In the neonate of either sex, the breasts may be enlarged and visible owing to maternal estrogen crossing the placenta. They may secrete a clear or white fluid, called "witch's milk." These signs are not significant and are resolved within a few days to a few weeks.

Note the position of the nipples on the prepubertal child. They should be symmetric, just lateral to the midclavicular line, between the fourth and fifth ribs. The nipple is flat, and the areola is darker pigmented.

ABNORMAL FINDINGS

Gynecomastia also occurs with some medications and some disease states. See Table 14–8.

NORMAL RANGE OF FINDINGS

The Adolescent

Adolescent breast development usually begins between 10 and 13 years of age. Expect some asymmetry during growth. (Distinguish breast development from extra adipose tissue present in obese children.) Record the stage of development using Tanner's sex maturity ratings described on p. 446. Use the chart to teach the adolescent normal developmental stages, and to assure her of her own normal progress.

With maturing adolescents, palpate the breasts as you would with the adult. The breasts normally feel firm and uniform. Note any mass.

Teach breast self-examination now, so that the technique will become a natural, comfortable habit by the time the girl becomes an adult and will be at higher risk. Teaching this age group has these advantages:

1. The population is easily accessible. Students entering high school seek health care for a required routine physical examination.
2. At a young age, you can encourage a girl that it is "all right" to touch her body, without guilt or embarrassment.
3. Positive health habits are established best at a young age. The earlier they become a habit, the more likely they will be complied with throughout life.
4. The teenager may take the information home to share with an older female family member who may be at higher risk (Harlin, 1980).

The Pregnant Female

A delicate blue vascular pattern is visible over the breasts. The breasts increase in size as do the nipples. Jagged linear stretch marks, or striae, may develop if the breasts have a large increase. The nipples also become darker and more erectile. The areolae widen, grow darker, and contain the small, scattered, elevated Montgomery's glands. On palpation, the breasts feel more nodular, and thick yellow colostrum can be expressed after the first trimester.

The Lactating Female

Colostrum changes to milk production around the third postpartum day. At this time, the breasts may become engorged, appearing enlarged, reddened, and shiny and feeling warm and hard. Frequent nursings help drain the ducts and sinuses and stimulate milk production. Nipple soreness is normal, appearing around the twentieth nursing, lasting 24 to 48 hours, then disappearing rapidly. The nipples may look red and irritated. They may even crack but will heal rapidly if kept dry and exposed to air. Again, frequent nursings are the best treatment for nipple soreness.

ABNORMAL FINDINGS

Note precocious development, occurring before age 8. It is usually normal, but also occurs with thyroid dysfunction, stilbestrol ingestion, or ovarian or adrenal tumor.

Note delayed development, occurring with hormonal failure, anorexia nervosa beginning before puberty, or severe malnutrition.

At this age, a mass is almost always a benign fibroadenoma, or a cyst (see Table 14–4).

One section of the breast surface appearing red and tender indicates a plugged duct (see Table 14–7).

NORMAL RANGE OF FINDINGS	ABNORMAL FINDINGS

The Aging Female

On inspection, the breasts look pendulous, flattened, and sagging. Nipples may be retracted but can be pulled outward. On palpation, the breasts feel more granular and the terminal ducts around the nipple feel more prominent and stringy. Thickening of the inframammary ridge at the lower breast is normal, and it feels more prominent with age.

Reinforce the value of the breast self-examination. Women over 50 years have an increased risk of breast cancer.

Abnormal findings: Since atrophy causes shrinkage of normal glandular tissue, cancer detection is somewhat easier. Any palpable lump that cannot be positively identified as a normal structure should be referred.

☑ SUMMARY CHECKLIST

1 ▶ Inspect breasts as the woman sits, raises arms overhead, pushes hands on hips, leans forward.

2 ▶ Inspect the supraclavicular and infraclavicular areas.

3 ▶ Palpate the axillae and regional lymph nodes.

4 ▶ With woman supine, palpate the breast tissue including tail of Spence, the nipples, and areolae.

5 ▶ Teach breast self-examination.

SAMPLE RECORDING

Female

Subjective

▶ States no breast pain, lump, discharge, rash, swelling, or trauma. No history of breast disease herself, does have mother with fibrocystic disease. No surgery. Never been pregnant. Performs breast self-examination monthly.

Objective

▶ Breasts symmetric. No retraction, no nipple discharge, no lesions. Contour and consistency firm and homogeneous. No masses or tenderness. No lymphadenopathy.

Male

Subjective

▶ No pain, lump, rash or swelling.

Objective

▶ No masses or tenderness. No lymphadenopathy.

SAMPLE CLINICAL PROBLEM 1

J.G. is a 32-year-old white female high-school teacher, married with no children. She reports good health until finding "lump in right breast 2 weeks ago."

Subjective

▶ 2 weeks PTA—Noticed lump in Rt. breast on self-examination. Lump firm, non-moveable area "the size of a quarter," in upper outer quadrant of breast, tender on touch only. No skin changes, no nipple discharge, on no medications. Last breast exam by MD 3 months before was reported normal. Did not notice lump on previous self-exam one month before. No history of breast disease in self or family.

2 days PTA—saw MD who confirmed presence of lump and recommended biopsy as outpatient. Last menstrual period 1/25/ (2 1/2 weeks PTA). States the last 2 days has been so nervous has been unable to sleep well or to concentrate at work. "I just know it's cancer."

Objective

▶ Voice trembling and breathless during history. Sitting posture stiff and rigid. B/P 148/78. 37°-92-16.

Breasts symmetric, nipples everted. No skin lesions, no dimpling, no retraction, no fixation.

Left breast firm, no mass, no tenderness, no discharge. Right breast firm, with 2 cm × 2 cm × 1 cm mass at 10:00 position, 5 cm from the nipple. Lump is firm, oval, with smooth discrete borders, nonmoveable, tender to palpation. No other mass. No discharge. No lymphadenopathy.

Assessment

▶ Lump in Rt. breast

Anxiety R/T threat to health status

SAMPLE CLINICAL PROBLEM 2

D.B. is a 62-year-old black female bank comptroller, married with no children. History of hypertension, managed by diuretic medication and diet. No other health problems until yearly company physical exam 3 days PTA, when MD "found a lump in my right breast."

Subjective

▶ 3 days PTA—MD noted lump in right breast during yearly physical exam. MD did not describe lump but told D.B. it was "serious" and needed immediate biopsy. D.B. has not felt it herself. States has noted no skin changes, no nipple discharge. No previous history of breast disease. Mother died age 54 of breast cancer, no other relative with breast disease. D.B. has had no full-term pregnancies; 2 spontaneous abortions, age 28, 31. Menopause completed at age 52.

Aware of breast self-examination but has never performed it. "I feel so bad. If only I had been doing it. I should have found this myself." Married 43 years. States husband supportive, but "I just can't talk to him about this. I can't even go near him now."

Objective

- Breasts symmetric when sitting, arms down. Nipples flat. No lesions, no discharge. As lifts arms, left breast elevates, right breast stays fixed. Dimple in right breast, 9:00, apparent at rest and with muscle contraction. Leaning forward reveals left breast falls free, right breast flattens.
  On palpation left breast feels soft and granular throughout, no mass. Right breast soft and granular, with large, stony hard mass in outer quadrant. Lump is 5 × 4 × 2 cm, at 9:00 position, 3 cm from nipple. Borders irregular, mass fixed to tissues, no pain with palpation. One firm, palpable lymph node in center of right axilla. No palpable nodes on the left.

Assessment

- Lump in Rt. breast
  Ineffective individual coping R/T effects of breast lump

NURSING DIAGNOSES COMMONLY ASSOCIATED WITH BREAST DISORDERS

Diagnosis	Related Factors (Etiology)	Defining Characteristics (Symptoms and Signs)
Ineffective breast-feeding	Prematurity Infant receiving supplemental feedings with artificial nipple Poor infant sucking reflex Nonsupportive partner/family Knowledge deficit Interruption of breast-feeding Maternal anxiety or ambivalence	Unsatisfactory breast-feeding process Actual or perceived inadequate milk supply Infant inability to attach onto maternal breast correctly Nonsustained suckling at the breast Persistence of sore nipples beyond first week of breast-feeding Observable signs of inadequate infant intake Insufficient emptying of each breast per feeding Insufficient opportunity for suckling at the breast Infant arching and crying at the breast, resisting latching on
Ineffective individual coping	Effects of acute or chronic illness Loss of control over body part or body system	Change in communication pattern Inability to meet or be responsible for basic needs

Diagnosis	Related Factors (Etiology)	Defining Characteristics (Symptoms and Signs)

	Lack of support systems
	Low self-esteem
	Major change in lifestyle
	Unrealistic perceptions
	Situational or maturational crisis
	Knowledge deficit about
	  disease process
	  therapeutic regimen
	  prognosis
	Separation from or loss of significant other
	Sensory overload
		Fear of pain, death
		Frequent headaches
		Emotional tension
		Insomnia
		Verbalizes inability to cope or inability to ask for help
		Inability to perform expected roles
		Insomnia
		Physical inactivity
		Stress-related disorders
		  Ulcers
		  Hypertension
		  Irritable bowel
		Substance abuse
		Inappropriate use of defense mechanisms
		  Withdrawal
		  Depression
		  Overeating
		  Blaming
		  Scapegoating
		  Manipulative behavior
		  Self-pity
		Chronic anxiety
		Indecisiveness

Knowledge deficit: breast self-examination	Lack of exposure or recall Information misinterpretation Unfamiliarity with information resources Lack of interest in learning Denial Effects of aging Sensory deficits Language barrier Cognitive limitations Inadequate economic resources	Expresses inaccurate perception of potential problem Repeatedly requests information Inadequate performance of examination Verbalizes the problem Inaccurate use of health-related vocabulary Inability to explain therapeutic regimen or describe personal health status

Other related nursing diagnosis:
Body image disturbance (see example in Chapter 10)

ABNORMAL FINDINGS

Table 14-3 ► Signs of Retraction and Inflammation in the Breast

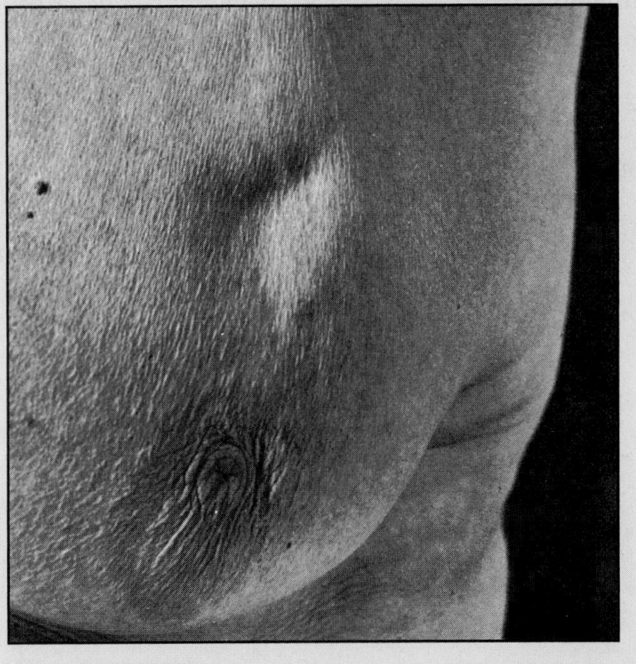

DIMPLING

The broad shallow dimple shown here is a sign of skin retraction. Cancer causes fibrosis, which contracts the suspensory ligaments. The dimple may be apparent at rest, with compression, or with lifting of the arms. Also, note the distortion of the areola here as the fibrosis pulls the nipple toward it.

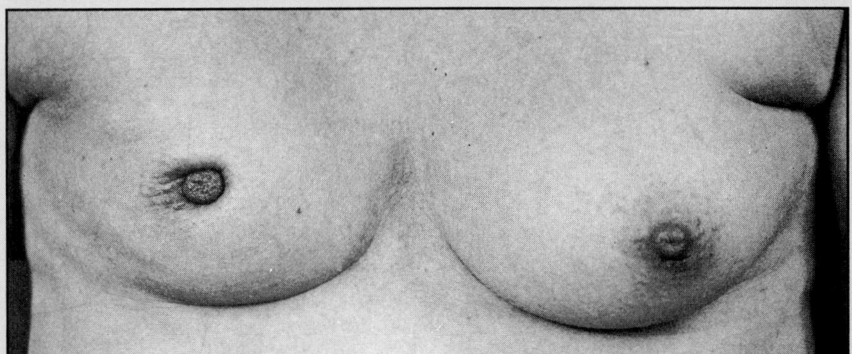

NIPPLE RETRACTION

The right nipple looks flatter and broader, like an underlying crater. A recent retraction suggests cancer directly under the nipple, which causes fibrosis of the whole duct system and pulls in the nipple. It also may occur with benign lesions such as ectasia of the ducts. Do not confuse retraction with the normal long-standing type of nipple inversion, which has no broadening and is not fixed.

Table 14-3 ▶ Signs of Retraction and Inflammation in the Breast *Continued*

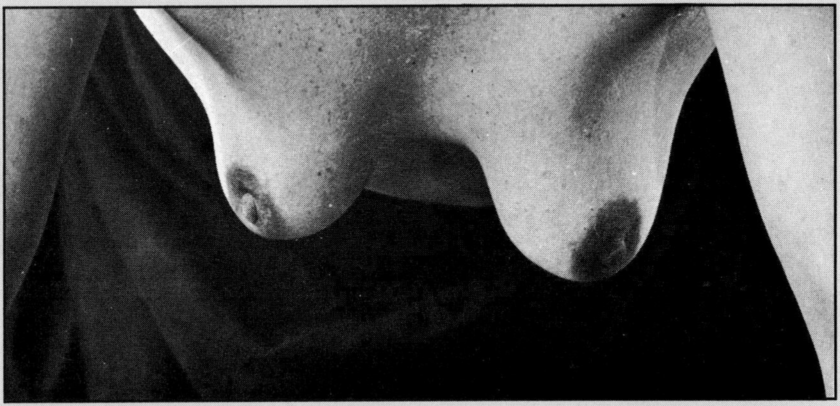

FIXATION

Asymmetry, distortion, or decreased mobility with the forward-bending maneuver. As cancer becomes invasive, the fibrosis fixes the breast to the underlying pectoral muscles. Here, note the right breast is held against the chest wall, with lateral deviation of the nipple and areola.

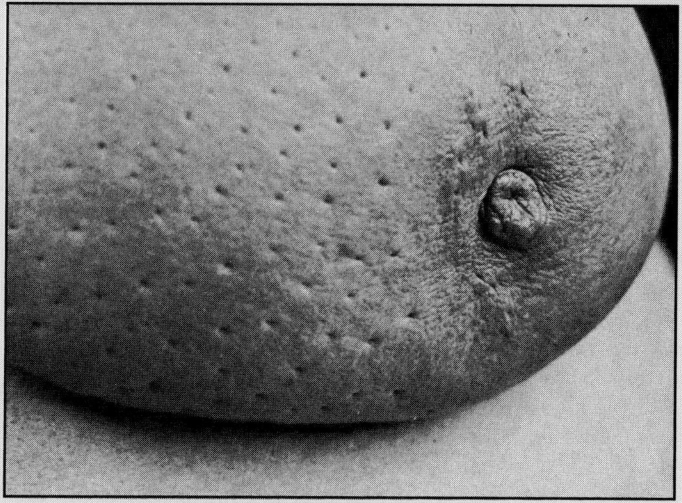

EDEMA (PEAU D'ORANGE)

Lymphatic obstruction produces edema. This thickens the skin and exaggerates the hair follicles, giving a pigskin or orange-peel look. This condition suggests cancer, here quite extensive. Edema usually begins in the skin around and beneath the areola, the most dependent area of the breast.

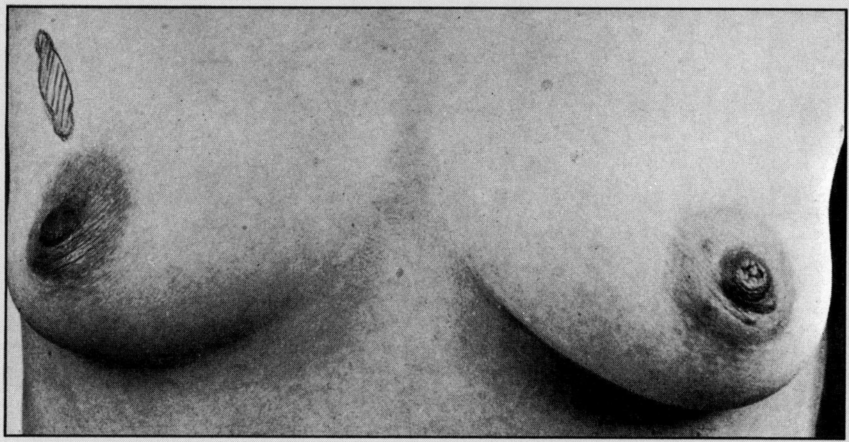

DEVIATION IN NIPPLE POINTING

An underlying cancer causes fibrosis in the mammary ducts, which pulls the nipple angle toward it. Here, note that the horizontal level of the right nipple is elevated and the nipple tilts upward and laterally.

PROMINENT VENOUS PATTERN (not illustrated)

An obvious venous pattern that is unilateral occurs with some types of breast tumors.

Table 14-4 ▸ Breast Lump

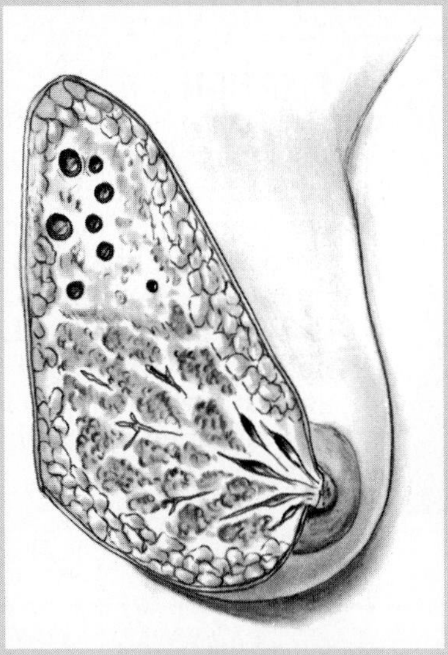

FIBROCYSTIC DISEASE (CYSTIC HYPERPLASIA, CHRONIC CYSTIC MASTOPATHY)

Multiple tender masses. These include a range of disorders that are the most common lesions of the breast. They occur bilaterally and are regular, firm nodules. They are also mobile and well demarcated. Usually, there is no dominant nodule and no fixation or retraction. The woman often feels dull heavy pain and fullness, just before menses as nodules enlarge. Most common in upper outer quadrant. Lesions feel rubbery, like small water balloons. Most common in women aged 30 to 55, frequently decreases after menopause. Not premalignant, but do produce difficulty in detecting other cancerous lumps.

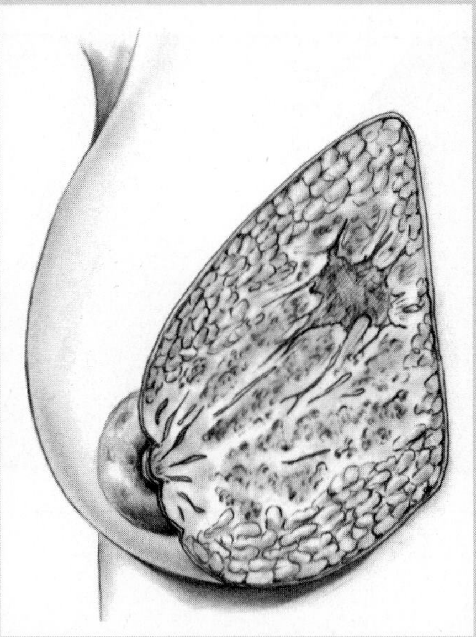

CANCER

Solitary unilateral nontender mass. Single focus in one area, although it may be interspersed with other nodules. Solid, hard, dense, and fixed to underlying tissues or skin as cancer becomes invasive. Borders are irregular and poorly delineated. Grows constantly. Often painless, although the person may have pain. Most common in upper outer quadrant. Usually found in women aged 30 to 80; increased risk in ages 40 to 44 and in women older than 50 years. As cancer advances, signs include firm or hard irregular axillary nodes, skin dimpling, nipple retraction, elevation, and discharge.

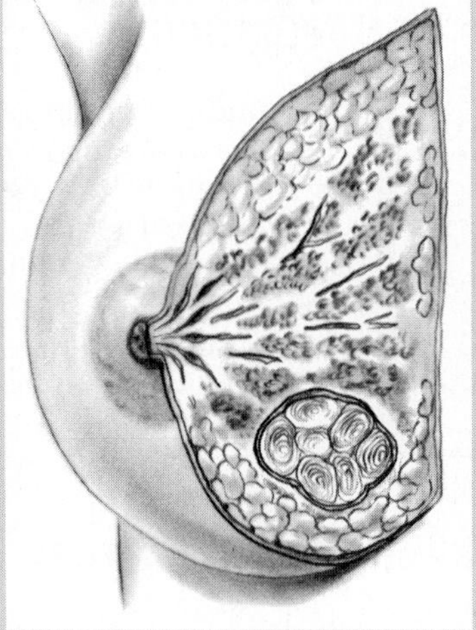

FIBROADENOMA

Solitary nontender mass. (Can be multiple or bilateral.) Solid, firm, and elastic. Round, oval, or lobulated; 1 to 5 cm. Freely moveable, slippery; fingers slide it easily through tissue. Most commonly found in younger women between 15 and 20 years, but can occur up to age 55 years. Grows quickly and constantly. Benign, although it must be diagnosed by biopsy.

Table 14-5 ► Differentiating Breast Lumps

	FIBROADENOMA	FIBROCYSTIC DISEASE	CANCER
Likely Age	15–20, can occur up to 55	30–55, decreases after menopause	30–80, risk increases after 50
Shape	Round, lobular	Round, lobular	Irregular, star-shaped
Consistency	Usually firm, can be soft	Firm to soft, rubbery	Firm to stony hard
Demarcation	Well demarcated, clear margins	Well demarcated	Poorly defined
Number	Usually single	Multiple usually, may be single	Single
Mobility	Very mobile, slippery	Mobile	Fixed
Tenderness	Usually none	Tender, increases before menses	Usually none, can be tender
Skin retraction	None	None	Usually
Pattern of growth	Grows quickly and constantly	Size may increase or decrease rapidly	Grows constantly
Risk to health	None; they are benign. Must diagnose by biopsy	Benign, though general lumpiness may mask other cancerous lump	Serious, needs early treatment

Table 14-6 ► Abnormal Nipple Discharge

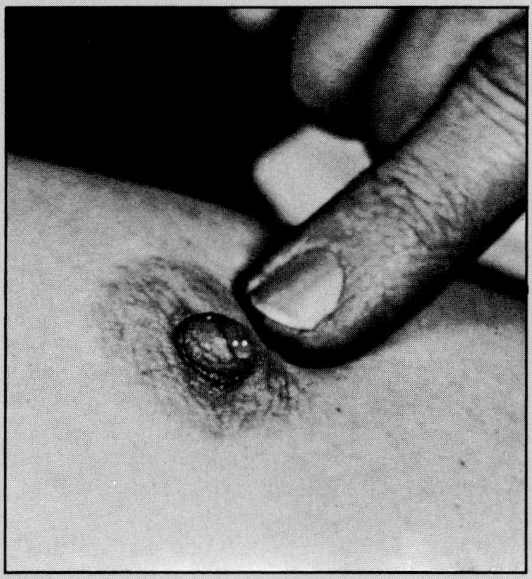

MAMMARY DUCT ECTASIA (not illustrated)

Pastelike matter in subareolar ducts produces multicolored sticky discharge. Bilateral, from multiple ducts. May have redness, itching around nipple. Also burning or drawing pain around nipple. Ducts are palpable, as rubbery twisted tubules under areola. May have palpable mass, soft or firm, poorly delineated. Not premalignant, but needs biopsy.

INTRADUCTAL PAPILLOMA

Serous or serosanguineous discharge, which is spontaneous, unilateral, and from a single duct. Lesion consists of tiny tumors, 2 to 3 mm, which are too small to palpate. Usually no palpable mass. If you can palpate mass, it is soft, poorly delineated. Moderate pain. Has increased risk for cancer. Treat by excision of involved duct.

Table continued on following page

Table 14-6 ► Abnormal Nipple Discharge *Continued*

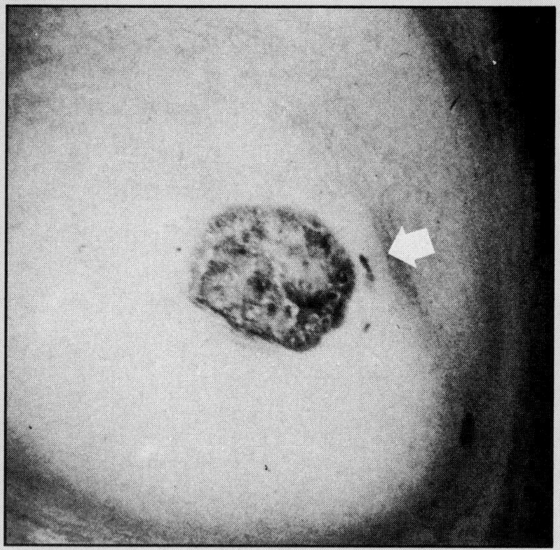

PAGET'S DISEASE (INTRADUCTAL CARCINOMA)

Early dry, scaling crusts, friable at nipple apex. Spreads to areola. Later nipple reddened, excoriated, ulcerated. Arrow indicates underlying invasive carcinoma.

Except for the redness and occasional cracking due to initial breast-feeding, any dermatitis of the nipple area must be carefully explored and referred.

Table 14-7 ► Disorders Occurring During Lactation

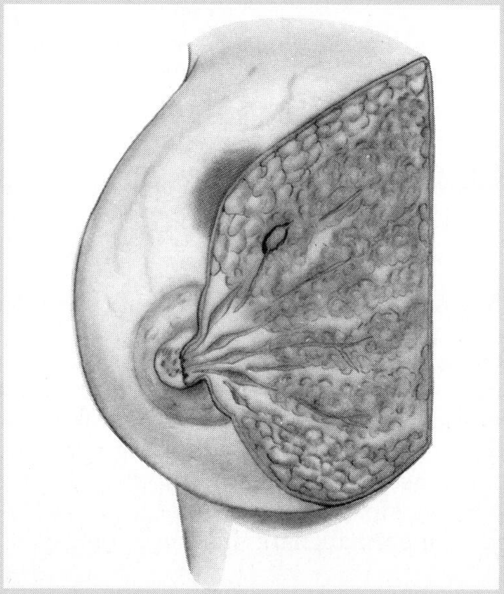

PLUGGED DUCT

A fairly common and not serious condition. One milk duct is clogged. One section of the breast is tender; may be reddened. No infection. It is important to keep breast as empty as possible and milk flowing. The woman should nurse her baby frequently, on affected side first to ensure complete emptying, and manually express any remaining milk. A plugged duct usually resolves in less than 1 day.

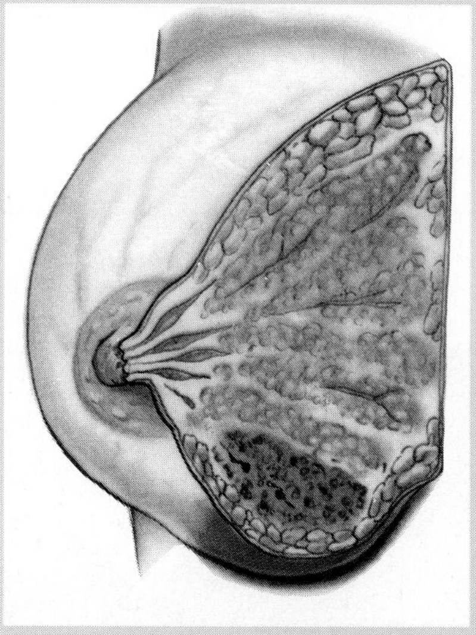

MASTITIS

This is uncommon; an inflammatory mass. Usually occurs in single quadrant. Area is red, swollen, tender, very hot and hard. Also, the woman has a headache, malaise, fever, chills and sweating, increased pulse, flulike symptoms. May occur during first 4 months of lactation from infection or from stasis due to plugged duct. Treat with rest, local heat to area, antibiotics, and frequent nursing to keep breast as empty as possible. Must not wean now or the breast will become engorged and the pain will increase. Mother's antibiotic not harmful to infant. Usually resolves in 2 to 3 days.

Table 14-7 ▸ Disorders Occurring During Lactation *Continued*

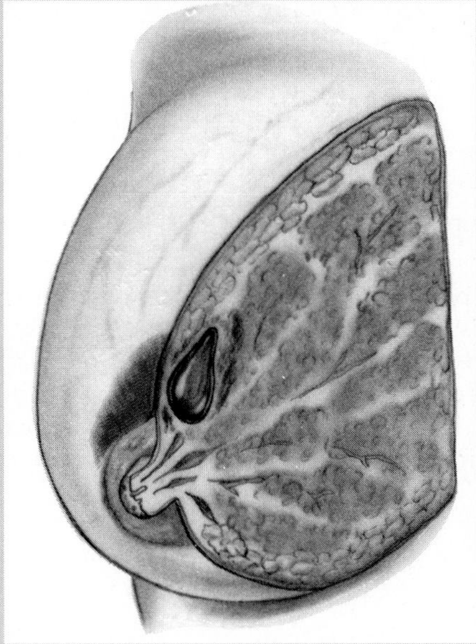

BREAST ABSCESS

A rare complication of generalized infection, e.g., mastitis if untreated. A pocket of pus accumulates in one local area. Must temporarily discontinue nursing on affected breast; manually express milk and discard. Continue to nurse on unaffected side. Treat with antibiotics, surgical incision, and drainage.

Table 14-8 ▸ Abnormalities in the Male Breast

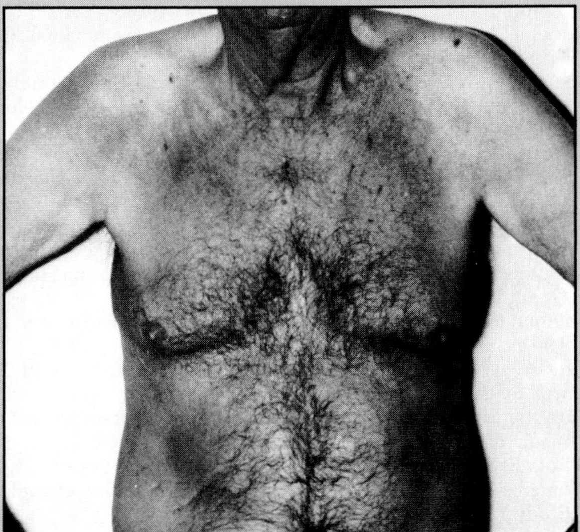

GYNECOMASTIA

Noninflammatory enlargement of male breast tissue. This is idiopathic at puberty, unilateral, usually mild and transient. Gynecomastia occurs commonly in aging males (here in a 72-year-old) owing to changing hormone levels. It is bilateral and may be tender. It also occurs bilaterally from: hormone stimulation, e.g., on estrogen for cancer of prostate, Cushing's syndrome; cirrhosis of liver as unable to metabolize estrogen completely; leukemia occasionally, and sometimes with medication—digitalis, isoniazid, spironolactone, phenothiazine.

Table continued on following page

Table 14-8 ▸ Abnormalities in the Male Breast *Continued*

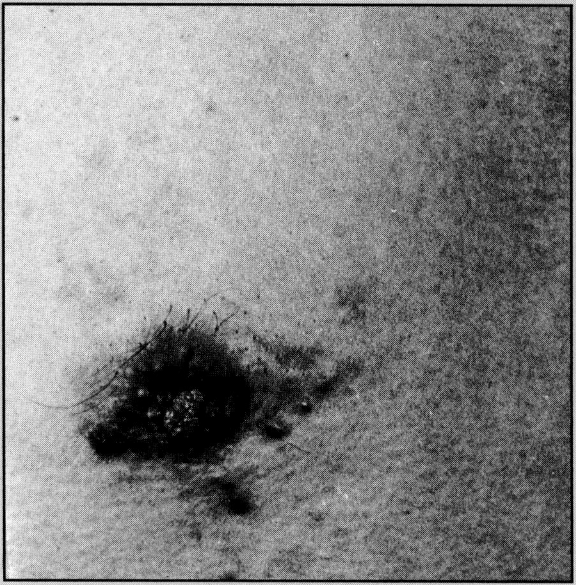

CARCINOMA

Only 1 to 2 percent of all breast cancer occurs in men. The lesion is a hard, irregular, nontender mass, most often directly under the areola. Fixed to the area; may have nipple retraction. Mass is noticeable early owing to minimal breast tissue. Also has early spread to axillary lymph nodes owing to minimal breast tissue.

Bibliography

American Cancer Society: Cancer Facts and Figures—1991. Atlanta, GA, The American Cancer Society, 1991.

Bennett SE, Lawrence RS, Fleishman KH, et al.: Profile of women practicing breast self-examination. J Am Med Assoc 249:488–491, 1983.

Bullough B: Discovery of the first signs and symptoms of breast cancer. Nurse Pract 5:31–32, 1980.

Bullough B, Hindi-Alexander M, Fetouh S: Methylxanthines and fibrocystic breast disease: A study of correlations. Nurs Pract 15(3):36–44, 1990.

Edwards V: Changing breast self-examination behavior. Nurs Res 29:301–306, 1980.

Haagensen, CD: Diseases of the Breast. 3rd ed. Philadelphia, WB Saunders, 1986.

Hallal JC: The relationship of health beliefs, health locus of control, and self-concept to the practice of breast self-examination in adult women. Nurs Res 31:137–142, 1982.

Hamwi DA: Screening mammography: Increasing the effort toward breast cancer detection. Nurs Pract 15(12):27–32, 1990.

Harlan WR, Harlan EA, Grillo GP: Secondary sex characteristics of girls 12 to 17 years of age: The U.S. Health Examination Survey. J Pediatr 96(6):1074–1078, 1980.

Harlin VK: Teaching breast self-examination in the high school. J School Health 47:243–247, 1977.

Harrison LL: Life-saving patient education: Breast self-examination. MCN 14(5):315, 1989.

Hortobagyi GN, McLelland R, Reed FM: Your key role in breast Ca screening. Patient Care 24(13):82–113, 1990.

Kushner R: Breast Cancer: A Personal History and an Investigative Report. New York, Harcourt Brace Jovanovich, 1975.

Ludwick R: Breast examination in the older adult. Cancer Nurs 11(2):99–102, 1988.

Nemcek M: Factors influencing black women's breast self-examination practice. Cancer Nurs 12(6):339–343, 1989.

Pawson IG, Petrakis NL: Comparisons of breast pigmentation among women of different racial groups. Hum Biol 47(4):441–450, 1975.

Public Awareness of Cancer Detection Tests: Results of a recent Gallup poll. Cancer 27:255–266, 1975.

Redeker NS: Health beliefs, health locus of control, and the frequency of practice of breast self-examination in women. JOGNN 18(1):45–51, 1989.

Rossman I: Clinical Geriatrics. 3rd ed. Philadelphia, JB Lippincott, 1986.

Rudolph A, McDermott RJ: The breast physical examination. Cancer Nurs 10(2):100–106, 1987.

Schuleter LA: Knowledge and beliefs about breast cancer and breast self-examination among athletic and nonathletic women. Nurs Res 31:348–353, 1982.

Secretary's Task Force on Black & Minority Health: Report. Volume III: Cancer. Washington, DC, U.S. Department of Health and Human Services, 1986.

Spuhler JN: Genetics of three normal morphological variations: patterns of superficial veins of the anterior thorax, peroneus tertius muscle and the number of vallate papillae. Cold Spring Harb Symp Quant Biol 15:175–189, 1950.

Stillman MJ: Women's health beliefs about breast cancer and breast self-examination. Nurs Res 26:121–127, 1977.

Tanner JM: Growth at Adolescence. 2nd ed. Oxford, England, Blackwell Scientific, 1962.

Turnbull EM: Effect of basic preventive health practices and mass media on the practice of BSE. Nurs Res 27:98–102, 1978.

Wilcox PM: Benign breast disorders. Am J Nurs 81:1644–1651, 1981.

Women's attitudes regarding breast cancer. (The Gallup Organization Study.) Occup Health Nurs 22:20–23, 1974.

CHAPTER

15 The Thorax and Lungs

STRUCTURE AND FUNCTION

POSITION AND SURFACE LANDMARKS

The thoracic cage is a bony structure with a conical shape, which is narrower at the top (Fig. 15–1). It is defined by the sternum, 12 pairs of ribs, and 12 thoracic vertebrae. Its "floor" is the diaphragm, a musculotendinous septum that separates the thoracic cavity from the abdomen. The first seven ribs attach directly to the sternum via their costal cartilages; ribs 8, 9, and 10 attach to the costal cartilage above; and ribs 11 and 12 are "floating," with free palpable tips. The costochondral junctions are the points at which the ribs join their cartilages. They are not palpable.

Surface landmarks on the thorax are signposts for underlying respiratory structures. Knowledge of landmarks will help you localize a finding and will facilitate communication of your findings to others.

Suprasternal Notch. Feel this hollow U-shaped depression just above the sternum, in between the clavicles.

Sternum. The "breastbone" has three parts—the manubrium, the body, and the xiphoid process. Walk your fingers down the manubrium a few centimeters until you feel a distinct bony ridge, the manubriosternal angle.

Manubriosternal Angle. Often called the "angle of Louis," this is the articulation of the manubrium and body of the sternum, and it is continuous with the second rib. The angle of Louis is a useful place to start counting ribs, which helps localize a respiratory finding horizontally. Identify the angle of Louis, palpate lightly to the second rib and slide down to the second intercostal space. Each intercostal space is numbered by the rib above it. Continue counting down the ribs in the middle of the hemithorax, not close to the sternum where the costal cartilages lie too close together to count. You can palpate easily down to the tenth rib.

The angle of Louis also marks the site of tracheal bifurcation into the right and left main bronchi; it corresponds with the upper border of the atria of the heart,

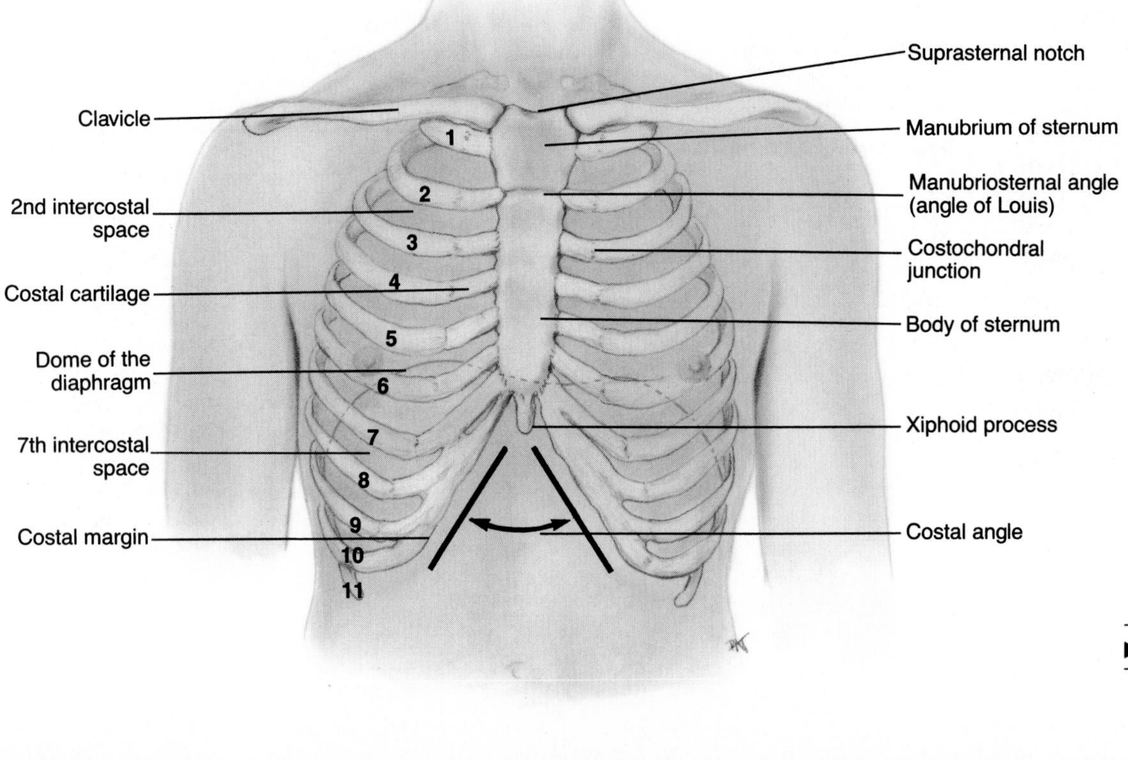

▶ Figure 15–1

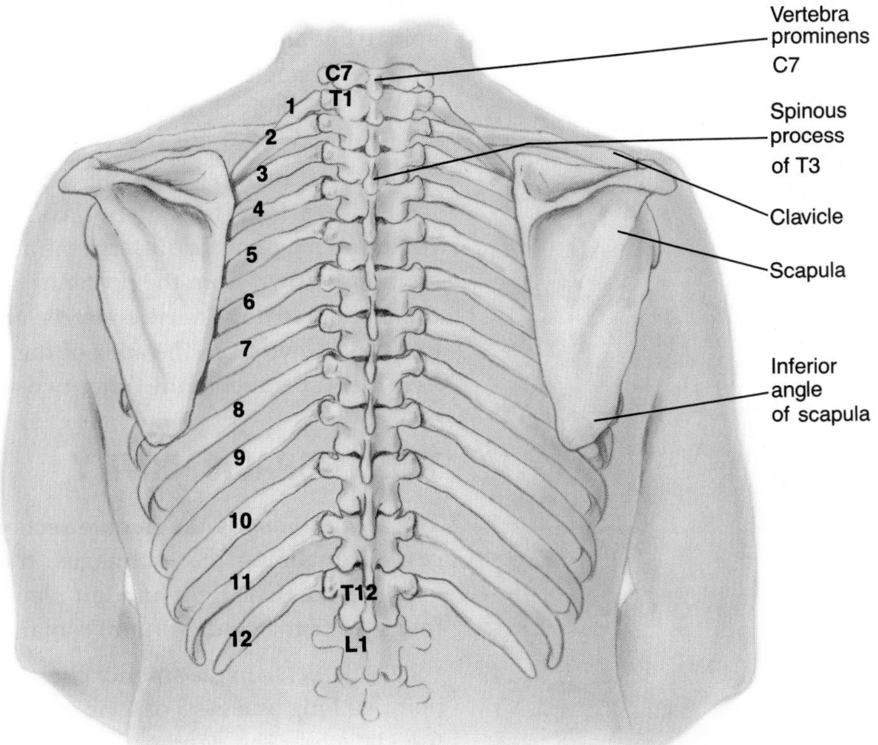

▶ **Figure 15-2**

and it lies above the fourth thoracic vertebra on the back.

Costal Angle. The right and left costal margins form an angle where they meet at the xiphoid process. Usually 90 degrees or less, this angle increases when the rib cage is chronically overinflated, as in emphysema.

Counting ribs and intercostal spaces on the back is a bit harder due to the muscles and soft tissue surrounding the ribs and spinal column (Fig. 15-2).

Vertebra Prominens. Start here. Flex your head and feel for the most prominent bony spur protruding at the base of the neck. This is the spinous process of C7. If two bumps seem equally prominent, the upper one is C7 and the lower one is T1.

Spinous Processes. Count down these knobs on the vertebrae, which stack together to form the spinal column. Note that the spinous processes align with their same numbered ribs only down to T4. After T4, the spinous processes angle downward from their vertebral body, and overlie the vertebral body and rib below.

Inferior Border of the Scapula. The scapulae are located symmetrically in each hemithorax. The lower tip is usually at the seventh or eighth rib.

Twelfth Rib. Palpate midway between the spine and the person's side to identify its free tip.

Reference Lines. Use these to pinpoint a finding vertically on the chest. On the anterior chest, note the *midsternal* line and the *midclavicular* line. The midclavicular line bisects the center of each clavicle at a point halfway between the palpated sternoclavicular and acromioclavicular joints (Fig. 15-3).

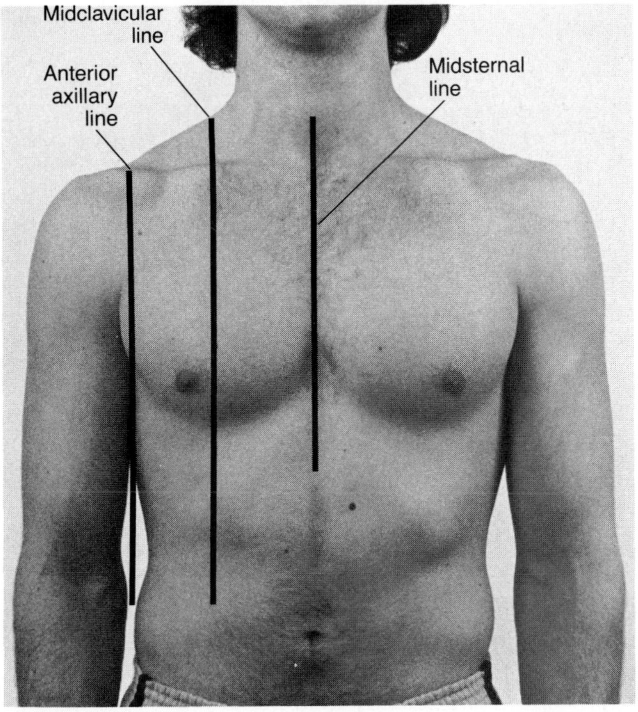

▶ **Figure 15-3**

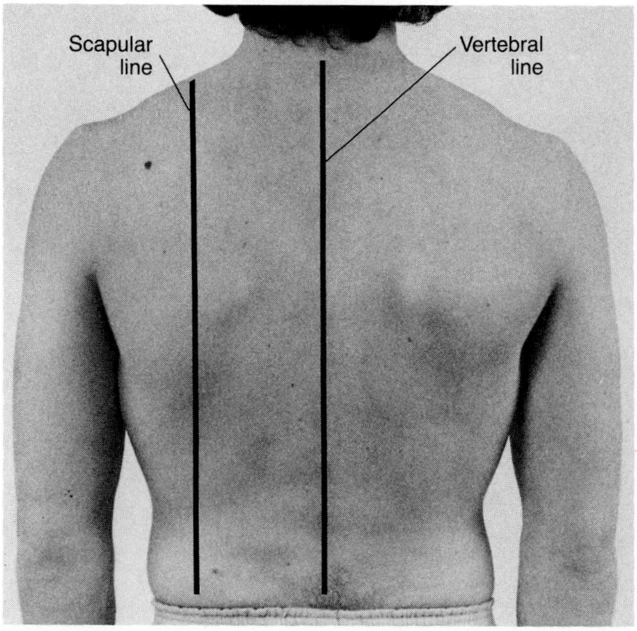

► **Figure 15-4**

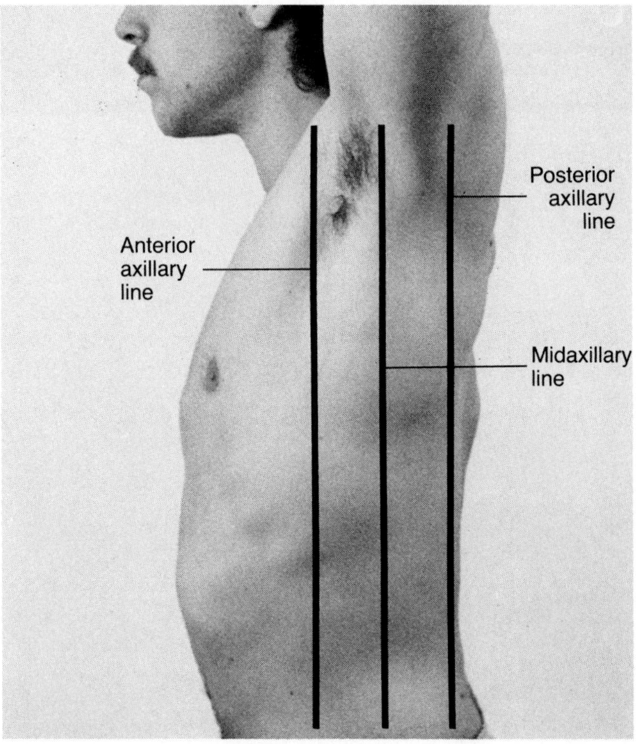

► **Figure 15-5**

The posterior chest wall has the *vertebral* (or midspinal) line and the *scapular* line, which extends through the inferior angle of the scapula when the arms are at the sides of the body (Fig. 15-4).

Lift up the person's arm 90 degrees, and divide the lateral chest by three lines: the *anterior axillary* line extends down from the anterior axillary fold where the pectoralis major muscle inserts; the *posterior axillary* line continues down from the posterior axillary fold where the latissimus dorsi muscle inserts; and the *midaxillary* line runs down from the apex of the axilla and lies between and parallel to the other two (Fig. 15-5).

THE THORACIC CAVITY

The *mediastinum* is the middle section of the thoracic cavity containing the esophagus, trachea, heart, and great vessels. The right and left pleural cavities, on either side of the mediastinum, contain the lungs.

Lung Borders. In the anterior chest the *apex,* or highest point, of lung tissue is 3 or 4 cm above the inner third of the clavicles. The *base,* or lower border, rests on the diaphragm at about the fifth intercostal space in the right midclavicular line and at the sixth rib in the left midclavicular line. Laterally, lung tissue extends from the apex of the axilla down to the seventh or eighth rib. Posteriorly, the location of C7 marks the apex of lung tissue, and T10 usually corresponds to the base. Deep inspiration expands the lungs and their lower border drops to the level of T12.

Lobes of the Lungs. The lungs are paired but not precisely symmetric structures. The right lung is shorter than the left lung because of the underlying liver. The left lung is narrower than the right lung because the heart bulges to the left. The right lung has three lobes, and the left lung has two lobes. These lobes are not arranged in horizontal bands like dessert layers in a parfait glass. Rather, they stack in diagonal sloping segments, and are separated by fissures that run obliquely through the chest.

On the anterior chest, the *oblique* (the major, or diagonal) fissure crosses the fifth rib in the midaxillary line and terminates at the sixth rib in the midclavicular line. The right lung also contains the *horizontal* (minor) fissure, which divides the right upper and middle lobes (Fig. 15-6). This fissure extends from the fifth rib in the right midaxillary line to the third intercostal space or fourth rib at the right sternal border.

The most remarkable point about the posterior chest is that it is almost all lower lobe (Fig. 15-7). The upper

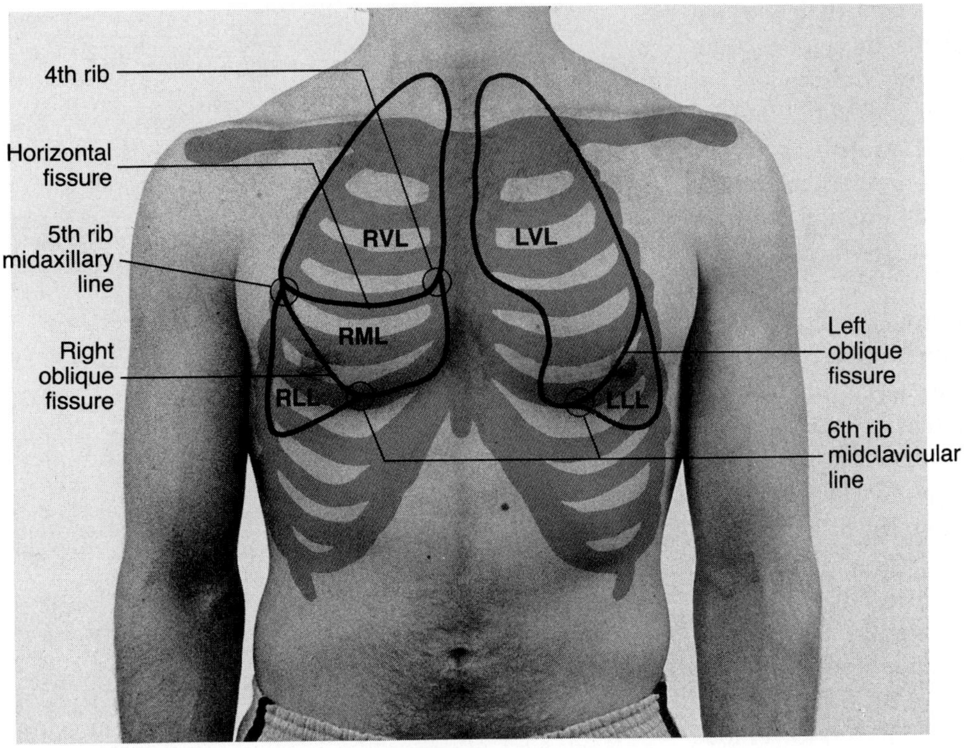

► Figure 15-6

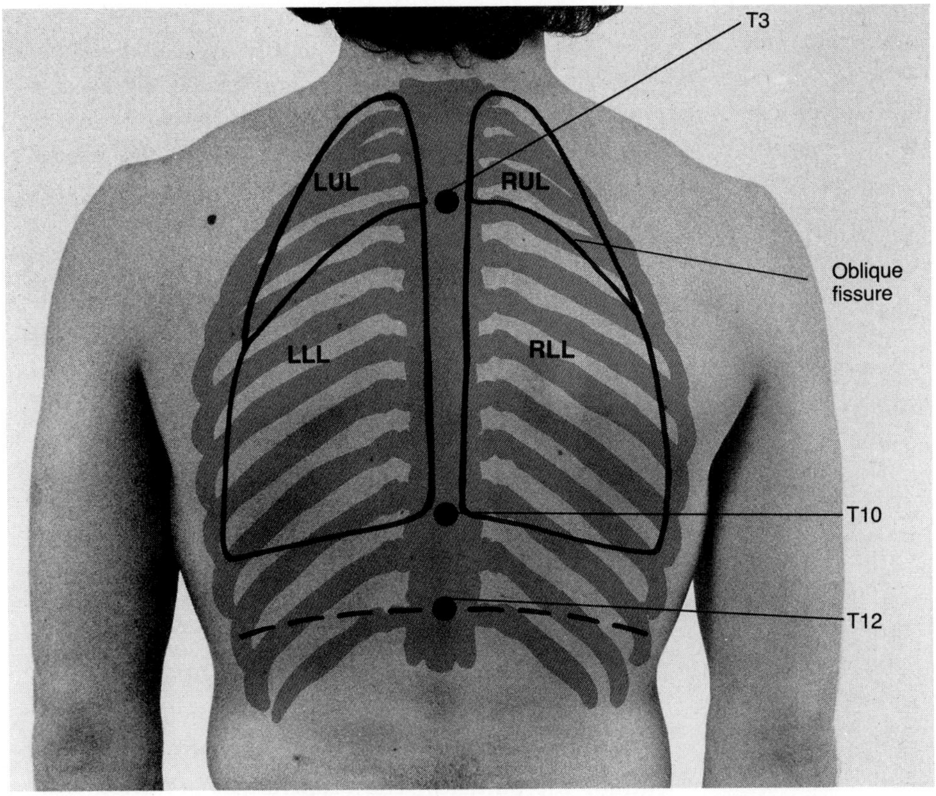

► Figure 15-7

lobes occupy a smaller band of tissue from their apices at T1 down to T3 or T4. At this level, the lower lobes begin and their inferior border reaches down to the level of T10 on expiration and to T12 on inspiration. Note the right middle lobe does not project onto the posterior chest at all. If the person abducts the arms and places the hands on the back of the head, the division between upper and lower lobes corresponds to the medial border of the scapulae.

Laterally, lung tissue extends from the apex of the axilla down to the seventh or eighth rib. The right upper lobe extends from the apex of the axilla down to the horizontal fissure at the fifth rib (Fig. 15–8). The right middle lobe extends from the horizontal fissure down and forward to the sixth rib at the midclavicular line. The right lower lobe continues from the fifth rib to the eighth rib in the midaxillary line.

The left lung contains only two lobes, upper and lower (Fig. 15–9). These are seen laterally as two triangular areas separated by the oblique fissure. The left upper lobe extends from the apex of the axilla down to the fifth rib at the midaxillary line. The left lower lobe continues down to the eighth rib in the midaxillary line.

Using these landmarks, take a grease pencil and try tracing the outline of each lobe on a willing partner. Take special note of the three points that commonly confuse beginning examiners:

1. The left lung has no middle lobe,
2. The anterior chest contains mostly upper and middle lobe with very little lower lobe,
3. The posterior chest contains almost all lower lobe.

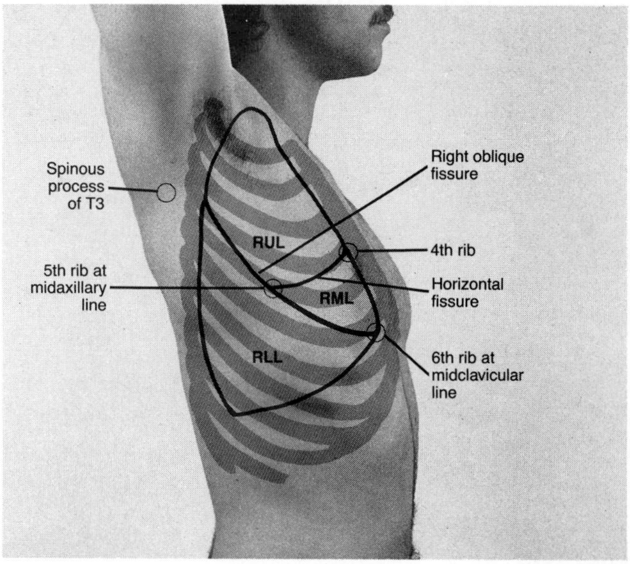

▶ **Figure 15–8**

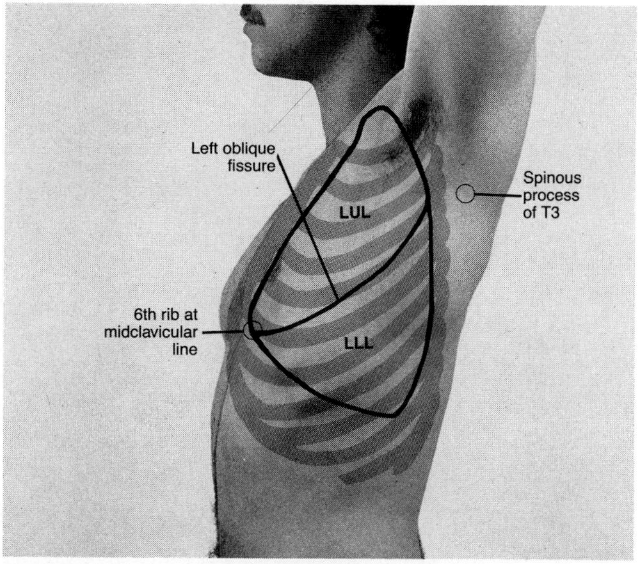

▶ **Figure 15–9**

Pleurae. The thin slippery pleurae form an envelope between the lungs and the chest wall (Fig. 15–10). The *visceral* pleura lines the outside of the lungs, dipping down into the fissures. It is continuous with the *parietal* pleura lining the inside of the chest wall and diaphragm. The inside of the envelope, the pleural cavity, is a potential space filled only with a few milliliters of lubricating fluid. It normally has a vacuum, or negative pressure, which holds the lungs tightly against the chest wall. The lungs slide smoothly and noiselessly up and down during respiration, lubricated by a few milliliters of fluid. The pleurae extend about 3 cm below the level of the lungs, forming the *costodiaphragmatic recess.* This is a potential space; when it abnormally fills with air or fluid, it compromises lung expansion.

Trachea and Bronchial Tree. The trachea lies anterior to the esophagus and is 10 to 11 cm long in the adult. It begins at the level of the cricoid cartilage in the neck and bifurcates just below the sternal angle into the right and left main bronchi. Posteriorly, tracheal bifurcation is at the level of T4 or T5. The right main bronchus is shorter, wider, and more vertical than the left main bronchus.

The trachea and bronchi transport gases between the environment and the lung parenchyma. They constitute the *dead space,* or space that is filled with air but is not available for gaseous exchange. This is about 150 ml in the adult. The bronchial tree also protects alveoli from small particulate matter in the inhaled air. The bronchi are lined with goblet cells, which secrete mucus that entraps the particles. The bronchi also are lined with

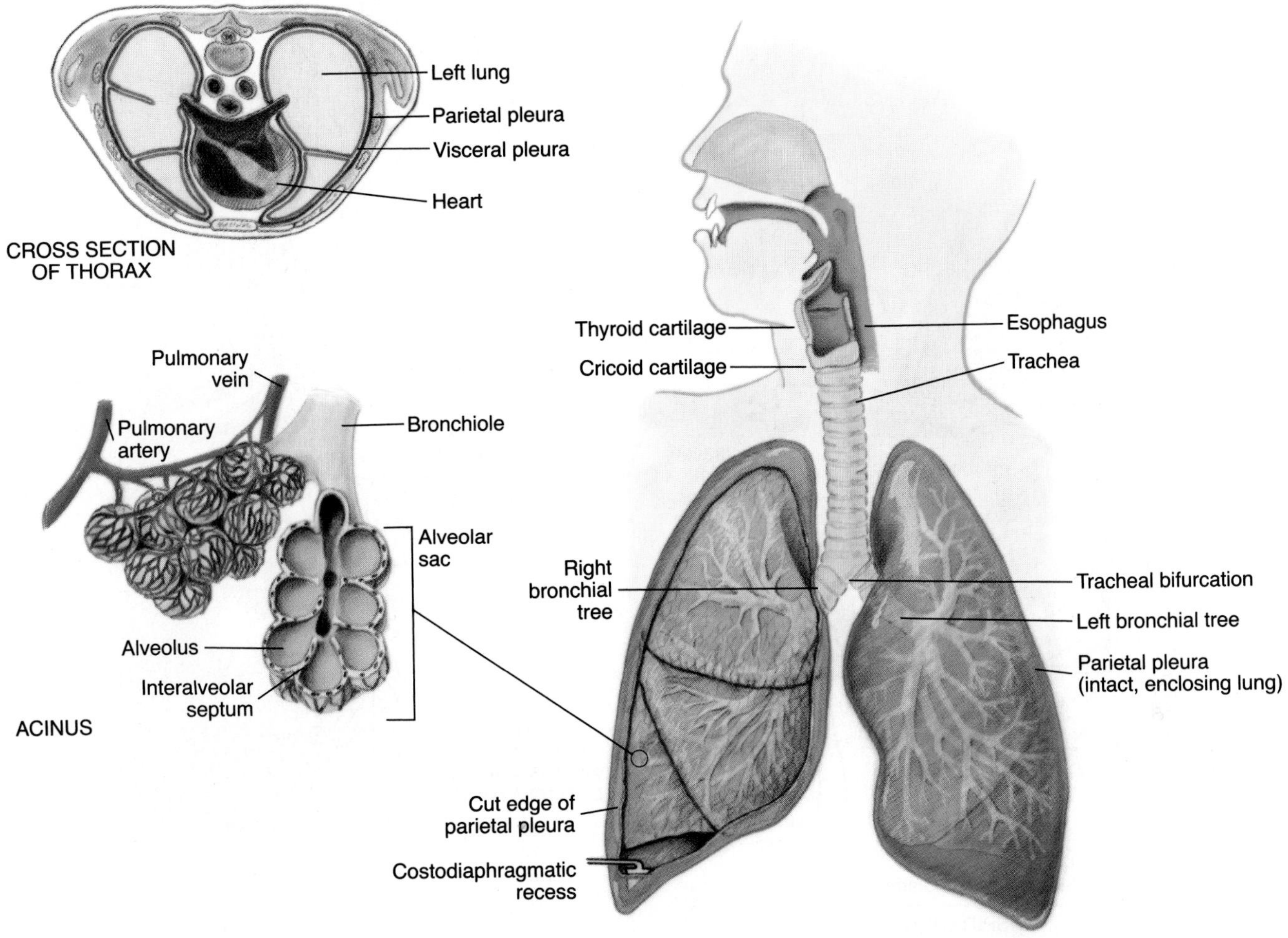

▶ **Figure 15-10**

cilia, which sweep particles upward where they can be swallowed or expelled.

An *acinus* is a functional respiratory unit and consists of the bronchioles, alveolar ducts, alveolar sacs, and the alveoli. Gaseous exchange occurs across the respiratory membrane in the alveolar duct and in the millions of alveoli. Note how the alveoli are clustered like grapes around each alveolar duct. This creates millions of interalveolar septa (walls) that increase tremendously the working space available for gas exchange. This bunched arrangement creates a surface area for gas exchange that is as large as a tennis court.

MECHANICS OF RESPIRATION

The purpose of the lungs is to maintain homeostasis of arterial blood. By supplying oxygen to the blood and eliminating excess carbon dioxide, respiration maintains the pH or the acid-base balance of the blood.

The body tissues are bathed by blood that normally has a narrow acceptable range of pH. Although a number of compensatory mechanisms regulate the pH, the lungs help maintain the balance by adjusting the level of carbon dioxide through respiration. That is, hypoventilation (slow, shallow breathing) causes carbon dioxide to build up in the blood, and hyperventilation (rapid, deep breathing) causes carbon dioxide to be blown off.

Respiration is the physical act of breathing; air rushes into the lungs as the chest size increases (inspiration) and is expelled from the lungs as the chest recoils (expiration). The mechanical expansion and contraction of the chest cavity alters the size of the thoracic container in two dimensions: (1) The vertical diameter lengthens or shortens; this is accomplished by downward or upward movement of the diaphragm. (2) The anteroposterior diameter increases or decreases; this is accomplished by elevation or depression of the ribs (Fig. 15-11).

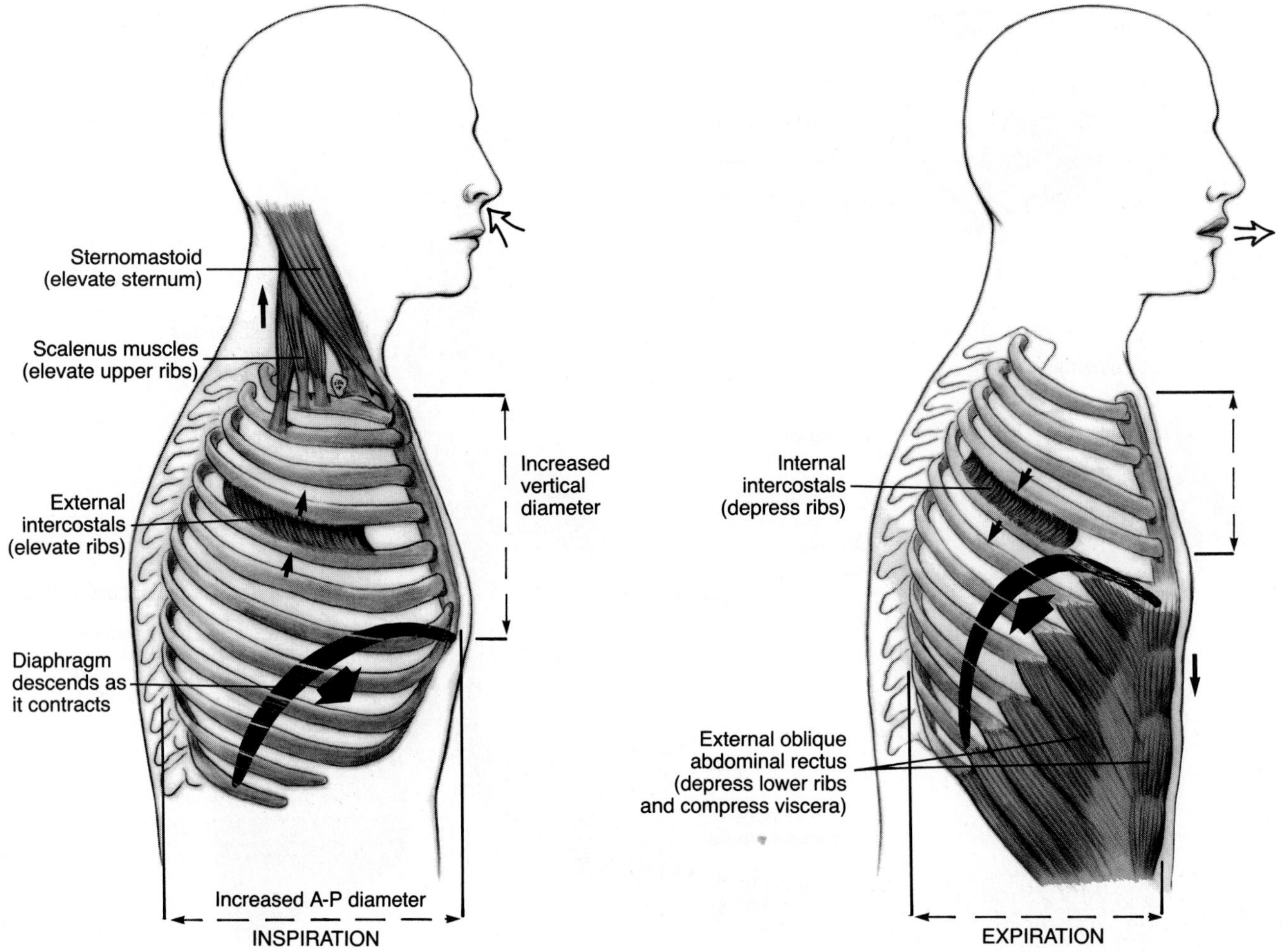

▶ Figure 15-11

In inspiration, increasing the size of the thoracic container creates a slightly negative pressure in relation to the atmosphere, so air rushes in. The major muscle responsible for this increase is the diaphragm. During inspiration, contraction of the bell-shaped diaphragm causes it to descend and flatten. This lengthens the vertical diameter. Intercostal muscles lift the sternum and elevate the ribs making them more horizontal. This increases the anteroposterior (AP) diameter.

Expiration is primarily passive. As the diaphragm relaxes, elastic forces within the lung, chest cage, and abdomen cause it to dome up. All this squeezing creates a relatively positive pressure within the alveoli, and the air flows out.

Forced inspiration, such as that following heavy exercise or occurring pathologically with respiratory distress, commands the use of the accessory neck muscles to heave up the sternum and rib cage. These neck muscles are the sternomastoids, the scaleni, and the trapezii. In forced expiration, the abdominal muscles contract powerfully to push the abdominal viscera forcefully in and up against the diaphragm, making it dome upward, and making it squeeze against the lungs.

Normally, our breathing pattern changes without our awareness in response to cellular demands. This involuntary control of respirations is mediated by the respiratory center in the brain stem (pons and medulla). The major feedback loop is humoral regulation, or the change in carbon dioxide and oxygen levels in the blood, and less importantly, the hydrogen ion level. The normal stimulus to breathe for most of us is an increase of carbon dioxide in the blood, or hypercapnia. A decrease of oxygen in the blood (hypoxemia) also increases respirations but is less effective than hypercapnia.

DEVELOPMENTAL CONSIDERATIONS

Infants and Children

During the first 5 weeks of fetal life, the primitive lung bud emerges; by 16 weeks, the conducting airways reach the same number as in the adult; at 32 weeks, *surfactant,* the complex lipid substance needed for sustained inflation of the air sacs, is present in adequate amounts; and by birth the lungs have 70 million primitive alveoli ready to start the job of respiration.

Breath is life. When the newborn inhales the first breath, the lusty cry that follows reassures straining parents that their baby is all right (Fig. 15–12). The baby's body systems all have been developing in utero, but the respiratory system alone has not been functional until now. Birth demands its instant performance.

When the cord is cut, blood is cut off from the placenta and it gushes into the pulmonary circulation. There is relatively less resistance in the pulmonary arteries than in the aorta, so the foramen ovale closes just after birth. (See the discussion of fetal circulation, Chapter 16, p. 543.) The ductus arteriosus contracts and closes some hours later, and pulmonary and systemic circulation are functional.

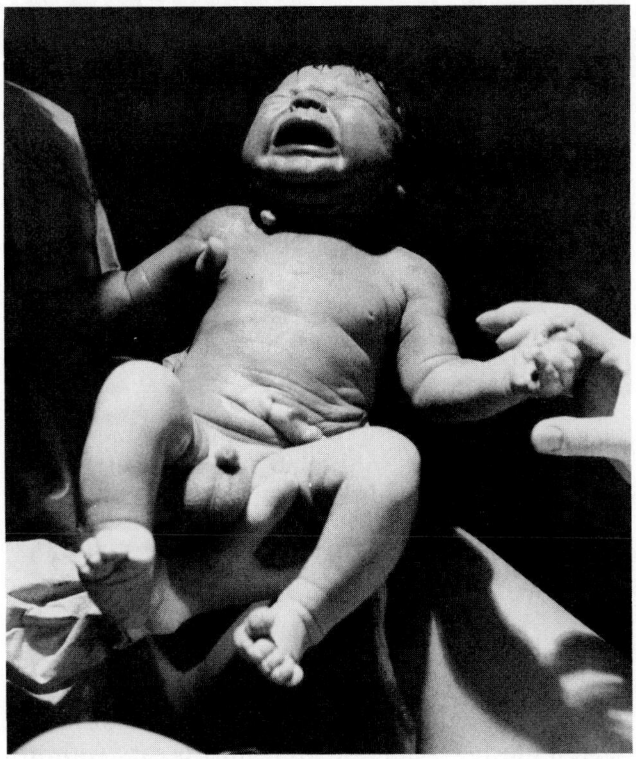

▶ **Figure 15–12**

Respiratory development continues throughout childhood, with increases in diameter and length of airways, and increases in size and number of alveoli, reaching the adult range of 300 million by adolescence.

The Pregnant Female

The enlarging uterus elevates the diaphragm 4 cm during pregnancy. This decreases the vertical diameter of the thoracic cage, but this decrease is compensated for by an increase in the horizontal diameter. The increase in estrogen level relaxes the chest cage ligaments. This allows an increase in the transverse diameter of the chest cage by 2 cm, and the costal angle widens. The total circumference of the chest cage increases by 6 cm. Although the diaphragm is elevated, it is not fixed. It moves with breathing even more during pregnancy, which results in an increase in tidal volume (Pritchard et al, 1985).

The growing fetus increases the oxygen demand on the mother's body. This is met easily by the increasing tidal volume (deeper breathing). There is little change in the respiratory rate. There is an increased awareness of the need to breathe, even early in pregnancy, and some pregnant women may interpret this as dyspnea even though structurally nothing is wrong (Milne et al, 1978).

The Aging Adult

The costal cartilages become calcified, which produces a less mobile thorax, and after age 40 there is some degeneration of respiratory muscles. A more significant change is the decrease in elastic properties within the lungs, making them less distensible and lessening their tendency to collapse and recoil. In all, the aging lung is a more rigid structure that is harder to inflate.

These changes result in an increase in small airway closure, and that yields a decreased vital capacity (the maximum amount of air that a person can expel from the lungs after first filling the lungs to maximum) and an increased residual volume (the amount of air remaining in the lungs even after the most forceful expiration).

With aging there are histologic changes, i.e., a gradual loss of intra-alveolar septa and a decreased number of alveoli, so less surface area is available for gas exchange. Also the lung bases become less ventilated due to closing off of a number of airways. This increases the older person's risk of dyspnea with exertion beyond his or her usual workload.

The histologic changes also increase the older person's risk of postoperative pulmonary complications. That is, the older person has a greater risk of postoperative atelectasis due to a decreased ability to cough, a loss of protective airway reflexes, and increased secretions (Duncalf and Kepes, 1986).

TRANSCULTURAL CONSIDERATIONS

Biocultural differences in the size of the thoracic cavity significantly influence pulmonary functioning as determined by vital capacity and forced expiratory volume (Oscherwitz et al, 1972; Lapp et al, 1974). In descending order, the largest chest volumes are found in whites, blacks, Asians, and Native Americans. Even when the shorter height of Asians is considered, their chest volume remains significantly lower than whites and blacks.

Some biocultural differences are present even before birth. The *lecithin/sphingomyelin ratio* is a laboratory measurement of the amniotic fluid that indicates fetal pulmonary maturation. The ratio is used to calculate the risk of respiratory distress syndrome in premature infants. This ratio differs between blacks and whites, as does the pulmonary maturity it predicts (Olowe and Akinkugbe, 1978). Blacks have higher ratios than whites from 23 to 42 weeks of gestation. Lung maturity, measured by a lecithin/sphingomyelin ratio of 2.0, is reached 1 week earlier in blacks than in whites, i.e., at 34 versus 35 weeks. The risk of respiratory distress syndrome is 40 to 50 percent for a ratio score between 1.5 and 1.9 for premature white infants but not for premature blacks. Premature black infants have a much lower risk of respiratory distress syndrome at the same low ratio scores. When the lecithin/sphingomyelin ratio is determined before induction of labor or elective cesarean section, the racial difference should be considered in making the decision (Overfield, 1985).

SUBJECTIVE DATA

- Cough
- Shortness of breath
- Chest pain with breathing
- Past history of respiratory infections
- Cigarette smoking
- Environmental exposure
- Self-care behaviors

EXAMINER ASKS:	RATIONALE:
1. Do you have a **cough?** When did it start? Was it gradual or sudden? How long have you had it? How often do you cough? Do you cough at any special time of day or just on arising? Does the cough wake you up at night?	Some conditions have a characteristic timing of a cough: Continuous throughout day—associated with acute illness, e.g., respiratory infection Afternoon/evening—may reflect exposure to irritants at work Night—postnasal drip, sinusitis Early morning—chronic bronchial inflammation of smokers.
Do you bring up any phlegm or cough up any sputum? How much do you cough up? What color is it?	Chronic bronchitis occurs with a history of productive cough for 3 months of the year for 2 years in a row.

EXAMINER ASKS:	RATIONALE:
Do you cough up any blood? Does this look like streaks or frank blood? Does the sputum have a foul odor?	Hemoptysis Although sputum is not diagnostic alone, some conditions have characteristic sputum production: white or clear mucoid—colds, bronchitis, viral infections; yellow or green—bacterial infections; rust colored—tuberculosis, pneumococcal pneumonia; pink, frothy—pulmonary edema, some sympathomimetic medications have a side effect of pink-tinged mucus.
How would you describe your cough: hacking, dry, barking, hoarse, congested, bubbling?	Though not mutually exclusive, some conditions have a characteristic cough: mycoplasma pneumonia—hacking; early congestive heart failure—dry; croup—barking; colds, bronchitis, pneumonia—congested.
Does the cough seem to come with anything: activity, position (lying), fever, congestion, talking, anxiety?	
Does activity make it better or worse?	
What treatment have you tried? Prescription or over-the-counter medications, vaporizer, rest, position change?	Assess effectiveness of coping strategies.
Does the cough bring on anything: chest pain, ear pain? Is it tiring? Are you concerned about it?	Note severity.
2. Ever had any **shortness of breath,** or hard breathing spells? What brings it on? How severe is it? How long does it last?	Determine exactly how much activity precipitates the shortness of breath—state specific number of blocks walked, number of stairs.
Is it affected by position, like lying down?	Orthopnea—difficulty breathing when supine. State number of pillows the person sleeps with to achieve comfort, e.g., "2-pillow orthopnea."
Does it occur at any specific time of day or night?	Paroxysmal nocturnal dyspnea—awakened from sleep with shortness of breath and needs to be upright to achieve comfort.
Are the shortness of breath episodes associated with night sweats? Or cough, chest pain, or bluish color around lips or nails? Wheezing sound?	Diaphoresis. Cyanosis.
Do the episodes seem to be related to food, pollen, dust, animals, season, or emotion?	Asthma attacks are associated with a specific allergen.
What do you do in a hard-breathing attack? Do you take a special position, or use pursed-lip breathing? Do you use any oxygen, inhalers, or medications?	Assess effect of coping strategies and the need for more teaching.
How does the shortness of breath affect your work or home activities? Do you think it is getting better or worse or staying about the same?	Assess effect on activities of daily living.
3. Do you have any **chest pain with breathing?** Please point to the exact location.	

EXAMINER ASKS:	RATIONALE:
When did it start? Is it constant or does it come and go? How would you describe the pain: burning, stabbing? Does it seem to be brought on by respiratory infection, coughing, or trauma? Is it associated with fever, deep breathing, unequal chest inflation? What have you done to treat it? Have you used medication or heat application?	
4. Any **past history** of breathing trouble, or lung diseases like bronchitis, emphysema, asthma, pneumonia?	Consider sequelae following these conditions.
Do you have any unusually frequent or unusually severe colds?	Since most people have had some colds, it is more meaningful to ask about excess number or severity.
Is there any family history of allergies, tuberculosis, or asthma?	Assess possible risk factors.
5. Do you **smoke** cigarettes or cigars? At what age did you start? How many packs per day do you smoke now? For how long?	State number of packs per day and the number of years.
Have you ever tried to quit? What helped? Why do you think it did not work? What activities do you associate with smoking?	Most people already know they should quit smoking. Instead of admonishing, assess smoking behavior and ways to modify daily smoking activities.
6. Are there any **environmental conditions** that may affect your breathing? Where do you work? At a factory, chemical plant, coal mine, farming, outdoors in a heavy traffic area?	Pollution exposure. Farmers may be at risk for grain inhalation, pesticide inhalation. Certain areas of North America have a risk of histoplasmosis exposure. Coal miners have a risk of pneumoconiosis. Stone cutters, miners, potters — silicosis. Other irritants: asbestos, beryllium.
Do you do anything to protect your lungs, such as wear a mask or have the ventilatory system checked at work? Do you do anything to monitor your exposure? Do you have periodic examinations, pulmonary function tests, x-ray examination?	Assess **self-care** measures.
Do you know what specific symptoms to note that may signal breathing problems?	General symptoms: cough, shortness of breath. Some gases have specific symptoms: Carbon monoxide — dizziness, headache, fatigue; sulfur dioxide — cough, congestion.
7. When did you last have tuberculosis skin test, chest x-ray study, influenza immunization?	Self-care measures.

ADDITIONAL QUESTIONS FOR INFANTS AND CHILDREN

Has the child had any frequent or very severe colds?	Limit of 4 to 6 uncomplicated upper respiratory infections per year is expected in early childhood.

EXAMINER ASKS:	RATIONALE:
Is there any history of allergy in the family?	
(For child under 2 years of age.) At what age were new foods introduced?	Consider new foods as possible allergens.
Was the child breast-fed or bottle-fed?	Consider formula as allergen.
Does the child have a cough? Does the child seem congested? Does the child have noisy breathing, or wheezing? (Further questions similar to those listed in the section on adults)	Screen for onset and follow course of childhood chronic respiratory problems: asthma, bronchitis.
What measures have you taken to child-proof your home? Yard? Is there any possibility of the child inhaling or swallowing toxic substances?	Self-care behaviors. Young child is at risk for accidental aspiration, poisoning, and injury.
Has anyone taught you emergency care measures in case of accidental choking or a hard-breathing spell?	Assess knowledge level of parent and care givers.

ADDITIONAL QUESTIONS FOR THE AGING ADULT

Have you noticed any shortness of breath or fatigue with your daily activities?	Some older adults have a less efficient respiratory system (decreased vital capacity, less surface area for gas exchange) so they experience less tolerance for activity.
Tell me about your usual amount of physical activity.	Assess self-care behaviors. May have reduced capacity to perform exercise because of pulmonary function deficits of aging. Sedentary or bedridden people are at risk for respiratory dysfunction.
For those with a history of chronic obstructive pulmonary disease (COPD), or lung cancer, or tuberculosis: How are you getting along each day? Have you had any weight change in the last 3 months? How much?	Assess coping strategies.
How about energy level? Do you tire more easily? How does your illness affect you at home? At work?	Activities may decrease because of increasing shortness of breath, or pain.
Do you have any chest pain with breathing?	Some older adults feel pleuritic pain less intensely than younger adults.
Have you had any chest pain after a bout of coughing? After a fall?	Precisely localized sharp pain (person points to it with one finger) —consider fractured rib or muscle injury.

OBJECTIVE DATA

Equipment Needed:

Stethoscope
Small ruler, marked in centimeters
Marking pen

Preparation

Ask the person to sit upright and the male to disrobe to the waist. On the female, leave the gown on and open at the back. When examining the anterior chest, lift up the gown and drape it on her shoulders rather than remove it completely. This promotes comfort by giving her the feeling of being somewhat clothed. These provisions will ensure further comfort: a warm room, a warm diaphragm endpiece, and a private examination time with no interruptions.

For smooth choreography in a complete examination, begin the respiratory examination just after palpating the thyroid gland when you are standing behind the person. Perform the inspection, palpation, percussion, and auscultation on the posterior and lateral thorax. Then move to face the person and repeat the four maneuvers on the anterior chest. This avoids repetitiously moving front-to-back around the person.

METHOD OF EXAMINATION

NORMAL RANGE OF FINDINGS	ABNORMAL FINDINGS
THE POSTERIOR CHEST	
Inspect the posterior chest.	
Note the *shape and configuration* of the chest wall. The spinous processes should appear in a straight line. The thorax is symmetric, in an elliptical shape, with downward sloping ribs, about 45 degrees relative to the spine. The scapulae are placed symmetrically in each hemithorax.	Skeletal deformities may limit thoracic cage excursion: scoliosis, kyphosis (see Table 15–5).
The anteroposterior diameter is less than the transverse diameter. The ratio of anteroposterior : transverse diameter is from 1 : 2 to 5 : 7.	Anteroposterior = transverse diameter, or "barrel chest." Ribs are horizontal, chest appears as if held in continuous inspiration. This occurs in chronic emphysema due to hyperinflation of the lungs (see Table 15–5).
The neck muscles and trapezius muscles should be developed normally for age and occupation.	Neck muscles are hypertrophied in chronic obstructive pulmonary

NORMAL RANGE OF FINDINGS

Note the *position* the person takes to breathe. This includes a relaxed posture and the ability to support one's own weight with arms comfortably at the sides or in the lap.

Assess the *skin color and condition.* Color should be consistent with person's genetic background, with allowance for sun-exposed areas on the chest and the back. There should be no cyanosis or pallor. Note any lesions. Inquire as to any change in a nevus on the back, for example, where the person may have difficulty monitoring (see Chapter 9, Assessing the Skin).

Palpate the posterior chest.

Symmetric Expansion

Confirm *symmetric chest expansion* by placing your warmed hands on the posterolateral chest wall with thumbs at the level of T9 or T10. Slide your hands medially to pinch up a small fold of skin between your thumbs (Fig. 15–13).

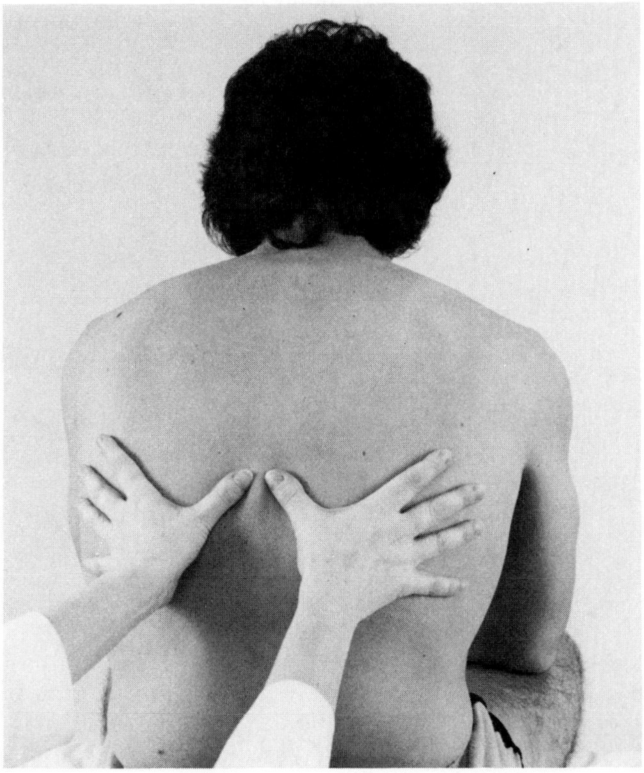

▸ **Figure 15–13**

ABNORMAL FINDINGS

disease from aiding in forced respirations.

People with chronic obstructive pulmonary disease often sit in a tripod position, leaning forward with arms braced against their knees, chair, or bed. This gives them leverage so that their rectus abdominis, intercostal, and accessory neck muscles all can aid in expiration.

NORMAL RANGE OF FINDINGS	ABNORMAL FINDINGS

Ask the person to take a deep breath. Your hands serve as mechanical amplifiers; as the person inhales deeply, your thumbs should move apart symmetrically. Note any lag in expansion.

Unequal chest expansion occurs with marked atelectasis or pneumonia; with thoracic trauma, such as fractured ribs; or pneumothorax.

Pain accompanies deep breathing when the pleurae are inflamed.

Tactile Fremitus

Assess *tactile (or vocal) fremitus.* Fremitus is a palpable vibration. Sounds generated from the larynx are transmitted through patent bronchi and through the lung parenchyma to the chest wall where you feel them as vibrations.

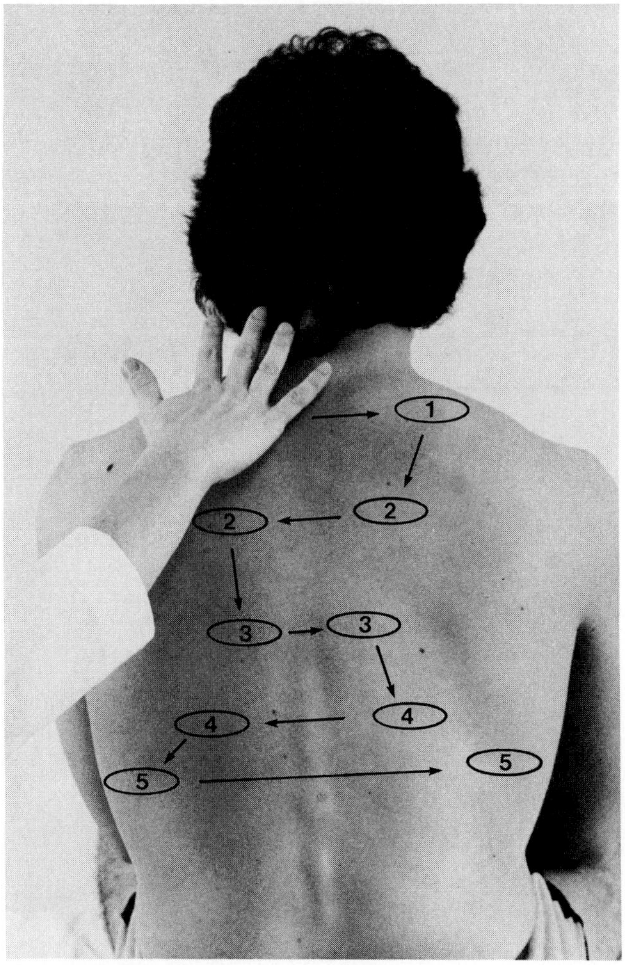

► **Figure 15–14**

NORMAL RANGE OF FINDINGS

Use the palmar base (the ball) of the fingers of one hand, and touch the person's chest while he or she repeats the words "ninety-nine" or "blue moon." These are resonant phrases that generate strong vibrations. Start over the lung apices and palpate from one side to another (Fig. 15–14). Fremitus varies among persons but symmetry is most important; the vibrations should feel the same in the corresponding area on each side. However, just between the scapulae, fremitus may feel stronger on the right side than on the left side. Avoid palpating over the scapulae because bone damps out sound transmission.

The following factors affect the normal intensity of tactile fremitus:

- Relative location of bronchi to the chest wall.

Normally, fremitus is most prominent between the scapulae and around the sternum, sites where the major bronchi are closest to the chest wall. Fremitus normally decreases as you progress down because more and more tissue impedes sound transmission.

- Thickness of the chest wall.

Fremitus feels greater over a thin chest wall than over an obese or heavily muscular one where thick tissue damps the vibration.

- Pitch and intensity.

A loud, low-pitched voice generates more fremitus than a soft, high-pitched one.

Note any areas of abnormal fremitus. Sound is conducted better through a uniformly dense structure than through a porous one, which changes in shape and solidity (as does the lung tissue during normal respiration). Thus, conditions that increase the density of lung tissue make a better conducting medium for sound vibrations and increase tactile fremitus.

Using the fingers, gently *palpate the entire chest* wall. This enables you to note any areas of tenderness, to note skin temperature and moisture, detect any superficial lumps or masses, and explore any skin lesions noted on inspection.

Percuss the posterior chest.

Lung Fields

Determine the *predominant note over the lung fields.* Start at the apices and percuss the band of normally resonant tissue across the tops of both

ABNORMAL FINDINGS

Decreased fremitus occurs when anything obstructs transmission of vibrations, e.g., obstructed bronchus, pleural effusion or thickening, pneumothorax, or emphysema. Any barrier that comes between the sound and your palpating hand will decrease fremitus.

Increased fremitus occurs with compression or consolidation of lung tissue, e.g., lobar pneumonia. This is present only when the bronchus is patent and when the consolidation extends to the lung surface. Note that only gross changes increase fremitus. Small areas of early pneumonia do not significantly affect fremitus.

Rhonchal fremitus is palpable with thick bronchial secretions.

Pleural friction fremitus is palpable with inflammation of the pleura (see Table 15–7, p. 517).

Crepitus is a coarse crackling sensation palpable over the skin surface. It occurs in subcutaneous emphysema when air escapes from the lung and enters the subcutaneous tissue, as following open thoracic injury or surgery.

NORMAL RANGE OF FINDINGS	ABNORMAL FINDINGS

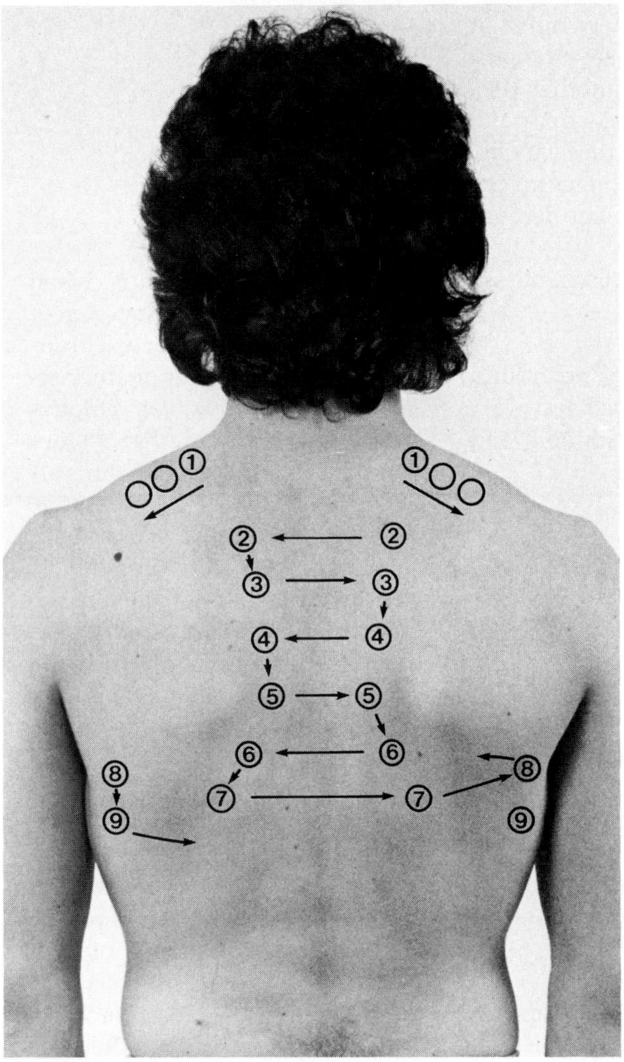

Sequence for percussion

► **Figure 15-15**

shoulders (Fig. 15-15). Then, percussing in the interspaces, make a side-to-side comparison all the way down the lung region. Percuss at 5-cm intervals. Avoid the damping effect of the scapulae and ribs.

Resonance predominates in healthy lung tissue in the adult (Fig. 15-16). However, resonance is a relative term and has no constant standard. The resonant note may be modified somewhat in the athlete with a heavily

Hyperresonance is found when too much air is present, as in emphysema or pneumothorax.

NORMAL RANGE OF FINDINGS

ABNORMAL FINDINGS

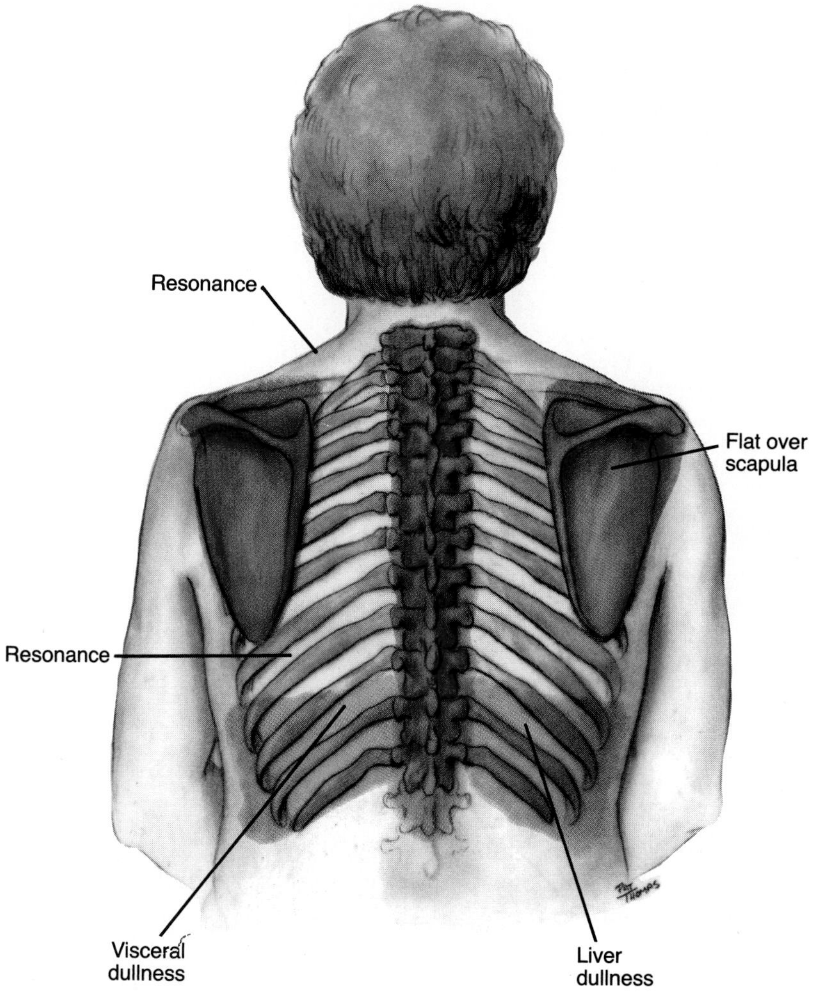

► **Figure 15–16**

muscular chest wall and in the heavily obese adult in whom subcutaneous fat produces scattered dullness.

A *dull* note signals abnormal density in the lungs, as with pneumonia, pleural effusion, atelectasis, or tumor.

There are limits to the depth of penetration of percussion. Percussion sets into motion only the outer 5 to 7 cm of tissue. It will not penetrate to reveal any change in density deeper than that. Also, an abnormal finding must be 2 to 3 cm wide to yield an abnormal percussion note. Lesions smaller than that are not detectable by percussion.

NORMAL RANGE OF FINDINGS | ABNORMAL FINDINGS

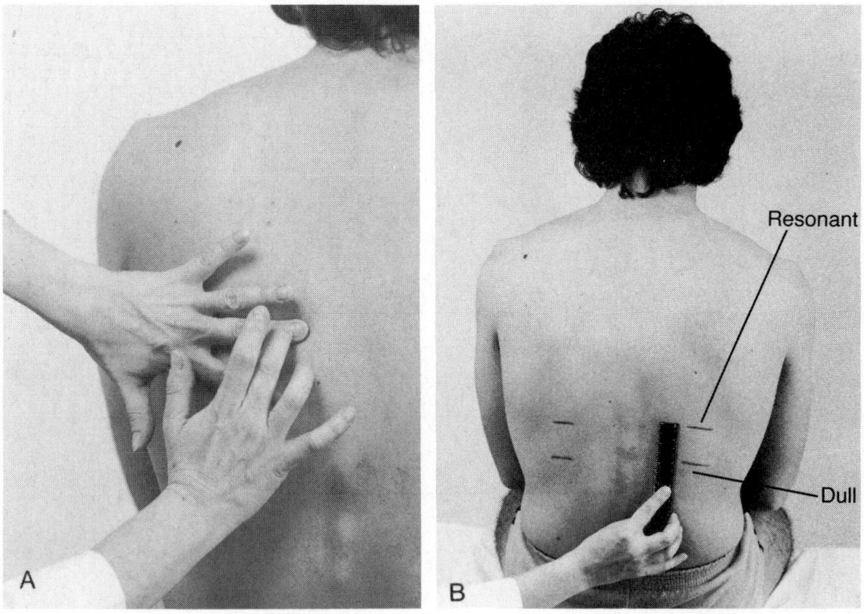

► Figure 15–17

Diaphragmatic Excursion

Determine *diaphragmatic excursion* (Fig. 15–17). Percuss to map out the lower lung border, both in expiration and in inspiration. First, ask the person to "exhale and hold it" briefly while you percuss down the scapular line until the sound changes from resonant to dull on each side. This estimates the level of the diaphragm separating the lungs from the abdominal viscera. It may be somewhat higher on the right side (about 1 to 2 cm) due to the presence of the liver. Mark the spot.

Now ask the person to "take a deep breath and hold it." Continue percussing down from your first mark and mark the level where the sound changes on this deep inspiration. Measure the difference. This *diaphragmatic excursion* should be equal bilaterally and measure about 3 to 5 cm in adults, although it may be up to 7 to 8 cm in well-conditioned people.

An abnormally high level of dullness, as well as absence of excursion occurs with pleural effusion or atelectasis of the lower lobes.

Often, the beginning examiner becomes so involved in the subtle differences of percussion notes that she or he extends the client's limits of breathholding. Always hold your own breath when you ask your client to. When you run out of air, the other person surely has too, especially if that person has a respiratory problem.

Auscultate the posterior chest.

The passage of air through the tracheobronchial tree creates a characteristic set of noises that are audible through the chest wall. These noises also may be modified by obstruction within the respiratory passageways or by changes in the lung parenchyma, the pleura, or the chest wall.

Breath Sounds

Evaluate the presence and quality of *normal breath sounds.* The person is sitting, leaning forward slightly, with arms resting comfortably across the lap. Instruct the person to breathe through the mouth, a little bit deeper

NORMAL RANGE OF FINDINGS

ABNORMAL FINDINGS

than usual, but to stop if he or she begins to feel dizzy. Be careful to monitor the breathing throughout the examination, and offer times for the person to rest and breathe normally. The person is usually willing to comply with your instructions in an effort to please you and to be a "good patient." Watch that he or she does not hyperventilate to the point of fainting.

Use the flat diaphragm endpiece of the stethoscope and hold it firmly on the person's chest wall. Listen to at least one full respiration in each location. Side-to-side comparison is most important.

Do not confuse background noise with lung sounds. Become familiar with these extraneous noises that may be confused with lung pathology if not recognized:

1. Examiner's breathing on stethoscope tubing
2. Stethoscope tubing bumping together
3. Client shivering
4. Client's hairy chest; movement of hairs under stethoscope sounds like crackles (rales) (see p. 518). Minimize this by pressing harder or by wetting the hair with a damp cloth.
5. Rustling of paper gown or paper drapes

While standing behind the person listen to the following lung areas—posterior from the apices at C7 to the bases (around T10), and laterally from the axilla down to the seventh or eighth rib. Use the sequence illustrated in Figure 15–18.

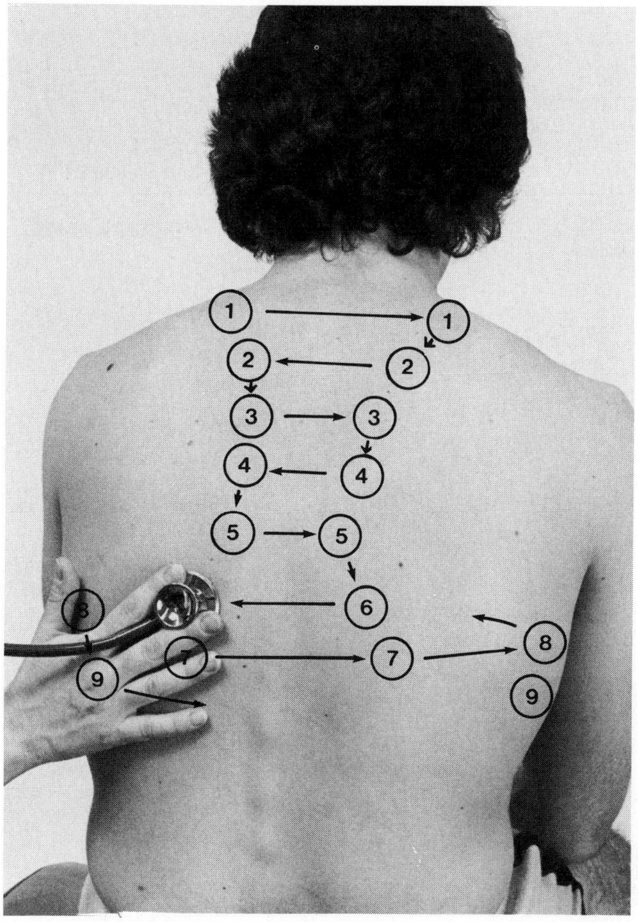

► **Figure 15–18**

NORMAL RANGE OF FINDINGS

Continue to visualize approximate locations of the lobes of each lung so that you correlate your findings to anatomic areas. As you listen, think, (1) What am I hearing over this spot, and (2) What should I EXPECT to be hearing? You should expect to hear three types of normal breath sounds in the adult and older child: bronchial (sometimes called tracheal or tubular), bronchovesicular, and vesicular (Table 15–1).

Note the normal location of the three types of breath sounds on the chest wall of the adult and older child (Figs. 15–19 and 15–20).

ABNORMAL FINDINGS

Decreased or absent breath sounds occur

1. When the bronchial tree is obstructed at some point by secretions, mucous plug or a foreign body
2. In emphysema due to loss of elasticity in the lung fibers and decreased force of inspired air. Also the lungs are already hyperinflated so the inhaled air does not make as much noise
3. When anything obstructs transmission of sound between the lung and your stethoscope, such as pleurisy or pleural

Table 15–1 ▶ Characteristics of Normal Breath Sounds

	PITCH	AMPLITUDE	DURATION	QUALITY	NORMAL LOCATION
Bronchial (Tracheal) 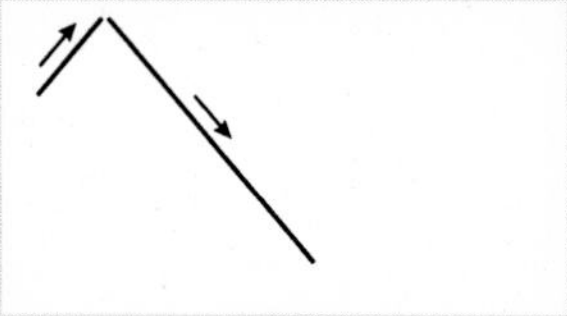	High	Loud	Inspiration < expiration	Harsh, hollow, tubular	Trachea and larynx
Bronchovesicular 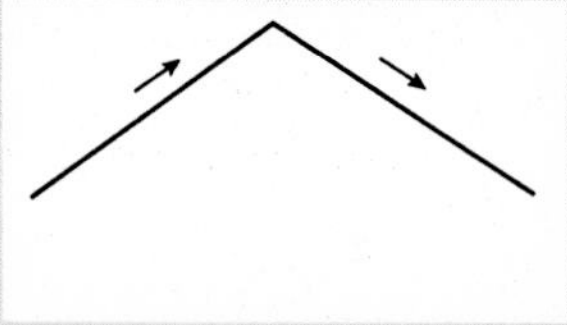	Moderate	Moderate	Inspiration = expiration	Mixed	Over major bronchi where fewer alveoli are located: posterior, between scapulae especially on right; anterior, around upper sternum in first and second intercostal spaces
Vesicular 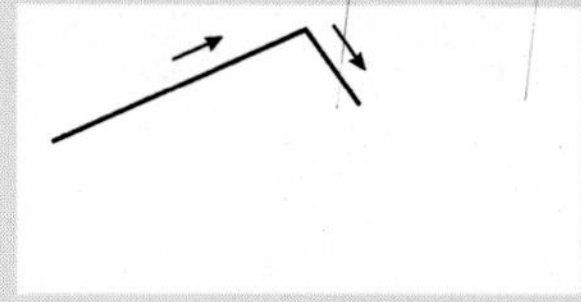	Low	Soft	Inspiration > expiration	Rustling, like the sound of the wind in the trees	Over peripheral lung fields where air flows through smaller bronchioles and alveoli

NORMAL RANGE OF FINDINGS

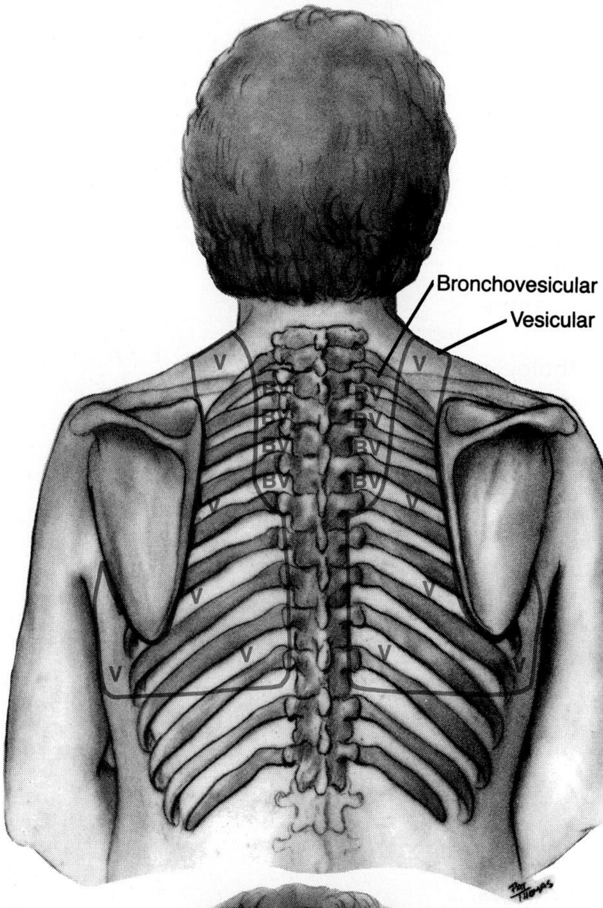

► **Figure 15-19**

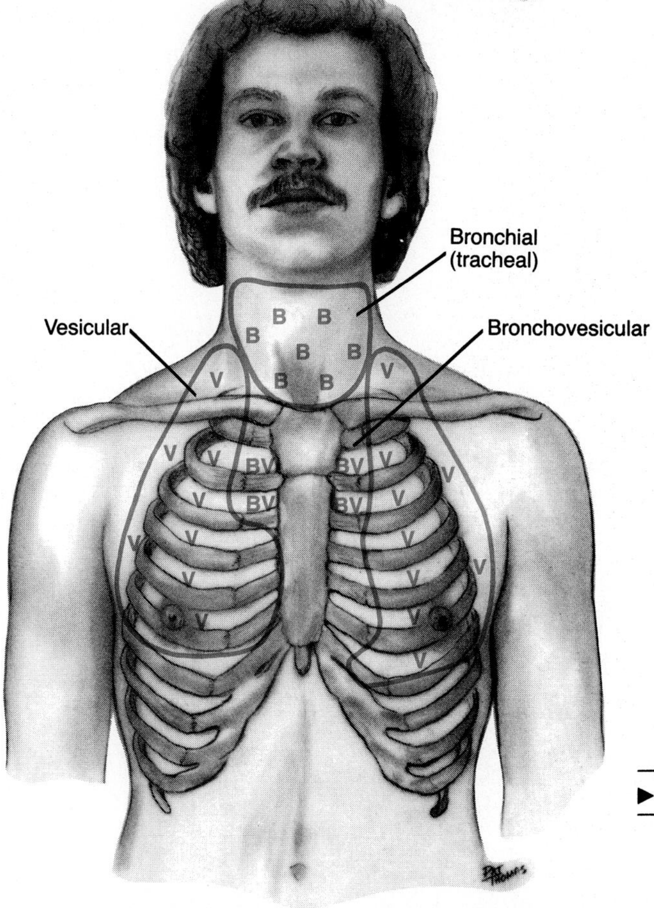

► **Figure 15-20**

ABNORMAL FINDINGS

thickening, or air (pneumothorax) or fluid (pleural effusion) in the pleural space.

A silent chest means no air is moving in or out, which is a serious sign.

Increased breath sounds—bronchial sounds are abnormal when they are heard over an abnormal location, the peripheral lung fields. They have a high-pitched tubular quality, with a prolonged expiratory phase and a distinct pause between inspiration and expiration. They sound very close to your stethoscope, as if they were right *in* the tubing close to your ear. They occur when consolidation (e.g., pneumonia) or compression yields a denser lung area that enhances the transmission of sound from the bronchi. When the inspired air reaches the alveoli, it hits solid lung tissue that conducts sound more efficiently to the surface.

NORMAL RANGE OF FINDINGS	ABNORMAL FINDINGS

Adventitious Sounds

Note the presence of any *adventitious sounds.* These are added sounds that are *not* normally heard in the lungs. If present, they are heard as being superimposed on the breath sounds. They are caused by moving air colliding with secretions in the tracheobronchial passageways, or by the popping open of previously deflated airways. Sources differ as to the classification and nomenclature of these sounds (see Table 15–8), but crackles (or rales) and wheeze (or rhonchi) are terms commonly used by many examiners.

One type of adventitious sound, *atelectatic crackles,* is not pathologic. They are short, popping, crackling sounds that sound like fine crackles but do not last beyond a few breaths. When sections of alveoli are not fully aerated (as in people who are asleep, or in the elderly), they deflate slightly and accumulate secretions. Crackles are heard when these sections are re-expanded by a few deep breaths. Atelectatic crackles are heard only in the periphery, usually in dependent portions of the lungs, and disappear after the first few breaths, or after a cough.

In the past, persons were asked to "take a deep breath and blow it out hard," in order to screen for the presence of wheezing. However, this maneuver is futile because it is now known that wheezing may occur on maximal forced exhalation in normal people (King et al, 1989).

During normal tidal flow, wheezing indicates asthma.

Voice Sounds

Determine the quality of *voice sounds or vocal resonance.* The spoken voice can be auscultated over the chest wall just as it can be felt in tactile fremitus described earlier. Ask the person to repeat a phrase while you listen over the chest wall. Normal voice transmission is soft, muffled, and indistinct; you can hear sound through the stethoscope but cannot distinguish exactly what is being said. Pathology that increases lung density enhances transmission of voice sounds.

Consolidation or compression of lung tissue will enhance the voice sounds.

Eliciting the voice sounds is usually not done in the routine examination. Rather, these are supplemental maneuvers that are performed if you suspect lung pathology based on earlier data. When they are performed, you are testing for possible presence of *bronchophony, egophony* and *whispered pectoriloquy* (Table 15–2).

Table 15-2 ▶ Voice Sounds

TECHNIQUE	NORMAL FINDING	ABNORMAL FINDING
Bronchophony Ask the person to repeat "ninety-nine" while you listen with the stethoscope over the chest wall. Listen especially if you suspect pathology.	Normal voice transmission is soft, muffled and indistinct; you can hear sound through the stethoscope but cannot distinguish exactly what is being said.	Pathology that increases lung density will enhance transmission of voice sounds. You auscultate a clear "ninety-nine." The words are more distinct than normal and sound close to your ear.
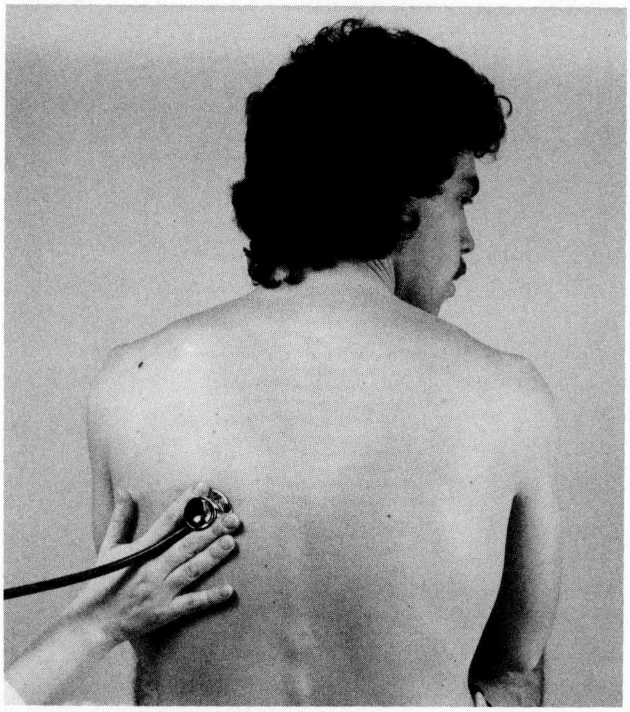		
Egophony (Greek: the voice of a goat) Auscultate the chest while the person phonates a long "ee-ee-ee-ee" sound.	Normally, you should hear "eeeeee" through your stethoscope.	Over areas of consolidation or compression, the spoken "eeee" sound changes to a bleating long "aaaaa" sound. If this is present, record, "E → A changes"
Whispered pectoriloquy Ask the person to whisper a phrase like "one-two-three" as you auscultate.	The normal response is faint, muffled and almost inaudible.	With only small amounts of consolidation, the whispered voice is transmitted very clearly and distinctly, although still somewhat faint. It sounds as if the person is whispering right into your stethoscope, "one-two-three."

NORMAL RANGE OF FINDINGS	ABNORMAL FINDINGS

THE ANTERIOR CHEST

Inspect the anterior chest.

Note the *shape and configuration* of the chest wall. The ribs are sloping downward with symmetric interspaces. The costal angle is within 90 degrees. Development of abdominal muscles is as expected for the person's age, weight, and athletic condition.

Barrel chest has horizontal ribs and costal angle > 90 degrees.

Hypertrophy of abdominal muscles occurs in chronic emphysema.

Note the person's *facial expression.* The facial expression should be relaxed and benign, indicating an unconscious effort of breathing.

Tense, strained, tired facies accompany chronic obstructive pulmonary disease.

The person may purse the lips in a whistling position. By exhaling slowly and against a narrow opening, the pressure in the bronchial tree remains positive and fewer airways collapse.

Assess the *level of consciousness.* The level of consciousness should be alert and cooperative.

Cerebral hypoxia may be reflected by excessive drowsiness or by anxiety, restlessness, and irritability.

Note *skin color and condition.* The lips and nail beds are free of cyanosis or unusual pallor. The nails are of normal configuration. Explore any skin lesions.

Clubbing of distal phalanx occurs with chronic respiratory disease.

Cutaneous angiomas (spider nevi) associated with liver disease or portal hypertension may be evident on the chest.

Assess the quality of *respirations.* Normal relaxed breathing is automatic and effortless, regular and even, and produces no noise. The chest expands symmetrically with each inspiration. Note any localized lag on inspiration.

Noisy breathing occurs with severe asthma or chronic bronchitis.

Unequal chest expansion occurs when part of the lung is obstructed or collapsed, as with pneumonia, or guarding to avoid postoperative incisional pain or the pain of pleurisy.

There should be no retraction or bulging of the interspaces on inspiration.

Retraction suggests obstruction of respiratory tract or increased inspiratory effort is needed as with atelectasis. Bulging indicates trapped air as in the forced expiration associated with emphysema or asthma.

Normally, accessory muscles are not used to augment respiratory effort. However, with very heavy exercise, the accessory neck muscles (scalene, sternomastoid, trapezius) are used momentarily to enhance inspiration.

Accessory muscles must be used in acute airway obstruction and massive atelectasis.

Rectus abdominis and internal intercostal muscles are used to force expiration in chronic obstructive pulmonary disease.

NORMAL RANGE OF FINDINGS

The respiratory rate is within normal limits for the person's age (see Chapter 8) and the pattern of breathing is regular. Occasional sighs normally punctuate breathing.

Palpate the anterior chest.

Palpate *symmetric chest expansion.* Place your hands on the anterolateral wall with the thumbs along the costal margins and pointing toward the xiphoid process (Fig. 15–21).

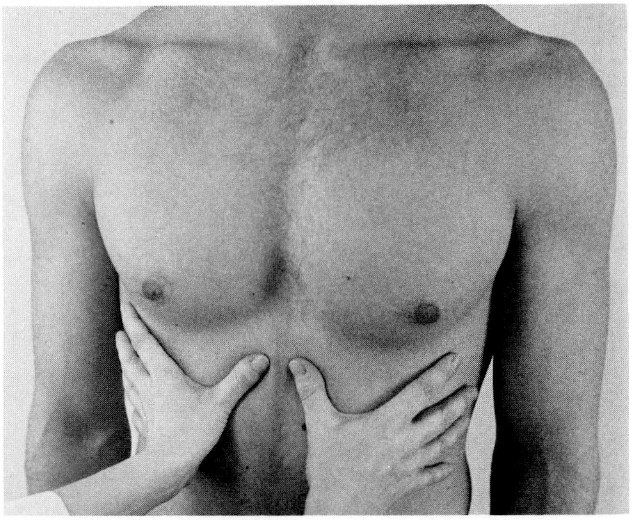

► Figure 15–21

Ask the person to take a deep breath. Watch your thumbs move apart symmetrically, and note smooth chest expansion with your fingers. Any limitation in thoracic expansion is easier to detect on the anterior chest because there is greater range of motion with breathing here.

ABNORMAL FINDINGS

Tachypnea and hyperventilation, bradypnea and hypoventilation, periodic breathing (see Table 15–6).

An abnormally wide costal angle with little inspiratory variation occurs with emphysema.

A lag in expansion occurs with atelectasis, pneumonia, and postoperative guarding.

A palpable grating sensation with breathing indicates pleural friction fremitus (see Table 15–7).

NORMAL RANGE OF FINDINGS	ABNORMAL FINDINGS

Assess *tactile (vocal) fremitus.* Begin palpating over the lung apices in the supraclavicular areas (Fig. 15–22). Compare vibrations from one side to the other as the person repeats "ninety-nine." Avoid palpating over female breast tissue because breast tissue normally damps the sound.

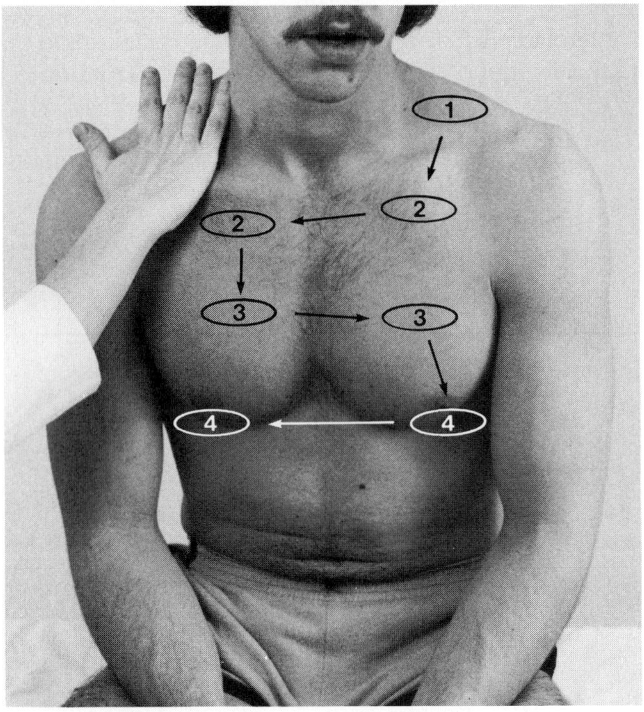

▶ **Figure 15–22**

Palpate the anterior chest wall to note any tenderness (normally there is none) and to detect any superficial lumps or masses (again, normally there are none). Note skin mobility and turgor, and note skin temperature and moisture.

Percuss the anterior chest.

Begin percussing the apices in the supraclavicular areas. Then, percussing the interspaces and comparing one side to the other, move down the anterior chest.

Interspaces are easier to palpate on the anterior chest than on the back. Do not percuss directly over female breast tissue because this would produce a dull note. Shift the breast tissue over slightly using the edge of your stationary hand. In females with large breasts, percussion may yield little useful data. With all people, use the sequence illustrated in Figure 15–23.

Note the borders of cardiac dullness normally found on the anterior chest and do not confuse these with suspected lung pathology (Fig. 15–24). In the right hemithorax, the upper border of liver dullness is located in the fifth intercostal space in the right midclavicular line. On the left, tympany is evident over the gastric space.

Lungs are hyperinflated with chronic emphysema, resulting in hyperresonance where you would expect cardiac dullness.

NORMAL RANGE OF FINDINGS

ABNORMAL FINDINGS

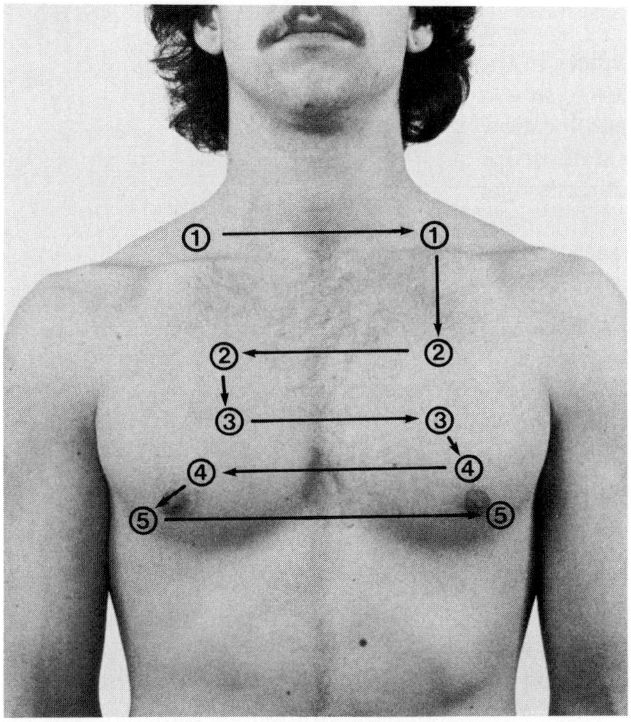

► **Figure 15-23**

Sequence for percussion and auscultation

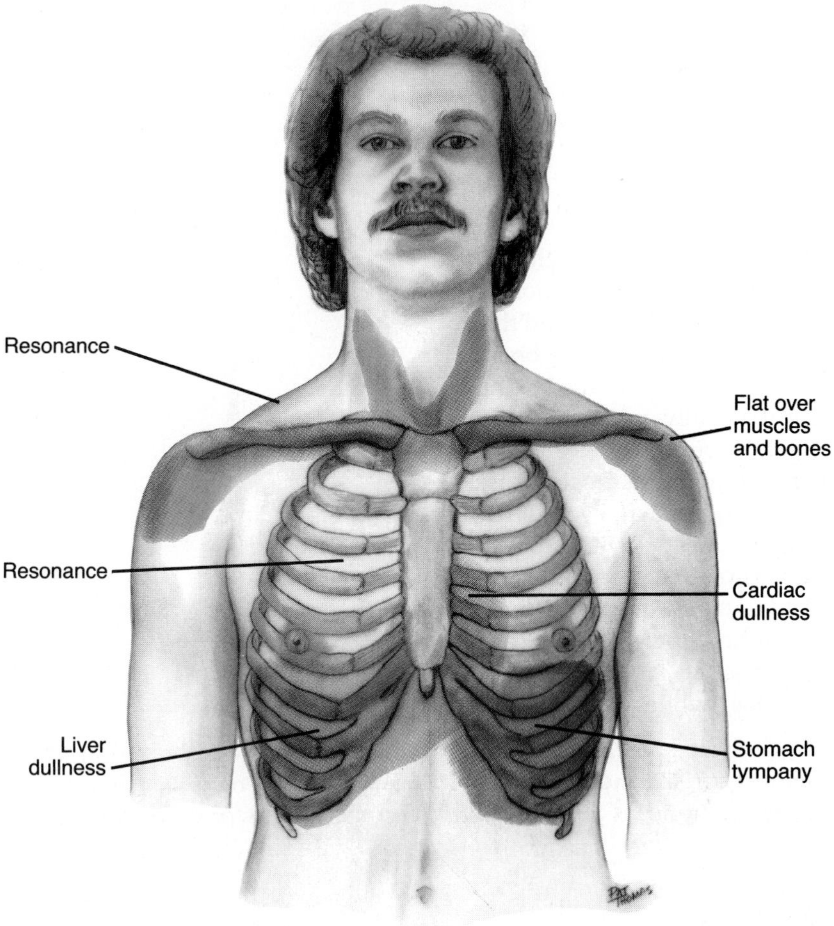

► **Figure 15-24**

NORMAL RANGE OF FINDINGS	ABNORMAL FINDINGS

Auscultate the anterior chest.

Auscultate the lung fields over the anterior chest from the apices in the supraclavicular areas down to the sixth rib. Progress from side to side as you move downward, and listen to one full respiration in each location. Use the sequence indicated for percussion. Do not place your stethoscope directly over the female breast. Displace the breast and listen directly over the chest wall.

Evaluate normal breath sounds, note any abnormal breath sounds and any adventitious sounds. If the situation warrants, assess the voice sounds on the anterior chest.

Measurement of Forced Expiratory Time

The *forced expiratory time* is the number of seconds it takes for the person to exhale from total lung capacity to residual volume. It is a screening measure of airflow obstruction. Although the test usually is not performed in the respiratory assessment, it is useful when you wish to screen for pulmonary function.

Ask the person to inhale the deepest breath possible and then to blow it all out hard, as quickly as possible, with the mouth open. Listen with your stethoscope over the sternum. The normal time for full expiration is 4 seconds or less.

A forced expiration of 6 seconds or more occurs with obstructive lung disease. Refer this person for more precise pulmonary function studies.

DEVELOPMENTAL CONSIDERATIONS

Infants and Children

To prepare, let the parent hold an infant supported against the chest or shoulder. Do not let the usual sequence of the physical examination restrain you; seize the opportunity with a sleeping infant to inspect and then to listen to lung sounds next. This way you can concentrate on the breath sounds before the baby wakes up and possibly cries. Infant crying does not have to be a problem for you though, because it actually enhances palpation of tactile fremitus and auscultation of breath sounds.

A child may sit upright on the parent's lap. Offer the stethoscope and let the child handle it. This reduces any fear of the equipment. Promote the child's participation; school-age children usually are delighted to hear their own breath sounds when you place the stethoscope properly. While listening to breath sounds, ask the young child to take a deep breath and "blow out" your penlight while you hold the stethoscope with your other hand. Time your letting go of the penlight button so the light goes off after the child blows. Or, ask the child to "pant like a dog" while you auscultate.

Inspection. The infant has a rounded thorax with an equal anteroposterior: transverse chest diameter (Fig. 15–25). By age 6, the thorax reaches the adult ratio of 1:2. The newborn's chest circumference is 30 to 36 cm

Note a barrel shape persisting after age 6, which may develop with chronic asthma or cystic fibrosis.

NORMAL RANGE OF FINDINGS | ABNORMAL FINDINGS

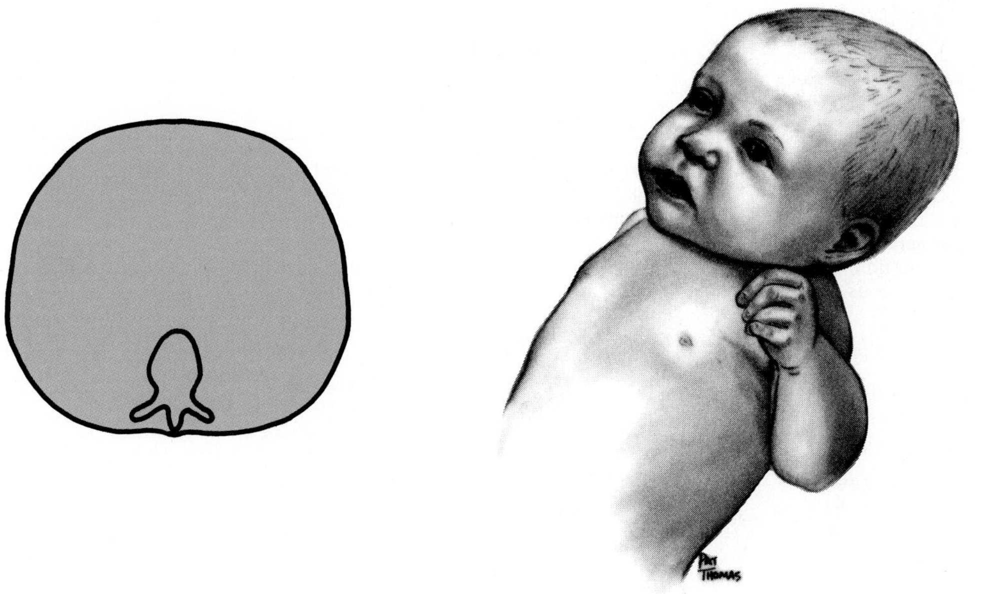

Round thorax in an infant

▶ Figure 15–25

and is 2 cm smaller than the head circumference until 2 years of age. The chest wall is thin with little musculature. The ribs and the xiphoid are prominent; you can see as well as feel the sharp tip of the xiphoid process. The thoracic cage is soft and flexible.

In newborn males and females the breasts may look enlarged by the second or third day due to maternal estrogen. Occasionally, a white fluid, called by the slang expression "witch's milk," can be expressed. This resolves within a week.

In some children, "Harrison's groove" occurs normally. This is a horizontal groove in the rib cage at the level of the diaphragm, extending from the sternum to the midaxillary line.

Harrison's groove also occurs with rickets.

The newborn's first respiratory assessment is part of the Apgar Scoring System to measure the successful transition to extrauterine life (Table 15–3). The five standard parameters are scored at 1 minute and at 5 minutes after birth. A 1-minute Apgar with a total score of 7 to 10 indicates a newborn in good condition, needing only suctioning of the nose and mouth and otherwise routine care.

In the immediate newborn period, depressed respirations are due to maternal drugs, interruption of the uterine blood supply, or obstruction of the tracheobronchial tree with mucus or fluid.

A 1-minute Apgar with a total score of 3 to 6 indicates a moderately depressed newborn needing more resuscitation and subsequent close observation. A score of 0 to 2 indicates a severely depressed newborn needing full resuscitation, ventilatory assistance, and subsequent intensive care.

NORMAL RANGE OF FINDINGS | **ABNORMAL FINDINGS**

Table 15-3 ▶ Apgar Scoring System

	2	1	0	
Heart rate	Over 100	Slow (below 100)	Absent	______
Respiratory effort	Good, sustained cry; regular respirations	Slow, irregular, shallow	Absent	______
Muscle tone	Active motion, spontaneous flexion	Some flexion of extremities; some resistance to extension	Limp, flaccid	______
Reflex irritability (response to catheter in nares)	Sneeze, cough, cry	Grimace, frown	No response	______
Color	Completely pink	Body pink, extremities pale	Cyanotic, pale	______
			Total Score	______

The infant breathes through the nose rather than the mouth, and is an obligatory nose-breather until 3 months. There may be slight flaring of the lower costal margins with respirations, but normally there is no flaring of the nostrils and no sternal retractions or intercostal retractions. The diaphragm is the newborn's major respiratory muscle. Intercostal muscles are not well developed. Thus you observe the abdomen bulge with each inspiration but see little thoracic expansion.

Marked retractions of sternum and intercostal muscles indicate increased inspiratory effort, as in atelectasis, pneumonia, asthma, acute airway obstruction.

Count the respiratory rate for 1 full minute. Normal rates for the newborn are 30 to 40 breaths per minute but may spike up to 60 per minute (Table 15-4). Obtain the most accurate respiratory rate by counting when the infant is asleep, because infants reach rapid rates with very little excitation when awake. The respiratory pattern may be irregular when there are extremes in room temperature, or with feeding or sleeping. Brief periods of apnea less than 10 or 15 seconds are common. This periodic breathing is more common in premature infants.

Rapid respiratory rates accompany pneumonia, fever, pain, heart disease, and anemia.

In an infant, tachypnea of 50 to 100 per minute during sleep may be an early sign of left-sided congestive heart failure.

Periodic breathing with persistent or prolonged apnea (>20 seconds) may signify an increased risk of sudden infant death syndrome (SIDS).

Table 15-4 ▶ Normal Respiratory Rates

AGE	BREATHS PER MINUTE
Neonate	30 to 40
1 year	20 to 40
2 years	25 to 32
4 years	23 to 30
6 years	21 to 26
8 years	20 to 26
10 years	20 to 26
12 years	18 to 22
14 years	18 to 22
16 years	16 to 20
18 years	12 to 20

NORMAL RANGE OF FINDINGS	ABNORMAL FINDINGS
Palpation. Palpate symmetric chest expansion by encircling the infant's thorax with both hands. Further palpation should yield no lumps, masses, or crepitus, although you may feel the costochondral junctions in some normal infants.	Asymmetric expansion occurs with diaphragmatic hernia or pneumothorax. Crepitus is palpable around a fractured clavicle, which may occur with difficult forceps delivery. Rachitic rosary—prominent round knobs at costochondral junctions, seen in infants with rickets or scurvy.
Percussion. Percussion is of limited usefulness in the newborn and especially in the premature newborn because the adult's fingers are too large in relation to the tiny chest. The percussion note of hyperresonance occurs normally in the infant and young child owing to the relatively thin chest wall. Anything less than hyperresonance would have the same clinical significance as would dullness in the adult. If measured, diaphragmatic excursion measures about 1 to 2 rib interspaces in children.	
Auscultation. Auscultation normally yields bronchovesicular breath sounds in the peripheral lung fields of the infant and young child up to age 5 to 6. Their relatively thin chest walls with underdeveloped musculature do not damp off the sound as do the thicker walls of adults, so breath sounds are louder and harsher.	Diminished breath sounds occur with pneumonia, atelectasis, pleural effusion, or pneumothorax.
Fine crackles are the adventitious sounds commonly heard in the immediate newborn period due to opening of the airways and clearing of fluid. Since the newborn's chest wall is so thin, transmission of sounds is enhanced and heard easily all over the chest, making localization of breath sounds a problem. Even bowel sounds are easily heard in the chest. Try using the smaller pediatric diaphragm endpiece, or place the bell over the infant's interspaces and not over the ribs.	Persistent fine crackles scattered over the chest occur with pneumonia, bronchiolitis, or atelectasis. Crackles only in upper lung fields occur with cystic fibrosis; crackles only in lower lung fields occur with heart failure. Expiratory wheezing occurs with asthma or bronchiolitis. Persistent peristaltic sounds with diminished breath sounds on the same side may indicate diaphragmatic hernia. Stridor is a high-pitched inspiratory crowing sound heard without the stethoscope, occurring with croup or acute epiglottitis.

The Pregnant Female

The thoracic cage may appear wider, and the costal angle may feel wider than in the nonpregnant state. Respirations may be deeper, although this can be quantified only with pulmonary function tests.

NORMAL RANGE OF FINDINGS	ABNORMAL FINDINGS

The Aging Adult

The chest cage commonly shows an increased anteroposterior diameter, giving a round barrel shape, and *kyphosis* or an outward curvature of the thoracic spine (see Table 15–5). The person compensates by holding the head extended and tilted back. You may palpate marked bony prominences because of decreased subcutaneous fat. Chest expansion may be somewhat decreased with the older person, although it still should be symmetric. The costal cartilages become calcified with aging, resulting in a less mobile thorax.

The older person may fatigue easily, especially during auscultation when deep mouth breathing is required. Take care that this person does not hyperventilate and become dizzy. Allow brief rest periods or quiet breathing. If the person does feel faint, holding the breath for a few seconds will restore equilibrium.

The Acutely Ill Person

Ask a second examiner to hold the person's arms and to support him or her in the upright position. If no one else is available, you need to roll the person from side to side, examining the uppermost half of the thorax. This obviously prevents you from comparing findings from one side to another. Also, side flexion of the trunk alters percussion findings because the ribs of the upward side may flex closer together.

☑ SUMMARY CHECKLIST

1 ▶ Inspection
- Thoracic cage
- Respirations
- Skin color and condition
- Person's position
- Facial expression
- Level of consciousness

2 ▶ Palpation
- Confirm symmetric expansion
- Tactile fremitus
- Detect any lumps, masses, tenderness

3 ▶ Percussion
- Percuss over lung fields
- Estimate diaphragmatic excursion

4 ▶ Auscultation
- Assess normal breath sounds
- Note any abnormal breath sounds
  - If so, perform bronchophony, whispered pectoriloquy, egophony
- Note any adventitious sounds

SAMPLE RECORDING

Subjective

- No cough, shortness of breath, or chest pain with breathing. No past history of respiratory diseases. Has "one or none" colds per year. Has never smoked. Works in well-ventilated office—smoking co-workers are restricted to smoke in lounge. Last Tb skin test 4 years PTA, negative. Never had chest x-ray.

Objective

- AP < transverse diameter. Respirations 16/min, relaxed and even. Chest expansion symmetric. Tactile fremitus equal bilaterally. Resonant to percussion over lung fields. Diaphragmatic excurion 5 cm and = bilaterally. Breath sounds clear. No adventitious sounds.

SAMPLE CLINICAL PROBLEM

Thomas G. is a 58-year-old, thin, white, male, traffic patrolman who appears older than stated age. Face is anxious and tense though at no acute distress at this time. Seeks care for "increasing SOB and fatigue in last couple months."

Subjective

- 1 year PTA—Noticed more "winded" than usual when walking > 3–4 blocks. Early morning cough present daily × 10 years, but now increased sputum production to 2 T, frothy white.
  6 mo. PTA—Had a "cold" with severe harsh coughing, productive of 1/2 cup thick white sputum/day. Noted midsternal chest pain (mild) with cough. Lasted 2 weeks. Treated self with humidifier and OTC cough syrup—minimal relief.
  3 mo. PTA—Noticed increasing SOB with less activity. Fatigue and SOB when working outside during traffic rush hours. Unable to take evening walks (usually 2–3 blocks) due to SOB and fatigue. Has 2-pillow orthopnea. Wakes 3–4 times during night.
  Now—Feels he is "worse and needs some help." Continues with 2-pillow orthopnea. Unable to walk > 2 blocks or climb > 1 flight stairs without resting. Unable to blow out birthday candles on cake last week. Morning cough productive of 1/4 cup thin white sputum, cough continues sporadically during day.
  No chest pain, hemoptysis, night sweats, or paroxysmal nocturnal dyspnea. No history of allergies, hospitalizations, or injuries to chest. No family history of Tb, allergies, asthma, or cancer. Smokes cigarettes 2 packs per day × 30 years. Alcohol < one 6-pack beer/week summer months only.

Objective

- Sitting on side of bed with arms propped on bedside table. Resp. resting 24/min, regular, shallow with prolonged expiration; resp. 34/min ambulating. Increased use of accessory muscles, AP = transverse diameter with widening of costal angle, slightly flushed face, tense expression.

Minimal but symmetric chest expansion. Tactile fremitus = bilaterally. No lumps, masses or tenderness to palpation.
Diaphragmatic excursion is 1 cm and = bilaterally. Hyperresonance over lung fields.
Breath sounds diminished. Expiratory wheeze throughout posterior chest, R > L. No crackles.

Assessment

▶ Chronic and increasing SOB
Activity intolerance R/T imbalance between oxygen supply and demand
Sleep pattern disturbance R/T dyspnea and decreased mobility

Nursing Diagnoses Commonly Associated with the Thorax and Lungs—Respiratory Disorders

Diagnosis	Related Factors (Etiology)	Defining Characteristics (Symptoms and Signs)
Activity intolerance	Imbalance between oxygen supply and demand Deconditioned status Pain Fatigue Bed rest Sedentary lifestyle Electrolyte imbalance Hypovolemia Malnourishment Interrupted sleep Impaired sensory or motor function Effects of aging Generalized weakness Side effects of sedatives, tranquilizers, or narcotics Immobility Depression Lack of motivation	Increased or decreased heart rate, blood pressure, respirations Exertional discomfort or dyspnea Redness, cyanosis, or pallor of skin during activity Dizziness during activity Requiring frequent rest periods Worried or uneasy facial expression Verbal report of fatigue or weakness Impaired ability to change position or stand or walk without support Weakness Confusion
Ineffective breathing pattern	Decreased energy, lung expansion Effect of Anesthesia Medication (narcotics, sedatives, tranquilizers)	Abnormal blood gases Altered chest excursion Assumption of three-point position Cough

Diagnosis	Related Factors (Etiology)	Defining Characteristics (Symptoms and Signs)
	Obesity Fatigue Immobility, inactivity Impairment Cognitive Musculoskeletal Neuromuscular Perceptual Inflammatory processes Pain Tracheobronchial obstruction Anxiety	Cyanosis Dyspnea Fremitus Nasal flaring Pursed-lip breathing and prolonged expiratory phase Respiratory rate, depth changes Shortness of breath Tachypnea Use of accessory muscles
Ineffective airway clearance	Decreased energy, fatigue Effects of Anesthesia Infection Medication (narcotics, sedatives, tranquilizers) Inability to cough effectively Perceptual or cognitive impairment Presence of artificial airway Tracheobronchial secretions or obstruction Aspiration of foreign matter Environmental pollutants Inhalation of toxic fumes or substances Trauma	Absent or adventitious sounds Air hunger Change in respiratory rate or depth Cough, effective or ineffective, with or without spasm Cyanosis Diaphoresis Dyspnea Fever Nasal flaring Restlessness Stridor Substernal, intercostal retraction Tachycardia Tachypnea Anxiety
Impaired gas exchange	Altered Blood flow Oxygen-carrying capacity of blood Oxygen supply Alveolar-capillary membrane changes Aspiration of foreign matter Decreased surfactant production	Clubbing of fingers Confusion Cyanosis Fatigue and lethargy Hypercapnia Hypoxia Inability to move secretions Irritability Restlessness

Table continued on following page

Diagnosis	Related Factors (Etiology)	Defining Characteristics (Symptoms and Signs)
	Effects of Anesthesia Medications (narcotics, sedatives, tranquilizers) Hypoventilation or hyperventilation Inhalation of toxic fumes or substances	Somnolence Tachycardia Use of accessory muscles
Fluid volume excess	Compromised regulatory mechanisms Aldosterone Antidiuretic hormone Renin-angiotensin Effects of Age extremes Medications Pregnancy Excessive fluid or sodium intake	Abnormal breath sounds, rales Changes in Respiratory pattern Blood pressure Central venous pressure Mental status Pulmonary artery pressure Specific gravity Edema Pulmonary congestion on x-ray study Shortness of breath, orthopnea Restlessness and anxiety Altered electrolytes Anasarca Azotemia Intake greater than output Jugular vein distention Nausea and/or vomiting Oliguria Positive finding of hepatojugular reflex S_3 heart sound Weight gain
Fatigue	Decreased/increased metabolic energy production Increased energy requirements to perform activities of daily living Overwhelming psychological or emotional demands Excessive social and/or role demands	Verbalization of an unremitting and overwhelming lack of energy Inability to maintain usual routines Increase in physical complaints Inability to concentrate Decreased performance

Diagnosis	Related Factors (Etiology)	Defining Characteristics (Symptoms and Signs)
	States of discomfort Altered body chemistry Medications Drug withdrawal Chemotherapy	Accident prone Lethargy or listlessness Disinterest in surroundings/introspection Decreased libido
Anxiety	Threat to or change in health status, relationships, role functioning, self-concept, socioeconomic status Threat of death Lack of knowledge Loss of control Actual or perceived loss of significant others Situational or maturational crises Unmet needs Unconscious conflict about essential values and goals of life Feelings of failure Disruptive family life Interpersonal transmission and contagion	Trembling Increased blood pressure Rapid respiration and pulse Feelings of helplessness, apprehensiveness, inadequacy, dread, worry Focus on self Irritability Restlessness Inability to concentrate Crying Change in appetite Diaphoresis Lack of eye contact Extraneous movements, foot shuffling, hand or arm movements Nausea Headache Increased wariness Lack of awareness of surroundings Regretful Uncertainty Change in sleeping patterns Agitated Worried Feeling of dread Difficulty expressing self Change in voice quality Fear of unspecific consequences Expressed concern regarding changes in life events

Other related nursing diagnoses

- Impaired home maintenance management (see Chapter 11)
- Pain (see Chapter 13)
- Sleep pattern disturbance

ABNORMAL FINDINGS

Table 15-5 ▸ Configurations of the Thorax

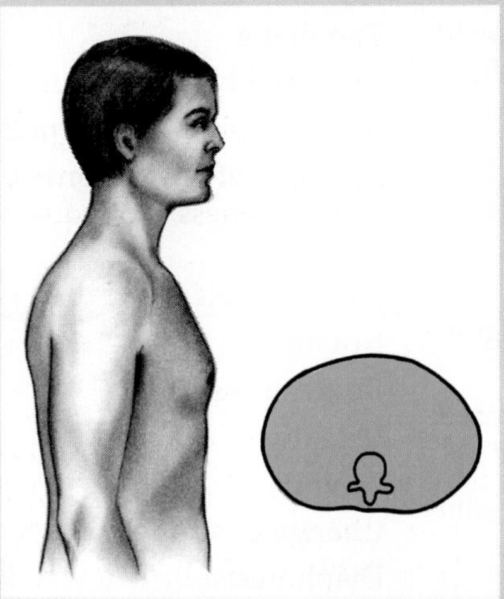

NORMAL ADULT (FOR COMPARISON)

The thorax has an elliptical shape with an anteroposterior : transverse diameter of 1 : 2 or 5 : 7.

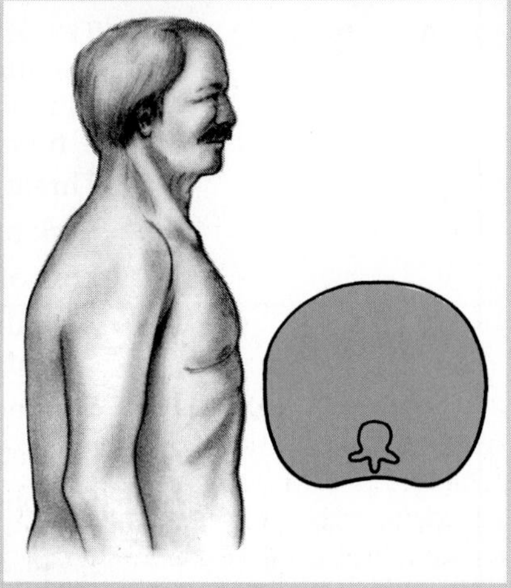

BARREL CHEST

Note anteroposterior = transverse diameter and that ribs are horizontal instead of the normal downward slope. This is associated with normal aging and also with chronic emphysema and asthma due to hyperinflation of lungs.

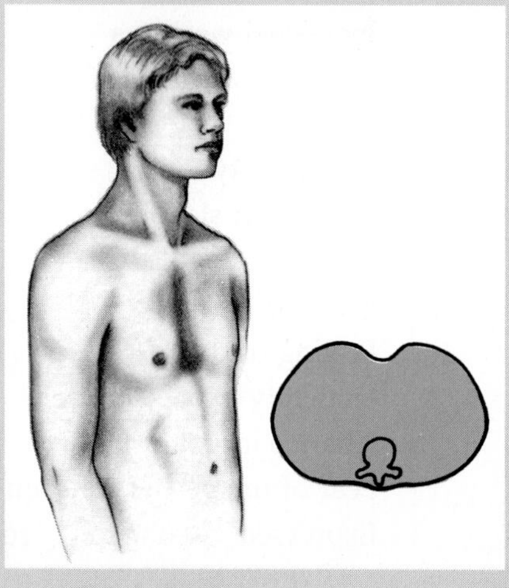

PECTUS EXCAVATUM

A markedly sunken sternum and adjacent cartilages (also called funnel breast). Depression begins at second intercostal space, becoming depressed most at junction of xiphoid with body of sternum. More noticeable on inspiration. Congenital, usually not symptomatic. When severe, sternal depression may cause embarrassment and a negative self-concept. Surgery may be indicated for cosmetic purposes.

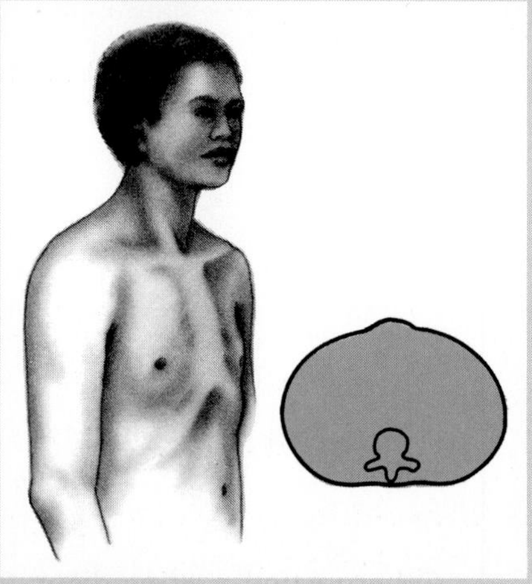

PECTUS CARINATUM

A forward protrusion of the sternum, with ribs sloping back at either side and vertical depressions along costochondral junctions (pigeon breast). Less common than pectus excavatum, this minor deformity requires no treatment. If severe, surgery may be indicated for cosmetic purposes.

Table 15-5 ▸ Configurations of the Thorax *Continued*

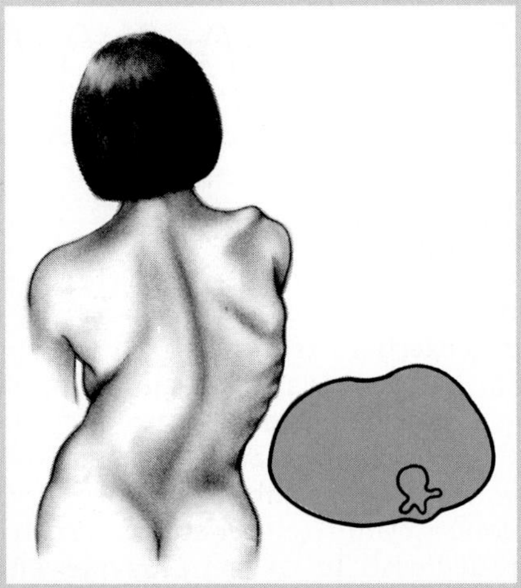

SCOLIOSIS

A lateral S-shaped curvature of the thoracic and lumbar spine, usually with involved vertebrae rotation. Note unequal shoulder and scapular height and unequal hip levels, rib interspaces flared on convex side. More prevalent in adolescent age groups, especially girls. Mild deformities are asymptomatic. If severe (> 45 degrees) deviation is present, scoliosis may reduce lung volume, then person is at risk for impaired cardiopulmonary function. Primary impairment is cosmetic deformity, negatively affecting self-image. Refer early for treatment, often surgery.

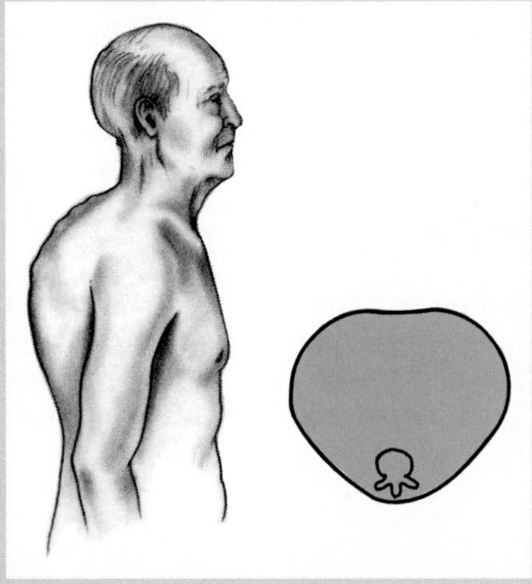

KYPHOSIS

An exaggerated posterior curvature of the thoracic spine (humpback). Mild deformities are asymptomatic. Severe deformities impair cardiopulmonary function. Also associated with aging. Compensation may occur by hyperextension of head to maintain level of vision.

Table 15-6 ▸ Respiratory Patterns*

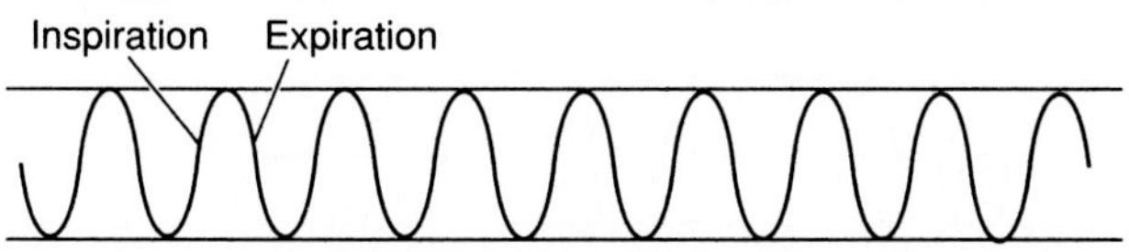

NORMAL ADULT (FOR COMPARISON)

Rate—10 to 20 breaths per minute
Depth—500 ml to 800 ml
Pattern—even
The ratio of pulse to respirations is fairly constant, about 4 : 1. Both values increase as a normal response to exercise, fear, or fever.
Depth—air moving in and out with each respiration.

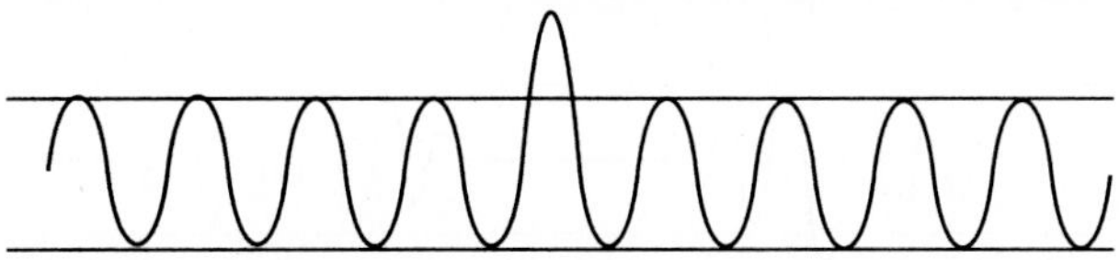

SIGH

Occasional sighs punctuate the normal breathing pattern and are purposeful to expand alveoli. Frequent sighs may indicate emotional dysfunction. Frequent sighs also may lead to hyperventilation and dizziness.

* Assess the (1) rate, (2) depth (tidal volume), and (3) pattern.

Table continued on following page

Table 15-6 ▸ Respiratory Patterns* *Continued*

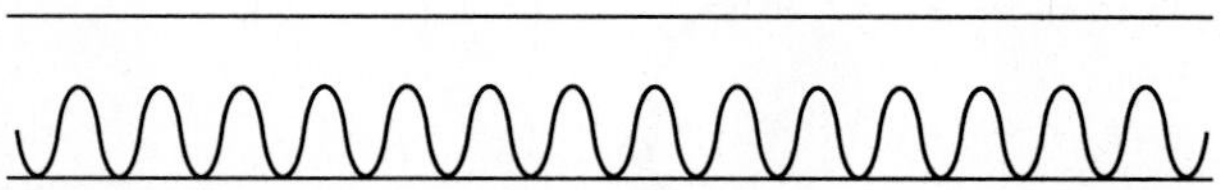

TACHYPNEA

Rapid shallow breathing. Increased rate > 24 per minute. This is a normal response to fever, fear, or exercise. Rate also increases with respiratory insufficiency, pneumonia, alkalosis, pleurisy, and lesions in the pons.

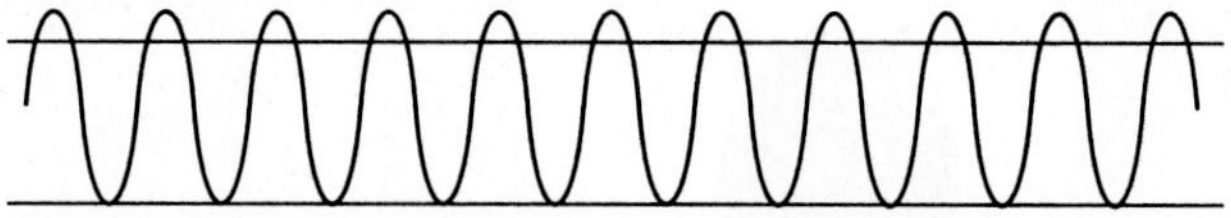

HYPERVENTILATION

Increase in both rate and depth. Normally occurs with extreme exertion, fear, or anxiety. Also occurs with diabetic ketoacidosis (Kussmaul's respirations), hepatic coma, salicylate overdose (producing a respiratory alkalosis to compensate for the metabolic acidosis), lesions of the midbrain, and alteration in blood gas concentration (either an increase in carbon dioxide or decrease in oxygen). Hyperventilation blows off carbon dioxide, causing a decreased level in the blood (alkalosis).

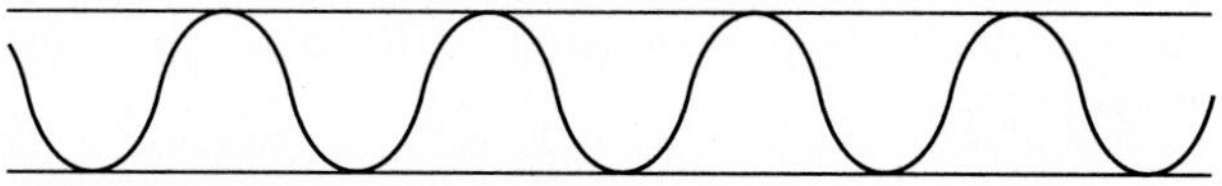

BRADYPNEA

Slow breathing. A decreased but regular rate (less than 10 per minute), as in drug-induced depression of the respiratory center in the medulla, increased intracranial pressure, and diabetic coma.

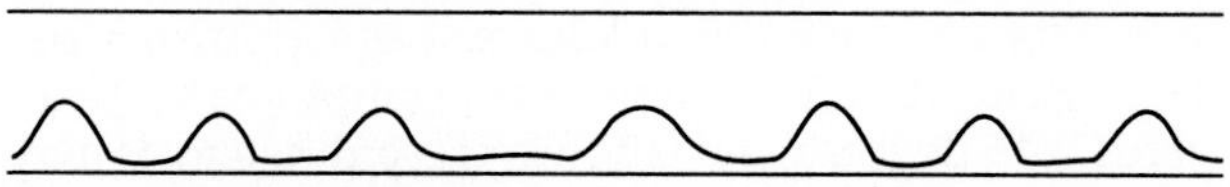

HYPOVENTILATION

An irregular shallow pattern caused by an overdose of narcotics or anesthetics. May also occur with prolonged bed rest or conscious splinting of the chest to avoid respiratory pain.

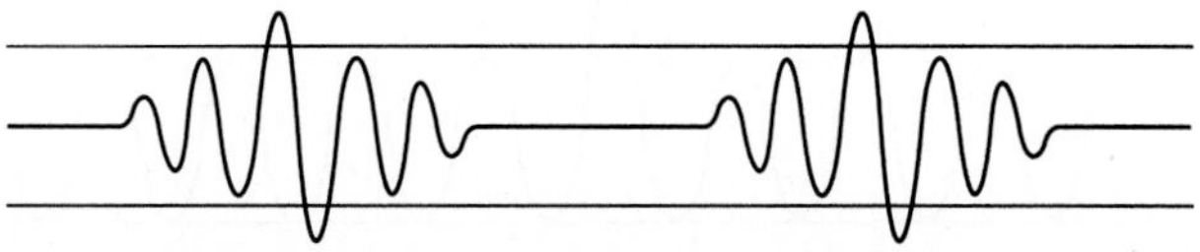

CHEYNE-STOKES RESPIRATION

A cycle in which respirations gradually wax and wane in a regular pattern, increasing in rate and depth and then decreasing. The breathing periods last 30 to 45 seconds, with periods of apnea (20 seconds) alternating the cycle. The most common cause is severe congestive heart failure; other causes are renal failure, meningitis, drug overdose, increased intracranial pressure. Occurs normally in infants and aging persons during sleep.

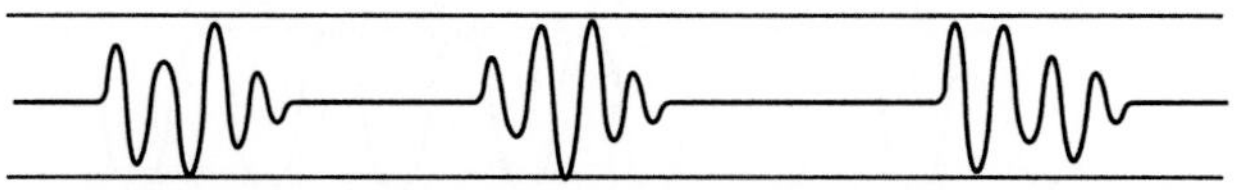

BIOT'S RESPIRATION

Similar to Cheyne-Stokes respiration, except that the pattern is irregular. A series of normal respirations (3 to 4) is followed by a period of apnea. The cycle length is variable, lasting anywhere from 10 seconds to 1 minute. Seen with head trauma, brain abscess, heat stroke, spinal meningitis, and encephalitis.

Table 15-6 ▶ Respiratory Patterns* *Continued*

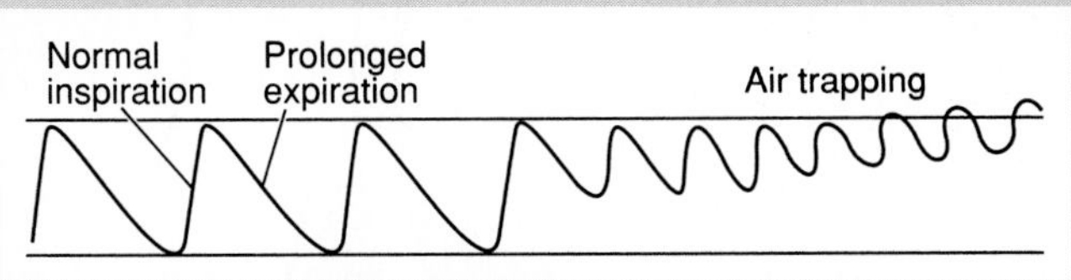

CHRONIC OBSTRUCTIVE BREATHING

Normal inspiration and prolonged expiration to overcome increased airway resistance. In a person with chronic obstructive lung disease, any situation calling for increased rate (exercise) may lead to dyspneic episode (air trapping), because then the person does not have enough time for full expiration.

Table 15-7 ▶ Abnormal Tactile Fremitus

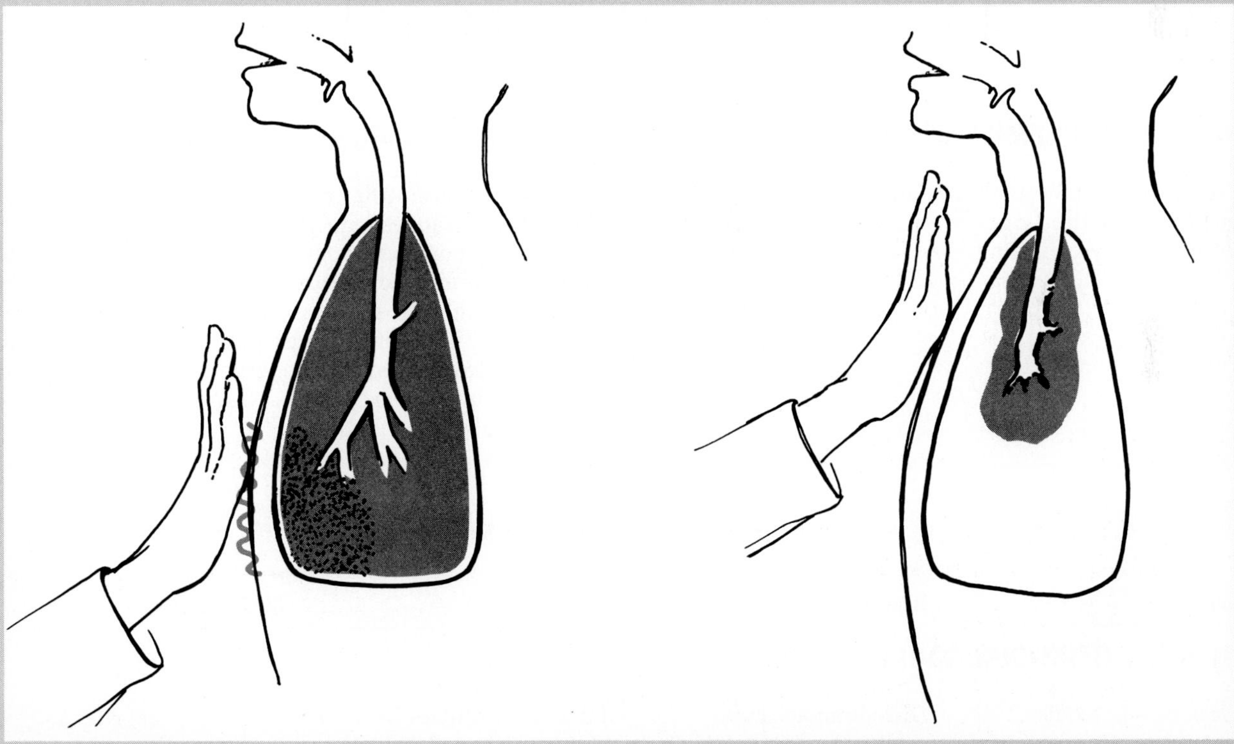

INCREASED TACTILE FREMITUS

Occurs with conditions that increase the density of lung tissue, thereby making a better conducting medium for vibrations, e.g., compression or consolidation (pneumonia). There must be a patent bronchus, and consolidation must extend to lung surface for increased fremitus to be apparent.

DECREASED TACTILE FREMITUS

Occurs when anything obstructs transmission of vibrations, e.g., an obstructed bronchus, pleural effusion or thickening, pneumothorax, and emphysema. Any barrier that gets in the way of the sound and your palpating hand decreases fremitus.

Table continued on following page

Table 15-7 ► Abnormal Tactile Fremitus *Continued*

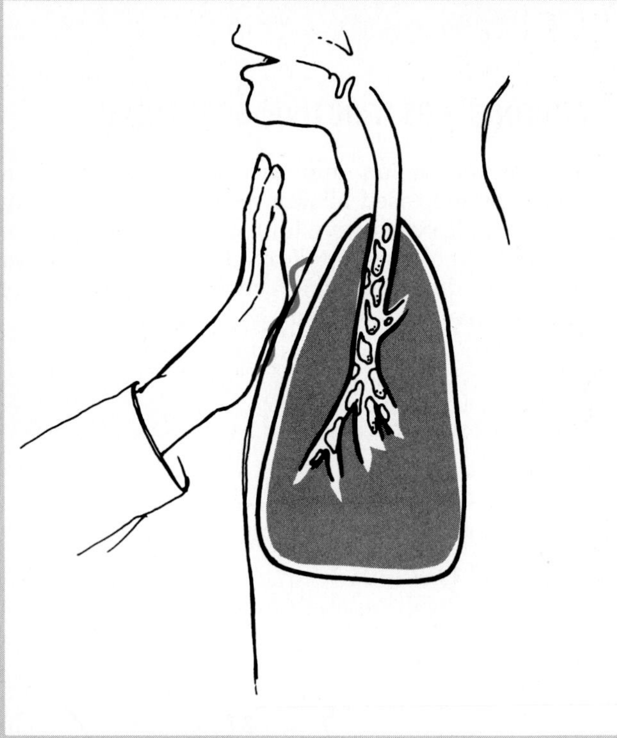

RHONCHAL FREMITUS

Vibration felt when inhaled air passes through thick secretions in the larger bronchi. This may decrease somewhat by coughing.

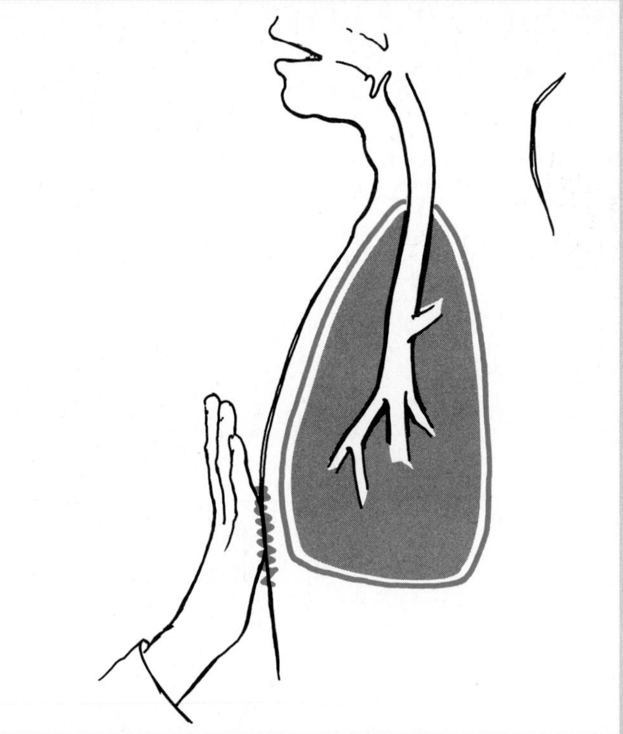

PLEURAL FRICTION FREMITUS

Produced when inflammation of the parietal or visceral pleura causes a decrease in the normal lubricating fluid. Then the opposing surfaces make a coarse grating sound when rubbed together during breathing. Although this sound is best detected by auscultation, it may sometimes be palpable and feels like two pieces of leather grating together. It is synchronous with respiratory excursion. Also called a palpable friction rub.

Table 15-8 ► Adventitious Sounds*

Sound	Description	Mechanism	Clinical Example
(1) DISCONTINUOUS SOUNDS			
Crackles—fine (rales, crepitations) 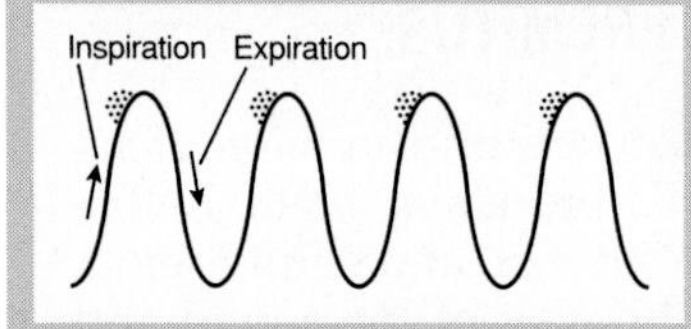	Discontinuous, high-pitched, short crackling, popping sounds heard during inspiration that are not cleared by coughing. You can simulate this sound by rolling a strand of hair between your fingers near your ear, or by moistening your thumb and index finger and separating them near your ear.	Inhaled air collides with previously deflated airways; airways suddenly pop open, creating crackling sound as gas pressures between the two compartments equalize (Forgacs, 1978).	*Late inspiratory crackles* occur with restrictive disease: pneumonia, congestive heart failure, and interstitial fibrosis. *Early inspiratory crackles* occur with obstructive disease: chronic bronchitis, asthma, and emphysema.

* Although nothing in clinical practice seems to differ more than the nomenclature of adventitious sounds, most authorities concur on two categories: (1) discontinuous, discrete crackling sounds, and (2) continuous, coarse, or musical sounds.

Table 15-8 ► Adventitious Sounds* *Continued*

Sound	Description	Mechanism	Clinical Example
Crackles—coarse (coarse rales) 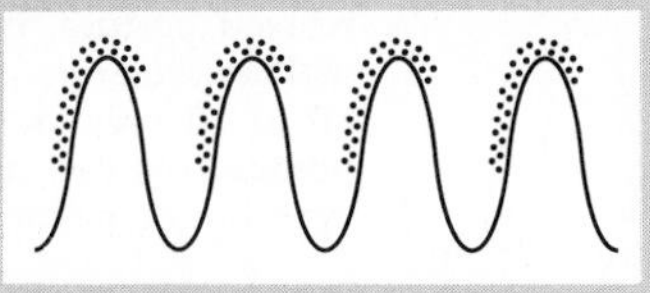	Loud, low-pitched, bubbling and gurgling sounds that start in early inspiration and may be present in expiration. May decrease somewhat by suctioning or coughing but will reappear shortly. Sounds like opening a Velcro fastener.	Inhaled air collides with secretions in the trachea and large bronchi.	Pulmonary edema, pneumonia, pulmonary fibrosis, and in the terminally ill who have a depressed cough reflex.
Atelectatic crackles (atelectatic rales) 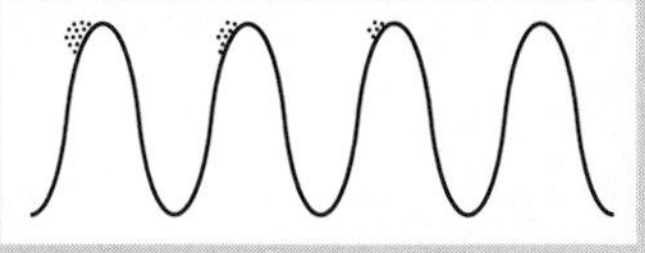	Sound like fine crackles, but do not last and are not pathologic. Disappear after the first few breaths. Heard in axillae and bases (usually dependent) of lungs.	When sections of alveoli are not fully aerated, they deflate and accumulate secretions. Crackles are heard when these sections re-expand with a few deep breaths.	In aging adults, bed-ridden persons, or in persons just aroused from sleep.
Pleural friction rub 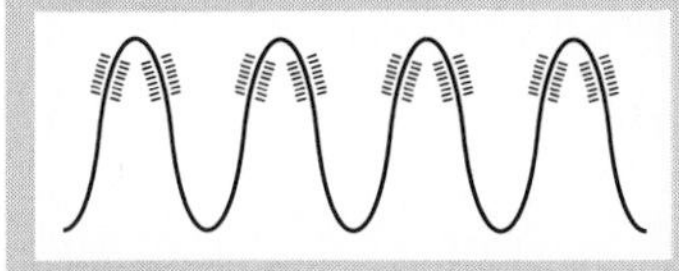	A very superficial sound that is coarse and low pitched; it has a grating quality as if two pieces of leather are being rubbed together. Sounds just like crackles, but *close* to the ear. Sounds louder if you push the stethoscope harder onto the chest wall. Sound is inspiratory and expiratory.	Caused when pleurae become inflamed and lose their normal lubricating fluid. Their opposing roughened pleural surfaces rub together during respiration. Heard best in anterolateral wall where there is greatest lung mobility.	Pleuritis, accompanied by pain with breathing. (Rub disappears after a few days if pleural fluid accumulates and separates pleurae.)

(2) CONTINUOUS SOUNDS

Sound	Description	Mechanism	Clinical Example
Wheeze—high-pitched (sibilant rhonchi) 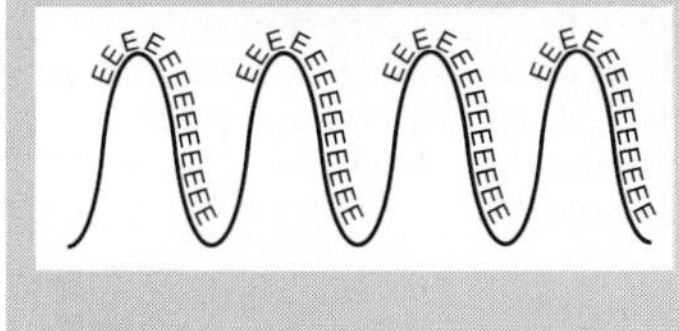	High-pitched, musical squeaking sounds that predominate in expiration but may occur in both expiration and inspiration.	Air squeezed or compressed through passageways narrowed almost to closure by collapsing, swelling, secretions, or tumors. The passageway walls oscillate in apposition between the closed and barely open positions. The resulting sound is similar to a vibrating reed (Forgacs, 1978).	Obstructive lung disease such as asthma or emphysema.
Wheeze—low-pitched (sonorous rhonchi) 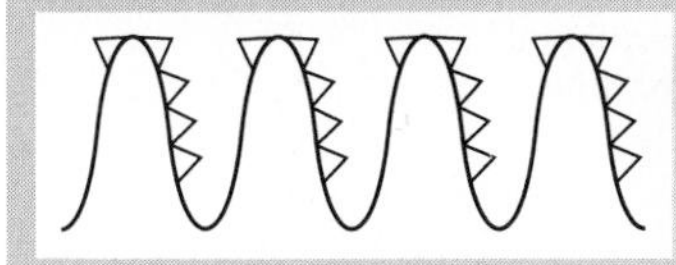	Low-pitched, musical snoring, moaning sounds. They are heard throughout the cycle, although they are more prominent on expiration. May clear somewhat by coughing.	Airflow obstruction as described by the vibrating reed mechanism above. The pitch of the wheeze cannot be correlated to the size of the passageway that generates it.	Bronchitis

Table 15–9 ► Assessment of Common Respiratory Conditions

NORMAL LUNG

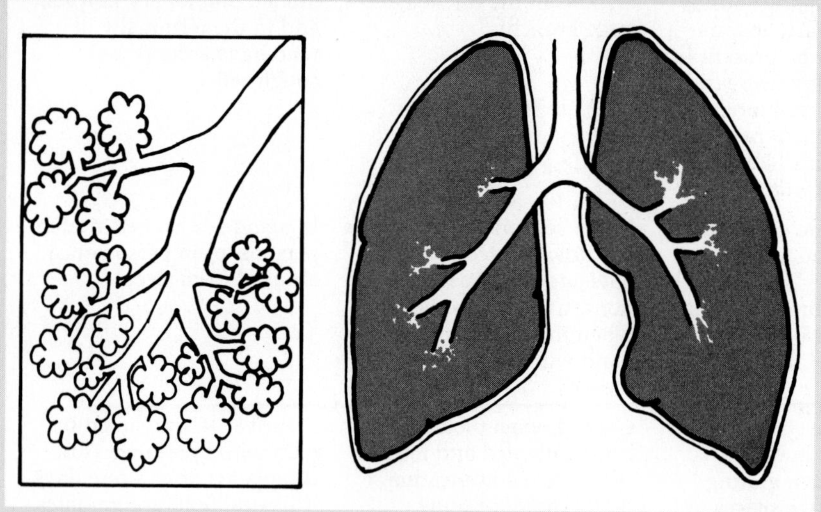

	CONDITION	INSPECTION
NORMAL LUNG		Anteroposterior < transverse diameter, relaxed posture, normal musculature. Rate 10 to 18 breaths per minute, regular, no cyanosis or pallor

ATELECTASIS

(impaired expansion)

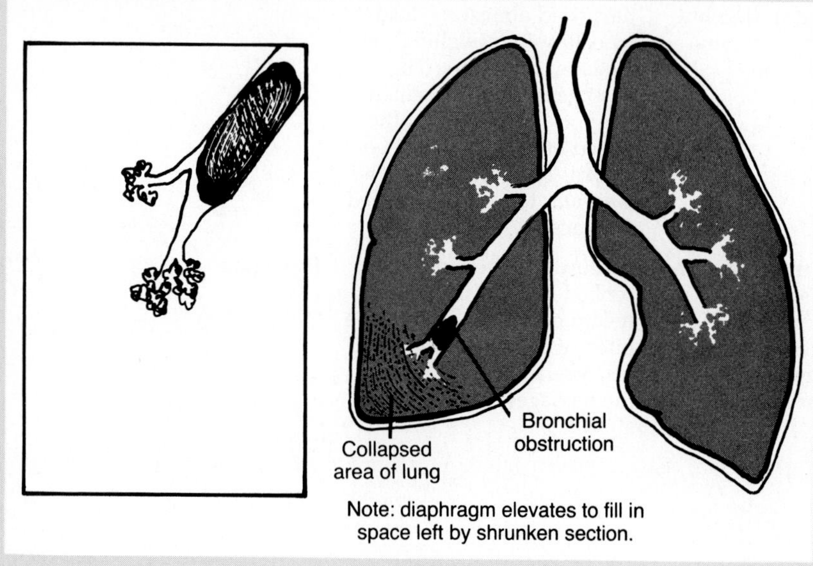
Bronchial obstruction
Collapsed area of lung
Note: diaphragm elevates to fill in space left by shrunken section.

	CONDITION	INSPECTION
ATELECTASIS	Collapsed shrunken section of alveoli, or an entire lung, due to (1) airway obstruction (e.g., the bronchus is completely blocked by thick exudate, aspirated foreign body or tumor), the alveolar air beyond it is gradually absorbed by the pulmonary capillaries, and the alveolar walls cave in; (2) compression on the lung; and (3) lack of surfactant (hyaline membrane disease).	Cough Lag on expansion on affected side Increased respiratory rate Increased pulse Possible cyanosis

Table 15-9 ▶ Assessment of Common Respiratory Conditions *Continued*

PALPATION	PERCUSSION	AUSCULTATION	ADVENTITIOUS SOUNDS
Symmetric chest expansion Tactile fremitus present and equal bilaterally, diminishing toward periphery No lumps, masses, or tenderness	Resonant Diaphragmatic excursion 3 to 5 cm and equal bilaterally	Vesicular over peripheral fields Bronchovesicular parasternally (anterior) and between scapulae (posterior) Infant and young child—bronchovesicular throughout	None
Chest expansion decreased on affected side Tactile fremitus decreased or absent over area With large collapse, tracheal shift *toward* affected side	Dull over area (remainder of thorax sometimes may have hyperresonant note)	Breath sounds decreased vesicular or absent over area Voice sounds variable, usually decreased or absent over affected area	None if bronchus is obstructed Occasional fine crackles if bronchus is patent

Table continued on following page

Table 15–9 ▸ Assessment of Common Respiratory Conditions *Continued*

LOBAR PNEUMONIA

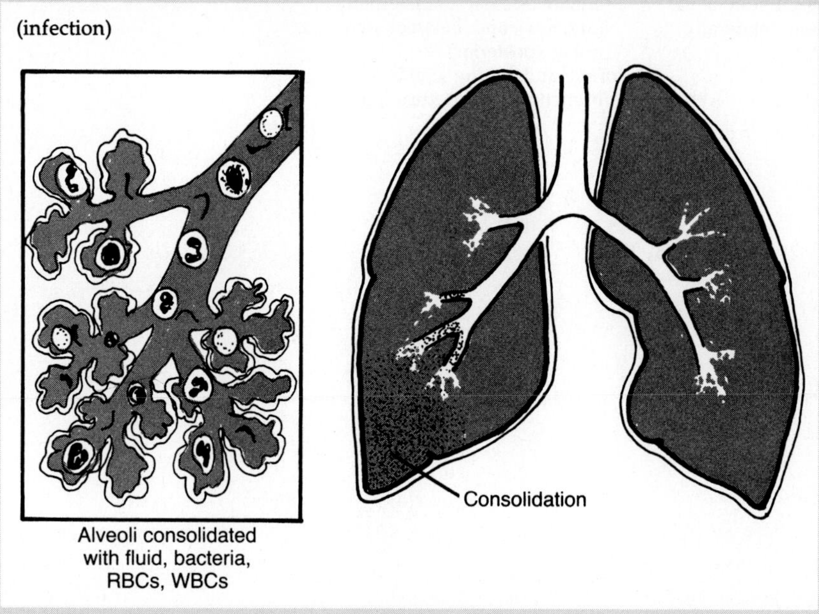

CONDITION	INSPECTION
Infection in lung parenchyma leaves alveolar membrane edematous and porous, so red blood cells and white blood cells pass from blood to alveoli. Alveoli progressively fill up (become consolidated) with bacteria, solid cellular debris, fluid, and blood cells, all of which replace alveolar air. This results in decreased surface area of the respiratory membrane, which causes hypoxemia.	Increased respiratory rate Guarding and lag on expansion on affected side Children—sternal retraction, nasal flaring

BRONCHITIS

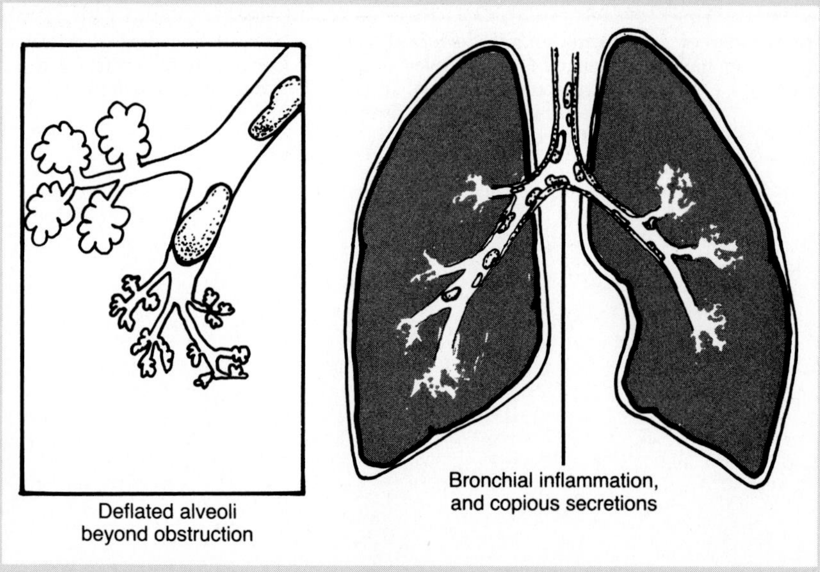

CONDITION	INSPECTION
Proliferation of mucous glands in the passageways, resulting in excessive mucus secretion. Inflammation of bronchi with partial obstruction of bronchi by secretions or constrictions. Sections of lung distal to obstruction may be deflated. Bronchitis may be acute or chronic with recurrent productive cough. Chronic bronchitis is usually caused by cigarette smoking.	Hacking, rasping cough productive of thick mucoid sputum Chronic—dyspnea, fatigue, cyanosis, possible clubbing of fingers

Table 15-9 ▸ Assessment of Common Respiratory Conditions *Continued*

PALPATION	PERCUSSION	AUSCULTATION	ADVENTITIOUS SOUNDS
Chest expansion decreased on affected side Tactile fremitus increased if bronchus patent, decreased if bronchus obstructed	Dull over lobar pneumonia	Breath sounds louder with patent bronchus, as if coming directly from larynx Voice sounds have increased clarity, bronchophony, egophony, whispered pectoriloquy present Children—diminished breath sounds may occur early in pneumonia	Crackles, fine to medium
Tactile fremitus normal	Resonant	Normal vesicular Voice sounds normal Chronic—prolonged expiration	Crackles over deflated areas May have wheeze

Table continued on following page

Table 15–9 ▸ Assessment of Common Respiratory Conditions *Continued*

	CONDITION	INSPECTION
EMPHYSEMA 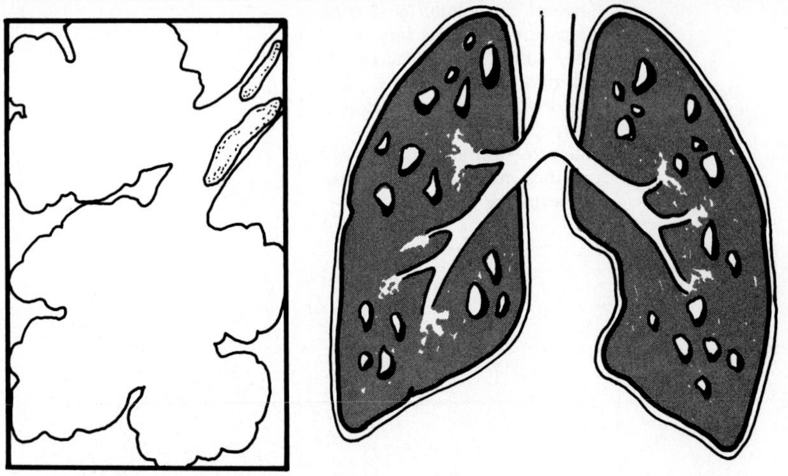 Overdistended alveoli with destruction of septa	Chronic obstruction of bronchioles due to hyperplasia and increased mucus secretion. Plug traps air in alveoli, causing overdistention of air sacs and rupture of interalveolar walls. Increased airway resistance, especially on expiration. Produces a hyperinflated lung and an increase in lung volume.	Increased anteroposterior diameter Barrel chest Use of accessory muscles to aid respiration Tripod position Shortness of breath, especially on exertion.
ASTHMA 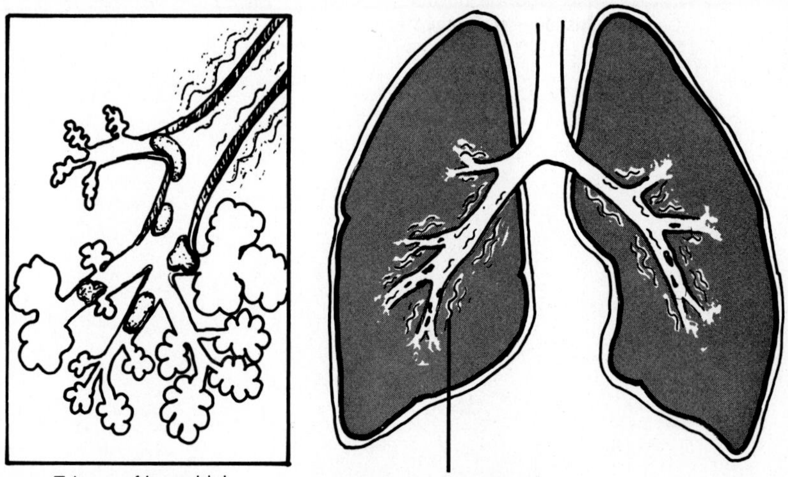 Edema of bronchial mucosa, thick mucus	An allergic hypersensitivity to certain inhaled particles (e.g., pollen) that produces inflammation and a reaction of bronchospasm, edema in walls of bronchioles, and thick mucus secreted into bronchial airways. All these factors greatly increase airway resistance, especially during expiration.	During severe attack: increased respiratory rate, shortness of breath with audible wheeze Use of accessory neck muscles Cyanosis Apprehension Retraction of intercostal spaces Expiration labored, prolonged When chronic may have barrel chest

Table 15-9 ► Assessment of Common Respiratory Conditions *Continued*

PALPATION	PERCUSSION	AUSCULTATION	ADVENTITIOUS SOUNDS
Tactile fremitus decreased Chest expansion decreased	Hyperresonant Decreased diaphragmatic excursion	Decreased vesicular May have prolonged expiration	Usually none Occasionally, you may hear wheeze
Tactile fremitus decreased	Resonant May be hyperresonant if chronic	Breath sounds decreased, with prolonged expiration Voice sounds decreased	Wheeze on expiration

Table continued on following page

Table 15-9 ▶ Assessment of Common Respiratory Conditions *Continued*

PLEURAL EFFUSION (FLUID) OR THICKENING

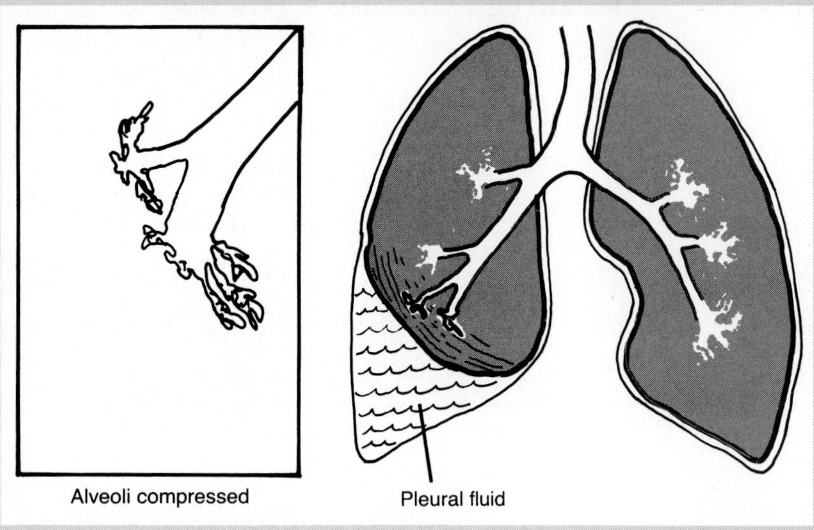

CONDITION	INSPECTION
Collection of fluid in the intrapleural space, with compression of overlying lung tissue. Fluid collects by gravity in dependent areas of the thorax. Presence of fluid subdues all sounds.	Increased respiratory rate Dyspnea

PNEUMOTHORAX

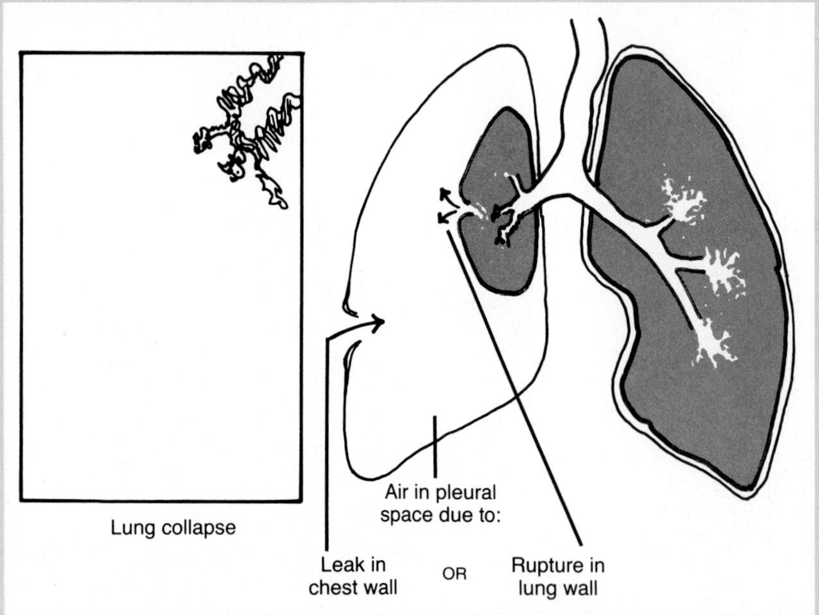

CONDITION	INSPECTION
Free air in pleural space causes partial or complete lung collapse. Air in pleural space neutralizes the usual negative pressure present, thus lung collapses. Usually unilateral. Pneumothorax can be (1) spontaneous (air enters pleural space through rupture in lung wall), (2) traumatic (air enters through opening or injury in chest wall), or (3) tension (trapped air in pleural space increases, compressing lung and shifting mediastinum to the unaffected side).	Unequal chest expansion If large, increased respiratory rate, cyanosis, apprehension, bulging in interspaces

Table 15–9 ▸ Assessment of Common Respiratory Conditions *Continued*

PALPATION	PERCUSSION	AUSCULTATION	ADVENTITIOUS SOUNDS
Tactile fremitus decreased or absent Tracheal shift away from affected side Chest expansion decreased on affected side	Dull to flat No diaphragmatic excursion on affected side	Breath sounds decreased or absent Voice sounds decreased or absent When remainder of lung is compressed near the effusion, may have bronchial breath sounds over the compression along with bronchophony, egophony, whispered pectoriloquy	None
Tactile fremitus decreased or absent Tracheal shift to opposite side (unaffected side) Chest expansion decreased on affected side	Hyperresonant Decreased diaphragmatic excursion	Breath sounds decreased or absent Voice sounds decreased or absent	None

Table continued on following page

Table 15-9 ► Assessment of Common Respiratory Conditions *Continued*

CONGESTIVE HEART FAILURE

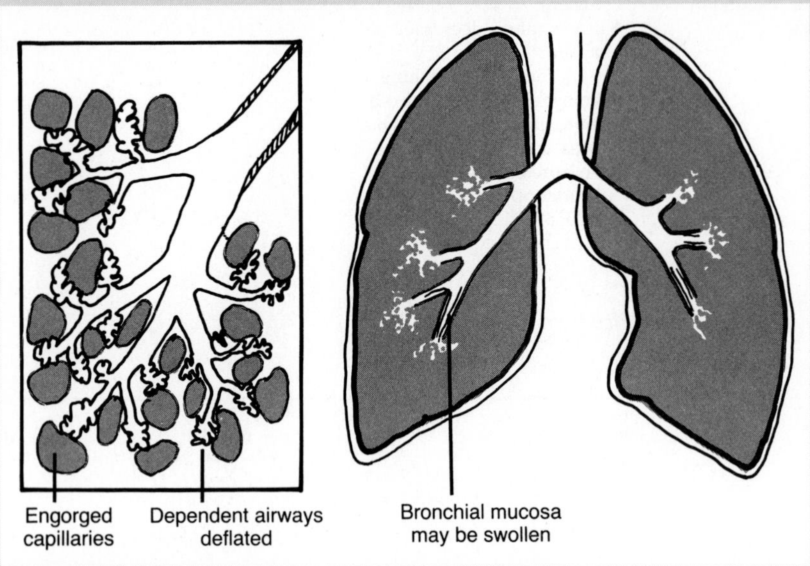

CONDITION	INSPECTION
Increasing pressure of cardiac overload causes pulmonary congestion, or an increased amount of blood present in pulmonary capillaries. Dependent air sacs are deflated. Pulmonary capillaries engorged. Bronchial mucosa may be swollen.	Increased respiratory rate Shortness of breath on exertion Orthopnea Paroxysmal nocturnal dyspnea Nocturia Ankle edema Pallor in light-skinned people

Table 15-9 ▶ Assessment of Common Respiratory Conditions *Continued*

PALPATION	PERCUSSION	AUSCULTATION	ADVENTITIOUS SOUNDS
Skin moist, clammy Tactile fremitus normal	Resonant	Normal vesicular Heart sounds include S3 gallop	Crackles at lung bases

Bibliography

Apgar V: A proposal for a new method of evaluating the newborn infant. Curr Res Anesth Analg Jul/Aug:260, 1953.

Cherniack RM, Cherniack L: Respiration in Health and Disease. 3rd ed. Philadelphia, WB Saunders, 1983.

Duncalf D, Kepes ER: Geriatric anesthesia. *In* Rossman I: Clinical Geriatrics. 3rd ed. Philadelphia, JB Lippincott, 1986.

Forgacs P: The functional basis of pulmonary sounds. Chest 73:399–405, 1978.

Forgacs P: Lung Sounds. London, Ballière Tindall, 1978.

King RP, Thompson BT, Johnson DC: Wheezing on maximal forced exhalation in the diagnosis of atypical asthma. Ann Intern Med 110(6):451–455, 1989.

Lapp NL: Lung volumes and flow rates in black and white subjects. Thorax 29:185–188, 1974.

Lehrer S: Understanding Lung Sounds. Philadelphia, WB Saunders, 1984.

Loudon RG: The lung exam. Clin Chest Med 8:265–272, 1987.

Milne JS, Howie AD, Pack AI: Dyspnoea during normal pregnancy. Br J Obstet Gynaecol 85:260, 1978.

Naylor CD, McCormack DG, Sullivan SN: The midclavicular line: A wandering landmark. Can Med Assoc J 136:48–50, 1987.

Olowe SA, and Akinkugbe A: Amniotic fluid lecithin/sphingomyelin ratio: Comparison between an African and a North American community. Pediatrics 62(1):38–41, 1978.

Oscherwitz R: Differences in pulmonary functions in various racial groups. Am J Epidemiol 96(5):319–327, 1972.

Overfield T: Biologic Variation in Health and Illness: Race, Age, and Sex Differences. Menlo Park, CA, Addison-Wesley, 1985.

Petty TL: ABCs of simple pulmonary function assessment. Nurse Pract 11(6):50–60, 1986.

Pritchard JA, MacDonald PC, Gant NF: Williams Obstetrics. 17th ed. Norwalk, CT, Appleton-Century-Crofts, 1985.

Smith J: Big differences in little people. Am J Nurs 88:458–462, 1988.

Stevens SA, Becker KL: How to perform picture-perfect respiratory assessment. Nursing 88 18:57–63, 1988.

CHAPTER

16 Heart and Neck Vessels

STRUCTURE AND FUNCTION

The cardiovascular system consists of the *heart,* a muscular pump, and the *blood vessels.* The blood vessels are arranged in two continuous loops, the *pulmonary circulation* and the *systemic circulation* (Fig. 16–1). When the heart contracts, it pumps blood simultaneously into both loops.

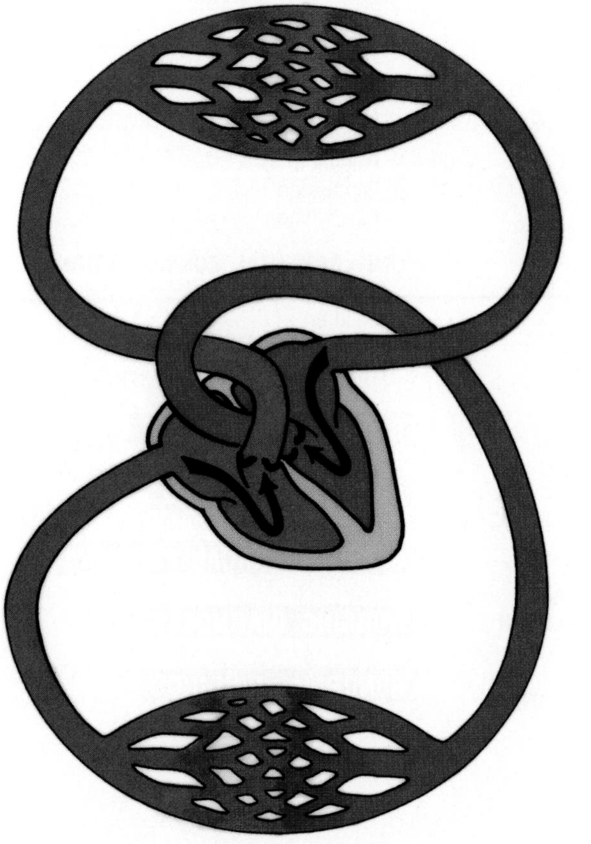

► **Figure 16–1**

POSITION AND SURFACE LANDMARKS

The *precordium* is the area on the anterior chest overlying the heart and great vessels. The great vessels are the major arteries and veins connected to the heart. The heart and the great vessels are located between the lungs in the middle third of the thoracic cage, called the *mediastinum.* The heart extends from the second to the fifth intercostal space, and from the right border of the sternum to the left midclavicular line (Fig. 16–2).

Think of the heart as an upside down triangle in the chest. The "top" of the heart is the broader *base,* and the "bottom" is the *apex,* which points down and to the left. During contraction, the apex beats against the chest wall, producing an apical impulse. This is palpable in most people, normally at the fifth intercostal space, 7 to 9 cm from the midsternal line.

Inside the body, the heart is rotated so that its right side is anterior and its left side is mostly posterior. Of the heart's four chambers, the right ventricle forms the greatest area of anterior cardiac surface (Fig. 16–3). The left ventricle lies behind the right ventricle and forms the apex and slender area of left border. The right atrium lies to the right and above the right ventricle and forms the right border. The left atrium is located posteriorly, with only a small portion, the left atrial appendage, showing anteriorly.

The great vessels lie bunched above the base of the heart. The *superior* and *inferior vena cavae* return unoxygenated venous blood to the right side of the heart. The *pulmonary artery* leaves the right ventricle, bifurcates, and carries the venous blood to the lungs. The *pulmonary veins* return the freshly oxygenated blood to the left side of the heart, and the *aorta* carries it out to the body. The aorta ascends from the left ventricle, arches back at the level of the sternal angle, and descends behind the heart.

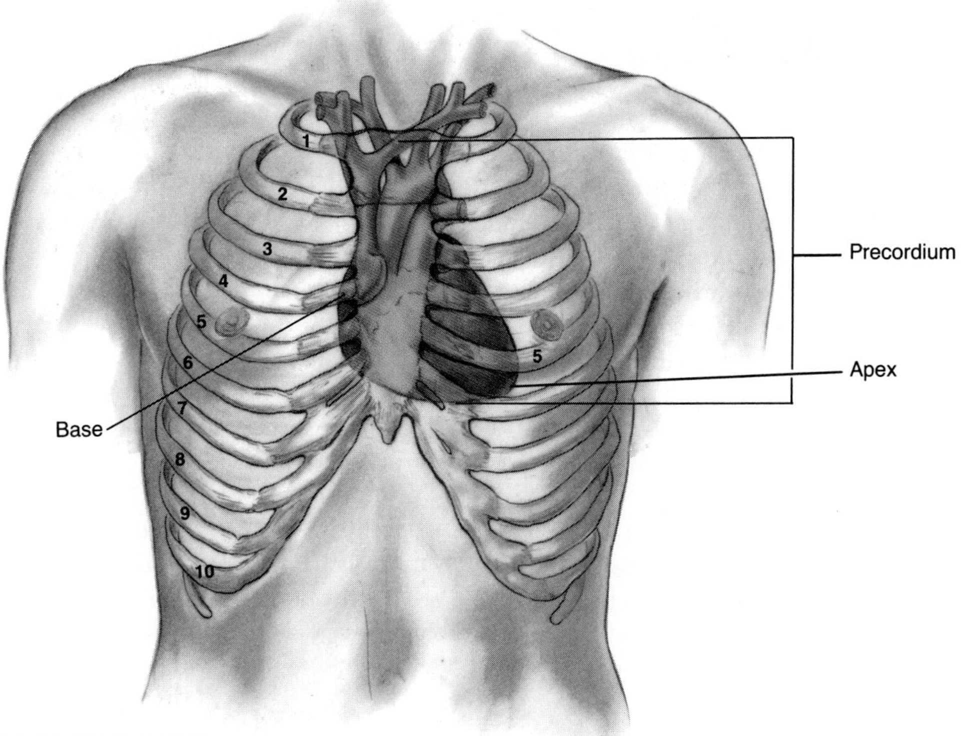

► **Figure 16-2**

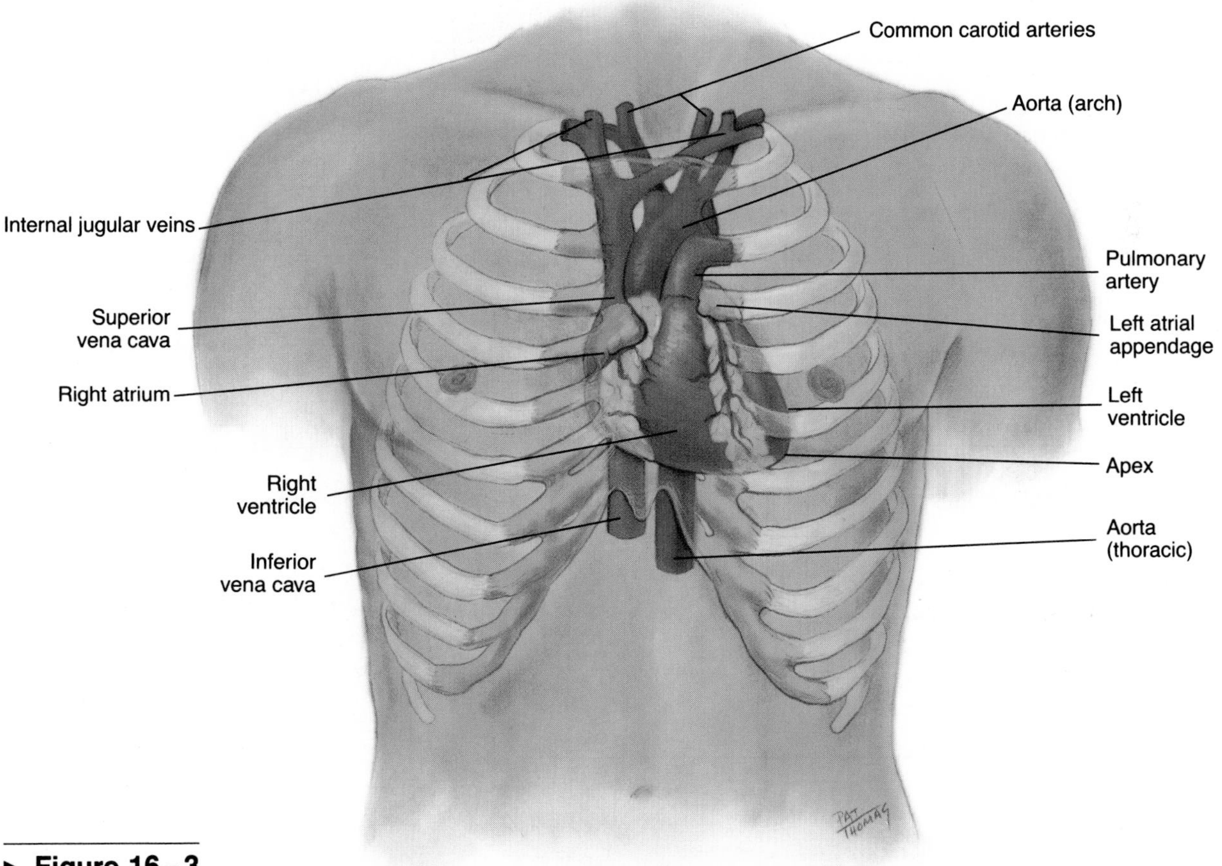

► **Figure 16-3**

HEART WALL, CHAMBERS, AND VALVES

The heart wall has numerous layers. The *pericardium* is a tough, fibrous, double-walled sac that surrounds and protects the heart. It has two layers that contain a few milliliters of serous *pericardial fluid.* This ensures smooth friction-free movement of the heart muscle. The pericardium is adherent to the great vessels, esophagus, sternum, and pleurae and is anchored to the diaphragm. The *myocardium* is the muscular wall of the heart; it does the pumping. The *endocardium* is the thin layer of endothelial tissue that lines the inner surface of the heart chambers and valves.

The common metaphor is to think of the heart as a pump. But consider that the heart actually is two pumps; the right side of the heart pumps blood into the lungs, and the left side of the heart simultaneously pumps blood into the body. The two pumps are separated by an impermeable wall, the septum. Each side has an *atrium* and a *ventricle.* The atrium (anteroom) is a thin-walled reservoir for holding blood, and the thick-walled ventricle is the muscular pumping chamber. (It is common to use the following abbreviations to refer to the chambers: RA, right atrium; RV, right ventricle; LA, left atrium; and LV, left ventricle.)

The four chambers are separated by swinging door–like structures, called *valves,* whose main purpose is to prevent backflow of blood. The valves are unidirectional; they can only open one way. The valves open and close *passively,* in response to pressure gradients in the moving blood.

There are four valves in the heart (Fig. 16–4). The two *atrioventricular* (AV) valves separate the atria and the ventricles. The right AV valve is the *tricuspid,* the left AV valve is the bicuspid or *mitral* valve (so named because it resembles a bishop's mitred cap). The valves' thin leaflets are anchored by collagenous fibers *(chordae tendin-*

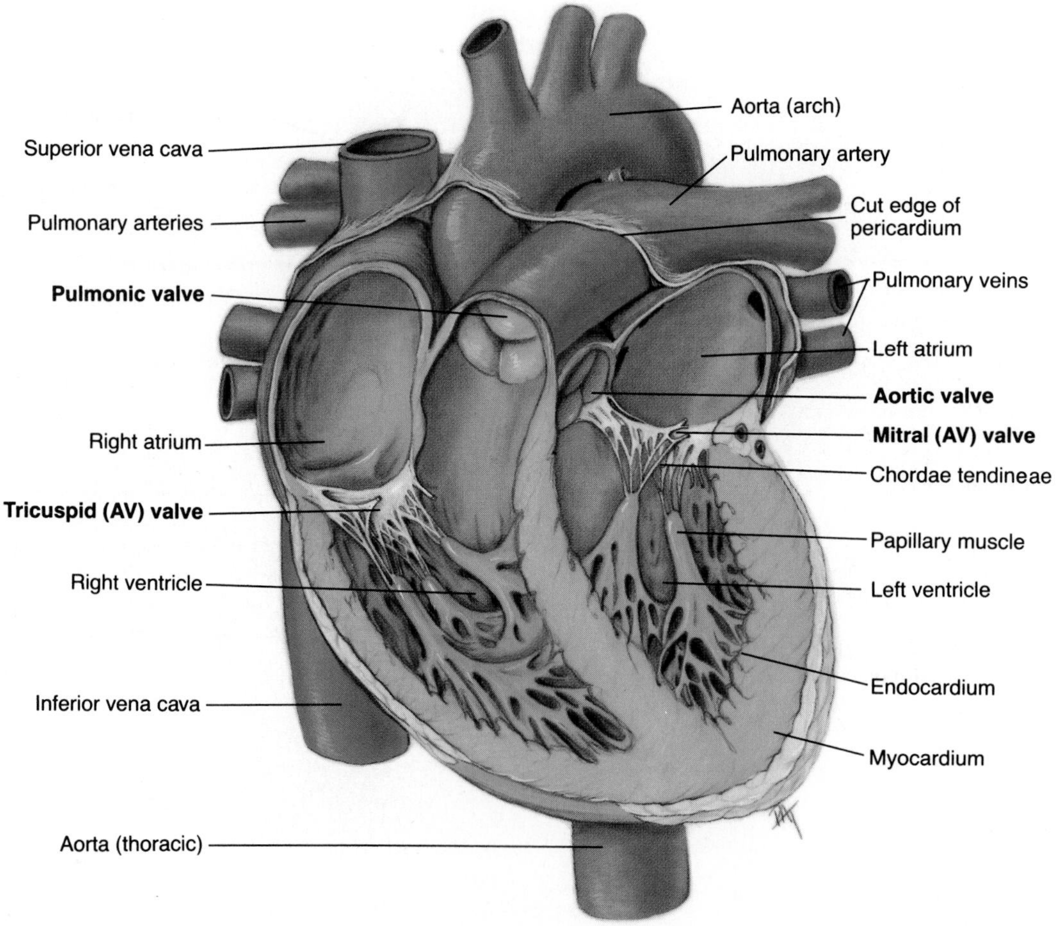

► **Figure 16–4**

eae) to papillary muscles embedded in the ventricle floor. The AV valves open during the heart's filling phase, or *diastole,* to allow the ventricles to fill with blood. During systole, AV valves close to prevent regurgitation of blood back up into the atria. The papillary muscles contract at this time, so that the valve leaflets meet and unite to form a perfect seal without turning themselves inside out.

The *semilunar* (SL) valves are set between the ventricles and the arteries. Each valve has three cusps that look like half-moons. The SL valves are the *pulmonic* valve in the right side of the heart and the *aortic* valve in the left side of the heart. They open during pumping, or *systole,* to allow blood to be ejected from the heart.

Note that there are no valves between the vena cavae and the right atrium, nor between the pulmonary veins and the left atrium. For this reason, abnormally high pressure in the left side of the heart gives a person symptoms of pulmonary congestion, and abnormally high pressure in the right side of the heart shows in the neck veins and abdomen.

DIRECTION OF BLOOD FLOW

Think of an unoxygenated red blood cell being drained downstream into the vena cava. It is swept along with the flow of venous blood and follows the route illustrated in Figure 16–5.

1. From liver to RA via inferior vena cava
   Superior vena cava drains venous blood from head and upper extremities
   From RA, venous blood travels through tricuspid valve to RV
2. From RV, venous blood flows through pulmonic valve to pulmonary artery
   Pulmonary artery delivers unoxygenated blood to lungs.
3. Lungs oxygenate blood.
   Pulmonary veins return fresh blood to LA.
4. From LA, aterial blood travels through mitral valve to LV.
   LV ejects blood through aortic valve into aorta.
5. Aorta delivers oxygenated blood to body.

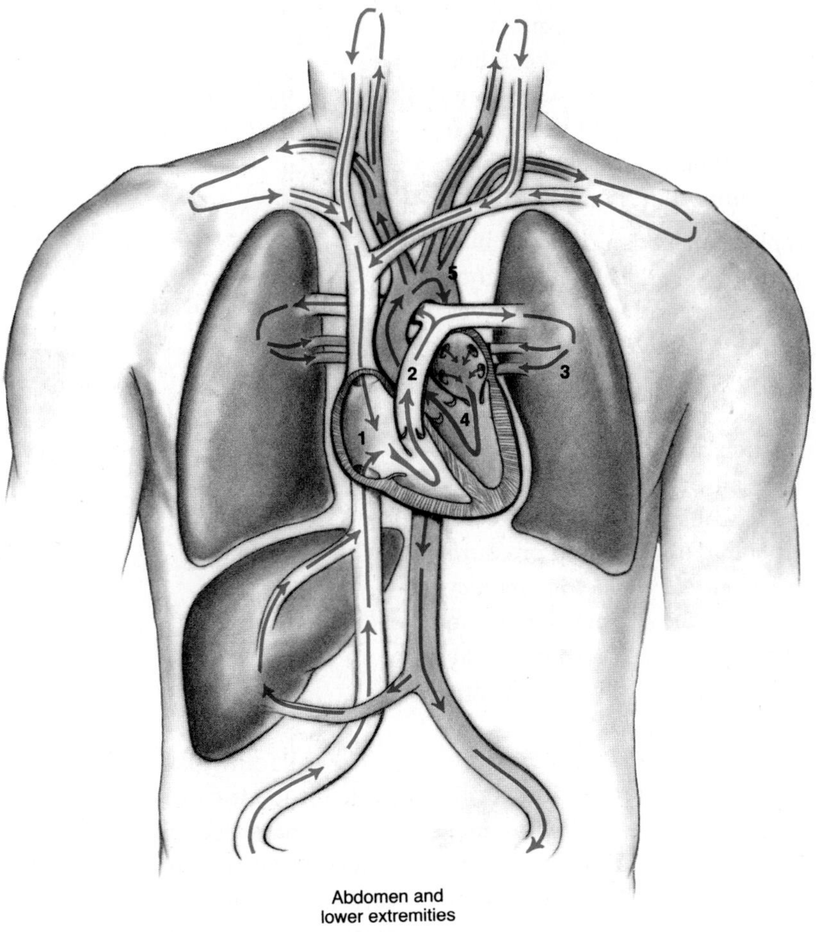

▸ Figure 16–5

Remember that the circulation is a continuous loop. The blood is kept moving along by continually shifting pressure gradients. The blood flows from an area of higher pressure to one of lower pressure.

CARDIAC CYCLE

The rhythmic movement of blood through the heart is the *cardiac cycle.* It has two phases, *diastole* and *systole.* In *diastole,* the ventricles relax and fill with blood. This takes up two-thirds of the cardiac cycle. The heart's contraction is *systole.* During systole, blood is pumped from the ventricles and fills the pulmonary and systemic arteries. This is one-third of the cardiac cycle.

Diastole. In diastole, the ventricles are relaxed and the AV valves, i.e., the tricuspid and mitral, are open (Fig. 16–6). (Opening of the normal valve is acoustically silent.) The pressure in the atria is higher than that in the ventricles, so blood pours rapidly into the ventricles. This first passive filling phase is called *early* or *protodiastolic filling.*

Toward the end of diastole, the atria contract and push the last amount of blood (about 25 percent of stroke volume) into the ventricles. This active filling phase is called *presystole,* or *atrial systole,* or sometimes the "atrial kick." It causes a small rise in left ventricular pressure. (Note that atrial systole occurs during ventricular diastole, a confusing but important point.)

Systole. Now so much blood has been pumped into the ventricles that ventricular pressure is finally higher than that in the atria, so the mitral and tricuspid valves swing shut. The closure of the AV valves contributes to the first heart sound (S_1) and signals the beginning of systole. The AV valves close to prevent any regurgitation of blood back up into the atria during contraction.

For a very brief moment, all four valves are closed (Fig. 16–7). The ventricular walls contract. This contraction against a closed system works to build pressure inside the ventricles to a high level *(isometric contraction).* Consider first the left side of the heart. When the pressure in the ventricle finally exceeds pressure in the aorta, the aortic valve opens and blood is ejected rapidly.

After the ventricle's contents are ejected, its pressure falls. When pressure falls below pressure in the aorta, some blood flows backward toward the ventricle, causing the aortic valve to swing shut. This closure of the semilunar valves causes the second heart sound (S_2) and signals the end of systole.

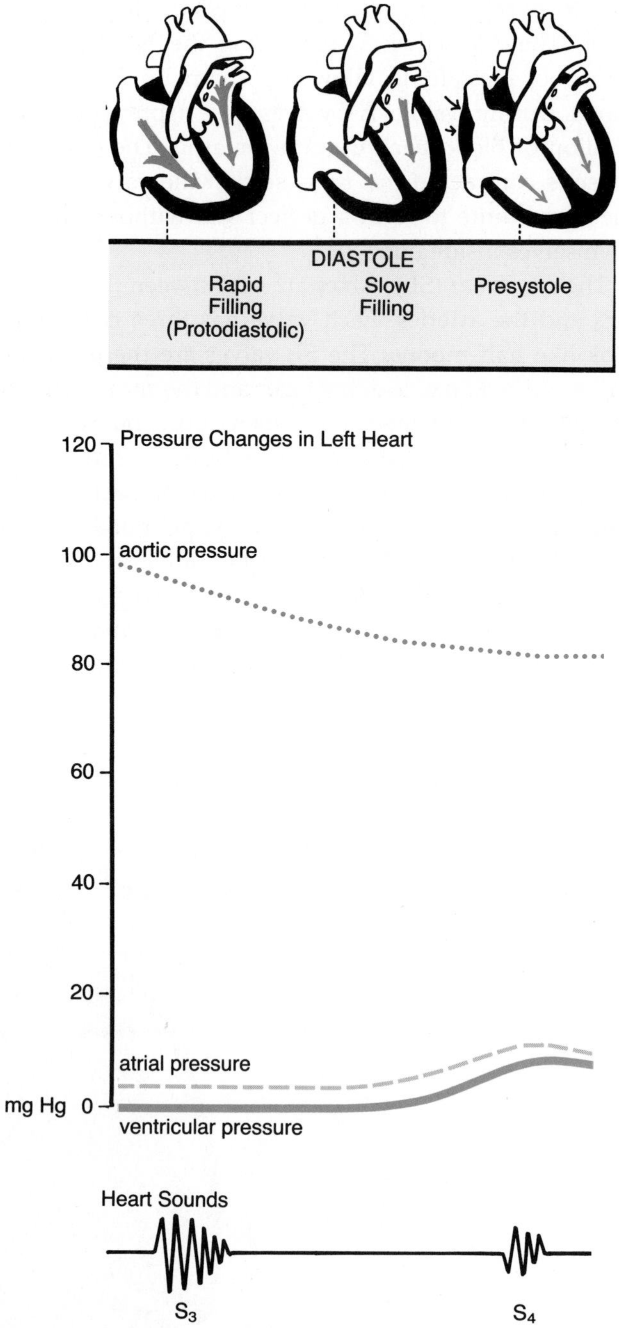

► **Figure 16–6**

Now all four valves are closed and the ventricles relax (called isometric or isovolumic relaxation). Meanwhile, the atria have been filling with blood delivered from the lungs. Atrial pressure is now higher than the relaxed ventricular pressure. The mitral valve drifts open and diastolic filling begins again.

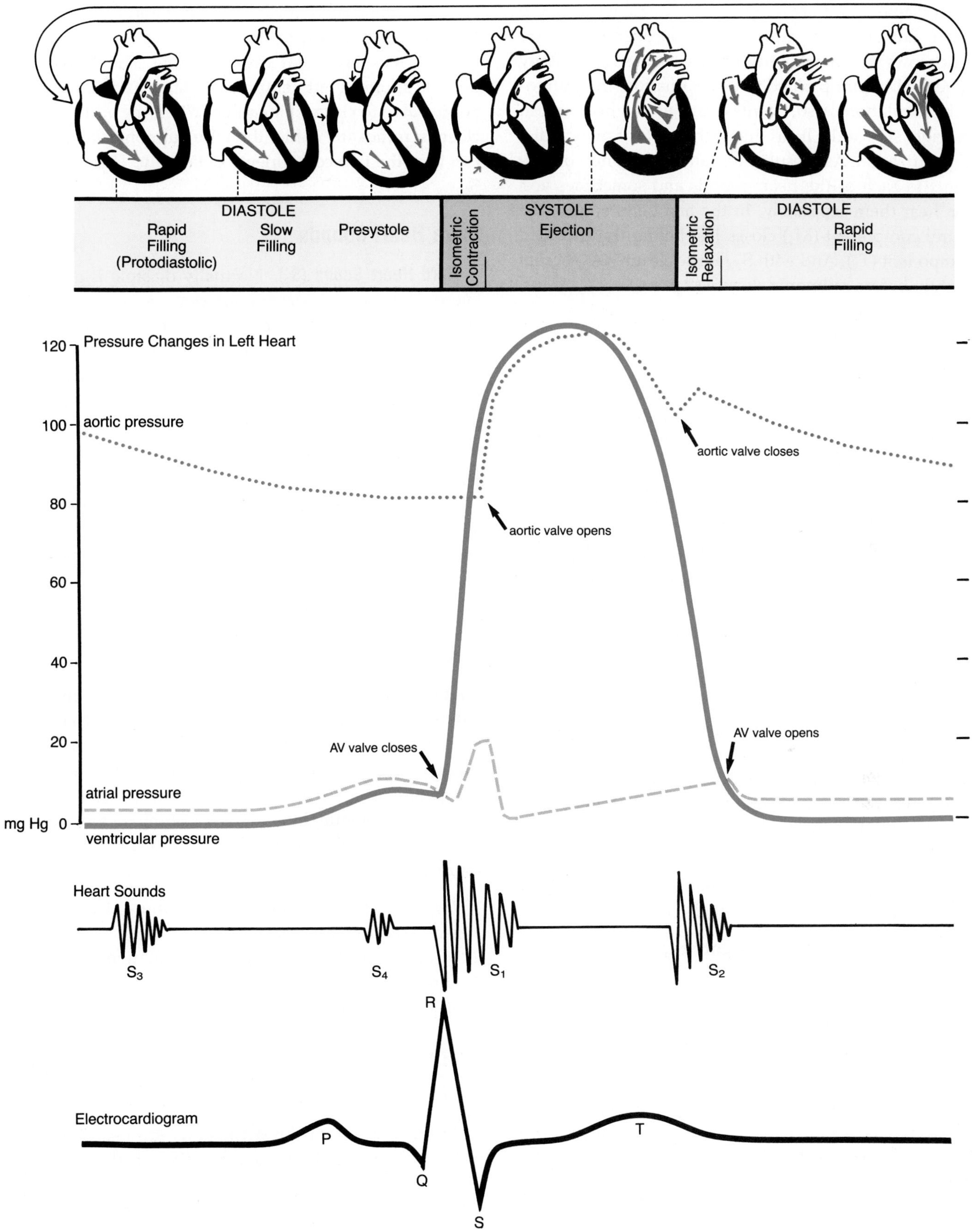

DIASTOLE
Rapid Filling (Protodiastolic)
Slow Filling
Presystole
Isometric Contraction
SYSTOLE
Ejection
Isometric Relaxation
DIASTOLE
Rapid Filling
Pressure Changes in Left Heart
120
100
80
60
40
20
mg Hg 0
aortic pressure
aortic valve closes
aortic valve opens
AV valve closes
AV valve opens
atrial pressure
ventricular pressure
Heart Sounds
S_3
S_4
S_1
S_2
Electrocardiogram
P
Q
R
S
T

▶ Figure 16-7

The same events are happening in the right side of the heart. But pressures in the right side of the heart are much lower than that of the left side because less energy is needed to pump blood to its destination, the pulmonary circulation. Also, events occur just slightly later in the right side of the heart due to the route of myocardial depolarization. As a result, there are two distinct components to each of the heart sounds and sometimes you can hear them separately. In the first heart sound, the mitral component (M_1) closes just before the tricuspid component (T_1). And with S_2, aortic closure (A_2) occurs slightly before pulmonic closure (P_2).

HEART SOUNDS

Events in the cardiac cycle generate sounds that can be heard through a stethoscope over the chest wall. These include normal heart sounds and, occasionally, extra heart sounds and murmurs.

Normal Heart Sounds

The *first heart sound* (S_1) occurs with closure of the AV valves and thus signals the beginning of systole. The mitral component of the first sound (M_1) slightly precedes the tricuspid component (T_1), but you usually hear these two components fused as one sound. You can hear S_1 over all the precordium, but usually it is loudest at the apex.

The *second heart sound* (S_2) occurs with closure of the semilunar valves and signals the end of systole. The aortic component of the second sound (A_2) slightly precedes the pulmonic component (P_2). Although it is heard over all the precordium, S_2 is loudest at the base.

Effect of Respiration. The volume of right and left ventricular systole is just about equal, but this can be affected by respiration. To learn this, consider the phrase:

More to the *r*ight heart,
Less to the *l*eft.

That means that during inspiration, intrathoracic pressure is decreased. This pushes more blood into the vena cavae, increasing venous return to the right side of the heart, which increases right ventricular stroke volume. The increased volume prolongs right ventricular systole and delays pulmonic valve closure. Meanwhile on the left side, a greater amount of blood is sequestered in the lungs during inspiration. This momentarily decreases the amount returned to the left side of the heart, decreasing left ventricular stroke volume. The decreased volume shortens left ventricular systole and allows the aortic valve to close a bit earlier. When the aortic valve closes significantly earlier than the pulmonic valve, you can hear the two components separately. This is a *split* S_2.

Extra Heart Sounds

Third Heart Sound (S_3). Normally diastole is a silent event. However, in some conditions, ventricular filling creates vibrations that can be heard over the chest. These vibrations are S_3. S_3 occurs when the ventricles are resistant to filling during the early rapid filling phase (protodiastole). This occurs immediately after S_2, when the AV valves open and atrial blood first pours into the ventricles. (See a complete discussion of S_3 in Table 16–6).

Fourth Heart Sound (S_4). S_4 occurs at the end of diastole, at presystole, when the ventricle is resistant to filling. The atria contract and push blood into a noncompliant ventricle. This creates vibrations that are heard as S_4. S_4 occurs just before S_1.

Murmurs

Blood circulating through normal cardiac chambers and valves usually makes no noise. However, some conditions create turbulent blood flow and collision currents. These result in a murmur, much like a pile of stones or a sharp turn in a stream creates a noisy water flow. A murmur is a gentle, blowing, swooshing sound which can be heard on the chest wall. Conditions resulting in a murmur are as follows:

1. Velocity of blood increases (flow murmur), e.g., in exercise, thyrotoxicosis
2. Viscosity of blood decreases, e.g., in anemia
3. Structural defects in the valves or unusual openings in the chambers.

Characteristics of Sound

All heart sounds are described by:

1. Frequency (pitch)—heart sounds are described as high-pitched or low-pitched, although these terms

are relative because all are low-frequency sounds, and you need a good stethoscope to hear them.
2. Intensity (loudness)—loud or soft
3. Duration—very short for heart sounds; silent periods are longer
4. Timing—systole or diastole

CONDUCTION

Of all organs, the heart has a unique ability—automaticity. The heart can contract by itself, independent of any signals or stimulation from the body. The heart contracts in response to an electrical current conveyed by a conduction system. Specialized cells in the sinoatrial (SA) node near the superior vena cava initiate an electrical impulse. (Because the SA node has an intrinsic rhythm, it is the "pacemaker.") The current flows in an orderly sequence (Fig. 16–8), first across the atria to the AV node low in the atrial septum. There, it is delayed slightly so that the atria have time to contract before the ventricles are stimulated. Then, the impulse travels to the bundle of His, the right and left bundle branches, and then through the ventricles.

The electrical impulse stimulates the heart to do its work, which is to contract. A small amount of electricity spreads to the body surface, where it can be measured and recorded on the electrocardiograph (ECG). The ECG waves are arbitrarily labeled PQRST, which stand for the following elements:

P wave—depolarization of the atria

PR interval—from the beginning of the P wave to the beginning of the QRS complex. (The time necessary for atrial depolarization plus time for the impulse to travel through the AV node to the ventricles.)

QRS complex—depolarization of the ventricles

T wave—repolarization of the ventricles

Electrical events slightly *precede* the mechanical events in the heart. The ECG juxtaposed on the cardiac cycle is illustrated in Figure 16–9.

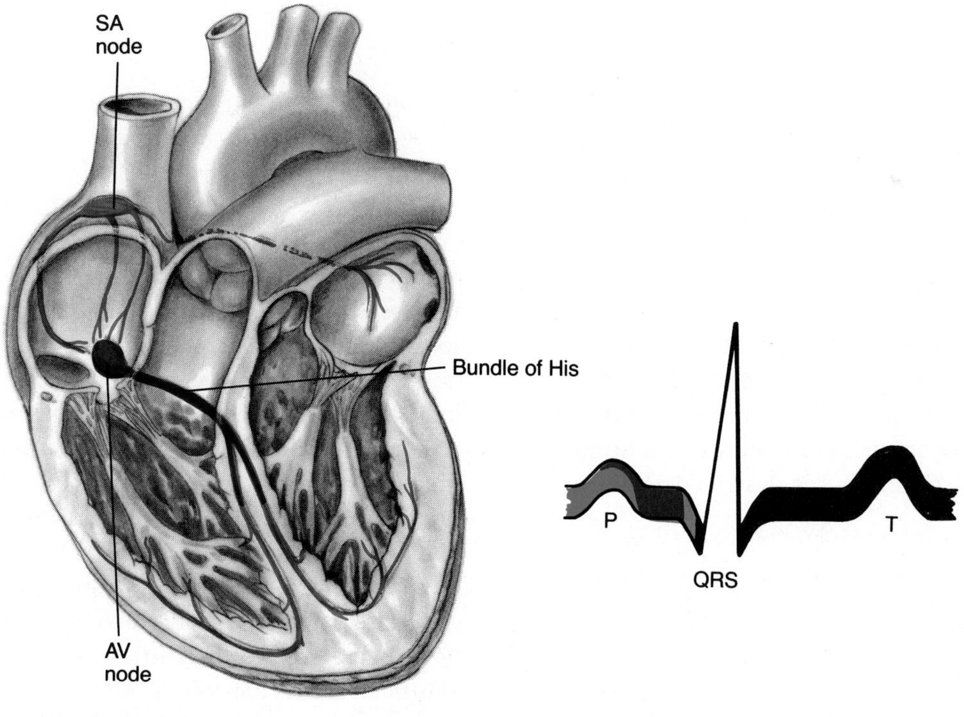

► **Figure 16–8**

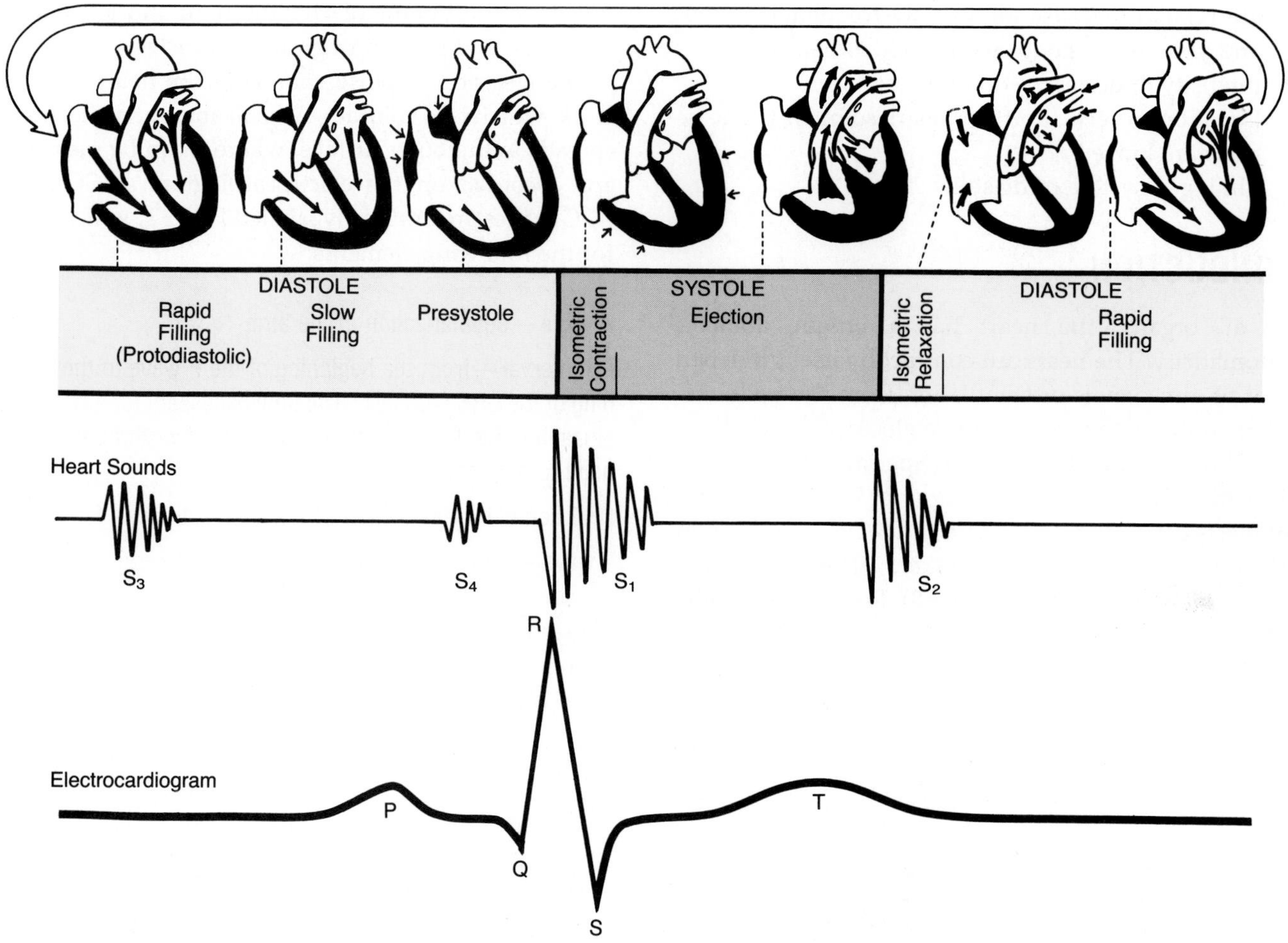

▶ **Figure 16–9**

PUMPING ABILITY

In the resting adult, the heart normally pumps between 4 and 6 liters of blood per minute throughout the body. This *cardiac output* equals the volume of blood in each systole (called the stroke volume) times the number of beats per minute (rate). This is described as:

$$CO = SV \times R$$

The heart can alter its cardiac output to adapt to the metabolic needs of the body. Preload and afterload affect the heart's ability to increase cardiac output.

Preload is the passive stretching force applied to the ventricular muscle at the end of diastole (Fig. 16–10). When the volume of blood returned to the ventricles is increased (as when exercise stimulates skeletal muscles to contract and force more blood back to the heart), the muscle bundles are stretched beyond their normal resting state to accommodate. The force of this stretch is the preload. According to the Frank-Starling law, the greater the stretch, the stronger is the heart's contraction. This increased contractility results in an increased volume of blood ejected (increased stroke volume).

Afterload is the opposing pressure the ventricle must generate to open the aortic valve against the higher aortic pressure. Once the ventricle is filled with blood, the ventricular end diastolic pressure is 5 to 10 mm Hg, whereas that in the aorta is 70 to 80 mm Hg. To over-

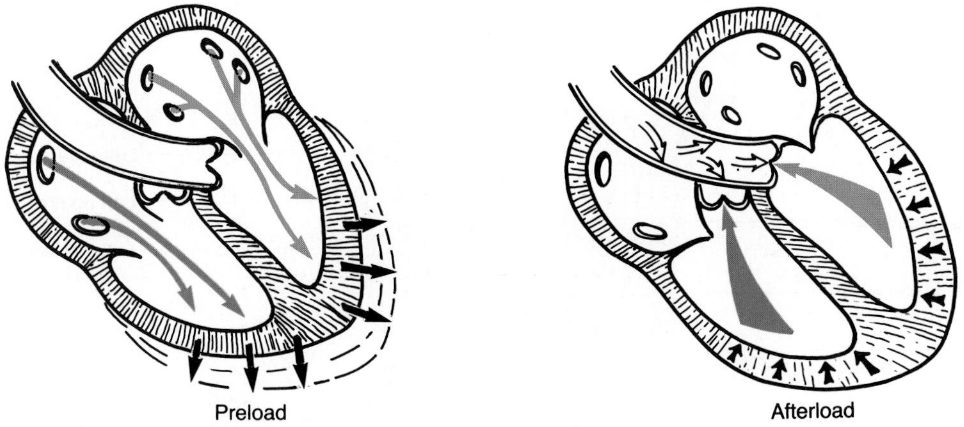

▶ **Figure 16–10**

come this difference, the ventricular muscle *tenses* (isovolumic contraction). After the aortic valve opens, rapid ejection occurs.

THE NECK VESSELS

Cardiovascular assessment includes the survey of vascular structures in the neck—the carotid artery and the jugular veins. These vessels reflect the efficiency of cardiac function.

The Carotid Artery Pulse

Chapter 8 describes the pulse as a pressure wave generated by each systole pumping blood into the aorta. The carotid artery is a central artery, i.e., it is close to the heart. Its timing closely coincides with ventricular systole. (Assessment of the peripheral pulses is found in Chapter 18, and blood pressure assessment is found in Chapter 8.)

The carotid artery is located in the groove between the trachea and the sternomastoid muscle, medial to and alongside that muscle. Note the characteristics of its waveform (Fig. 16–11): a smooth rapid upstroke, a summit that is rounded and smooth, and a downstroke that is more gradual and that has a dicrotic notch caused by closure of the aortic valve (marked D in the Figure).

Jugular Venous Pulse and Pressure

The jugular veins empty unoxygenated blood directly into the superior vena cava. Since there is no cardiac valve separating the superior vena cava from the right atrium, the jugular veins give information about activity on the right side of the heart. Specifically, they reflect filling pressure and volume changes. Since volume and pressure increase when the right side of the heart fails to pump efficiently, the jugular veins expose this.

There are two jugular veins in each side of the neck (Fig. 16–12). The larger *internal* jugular lies deep and medial to the sternomastoid muscle. It is usually not visible, although its diffuse pulsations may be seen in the sternal notch when the person is supine. The *external* jugular vein is more superficial; it lies lateral to the sternomastoid muscle, above the clavicle.

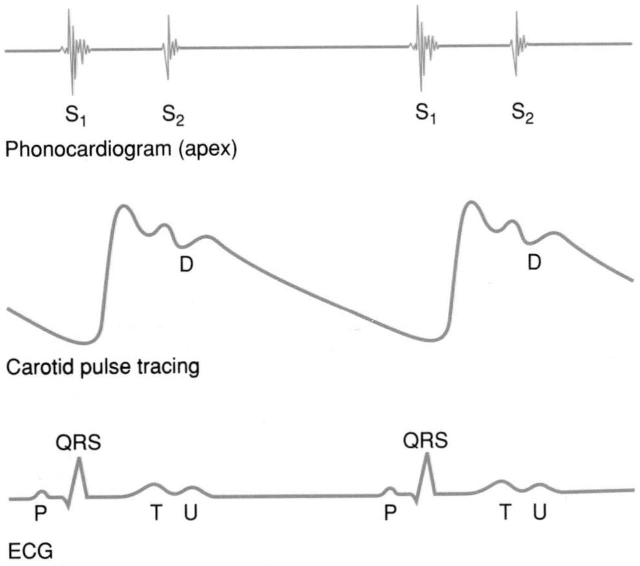

▶ **Figure 16–11**

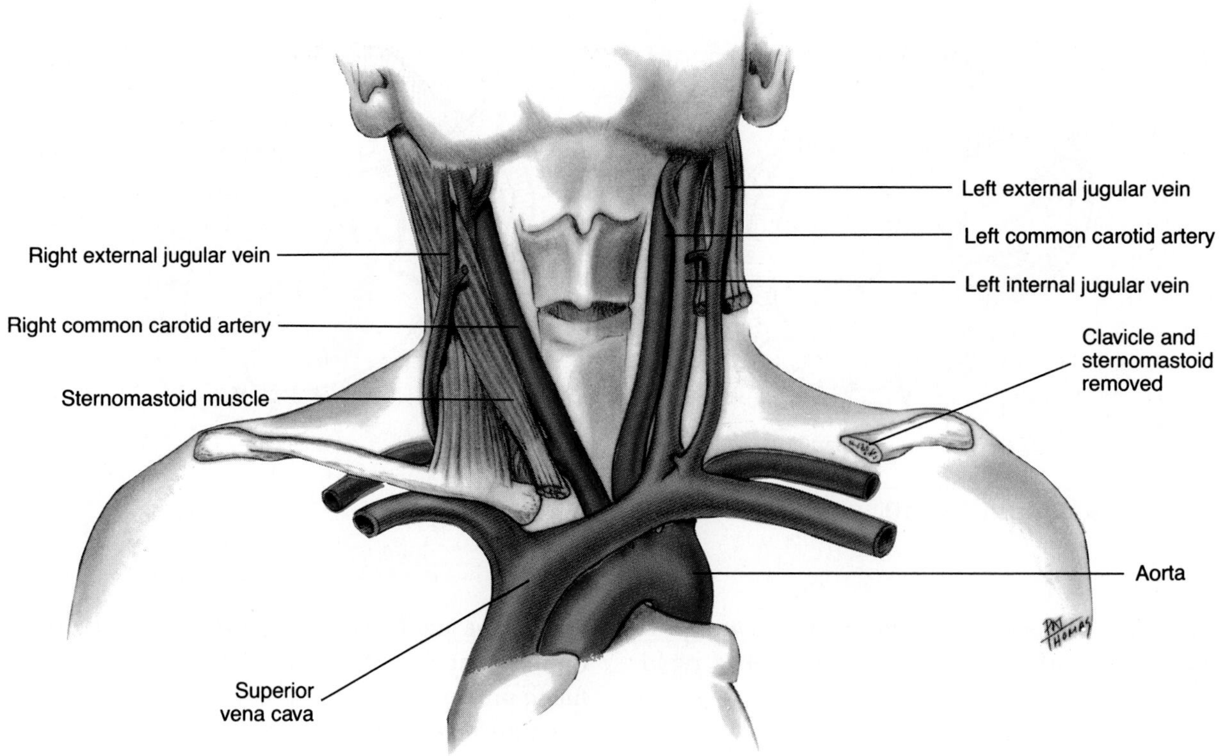

► **Figure 16–12**

Although an arterial pulse is caused by a forward propulsion of blood, the jugular pulse is different. The jugular pulse results from a backwash, a waveform moving backward caused by events upstream. The jugular pulse has five components (Fig. 16–13):

	REFLECTS	RESULTS FROM
a wave	atrial contraction	some blood flows backward to the vena cava during right atrial contraction
c wave	ventricular contraction	backflow from bulging upward of tricuspid valve when it closes at beginning of ventricular systole (not from neighboring carotid artery pulsation)
x descent	atrial relaxation	right ventricle contracts (systole) and pulls bottom of atria downward
v wave	passive atrial filling	increasing volume of atrial filling and increased pressure
y descent	passive ventricular filling	tricuspid valve opens and blood flows from RA to RV

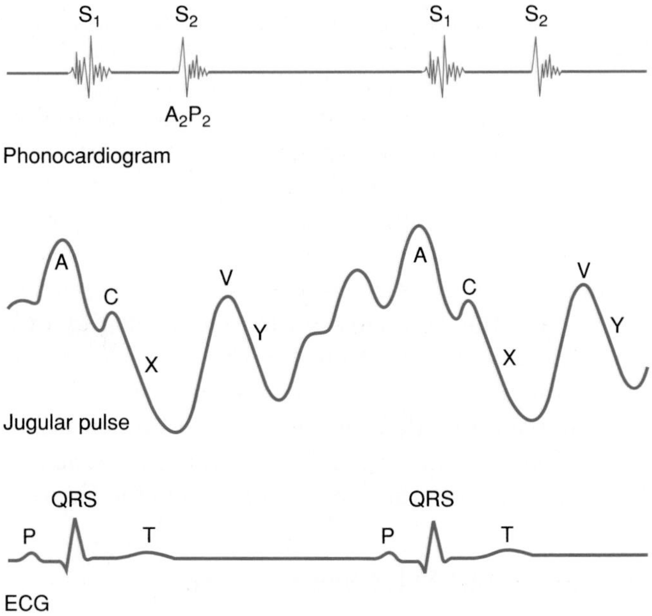

► **Figure 16–13**

DEVELOPMENTAL CONSIDERATIONS

Infants and Children

The fetal heart functions early; it begins to beat at the end of 3 weeks' gestation. The lungs are nonfunctional, but the fetal circulation compensates for this (Fig. 16–14). Oxygenation takes place at the placenta, and the arterial blood is returned to the right side of the heart. There is no point in pumping all this freshly oxygenated blood through the lungs, so it is rerouted in two ways. First, about two-thirds of it is shunted through an opening in the atrial septum, the *foramen ovale,* into the left side of the heart, where it is pumped out through the aorta. Second, the rest of the oxygenated blood is pumped by the right side of the heart out the pulmonary artery, but it is detoured through the *ductus arteriosus* to the aorta. Because they are both pumping into the systemic circulation, the right and left ventricles are equal in weight and muscle wall thickness.

Inflation and aeration of the lungs at birth produces circulatory changes. Now the blood is oxygenated through the lungs rather than through the placenta. The foramen ovale closes within the first hour because of the

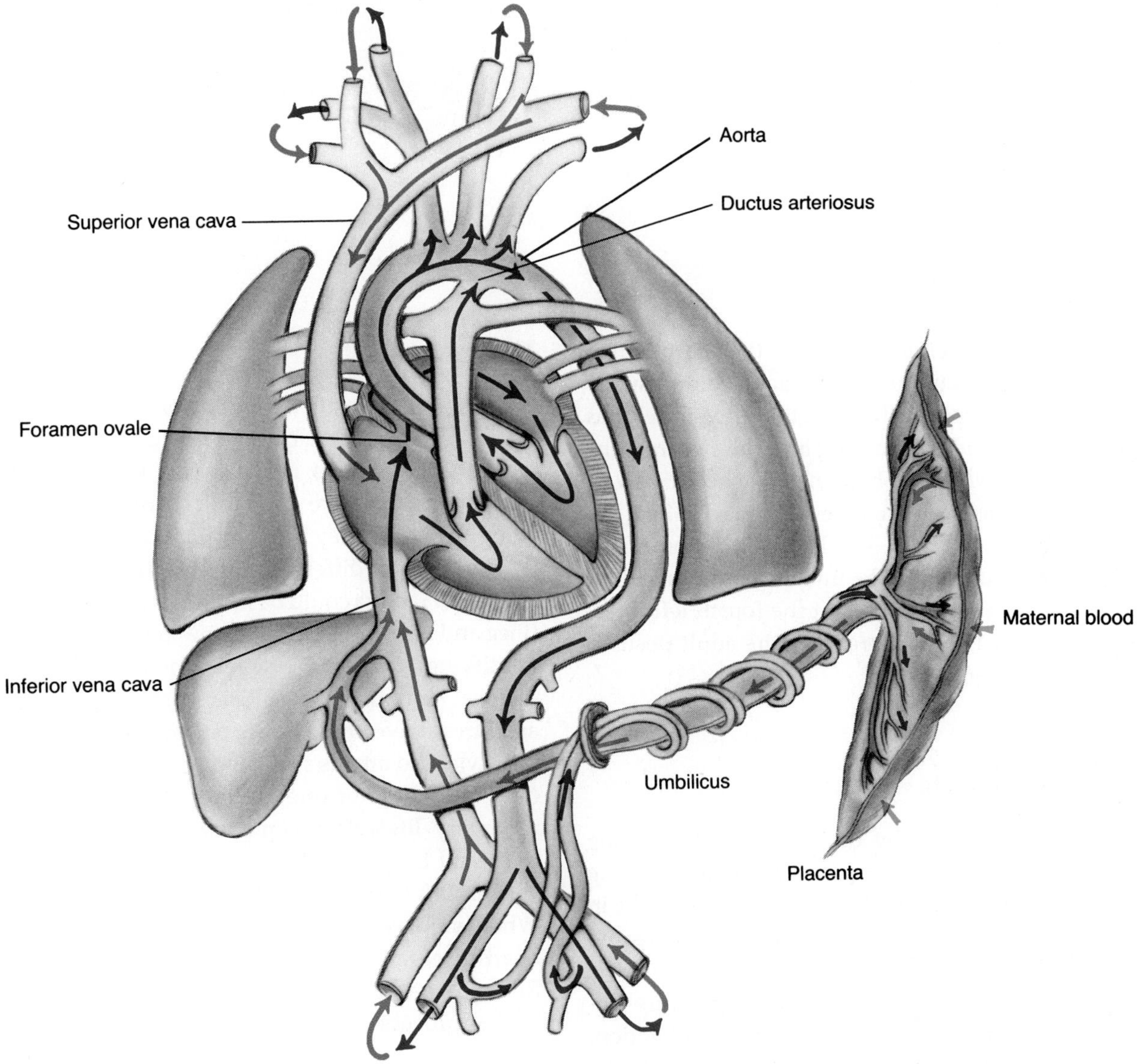

▶ **Figure 16–14**

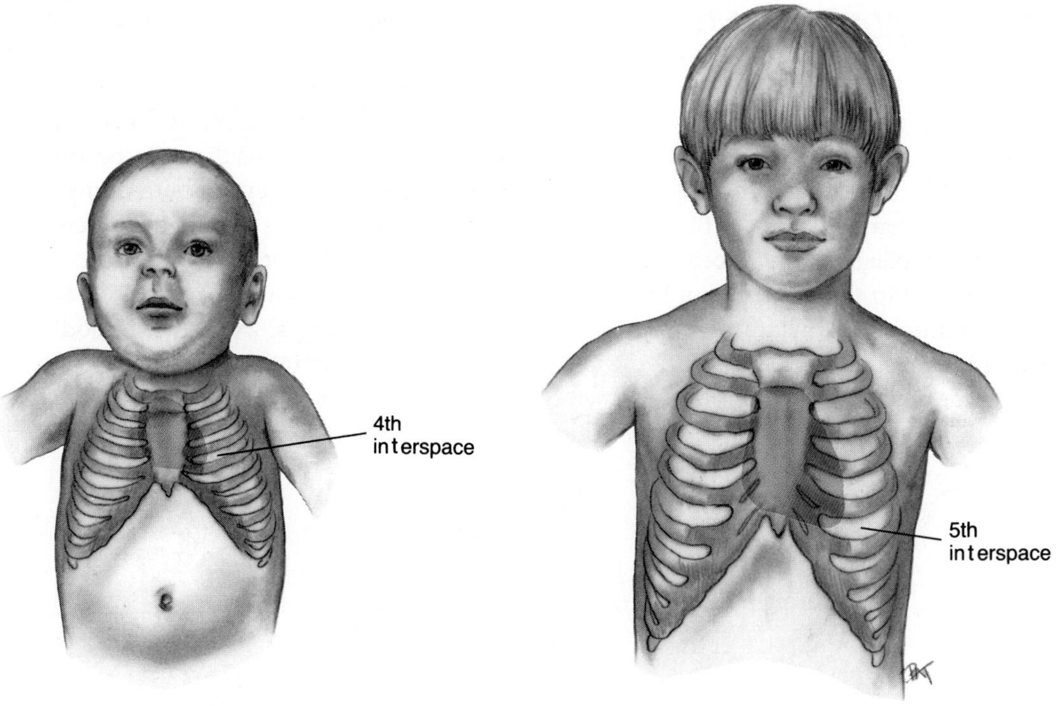

► Figure 16–15

new lower pressure in the right side of the heart than in the left side. The ductus arteriosus closes later, usually within 10 to 15 hours of birth. Now, the left ventricle has the greater workload of pumping into the systemic circulation, so that when the baby has reached 1 year of age its mass increases to reach the adult ratio of 2 : 1, left ventricle to right ventricle. The heart's position in the chest is more horizontal in the infant than in the adult; thus the apex is higher, located at the fourth left intercostal space (Fig. 16–15). It reaches the adult position when the child reaches age 7.

The Pregnant Female

Blood volume increases by 30 to 40 percent during pregnancy, with the most rapid expansion occurring during the second trimester. This creates an increase in stroke volume and cardiac output, and an increased pulse rate of 10 to 15 beats per minute. Despite the increased cardiac output, arterial blood pressure decreases in pregnancy, due to peripheral vasodilatation. The blood pressure drops to its lowest point during the second trimester, then rises after that. The blood pressure varies with the person's position, as described on p. 565.

The Aging Adult

It is difficult to isolate the "aging process" of the cardiovascular system *per se* because it is so closely interrelated with lifestyle, habits, and diseases. Earlier studies suggested a progressive decline in cardiac function with aging, but also they were dramatically varied in their results among different populations. This suggested that other factors could be modifiers in the aging process (Fleg and Lakatta, 1986). We now know that lifestyle is a modifying factor in the development of cardiovascular disease; smoking, diet, alcohol use, exercise patterns, and stress have an influence on coronary artery disease. Lifestyle also affects the aging process; cardiac changes once thought to be due to aging are partially due to the sedentary lifestyle accompanying aging (Fig. 16–16) (Fleg and Lakatta, 1986).

What is left to be attributed to the aging process alone? When studies exclude people with clinical or occult heart disease (Gerstenblith et al, 1977; Berman, 1982; Rodenheffer et al, 1984), the following hemodynamic "aging process" emerges.

Hemodynamic Changes

- From age 20 to 80, systolic blood pressure tends to increase within the normal range by 25 to 30 percent.

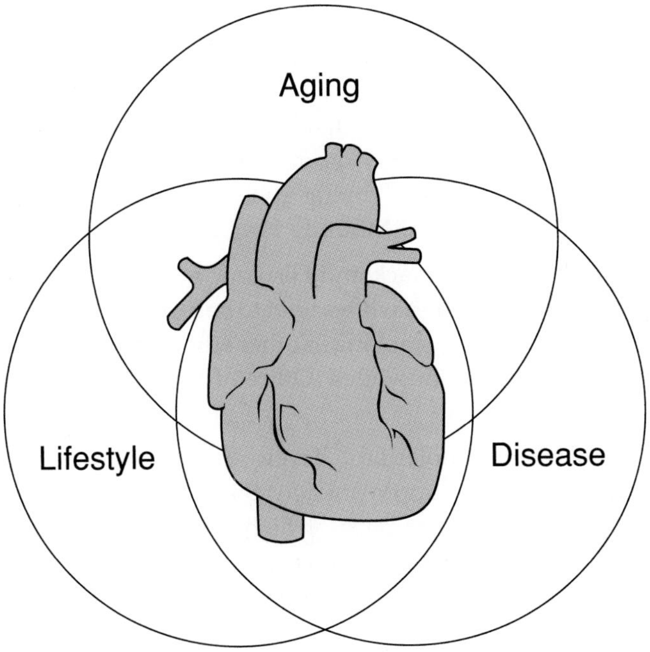

► **Figure 16-16**

This is due to stiffening of the large arteries, which, in turn, is due to calcification of vessel walls (arteriosclerosis). This stiffening creates an increase in pulse wave velocity because the less compliant arteries cannot store the volume ejected.

- From age 20 to 80, left ventricular wall thickness increases by about 25 percent, which is still within normal range. This is an adaptive mechanism to accommodate the vascular stiffening mentioned earlier that creates an increased work load on the heart.
- There is no significant change in diastolic pressure with age. A rising systolic pressure with a relatively constant diastolic results in an increase in pulse pressure (the difference between the two).
- There is no change in resting heart rate with aging.
- Cardiac output at rest is not changed with aging.
- Cardiac output during aerobic exercise does not decrease significantly either; maximal heart rate attained does decrease but is compensated for by an increase of stroke volume due to increased end-diastolic filling volume.

Arrhythmias. The presence of supraventricular and ventricular arrhythmias increases with age. Ectopic beats are common in aging people, and the mere presence of an arrhythmia is not an accurate indicator of underlying organic heart disease (Fleg and Kennedy, 1982).

Tachyarrhythmias may not be tolerated as well in older people. The myocardium is thicker and less compliant, and early diastolic filling is impaired at rest. Thus, it may not tolerate a tachycardia as well because of shortened diastole (Fleg and Lakatta, 1986). Another consequence is that tachyarrhythmias may further compromise a vital organ whose function already has been affected by aging or disease. For example, a ventricular tachycardia produces a 40 to 70 percent decrease in cerebral blood flow. Although a younger person may tolerate this, an older person with cerebrovascular disease may experience syncope (Fleg and Lakatta, 1986).

ECG. Age-related changes in the ECG occur due to histologic changes in the conduction system. These include:

- prolonged P-R interval (first-degree AV block) and prolonged Q-T interval, but the QRS interval is unchanged;
- left axis deviation due to age-related mild LV hypertrophy and fibrosis in left bundle branch;
- increased incidence of bundle branch block (Fleg and Lakatta, 1986).

Although the hemodynamic changes associated with aging alone do not seem severe or portentous, the fact remains that the incidence of cardiovascular disease increases with age. The incidence of coronary artery disease increases sharply with advancing age and accounts for about half of the deaths of older people. Mixed hypertension (systolic > 160 mm Hg and diastolic > 95 mm Hg) also increases with age (Fleg and Lakatta, 1986). Certainly, lifestyle habits (smoking, lack of exercise, diet) play a significant role in the acquisition of heart disease. Also, current studies suggest that aerobic exercise may help to retard the development of heart disease, even in the geriatric population (Kavanagh and Shepard, 1990). Both points underscore the need for health teaching as an important treatment parameter.

TRANSCULTURAL CONSIDERATIONS

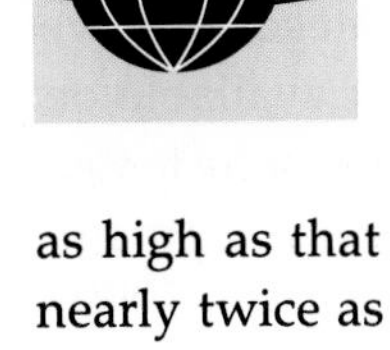

Heart disease and stroke account for more than one-third of all deaths among individuals from culturally diverse backgrounds (Fig. 16-17). Under age 35, heart disease mortality for Native Americans is approximately twice as high as that for all other Americans. Black men are nearly twice as likely to die from stroke as white men,

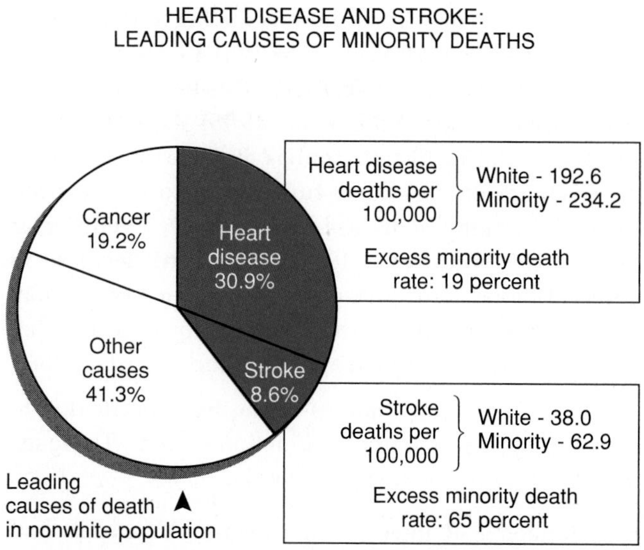

► **Figure 16–17**

and their death rate from stroke is more than double that of other ethnic groups (Office of Minority Health, 1990).

Among blacks 20 to 64 years of age, there is a greater number of deaths from coronary artery disease compared with whites. The incidence of mortality from coronary disease is greater in black women than in black men.

A *risk factor* is anything that increases a person's chance of developing a disease. The major risk factors for heart disease and stroke are high blood pressure, smoking, high cholesterol levels, obesity, and diabetes.

Research on risk factors reveals the following data concerning individuals from the federally defined ethnic minority groups as reported by the Office of Minority Health, United States Public Health Service, Department of Health and Human Services.

Hypertension. Blacks, Puerto Ricans, Cubans, and Mexicans have a higher incidence of hypertension than whites. The prevalence of hypertension in blacks is 1.4 times greater than in whites despite a decline in mean blood pressure in blacks between 1960 and 1980. Reduction of blood pressure can reduce the incidence of coronary heart disease among both whites and blacks. Although data pertaining to Asian Americans are scarce, Filipinos of all gender and age categories have higher blood pressure than whites. Data available on Japanese Americans and Native Americans indicate that there is a lower prevalence of hypertension among members of these groups (Office of Minority Health, 1990).

Blacks and individuals with lower educational and income levels tend to have higher blood pressures. Although the exact reason for this is unknown, the Secretary's Task Force reports that hypertension is related to living in "areas of high social stress and instability as well as to education, coping styles, and occupational insecurity" (Office of Minority Health, 1990).

Smoking. More black and Hispanic men smoke than white men, although whites tend to be heavier smokers. The prevalence of smoking in other ethnic groups tends to be lower than in whites (Office of Minority Health, 1990).

Cholesterol. Cholesterol levels among black and white adults are approximately the same. Black men tend to have higher rates of high density lipoprotein (HDL), which reduces cardiovascular risks. Certain Hispanic subgroups, such as Mexican Americans and Puerto Ricans, exhibit higher cholesterol levels than whites. Both Native Americans and Japanese Americans show lower cholesterol levels than whites (Office of Minority Health, 1990).

Obesity. Obesity is defined as an excess of 20 percent of standard weight for age and height. This risk factor for cardiovascular disease is more common among black women than other groups, but obesity is also problematic among many Hispanic women.

Diabetes. Diabetes is a contributing factor to 300,000 deaths per year. It has been ranked seventh among leading causes of death in the United States. In many Native American tribes, more than 20 percent of members have diabetes, ten times the incidence found among the general population. A dramatic increase in obesity among Native Americans has accompanied the increase in diabetes that has been documented during the past 50 years. In one tribe, the Pima Indians, nearly 50 percent of those over 35 years of age are affected. The complications of diabetes, especially kidney disease, blindness, and amputation, are known to have increased severity in Native Americans (Office of Minority Health, 1990).

Diabetes is 33 percent more common among blacks than among whites, with black women having an incidence of 50 percent more cases of diabetes than white women. Obesity among diabetic black women is also higher than the incidence found among non-black women. The complications of diabetes, such as blindness and kidney disease, are more frequent in blacks than in whites. Unfortunately, the infants of pregnant diabetic black women also are at greater risk, with the death rate being three times higher for infants born to black diabetic mothers than to white diabetic mothers (Office of Minority Health, 1990).

Hispanics in the United States have three times the risk of developing diabetes as do non-Hispanic whites. Research-based data on Hispanics are scarce because early studies included Hispanics as part of the white population.

Among Japanese men in the United States aged 40 or older, researchers find the diabetes rate to be as high as 10 to 14 percent, and Japanese living in the United States have, as a group, more than twice the incidence of diabetes as Japanese living in Japan. Japanese, Chinese, and Filipino Americans who are born in the United States have higher death rates from diabetes than their native-born counterparts. The blame for what these statistics reveal is being placed on the high fat content of a typical American diet. Japanese diets in the United States, for example, are much higher in both animal and total fat content than in Japan.

SUBJECTIVE DATA

- Chest pain
- Dyspnea
- Orthopnea
- Cough
- Fatigue
- Cyanosis or pallor
- Edema
- Nocturia
- Past history
- Family history
- Personal habits

EXAMINER ASKS:	RATIONALE:
1. Have you been having any **chest pain** or tightness? Onset: When did it start? How long have you had it *this* time? Have you had this type of pain before? How often?	Angina, an important cardiac symptom, occurs when heart's vascular supply cannot keep up with metabolic demand.
Location: where did the pain start? Does the pain radiate to any other spot? Character: How would you describe it? (crushing, stabbing, burning, vise-like. Allow the person to offer adjectives before you suggest them.) (Note if uses clenched fist to describe pain.)	Chest pain also may have pulmonary, musculoskeletal, or gastrointestinal origin; it is important to differentiate. "Clenched fist" sign is characteristic of angina.
Was the pain brought on by: activity—what type; rest; emotional upset; after eating; during sexual intercourse; with cold weather?	
Are there any associated symptoms: sweating, ashen gray or pale skin, heart skips beat, shortness of breath, nausea or vomiting, racing of heart?	Diaphoresis. Pallor, palpitations dyspnea, nausea, tachycardia.
Is the pain made worse by moving the arms or neck, breathing, lying flat? Is the pain relieved by rest, nitroglycerin? How many tablets?	

EXAMINER ASKS:	RATIONALE:
2. Shortness of breath What type of activity brings on shortness of breath? How much activity brings it on now? How much activity brought it on 6 months ago?	**Dyspnea** (Also a pulmonary symptom, see Chapter 15). Dyspnea on exertion (DOE)—quantify exactly, e.g., DOE after walking two level blocks.
Onset: Does the shortness of breath come on unexpectedly?	Paroxysmal
Duration: Is it constant or does it come and go?	Constant or intermittent
Does it seem to be affected by position: lying down?	Recumbent
Does it awaken you from sleep at night?	Paroxysmal nocturnal dyspnea (PND) occurs with congestive heart failure. Lying down increases volume of intrathoracic blood, and the weakened heart cannot accommodate the increased load. Classically, the person awakens after 2 hours of sleep, arises, and flings open a window with the perception of needing fresh air.
Does the shortness of breath interfere with activities of daily living?	
3. How many pillows do you use when sleeping or lying down?	**Orthopnea** is the need to assume a more upright position in order to breathe. Note the exact number of pillows used.
4. Do you have a **cough?** Duration: How long have you had it? Frequency: Is it related to time of day? Type: Is the cough dry, hacking, barky, hoarse, or congested?	
Do you cough up mucus? What color is it? Does the mucus have an odor? Is it blood tinged?	Sputum production, mucoid or purulent. Hemoptysis is often of a pulmonary disorder but also occurs with mitral stenosis.
Is the cough associated with: activity, position (lying down), anxiety, talking? Does activity make it better or worse (sit, walk, exercise)? Is it relieved by rest or medication?	
5. **Fatigue:** Do you seem to tire easily? Are you able to keep up with your family and co-workers? Onset: When did fatigue start? Was it sudden or gradual? Has there been any *recent* change in energy level?	
Is your fatigue related to time of day: all day, morning, evening?	Fatigue due to decreased cardiac output is worse in the evening, whereas fatigue from anxiety or depression occurs all day or is worse in the morning.
6. Have you noted your facial skin turn blue or turn ashen?	**Cyanosis** or **pallor** (see Chapter 9).
7. Have you noticed any swelling of your feet and legs?	**Edema** is dependent when due to congestive heart failure.
Onset: When did you first notice this? Has there been any recent change? What time of day does the swelling occur? Do your shoes feel tight at the end of day?	Cardiac edema is worse at evening

EXAMINER ASKS: | **RATIONALE:**

How much swelling would you say there is? Are both legs equally swollen?
Does the swelling go away with: rest, elevation, after a night's sleep?
Are there any associated symptoms, such as shortness of breath? If so, does the shortness of breath occur before leg swelling or after?

and better in morning after elevating legs all night.

8. Do you awaken at night with an urgent need to urinate? For how long has this been occurring? Has there been any recent change?

Nocturia—recumbency at night promotes fluid reabsorption and excretion; this occurs with heart failure in the person who is ambulatory during the day.

9. Do you have any **past history** of hypertension, elevated blood cholesterol or triglycerides, heart murmur, congenital heart disease, rheumatic fever or unexplained joint pains as child or youth, recurrent tonsillitis, anemia?
   Have you ever had heart disease? When was this? Was it treated by medication, or heart surgery? When was your last ECG, stress ECG, other heart tests?
10. Do you have any **family history** of: hypertension, obesity, diabetes, coronary artery disease, sudden death at younger age?
11. **Personal history**
    a. Nutrition: Please describe your usual daily diet. (Note if this diet is representative of the basic food groups, the amount of calories, cholesterol, and any additives such as salt.)
       What is your usual weight? Has there been any recent change?
    b. Smoking: Do you smoke cigarettes or other tobacco? At what age did you start? How many packs per day? For how many years have you smoked this amount?
       Have you ever tried to quit? If so, how did this go?
    c. Alcohol: How much alcohol do you usually drink each week, or each day? When was your last drink? What was the number of drinks that episode? Have you ever been told you had a drinking problem?
    d. Exercise: What is your usual amount of exercise each day or week? What type of exercise (state type or sport)? If a sport, what is your usual amount (light, moderate, heavy)?
    e. Drugs: Do you take any antihypertensives, beta-blockers, digoxin, diuretics, aspirin/anti-coagulants, over-the-counter, or street drugs?

ADDITIONAL QUESTIONS FOR INFANTS

How was the mother's health during pregnancy: any unexplained fever, rubella first trimester, other infection, hypertension, drugs taken?

Have you noted any cyanosis while nursing, crying? Is the baby able to eat, nurse or finish bottle without tiring?

To screen for heart disease in infant, focus on feeding. Note fatigue during feeding. Infant with congestive heart failure takes fewer ounces each feeding; be-

EXAMINER ASKS:	RATIONALE:
	comes dyspneic with sucking; may be diaphoretic, then falls into exhausted sleep; awakens after a short time hungry again.
Growth: Has this baby grown as expected by growth charts, and about the same as siblings or peers?	Poor weight gain.
Activity: Were this baby's motor milestones achieved as expected? Is the baby able to play without tiring? How many naps does the baby take each day? How long does a nap last?	

ADDITIONAL QUESTIONS FOR CHILDREN

Growth: Has this child grown as expected by growth charts?	Poor weight gain.
Activity: Is this child able to keep up with siblings or age-mates? Is the child willing or reluctant to go out to play? Is the child able to climb stairs, ride a bike, walk a few blocks? Does the child squat to rest during play or to watch television, or assume a knee-chest position while sleeping?	Fatigue. Record specific limitations.
Have you noted "blue spells" during exercise?	Cyanosis.

Has the child had any unexplained joint pains, or unexplained fever?

Does the child have frequent headaches, nosebleeds?

Does the child have frequent respiratory infections? How many per year? How are they treated? Have any of these proved to be streptococcal infections?

Family history: Does the child have a sibling with heart defect?

Past history: Is anyone in the child's family known to have chromosomal abnormalities, e.g., Down syndrome?

ADDITIONAL QUESTIONS FOR THE PREGNANT FEMALE

1. Have you had any hypertension during this or earlier pregnancies? What was your usual blood pressure level before pregnancy? How has your blood pressure been monitored during the pregnancy?
If high blood pressure, what treatment has been started?
Have you had any associated symptoms: weight gain, protein in urine, swelling in feet, legs, or face?
2. Have you experienced any faintness or dizziness with this pregnancy?

ADDITIONAL QUESTIONS FOR THE AGING ADULT

1. Do you have any known heart or lung disease: hypertension, coronary artery disease, chronic emphysema or bronchitis?
What efforts to treat this have been started?
Have your usual symptoms changed recently? Does your illness interfere with activities of daily living?
Do you take any medications for your illness? Are you aware of side effects? Do you take any type of digitalis medication?
2. Environment: Are there any stairs at home? How often do you need to climb them? Does this have any effect on activities of daily living?

Equipment Needed:

Marking pen
Small centimeter ruler
Stethoscope with diaphragm and bell endpieces

Preparation

To evaluate the carotid arteries, the person can be sitting up. To assess the jugular veins and the precordium, the person should be supine with the head and chest slightly elevated. Stand on the person's right side; this will facilitate your hand placement and auscultation of the precordium. The room must be warm — chilling makes the person uncomfortable, and shivering interferes with heart sounds. Take scrupulous care to ensure *quiet;* heart sounds are very soft and any ambient room noise masks them.

Ensure the female's privacy by keeping her breasts draped. The female's left breast overrides part of the area you will need to examine. Gently displace the breast upward, or ask the woman to hold it out of the way.

When performing a regional cardiovascular assessment, use this order:

1. Pulse and blood pressure (see Chapter 8)
2. Extremities (see Peripheral Vascular Assessment, Chapter 18)
3. Neck vessels
4. Precordium

The logic of this order is that you will begin observations peripherally and move in toward the heart. For choreography of these steps in the complete physical examination, see Chapter 24.

METHOD OF EXAMINATION

NORMAL RANGE OF FINDINGS	ABNORMAL FINDINGS

THE NECK VESSELS

The Carotid Arteries

Palpate the carotid artery.

Located central to the heart, the carotid artery yields important information on cardiac function.

Palpate each carotid artery medial to the sternomastoid muscle in the lower third of the neck (Fig. 16–18). Avoid the carotid sinus area higher in the neck; excessive vagal stimulation here could slow down the heart rate, especially in older adults. Take care to palpate gently. Palpate only one carotid artery at a time to avoid compromising arterial blood to the brain.

Feel the contour and amplitude of the pulse. Normally the contour is smooth with a rapid upstroke and slower downstroke, and the normal strength is 2+ or moderate (see Chapter 18). Your findings should be the same bilaterally.

Abnormal findings: Diminished pulse feels small and weak; occurs with decreased stroke volume.

NORMAL RANGE OF FINDINGS

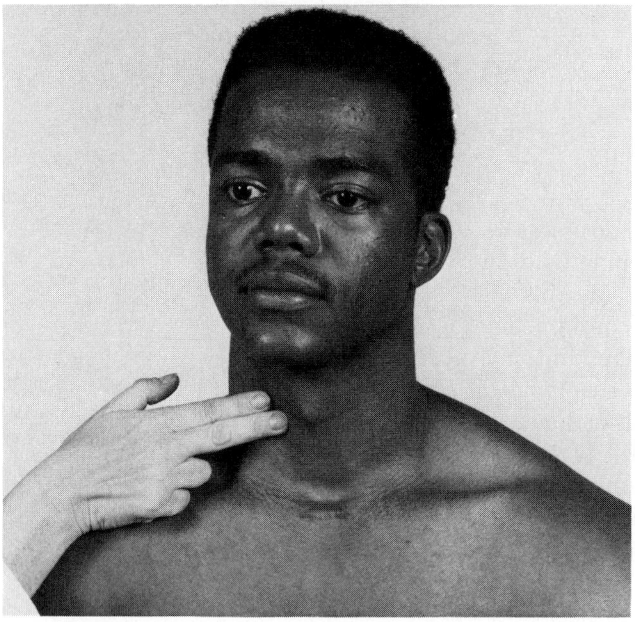

► **Figure 16–18**

Auscultate the carotid artery.

For persons older than middle age or who show symptoms or signs of cardiovascular disease, auscultate each carotid artery for the presence of a *bruit* (Fig. 16–19). This is a blowing, swishing sound indicating blood flow

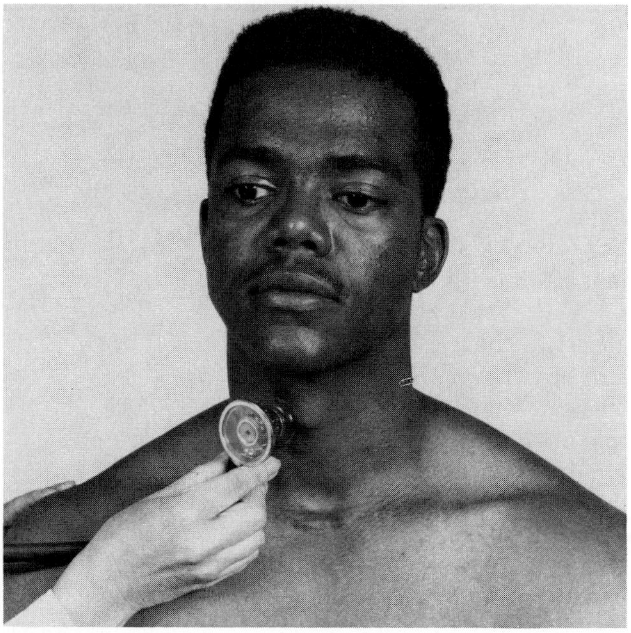

► **Figure 16–19**

ABNORMAL FINDINGS

Increased pulse feels full and strong; occurs with hyperkinetic states (see Table 18–2).

A bruit indicates turbulence due to a local vascular cause, e.g., atherosclerotic narrowing.

A murmur sounds much the same but is caused by a cardiac disorder. Some aortic valve murmurs radiate to the neck and must be distinguished from a local bruit.

NORMAL RANGE OF FINDINGS	ABNORMAL FINDINGS

turbulence; normally there is none. Ask the person to hold his or her breath while you listen so that tracheal breath sounds do not mask or mimic a carotid artery bruit. Sometimes you can hear normal heart sounds transmitted to the neck; do not confuse these with a bruit.

The Jugular Veins

Inspect the jugular venous pulse.

From the jugular veins you can assess the central venous pressure (CVP) and thus the heart's efficiency as a pump. Although the external jugular vein is easier to see, the internal (especially the right) is attached more directly to the superior vena cava and thus is more reliable for assessment. You cannot see the internal jugular vein itself but you can see its pulsation.

Position the person anywhere from a 30- to a 45-degree angle, wherever you can best see the pulsations. In general the higher the venous pressure, the higher the position you need. Remove the pillow to avoid flexing the neck; the head should be in the same plane as the trunk. Turn the person's head slightly away from the examined side, and direct a strong light tangentially onto the neck to highlight pulsations and shadows.

Note the external jugular veins overlying the sternomastoid muscle. In some persons, the veins are not visible at all; whereas in others, they are full in the supine position. As the person is raised to a sitting position, these external jugulars flatten and disappear, usually at 45 degrees.

Unilateral distention of external jugular veins is due to local cause, e.g., kinking or aneurysm.

Full distended external jugular veins above 45 degrees signify increased CVP.

Now look for pulsations of the internal jugular veins in the area of the suprasternal notch or around the origin of the sternomastoid muscle around the clavicle. You must be able to distinguish internal jugular vein pulsation from that of the carotid artery. It is easy to confuse them because they lie close together. Use the guidelines shown in Table 16–1.

Table 16–1 ► Characteristics of Jugular Versus Carotid Pulsations

	INTERNAL JUGULAR PULSE	CAROTID PULSE
1. Location	Lower, more lateral, under or behind the sternomastoid muscle	Higher and medial to this muscle
2. Quality	Undulant and diffuse, two visible waves per cycle	Brisk and localized; one wave per cycle
3. Respiration	Varies with respiration. Its level descends during inspiration when intrathoracic pressure is decreased	Does not vary
4. Palpable	No	Yes
5. Pressure	Light pressure at the base of the neck easily obliterates	No change
6. Position of person	Level of pulse drops and disappears as the person is brought to a sitting position	Unaffected

NORMAL RANGE OF FINDINGS	ABNORMAL FINDINGS

Estimate the jugular venous pressure.

Think of the jugular veins as a CVP manometer attached directly to the right atrium. You can "read" the CVP at the highest level of pulsations (Fig. 16–20). Use the angle of Louis (sternal angle) as an arbitrary reference point, and compare it with the highest level of venous pulsation. Hold a vertical ruler on the sternal angle. Align a straight edge on the ruler like a T-square, and adjust the level of the horizontal straight edge to the level of pulsation. Read the level of intersection on the vertical ruler; normal jugular venous pulsation is 2 cm or less above the sternal angle. Also state the person's position.

Elevated pressure is more than 3 cm above the sternal angle while at 45 degrees, and occurs with right-sided congestive heart failure.

If you cannot find the internal jugular veins, use the external jugular veins and note the point where they look collapsed. Be aware that the technique of estimating venous pressure is difficult and is not always a reliable predictor of CVP. Consistency in grading among examiners is difficult to achieve.

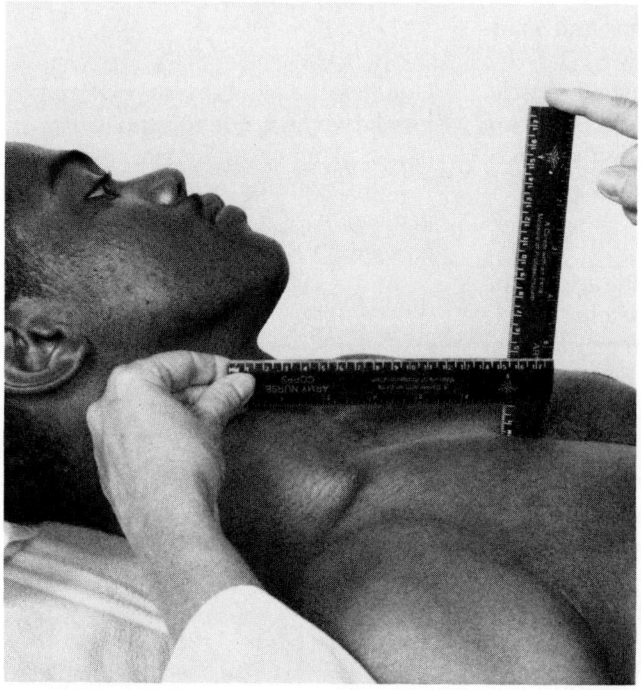

▶ **Figure 16–20**

If venous pressure is elevated, or if you suspect congestive heart failure, perform *hepatojugular reflux* (Fig. 16–21). Position the person comfortably supine and instruct him or her to breathe quietly through an open mouth. Hold your right hand on the right upper quadrant of the person's abdomen just below the rib cage. Watch the level of jugular

NORMAL RANGE OF FINDINGS | **ABNORMAL FINDINGS**

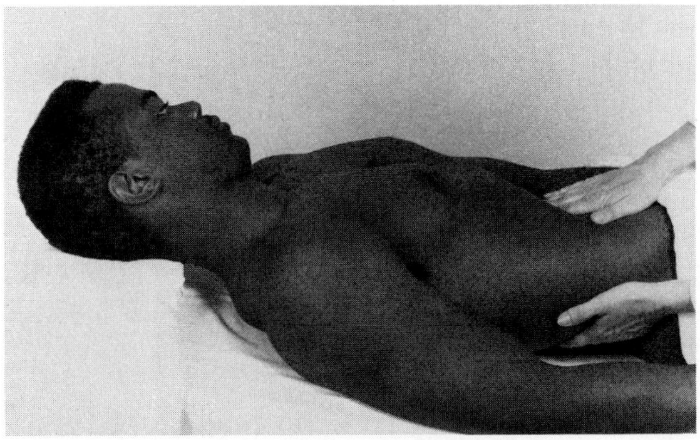

► Figure 16-21

pulsation as you push in with your hand. Exert firm sustained pressure for 30 seconds. This empties venous blood out of the liver sinusoids and adds its volume to the venous system. If the right side of the heart is able to pump this additional volume (i.e., if there is no elevated CVP), the jugular veins will rise for a few seconds, then recede back to previous level.

If right-sided congestive heart failure does exist, the jugular veins will elevate and stay elevated as long as you push.

THE PRECORDIUM

Inspection

Inspect the anterior chest.

Arrange tangential lighting to accentuate any flicker of movement.

Pulsations. You may or may not see the *apical impulse,* the pulsation created as the left ventricle rotates against the chest wall during systole. When visible, it occupies the fourth or fifth intercostal space, at or inside the midclavicular line. It is easier to see in children or those with thinner chest walls.

A *heave* or *lift* is a sustained forceful thrusting of the ventricle during systole. It occurs with ventricular hypertrophy due to increased workload. A right ventricular heave is seen at the sternal border; a left ventricular heave is seen at the apex (see Table 16-7).

Palpation

Palpate the apical impulse.

(This used to be called the point of maximal impulse or PMI. Since some abnormal conditions may cause a maximal impulse to be felt elsewhere on the chest, use the term apical impulse specifically for the apex beat.)

Localize the apical impulse precisely using one finger pad (Fig. 16-

NORMAL RANGE OF FINDINGS	ABNORMAL FINDINGS

22). Asking the person to "exhale and then hold it" aids the examiner in locating the pulsation. You may need to roll the person midway to the left to find it; note that this also displaces the apical impulse farther to the left.

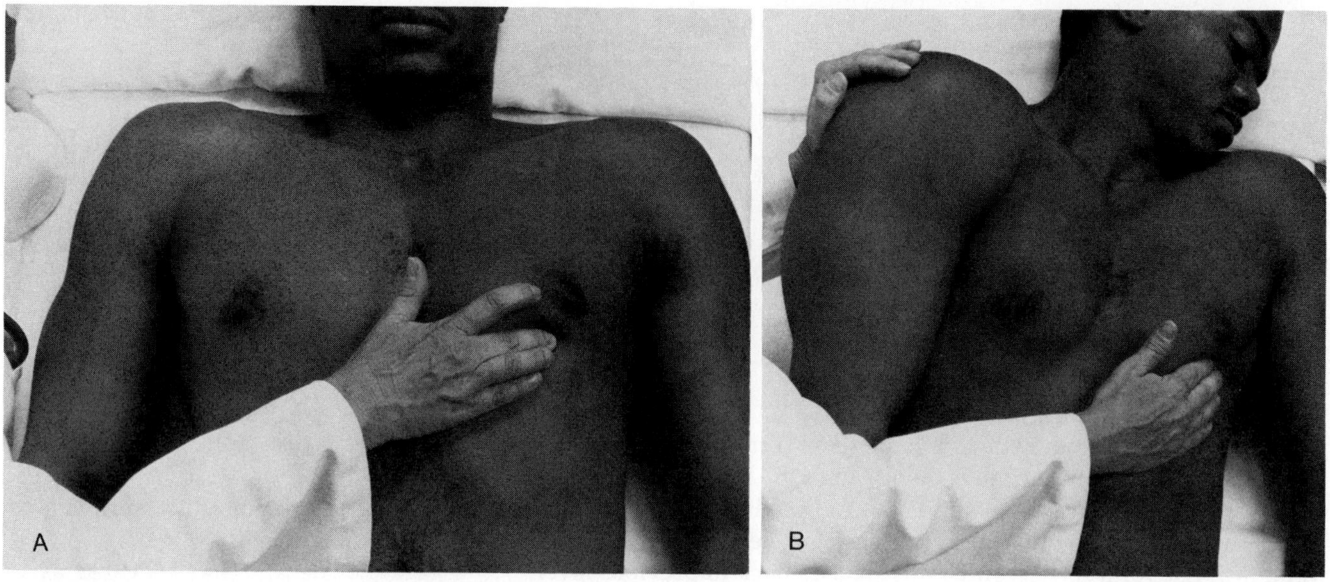

▶ **Figure 16-22**

Note

- Location—the apical impulse should occupy only one interspace, the fourth or fifth, and be at or medial to the midclavicular line.
- Size—normally 1 cm × 2 cm.
- Amplitude—normally a short gentle tap.
- Duration—short, normally occupies only first half of systole.

Cardiac enlargement:

- Left ventricular dilatation (volume overload) displaces impulse down and to left, and increases size more than 1 space.
- Increased force and duration but no change in location occurs with left ventricular hypertrophy and no dilatation (pressure overload) (see Table 16-7).

The apical impulse is palpable in about half of adults. It is not palpable with obese persons or persons with thick chest walls. With high cardiac output states (anxiety, fever, hyperthyroidism, anemia), the apical impulse increases in amplitude and duration.

Not palpable with pulmonary emphysema due to overriding lungs.

Palpate across the precordium.

Using the palmar aspects of your four fingers, gently palpate the apex, the left sternal border, and the base, searching for any other pulsations (Fig. 16-23). Normally there are none. If any are present, note the timing. Use the carotid artery pulsation as a guide or auscultate as you palpate.

A *thrill* is a palpable vibration. It feels like the throat of a purring cat. The thrill signifies turbulent blood flow, and accompanies loud murmurs. Absence of a thrill, however, does not necessarily rule out the presence of a murmur.

NORMAL RANGE OF FINDINGS

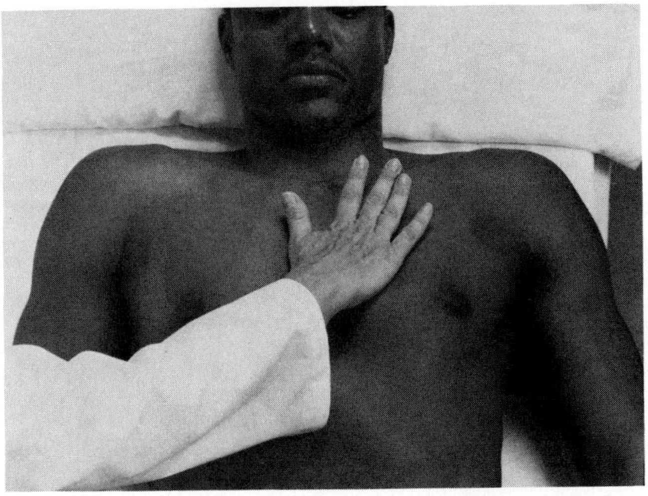

► **Figure 16–23**

Percussion

Percussion has been used to outline the heart's borders, but it has been displaced by the chest x-ray study. The x-ray study is much more accurate in detecting heart enlargement. When the right ventricle enlarges, it does so in the AP diameter, which is better seen on x-ray film. Also, percussion is of limited usefulness with the female breast tissue or in an obese person or a person with a muscular chest wall.

However, there are times when your percussing hands are the only tools you have with you, such as in an outpatient setting, extended care facility, or the person's home. When you need to search for cardiac enlargement, place your stationary finger in the person's fifth intercostal space over on the left side of the chest near the anterior axillary line. Slide your stationary hand toward yourself, percussing as you go, and note the change of sound from resonance over the lung to dull (over the heart). Normally, the left border of cardiac dullness is at the midclavicular line in the fifth interspace and slopes in toward the sternum as you progress upward so that by the second interspace the border of dullness coincides with the left sternal border. The right border of dullness normally matches the sternal border.

Auscultation

Identify the auscultatory areas where you will listen. These include the four traditional valve "areas" (Fig. 16–24). The valve areas are not over the actual anatomic locations of the valves but are the sites on the chest wall where sounds produced by the valves are best heard. The sound radiates with the direction of blood flow.

- Second right interspace—Aortic valve area.
- Second left interspace—Pulmonic valve area.
- Left lower sternal border—Tricuspid valve area.
- Fifth interspace at around left midclavicular line—Mitral valve area.

ABNORMAL FINDINGS

Accentuated first and second heart sounds and extra heart sounds also may cause abnormal pulsations.

NORMAL RANGE OF FINDINGS | **ABNORMAL FINDINGS**

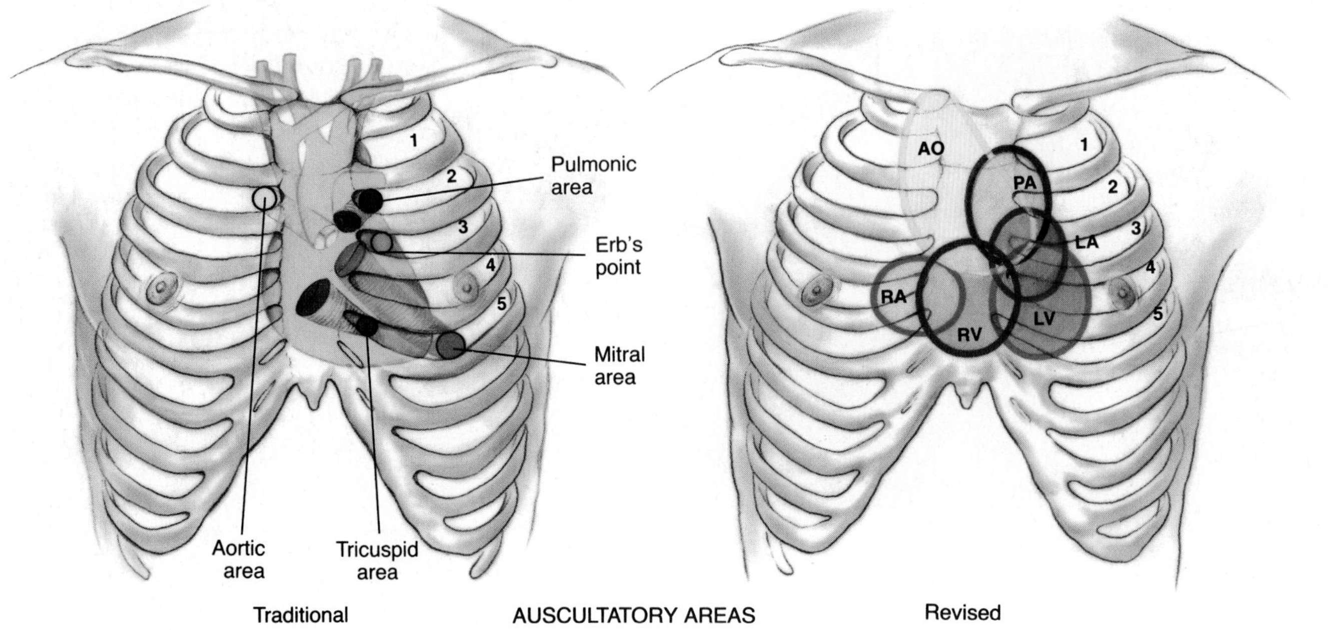

▶ **Figure 16–24**

Do not limit your auscultation to only four locations. Sounds produced by the valves may be heard all over the precordium. (For this reason, many experts even discourage the naming of the valve areas.) Thus, learn to inch your stethoscope in a "Z" pattern, from the base of the heart across and down, then over to the apex. Or, start at the apex and work your way up. Include the sites shown in Figure 16–24.

Recall the characteristics of a good stethoscope (see Chapter 7). You will use both endpieces. Although all heart sounds are low frequency, the diaphragm is for relatively higher pitched sounds and the bell is for relatively lower pitched ones.

Before you begin, alert the person, "I always listen to the heart in a number of places on the chest. Just because I am listening a long time, it does not necessarily mean that something is wrong."

Concentrate, and listen selectively to *one sound at a time.* Consider that at least two, and perhaps three or four, sounds may be happening in less than one second. You cannot process everything at once. Begin with the diaphragm endpiece and use the following routine: (1) Note the rate and rhythm, (2) identify S_1 and S_2, (3) assess S_1 and S_2 separately, (4) listen for extra heart sounds, and (5) listen for murmurs.

Note the rate and rhythm. The rate ranges normally from 60 to 100 beats per minute. (Review the full discussion of the pulse in Chapter 8, and the normal rates across age groups.) The rhythm should be regular, although *sinus arrhythmia* occurs normally in young adults and children. With sinus arrhythmia, the rhythm varies with the person's breathing, increasing at the peak of inspiration, and slowing with expiration. Note any other irregular rhythm. If one occurs, check if there is any pattern to it, or if it is totally irregular.

Premature beat—an isolated beat is early, or a pattern occurs in which every third or fourth beat sounds early.

Irregularly-irregular —no pattern to the sounds; beats come rapidly and at random intervals.

NORMAL RANGE OF FINDINGS

Identify S_1 and S_2. This is important because S_1 is the start of systole and thus serves as the reference point for the timing of all other cardiac sounds. Usually, you can identify S_1 instantly, because you hear a pair of sounds close together (lub-dup) and S_1 is the first of the pair. This guideline works, except in the cases of the tachyarrhythmias (rates > 100 per minute). Then the diastolic filling time is shortened, and the beats are too close together to distinguish. Other guidelines to distinguish S_1 from S_2 are:

- S_1 is louder than S_2 at the apex; S_2 is louder than S_1 at the base.
- S_1 coincides with the carotid artery pulse. Feel the carotid gently as you auscultate at the apex; the sound you hear as you feel each pulse is S_1 (Fig. 16–25).
- S_1 coincides with the R wave (the upstroke of the QRS complex) if the person is on an ECG monitor.

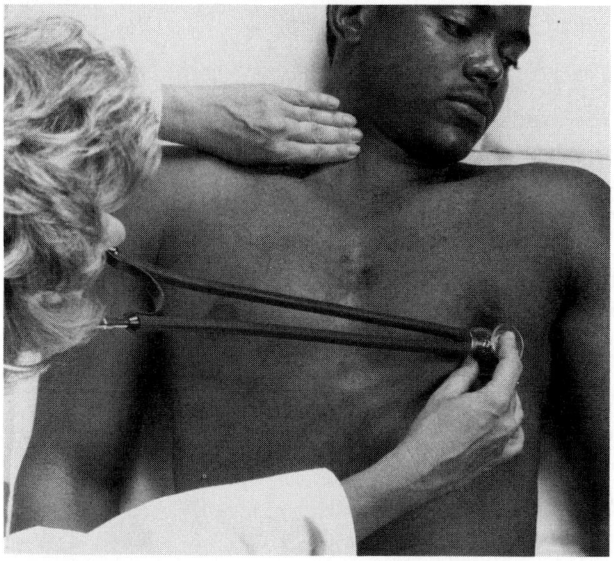

► **Figure 16–25**

Listen to S_1 and S_2 separately. Note whether each heart sound is normal, accentuated, diminished, or split. Inch your diaphragm across the chest as you do this.

First Heart Sound (S_1). Caused by closure of the AV valves, S_1 signals the beginning of systole. You can hear it over the entire precordium, though it is loudest at the apex (Fig. 16–26). (Sometimes the two sounds are equally loud at the apex, because S_1 is lower pitched than S_2.)

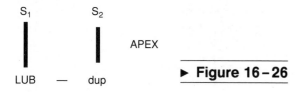

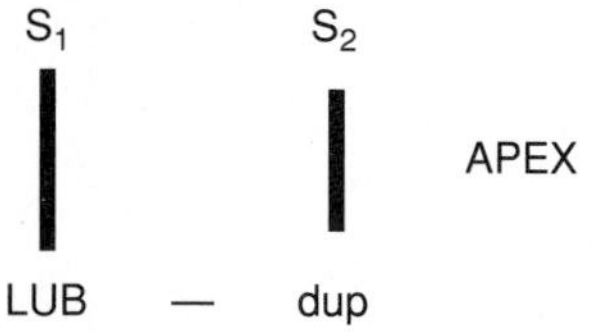

► **Figure 16–26**

ABNORMAL FINDINGS

Causes of accentuated or diminished S_1 (see Table 16–2).

Both heart sounds are diminished with conditions that place an increased amount of tissue between the heart and your stethoscope: emphysema (hyperinflated lungs), obesity, pericardial fluid.

NORMAL RANGE OF FINDINGS

ABNORMAL FINDINGS

You can hear S_1 with the diaphragm, with the person in any position, and equally well in inspiration and expiration. A split S_1 is normal, but it occurs rarely. A split S_1 means you are hearing the mitral and tricuspid components separately. It is audible in the tricuspid valve area, the left lower sternal border. The split is very rapid, with the two components only 0.03 second apart.

Second Heart Sound (S_2). S_2 is associated with closure of the semilunar valves. You can hear it with the diaphragm, over the entire precordium, though S_2 is loudest at the base (Fig. 16–27).

Accentuated or diminished S_2 (see Table 16–3).

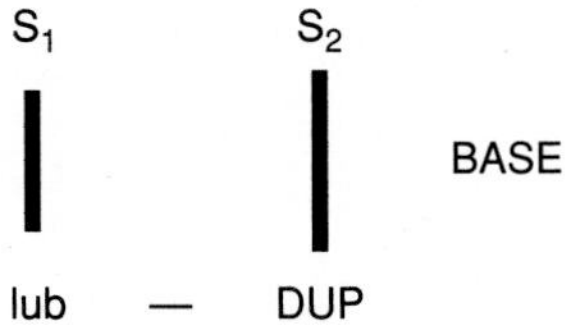

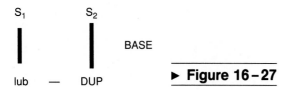

► **Figure 16–27**

Splitting of S_2. A split S_2 is a normal phenomenon that occurs toward the end of inspiration in some people. Recall that closure of the aortic and pulmonic valves is nearly synchronous. Because of the effects of respiration on the heart described earlier, inspiration separates the timing of the two valves' closure, and the aortic valve closes 0.06 second before the pulmonic valve. Instead of one DUP, you hear a split sound—T-DUP (Fig. 16–28). During expiration, synchrony returns and the aortic and pulmonic components fuse together. A split S_2 is heard only in the pulmonic valve area, the second left interspace.

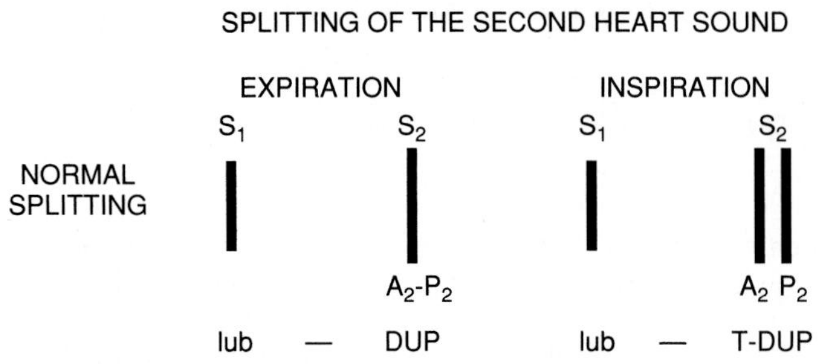

► **Figure 16–28**

When you first hear the split S_2, do *not* be tempted to ask the person to hold his or her breath so that you can concentrate on the sounds. Breath holding will only equalize ejection times in the right and left sides of the heart, and the split goes away. Instead, concentrate on the split as you watch the person's chest rise up and down with breathing. The split S_2 occurs about every fourth heartbeat, fading in with inhalation and fading out with exhalation.

A fixed split is unaffected by respiration; the split is always there.

A paradoxical split is the opposite of what you would expect; the sounds fuse on inspiration and split on expiration (see Table 16–4).

Focus on systole, then on diastole, and listen for any *extra heart sounds.* Listen with the diaphragm, then switch to the bell, covering all auscultatory areas (Fig. 16–29). Usually, these are silent periods. When you do detect an extra heart sound, listen carefully to note its timing and

NORMAL RANGE OF FINDINGS

ABNORMAL FINDINGS

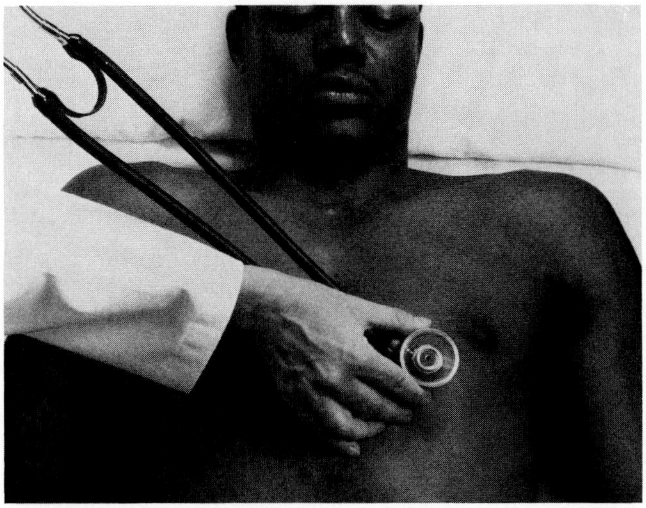

► **Figure 16-29**

characteristics. During systole, the midsystolic click is the most common extra sound (see Table 16–5). The third heart sound and fourth heart sound occur in diastole; either may be normal or abnormal (see Table 16–6).

Listen for murmurs. A murmur is a blowing, swooshing sound that occurs with turbulent blood flow in the heart or great vessels. If you hear a murmur, describe it by indicating these characteristics:

Timing. It is crucial to define the murmur by its occurrence in systole or diastole. You must be able to identify S_1 and S_2 accurately to do this. Try to further describe the murmur as being early, mid, or late in systole or diastole; throughout the cardiac event (termed pansystolic or holosystolic/pandiastolic or holodiastolic); and whether it obscures or muffles the heart sounds.

Loudness. Describe the intensity in terms of six "grades." For example, note a grade ii murmur as "ii/vi."

Grade i—barely audible, heard only in a quiet room and then with difficulty

Grade ii—clearly audible, but faint

Grade iii—moderately loud

Grade iv—loud, associated with a thrill palpable on the chest wall

Grade v—very loud, heard with one corner of the stethoscope lifted off the chest wall

Grade vi—loudest, still heard with entire stethoscope lifted just off the chest wall

Pitch. Describe the pitch as high, medium, or low. The pitch depends on the pressure and the rate of blood flow producing the murmur.

Pattern. The intensity may follow a pattern during the cardiac phase, growing louder (crescendo), tapering off (decrescendo), or increasing to a

NORMAL RANGE OF FINDINGS	ABNORMAL FINDINGS

peak and then decreasing (crescendo-decrescendo, or diamond shaped). Since the whole murmur is just milliseconds long, it takes practice to diagnose any pattern.

Quality. Describe the quality as musical, blowing, harsh, or rumbling.

The murmur of mitral stenosis is rumbling, whereas that of aortic stenosis is harsh (see Table 16–9).

Location. Describe the area of maximum intensity of the murmur (where it is best heard) by noting the valve area or intercostal spaces.

Radiation. The murmur may be transmitted downstream in the direction of blood flow, and may be heard in another place on the precordium, the neck, the back, or the axilla.

Posture. Some murmurs disappear or are enhanced by a change in position.

Some murmurs are common in healthy children or adolescents and are termed *innocent* or *functional.** The contractile force of the heart is greater in children. This increases blood flow velocity. The increased velocity plus a smaller chest measurement makes an audible murmur. The innocent murmur is generally soft (grade ii), midsystolic, short, crescendo-decrescendo, and with a vibratory or musical quality ("vooot" sound like fiddle strings). Also, the innocent murmur is heard at the second or third left intercostal space and disappears with sitting, and the young person has no associated signs of cardiac dysfunction.

Although it is important to distinguish innocent murmurs from pathologic ones, it is best to suspect all murmurs as pathologic until they are proved otherwise. Diagnostic tests such as ECG, phonocardiogram, and echocardiogram are needed to establish an accurate diagnosis.

Change position. After auscultating in the supine position, roll the person toward his or her left side. Listen with the bell at the apex for the presence of any diastolic filling sounds (Fig. 16–30).

S_3 and S_4, and the murmur of mitral stenosis sometimes may be heard only when on the left side.

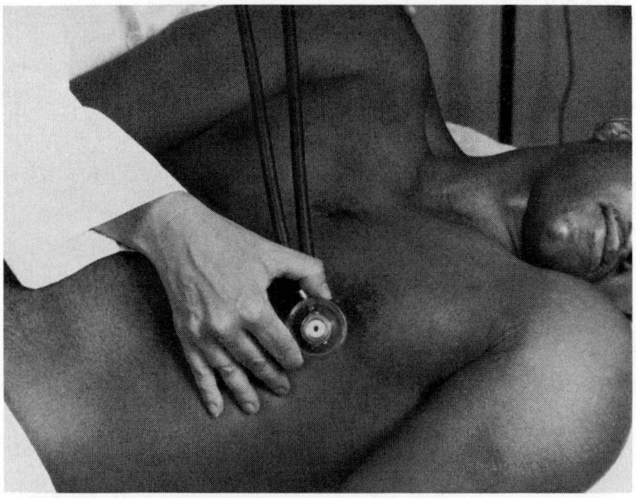

► **Figure 16–30**

* *Innocent* (no valvular or other pathologic cause), *functional* (due to increased blood flow in the heart, e.g., in anemia, fever, pregnancy, hyperthyroidism)

NORMAL RANGE OF FINDINGS	ABNORMAL FINDINGS

Ask the person to sit up and lean forward slightly. Listen with the diaphragm at the base, right and left sides. Check for the high-pitched diastolic murmur of aortic or pulmonic regurgitation (Fig. 16–31).

Murmur of aortic regurgitation sometimes may be heard only when the person is leaning forward in the sitting position.

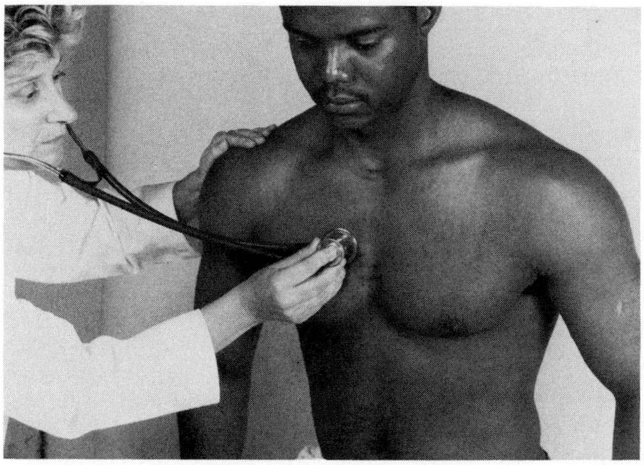

► **Figure 16–31**

DEVELOPMENTAL CONSIDERATIONS

Infants

The transition from fetal to pulmonic circulation occurs in the immediate newborn period. Fetal shunts normally close within 10 to 15 hours but may take up to 48 hours. Thus, you should assess the cardiovascular system during the first 24 hours, and again in 2 to 3 days.

Failure of shunts to close, e.g., PDA, ASD (see Table 16–8).

Note any extracardiac signs that may reflect heart status, particularly in the skin, liver size, and respiratory status. The skin color should be pink to pinkish brown, depending on the infant's genetic heritage. If cyanosis occurs, determine its first appearance—at or shortly after birth versus after the neonatal period. Normally, the liver is not enlarged, nor are the respirations labored. Also, note the expected parameters of weight gain throughout infancy.

Cyanosis signals oxygen desaturation of congenital heart disease. Cyanosis at or just after birth suggests Fallot tetralogy, transposition of great vessels, severe septal defect, severe pulmonic stenosis, or tricuspid atresia.

The most important signs of congestive heart failure in an infant are persistent tachycardia, tachypnea, and liver enlargement. Engorged veins, gallop rhythm and pulsus alternans also are signs. Respiratory crackles (rales) is an important sign in adults but not in infants.

Failure to thrive occurs with cardiac disease.

NORMAL RANGE OF FINDINGS	ABNORMAL FINDINGS

Palpate the apical impulse to determine the size and position of the heart. Since the infant's heart has a more horizontal placement, expect to palpate the apical impulse at the fourth intercostal space just lateral to the midclavicular line. It may or may not be visible.

The apex is displaced with:

- cardiac enlargement, shifts to the left;
- pneumothorax, shifts away from affected side;
- diaphragmatic hernia, shifts usually to right because this hernia occurs more often on the left;
- dextrocardia, a rare anomaly in which the heart is located on right side of chest.

The heart rate is best auscultated because radial pulses are hard to count accurately. Use the small (pediatric size) diaphragm and bell. The heart rate may range from 100 to 180 per minute immediately after birth, then stabilize to an average of 120 to 140 per minute. Infants normally have wide fluctuations with activity, from 170 per minute or more with crying or being active to 70 to 90 per minute with sleeping. Variations are greatest at birth, and even more so with premature babies (see Table 8–3).

Persistent tachycardia,

- >200 per minute in newborns or
- >150 per minute in infants,

Bradycardia, some state

- <90 per minute—all warrant further investigation.

Expect the heart rhythm to have sinus arrhythmia, the phasic speeding up or slowing down with the respiratory cycle.

Investigate any irregularity except sinus arrhythmia.

Rapid rates make it more challenging to evaluate heart sounds. Expect heart sounds to be louder in infants than in adults because of the infant's thinner chest wall. Also S_2 has a higher pitch and is sharper than S_1. Splitting of S_2 just after the height of inspiration is common, not at birth but beginning a few hours after birth.

Fixed split S_2 indicates atrial septal defect (ASD) (see Table 16–8).

Murmurs in the immediate newborn period do not necessarily indicate congenital heart disease. Murmurs are relatively common in the first 2 to 3 days because of fetal shunt closure. These murmurs are usually grade i or ii, systolic, accompany no other signs of cardiac disease, and disappear in 2 to 3 days. The murmur of patent ductus arteriosus (PDA) is a continuous machinery murmur, which disappears by 2 to 3 days. On the other hand, absence of a murmur in the immediate newborn period does not ensure a perfect heart; congenital defects can be present that are not signaled by an early murmur. It is best to listen frequently and to note and describe any murmur according to the characteristics listed on pp. 561–563.

Persistent murmur after 2 to 3 days, holosystolic murmurs or those that last into diastole, and those that are loud all warrant further evaluation.

Children

Note any extracardiac or cardiac signs that may indicate heart disease: poor weight gain, developmental delay, persistent tachycardia, tachypnea, dyspnea on exertion, cyanosis, and clubbing. Note that clubbing of fingers and toes usually does not appear until late in the first year, even with severe cyanotic defects.

The apical impulse is sometimes visible in children with thin chest walls. Note any obvious bulge or any heave—these are not normal.

A precordial bulge to the left of the sternum with a hyperdynamic precordium signals cardiac enlargement. The bulge occurs because the cartilaginous rib cage is more compliant.

NORMAL RANGE OF FINDINGS

ABNORMAL FINDINGS

A substernal heave occurs with right ventricular enlargement, and an apical heave occurs with left ventricular hypertrophy.

Palpate the apical impulse: in the fourth intercostal space to the left of the midclavicular line until age 4; at the fourth interspace at the midclavicular line from age 4 to age 6; and in the fifth interspace to the right of the midclavicular line at age 7.

The apical impulse moves laterally with cardiac enlargement.

Thrill, palpable vibration.

The average heart rate slows as the child grows older, although it is still variable with rest or activity (see Table 8–3).

The heart rhythm remains characterized by sinus arrhythmia. Physiologic S_3 is common in children (see Table 16–6). It occurs in early diastole, just after S_2, and is a dull soft sound that is best heard at the apex.

A *venous hum,* due to turbulence of blood flow in the jugular venous system, is common in normal children and has no pathologic significance. It is a continuous, low-pitched, soft hum, heard throughout the cycle, although it is loudest in diastole. Listen with the bell over the supraclavicular fossa at the medial third of the clavicle, especially on the right, or over the upper anterior chest. The venous hum is usually not affected by respiration, may sound louder when the child stands, and is easily obliterated by occluding the jugular veins in the neck with your fingers. The latter maneuver helps differentiate the insignificant venous hum from other organic cardiac murmurs, e.g., PDA.

Heart murmurs that are innocent (or functional) in origin are very common through childhood. Some authors say they have a 30 percent occurrence, and some authors say nearly all children may demonstrate a murmur at some time. Most innocent murmurs have these characteristics: soft, relatively short systolic ejection murmur; medium pitch; vibratory; best heard at the left lower sternal or midsternal border, with no radiation to the apex, base, or back.

It is important to distinguish innocent murmurs from pathologic ones. This may involve referral to another examiner or the performance of diagnostic tests such as the ECG or echocardiogram.

For the child whose murmur has been shown to be innocent, it is very important that the parents understand this completely. They need to believe that this murmur is just a "noise" and has no pathologic significance (Behrman, 1983). Otherwise, the parents may become overprotective and limit activity for the child, which may result in the child developing a negative self-concept.

The Pregnant Female

The vital signs usually yield an increase in resting pulse rate of 10 to 15 beats per minute, and a drop in blood pressure from the normal prepregnancy level. The blood pressure decreases to its lowest point during the second trimester and then slowly rises during the third trimester. The blood pressure varies with position. It is usually lowest in left lateral recumbent position, a bit higher when supine (except for some who experience hypotension when supine), and highest when sitting (Pritchard, 1985).

Suspect pregnancy-induced hypertension with a sustained rise of 30 mm Hg systolic or 15 mm diastolic under basal conditions.

NORMAL RANGE OF FINDINGS	ABNORMAL FINDINGS

Inspection of the skin often shows a mild hyperemia in light-skinned women, because the increased cutaneous blood flow tries to eliminate the excess heat generated by the increased metabolism. Palpation of the apical impulse is higher and lateral as compared with the normal position, as the enlarging uterus elevates the diaphragm and displaces the heart up and to the left and rotates it on its long axis.

Auscultation of the heart sounds shows changes due to the increased blood volume and workload:

Heart sounds

- exaggerated splitting of S_1 and increased loudness of S_1
- a loud, easily heard S_3

Heart murmurs

- a systolic murmur in 90 percent, which disappears soon after delivery
- a soft, diastolic murmur heard transiently in 19 percent
- a continuous murmur arising from breast vasculature in 10 percent (Cutforth and MacDonald, 1966).

The last-mentioned murmur is termed a *mammary souffle,* (pronounced SOOF′ f′l) which occurs near term or when the mother is lactating and is due to increased blood flow through the internal mammary artery. The murmur is heard in the second, third, or fourth intercostal space, and it is continuous, although it is accented in systole. You can obliterate it by pressure with the stethoscope or one finger lateral to the murmur. This distinguishes it from the murmur of aortic stenosis, aortic insufficiency, or PDA.

The ECG has no changes except for a slight left axis deviation due to the change in the heart's position.

The Aging Adult

A gradual rise in systolic blood pressure is common with aging; the diastolic blood pressure stays fairly constant with a resulting widening of pulse pressure. Some older adults experience *orthostatic hypotension,* a sudden drop in blood pressure when rising to sit or stand.

The chest often increases in anteroposterior diameter with aging. This makes it more difficult to palpate the apical impulse and to hear the splitting of S_2. The S_4 often occurs in older people with no known cardiac disease.

Occasional ectopic beats are common and do not necessarily indicate underlying heart disease. When in doubt, obtain an ECG. However, consider that the ECG only records for one isolated minute in time, and may need to be supplemented by a test of 24-hour ambulatory heart monitoring.

☑ SUMMARY CHECKLIST

Cardiovascular Examination

1 ▶ Neck
   A. Carotid pulse—observe and palpate
   B. Observe jugular venous pulse
   C. Estimate jugular venous pressure

2 ▶ Precordium
   A. Inspection and palpation
      (1) Describe location of apical impulse
      (2) Note any heave (lift) or thrill
   B. Auscultation
      (1) Identify anatomic areas where you listen
      (2) Note rate and rhythm of heartbeat
      (3) Identify S_1 and S_2 and note any variation
      (4) Listen in systole and diastole for any extra heart sounds
      (5) Listen in systole and diastole for any murmurs
      (6) Repeat sequence with bell
      (7) Listen at the apex with person in left lateral position
      (8) Listen at the base with person in sitting position

SAMPLE RECORDING

Subjective

▶ No chest pain, dyspnea, orthopnea, cough, fatigue or edema. No past history of hypertension, abnormal blood tests, heart murmur, or rheumatic fever in self. Last ECG 2 yrs. PTA, result normal. No stress ECG or other heart tests. Family history: father with obesity, smoking, and hypertension, treated c̄ diuretic medication. No other family history significant for cardiovascular disease. Personal habits: Diet balanced in 4 food groups, 2 to 3 c. regular coffee/day; no smoking; alcohol, 1 to 2 beers occasionally on weekend; exercise, runs 2 miles, 3 to 4 ×/week; no prescription or OTC medications or street drugs.

Objective

▶ *Neck* Carotids 2+ & = bilaterally, internal jugular pulsations disappear @ 45°.
Precordium Apical impulse 5th ics @ left MCL, no heave or thrill, rate 68/min. & regular, S_1–S_2 normal, no extra sounds, no murmurs.

SAMPLE CLINICAL PROBLEM

Mr. N.V. is a 53-year-old white male woodcutter admitted to the CCU at University Medical Center (UMC) with chest pain

Subjective

► 1 year PTA—NV admitted to UMC with crushing substernal chest pain, radiating to L shoulder, accompanied by N & V, diaphoresis.
Diagnosed as MI, hospitalized 7 days, discharged with nitroglycerin prn for anginal pain. Did not return to work. Activity included walking 1 mile/day, hunting. Had occasional episodes of chest pain with exercise, relieved by rest.
1 day PTA—had increasing frequency of chest pain, about every 2 hours, lasting few minutes, saw pain as warning to go to MD
Day of admission—severe substernal chest pain ("like someone sitting on my chest") unrelieved by rest. Saw personal MD, while in office had episode of chest pain as last year's, accompanied by diaphoresis, no N & V or SOB, relieved by 1 nitroglycerin. Transferred to UMC by MD. No further pain since admission 2 hours ago.
Family hx. Mother died of MI at age 57.
Personal habits—Smokes 1 1/2 pack cigarettes daily × 34 years, no alcohol, diet—trying to limit fat and fried food, still high in added salt.

Objective

► *Extremities* Skin pink, no cyanosis. Upper extrem.—capillary refill sluggish, no clubbing. Lower extrem.—no edema, no hair growth 10 cm below knee bilaterally. Pulses—

Carotid	brachial	radial	femoral	popliteal	P.T.	D.P.	
2+	2+	2+	2+	0	0	1+	all = bilaterally.

B/P R arm 104/66

Neck External jugulars flat and internal jugular pulsations absent at 45°
Precordium Apical impulse visible 5th ics, 7 cm left of mid sternal line, no heave or thrill. Apical rate 92 regular, S_1—S_2 normal, no S_3 or S_4, grade iii/vi systolic murmur, at left lower sternal border

Assessment

► Substernal chest pain
Systolic murmur
Alteration in tissue perfusion R/T interruption in flow
Decreased cardiac output R/T reduction in stroke volume

NURSING DIAGNOSES COMMONLY ASSOCIATED WITH CIRCULATORY DISORDERS

Diagnosis	Related Factors (Etiology)	Defining Characteristics (Symptoms and Signs)
Decreased cardiac output	Reduction in stroke volume as a result of Electrical malfunction (alteration in conduction, rate, or rhythm) Mechanical malfunction (alteration in afterload, inotropic changes in heart, or preload) Structural problems secondary to congenital abnormalities, trauma	Abnormal heart sounds Altered blood gases Changes in mental status Cool clammy skin Cough Crackles (rales) Cyanosis or pallor Decreased peripheral pulses Dyspnea Dysrhythmias, electrocardiographic changes Edema, dependent Fatigue Frothy sputum Jugular vein distention Orthopnea Restlessness Syncope Tachycardia Urine output decreased Variations in hemodynamic readings Weight gain, sudden
Alteration in tissue perfusion	Exchange problems Hypervolemia Hypovolemia Interruption of flow	Cardiopulmonary Chest pain (relieved by rest) Increased heart rate Increased respiratory rate Shortness of breath Cerebral Alteration in thought processes Blurred vision Changes in level of consciousness Confusion Restlessness Syncope/vertigo

Table continued on following page

Diagnosis	Related Factors (Etiology)	Defining Characteristics (Symptoms and Signs)
Dysfunctional grieving	Effects of loss of function or body part Absence of anticipatory grieving Actual or perceived loss of health or social status, significant other, or valued object Multiple losses or crises Changes in lifestyle Decreased support system Thwarted grieving in response to a loss Lack of resolution of previous grieving response Ambivalent feelings toward loss	Changes in sleep patterns Feelings of anger, guilt, worthlessness, denial, sorrow Decreased interest in personal appearance Interference with life functioning Difficulty in expressing loss Fear of future Absence of emotion Suicidal thoughts Social withdrawal Weight loss Amenorrhea Decreased level of activity Reliving of past experiences Alteration in concentration Developmental regression Hyperactivity

Other related nursing diagnoses:

- Impaired home maintenance management (See Chapter 11)
- Pain (See Chapter 13)
- Activity intolerance (see Chapter 15)
- Anxiety (See Chapter 15)

ABNORMAL FINDINGS

Table 16-2 ▶ Variations in S_1*

	FACTOR	EXAMPLES
LOUD (ACCENTUATED) S_1 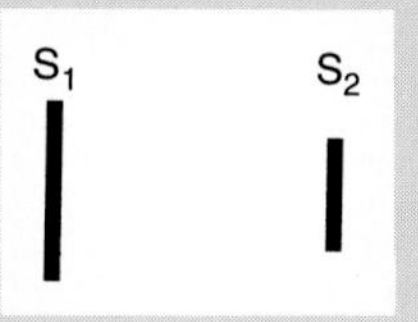	1. Position of AV valve at start of systole—wide open and no time to drift together	Hyperkinetic states where blood velocity is increased: exercise, fever, anemia, hyperthyroidism
	2. Change in valve structure—calcification of valve, needs increasing ventricular pressure to close the valve against increased atrial pressure	Mitral stenosis with leaflets still mobile
FAINT (DIMINISHED) S_1 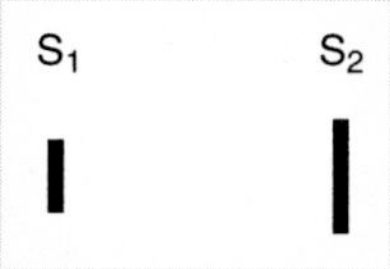	1. Position of AV valve—delayed conduction from atria to ventricles. Mitral valve drifts shut before ventricular contraction closes it	First-degree heart block (prolonged PR interval)
	2. Change in valve structure—extreme calcification, which limits mobility	Mitral insufficiency
	3. More forceful atrial contraction into noncompliant ventricle; delays or diminishes ventricular contraction	Severe hypertension—systemic or pulmonary
VARYING INTENSITY OF S_1 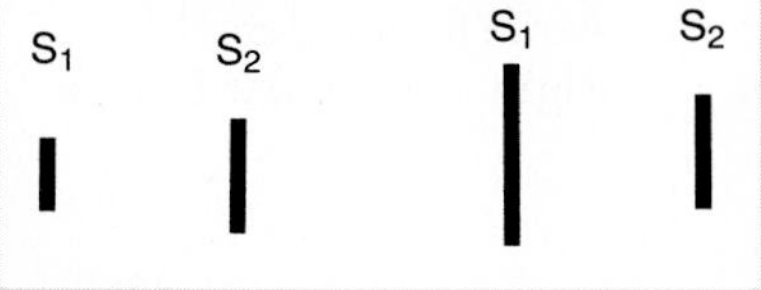	1. Position of AV valve varies before closing from beat to beat	Atrial fibrillation—irregularly-irregular rhythm
	2. Atria and ventricles beat independently	Complete heart block with changing P-R interval
SPLIT S_1 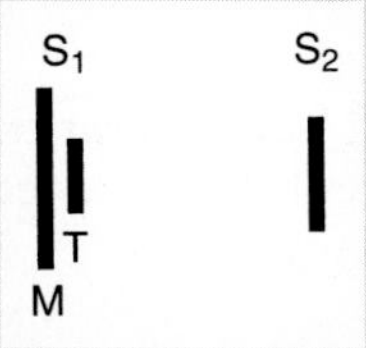	Mitral and tricuspid components are heard separately	Normal but uncommon

* The intensity of S_1 depends on three factors: (1) Position of AV valve at the start of systole, (2) structure of the valve leaflets, and (3) how quickly pressure rises in the ventricle.

Table 16–3 ▶ Variations in S_2

ACCENTUATED S_2

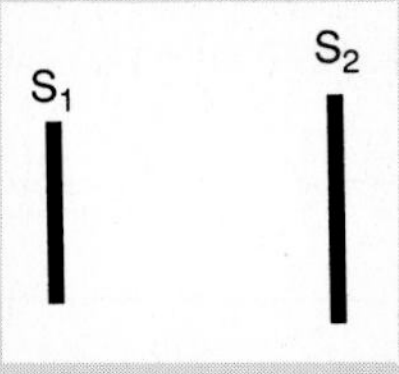

a

CONDITION	EXAMPLE
1. Higher closing pressure	Systemic hypertension, ringing or booming S_2
2. Exercise and excitement increase pressure in aorta	
3. Pulmonary hypertension	Mitral stenosis, congestive heart failure
4. Semilunar valves calcified but still mobile	Aortic or pulmonic stenosis

DIMINISHED S_2

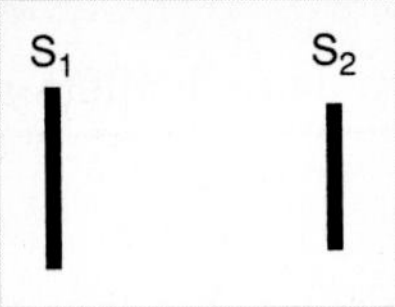

b

CONDITION	EXAMPLE
1. A fall in systemic blood pressure causes a decrease in valve strength	Shock
2. Semilunar valves thickened and calcified, with decreased mobility	Aortic or pulmonic stenosis

Table 16–4 ▶ Variations in Split S_2

NORMAL SPLITTING

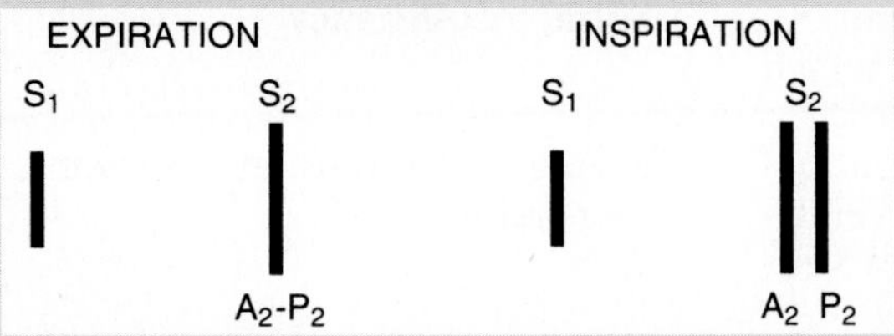

FIXED SPLIT

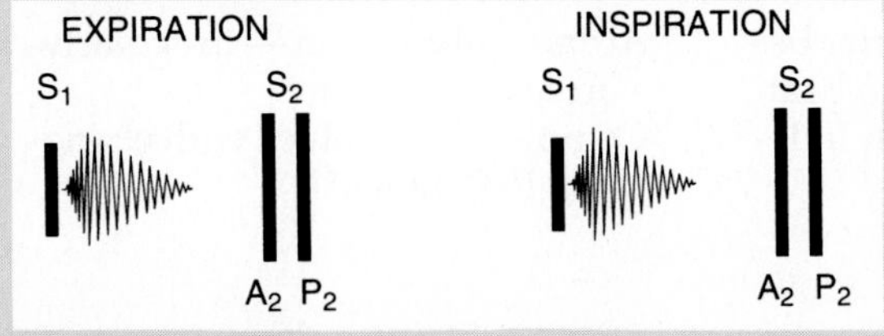

PARADOXICAL SPLIT

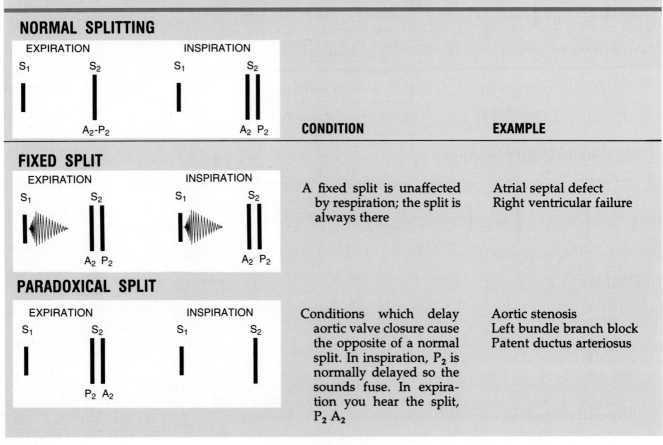

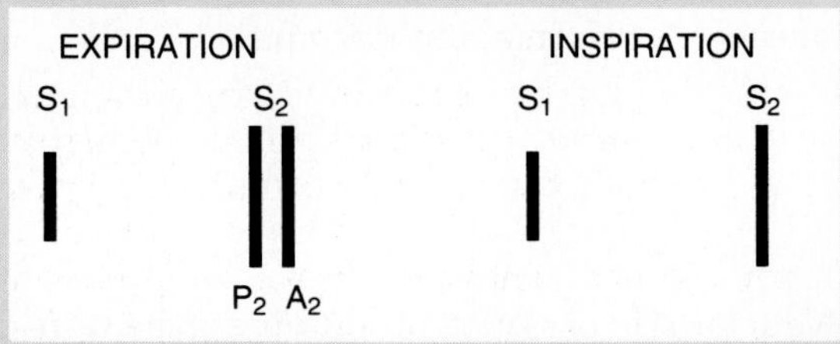

	CONDITION	EXAMPLE
FIXED SPLIT	A fixed split is unaffected by respiration; the split is always there	Atrial septal defect Right ventricular failure
PARADOXICAL SPLIT	Conditions which delay aortic valve closure cause the opposite of a normal split. In inspiration, P_2 is normally delayed so the sounds fuse. In expiration you hear the split, P_2 A_2	Aortic stenosis Left bundle branch block Patent ductus arteriosus

Table 16-4 ► Variations in Split S_2 *Continued*

WIDE SPLIT

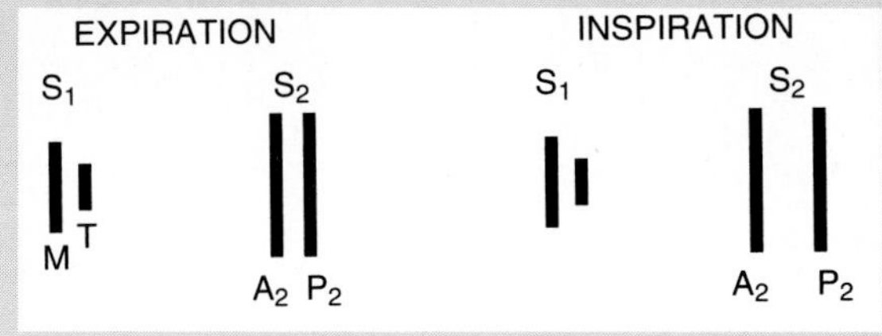

When right ventricle has delayed electrical activation, the split is very wide on inspiration and is still there on expiration

Right bundle branch block (which delays P_2)

Table 16-5 ► Systolic Extra Sounds

Early Systolic
- Ejection Click
- Aortic Prosthetic Valve Sounds

Mid/Late Systolic
- Midsystolic (mitral) Click

Aortic ejection click (apex and base)

Pulmonic ejection click (base only)

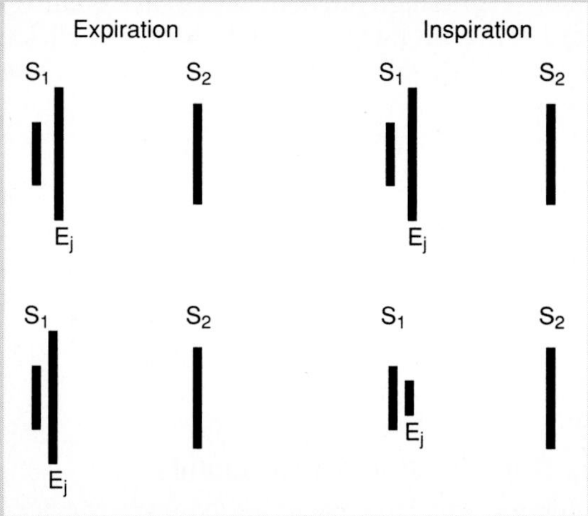

EJECTION CLICK

The ejection click occurs early in systole at the start of ejection, because it results from opening of the semilunar valves. Normally, the SL valves open silently, but in the presence of stenosis (e.g., aortic stenosis, pulmonic stenosis) their opening makes a sound. It is short and high pitched, with a click quality, and is heard better with the diaphragm. The aortic ejection click is heard at the second right interspace and apex, and may be loudest at the apex. Its intensity does not change with respiration. The pulmonic ejection click is best heard in the second left interspace and often grows softer with inspiration.

Table continued on following page

Table 16-5 ▶ Systolic Extra Sounds *Continued*

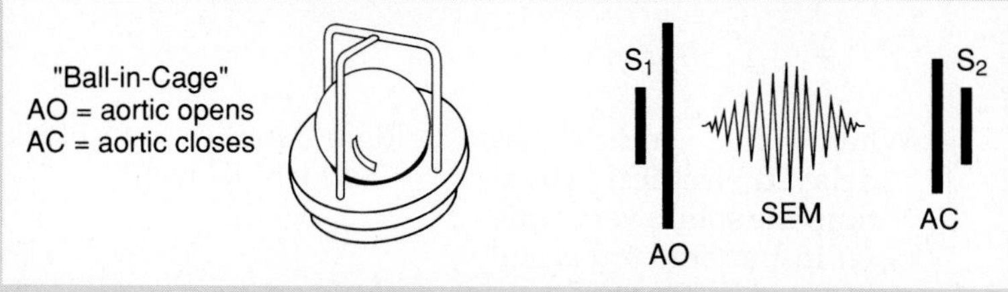

AORTIC PROSTHETIC VALVE SOUNDS

As a sequela of modern techologic intervention for heart problems, some people now have *iatrogenically* induced heart sounds. The opening of an aortic ball-in-cage prosthesis (e.g., Starr-Edwards prosthesis) produces an early systolic sound. This sound is less intense with a tilting disc prosthesis (e.g., Bjork-Shiley prosthesis), and is absent with a tissue prosthesis (e.g., porcine).

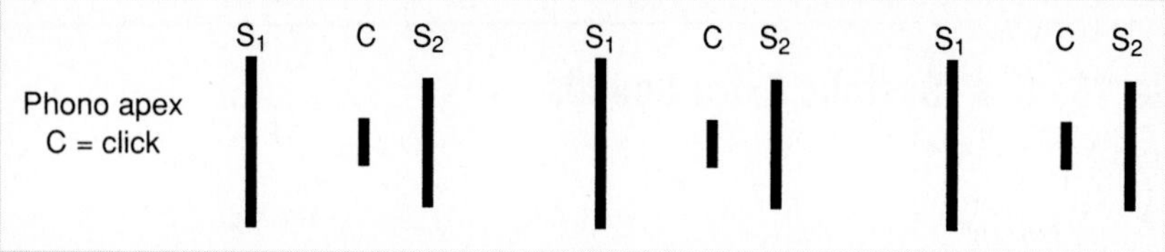

MIDSYSTOLIC CLICK

Although it is systolic, this is not an ejection click. It is associated with *mitral valve prolapse,* in which the mitral valve leaflets not only close with contraction but balloon back up into the left atrium. During ballooning, the sudden tensing of the valve leaflets and the chordae tendineae creates the click.

The sound occurs mid to late systole, and is short and high pitched, with a click quality. It is best heard with the diaphragm, at the apex, but also may be heard at the left lower sternal border. The click usually is followed by a systolic murmur. When the person assumes a squatting position, the click may move closer to S_2 and the murmur may sound louder and delayed.

Table 16-6 ▶ Diastolic Extra Sounds

Early diastole

- Opening snap
- Mitral prosthetic valve sound

Mid-diastole

- Third heart sound
- Summation sound (S3 + S4)

Late diastole

- Fourth heart sound
- Pacemaker-induced sound

Table 16-6 ► Diastolic Extra Sounds *Continued*

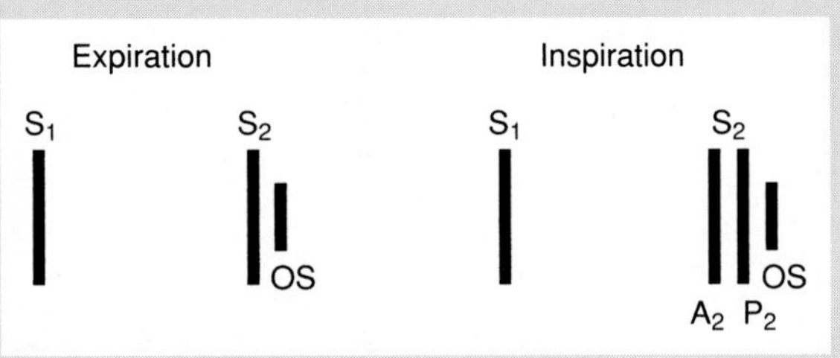

OPENING SNAP

Normally, the opening of the AV valves is silent. In the presence of stenosis, increasingly higher atrial pressure is required to open the valve. The deformed valve opens with a noise, the opening snap. It is sharp, high pitched, with a snapping quality. It sounds after S_2 and is best heard with the diaphragm at the third or fourth left interspace at the sternal border, less well at the apex.

The opening snap usually is not an isolated sound. As a sign of mitral stenosis, the opening snap usually ushers in the low-pitched diastolic rumbling murmur of that condition.

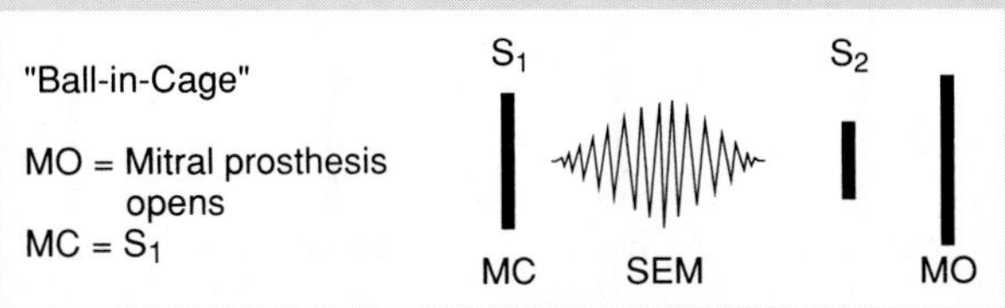

MITRAL PROSTHETIC VALVE SOUND

An iatrogenic sound, the opening of a ball-in-cage mitral prosthesis gives an early diastolic sound, an opening click just after S_2. It is loud, is heard over the whole precordium, and is loudest at the apex and left lower sternal border.

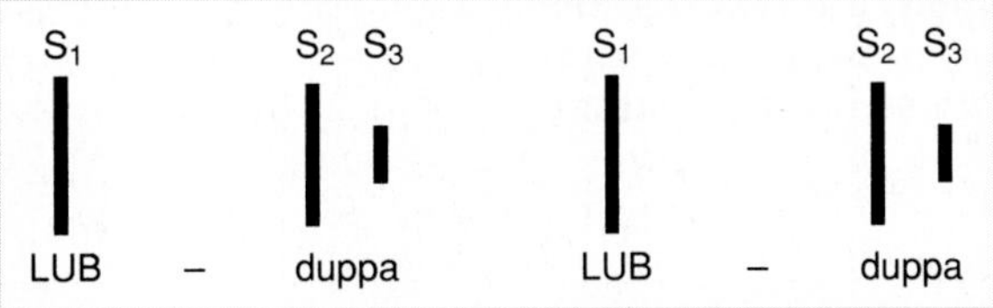

THIRD HEART SOUND

The S_3 is a ventricular filling sound. It occurs in early diastole during the rapid filling phase. Your hearing quickly accommodates to the S_3, so it is best heard when you listen initially. It sounds after S_2, but later than an opening snap would be. It is a dull, soft sound, and it is low pitched, like "distant thunder." It is heard best in a quiet room, at the apex, with the bell held lightly (just enough to form a seal), and with the person in the left lateral position.

The S_3 can be confused with a split S_2. Use these guidelines to distinguish the S_3:

- Location—the S_3 is heard at the apex or left lower sternal border; the split S_2 at the base.
- Respiratory variation—the S_3 does not vary in timing with respirations; the split S_2 does.
- Pitch—the S_3 is lower pitched; the pitch of the split S_2 stays the same.

The S_3 may be normal (physiologic) or abnormal (pathologic). The *physiologic* S_3 is heard frequently in children and young adults; it occasionally may persist after age 40, especially in women. The normal S_3 usually disappears when the person sits up.

In adults, the S_3 is usually abnormal. The *pathologic* S_3 is also called a *ventricular gallop* or an *S_3 gallop,* and it persists when sitting up. The S_3 indicates decreased compliance of the ventricles, as in congestive heart failure. The S_3 may be the earliest sign of heart failure. The S_3 may originate from either the left or the right ventricle; a left-sided S_3 is heard at the apex in the left lateral position, and a right-sided S_3 is heard at the left lower sternal border with the person supine and is louder in inspiration.

The S_3 occurs also with conditions of volume overload, e.g., mitral regurgitation, aortic or tricuspid regurgitation. The S_3 is also found in high cardiac output states in the absence of heart disease, such as hyperthyroidism, anemia, and pregnancy. When the primary condition is corrected, the gallop disappears.

Table continued on following page

Table 16–6 ▸ Diastolic Extra Sounds *Continued*

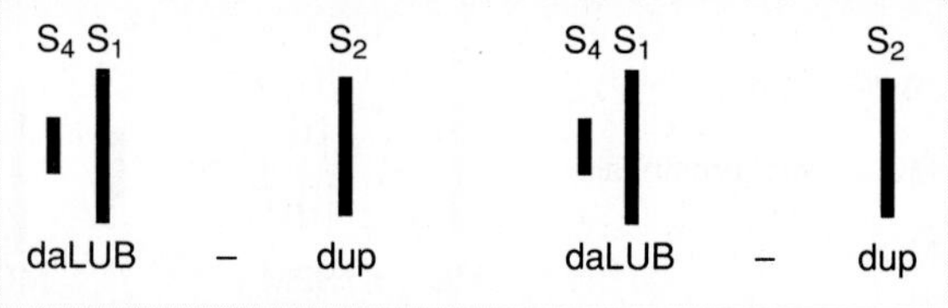

FOURTH HEART SOUND

S_4 is a ventricular filling sound. It occurs when the atria contract late in diastole. It is heard immediately before S1. This is a very soft sound, of very low pitch. You need a good bell, and you must listen for it. It is heard best at the apex, with the person in left lateral position.

A *physiologic S_4* may occur in adults older than 40 or 50 with no evidence of cardiovascular disease, especially after exercise.

A *pathologic S_4* is termed an *atrial gallop* or an *S_4 gallop.* It occurs with decreased compliance of the ventricle, e.g., coronary artery disease, cardiomyopathy, and with systolic overload (afterload), including outflow obstruction to the ventricle (aortic stenosis) and systemic hypertension. A left-sided S_4 occurs with these conditions. It is heard best at the apex, in the left lateral position.

A right-sided S_4 is less common. It is heard at the left lower sternal border and may increase with inspiration. It occurs with pulmonary stenosis or pulmonary hypertension.

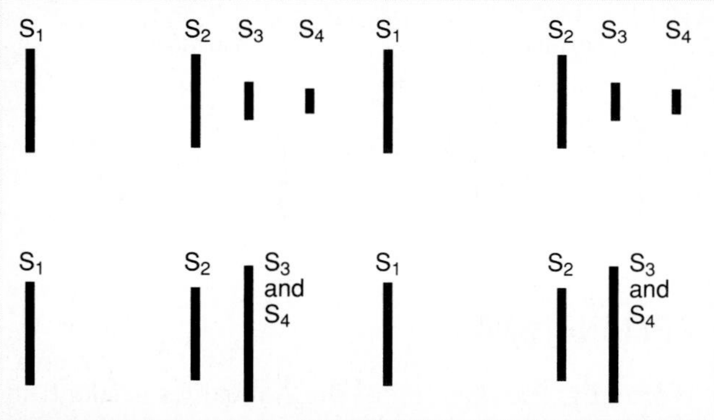

SUMMATION SOUND

When both the pathologic S3 and S4 are present, a quadruple rhythm is heard. Often, in cases of cardiac stress, one response is tachycardia. During rapid rates, the diastolic filling time shortens and the S_3 and S_4 move closer together. They sound superimposed in mid-diastole, and you hear one loud, prolonged, summated sound, often louder than either S_1 or S_2.

EXTRACARDIAC SOUNDS

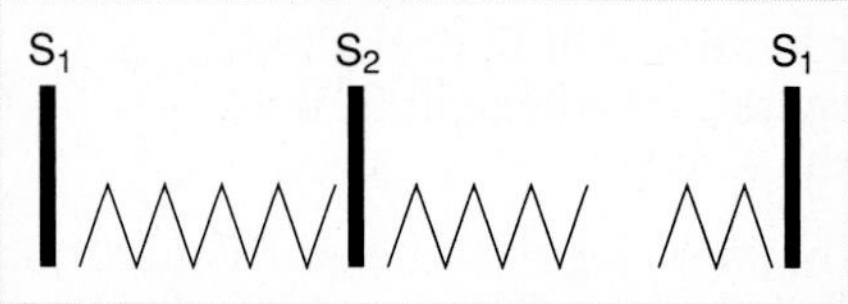

Pericardial Friction Rub

Inflammation of the precordium gives rise to a friction rub. The sound is high pitched and scratchy, like sandpaper being rubbed. It is best heard with the diaphragm, with the person sitting up and leaning forward, and with the breath held in expiration. A friction rub can be heard any place on the precordium but usually is best heard at the apex and left lower sternal border, places where the pericardium comes in close contact with the chest wall. Timing may be systolic and diastolic. The friction rub of pericarditis is common during the first week following a myocardial infarction, and may last only a few hours.

Table 16-6 ▶ Diastolic Extra Sounds *Continued*

Pacemaker-Induced Sound (not illustrated)

A cardiac pacemaker is placed to initiate a heartbeat in heart block. It may have a sound of high pitch, with a click quality, which is best heard at the apex or left lower sternal border. It is presystolic, just before S1.

The origin is not cardiac, but is due to skeletal muscle contraction. The pacemaker induced sound was described in 1965, but rarely is heard today because of improvements in pacemaker design.

Table 16-7 ▶ Abnormal Pulsations on the Precordium

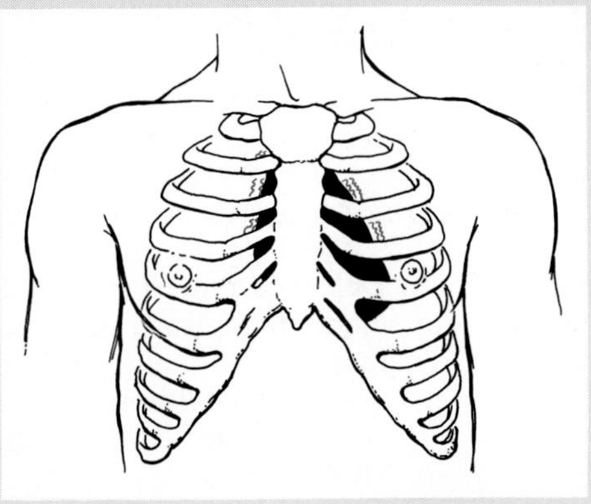

Base. A *thrill* in the second and third right interspaces occurs with severe aortic stenosis and systemic hypertension.

A thrill in the second and third left interspaces occurs with pulmonic stenosis and pulmonic hypertension.

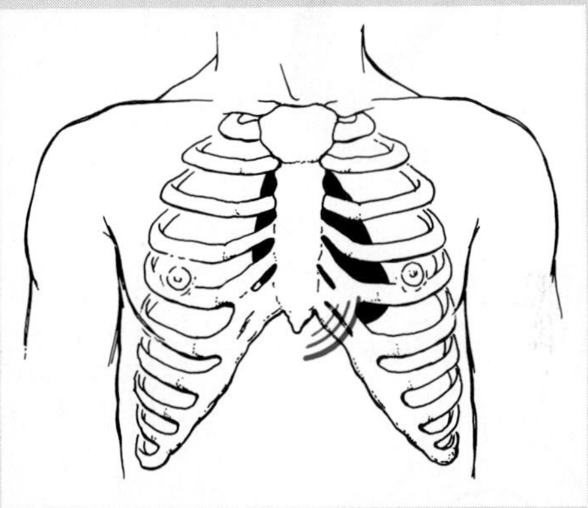

Left Sternal Border. A *lift (heave)* occurs with right ventricular hypertrophy, as found in pulmonic valve disease, pulmonic hypertension, and chronic lung disease. You feel a diffuse lifting impulse during systole at the left lower sternal border. It may be associated with retraction at the apex, because the left ventricle is rotated posteriorly by the enlarged right ventricle.

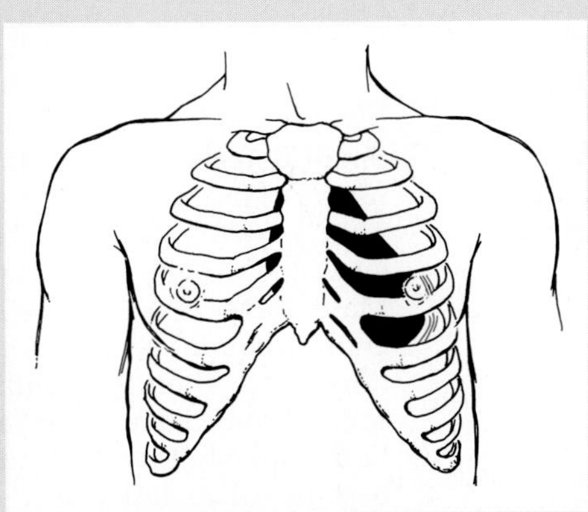

Apex. Cardiac enlargement displaces the apical impulse laterally and over a wider area when left ventricular hypertrophy and dilatation are present. This is *volume overload,* as in mitral regurgitation, aortic regurgitation, and left-to-right shunts.

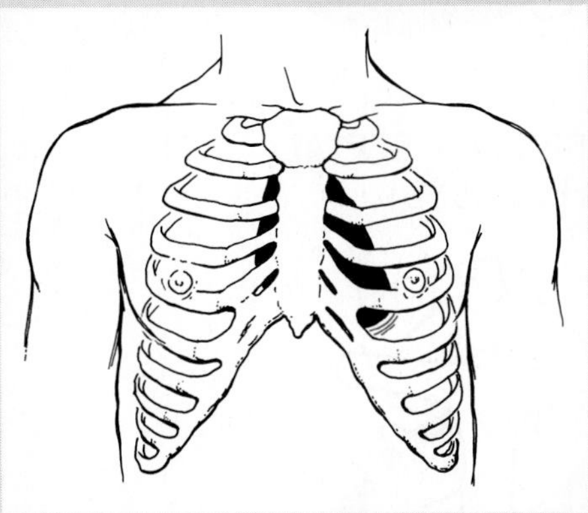

Apex. The apical impulse is increased in force and duration but is not necessarily displaced to the left when left ventricular hypertrophy occurs alone without dilatation. This is *pressure overload,* as found in aortic stenosis or systemic hypertension.

Table 16–8 ▸ Congenital Heart Defects

	DESCRIPTION	CLINICAL DATA
PATENT DUCTUS ARTERIOSUS (PDA) 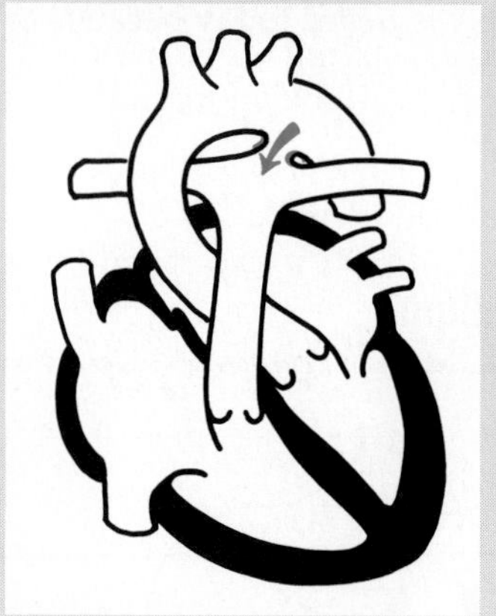	Persistence of channel joining left pulmonary artery to aorta. Normal in fetus, usually closes spontaneously within hours of birth.	S: Usually no symptoms in early childhood; growth and development are normal. O: Blood pressure has wide pulse pressure and bounding peripheral pulses owing to rapid runoff of blood into low resistance pulmonary bed during diastole. Thrill often palpable at left upper sternal border. The continuous murmur heard in systole and diastole is called a machinery murmur.
ATRIAL SEPTAL DEFECT (ASD) 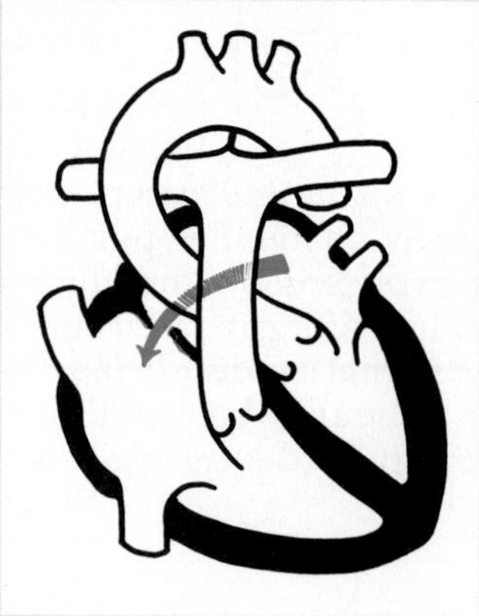	Abnormal opening in atrial septum, resulting usually in left-to-right shunt, and causing large increase in pulmonary blood flow.	S: Defect is remarkably well tolerated. Symptoms in infant are rare; growth and development normal. Children and young adults have mild fatigue and DOE. O: Sternal lift often present. S_2 has fixed split, with P_2 often louder than A_2. Murmur is systolic, ejection, medium pitch, best heard at base in second left interspace. Murmur caused not by shunt itself but by increased blood flow through pulmonic valve.
VENTRICULAR SEPTAL DEFECT (VSD) 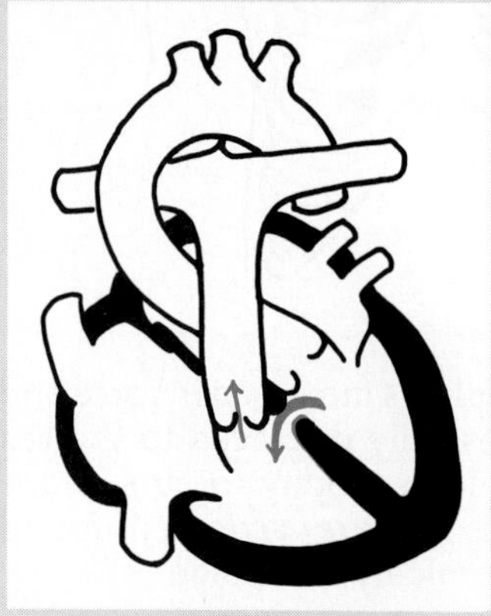	Abnormal opening in septum between ventricles, usually subaortic area. The size and exact position vary considerably.	S: Small defects asymptomatic. Infants with large defects have poor growth, slow weight gain, later look pale, thin, delicate. May have feeding problems, DOE, frequent respiratory infections, and when the condition is severe, congestive heart failure. O: Loud harsh holosystolic murmur, best heard at left lower sternal border, may be accompanied by thrill. Large defects also have soft diastolic murmur at apex (mitral flow murmur) owing to increased blood flow through mitral valve.

S, subjective data; O, objective data.

Table 16–8 ▸ Congenital Heart Defects *Continued*

TETRALOGY OF FALLOT 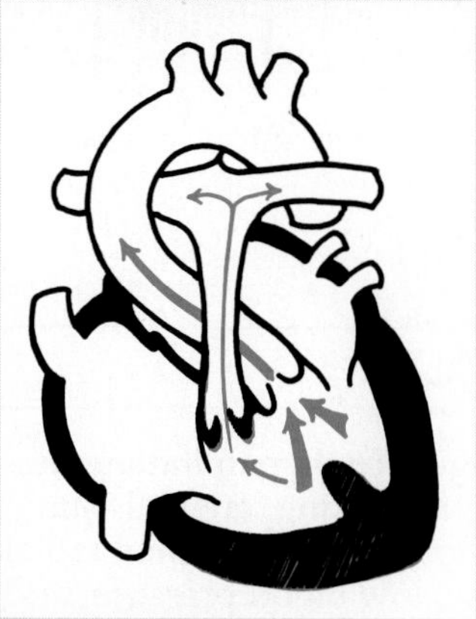	Four components: (1) right ventricular outflow stenosis, (2) VSD, (3) right ventricular hypertrophy, and (4) overriding aorta. Result: shunts a lot of venous blood directly into aorta away from pulmonary system, so blood never gets oxygenated.	S: Severe cyanosis, not in first months of life but develops as infant grows and RV outflow (i.e., pulmonic) stenosis gets worse. Cyanosis with crying and exertion at first, then at rest. Uses squatting posture after starts walking. DOE common. Development slowed. O: Thrill palpable at left lower sternal border, S_1 normal, S_2 has A_2 loud and P_2 diminished or absent. Murmur is systolic, loud, crescendo-decrescendo.
COARCTATION OF THE AORTA 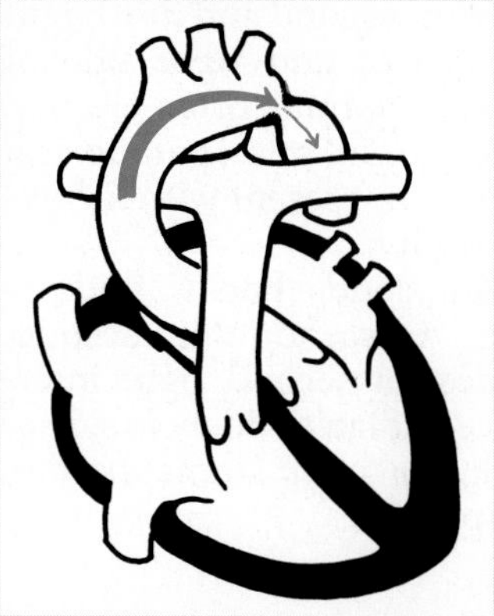	Severe narrowing of descending aorta. Results in increased workload on left ventricle. Associated with defects of aortic valve in 80 percent of cases.	S: No symptoms in childhood; growth and development are normal. Diagnosis usually accidental due to blood pressure findings. O: Blood pressure may be 10 to 15 mm Hg higher in right arm than in the left. Most important sign—absent or greatly diminished femoral pulses, a pathognomonic sign in children and young adults.

S, subjective data; O, objective data.

Table 16-9 ▸ Murmurs Due to Valvular Defects

MIDSYSTOLIC EJECTION MURMURS

(due to forward flow through semilunar valves)

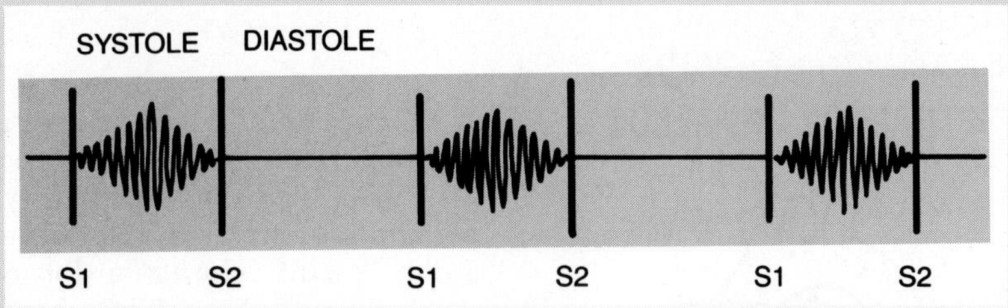

	DESCRIPTION	CLINICAL DATA
Aortic Stenosis 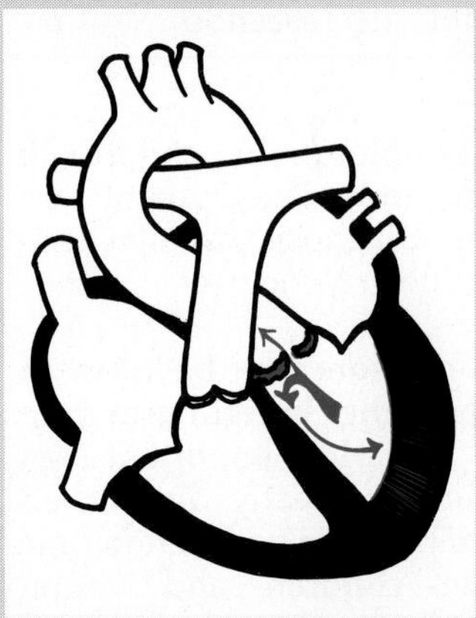	Calcification of aortic valve cusps restricts forward flow of blood during systole; LV hypertrophy develops.	S: Fatigue, DOE, palpitation, dizziness, fainting, anginal pain O: Pallor, slow diminished radial pulse, low blood pressure, and auscultatory gap are common. Apical impulse sustained and displaced to left. Thrill in systole over second and third right interspaces and right side of neck. S_1 normal, often ejection click present, often paradoxical split S_2, S_4 present with LV hypertrophy. Murmur: loud, harsh, midsystolic, crescendo-decrescendo, loudest at second right interspace, radiates widely to side of neck, down left sternal border, or apex.
Pulmonic Stenosis 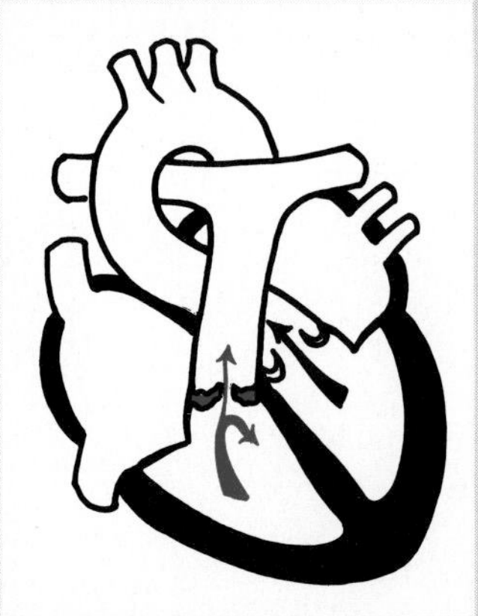	Calcification of pulmonic valve restricts forward flow of blood.	O: Thrill in systole at second and third left interspace, ejection click often after S_1, diminished S_2 and usually with wide split, S_4 common with RV hypertrophy. Murmur: systolic, medium pitch, coarse, crescendo-decrescendo (diamond shape), best heard at second left interspace, radiates to left and neck.

S, subjective data; O, objective data.

Table 16–9 ▸ Murmurs Due to Valvular Defects *Continued*

PANSYSTOLIC REGURGITANT MURMURS

(due to backward flow of blood from area of higher pressure to one of lower pressure.)

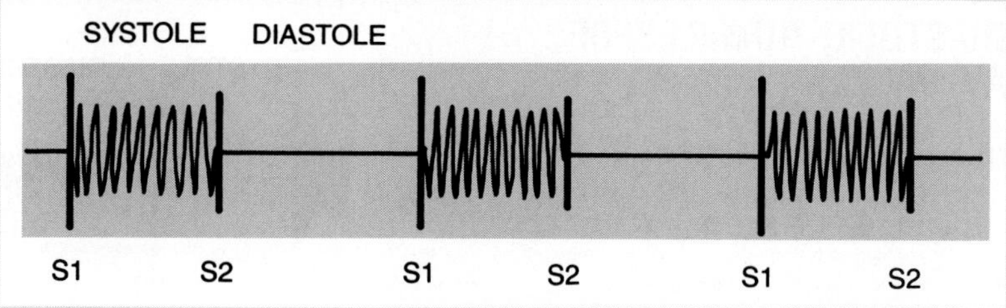

	DESCRIPTION	CLINICAL DATA
Mitral Regurgitation 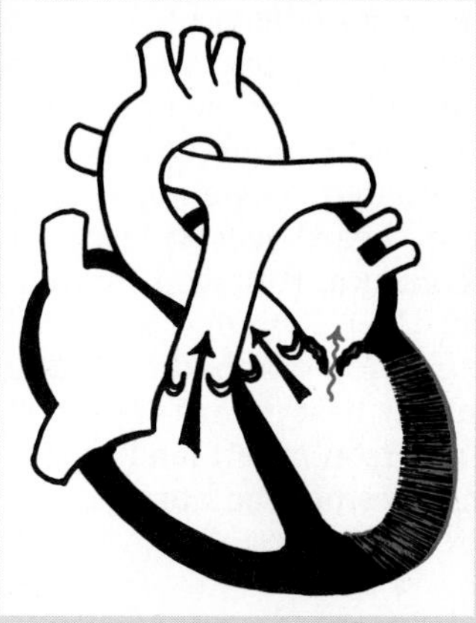	Stream of blood regurgitates back into LA during systole through incompetent mitral valve. In diastole blood passes back into LV again along with new flow; results in LV dilatation and hypertrophy.	S: Fatigue, palpitation, orthopnea, PND O: Thrill in systole at apex. Lift at apex. Apical impulse displaced down and to left. S_1 diminished, S_2 accentuated, S_3 at apex often present. Murmur: pansystolic, often loud, blowing, best heard at apex, radiates well to left axilla.
Tricuspid Regurgitation 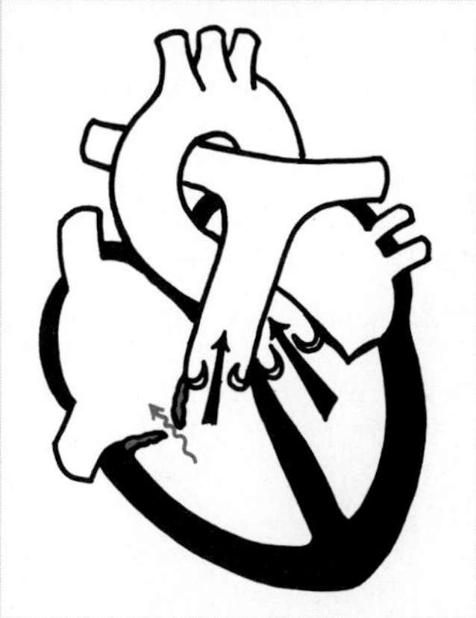	Backflow of blood through incompetent tricuspid valve into RA.	O: Engorged pulsating neck veins, liver enlarged. Lift at sternum if RV hypertrophy present, often thrill at left lower sternal border. Murmur: soft, blowing, pansystolic, best heard at left lower sternal border, increases with inspiration.

S, subjective data; O, objective data.

Table continued on following page

Table 16-9 ▸ Murmurs Due to Valvular Defects *Continued*

DIASTOLIC RUMBLES OF AV VALVES

(filling murmurs at low pressures, best heard with bell lightly touching skin.)

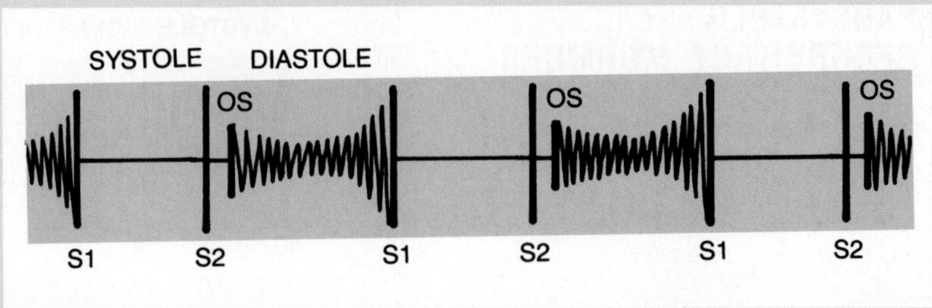

	DESCRIPTION	CLINICAL DATA
Mitral Stenosis 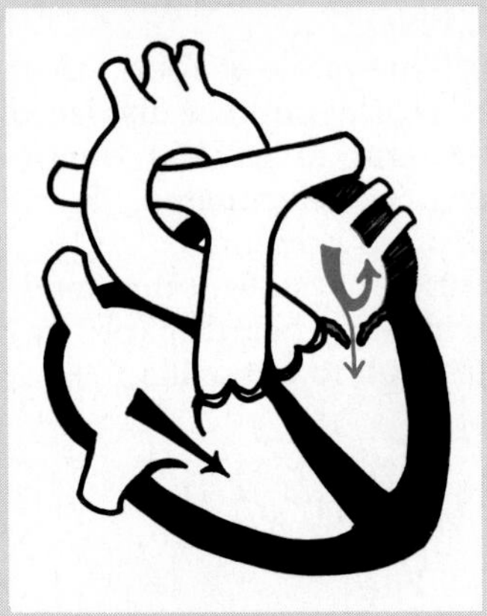	Calcified mitral valve will not open properly, impedes forward flow of blood into LV during diastole. Results in LA enlarged and LA pressure increased.	S: Fatigue, palpitations, DOE, orthopnea, occasional PND or pulmonary edema O: Diminished, often irregular arterial pulse. Lift at apex, diastolic thrill common at apex. S_1 accentuated, opening snap after S_2 heard over wide area of precordium, followed by murmur. Murmur: low-pitched diastolic rumble, best heard at apex, with person in left lateral position; does not radiate.
Tricuspid Stenosis 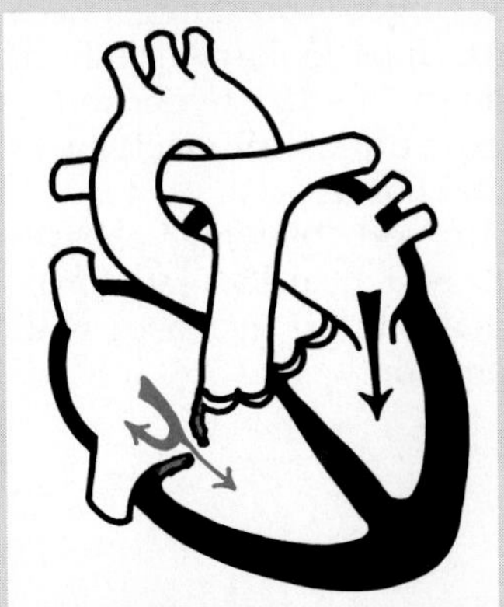	Calcification of tricuspid valve impedes forward flow into RV during diastole.	O: Diminished arterial pulse, jugular venous pulse prominent. Murmur: diastolic rumble; best heard at left lower sternal border; louder in inspiration.

S, subjective data; O, objective data.

Table 16-9 ▶ Murmurs Due to Valvular Defects *Continued*

EARLY DIASTOLIC MURMURS

(due to SL valve incompetence)

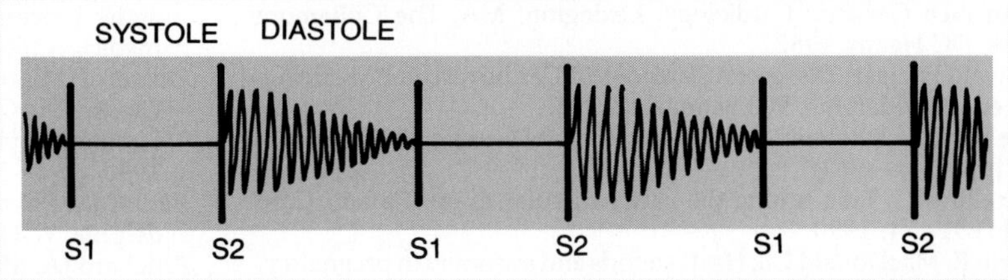

	DESCRIPTION	CLINICAL DATA
Aortic Regurgitation 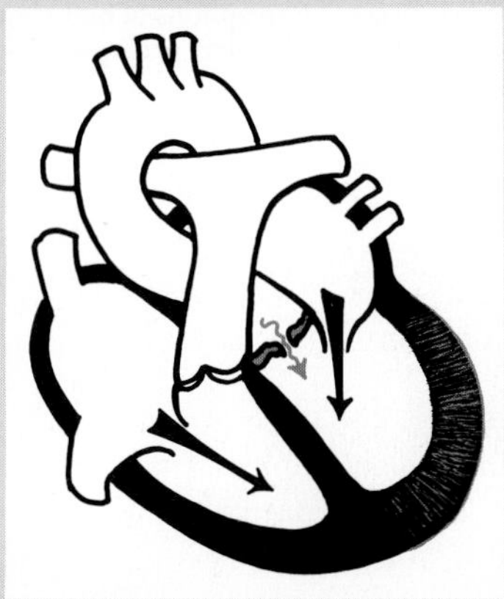	Stream of blood regurgitates back through incompetent aortic valve into LV during diastole; LV dilatation and hypertrophy due to increased LV stroke volume. Rapid ejection of large stroke volume into poorly filled aorta, then rapid runoff in diastole as part of blood pushed back into LV.	S: Only minor symptoms for many years, then rapid deterioration: DOE, PND, angina, dizziness O: Bounding "water-hammer" pulse in carotid, brachial and femoral arteries. Blood pressure has wide pulse pressure. Pulsations in cervical and suprasternal area, apical impulse displaced to left and down, apical impulse feels *brief.* Murmur starts almost simultaneously with S_2: soft, high pitched, blowing diastolic, decrescendo, best heard at third left interspace at base, as person sits up and leans forward, radiates down.
Pulmonic regurgitation 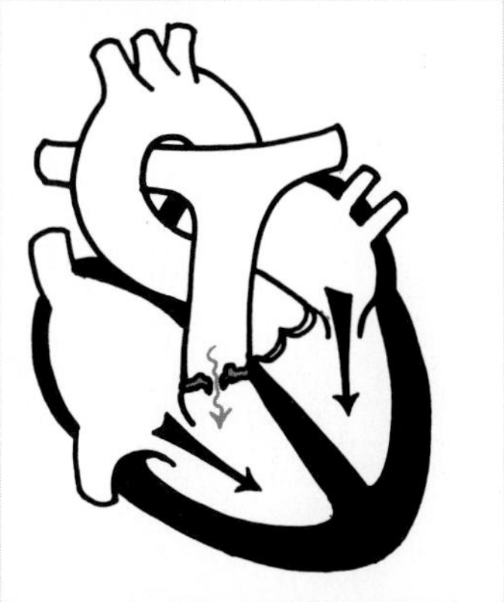	Backflow of blood through incompetent pulmonic valve, from pulmonary artery to RV.	Murmur has same timing and characteristics as that of aortic regurgitation, and is hard to distinguish on physical examination.

S, subjective data; O, objective data.

Bibliography

Behrman RE, Vaughan VC (Eds): Nelson Textbook of Pediatrics, 13th ed. Philadelphia, WB Saunders, 1987.

Berman ND: Geriatric Cardiology. Lexington, MA, The Collamore Press, DC Heath, 1982.

Braunwald E: Heart Disease: A Textbook of Cardiovascular Medicine. 3rd ed. Philadelphia, WB Saunders, 1988.

Chung EK: Quick Reference to Cardiovascular Diseases. Philadelphia, JB Lippincott, 1983.

Criscitiello MG: Fine-tuning the cardiovascular exam. Patient Care 24(11):51–74, 1990.

Cutforth R, MacDonald CB: Heart sounds and murmurs in pregnancy. Am Heart J 71:741, 1966.

DeLeon AC: Fine-tuning the examination of the heart. Consultant 29(4):51–61, 1989.

Fleg JL, Lakatta EG: Cardiovascular disease in old age. *In* Rossman I: Clinical Geriatrics. 3rd ed. Philadelphia, JB Lippincott, 1986.

Fleg JL, Kennedy HL: Cardiac arrhythmias in a healthy elderly population: Detection by 24-hour ambulatory electrocardiography. Chest 81:302, 1982.

Gerstenblith G, Frederiksen J, Yin FCP, et al: Echocardiographic assessment of a normal adult aging population. Circulation 56:273, 1977.

Henkind SJ, Benis AM, Teichholz LE: The paradox of pulsus paradoxus. Am Heart J 114:198, 1987.

Hunt AH: Mitral valve prolapse: Physical assessment, complications and management. Nurse Pract 10:15–21, 1985.

Huston TP, Puffer JC, Rodney WM: The athletic heart syndrome. N Engl J Med 313:24, 1985.

Kavanagh T, Shephard RJ: Can regular sports participation slow the aging process? Data on Masters athletes. Physician and Sportsmedicine 18(6):94–104, 1990.

Office of Minority Health: Heart Disease, Stroke, and Minorities. Closing the Gap. Public Health Service, Department of Health and Human Services. Washington, DC, Government Printing Office, 1990, pp 1–5.

Perloff JK: Physical Examination of the Heart and Circulation. Philadelphia, WB Saunders, 1982.

Pritchard JA, MacDonald PC, Gant NF: Williams Obstetrics. 17th ed. Norwalk, CT, Appleton-Century-Crofts, 1985.

Rodenheffer RJ, Gerstenblith G, Becker LC, et al: Exercise cardiac output is maintained with advancing age in healthy human subjects. Circulation 69:203, 1984.

Rothman A, Goldberger AL: Aids to cardiac auscultation. Ann Intern Med 99:346, 1983.

Saul L: Heart sounds and common murmurs. Am J Nursing 83:1679–1689, 1983.

Tilkian AG, Conover MB: Understanding Heart Sounds and Murmurs. 2nd ed. Philadelphia, WB Saunders, 1984.

Utz SW, Hammer J, Whitmire VM, Grass S: Perceptions of body image and health status in persons with mitral valve prolapse. Image 22(1):18–22, 1990.

CHAPTER

17 Abdomen

STRUCTURE AND FUNCTION

SURFACE LANDMARKS

The abdomen is a large oval cavity extending from the diaphragm down to the brim of the pelvis. It is bordered in back by the vertebral column and paravertebral muscles, and at the sides and front by the lower rib cage and abdominal muscles (Fig. 17–1). Four layers of large, flat muscles form the ventral abdominal wall. These are joined at the midline by a tendinous seam, the *linea alba.* One set, the *rectus abdominis,* forms a strip extending the length of the midline and its edge is often palpable.

For convenience in description, the abdominal wall is divided into four quadrants by a vertical and a horizontal line bisecting the umbilicus (Fig. 17–2). (An older, more complicated scheme divided the abdomen into nine regions. Although the old system generally is not used, some regional names persist, such as *epigastric* for the area between the costal margins, *umbilical* for the area around the umbilicus, and *hypogastric* or *suprapubic* for the area above the pubic bone.)

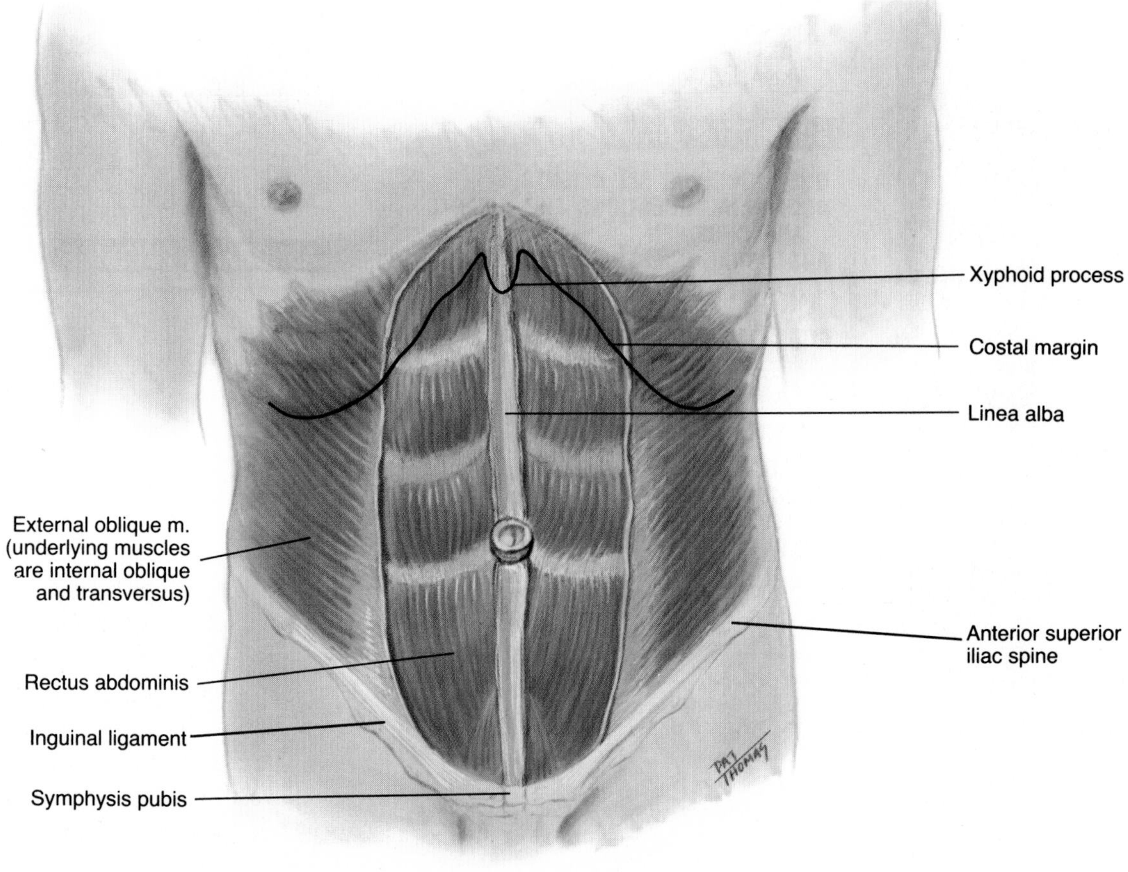

► **Figure 17–1**

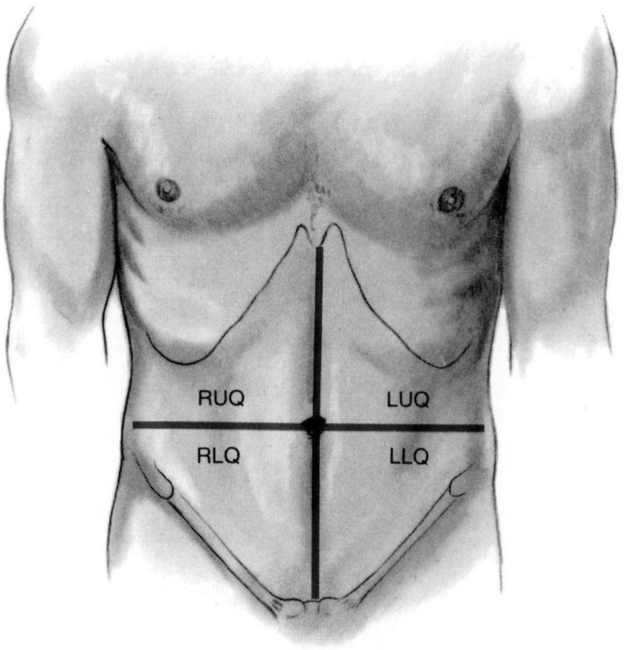

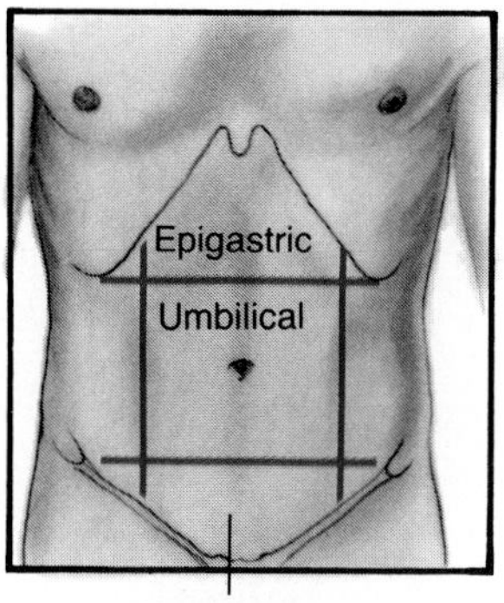

► **Figure 17-2**

INTERNAL ANATOMY

RIGHT UPPER QUADRANT (RUQ)	LEFT UPPER QUADRANT (LUQ)
Liver	Stomach
Gallbladder	Spleen
Duodenum	Left lobe of liver
Head of pancreas	Body of pancreas
Right kidney and adrenal	Left kidney and adrenal
Hepatic flexure of colon	Splenic flexure of colon
Part of ascending and transverse colon	Part of transverse and descending colon

RIGHT LOWER QUADRANT (RLQ)	LEFT LOWER QUADRANT (LLQ)
Cecum	Part of descending colon
Appendix	Sigmoid colon
Right ovary and tube	Left ovary and tube
Right ureter	Left ureter
Right spermatic cord	Left spermatic cord

MIDLINE
Aorta
Uterus (if enlarged)
Bladder (if distended)

The abdominal cavity contains the *viscera.* It is important that you know the location of these organs so well that you could draw a roadmap on the skin (Fig. 17-3). You must be able to visualize each organ that you listen to or palpate through the abdominal wall.

The solid viscera are those that maintain a characteristic shape (liver, pancreas, spleen, adrenal glands, kidneys, ovaries, and uterus). The liver fills most of the RUQ and extends over to the left midclavicular line. The lower edge of the liver and the right kidney may be palpable normally. The ovaries normally are palpable only on bimanual examination during the pelvic examination.

The shape of the hollow viscera (stomach, gallbladder, small intestine, colon, and bladder) depends on the contents. They usually are not palpable, although you may feel a colon distended with feces or a bladder distended with urine. The stomach is just below the diaphragm, between the liver and spleen. The gallbladder rests under the posterior surface of the liver, just lateral to the right midclavicular line. Note that the small intestine is located in all four quadrants. It extends from the stomach's pyloric valve to the ileocecal valve in the RLQ where it joins the colon.

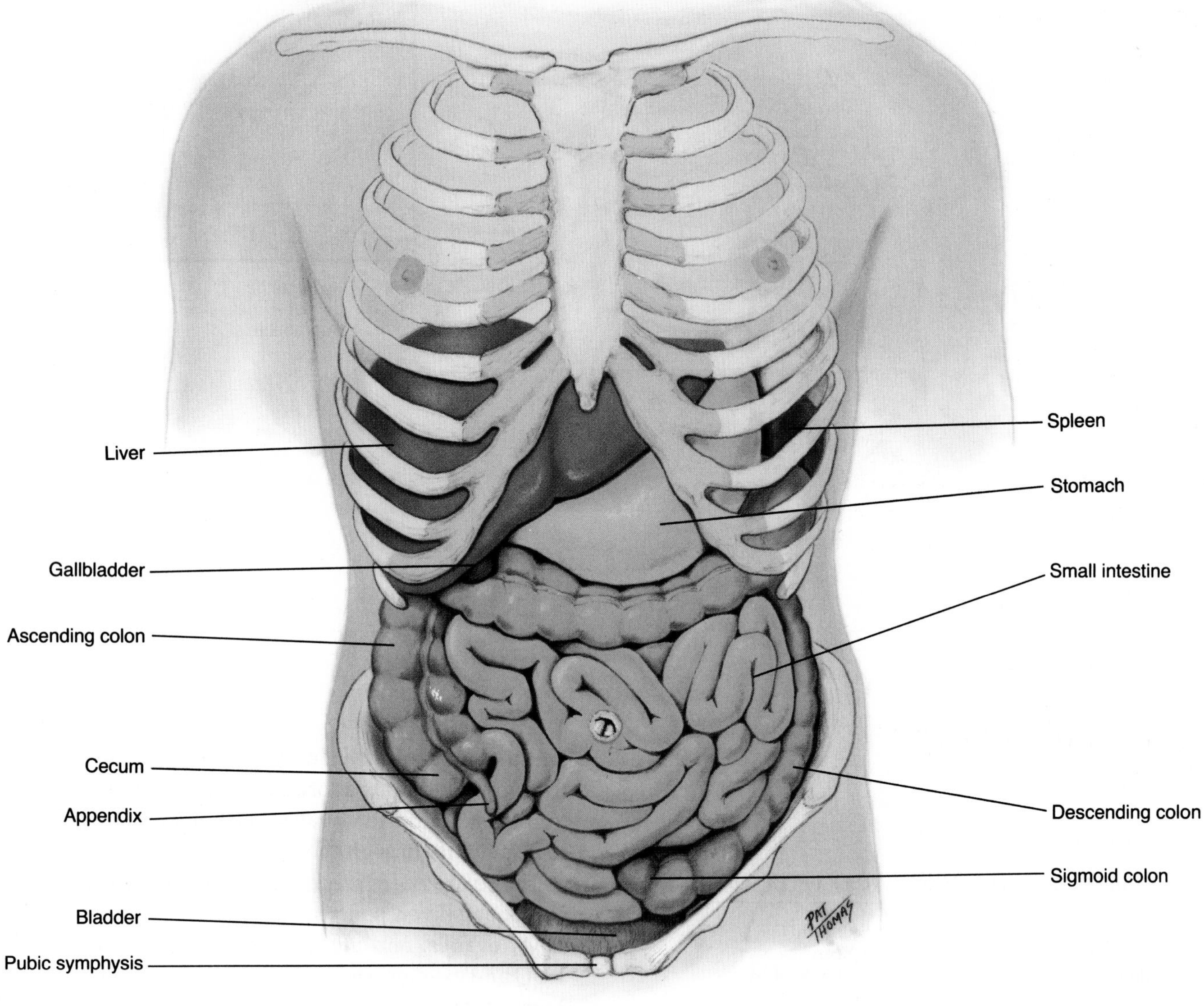

▶ **Figure 17-3**

The aorta is just to the left of midline in the upper abdomen (Fig. 17–4). At 2 cm below the umbilicus, it bifurcates into the right and left iliac arteries, which become the femoral arteries in the groin area.

The spleen is on the posterolateral wall of the abdominal cavity, immediately under the diaphragm (Fig. 17–5). It lies obliquely with its long axis behind and parallel to the 10th rib, lateral to the midaxillary line. Its width extends from the 9th to the 11th rib, about 7 cm. It is not palpable normally. If it becomes enlarged, its lower pole moves downward and toward the midline.

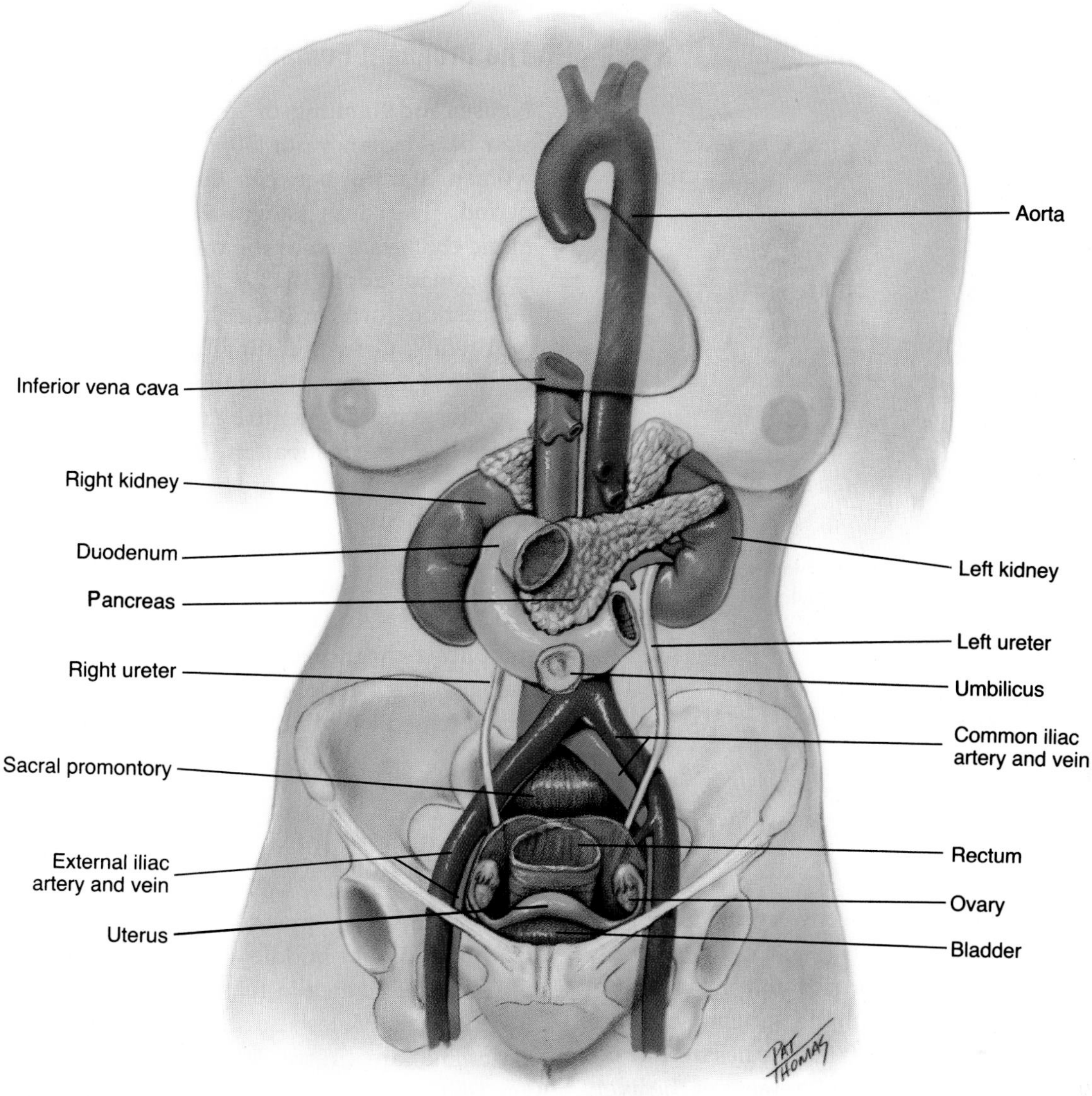

► **Figure 17 - 4**

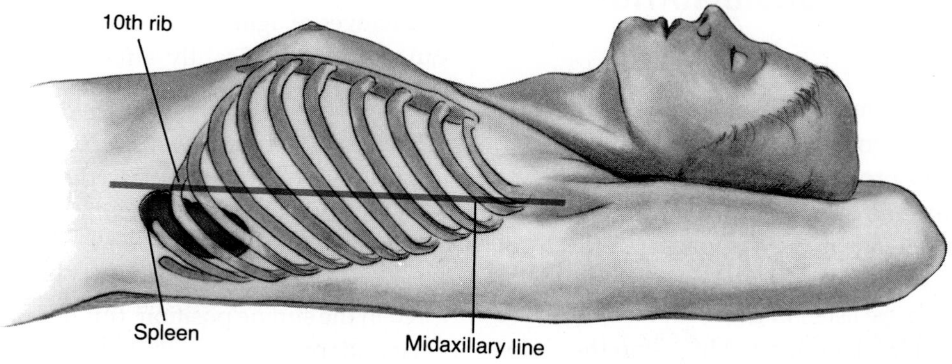

► **Figure 17 - 5**

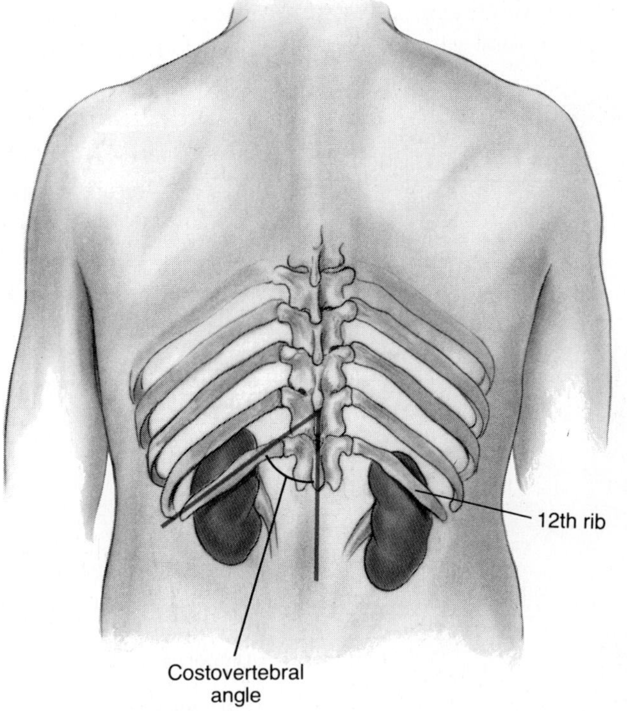

▶ **Figure 17-6**

The bean-shaped kidneys are retroperitoneal, or posterior to the abdominal contents (Fig. 17-6). They are well protected by the posterior ribs and musculature. The 12th rib forms an angle with the vertebral column, the costovertebral angle. The left kidney lies here at the 11th and 12th rib. Because of the placement of the liver, the right kidney rests 1 to 2 cm lower than the left kidney, and sometimes may be palpable.

DEVELOPMENTAL CONSIDERATIONS

Infants and Children

In the newborn, the umbilical cord shows prominently on the abdomen. It contains two arteries and one vein. The liver takes up proportionately more space in the abdomen at birth than in later life. In normal full-term neonates, the lower edge may be palpated 0.5 to 2.5 cm below the right costal margin. Age-related values of expected liver span are listed in the section on objective data. The urinary bladder is located higher in the abdomen than in the adult. It lies between the symphysis and umbilicus. Also during early childhood, the abdominal wall is less muscular, so the organs may be easier to palpate.

The Pregnant Female

Nausea and vomiting, or "morning sickness," is an early sign of pregnancy for 50 to 75 percent of pregnant women, starting between the first and second missed periods. The cause is unknown but may be due to hormone changes such as the production of human chorionic gonadotropin (hCG). Another symptom is "acid indigestion" or heartburn (pyrosis) caused by esophageal reflux. Gastrointestinal motility decreases, which prolongs gastric emptying time. The decreased motility also causes more water to be reabsorbed from the colon, which leads to constipation. The constipation, as well as increased venous pressure in the lower pelvis, may lead to hemorrhoids.

The enlarging uterus displaces the intestines upward and posteriorly. Bowel sounds are diminished. The appendix is displaced upward and to the right, which may complicate diagnosis of a possible appendicitis. Skin changes on the abdomen, such as striae and linea nigra, are discussed later in this chapter and in Chapter 9.

The Aging Adult

Aging alters the appearance of the abdominal wall. During and after middle age, some fat accumulates in the suprapubic area in females owing to decreased estrogen levels. Males also show some fat deposits in the abdominal area, resulting in the "spare tire," or "bay window." This is accentuated in adults with a more sedentary lifestyle.

With further aging, adipose tissue is redistributed away from the face and extremities and to the abdomen and hips. The abdominal musculature relaxes.

Changes of aging occur in the gastrointestinal system but do not significantly affect function as long as no disease is present.

- Salivation decreases, causing the aging person to have a dry mouth and a decreased sense of taste. Further changes involving the mouth and dentition are discussed in Chapter 13.
- Esophageal emptying is delayed. If an aging person is fed in the supine position, this may increase the risk of aspiration.
- Gastric acid secretion decreases with aging. This may cause pernicious anemia (because it interferes with vitamin B_{12} absorption), iron deficiency anemia, and malabsorption of calcium.

- The incidence of gallstones increases with age, occurring in more than 40 percent of people over 70 (Steinberg, 1983).
- Liver size decreases with age, particularly after 80 years, although most liver function remains normal. Drug metabolism by the liver may be impaired, particularly with anticonvulsant, psychotropic, and oral anticoagulants. Metabolism of alcohol seems unchanged (Steinberg, 1983).
- Aging persons frequently report constipation. It is commonly assumed that this condition is due to decreased peristalsis, but there is a lack of research to support that motility decreases solely because of aging. Rather, constipation is due to external factors, such as decreased bulk in the diet, decreased fluid intake, or laxative abuse, rather than organic factors (Steinberg, 1983).

SUBJECTIVE DATA

Appetite
Dysphagia
Food intolerance
Abdominal pain
Nausea/Vomiting
Bowel habits
Rectal conditions
Past abdominal history
Medications
Nutritional assessment

EXAMINER ASKS:	RATIONALE:
1. Have you experienced any change in **appetite?** Is this a loss of appetite? Have you had any change in weight? How much weight have you gained or lost? Over what time period? Is the weight loss due to diet?	Anorexia is a loss of appetite for food that occurs with gastrointestinal disease as well as a side effect to some medications, with pregnancy, or with psychological disorders.
2. Have you had any difficulty swallowing? When did you first notice this?	**Dysphagia** occurs with disorders of the throat or esophagus.
3. Are there any foods you cannot eat? What happens if you do eat them: allergic reaction, heartburn, belching, indigestion? Do you use antacids? How often?	**Food intolerance,** e.g., lactase deficiency resulting in bloating or excessive gas after taking milk products. Pyrosis (heartburn), a burning sensation in esophagus and stomach, owing to reflux of gastric acid. Eructation (belching).
Does your stomach feel swollen or bloated after eating?	Abdominal fullness.

EXAMINER ASKS:	RATIONALE:
4. Do you have any **abdominal pain?** Please point to it. Is the pain in one spot or does it move around? How did it start? How long have you had it? Is it constant or does it come and go? Does it occur before or after meals? Does it peak? When? How would you describe the character: cramping (colic type), burning in pit of stomach, dull, stabbing, aching?	Abdominal pain may be *visceral* from an internal organ (dull, general, poorly localized), *parietal* from inflammation of overlying peritoneum (sharp, precisely localized, aggravated by movement), or *referred* from a disorder in another site (see Table 17–2).
Is the pain affected by food: relieved by food, or worse after eating?	
Is the pain associated with: menstrual period or irregularities, stress, dietary indiscretion, fatigue, nausea and vomiting, gas, fever, rectal bleeding, frequent urination, vaginal or penile discharge?	
What makes the pain worse: food, position, stress, medication, activity?	Aggravating factors.
What have you tried to relieve pain: rest, heating pad, change in position, medication?	Alleviating factors.
5. Do you have any **nausea** or **vomiting?** How often does this occur? If you vomit, how much comes up? What is the color? Is there an odor?	Nausea/vomiting is a common side effect of many medications and occurs with gastrointestinal disease as well as early pregnancy.
Is it bloody?	Hematemesis occurs with ulcers of the stomach or duodenum and esophageal varices.
Is the nausea and vomiting associated with colicky pain, diarrhea, fever, chills?	
What foods did you eat in the last 24 hours? Where? At home, school, restaurant? Is there anyone else in the family with same symptoms in last 24 hours?	Consider food poisoning.
6. How often do you have a **bowel movement?**	Assess usual **bowel habits.**
What is the color? What is the consistency? Do you have any diarrhea, or constipation? How long have you had this? Have you had any recent change in bowel habits? Do you use laxatives? Which ones? How often do you use them?	Black stools may be tarry due to passage of occult blood (melena) from gastrointestinal bleeding or nontarry from injection of iron medications. Red blood in stools occurs with gastrointestinal bleeding or localized bleeding around the anus.
7. Do you have any **rectal problems:** itching, hemorrhoids, fissures?	Pruritus.
8. Do you have any **past history** of gastrointestinal problems: ulcer, gallbladder disease, hepatitis/jaundice, appendicitis, colitis, hernia? Have you ever had any operations in the abdomen? Please describe. Did you have any problems after surgery?	

EXAMINER ASKS:	RATIONALE:
Have you ever had any abdominal x-ray studies? How were the results?	
9. What **medications** are you currently taking?	Consider gastrointestinal side effects of certain medications, e.g., aspirin.
How about alcohol—how much would you say you drink each day? Each week? When was your last alcoholic drink?	
How about cigarettes—do you smoke? How many packs per day? For how long?	Cigarette smoking is a common cause of gastric ulcers.
10. Now I would like to ask you about your diet. Please tell me all the food you ate yesterday, starting with breakfast.	**Nutritional assessment,** via 24-hour recall (see Chapter 6 for a complete discussion).

ADDITIONAL QUESTIONS FOR INFANTS AND CHILDREN

Are you breast- or bottle-feeding the baby? If bottle-feeding, how does baby tolerate the formula?	
What table foods have you introduced? How does the infant tolerate the food?	Consider a new food as a possible allergen. Adding only one new food at a time to the infant's diet helps identify any possible allergies.
How often does your toddler/child eat? Does he or she eat regular meals? How do you feel about your child's eating patterns? Please describe all that your child had to eat yesterday, starting with breakfast. What foods does the child eat for snacks?	Irregular eating patterns, though common at this age, can be a source of parental anxiety. As long as child shows normal growth and development, and only nutritious foods are offered, parents may be reassured.
Does toddler/child ever eat nonfoods: grass, dirt, paint chips?	Pica—While a toddler may attempt nonfoods at some time, he or she should recognize edibles by age 2.
Does your child have constipation: How long has this been a problem? What are the number of stools/day? /week? How much water, juice is in the diet? Does the constipation seem to be associated with toilet training? What have you tried to treat the constipation?	
Does the child have abdominal pain? Please describe what you have noticed and when it started.	This symptom is hard to assess with young children. Many conditions of unrelated organ systems are associated with vague abdominal pain (e.g., otitis media). Young children do not have the capacity to articulate specific symptoms, and often focus on "the tummy." Abdominal pain accompanies inflammation of the bowel, as well as

EXAMINER ASKS:	RATIONALE:
	constipation, urinary tract infection, and anxiety.
For the child with obesity: How long has weight been a problem? At what age did the child first seem overweight? Was there any change in diet pattern then? Describe the diet pattern now.	Alteration in nutrition: more than body requirements.
Are there any others in family with similar problem?	Family history of obesity.
How does child feel about his or her own weight?	Assess body image.
For the adolescent: What do you eat at regular meals? Do you eat breakfast? What do you eat for snacks?	Adolescent takes control of eating and may reject family values, e.g., skipping breakfast, consuming junk foods, soda pop. The only control parents have is what is in the house.
How many calories do you figure you consume?	Probably the health professional cannot change adolescent eating pattern, but you can supply nutritional facts.
What is your exercise pattern?	Boys need an average 4000 cal/day to maintain weight; more calories are needed if exercise is pursued. Girls need 20 percent fewer calories, and the same nutrients. Fast food is a problem because it is high in fat, calories, salt, and has no fiber.
If weight is less than body requirements: How much have you lost? By diet, exercise, or how?	Screen any extremely thin teenage girl for *anorexia nervosa,* a serious psychosocial disorder that includes loss of appetite, voluntary starvation, and grave weight loss. This person may augment weight loss by purging (self-induced vomiting) and use of laxatives.
How do you feel? Tired, hungry? How do you think your body looks?	Denial of these feelings is common. Though thin, this person insists she looks fat, "disgusting." Distorted body image.
What is your activity pattern?	The anorectic may participate in normal activity and exercise but often is hyperactive.
Is the weight loss associated with any other body change, such as menstrual irregularity?	Amenorrhea is common with anorexia nervosa.
What do your parents say about your eating? Your friends?	This is a family problem involving control issues. Anyone at risk warrants immediate referral to a physician or psychologist.

EXAMINER ASKS:	RATIONALE:

ADDITIONAL QUESTIONS FOR THE AGING ADULT

How do you acquire your groceries and prepare your meals?	Assess if at risk for nutritional deficit due to limited access to grocery store, limited income, limited cooking facility, physical disability (impaired vision, decreased mobility, decreased strength, neurologic deficit).
Do you eat alone, or share meals with others?	Assess if at risk for nutritional deficit if living alone; may not bother to prepare all meals; social isolation; depression.
Please tell me all that you had to eat yesterday, starting with breakfast.	Note: 24-hour recall may not be sufficient because pattern may vary from day to day. Attempt week-long diary of intake. Food pattern may be different at the end of the month if monthly income, i.e. social security check, runs out.
Do you have any trouble swallowing these foods?	
What do you do right after eating: walk, take a nap?	
How often do your bowels move?	
If the person reports constipation: What do you mean by constipation? How much liquid is in your diet? How much bulk or fiber?	
Do you take anything for constipation, such as laxatives? Which ones? How often do you take laxatives?	
What medications do you take?	Consider gastrointestinal side effects: e.g., nausea, upset stomach, anorexia, dry mouth.

OBJECTIVE DATA

Equipment Needed

Stethoscope
Small centimeter ruler
Skin marking pen

Preparation

The lighting should include a strong overhead light, and a secondary stand light. Expose the abdomen so that it is fully visible. Drape the genitalia and female breasts.

The following measures will enhance abdominal wall relaxation. The person should have emptied the bladder, saving a urine specimen if needed. Keep the room warm to avoid chilling and tensing of muscles. Position the person supine, with the head on a pillow, the knees bent or on pillow, and the arms at the sides or across the chest. (Note: Discourage the person placing his or her arms over the head because this tenses abdominal musculature.) To avoid abdominal tensing, the stethoscope endpiece must be warm, your hands must be warm, and your fingernails very short. Inquire about any painful areas. Examine such an area last to avoid any muscle guarding. Finally, learn to use distraction: enhance muscle relaxation through breathing exercises; emotive imagery; your low, soothing voice; and the person relating his or her abdominal history while you palpate.

METHOD OF EXAMINATION

NORMAL RANGE OF FINDINGS

INSPECTION

Inspect contour, symmetry, umbilicus, skin, pulsation or movement, and hair distribution.

Contour. Stand on the person's right side and look down on the abdomen. Then stoop to gaze across the abdomen, or sit in a chair. Your head should be slightly higher than the abdomen. Determine the profile from the rib margin to the pubic bone. The contour describes the nutritional state, and normally ranges from flat to rounded (Fig. 17–7).

ABNORMAL FINDINGS

Protuberant abdomen, abdominal distention (see Table 17–3).

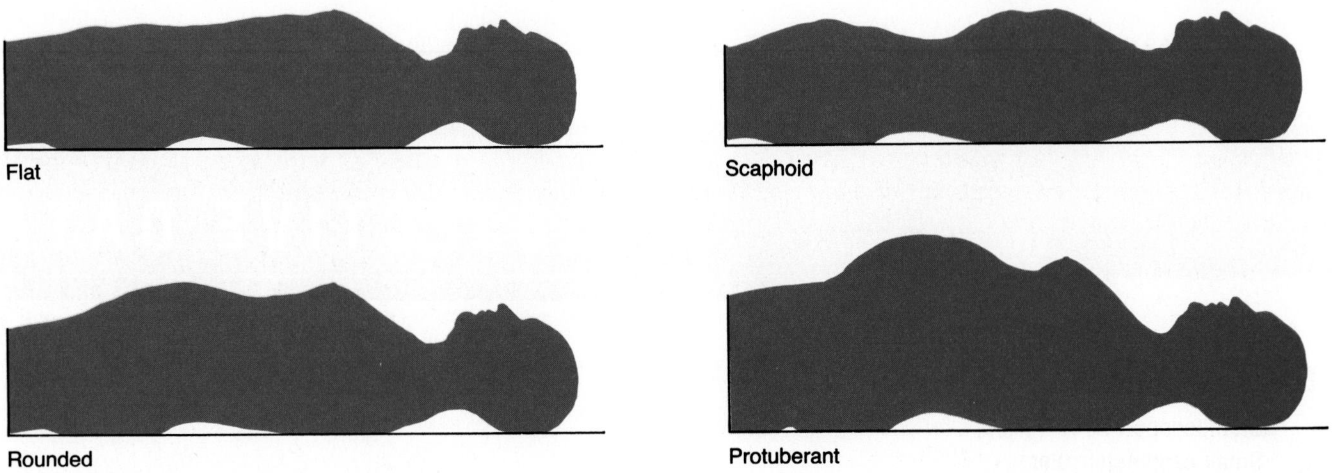

▶ **Figure 17–7**

NORMAL RANGE OF FINDINGS	ABNORMAL FINDINGS
Symmetry. Shine a light across the abdomen toward you, or shine it lengthwise across the person. The abdomen should be symmetric bilaterally (Fig. 17–8). Note any localized bulging, visible mass, or asymmetric shape. Even small bulges are highlighted by shadow. Step to the foot of the examination table to recheck symmetry.	Bulges, masses. Hernia—protrusion of abdominal viscera through abnormal opening in muscle wall (see Table 17–4).

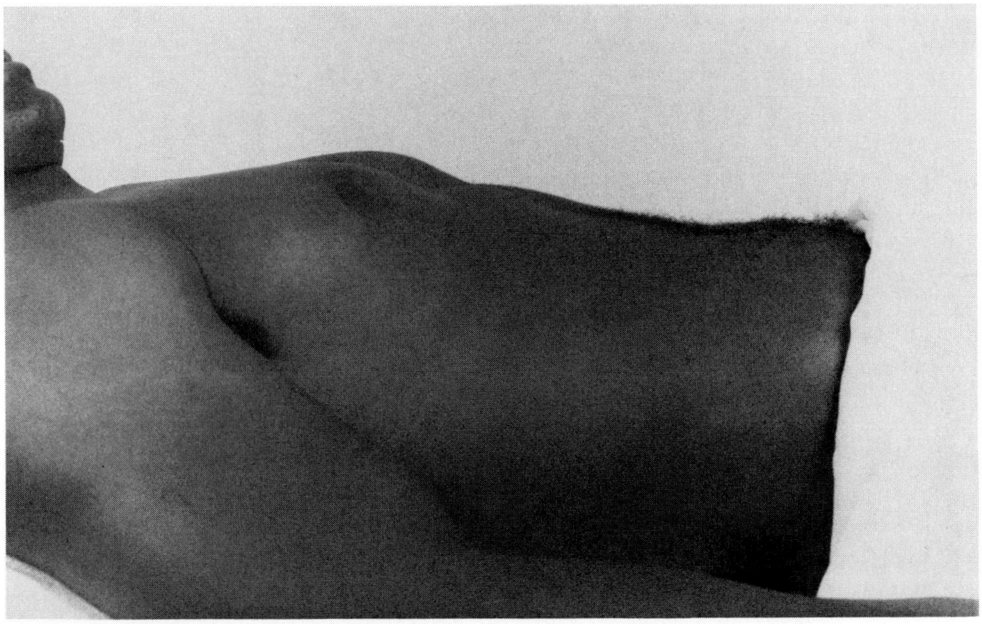

▶ **Figure 17–8**

Ask the person to take a deep breath to further highlight any change. The abdomen should stay smooth and symmetric. Or, ask the person to perform a sit-up without using the hands.	Note any localized bulging. Enlarged liver or spleen may show.
Umbilicus. Normally it is midline and inverted, with no sign of discoloration, inflammation, or hernia. It becomes everted and pushed upward with pregnancy.	Everted with acites, or underlying mass (see Table 17–3). Deeply sunken with obesity. Enlarged and everted with umbilical hernia. Bluish periumbilical color occurs with intra-abdominal bleeding (Cullen's sign).
Skin. The surface is smooth and even, with homogenous color. This is a good area to judge pigment because it is often protected from sun.	Redness with localized inflammation. Jaundice (shows best in natural daylight). Skin glistening and taut occurs with ascites.

NORMAL RANGE OF FINDINGS

One common pigment change is *striae* (linea albicantes), silvery-white, linear, jagged marks about 1 to 6 cm long (Fig. 17–9). They occur when elastic fibers in the reticular layer of the skin are broken following rapid or prolonged stretching, as in pregnancy or excessive weight gain. Recent striae are pink or blue, then they turn silvery white.

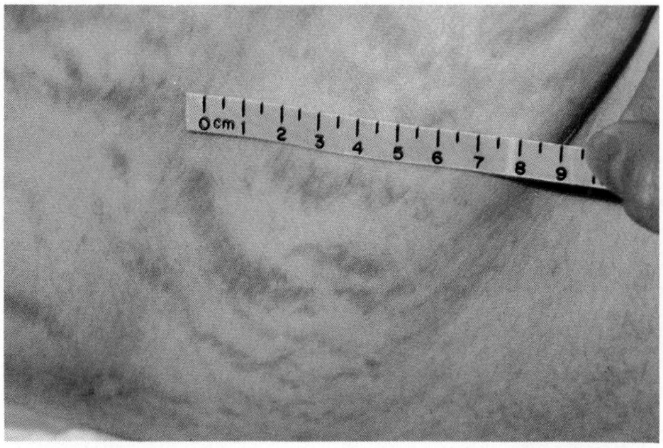

► **Figure 17–9**

Moles, circumscribed brown macular or papular areas, are common on the abdomen.

Normally, there are no lesions, although sometimes well-healed surgical scars are present. If a scar is present, draw its location in the person's record, indicating the length in centimeters (Fig. 17–10). (Not infre-

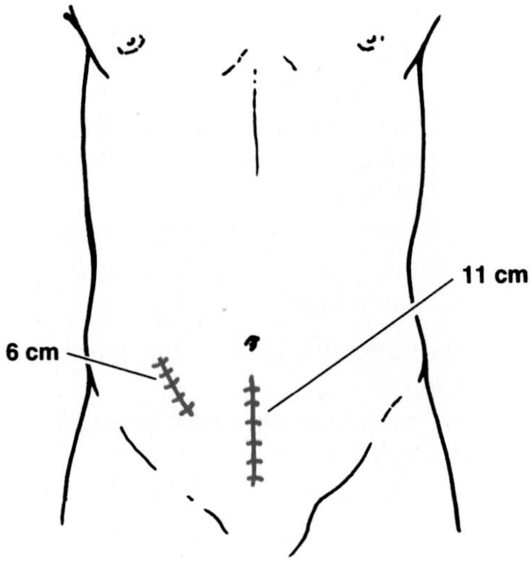

► **Figure 17–10**

ABNORMAL FINDINGS

Striae also occur with ascites.

Striae look purple-blue with Cushing's syndrome (excess adrenocortical hormone causes the skin to be fragile and easily broken from normal stretching).

Unusual color or change in shape of mole (see Chapter 9).

Petechiae.

Cutaneous angiomas (spider nevi) occur with portal hypertension or liver disease.

Lesions, rashes (see Chapter 9).

NORMAL RANGE OF FINDINGS	ABNORMAL FINDINGS
quently, a person forgets a past operation while providing the history. If you note a scar now, ask about it.) A surgical scar alerts you to the possible presence of underlying adhesions and excess fibrous tissue.	
Veins are usually not seen, but a fine venous network may be visible in thin persons.	Prominent, dilated veins occur with portal hypertension, cirrhosis, ascites, or venacaval obstruction. Veins are more visible with malnutrition due to thinned adipose tissue.
Good skin turgor reflects healthy nutrition. Gently pinch up a fold of skin; then release to note the skin's immediate return to original position.	Poor turgor occurs with dehydration, which often accompanies gastrointestinal disease.
Pulsation or Movement. Normally, you may see the pulsations from the aorta beneath the skin in the epigastric area, particularly in thin persons with good muscle wall relaxation. Respiratory movement also shows in the abdomen, particularly in males. Finally, waves of peristalsis sometimes are visible in very thin persons. They ripple slowly and obliquely across the abdomen.	Marked pulsation of the aorta occurs with widened pulse pressure (e.g., hypertension, aortic insufficiency, thyrotoxicosis) and with aortic aneurysm. Marked visible peristalsis, together with a distended abdomen, indicates intestinal obstruction.
Hair Distribution. The pattern of pubic hair growth normally has a diamond shape in adult males and an inverted triangle shape in adult females (see Chapters 21 and 22).	Patterns alter with endocrine or hormone abnormalities and chronic liver disease.
Demeanor. A comfortable person is relaxed quietly on the examining table and has a benign facial expression and slow, even respirations.	Restlessness and constant turning to find a comfortable position occur with the colicky pain of gastroenteritis or bowel obstruction. Absolute stillness, resisting any movement, is demonstrated with the pain of peritonitis. Knees flexed up, facial grimacing, and rapid, uneven respirations also indicate pain.

AUSCULTATION

Auscultate bowel sounds and vascular sounds.

Depart from the usual examination sequence and auscultate the abdomen next. This is done because percussion and palpation can increase peristalsis, which would give a false interpretation of bowel sounds. Use the diaphragm endpiece because bowel sounds are relatively high pitched. Hold the stethoscope lightly against the skin; pushing too hard may stimulate more bowel sounds (Fig. 17–11). Begin in the LRQ at the ileocecal valve area, because bowel sounds are always present here normally.

NORMAL RANGE OF FINDINGS | **ABNORMAL FINDINGS**

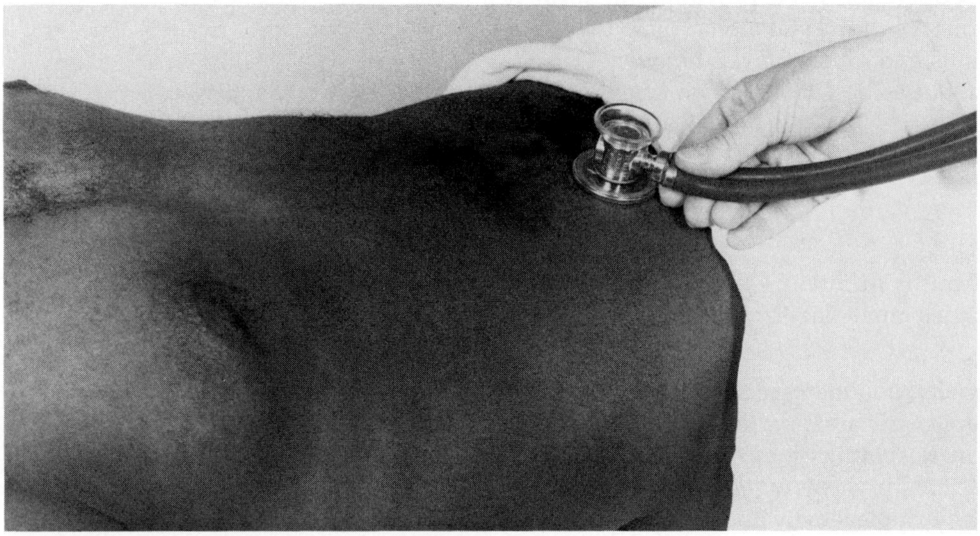

► **Figure 17-11**

Bowel Sounds. Note the character and frequency of bowel sounds. Bowel sounds originate from the movement of air and fluid through the small intestine. Depending on the time elapsed since eating, there can be a wide range of normal sounds. They are high-pitched, gurgling, cascading sounds, occurring irregularly anywhere from 5 to 30 times per minute. Do not bother to count them. Judge if they are normal, hypoactive or hyperactive. One type of hyperactive bowel sounds is fairly common. This is the hyperperistalsis when you feel your "stomach growling," termed *borborygmi.* A perfectly "silent abdomen" is uncommon; you must listen for 5 minutes by your watch before deciding bowel sounds are completely absent.

Two distinct patterns of abnormal bowel sounds may occur:

1. *Hyperactive* sounds are loud, high-pitched, rushing, tinkling sounds.
2. *Hypoactive* or *absent* sounds follow abdominal surgery or with inflammation of the peritoneum. (see Table 17-5).

Vascular Sounds. As you listen to the abdomen, note the presence of any vascular sounds or *bruits.* Using firmer pressure, check over the aorta, renal arteries, iliac and femoral arteries, especially in people with hyper-

Note location, pitch, and timing of a vascular sound.

A systolic bruit is a pulsatile blowing sound.

Venous hum.

Peritoneal friction rub (see Table 17-6).

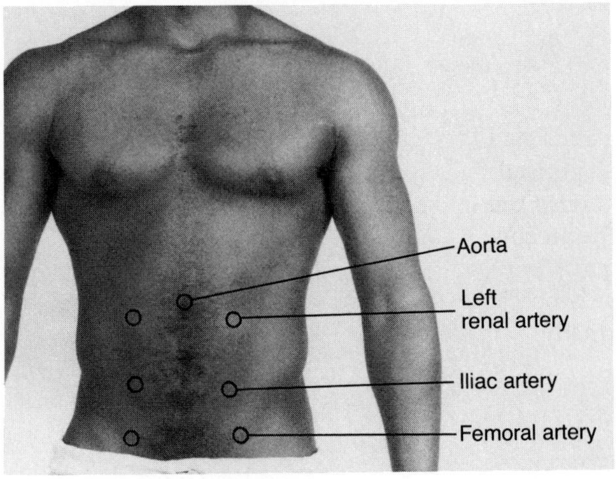

► **Figure 17-12**

NORMAL RANGE OF FINDINGS | ABNORMAL FINDINGS

tension (Fig. 17–12). Usually, there is no such sound. An upper abdominal bruit occasionally is heard in normal persons, especially young adults. (Julius and Stewart, 1967).

PERCUSSION

Percuss general tympany, liver span, and splenic dullness.

Percuss to assess the relative density of abdominal contents, to locate organs, and to screen for abnormal fluid or masses.

General Tympany. First, percuss lightly in all four quadrants to determine the prevailing amount of tympany and dullness (Fig. 17–13). Tympany should predominate because air in the intestines rises to the surface when the person is supine.

Dullness occurs over a distended bladder, adipose tissue, fluid, or a mass.

Hyperresonance is present with gaseous distention.

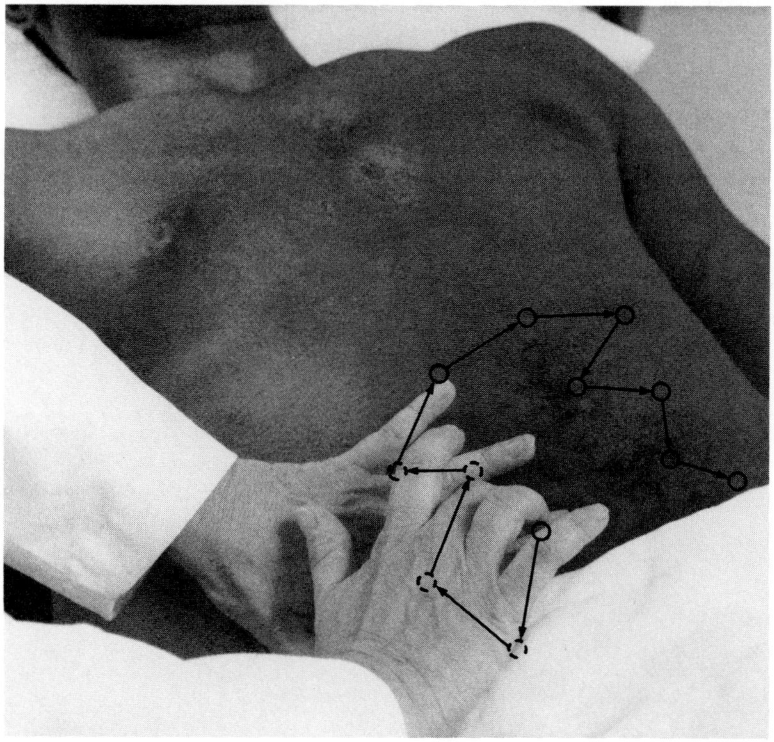

▶ **Figure 17–13**

Liver Span. Next, percuss to map out the boundaries of certain organs. Measure the height of the liver in the right midclavicular line. (For a consistent placement of the midclavicular line landmark, remember to palpate the acromioclavicular and the sternoclavicular joints and judge the

NORMAL RANGE OF FINDINGS	ABNORMAL FINDINGS

line at a point midway between the two.) Begin in the area of lung resonance, and percuss down the interspaces until the sound changes to a dull quality (Fig. 17–14a). Mark the spot, usually in the fifth intercostal space. Then find abdominal tympany, and percuss up in the midclavicular line. Mark where the sound changes from tympany to a dull sound, normally at the right costal margin.

Measure the distance between the two marks; the normal liver span in the adult ranges from 6 to 12 cm (Fig. 17–14b). The height of the liver span correlates with the height of the person; taller people have longer livers. Also males have a larger liver span than females of the same height. Overall, the mean liver span is 10.5 cm for males and 7 cm for females.

An enlarged liver span indicates liver enlargement or *hepatomegaly.*

Accurate detection of liver borders is confused by dullness above fifth intercostal space, which occurs with lung disease, e.g., pleural effusion or consolidation; lower border of dullness pushed up with ascites or pregnancy; gas distention in colon, which obscures lower border.

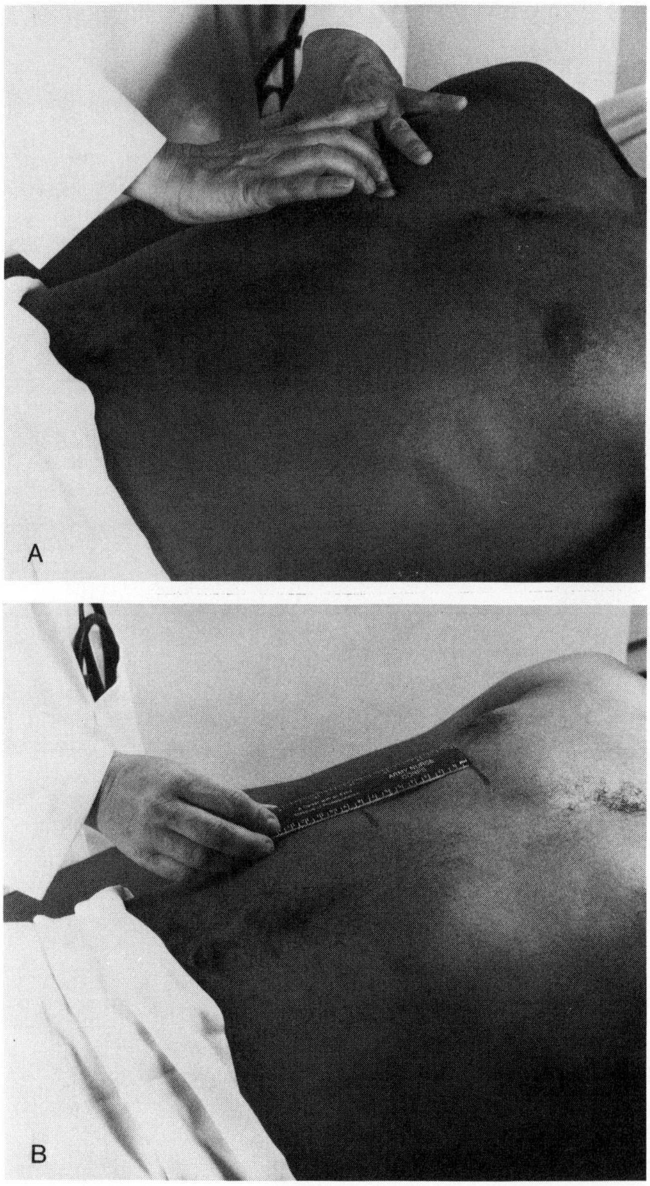

► Figure 17–14

NORMAL RANGE OF FINDINGS

One variation occurs in people with chronic emphysema, in which the liver is displaced downward by the hyperinflated lungs. Although you hear a dull percussion note well below the right costal margin, the overall span is still within normal limits.

Clinical estimation of liver span is important to screen for hepatomegaly and to monitor changes in liver size. However, this measurement is a gross estimate; one study showed the liver span was underestimated by more than 2 cm in 50 percent of the cases (Sullivan, 1976). The major problem was accurate detection of the upper border. A more recent study recommends *direct* percussion, lightly tapping the body surface directly with the index finger, as more sensitive to changes in pitch and vibration than the traditional method of indirect percussion (Skrainka et al, 1986). The bedside estimate of liver span by this direct percussion method was confirmed to be as accurate as ultrasound study.

Splenic Dullness. Often the spleen is obscured by stomach contents, but you may locate it by a dull note from the 9th to 11th intercostal space just behind the left midaxillary line (Fig. 17–15). The area of splenic dullness normally is not wider than 7 cm in the adult, and should not encroach on the normal tympany over the gastric air bubble.

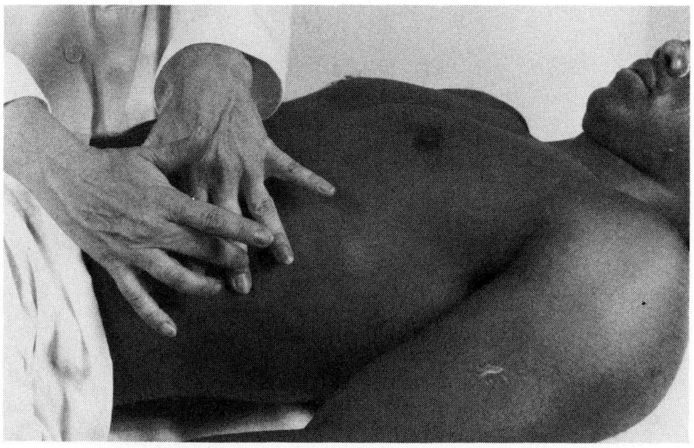

► **Figure 17–15**

Now percuss in the lowest interspace in the left *anterior* axillary line. Tympany should result. Ask the person to take a deep breath. Normally, tympany remains through full inspiration.

ABNORMAL FINDINGS

A dull note forward of the midaxillary line indicates enlargement of the spleen, as occurs with mononucleosis, trauma, and infection.

In this site, the *anterior* axillary line, a change in percussion from tympany to a dull sound with full inspiration is a *positive* spleen percussion sign. This method will detect mild to moderate splenomegaly before the spleen becomes palpable, as in mononucleosis, malaria, or hepatic cirrhosis (Castell, 1967).

NORMAL RANGE OF FINDINGS	ABNORMAL FINDINGS

Costovertebral Angle Tenderness. Indirect fist percussion causes the tissues to vibrate instead of producing a sound. To assess the kidney, place one hand over the 12th rib at the costovertebral angle on the back (Fig. 17–16). Thump that hand with the ulnar edge of your other fist. The person normally feels a thud but no pain.

Sharp pain occurs with inflammation of the kidney or paranephric area.

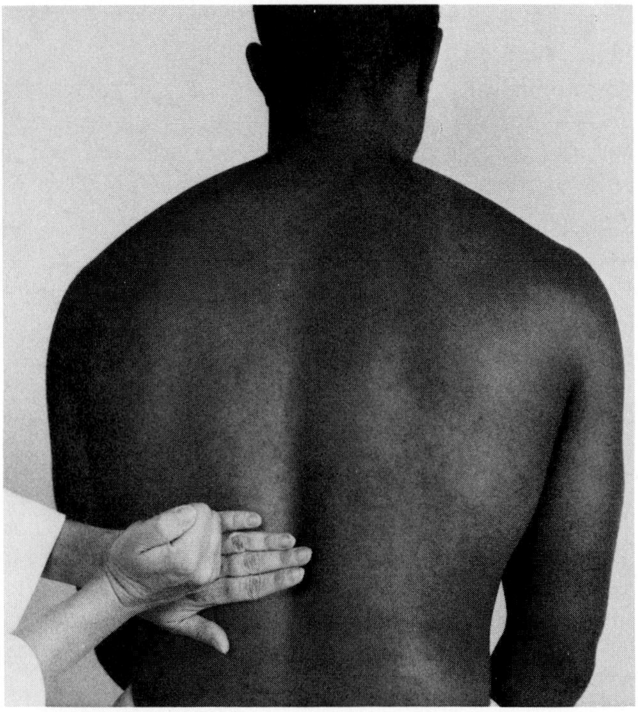

► **Figure 17–16**

(Although this step is explained here with percussion techniques, its usual sequence in a complete examination is with thoracic assessment, when the person is sitting up and you are standing behind.)

Special Procedures. At times, you may suspect a person has ascites (free fluid in the peritoneal cavity) because of a distended abdomen, bulging flanks, and an umbilucus that is protruding and displaced downward. You can differentiate ascites from gaseous distention by performing two percussion tests.

Ascites occurs with congestive heart failure, portal hypertension, cirrhosis, hepatitis, pancreatitis, and cancer.

First, test for a *fluid wave* by standing on the person's right side. Place the ulnar edge of another examiner's hand or the client's own hand firmly on the abdomen in the midline (Fig. 17–17). (This will stop transmission across the skin of the upcoming tap.) Place your left hand on the person's right flank. With your right hand, reach across the abdomen and give the left flank a firm strike. If acites is present, the blow will generate a fluid wave through the abdomen and you will feel a distinct tap on your left hand. If the abdomen is distended from gas or adipose tissue, you will feel no change.

A positive fluid wave test occurs with large amounts of ascitic fluid.

NORMAL RANGE OF FINDINGS

ABNORMAL FINDINGS

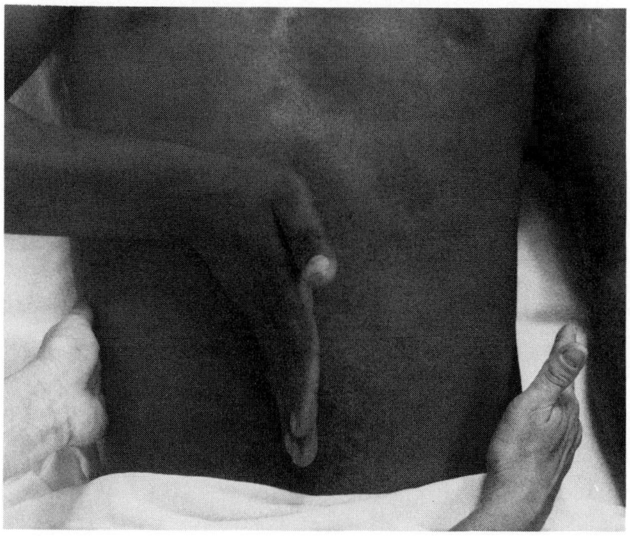

Fluid wave

► **Figure 17-17**

The second test for ascites is percussing for *shifting dullness.* In a supine person, ascitic fluid settles by gravity into the flanks, displacing the air-filled bowel upward. You will hear a tympanitic note as you percuss over the top of the abdomen because gas-filled intestines float over the fluid (Fig. 17-18). Then percuss down the side of the abdomen. If fluid is present, the note will change from tympany to dull as you reach its level. Mark this spot.

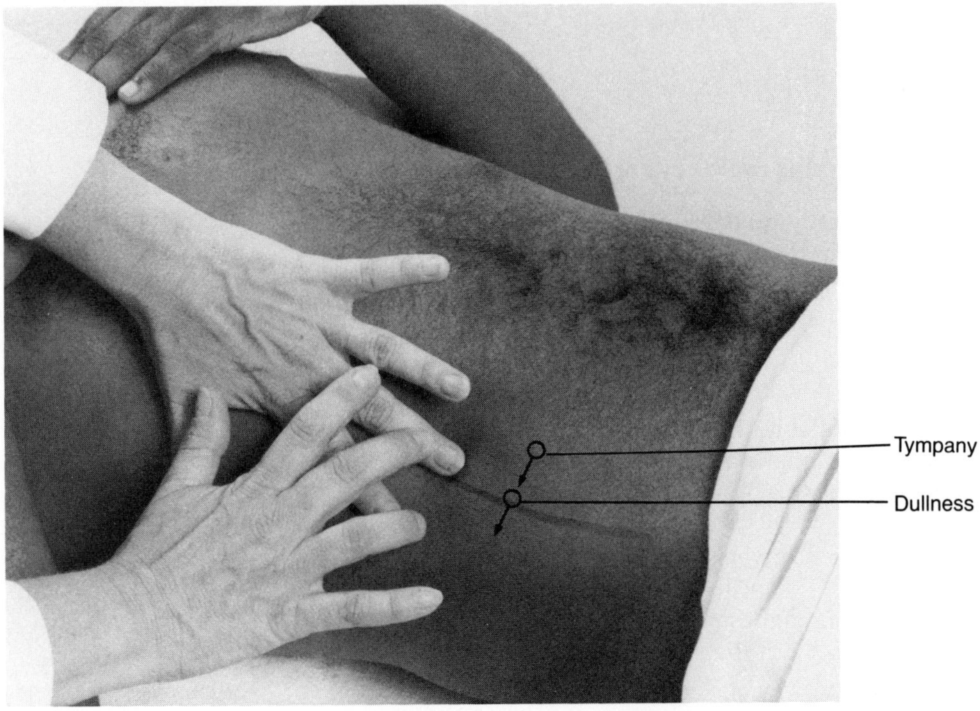

► **Figure 17-18**

NORMAL RANGE OF FINDINGS	ABNORMAL FINDINGS

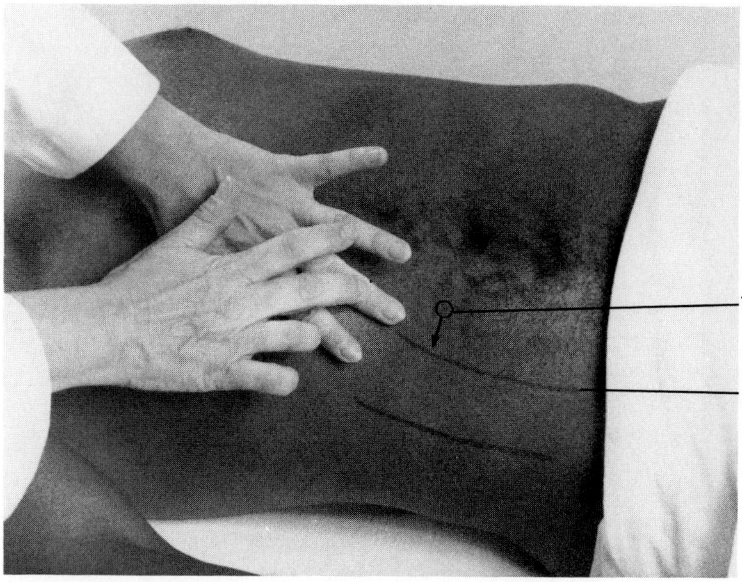

► Figure 17–19

Now turn the person onto the right side (roll the person toward you) (Fig. 17–19). The fluid will gravitate to the dependent (in this case, right) side, displacing the lighter bowel upward. Begin percussing the upper side of the abdomen and move downward. The sound changes from tympany to a dull sound as you reach the fluid level, but this time the level of dullness is higher, upward toward the umbilicus. This *shifting level of dullness* indicates the presence of fluid.

Both tests, fluid wave and shifting dullness, are not reliable. Ultrasound study is the definitive tool.

Shifting dullness is positive with a large volume of ascitic fluid: It will not detect less than 500 ml of fluid.

PALPATION

Palpate surface and deep areas, liver edge, spleen, and kidneys.

Perform palpation to judge the size, location, and consistency of certain organs and to screen for an abnormal mass or tenderness. Review comfort measures on p. 596. Since most people are naturally inclined to protect the abdomen, you need to use additional measures to enhance complete muscle relaxation.

1. Bend the person's knees.
2. Keep your palpating hand low and parallel to the abdomen. Holding the hand high and pointing down would make anyone tense up.
3. Teach the person to breathe slowly (in through the nose, and out through the mouth).
4. Keep your own voice low and soothing. Conversation may relax the person.
5. Try "emotive imagery." For example, you might say, "Now I want you to imagine you are dozing on the beach, with the sun warming your

NORMAL RANGE OF FINDINGS

ABNORMAL FINDINGS

muscles and the sound of the waves lulling you to sleep. Let yourself relax."

6. With a very ticklish person, keep the person's hand under your own with your fingers curled over his or her fingers. Move both hands around as you palpate; people are not ticklish to themselves.
7. Alternatively, perform palpation just after auscultation. Keep the stethoscope in place and curl your fingers around it, palpating as you pretend to auscultate. People do not perceive a stethoscope as a ticklish object. You can slide the stethoscope out when the person is used to being touched.

Light and Deep Palpation. Begin with **light palpation.** With the first four fingers close together, depress the skin about 1 cm (Fig. 17–20). Make a gentle rotary motion, sliding the fingers and skin together. Then lift the fingers (do not drag them) and move clockwise to the next location around the abdomen. The objective here is not to search for organs but to form an overall impression of the skin surface and superficial musculature. Save the examination of any identified tender areas until last. This method avoids pain and the resulting muscle rigidity that would obscure deep palpation later in the examination.

Muscle guarding.
Rigidity.
Large masses.
Tenderness.

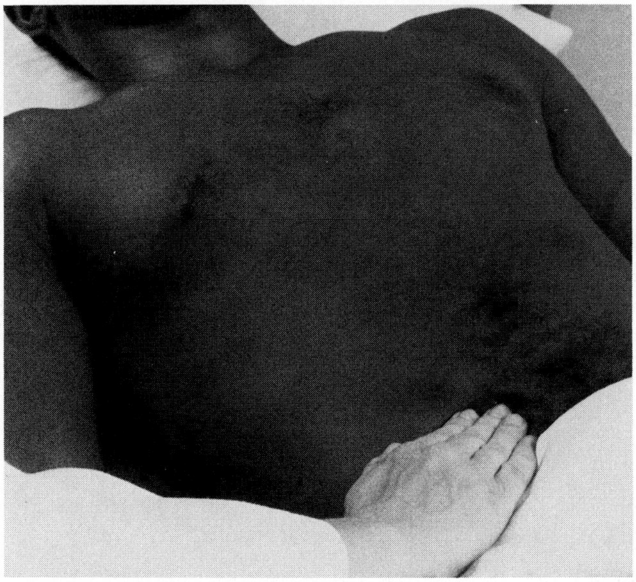

► **Figure 17–20**

As you circle the abdomen, discriminate between voluntary muscle guarding and involuntary rigidity. Voluntary *guarding* occurs when the person is cold, tense, or ticklish. It is bilateral, and you will feel the muscles relax slightly during exhalation. Use the relaxation measures to try to eliminate this type of guarding, or it will interfere with deep palpation. If the rigidity persists, it is probably involuntary.

Involuntary *rigidity* is a constant boardlike hardness of the muscles. It is a protective mechanism accompanying acute inflammation of the peritoneum. It may be unilateral, and the same area usually becomes painful when the person increases intra-abdominal pressure by attempting a sit-up.

NORMAL RANGE OF FINDINGS	ABNORMAL FINDINGS

Now perform **deep palpation,** using the same technique described earlier, but push down about 5 – 8 cm (2 – 3 inches) (Fig. 17 – 21a). Moving clockwise, explore the entire abdomen.

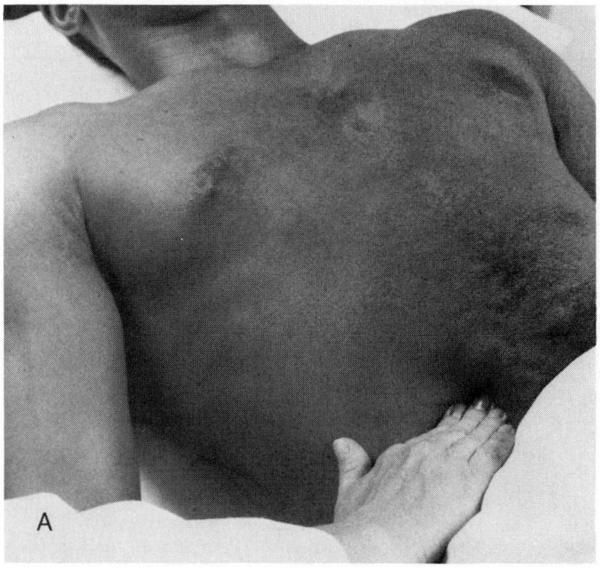

To overcome the resistance of a very large or obese abdomen, use a bimanual technique. Place your two hands on top of each other (Fig. 17 – 21b). The top hand does the pushing; the bottom hand is relaxed and can concentrate on the sense of palpation. With either technique, note the location, size, consistency, and mobility of any palpable organs and the presence of any abnormal enlargement, tenderness, or masses.

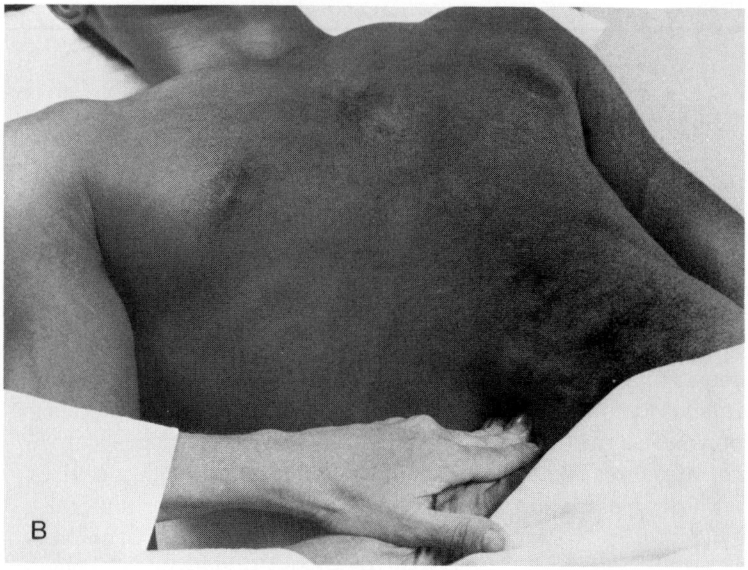

► **Figure 17 – 21**

NORMAL RANGE OF FINDINGS	ABNORMAL FINDINGS

Making sense of what you are feeling is more difficult than it looks. Inexperienced examiners complain that the abdomen "all feels the same," as if they are pushing their hand into a soft sofa cushion. It helps to memorize the anatomy and visualize what is under each quadrant as you palpate. Also remember that some structures are normally palpable, as illustrated in Figure 17–22.

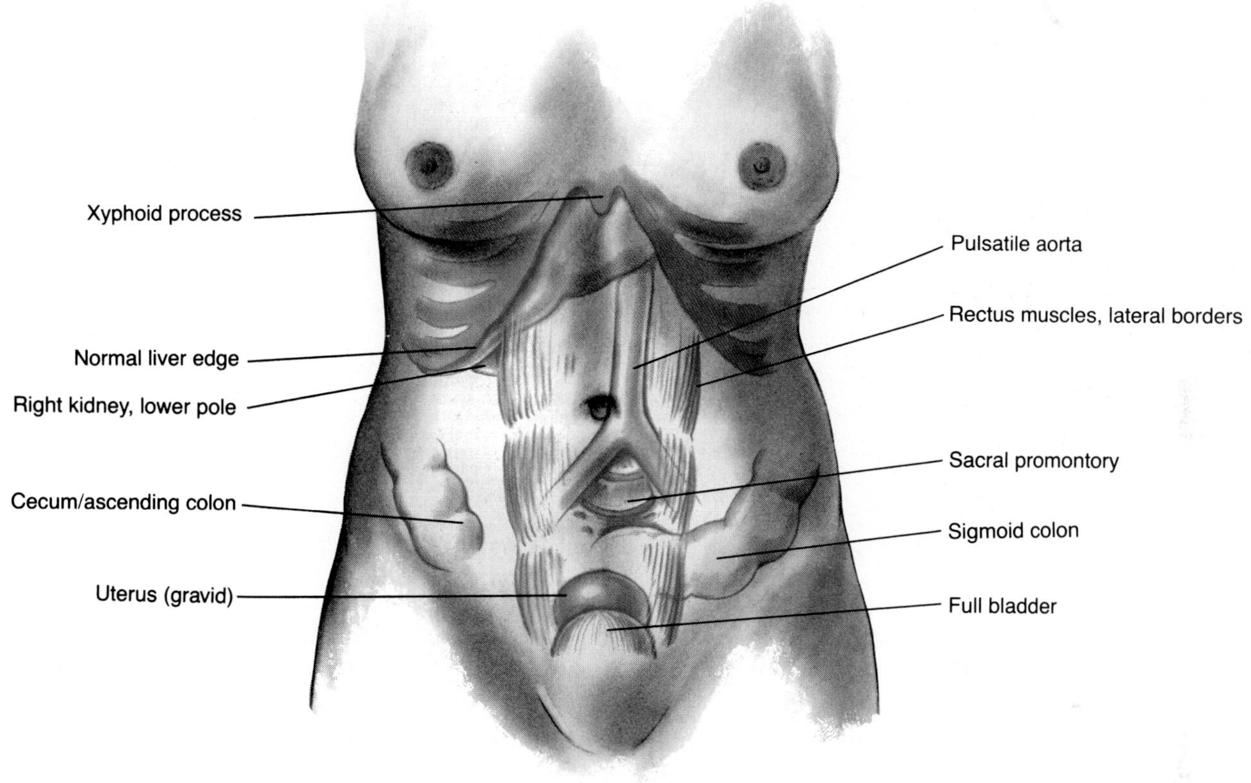

► **Figure 17–22**

There is normally mild tenderness when palpating the sigmoid colon. Any other tenderness should be investigated.

Abnormal findings: Tenderness occurs with local inflammation, inflammation of the peritoneum or underlying organ, and with an enlarged organ whose capsule is stretched.

If you identify a mass, first distinguish it from a normally palpable structure or an enlarged organ. Then note its:

1. Location
2. Size
3. Shape
4. Consistency (soft, firm, hard)
5. Surface (smooth, nodular)
6. Mobility (including movement with respirations)
7. Pulsatility
8. Tenderness

NORMAL RANGE OF FINDINGS

Liver. Next, palpate for specific organs beginning with the liver in the RUQ (Fig. 17–23). Place your left hand under the person's back parallel to the 11th and 12th ribs, and lift up to support the abdominal contents. Place your right hand on the RUQ, with fingers parallel to the midline. Push deeply down and under the right costal margin. Ask the person to take a deep breath. It is normal to feel the edge of the liver bump your fingertips as the diaphragm pushes it down during inhalation. It feels like a firm regular ridge. Often, the liver is not palpable and you feel nothing firm.

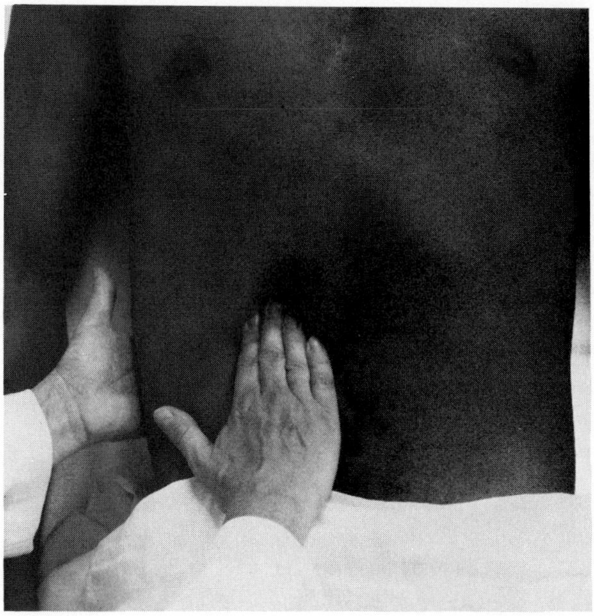

► **Figure 17–23**

Hooking Technique. An alternative method of palpating the liver is to stand up at the person's shoulder and swivel your body to the right so that you face the person's feet (Fig. 17–24). Hook your fingers over the costal margin from above. Ask the person to take a deep breath. Try to feel the liver edge bump your fingertips.

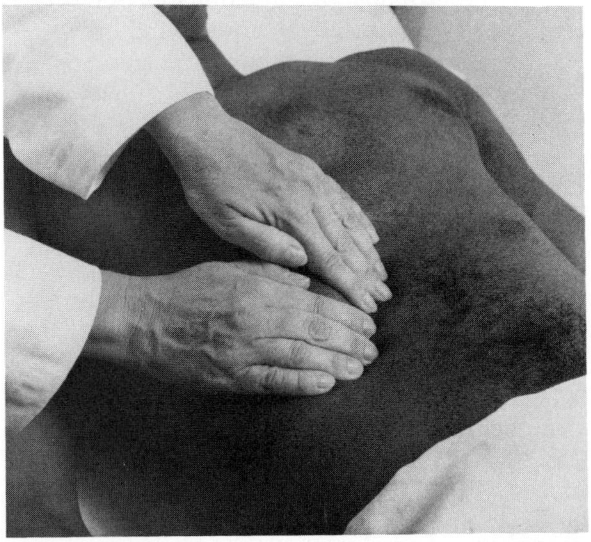

► **Figure 17–24**

ABNORMAL FINDINGS

Except with a depressed diaphragm, a liver palpated more than 1 to 2 cm below the right costal margin is enlarged. Record the number of centimeters it descends, and note its consistency (hard, nodular) and tenderness (see Table 17–7).

NORMAL RANGE OF FINDINGS	ABNORMAL FINDINGS

Spleen. Normally, the spleen is not palpable and must be enlarged three times its normal size to be felt. To search for it, reach your left hand over the abdomen and behind the left side at the 11th and 12th ribs (Fig. 17–25a). Lift up for support. Place your right hand obliquely on the LUQ with the fingers pointing toward the left axilla and just inferior to the rib margin. Push your hand deeply down and under the left costal margin and ask the person to take a deep breath. You should feel nothing firm.

The spleen enlarges with mononucleosis and trauma (see Table 17–7). If you feel an enlarged spleen, refer the person but do not continue to palpate it. An enlarged spleen is friable and can rupture easily with overpalpation.

Describe the number of cm it extends below the left costal margin.

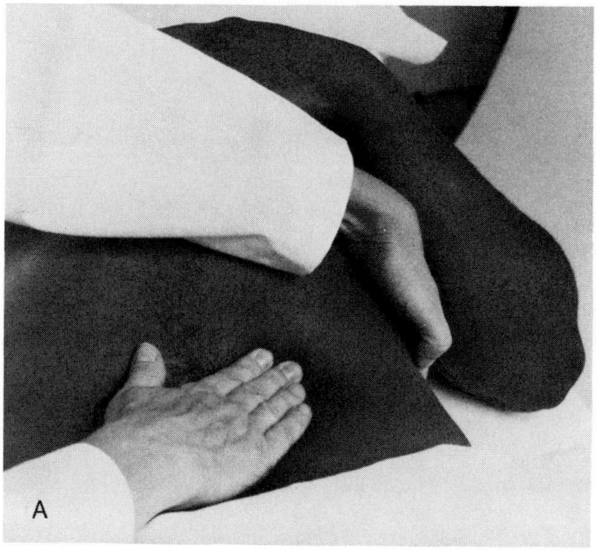

When enlarged, the spleen slides out and bumps your fingertips. It can grow so large that it extends into the lower quadrants. When this condition is suspected, start low so you will not miss it. An alternative position is to roll the person onto his or her right side to displace the spleen more forward and downward (Fig. 17–25b). Then palpate as described earlier.

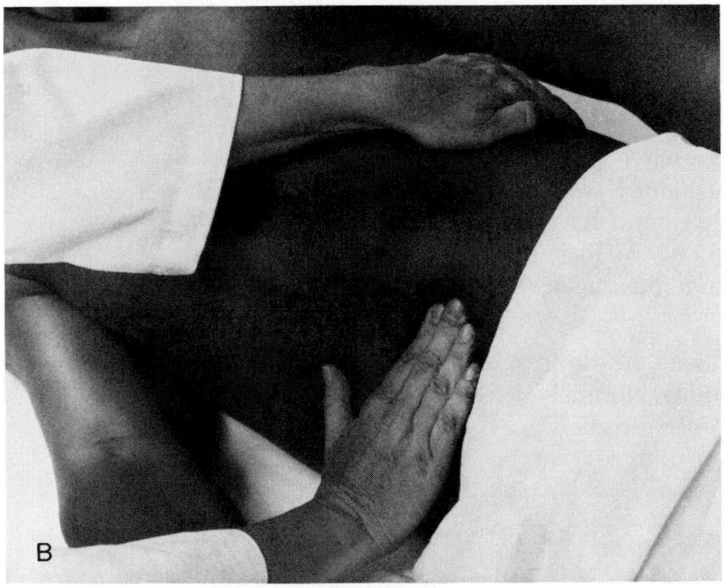

► **Figure 17–25**

NORMAL RANGE OF FINDINGS	ABNORMAL FINDINGS

Kidneys. Search for the right kidney by placing your hands together in a "duckbill" position at the person's right flank (Fig. 17–26a). Press your two hands together firmly (you need deeper palpation than that used with the liver or spleen) and ask the person to take a deep breath. In most people, you will feel no change. Occasionally, you may feel the lower pole of the right kidney as a round, smooth mass slide between your fingers. Either condition is normal.

Abnormal findings: Enlarged kidney. Kidney mass.

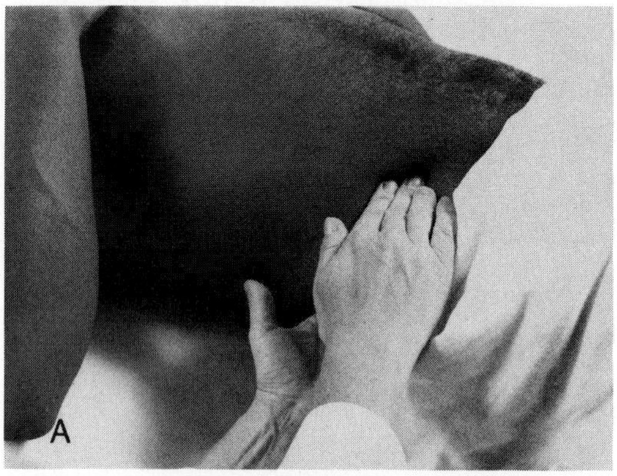

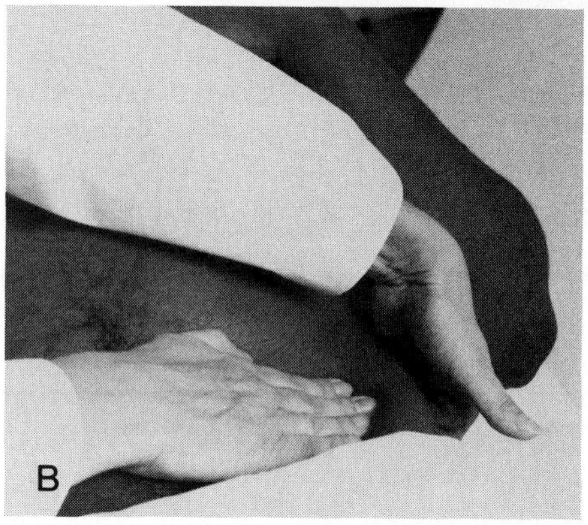

▶ **Figure 17–26**

The left kidney sits 1 cm higher than the right kidney and is not palpable normally. Search for it by reaching your left hand across the abdomen and behind the left flank for support (Fig. 17–26b). Push your right hand deep into the abdomen and ask the person to breathe deeply. You should feel no change with the inhalation.

Aorta. Using your opposing thumb and fingers, palpate the aortic pulsation in the upper abdomen slightly to the left of midline. Normally, it is 2.5 to 4 cm wide in the adult, and pulsates in an anterior direction.

Abnormal findings: Widened with aneurysm (see Tables 17–6 and 17–7). Prominent lateral pulsation with aortic aneurysm.

NORMAL RANGE OF FINDINGS

Special Procedures

Rebound Tenderness. Assess rebound tenderness when the person reports abdominal pain or when you elicit tenderness during palpation. Choose a site away from the painful area. Hold your hand 90 degrees or perpendicular to the abdomen. Push down slowly and deeply; then lift up *quickly* (Fig. 17–27a and b). This makes structures that are indented by palpation rebound suddenly. A normal, or negative, response is no pain on release of pressure. Perform this test at the end of the examination, because it can cause severe pain and muscle rigidity.

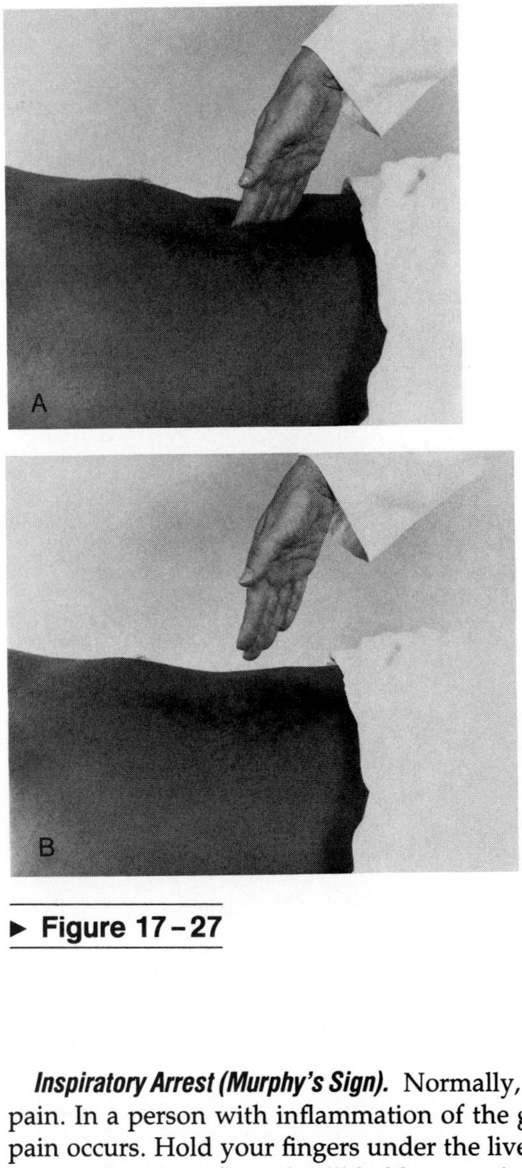

▶ **Figure 17–27**

Inspiratory Arrest (Murphy's Sign). Normally, palpating the liver causes no pain. In a person with inflammation of the gallbladder or choleycystitis, pain occurs. Hold your fingers under the liver border. As the descending liver pushes the inflamed gallbladder onto the examining hand, the person feels sharp pain and *abruptly* stops inspiration midway.

ABNORMAL FINDINGS

Pain on release of pressure confirms rebound tenderness, which is a reliable sign of peritoneal inflammation.

NORMAL RANGE OF FINDINGS	ABNORMAL FINDINGS

Iliopsoas Muscle Test. Perform the iliopsoas muscle test when the acute abdominal pain of appendicitis is suspected. With the person supine, lift the right leg straight up, flexing at the hip (Fig. 17–28); then push down over the lower part of the right thigh as the person tries to hold the leg up. When the test is negative, the person feels no change.

When the iliopsoas muscle is inflamed (which occurs with an inflamed or perforated appendix), pain is felt in the right lower quadrant.

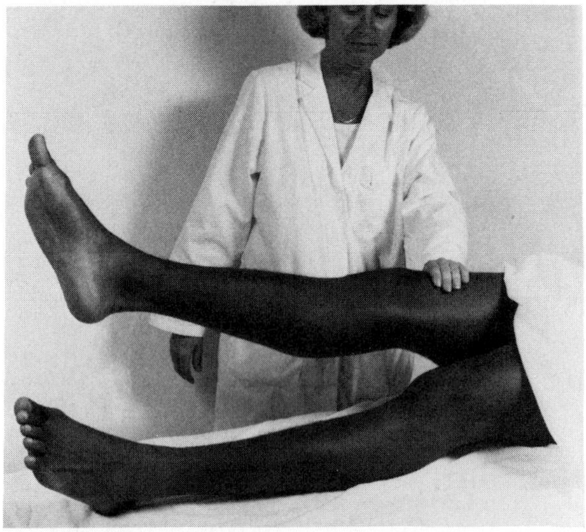

► **Figure 17–28**

Obturator Test. The obturator test also is performed when appendicitis is suspected. With the person supine, lift the right leg, flexing at the hip and 90 degrees at the knee (Fig. 17–29). Hold the ankle, and rotate the leg internally and externally. A negative or normal response is no pain.

A perforated appendix irritates the obturator muscle, producing pain.

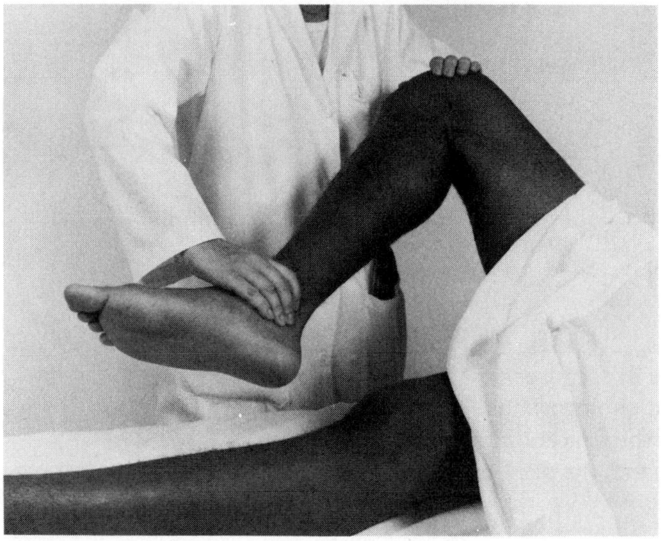

► **Figure 17–29**

NORMAL RANGE OF FINDINGS	ABNORMAL FINDINGS

DEVELOPMENTAL CONSIDERATIONS

The Infant

The contour of the abdomen is protuberant because of the immature abdominal musculature (Fig. 17–30). The skin contains a fine, superficial venous pattern. This may be visible in children up to the age of puberty.

Scaphoid shape.
Dilated veins.

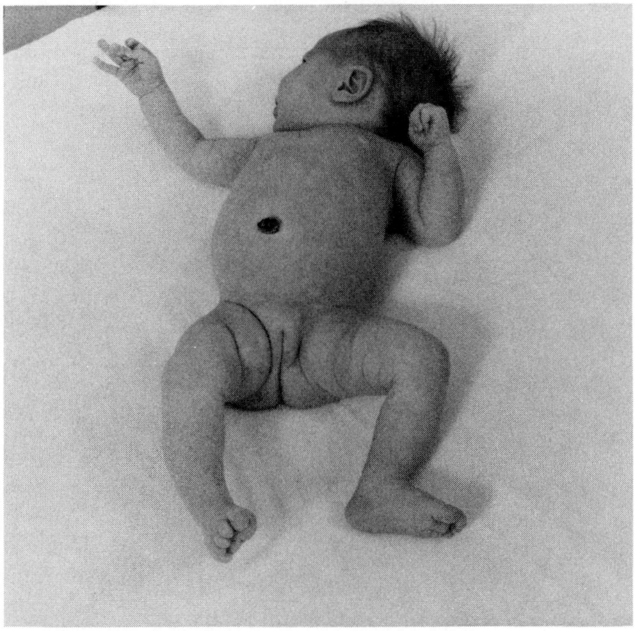

▶ **Figure 17–30**

Inspect the umbilical cord throughout the neonatal period. At birth, it is white and contains two umbilical arteries and one vein inside the Wharton's jelly. The umbilical stump dries within a week, hardens, and falls off by 10 to 14 days. Skin covers the area by 3 to 4 weeks.

The abdomen should be symmetric, although two bulges are common. You may note an *umbilical hernia*. It appears at 2 to 3 weeks and is especially prominent when the infant cries. The hernia reaches maximum size at 1 month (up to 2.5 cm or 1 inch), and usually disappears by 1 year. Another common variation is *diastasis recti*, a separation of the rectus muscles with a visible bulge along the midline. The condition is more common with black infants, and it usually disappears by early childhood.

The abdomen shows respiratory movement. The only other abdominal movement you should note is occasional peristalsis, which may be visible because of the thin musculature.

Auscultation yields only bowel sounds, the metallic tinkling of peristalsis. There should be no vascular sounds.

The presence of only one artery signals the risk of congenital defects.
Inflammation.
Drainage after cord falls off.
Refer any umbilical hernia: larger than 2.5 cm; that continues to grow after 1 month; lasting for more than 2 years in a white child, or for more than 7 years in a black child.

Refer diastasis recti lasting more than 6 years.
Marked peristalsis with pyloric stenosis (see Table 17–4).

Bruit
Venous hum

NORMAL RANGE OF FINDINGS

Percussion finds tympany over the stomach (the infant swallows some air with feeding) and dullness over the liver. Percussing the spleen is not done. The abdomen sounds tympanitic, though it is normal to percuss dullness over the bladder. This dullness may extend up to the umbilicus.

Aid palpation by flexing the baby's knees with one hand while palpating with the other (Fig. 17–31). Alternatively, you may hold the upper back and flex the neck slightly with one hand. Offer a pacifier to a crying baby.

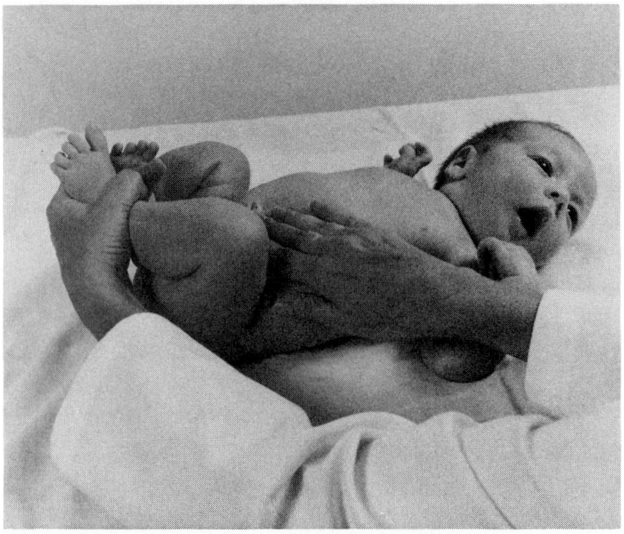

► **Figure 17–31**

The liver fills the RUQ. It is normal to feel the liver edge at the right costal margin or 1 to 2 cm below. Normally, you may palpate the spleen tip and both kidneys as well as the bladder. Also easily palpated are the cecum in the RLQ, and the sigmoid colon, which feels like a sausage in the left inguinal area.

Make note of the newborn's first stool, a sticky, greenish-black meconium stool within 24 hours of birth. By the fourth day, stools of breast-fed babies are golden-yellow, pasty, and smell like sour milk, whereas those of formula-fed babies are brown-yellow, firmer, and more fecal smelling.

The Child

Under age 4 years, the abdomen looks protuberant when the child is both supine and standing. After age 4 years, the potbelly remains when standing because of lumbar lordosis, but the abdomen looks flat when supine. Normal movement on the abdomen includes respirations, which remain abdominal until 7 years of age.

ABNORMAL FINDINGS

A scaphoid abdomen is associated with dehydration or malnutrition.

Under 7 years of age, the absence of abdominal respirations occurs with inflammation of the peritoneum.

NORMAL RANGE OF FINDINGS

ABNORMAL FINDINGS

To palpate the abdomen, position the young child on the parent's lap as you sit knee-to-knee with the parent (Fig. 17–32). Flex the knees up, and elevate the head slightly. The child can "pant like a dog" to further relax abdominal muscles. Hold your entire palm flat on the abdominal surface for a moment before starting palpation. This accustoms the child to being touched. If the child is very ticklish, hold his or her hand under your own as you palpate.

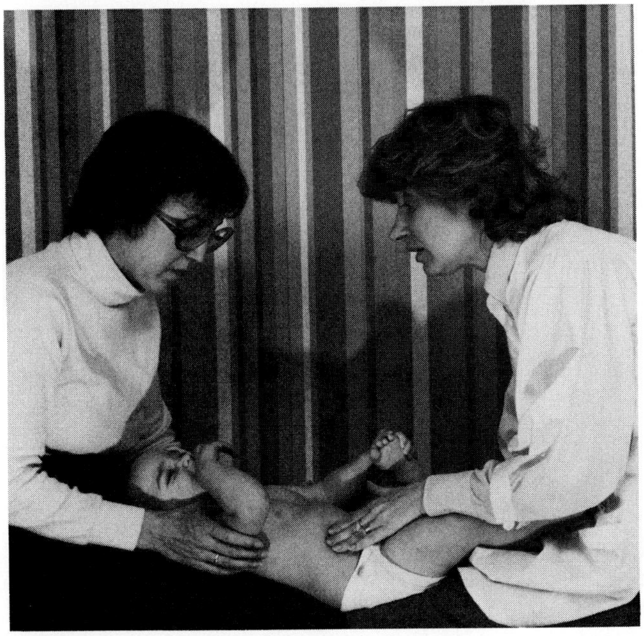

► **Figure 17–32**

The liver remains easily palpable 1 to 2 cm below the right costal margin. The edge is soft and sharp, and moves easily. On the left, the spleen also is easily palpable with a soft, sharp, movable edge. Usually you can feel 1 to 2 cm of the right kidney and the tip of the left kidney.

In assessing abdominal tenderness, remember that the young child often answers this question affirmatively no matter how the abdomen actually feels. Use objective signs to aid assessment, such as a cry changing in pitch as you palpate, facial grimacing, moving away from you, and guarding.

The school-aged child has a slim abdominal shape as she or he loses the potbelly. This slimming trend continues into adolescence. See Table 17–1 for age-related values of liver span by percussion.

The adolescent easily is embarrassed with exposure of the abdomen, and adequate draping is necessary. The physical findings are the same as those listed for the adult.

NORMAL RANGE OF FINDINGS | **ABNORMAL FINDINGS**

Table 17-1 ▶ Expected Liver Span by Percussion through Childhood and Adolescence

	MEAN ESTIMATED LIVER SPAN IN CM	
Age	**Males**	**Females**
6 mo	2.4	2.8
1	2.8	3.1
2	3.5	3.6
3	4.0	4.0
4	4.4	4.3
5	4.8	4.5
6	5.1	4.8
8	5.6	5.1
10	6.1	5.4
12	6.5	5.6
14	6.8	5.8
16	7.1	6.0
18	7.4	6.1
20	7.7	6.3

(Adapted from Lawson EE, Grand RJ, Neff RK, Cohen LF: Clinical estimation of liver span in infants and children. Am J Dis Child 132:474–476, 1978. Copyright 1978, American Medical Association.)

The Aging Adult

On inspection, you may note increased deposits of subcutaneous fat on the abdomen and hips as it is redistributed away from the extremities. The abdominal musculature is thinner and has less tone than that of the younger adult, so in the absence of obesity you may note peristalsis.

Owing to the thinner, softer abdominal wall, the organs may be easier to palpate (in the absence of obesity). The liver is easier to palpate. Normally, you will feel the liver edge at or just below the costal margin. With distended lungs and a depressed diaphragm, the liver is palpated lower, descending 1 to 2 cm below the costal margin with inhalation. The kidneys are easier to palpate.

Abdominal rigidity with acute abdominal conditions is less common in aging persons.

With an acute abdomen, the aging person often complains of less pain than a younger person would.

☑ SUMMARY CHECKLIST

1 ▶ Inspection
- Contour
- Symmetry
- Umbilicus
- Skin
- Pulsation or movement
- Hair distribution
- Demeanor

2 ▶ Auscultation
- Bowel sounds
- Note any vascular sounds

3 ▶ Percussion
- Percuss all four quadrants
- Percuss borders of liver, spleen

4 ▶ Palpation
- Light palpation in all four quadrants
- Deeper palpation in all four quadrants
- Palpate for liver, spleen, kidneys

SAMPLE RECORDING

Subjective

- States appetite good with no recent change, no dysphagia, no food intolerance, no pain, no nausea/vomiting. Has 1 formed BM/day. Takes vitamins, no other prescribed or over-the-counter medication. No history of abdominal disease, injury or surgery. Diet recall of last 24 hours listed at end of history.

Objective

- Insp. Abdomen flat, symmetric with no apparent masses. Skin smooth with no striae, scars, or lesions.
  Aus. Bowel sounds present, no bruits.
  Perc. Tympany in all 4 quadrants, liver span 8 cm in right midclavicular line, splenic dullness at 10th intercostal space in left midaxillary line.
  Palp. Abdomen soft, no organomegaly, no masses, no tenderness.

SAMPLE CLINICAL PROBLEM 1

George E. is a 58-year-old unemployed, divorced, white male with chronic alcoholism, who enters the Chemical Dependency Treatment Center.

Subjective

- States last 6 months has been drinking 1 pint whiskey/day. Last alcohol use 1 week PTA, with "5 or 6" drinks that episode. Estranged from family, lives alone, has hot plate, makes few meals. States never has appetite, also has fatigue and weakness.

Objective

- Insp. Appears older than stated age. Oriented, although verbal response time slowed. Weight loss of 12 lb in last 3 mo.
  Abdomen protuberant, symmetric, no visible masses. Poor skin turgor. Dilated venous pattern over abdominal wall. Hair sparse in axillary, pubic area.
  Aus. Bowel sounds present. No vascular sounds.
  Perc. Tympany over abdomen. Liver span 16 cm in right midclavicular line. No fluid wave. No shifting dullness.
  Palp. Soft. Liver palpable 10 cm below right costal margin, smooth and nontender. No other organomegaly or masses.

Assessment

- Alcohol dependence, severe
  Altered nutrition: less than body requirements R/T impaired absorption
  Ineffective individual coping R/T effects of chronic alcoholism

SAMPLE CLINICAL PROBLEM 2

Edith J. is a 63-year-old retired homemaker with a history of lung cancer with metastases to the liver.

Subjective

▶ Feeling "puffy and bloated" for the past week. States unable to get comfortable. Also short of breath "all the time now."

Objective

▶ Insp. Weight increase of 8 lb in one week. Abdomen distended with everted umbilicus and bulging flanks. Girth at umbilicus 85 cm. Prominent dilated venous pattern over abdomen.
Aus. Bowel sounds present, no vascular sounds.
Perc. When supine, tympany at dome of abdomen, dullness over flanks. Shifting dullness present. Positive fluid wave. Liver span 12 cm in right midclavicular line.
Palp. Abdominal wall firm, able to feel liver with deep palpation at 6 cm below right costal margin. Liver feels firm, nodular, nontender. 4+ pitting edema in ankles.

Assessment

▶ Ascites
Ineffective breathing pattern R/T increased intra-abdominal pressure
Pain R/T distended abdomen
Impaired skin integrity: potential R/T ascites, edema, and faulty metabolism

SAMPLE CLINICAL PROBLEM 3

Dan G. is a 17-year-old black male high school student who enters the emergency department with abdominal pain for 2 days.

Subjective

▶ 2 days PTA noted general abdominal pain in umbilical region. Now pain is sharp and Dan points to location in right lower quadrant. No BM for 2 days. Nausea and vomiting off and on 1 day.

Objective

▶ Insp. BP 112/70 Temp 38° C, pulse 116, resp 18.
Lying on side with knees drawn up under chin. Resists any movement. Face tight and occasionally grimacing. Cries out with any sudden movement.
Ausc. No bowel sounds present. No vascular sounds.
Perc. Tympany. Percussion over RLQ leads to tenderness.
Palp. Abdominal wall rigid. Tender to palpation in RLQ.
Rebound tenderness present to RLQ. Positive iliopsoas muscle test.

Assessment

▶ Acute abdominal pain in RLQ

NURSING DIAGNOSES COMMONLY ASSOCIATED WITH ABDOMINAL DISORDERS

Diagnosis	Related Factors (Etiology)	Defining Characteristics (Symptoms and Signs)
Constipation	Less than adequate dietary intake and bulk Neuromuscular or musculoskeletal impairment Pain/discomfort on defecation Effects of Diagnostic procedures Pregnancy Aging Medication Stress or anxiety Weak abdominal musculature Immobility or less-than-adequate physical activity Chronic use of laxatives and enemas Gastrointestinal lesions Ignoring urge to defecate Fear of rectal or cardiac pain	Frequency less than usual pattern Hard, formed stools Palpable mass Straining at stool Less than usual amount of stool Decreased bowel sounds Gas pain and flatulence Abdominal or back pain Reported feeling of abdominal or rectal fullness or pressure Impaired appetite Headache Nausea Irritability Palpable hard stool on rectal examination
Diarrhea	Effects of medications Radiation Surgical intervention Infectious process Inflammatory process Malabsorption syndrome Stress and anxiety Dietary alterations Food intolerances Increased caffeine consumption Excessive use of laxatives Allergies Nutritional disorders Ingestion of contaminated water or food Hyperosmolar tube feeding	Abdominal pain Anorexia Change in color or odor of stool Chills Cramping Fatigue Increased frequency of bowel sounds Loose, liquid stools Increased frequency of stool Irritated anal area Fever Malaise Muscle weakness Thirst Urgency Weight loss

Table continued on following page

Diagnosis	Related Factors (Etiology)	Defining Characteristics (Symptoms and Signs)
Urinary retention	Diminished or absent sensory and/or motor impulses Effects of some medications Anesthetics Opiates Psychotropics Strong sphincter Urethral blockage associated with fecal impaction, postpartum edema, prostate hypertrophy, or surgical swelling Anxiety (fear of postoperative pain)	Bladder distention Diminished force of urinary stream Dribbling Dysuria Hesitancy High residual urine Nocturia Sensation of bladder fullness Small, frequent voiding or absence of urine output
Alteration in tissue perfusion: renal and gastrointestinal	Exchange problems Hypervolemia Hypovolemia Interruption of flow	Renal Diminished urine output Edema Gastrointestinal Constipation Nausea and vomiting Pain

Other related nursing diagnoses:

- Pain (see Chapter 13)
- Perceived constipation
- Colonic constipation

ABNORMAL FINDINGS

Table 17–2 ► Common Sites of Referred Abdominal Pain

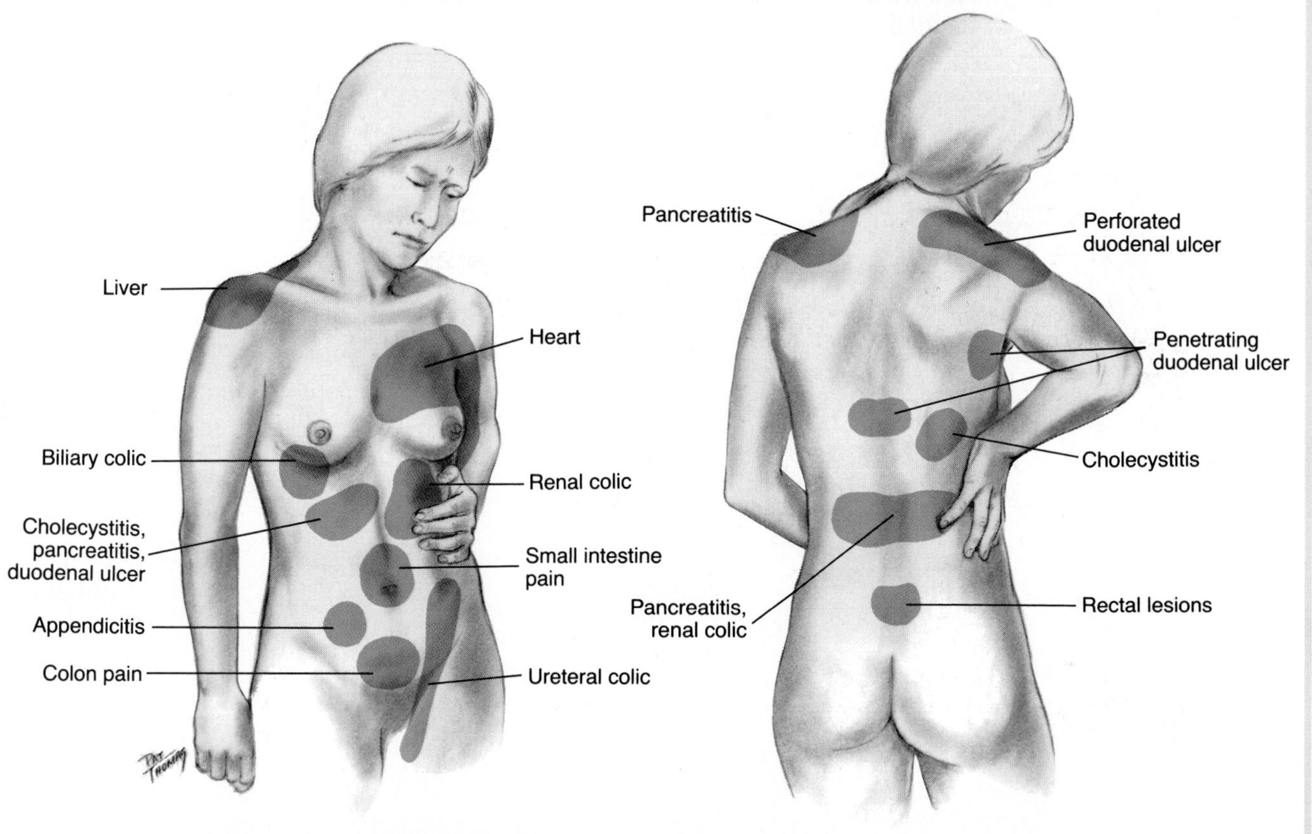

When a person gives a history of abdominal pain, the pain's location may not necessarily be directly over the involved organ. That is because the human brain has no felt image for internal organs. Rather, pain is referred to a site where the organ was located in fetal development. Although the organ migrates during fetal development, its nerves persist in referring sensations from the former location.

Table 17–3 ▶ Abdominal Distention*

	INSPECTION	AUSCULTATION	PERCUSSION	PALPATION
OBESITY	Uniformly rounded. Umbilicus sunken (it adheres to peritoneum, and layers of fat are superficial to it).	Normal	Tympany. Scattered dullness over adipose tissue.	Normal. May be hard to feel through thick abdominal wall.
AIR OR GAS	Single round curve.	Depends on cause of gas, e.g., decreased or absent with ileus; hyperactive with early intestinal obstruction.	Tympany over large area.	May have muscle spasm of abdominal wall.

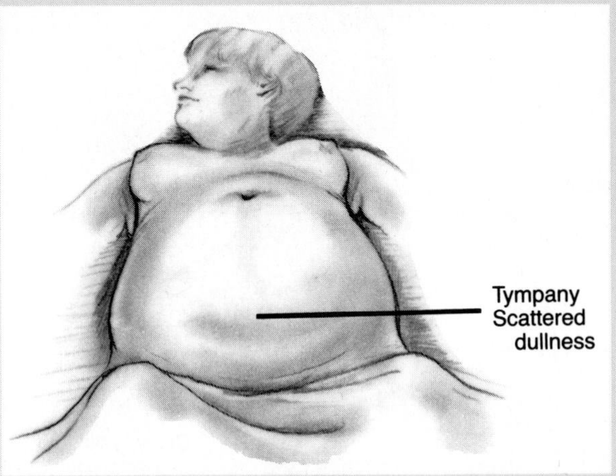

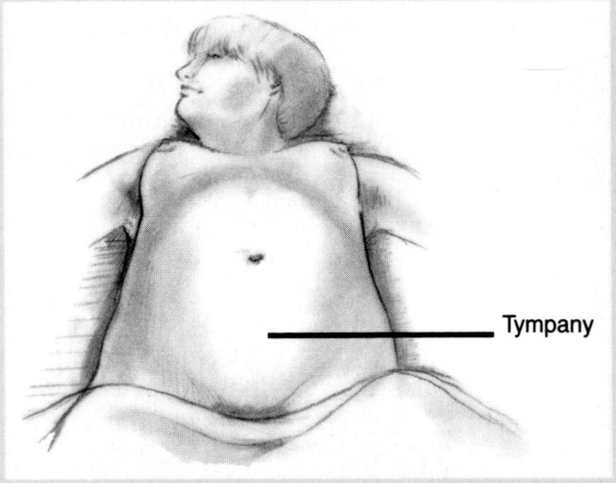

* A mnemonic device to recall the common causes of abdominal distention is the 7 Fs: Fat, flatus, fluid, fetus, feces, fatal growth, and fibroid.

Table 17–3 ▸ Abdominal Distention *Continued*

	INSPECTION	AUSCULTATION	PERCUSSION	PALPATION
ASCITES	Single curve. Everted umbilicus. Bulging flanks when supine. Taut, glistening skin.	Normal over intestines. Diminished over ascitic fluid.	Tympany at top where intestines float. Dull over fluid. Produces fluid wave and shifting dullness.	Taut skin and increased intra-abdominal pressure limit palpation.

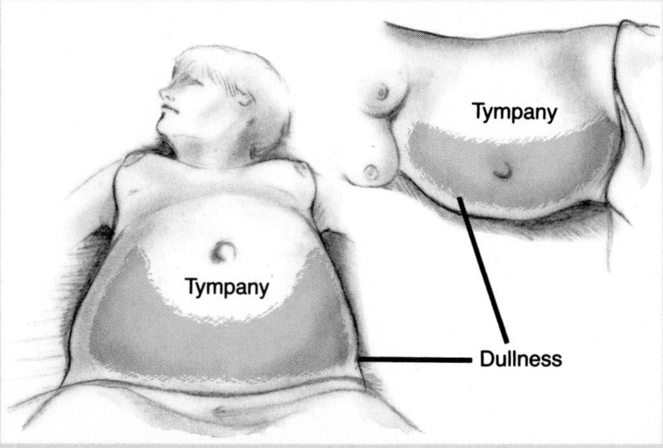

	INSPECTION	AUSCULTATION	PERCUSSION	PALPATION
OVARIAN CYST (LARGE)	Curve in lower half of abdomen, midline. Everted umbilicus.	Normal over upper abdomen where intestines pushed superiorly.	Top dull over fluid. Intestines pushed superiorly. Large cyst produces fluid wave and shifting dullness.	Transmits aortic pulsation while ascites does not.

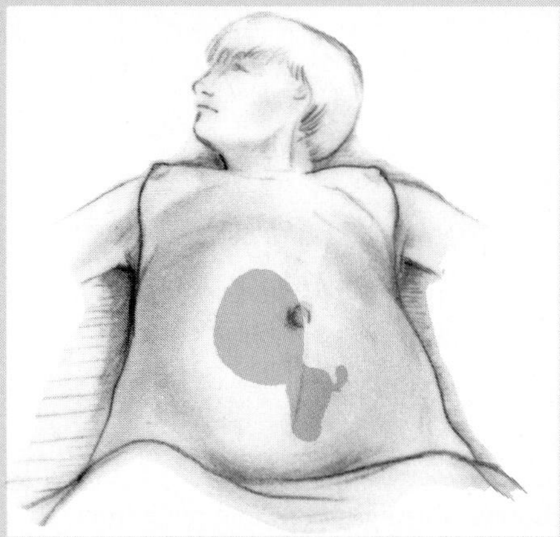

Table continued on following page

Table 17-3 ▶ Abdominal Distention *Continued*

	INSPECTION	AUSCULTATION	PERCUSSION	PALPATION
PREGNANCY†	Single curve. Umbilicus protruding. Breasts engorged.	Fetal heart tones. Bowel sounds diminished.	Tympany over intestines. Dull over enlarging uterus.	Fetal parts. Fetal movements.

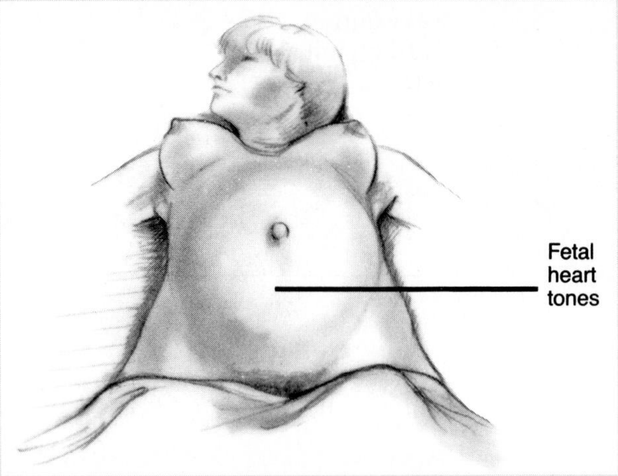

	INSPECTION	AUSCULTATION	PERCUSSION	PALPATION
FECES	Localized distention.	Normal.	Tympany predominates. Scattered dullness over fecal mass.	Plastic- or ropelike mass with feces in intestines.

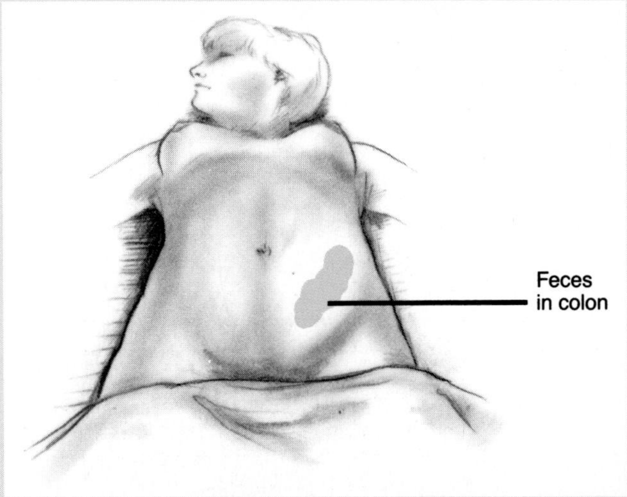

† Obviously a normal finding, pregnancy is included for comparison of conditions causing abdominal distention.

Table 17-3 ▸ Abdominal Distention *Continued*

	INSPECTION	AUSCULTATION	PERCUSSION	PALPATION
TUMOR	Localized distention.	Normal.	Dull over mass if reaches up to skin surface.	Define borders. Distinguish from enlarged organ or normally palpable structure.

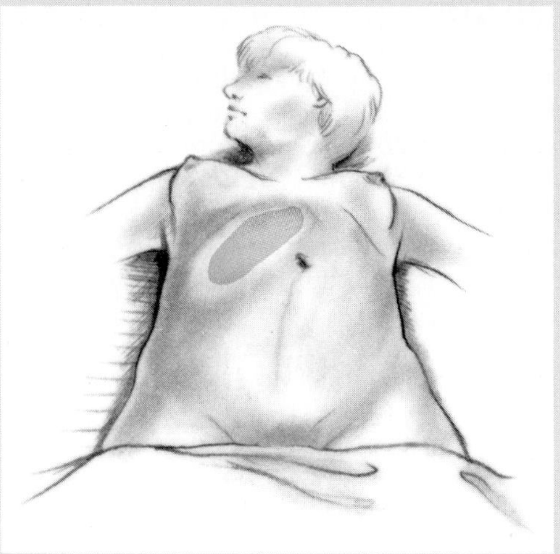

Table 17-4 ▸ Abnormalities on Inspection

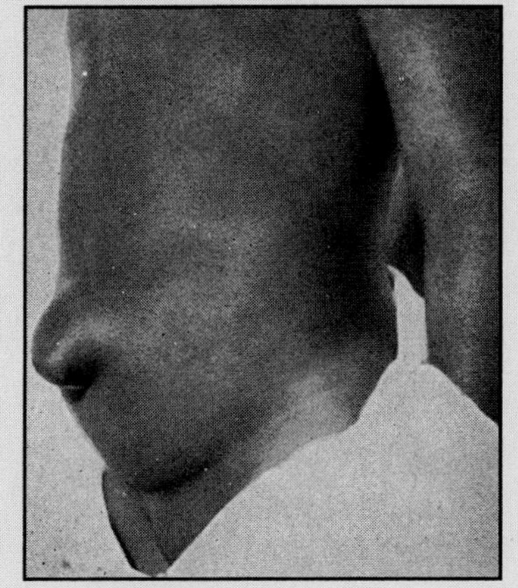

UMBILICAL HERNIA

Umbilical hernia, or a protrusion of part of the intestine at the navel, may show with relaxation or when person performs a sit-up. In a child, it is congenital, at umbilicus, with a central location in linea alba, and one can palpate a complete fibrous ring. In an adult, it is above an incomplete umbilical ring, covered only by skin and feels soft. Occurs with pregnancy, chronic ascites, or from chronic intrathoracic pressure (e.g., asthma, chronic bronchitis.)

Table continued on following page

Table 17-4 ► Abnormalities on Inspection *Continued*

EPIGASTRIC HERNIA

A small, fatty nodule at epigastrium in midline, through the linea alba. Usually one can feel it rather than observe it. May be palpable only when standing.

MARKED PERISTALSIS

Together with projectile vomiting in the newborn, this condition suggests pyloric stenosis, an obstruction of the stomach's pyloric valve. Pyloric stenosis is a congenital defect and appears in the second or third week. After feeding, pronounced peristaltic waves cross from left to right, leading to projectile vomiting. Then one can palpate an olive-sized mass in RUQ midway between the right costal margin and umbilicus. Refer promptly because of the risk of weight loss.

INCISIONAL HERNIA

A bulge near an old operative scar that may not show when person is supine, but is apparent when the person increases intra-abdominal pressure by a sit-up, stand, or a Valsalva maneuver.

DIASTASIS RECTI

Diastasis recti, or a midline longitudinal ridge, is a separation of the abdominal rectus muscles. Ridge is revealed when intra-abdominal pressure is increased by raising head while supine. Occurs congenitally and as a result of pregnancy or marked obesity in which prolonged distention or a decrease in muscle tone has occurred. It is not clinically significant.

Table 17-5 ► Abnormal Bowel Sounds

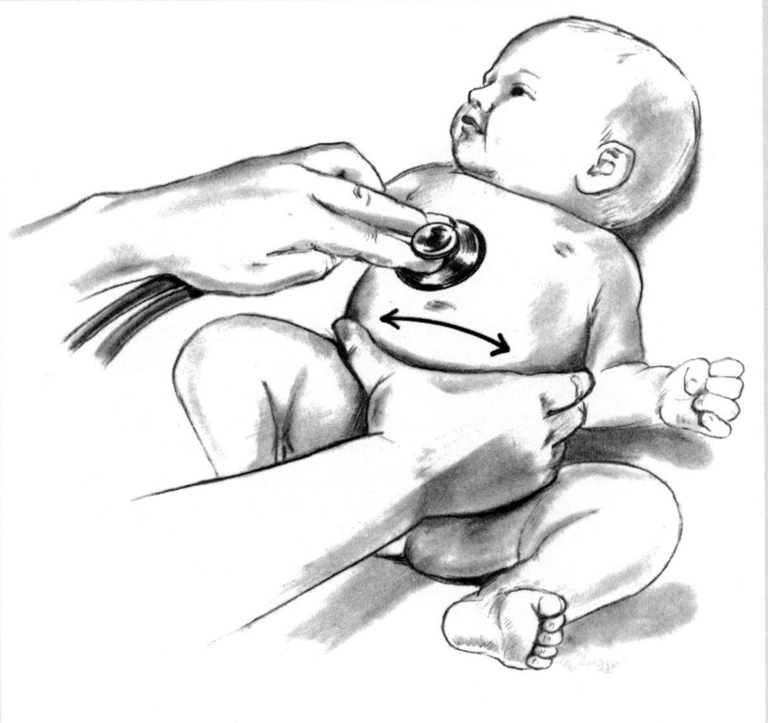

SUCCUSSION SPLASH

Unrelated to peristalsis, this is a very loud splash auscultated over the upper abdomen when the infant is rocked side to side. It indicates increased air and fluid in the stomach as seen with pyloric obstruction or large hiatus hernia.

Table 17-5 ▸ Abnormal Bowel Sounds *Continued*

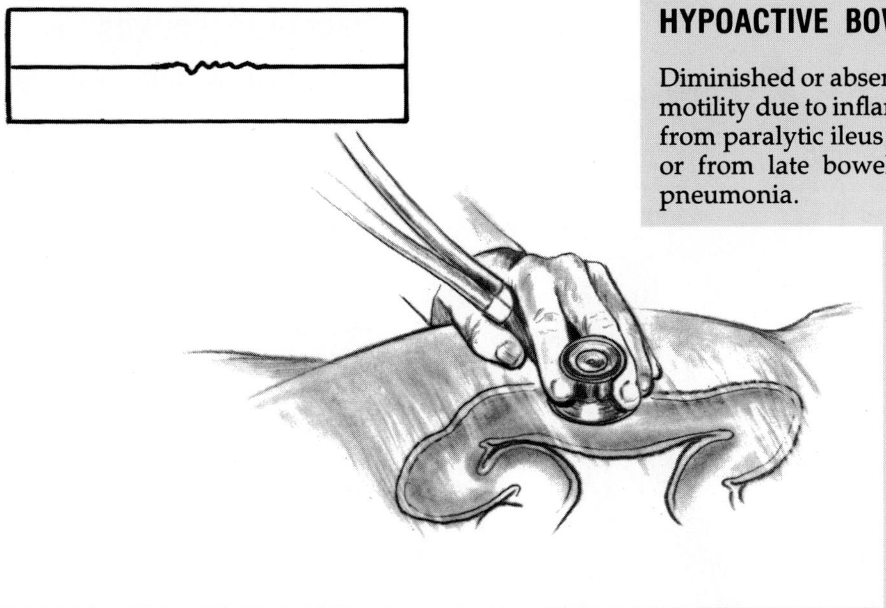

HYPOACTIVE BOWEL SOUNDS

Diminished or absent bowel sounds signal decreased motility due to inflammation as seen with peritonitis, from paralytic ileus as following abdominal surgery, or from late bowel obstruction. Occurs also with pneumonia.

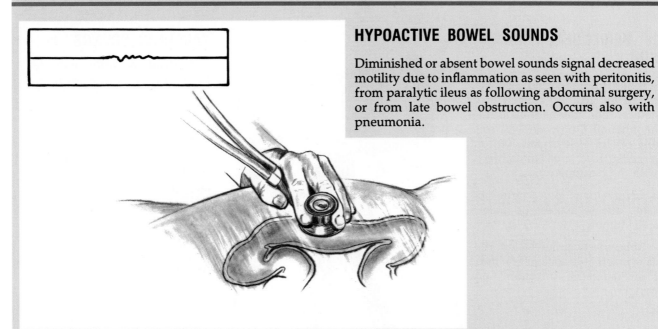

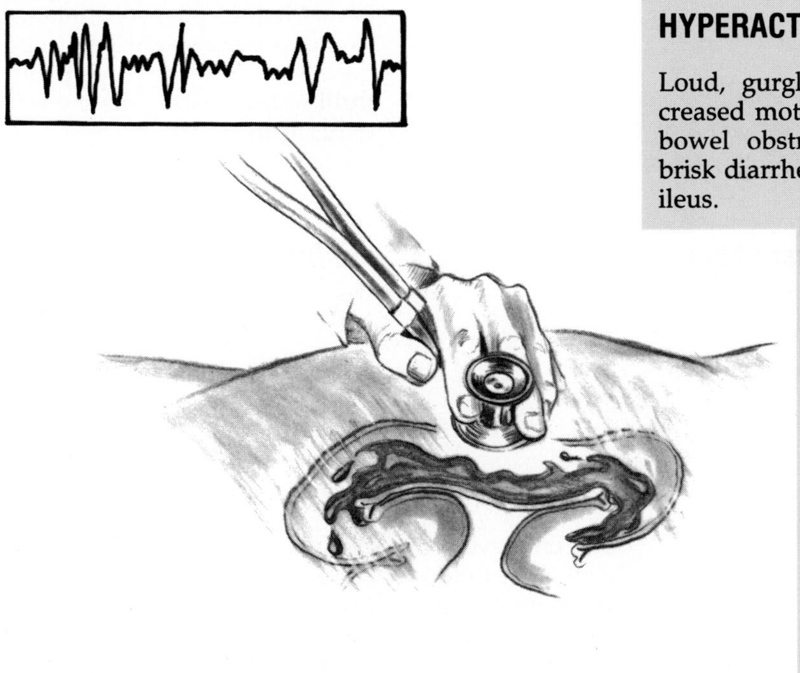

HYPERACTIVE BOWEL SOUNDS

Loud, gurgling sounds, "borborygmi," signal increased motility. They occur with early mechanical bowel obstruction (high pitched), gastroenteritis, brisk diarrhea, laxative use, and subsiding paralytic ileus.

Table 17-6 ► Abdominal Friction Rubs and Vascular Sounds

▷ PERITONEAL FRICTION RUB

A rough, grating sound, like two pieces of leather rubbed together, indicates peritoneal inflammation. Occurs rarely. Usually occurs over organs with a large surface area in contact with the peritoneum:

Liver—over lower right rib cage, due to abscess or metastatic tumor.

Spleen—over lower left rib cage in left anterior axillary line, from abscess, infection, or tumor.

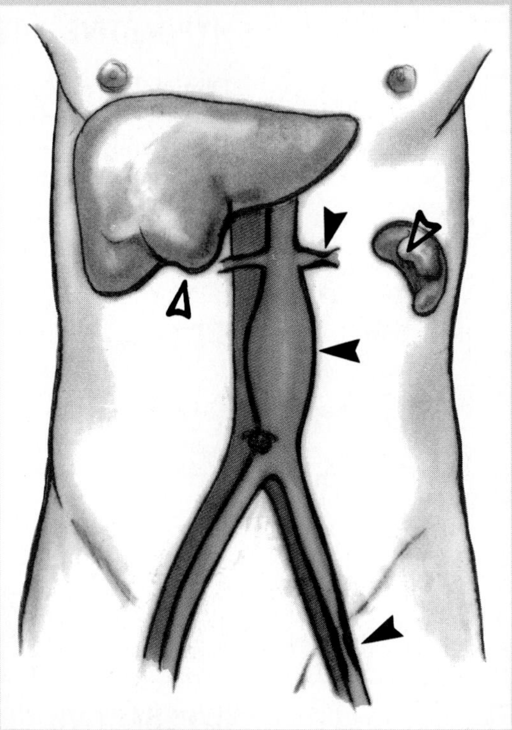

VASCULAR SOUNDS ►

Arterial. A bruit indicates turbulent blood flow, as found in constricted, abnormally dilated, or tortuous vessels. Use bell. Occurs with the following conditions.

Aortic Aneurysm. Murmur harsh, systolic, or continuous and accentuated with systole. Note in person with hypertension.

Renal Artery Stenosis. Murmur midline or toward flank, soft, low-to-medium pitch.

Partial Occlusion of Femoral Arteries.

Venous Hum. Occurs rarely. Heard in periumbilical region. Originates from inferior vena cava. Medium pitch, continuous sound, pressure on bell may obliterate it. May have palpable thrill. Occurs with portal hypertension and cirrhotic liver.

Table 17-7 ► Abnormalities on Palpation of Enlarged Organs

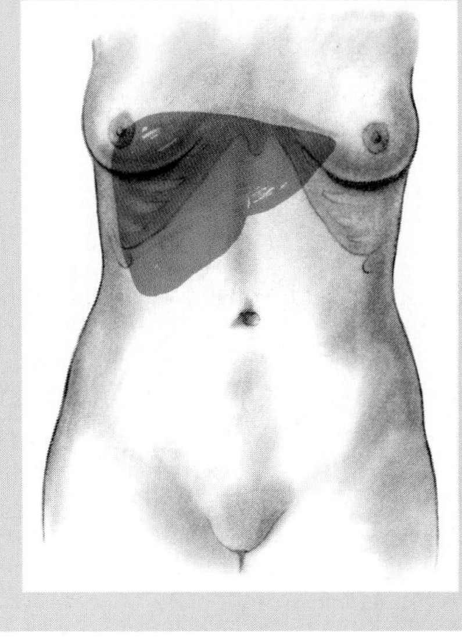

ENLARGED LIVER

An enlarged, smooth, and nontender liver occurs with fatty infiltration, portal obstruction or cirrhosis, high obstruction of inferior vena cava, and lymphocytic leukemia.

The liver feels the same but is tender to palpation with early congestive heart failure, acute hepatitis, or hepatic abscess.

Table 17-7 ► Abnormalities on Palpation of Enlarged Organs *Continued*

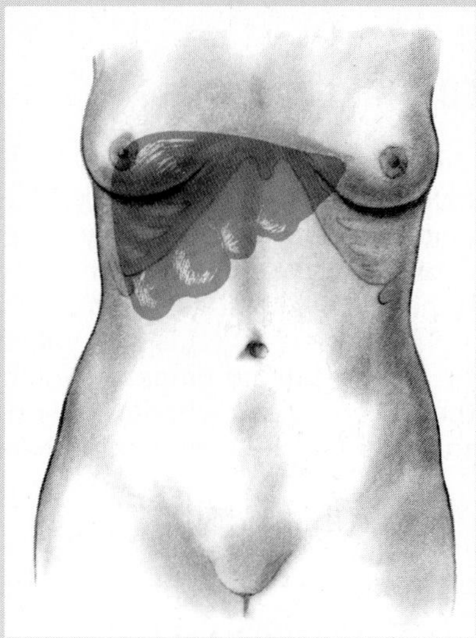

ENLARGED NODULAR LIVER

An enlarged and nodular liver occurs with late portal cirrhosis, metastatic cancer, or tertiary syphilis.

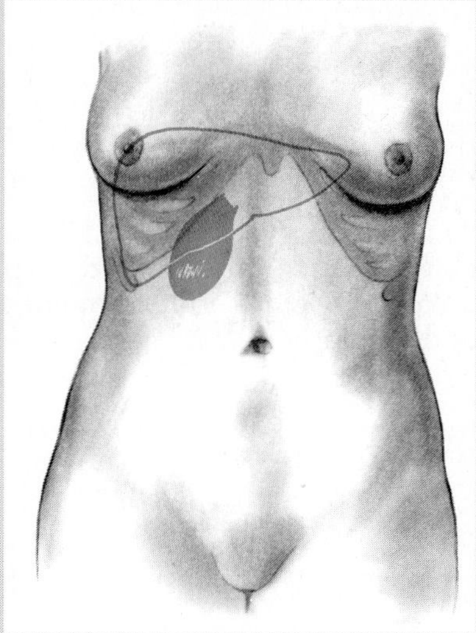

ENLARGED GALLBLADDER

An enlarged, tender gallbladder suggests acute cholecystitis. Feel it behind the liver border as a smooth and firm mass like a sausage, although it may be difficult to palpate due to involuntary rigidity of abdominal muscles. The area is exquisitely painful to fist percussion, and inspiratory arrest (Murphy's sign) is present.

An enlarged, nontender gallbladder also feels like a smooth sausage-like mass. It occurs when the gallbladder is filled with stones, as with common bile duct obstruction.

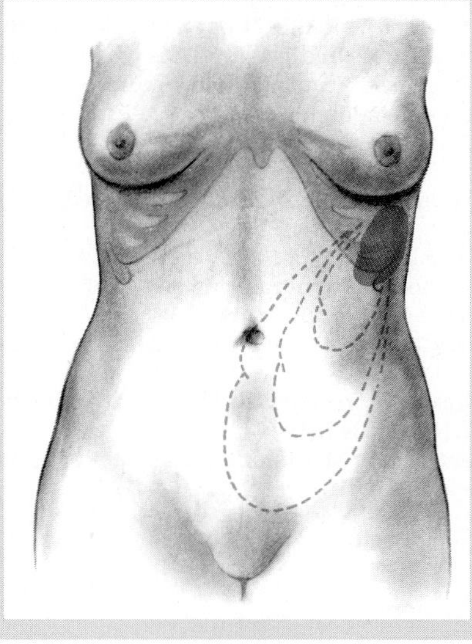

ENLARGED SPLEEN

Since any enlargement superiorly is stopped by the diaphragm, the spleen enlarges down and to the midline. When extreme, it can extend down to the left pelvis. It retains the splenic notch on the medial edge. When splenomegaly occurs with acute infections (mononucleosis), it is moderately enlarged and soft, with rounded edges. When due to a chronic cause, the enlargement is firm or hard, with sharp edges. An enlarged spleen is usually not tender to palpation; it is tender only if the peritoneum is also inflamed.

Table continued on following page

Table 17-7 ► Abnormalities on Palpation of Enlarged Organs *Continued*

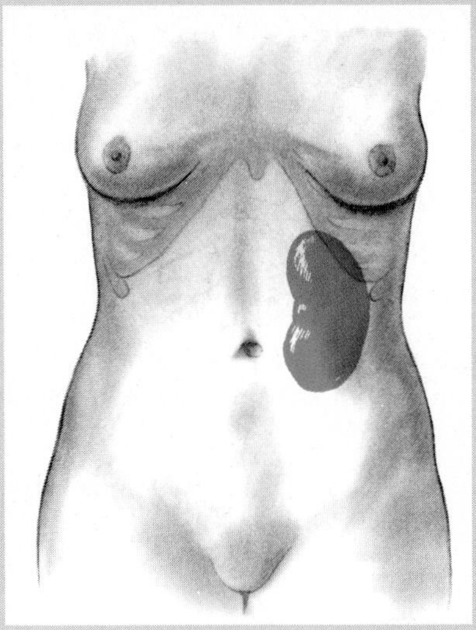

ENLARGED KIDNEY

Enlarged with hydronephrosis, cyst, or neoplasm. May be difficult to distinguish an enlarged left kidney from an enlarged spleen because they have a similar shape. Both extend forward and down. However, the spleen may have a sharp edge, whereas the kidney never does. The spleen retains the splenic notch, whereas the kidney has no palpable notch. Percussion over the spleen is dull, whereas over the kidney it is tympanitic due to the overriding bowel.

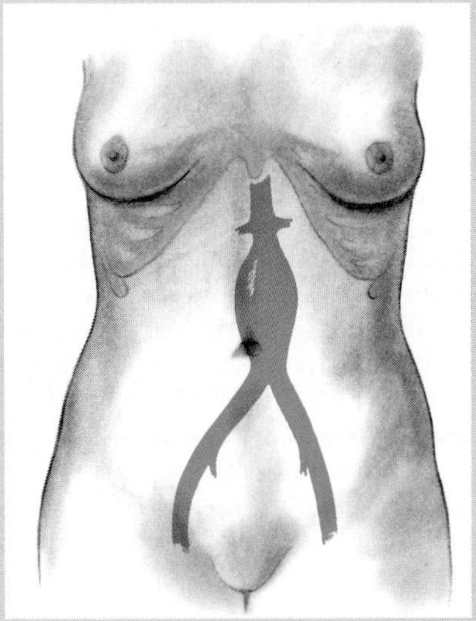

AORTIC ANEURYSM

Most aortic aneurysms (more than 95 percent) are located below the renal arteries and extend to the umbilicus. You will hear a bruit. Femoral pulses are present but decreased.

Bibliography

Buschiazzo L, Naab GA: Careful assessment of abdominal pain. J Emerg Nurs 12(2):72–75, 1986.

Castell DO: The spleen percussion sign. Ann Intern Med 67:1265–1267, 1967.

Castell DO, O'Brien KD, Muench H, Chalmers TC: Estimation of liver size by percussion in normal individuals. Ann Intern Med 70:1183–1189, 1969.

Castell DO, Frank B: Abdominal examination—role of percussion and auscultation. Postgrad Med 62:131–134, 1977.

Cope Z: The Early Diagnosis of the Acute Abdomen. London, Oxford University Press, 1979.

Fredette SL: When the liver fails. Am J Nurs 84:64–67, 1984.

GI Series: Physical Examination of the Abdomen. Richmond, VA, AH Robbins, 1974.

Julius S, Stewart BH: Diagnostic significance of abdominal murmurs. N Engl J Med 276:1175–1178, 1967.

Lawson EE, Grand RJ, Neff RK, Cohen LF: Clinical estimation of liver span in infants and children. Am J Dis Child 132:474–476, 1978.

Munn NE: Diagnosis: Acute abdomen. Nursing 18(9):34–41, 1988.

Nolan J: Infectious mononucleosis. Nurse Pract 4:12–14, 1979.

Plehn KW: Anorexia nervosa and bulimia: Incidence and diagnosis. Nurs Pract 15(4):22–31, 1990.

Rossman I: Clinical Geriatrics. 3rd ed. Philadelphia, J.B. Lippincott, 1986.

Skrainka B, Stahlhut J, Fulbeck CL, et al: Measuring liver span: Bedside examination versus ultrasound and scintiscan. J Clin Gastroenterol 8(3):267–270, 1986.

Steinberg FU: Care of the Geriatric Patient. St. Louis: C.V. Mosby, 1983.

Sullivan S, Krasner N, Williams R: The clinical estimation of liver size. Br Med J 2:1042–1043, 1976.

Walzer A, Koenigsberg M: Examining the anterior right kidney. JAMA 242:2320–2321, 1979.

CHAPTER

18 Peripheral Vascular System and Lymphatics

STRUCTURE AND FUNCTION

The vascular system consists of the vessels of the body. Vessels are tubes for transporting fluid, such as the blood or lymph.

ARTERIES

The heart pumps blood through the arteries to all body tissues. The pumping heart makes this a high-pressure system. The artery walls are strong, tough, and tense to withstand pressure demands. Each heartbeat creates a pressure wave, which makes the arteries expand and recoil. All arteries have this pressure wave, or *pulse,* throughout their length, but you can feel it only at body sites where the artery lies close to the skin and over a bone. The following arteries are accessible to examination.

Temporal Artery. Examination of the temporal artery is discussed in Chapter 10.

Carotid Artery. Examination of the carotid artery is covered in Chapter 16.

Aorta. Examination of the aorta is in Chapter 17.

Arteries in the Arm. The major artery supplying the arm is the *brachial* artery, which runs in the biceps-triceps furrow of the upper arm and surfaces at the antecubital fossa in the elbow medial to the biceps tendon (Fig. 18–1). Immediately below the elbow, the brachial artery bifurcates into the *ulnar* and *radial* arteries. These run distally and form two arches supplying the hand, called the superficial and deep palmar arches. The radial pulse lies just medial to the radius at the wrist; the ulnar artery is in the same relation to the ulna, but it is deeper and often difficult to feel.

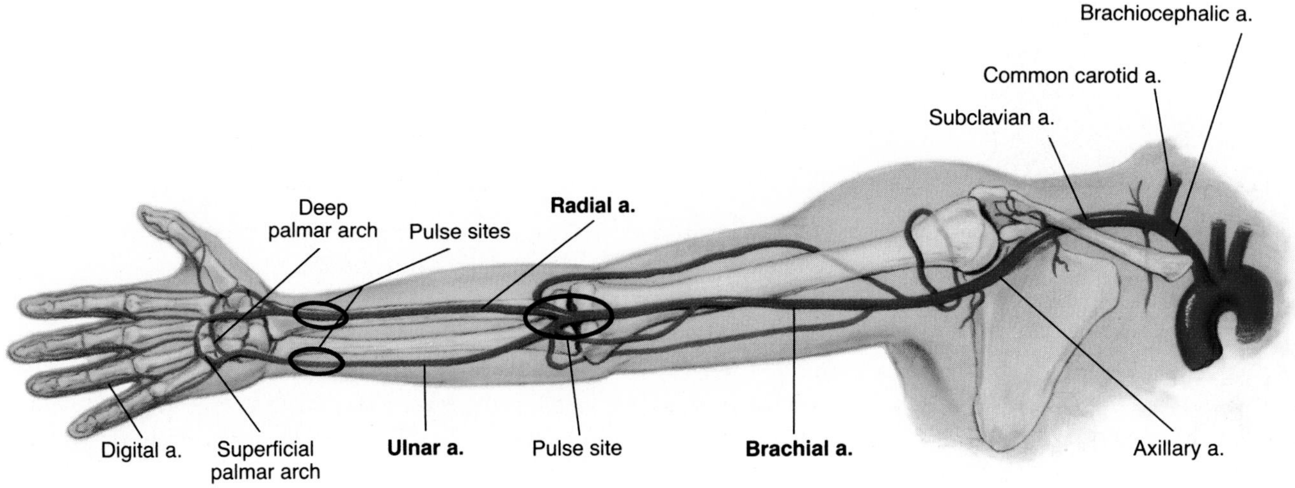

▶ **Figure 18–1**

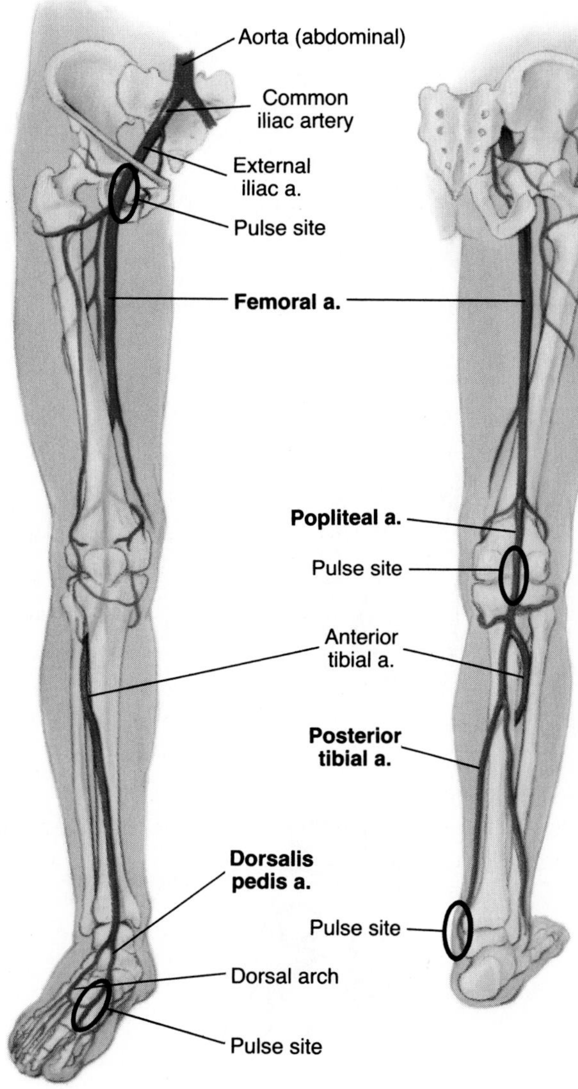

► **Figure 18-2**

Arteries in the Leg. The major artery to the leg is the *femoral artery,* passing under the inguinal ligament (Fig. 18-2). The femoral artery travels down the thigh; at the lower thigh, it courses posteriorly, then it is termed the *popliteal artery.* Below the knee, the popliteal artery divides. The anterior tibial artery travels down the front of the leg on to the dorsum of the foot, where it becomes the *dorsalis pedis.* In back of the leg, the *posterior tibial* artery travels down behind the medial malleolus, and in the foot, forms the plantar arteries.

Ischemia is a deficient supply of oxygenated arterial blood to a tissue due to obstruction of a blood vessel. A complete blockage leads to death of the distal tissue. A partial blockage creates an insufficient supply, and the ischemia may only be apparent at exercise when oxygen needs increase.

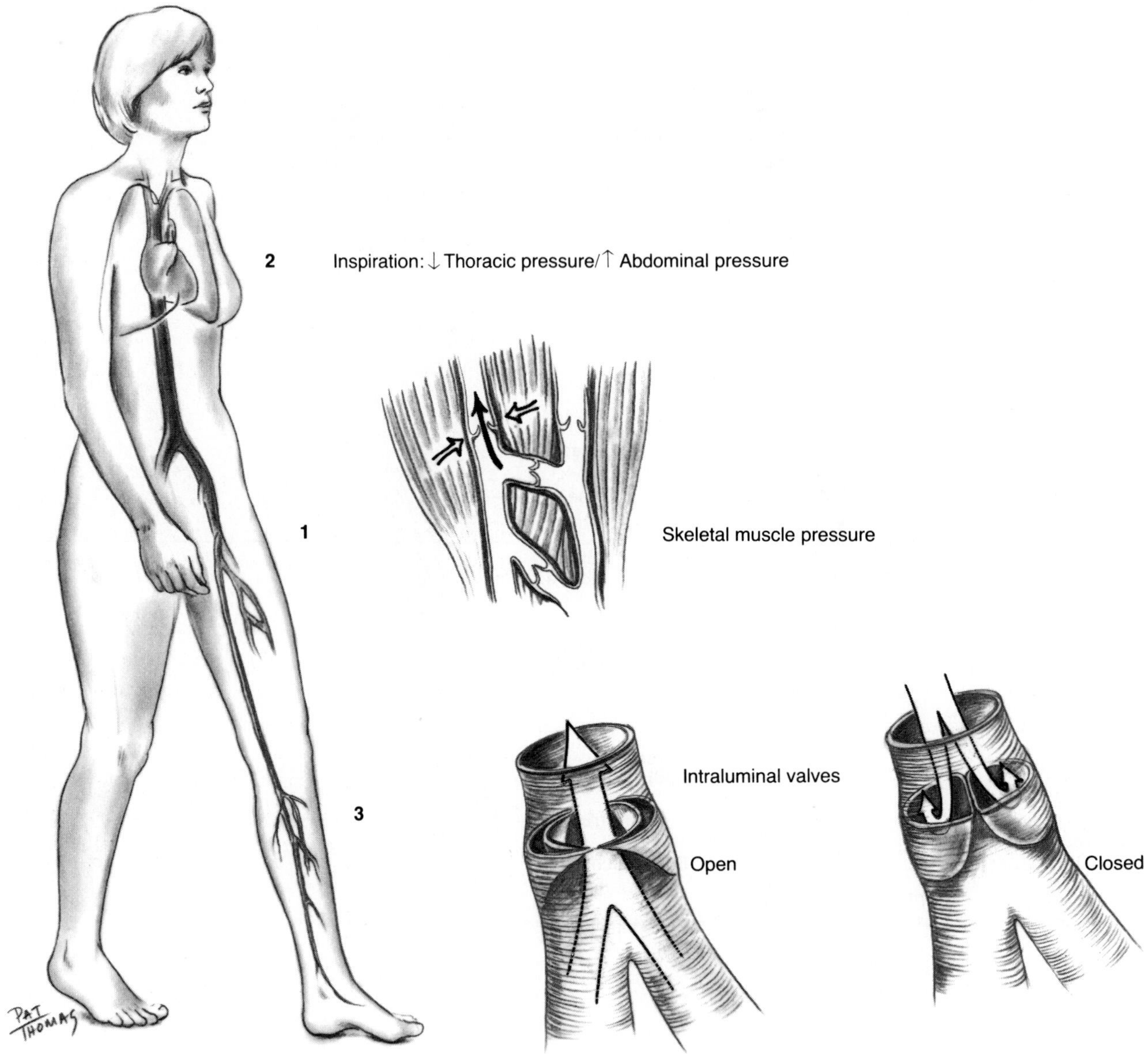

► **Figure 18–3 Mechanisms of venous flow**

VEINS

Veins drain the blood from the tissues and return it to the heart. Unlike the arteries, veins are a low-pressure system. Since there is no pump to generate blood flow, the veins need a mechanism to keep blood moving (Fig. 18–3). This is accomplished by (1) the contracting skeletal muscles that milk the blood proximally; (2) the pressure gradient caused by breathing, in which inspiration makes the thoracic pressure decrease and the abdominal pressure increase; and (3) the intraluminal valves, which ensure unidirectional flow. Each valve is a paired semilunar pocket that opens toward the heart and closes tightly when filled to prevent backflow.

Besides the presence of intraluminal valves, venous structure differs from arterial structure. Because venous

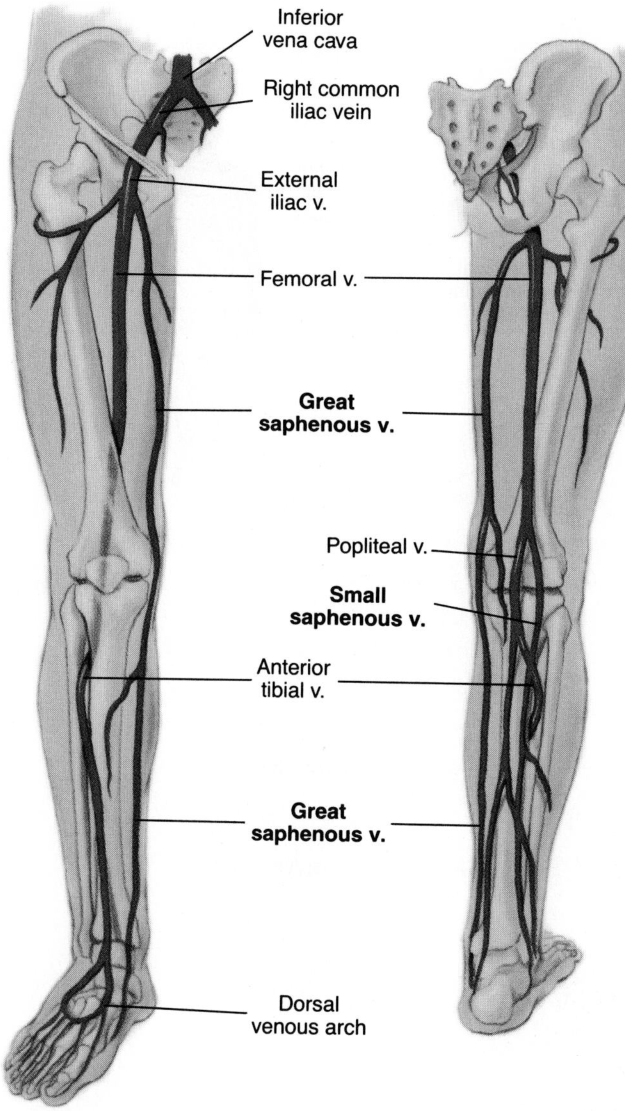

▶ **Figure 18–4**

pressure is lower, walls of the veins are thinner than those of the arteries. Veins have a larger diameter and are more distensible; they can expand and hold more blood when blood volume increases. This is a compensatory mechanism to reduce stress on the heart.

The course of veins parallels that of arteries, but there are more veins. The following veins are accessible to examination in the normal person.

Jugular Veins. Assessment of the jugular veins is presented in Chapter 16.

Veins in the Arm. There are two sets of veins in each arm, superficial and deep. The superficial veins are in the subcutaneous tissue and are responsible for most of the venous return.

Veins in the Leg. The legs have three types of veins (Fig. 18–4). (1) The deep veins run alongside the deep arteries and conduct most of the venous return from the legs. These are the *femoral* and *popliteal* veins. As long as these veins remain intact, the superficial veins can be excised without harming the circulation. (2) The superficial veins are the *great* and *small saphenous* veins. The great saphenous vein, inside the leg, starts at the medial side of the dorsum of the foot. You can see it ascend in front of the medial malleolus, then it crosses the tibia obliquely and ascends along the medial side of the thigh. The small saphenous vein, outside the leg, starts on the lateral side of the dorsum of the foot, ascends behind the lateral malleolus, up the back of the leg, where it joins the popliteal vein. (3) Perforators (not illustrated) are connecting veins that join the two sets and route blood from the superficial into the deep veins.

Efficient venous return is dependent on contracting skeletal muscles, competent valves in the veins, and patent lumen. Problems with any of these three elements lead to venous stasis. At risk for venous disease are people who undergo prolonged standing, sitting, or bedrest because they do not benefit from the milking action that walking accomplishes. Hypercoagulable states and vein wall trauma also place the person at risk for venous disease. Also, dilated and tortuous (varicose) veins create incompetent valves—the lumen is so wide the valve cusps cannot approximate. This condition increases venous pressure, which further dilates the vein. Some people have a genetic predisposition to varicose veins, but obesity and pregnancy are increased risk factors.

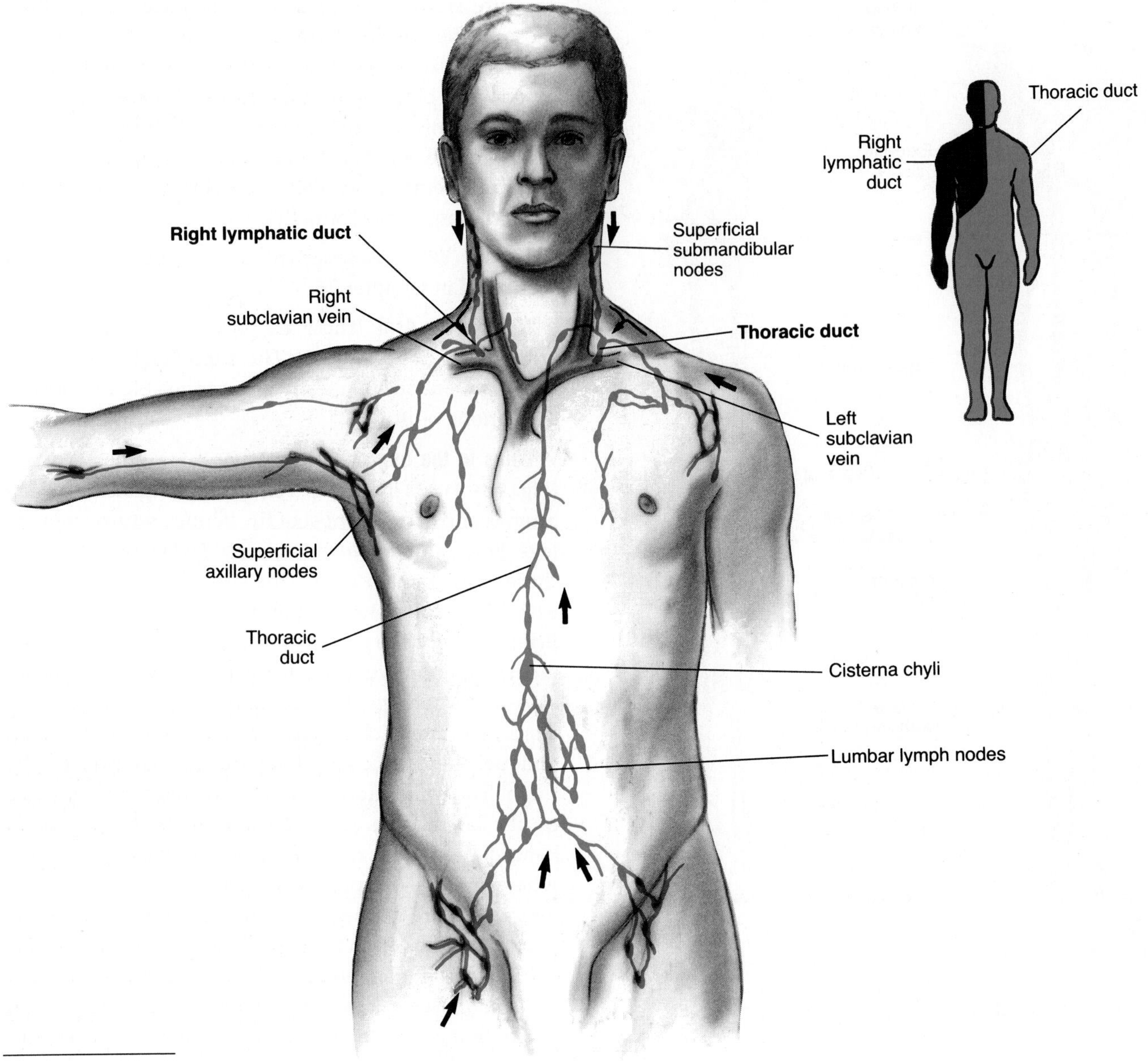

▶ **Figure 18–5**

LYMPHATICS

The lymphatics form a completely separate vessel system, which retrieves excess fluid from the tissue spaces and returns it to the blood stream. During circulation of the blood, somewhat more fluid leaves the capillaries than the veins can absorb. Without lymphatic drainage, fluid would build up in the interstitial spaces and produce edema.

The functions of the lymphatic system are (1) to conserve fluid and plasma proteins that leak out of the capillaries, (2) to form a major part of the immune system that defends the body against disease, and (3) to absorb lipids from the intestinal tract.

The processes of the immune system are complicated and not fully understood. The immune system detects and eliminates foreign substances, both those that come in from the environment and those arising from inside (abnormal or mutant cells). It accomplishes this by phagocytosis (digestion) of the substances and by production of specific antibodies or specific immune responses by the lymphocytes.

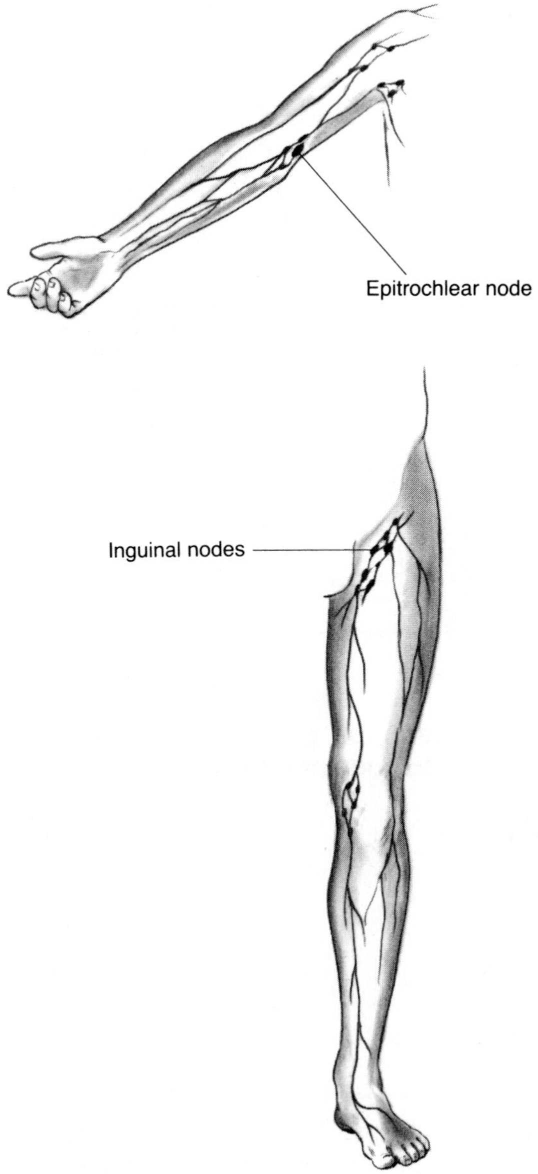

► **Figure 18-6**

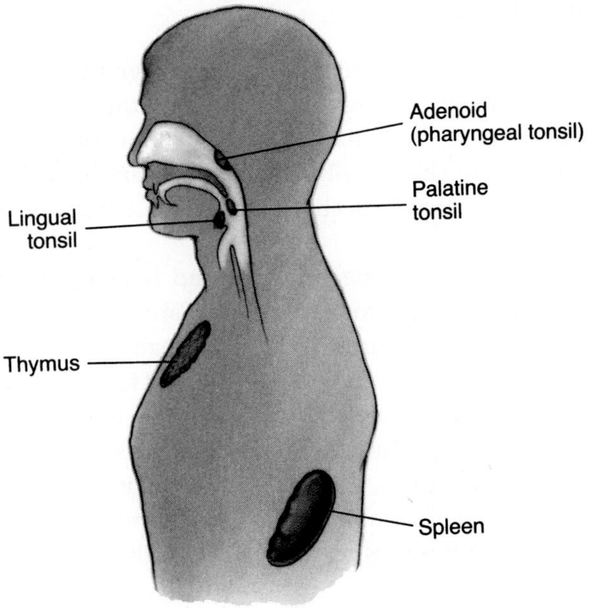

► **Figure 18-7**

The lymphatic vessels have a unique structure. Lymphatic capillaries start as microscopic open-ended tubes, which siphon interstitial fluid. The capillaries converge to form vessels. The vessels have valves, so flow is one-way from the tissue spaces into the blood stream. The many valves make the vessels look beaded. The flow of lymph is slow compared with that of the blood. Lymph flow is propelled by contracting skeletal muscles, pressure changes secondary to breathing, and contraction of the vessel walls themselves.

The vessels drain into two main trunks, which empty into the venous system at the subclavian veins (Fig. 18-5). (1) The *right lymphatic duct* empties into the right subclavian vein. It drains the right side of the head and neck, right arm, right side of thorax, right lung and pleura, right side of the heart, and right upper section of the liver. (2) The *thoracic duct* drains the rest of the body. It empties into the left subclavian vein.

Lymph nodes are small oval clumps of lymphatic tissue located at intervals along the vessels. Most nodes are arranged in groups, both deep and superficially in the body. Nodes filter the fluid before it is returned to the blood stream and filter out microorganisms that could be harmful to the body. With local inflammation, the nodes in that area become swollen and tender.

The superficial groups of nodes are accessible to inspection and palpation, and give clues to the status of the lymphatic system:

- Cervical nodes drain the head and neck, and are described in Chapter 10.
- Axillary nodes drain the breast and upper arm. They are described in Chapter 14.
- The epitrochlear node is in the antecubital fossa and drains the hand and lower arm (Fig. 18-6).
- The inguinal nodes in the groin drain most of the lymph of the lower extremity, the external genitalia, and the anterior abdominal wall.

Related Organs

The spleen, tonsils, and thymus aid the lymphatic system (Fig. 18–7). The spleen is located in the left upper quadrant of the abdomen. It has four functions: (1) to destroy old red blood cells, (2) to produce antibodies, (3) to store red blood cells and (4) to filter microorganisms from the blood.

The tonsils (palatine, adenoid, and lingual) are located at the entrance to the respiratory and gastrointestinal tracts and respond to local inflammation.

The thymus is the flat, pink-gray gland located in the superior mediastinum behind the sternum and in front of the aorta. It is relatively large in the fetus and young child, and atrophies after puberty. It is important in developing the T-lymphocytes of the immune system in children, but it serves no function in adults.

DEVELOPMENTAL CONSIDERATIONS

Infants and Children

The lymphatic system has the same function in children as in adults. Lymphoid tissue has a unique growth pattern when compared with other body systems (Fig. 18–8). It is well developed at birth and grows rapidly until age 10 or 11. By age 6, the lymphoid tissue reaches adult size, it surpasses adult size by puberty, and then it slowly atrophies. It is possible that the excessive antigen stimulation in children causes the early rapid growth.

Lymph nodes are relatively large in children, and the superficial ones often are palpable even when the child is healthy. With infection, there is excessive swelling and hyperplasia. Enlarged tonsils are familiar signs in respiratory infections. The excessive lymphoid response also may account for the common childhood symptom of abdominal pain with seemingly unrelated problems such as upper respiratory infections (Johnson et al, 1978). Possibly the inflammation of mesenteric lymph nodes produces the abdominal pain.

The Pregnant Female

Hormonal changes cause vasodilatation and the resulting drop in blood pressure described in Chapter 16. The growing uterus obstructs drainage of the iliac veins and the inferior vena cava. This condition causes low blood flow and increases venous pressure. This, in turn, causes dependent edema, varicosities in the legs and vulva, and hemorrhoids.

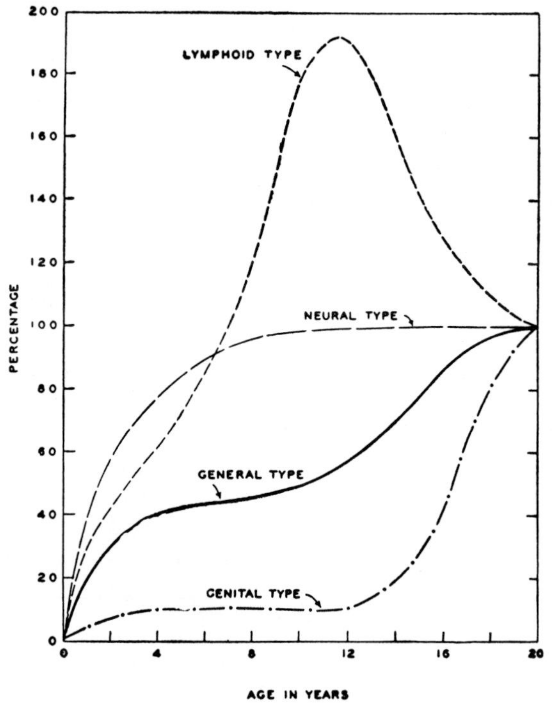

Comparison of growth rates of three types of tissues and the body as a whole

► **Figure 18–8**

The Aging Adult

Peripheral blood vessels grow more rigid with age, resulting in a condition called arteriosclerosis. This condition produces the rise in systolic blood pressure discussed in Chapter 8. Do not confuse this process with another one, atherosclerosis, or the deposition of fatty plaques on the intima of the arteries.

Aging produces a progressive enlargement of the intramuscular calf veins. This correlates with the increased frequency of leg vein thrombosis and pulmonary embolism in the aging population. Also, the technological growth of the health care field has prolonged the life of more critically ill people and has led to more extensive surgery for older people. Both of these factors increase the risk for thromboembolism (Haimovici, 1986).

Loss of lymphatic tissue leads to fewer numbers of lymph nodes in older people, and a decrease in the size of remaining nodes.

SUBJECTIVE DATA

- Leg pain or cramps
- Skin changes on arms or legs
- Swelling
- Lymph node enlargement

EXAMINER ASKS:	RATIONALE:
1. Do you have any **leg pain (cramps)?** Where? Describe the type of pain. Did this come on gradually or suddenly? Is it aggravated by activity, walking?	Peripheral vascular disease — see Table 18-3, History Profiles.
How many blocks (stairs) does it take to produce this pain?	*Claudication distance* — is number of blocks walked, stairs climbed to produce pain.
Has this amount changed recently?	Note sudden decrease in claudication distance, or pain suddenly not relieved by rest.
Is the pain worse with elevation? Is it worse with cool temperatures? Does the pain wake you up at night?	
Have you experienced any recent change in exercise, a new exercise, increasing exercise?	Pain of musculoskeletal origin rather than vascular.
What relieves this pain: dangling, walking, rubbing? Is the leg pain associated with any skin changes?	
Is it associated with any change in sexual function (males)?	Aortoiliac occlusion associated with impotence (Leriche's syndrome)
Do you have any past history of: vascular problems, heart problems, diabetes, obesity, pregnancy, smoking, trauma, prolonged standing, or bedrest?	
2. Have you noted any **skin changes** in arms or legs? What color: redness, pallor, blueness, brown discolorations?	
Have you noticed any change in temperature — excess warmth or coolness?	Coolness is associated with arterial disease.
Do your leg veins look bulging and tortuous? How have you treated these? Do you use support hose?	Varicose veins
Do you have any leg sores or ulcers? Where on the leg? Do you have any pain with the leg ulcer?	Leg ulcers occur with chronic arterial and chronic venous disease.
3. Have you noticed any **swelling** in the legs? Is it in one or both legs? When did this swelling start? What time of day is the swelling at its worse: morning, or after up most of day? Does the swelling come and go, or is it constant? What seems to bring it on: trauma, standing all day, sitting? What relieves swelling: elevation, support hose? Is swelling associated with: pain, heat, redness, ulceration, hardened skin?	
4. Have you noticed any "swollen glands" (lumps, kernels)? Where in body? How long have you had them? Have you noticed any recent change? How do they feel to you: hard, soft? Are the swollen glands associated with: pain, local infection?	**Enlarged lymph nodes**
5. What medications are you taking, e.g., oral contraceptives?	

OBJECTIVE DATA

Equipment Needed:

Occasionally need: Paper tape measure
Tourniquet or B/P cuff
Stethoscope

Preparation

During a complete physical examination, examine the arms at the very beginning when you are checking the vital signs—the person is sitting. Examine the legs directly after the abdominal examination while the person is still supine. Then stand the person up to evaluate the leg veins.

Examination of the arms and legs includes peripheral vascular characteristics (following here), the skin (see Chapter 9), musculoskeletal findings (Chapter 19), and neurologic findings (Chapter 20). A method of integrating these steps is discussed in Chapter 24.

Room temperature should be about 22°C (72°F) and draftless to prevent vasodilatation or vasoconstriction.

Use inspection and palpation. Compare your findings with the opposite extremity.

METHOD OF EXAMINATION

NORMAL RANGE OF FINDINGS	ABNORMAL FINDINGS

THE ARMS

Inspect and palpate the arms.

Lift both the person's hands in your hands. Inspect, then turn the person's hands over, noting color of skin and nailbeds, temperature, texture, and turgor of skin, and the presence of any lesions, edema, or clubbing. Use the *profile sign* (viewing the finger from the side) to detect early clubbing. The normal nail bed angle is 160 degrees. (See Chapter 9, Assessment of Skin, Hair, Nails, for a full discussion of skin color, lesions, and clubbing.)

With the person's hands near the level of his or her heart, check capillary refill. This is an index of peripheral perfusion and cardiac output. Depress and blanch the nail beds; release and note the time for color return. Usually, the vessels refill within a fraction of a second. Consider it normal if the color returns in less than 1 or 2 seconds. Note these conditions that can skew your findings: a cool room, decreased body temperature, cigarette smoking, peripheral edema, and anemia.

Flattening of angle, and clubbing (diffuse enlargement of terminal phalanges) occurs with congenital cyanotic heart disease, cor pulmonale and subacute bacterial endocarditis.

Refill lasting more than 1 or 2 seconds signifies vasoconstriction or decreased cardiac output (hypovolemia, congestive heart failure, shock). The hands are cold, clammy, and pale.

NORMAL RANGE OF FINDINGS	ABNORMAL FINDINGS
The two arms should be symmetric in size.	Edema of upper extremities is uncommon but does occur when lymphatic drainage is obstructed, as seen following some types of breast surgery.
Note the presence of any scars on hands and arms. Many occur normally with usual childhood abrasions, or with occupations involving hand tools.	Needle tracks in antecubital fossae occur with intravenous drug use; linear scars in wrists may signify past self-inflicted injury.
Palpate both radial pulses, noting rate, rhythm, elasticity of vessel wall, and equal force (Fig. 18–9). Grade the force (amplitude) on a four-point scale:	See Table 18–1.

4+, bounding

3+, increased

2+, **normal**

1+, weak

0, absent

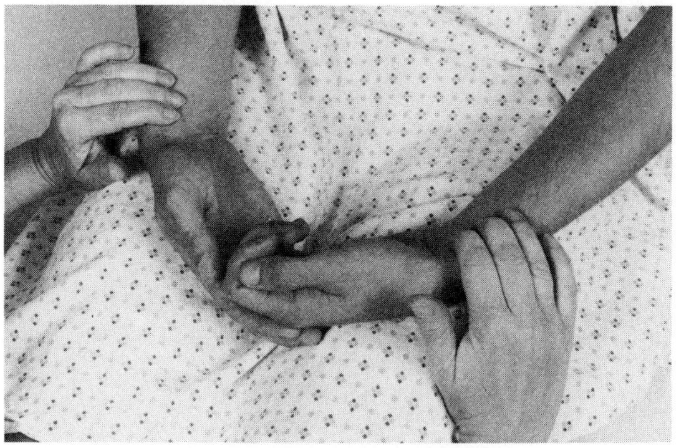

► **Figure 18–9**

It is not necessary to palpate the ulnar pulses. If indicated, palpate along the medial side of the inner forearm, although the ulnar pulses often are not palpable in the normal person (Fig. 18–10).

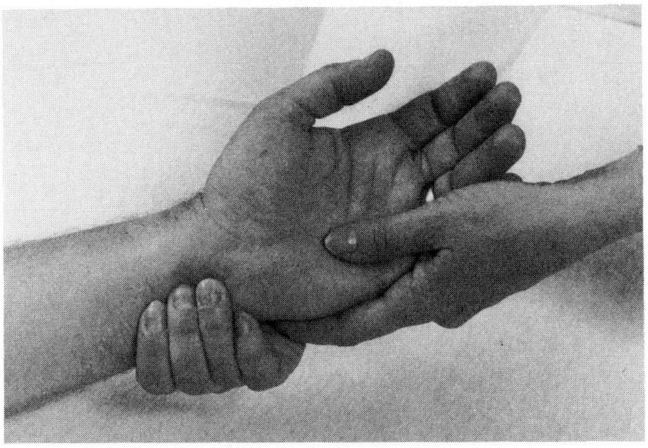

► **Figure 18–10**

NORMAL RANGE OF FINDINGS	ABNORMAL FINDINGS

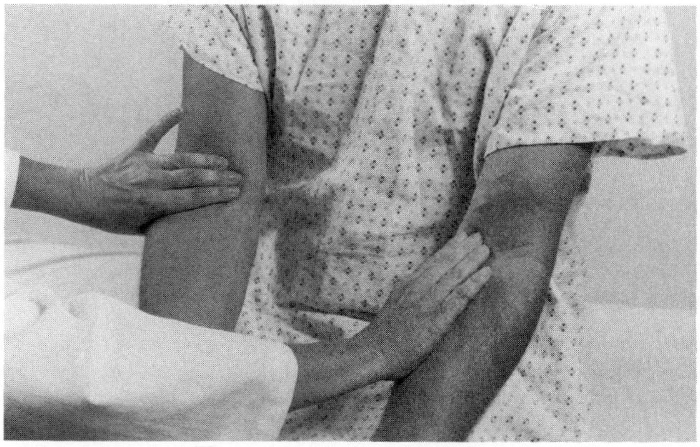

► **Figure 18–11**

Palpate the brachial pulses—their force should be equal bilaterally (Fig. 18–11). Check the epitrochlear lymph node in the depression above and behind the medial condyle of the humerus. Do this by "shaking hands" with the person and reaching your other hand under the person's elbow to the groove between the biceps and triceps muscles (Fig. 18–12).

An enlarged epitrochlear node occurs with infection of the hand or forearm.

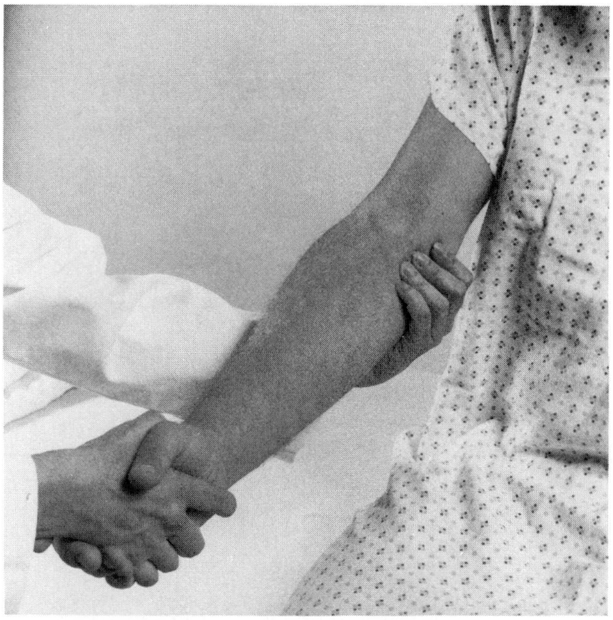

► **Figure 18–12**

NORMAL RANGE OF FINDINGS | **ABNORMAL FINDINGS**

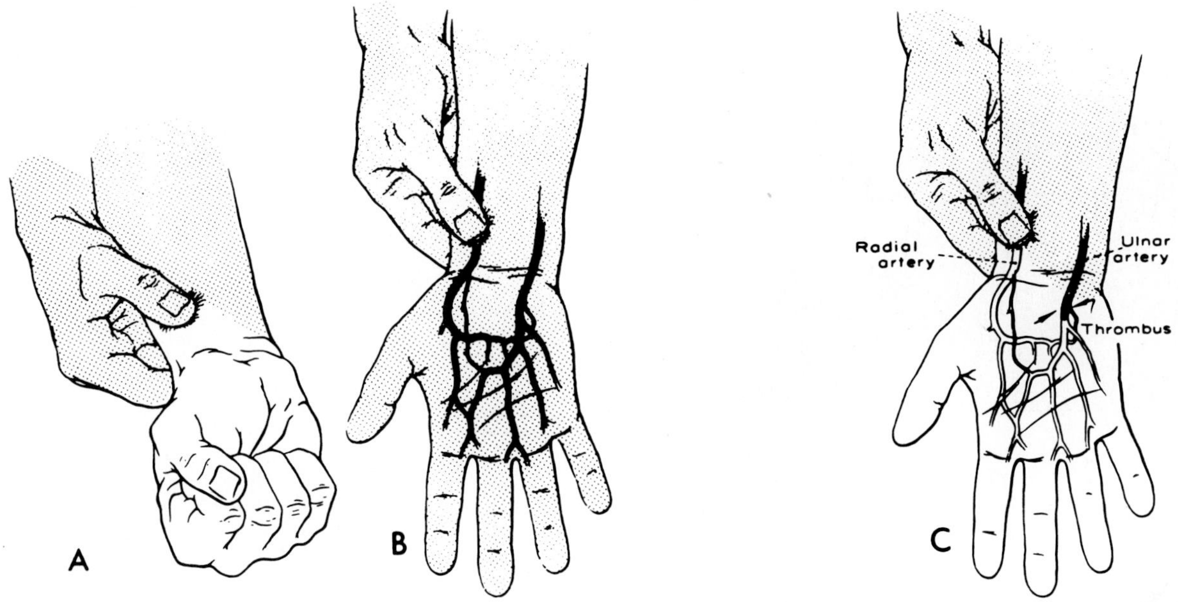

► **Figure 18-13** **Allen test**

The Allen Test. Determine the patency of the radial and ulnar arteries by performing the Allen test (Fig. 18-13). Ask the person to rest the hands on the knees, palms up. (A) Compress both radial arteries with your thumbs, and ask the person to open and close the fists several times. (B) Continue to compress the arteries and have the person open the hands (without hyperextending them). Look at the palms; they should turn pink promptly, as long as the ulnar artery is patent. Repeat the test while occluding the ulnar arteries.

(C) Pallor persists if ulnar artery or its arch is occluded.

THE LEGS

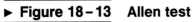

Inspect and palpate the legs.

Uncover the legs while keeping the genitalia draped. Inspect both legs together, noting skin color, hair distribution, venous pattern, size (swelling or atrophy), and any skin lesions or ulcers.

Normally hair covers the legs. Even if leg hair is shaved, you will still note hair on the dorsa of the toes.

Pallor with vasoconstriction; erythema with vasodilatation; cyanosis.

Malnutrition: thin, shiny atropic skin, thick-ridged nails, loss of hair, ulcers, gangrene. Malnutrition, pallor, and coolness occur with arterial insufficiency.

The venous pattern normally is flat and barely visible. Note obvious varicosities, although these are best assessed while standing.

Both legs should be symmetric in size without any swelling or atrophy. If the lower legs look asymmetric, measure the calf circumference

Diffuse bilateral edema occurs with systemic illnesses.

NORMAL RANGE OF FINDINGS	ABNORMAL FINDINGS

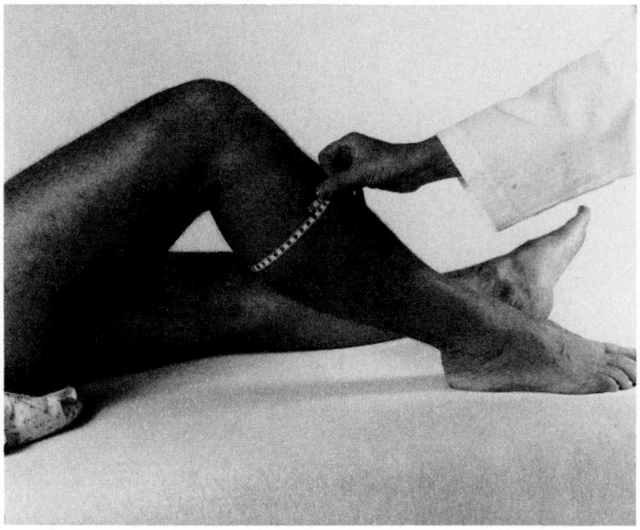

► **Figure 18–14**

with a nonstretchable tape measure (Fig. 18–14). Measure at the widest point, taking care to measure the other leg in exactly the same place, the same number of centimeters down from the patella or other landmark. Record your findings in centimeters.

Unilateral swelling indicates a local acute problem.

In the presence of skin discoloration, skin ulcers, or gangrene, note the size and the exact location.

Brown discoloration occurs with chronic venous stasis from capillary dilatation and damage.

Venous ulcers occur usually at medial malleolus due to bacterial invasion of poorly drained tissues (see Table 18–4).

With arterial deficit, ulcers occur on tips of toes, metatarsal heads, and lateral malleoli.

Using the dorsa of your hands, palpate for temperature from the feet up along the legs, comparing symmetric spots. The skin should be warm and equal bilaterally. Bilateral cool feet may be due to environmental factors such as cool room temperature, apprehension, and cigarette smoking. If there is any increase in temperature up the leg, note if it is gradual or abrupt.

A unilateral cool foot or leg occurs with arterial deficit.

Flex the person's knee, then gently compress the gastrocnemius (calf) muscle anteriorly against the tibia; there should be no tenderness. Or, you may sharply dorsiflex the foot against the calf. Flexing the knee first exerts pressure on the posterior tibial vein. Normally this does not cause pain.

Calf pain with these maneuvers is a positive *Homan's sign,* which occurs in about 35% of cases of deep vein thrombosis. It is not specific for this condition because it occurs also with superficial phlebitis, Achilles tendinitis, gastrocnemius, and plantal muscle injury.

Palpate the inguinal lymph nodes. It is not unusual to find palpable nodes that are small (1 cm or less), movable, and nontender.

Enlarged nodes, tender or fixed in area.

NORMAL RANGE OF FINDINGS

Palpate these peripheral arteries in both legs: femoral, popliteal, dorsalis pedis, and posterior tibial. Grade the force on the four-point scale. Locate the femoral arteries just below the inguinal ligament halfway between the pubis and anterior superior iliac spines (Fig. 18–15). To help expose the femoral area, particularly in obese people, ask the person to bend his or her knees to the side in a froglike position. Press firmly, and then slowly release, noting the pulse tap under your fingertips. Should this pulse be weak or diminished, auscultate the site for a bruit.

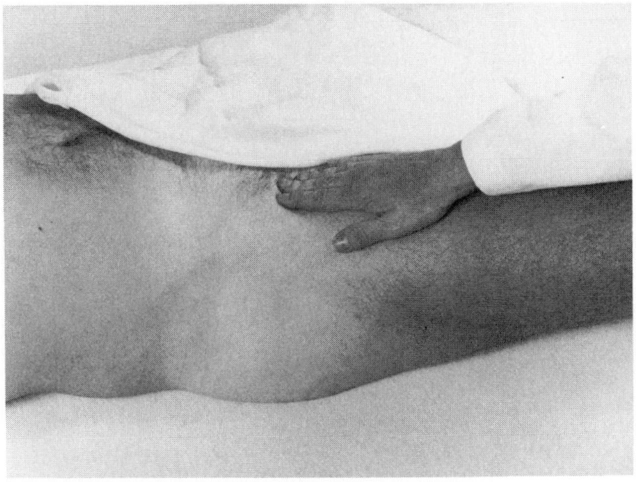

▶ **Figure 18–15**

The popliteal pulse is a more diffuse pulse and can be difficult to localize. Bend the knees up a little, anchor your thumbs on the knee, and curl your fingers around into the fossa (Fig. 18–16). Push forward against

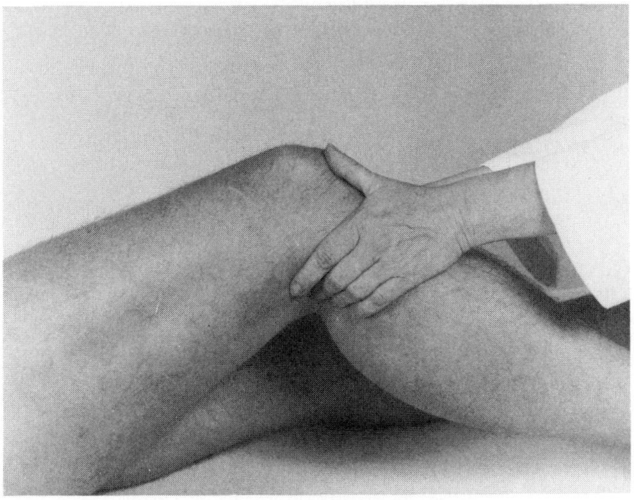

▶ **Figure 18–16**

ABNORMAL FINDINGS

A bruit occurs with turbulent blood flow, indicating partial occlusion.

NORMAL RANGE OF FINDINGS | **ABNORMAL FINDINGS**

the bone. Use a light touch and search the area. Often it is just lateral to the medial tendon. If you have difficulty, turn the person prone and lift up the lower leg (Fig. 18–17). Often, a normal popliteal pulse is impossible to palpate.

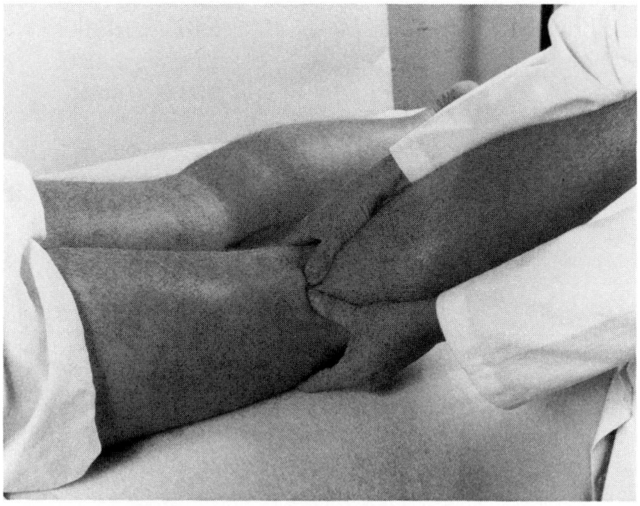

► **Figure 18–17**

For the posterior tibial pulse, curve your fingers around the medial malleolus (Fig. 18–18). You will feel the tapping right behind it in the groove between the malleolus and the Achilles tendon.

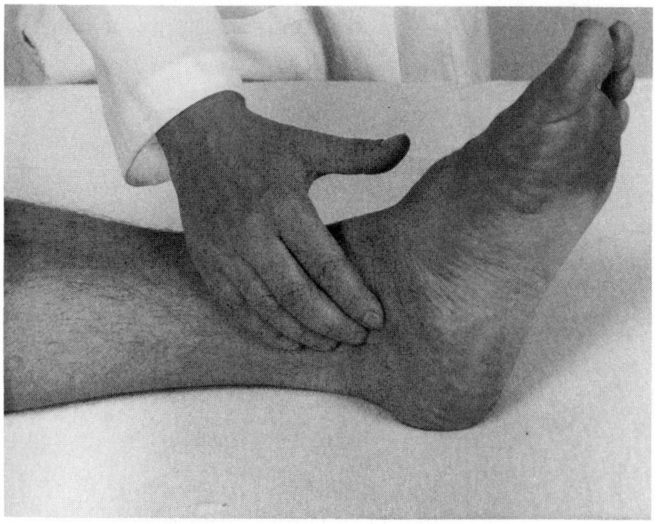

► **Figure 18–18 Posterior tibial pulse**

NORMAL RANGE OF FINDINGS

The dorsalis pedis pulse requires a very light touch. Normally it is just lateral to and parallel with the extensor tendon of the big toe (Fig. 18–19).

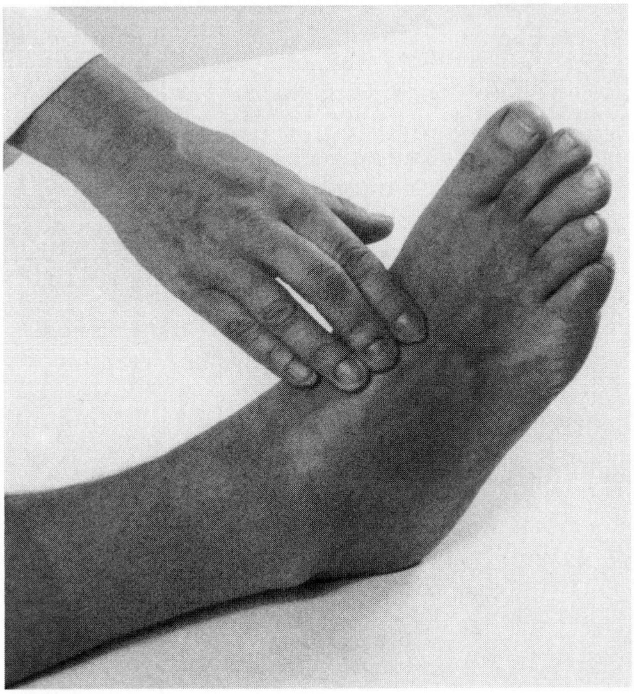

► **Figure 18–19 Dorsalis pedis pulse**

Check for pretibial edema. Firmly depress the skin over the tibia or the medial malleolus for 5 seconds and release (Fig. 18–20*A*). Normally, your finger should leave no indentation, although a pit commonly is seen if the

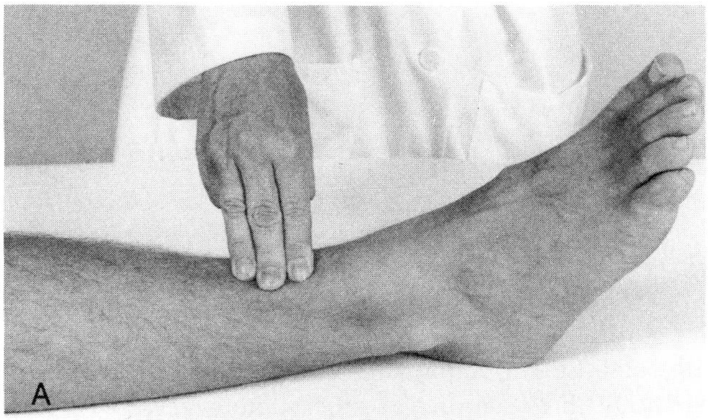

► **Figure 18–20**

ABNORMAL FINDINGS

Bilateral, dependent, pitting edema occurs with congestive heart failure and hepatic cirrhosis (see Fig. 18–20*B*).

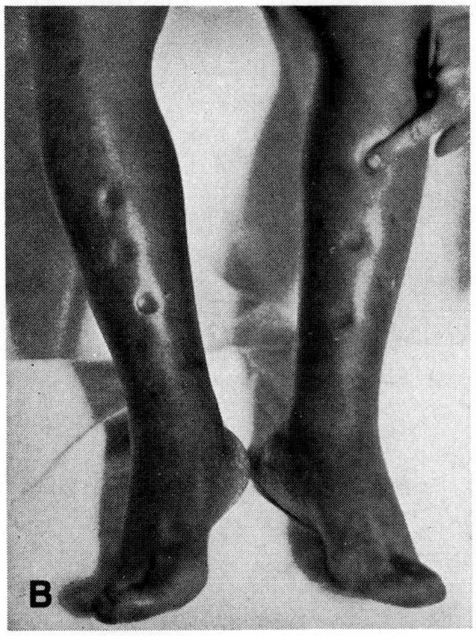

NORMAL RANGE OF FINDINGS	ABNORMAL FINDINGS

person has been standing all day or during pregnancy. If pitting edema is present, grade it on this scale:

1+ mild, slight depression
to
4+ severe, deep depression

This scale is subjective.

Unilateral edema occurs with occlusion of a deep vein and unilaterally or bilaterally with lymphatic obstruction. With these factors, it is "brawny" or nonpitting and feels hard to the touch.

Ask the person to stand so that you can assess the venous system. Note any visible, dilated and tortuous veins.

Varicosities occur in the saphenous veins (see Table 18–4).

Manual Compression Test. While the person is still standing, test the length of the varicose vein to determine if its valves are competent (Fig. 18–21). Place one hand on the lower part of the varicose vein, and compress the vein with your other hand about 15 to 20 cm higher. Competent valves will prevent a wave transmission and your distal fingers will feel nothing.

A palpable wave transmission occurs when the valves are incompetent.

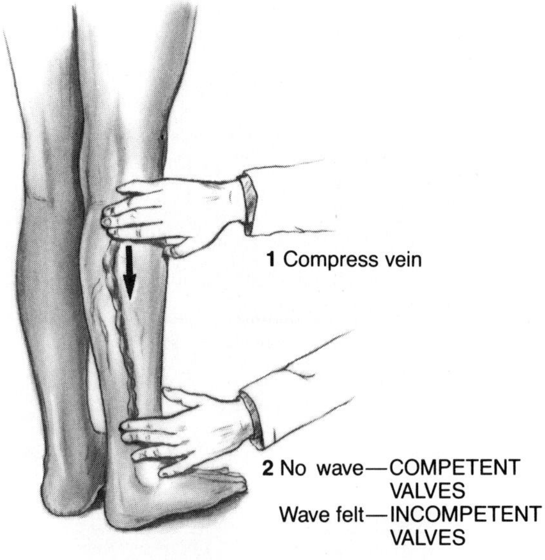

Manual compression test

► **Figure 18–21**

ADDITIONAL TECHNIQUES

The Trendelenburg Test. When varicosities are present in the legs, use the Trendelenburg test to determine valve competence (Fig. 18–22). Return the person to supine position, elevate the involved leg 90 degrees until the veins empty, and place a tourniquet high on the thigh. Help the person to stand up, and watch for venous filling. The saphenous veins should fill slowly from below in about 30 seconds.

Rapid filling of veins from above indicates incompetent valves.

After 30 seconds, take the tourniquet off. Now observe whether or not the varicose veins fill suddenly from above. Normally there is no sudden filling.

Sudden filling after removing the tourniquet indicates retrograde flow past incompetent saphenous valves.

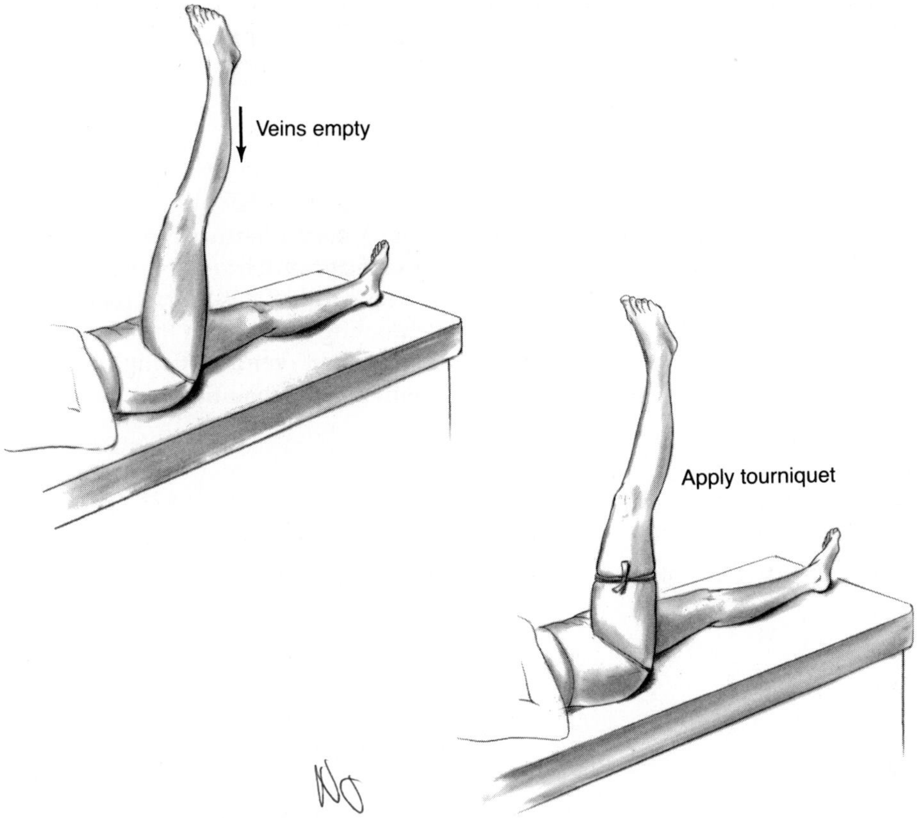

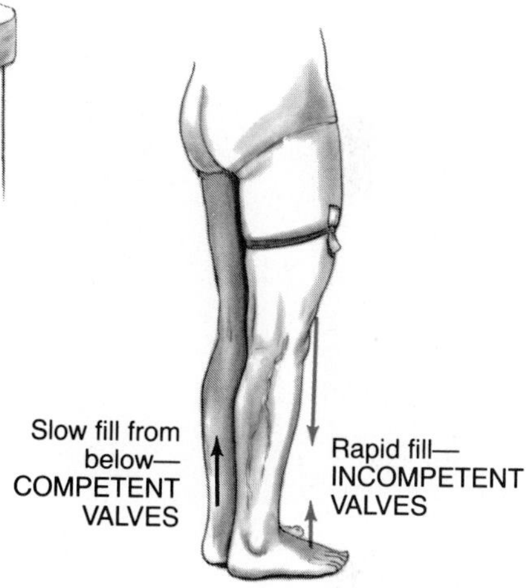

► **Figure 18-22 Trendelenburg test**

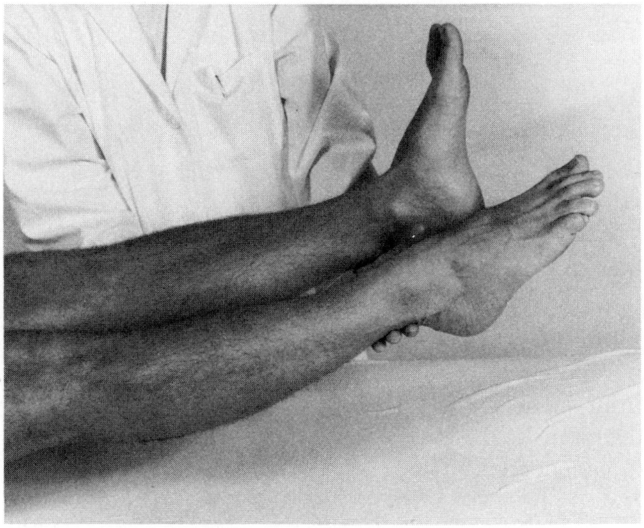

► **Figure 18-23**

Color Changes. If you suspect an arterial deficit, raise the legs about 30 cm (12 inches) and wag the feet to drain off venous blood (Fig. 18-23). The skin color now reflects only the contribution of arterial blood. A

Elevational pallor (marked) indicates arterial insufficiency.

NORMAL RANGE OF FINDINGS | **ABNORMAL FINDINGS**

light-skinned person's feet will look a little pale but still should be pink. A dark-skinned person's feet are more difficult to evaluate, but the soles should reveal extreme color change.

Now have the person sit up and dangle the legs over the side of the table (Fig. 18–24). Compare the color of both feet. Note the time it takes for color to return to the feet. Normally, this is 10 seconds or less. Note also the time it takes for the superficial veins around the feet to fill—the normal time is about 15 seconds. This test is unreliable if there is concomitant venous disease with incompetent valves.

Dependent rubor (deep blue-red color) occurs with severe arterial insufficiency. Chronic hypoxia produces a loss of vasomotor tone and a pooling of blood in the veins.

Delayed venous filling occurs with arterial insufficiency.

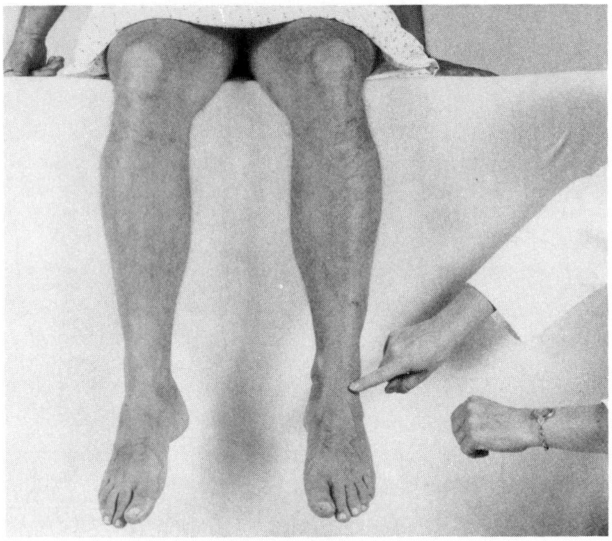

► **Figure 18–24**

Test the lower legs for strength (see Chapter 19). Test the lower legs for sensation (see Chapter 20).

Motor loss occurs with severe arterial deficit.

Sensory loss occurs with arterial deficit, especially with diabetes.

The Doppler Ultrasonic Flowmeter. Use this device to detect a weak peripheral pulse, to monitor blood pressure in infants or children, or to measure a low blood pressure or blood pressure in a lower extremity (Fig. 18–25). The Doppler flowmeter magnifies pulsatile sounds from the heart and blood vessels. Place a drop of coupling gel on the end of the hand-held transducer. Place the transducer over a pulse site, tilted at a 45-degree angle. Locate the pulse site by the swishing whooshing sound.

NORMAL RANGE OF FINDINGS | ABNORMAL FINDINGS

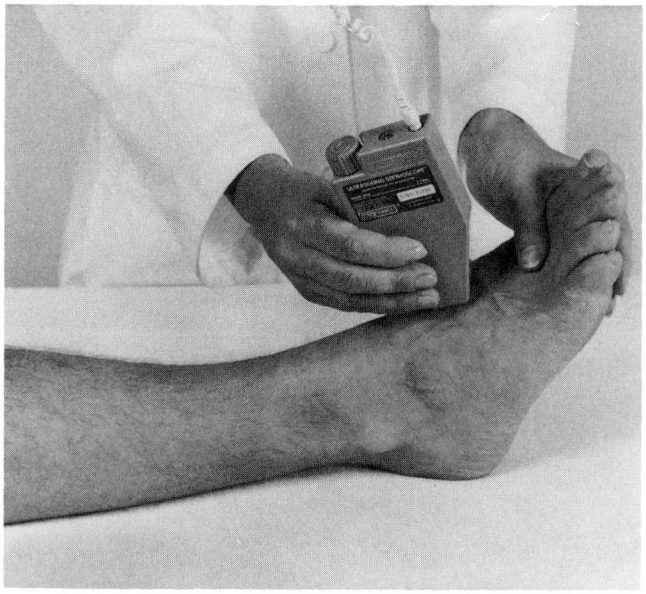

▶ **Figure 18-25**

DEVELOPMENTAL CONSIDERATIONS

Infants and Children

Transient acrocyanosis and skin mottling at birth are discussed in Chapter 9. Pulse force should be normal and symmetric. Pulse force also should be the same in the upper and lower extremities.

Weak pulses occur with vasoconstriction or diminished cardiac output.

Full bounding pulses occur with patent ductus arteriosus due to the large left-to-right shunt.

Diminished or absent femoral pulses while upper extremity pulses are normal suggests coarctation of aorta.

Palpable lymph nodes occur often in normal infants and children. They are small, firm (shotty), mobile, and nontender. They may be the sequelae of past infection, e.g., inguinal nodes from a diaper rash or cervical nodes from a respiratory infection. Vaccinations also can produce local lymphadenopathy. Note characteristics of any palpable nodes and whether they are local or generalized.

Enlarged, warm, tender nodes indicate current infection. Look for source.

The Pregnant Female

Expect diffuse bilateral pitting edema in the lower extremities, especially at the end of the day, and into the third trimester. Varicose veins in the legs also are common in the third trimester.

NORMAL RANGE OF FINDINGS	ABNORMAL FINDINGS
The Aging Adult The dorsalis pedis and posterior tibial pulses may become more difficult to find. Trophic changes associated with arterial insufficiency (thin shiny skin, thick-ridged nails, loss of hair on lower legs) also occur normally with aging.	

☑ SUMMARY CHECKLIST

1 ► Inspect arms for color, size, any lesions
2 ► Palpate pulses: radial, brachial
3 ► Check epitrochlear node
4 ► Inspect legs for color, size, any lesions, trophic skin changes
5 ► Palpate temperature of feet and legs
6 ► Palpate inguinal nodes
7 ► Palpate pulses: femoral, popliteal, posterior tibial, dorsalis pedis

SAMPLE RECORDING

Subjective

► No leg pain, no skin changes, no swelling or lymph node enlargement. No past history of heart or vascular problems, diabetes, or obesity. Does not smoke. On no medications.

Objective

► Extremities have pink-tan color without redness, cyanosis, or any skin lesions. Extremity size symmetric without swelling or atrophy. Temperature warm and = bilaterally. All pulses present, 2+ and = bilaterally. No lymphadenopathy.

SAMPLE CLINICAL PROBLEM

James K. is a 43-year-old married white male, city sanitation worker, admitted to University Medical Center today for "bypass surgery tomorrow to fix my aorta and these black toes."

Subjective

► 6 yrs PTA: Motorcycle accident with handle bars jammed into groin. Treated and released at local hospital. No apparent injury, although MD now thinks accident may have precipitated present stenosis of aorta.
1 yr PTA: Radiating pain in right calf on walking one mile. Pain relieved by stopping walking.
3 months PTA: Problems with sex, unable to maintain erection during intercourse.
1 month PTA: Leg pain present after walking 2 blocks. Numbness and tingling in right foot and calf. Tips of 3 toes on right foot look black. Saw MD. Diagnostic studies showed stenosis of aorta "below vessels that go to my kidneys."
Present: Leg pain at rest, constant and severe, worse at night, partially relieved by dangling leg over side of bed.
Past hx. No hx. of heart or vessel disease, hypertension, diabetes, obesity.
Personal habits: Smokes cigarettes 3 packs/day × 23 years. Now cut down to 1 ppd. Walking is part of occupation, although has been driving city truck last 3 months due to leg pain. On no medications.

Objective

► Lower extremity size = bilaterally with no swelling or atrophy. No varicosities. Color L leg pink, R leg pink when supine, but marked pallor to R foot on elevation. Black gangrene at tips of R 2nd, 3th, 4th toes. Leg hair present but absent on involved toes. Right foot cool and temperature gradually warms as proceed up R leg.
Pulses: femorals 1+; popliteals 0; posterior tibial 0 but present with Doppler; dorsalis pedis 0 but L present with Doppler and right not present with Doppler.

Assessment

► Ischemic rest pain R leg
Altered peripheral tissue perfusion R/T interruption of flow
Impaired tissue integrity R/T altered circulation
Activity intolerance R/T leg pain
Sexual dysfunction R/T effects of disease

NURSING DIAGNOSES COMMONLY ASSOCIATED WITH PERIPHERAL VASCULAR SYSTEM AND LYMPHATIC DISORDERS

Diagnosis	Related Factors (Etiology)	Defining Characteristics (Symptoms and Signs)
Altered tissue perfusion: peripheral	Exchange problems Hypervolemia Hypovolemia Interruption of flow	Altered sensory or motor function Burning Changes in hair pattern Claudication Coolness of skin Diminished pulse quality Edema Erythema Extremity pain Inflammation Pallor Positive Homan's sign Tissue necrosis Trophic skin changes Ulcerated skin/poorly healing areas
Sensory perceptual alteration: tactile	Circulatory impairment Inflammation Effects of anesthesia Nutritional deficiencies Effects of aging Effects of burns Neurologic impairment Pain Persistent tactile stimulation	Paresthesias Hyperesthesias Anesthesias

Other related nursing diagnoses:

- Activity intolerance (see Chapter 15)
- Altered tissue integrity
- Body image disturbance
- Fatigue (see Chapter 15)
- Pain (see Chapters 13 and 19)
- Sleep pattern disturbance
- Sexual dysfunction (see Chapter 22)

ABNORMAL CONDITIONS

Table 18-1 ► Variations in Arterial Pulse

DESCRIPTION	ASSOCIATED WITH
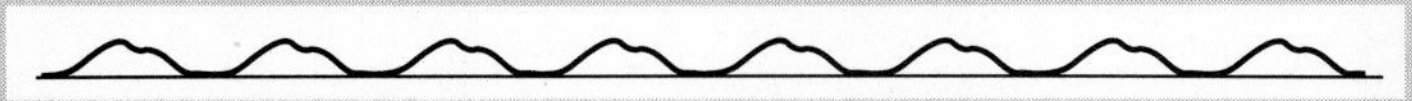 **Weak "Thready" Pulse—1+.** Hard to palpate, need to search for it, may fade in and out, easily obliterated by pressure.	Decreased cardiac output; peripheral arterial disease; aortic valve stenosis.
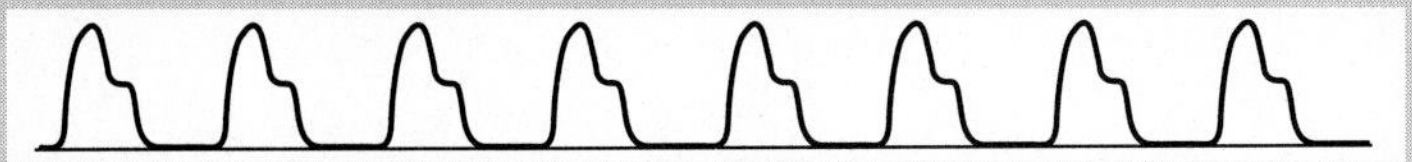 **Full Bounding Pulse—3+ or 4+.** Easily palpable, pounds under your fingertips.	Hyperkinetic states (exercise, anxiety, fever), anemia, hyperthyroidism.
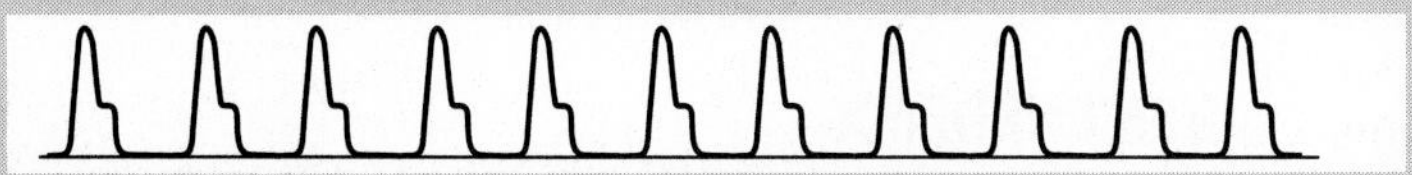 **Water-Hammer (Corrigan's) Pulse—4+.** Greater than normal force, then collapses suddenly.	Aortic valve regurgitation; patent ductus arteriosus.
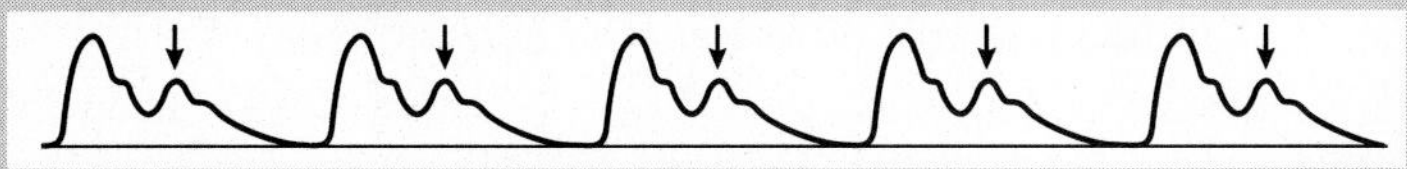 **Pulsus Bigeminus.** Rhythm is coupled, every other beat comes early, or normal beat followed by premature beat. Force of premature beat is decreased due to shortened cardiac filling time.	Conduction disturbance, e.g., premature ventricular contraction, premature atrial contraction.
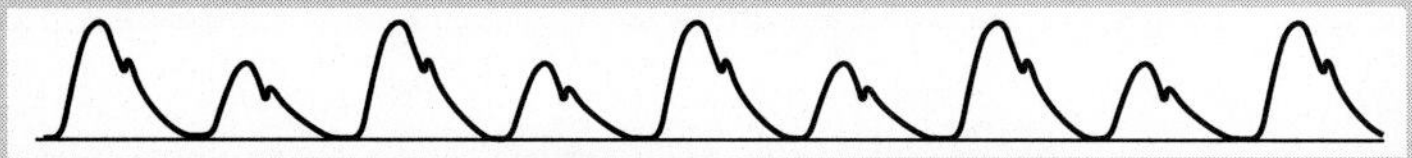 **Pulsus Alternans.** Rhythm is regular but force varies with alternating beats of large and small amplitude.	Left-sided congestive heart failure.
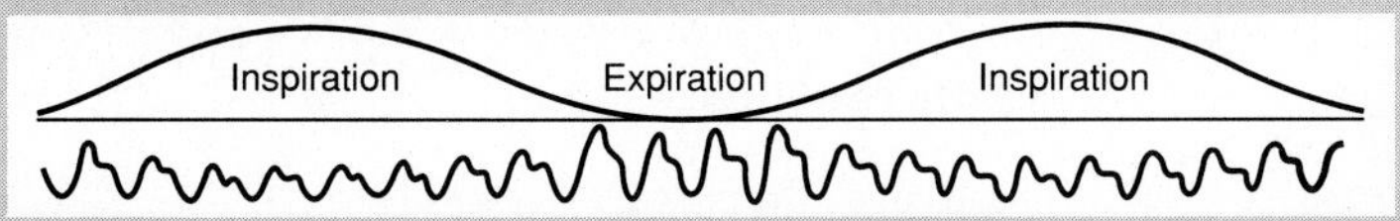 **Pulsus Paradoxus.** Beats have weaker amplitude with inspiration, stronger with expiration. Best determined during blood pressure measurement; reading decreases (>10 mm Hg) during inspiration and increases with expiration.	Cardiac tamponade; constrictive pericarditis.
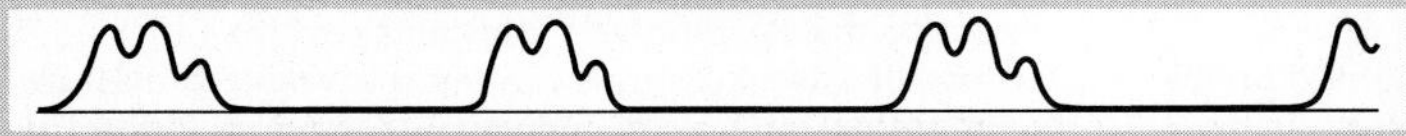 **Pulsus Bisferiens.** Each pulse has two strong systolic peaks, with a dip in between. Best assessed at the carotid artery.	Aortic valve stenosis plus regurgitation.

Table 18-2 ▸ Peripheral Vascular Disease in the Arms

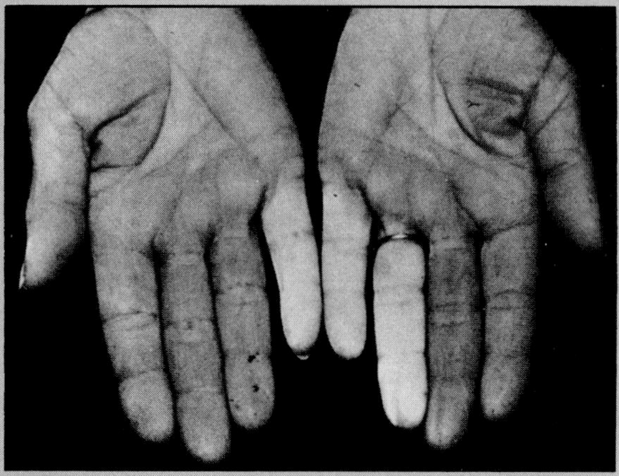

RAYNAUD'S DISEASE OR PHENOMENON

Episodes of abrupt color changes in fingers due to vasospasm: white (pallor) from arteriospasm and resulting deficit in supply; then blue (cyanosis) due to increased oxygen extraction from hemoglobin; then red (rubor) due to return of blood or reactive hyperemia. May have cold, numbness, or pain along with pallor or cyanosis stage; then burning, throbbing pain, swelling along with rubor. Lasts minutes to hours; occurs bilaterally.

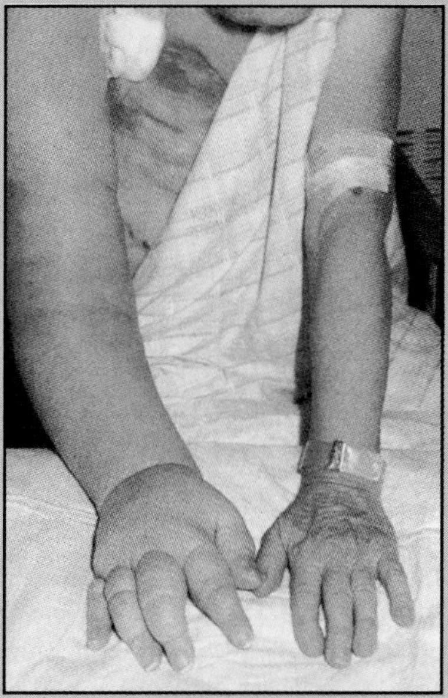

LYMPHEDEMA

Unilateral arm swelling from obstructed lymph channels, acquired condition from removal of axillary nodes with radical mastectomy. Overlying skin is indurated and lymphedema is nonpitting.

Table 18-3 ▸ History Profiles of Pain of Peripheral Vascular Disease

SYMPTOM ANALYSIS	CHRONIC ARTERIAL SYMPTOMS	ACUTE ARTERIAL SYMPTOMS
Location	Deep muscle pain, usually in calf, may be lower leg or dorsum of foot	Varies, distal to occlusion, may involve entire leg
Character	Intermittent claudication, feels like "cramp," "numbness and tingling," "feeling of cold"	Throbbing
Onset and duration	Chronic pain, onset gradual following exertion	Sudden onset (within 1 hour)
Aggravating factors	Activity (walking, stairs) "Claudication distance" is specific number of blocks, stairs it takes to produce pain. Elevation (Rest pain indicates severe involvement)	
Relieving factors	Rest (usually within 2 minutes) (e.g., standing) Dangling (severe involvement)	
Associated symptoms	Cool pale skin	6 Ps: pain, pallor, pulselessness, paresthesia, poikilothermia (coldness), paralysis (indicates severe)
Those at risk	Older adults, more males than females, inherited predisposition, history of hypertension, smoking, diabetes, hypercholesterolemia, obesity, vascular disease	History of vascular surgery, arterial invasive procedure, abdominal aneurysm (emboli), trauma including injured arteries, chronic atrial fibrillation

Table 18-3 ► History Profiles of Pain of Peripheral Vascular Disease *Continued*

	CHRONIC VENOUS SYMPTOMS	ACUTE VENOUS SYMPTOMS
Location	Calf, lower leg	Calf
Character	Aching, tiredness, feeling of fullness	Intense, sharp; deep muscle tender to touch
Onset and duration	Chronic pain, increases at end of day	Sudden onset (within 1 hour)
Aggravating factors	Prolonged standing, sitting	Pain may increase with sharp dorsiflexion of foot
Relieving factors	Elevation, lying, walking	
Associated symptoms	Edema, varicosities, weeping ulcers at ankles	Red, warm, swollen leg
Those at risk	Job with prolonged standing, sitting, obesity, pregnancy, prolonged bedrest, history of congestive heart failure, varicosities, or thrombophlebitis, veins crushed by trauma or surgery	

Table 18-4 ► Peripheral Vascular Disease in the Legs

CHRONIC ARTERIAL INSUFFICIENCY

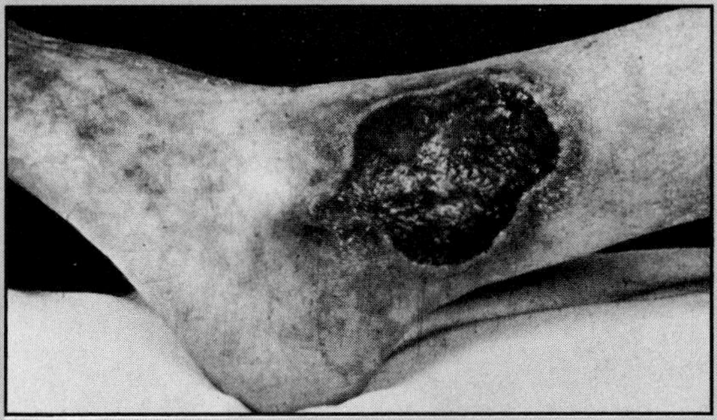

Ischemic Ulcer at Lateral Ankle + Mostly on toes

Build-up of fatty plaques on intima (atherosclerosis) plus calcification of arterial wall (arteriosclerosis).

S: See history profiles, p 658.

O: Coolness, pallor, elevational pallor, and dependent rubor; diminished pulses; signs of malnutrition (thin shiny skin, thick ridged nails, absence of hair). Ulcers occur at toes, metatarsal heads, heels, lateral malleolus, and are characterized by pale ischemic base, well-defined edges, and no bleeding.

Peripheral Vascular Disease Due to Diabetes Mellitus

Diabetes hastens changes described above, with generalized dysfunction in all arterial areas: peripheral, coronary, cerebral, retina, kidney. Peripheral involvement is associated with diabetic neuropathy and local infection.

CHRONIC VENOUS INSUFFICIENCY

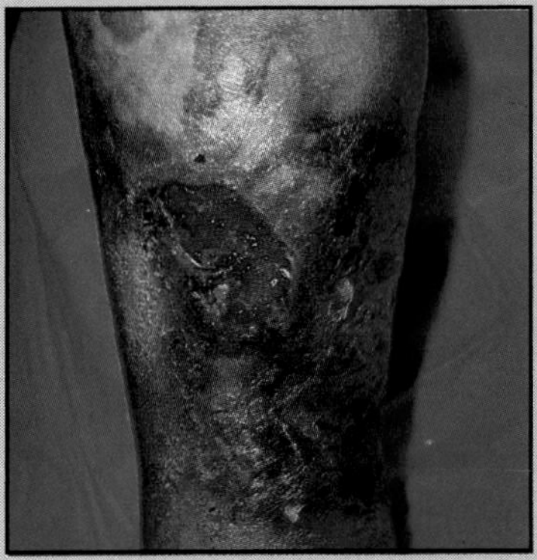

Stasis Ulcer

Following acute deep vein thrombosis, or chronic incompetent valves in deep veins.

S: See history profiles, on this page.

O: Firm brawny edema, coarse thickened skin, pulses normal, brown discoloration, petechiae, dermatitis.

Ulcers occur at medial malleolus and are characterized by bleeding, uneven edges.

on inside Ankle

Table continued on following page

Table 18-4 ▸ Peripheral Vascular Disease in the Legs *Continued*

CHRONIC VENOUS

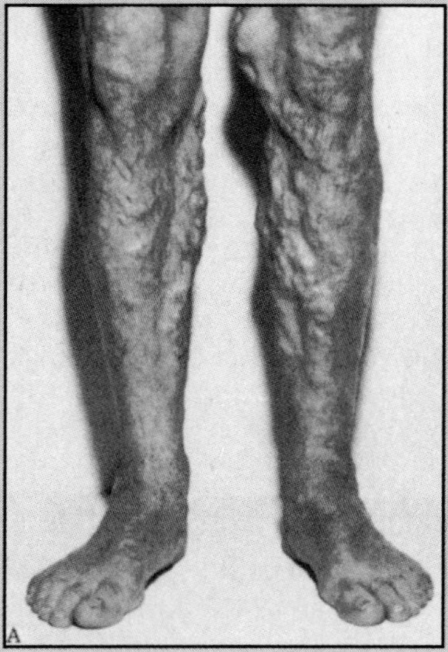

Superficial Varicose Veins

Incompetent valves permit reflux of blood, producing dilated, tortuous veins. Unremitting hydrostatic pressure causes distal valves to be incompetent and worsening of the varicosity.

S: Aching, heaviness in calf, easy fatigability, night leg or foot cramps.

O: Dilated, tortuous veins

ACUTE VENOUS

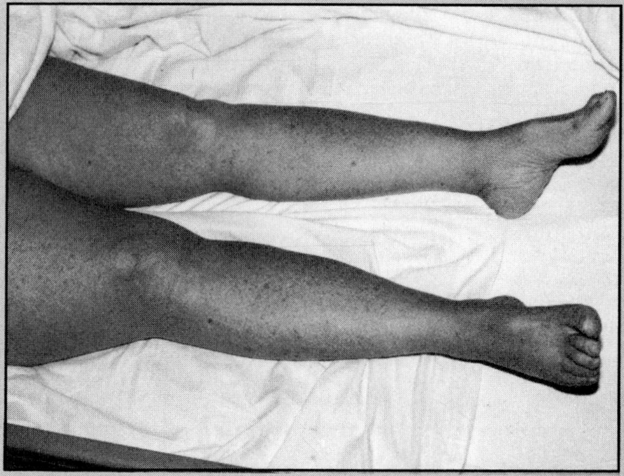

Deep Vein Thrombosis

S: See history profiles, p 659.

O: Increased warmth; swelling; redness; dependent cyanosis is mild or may be absent; tender to palpation; Homan's sign present only in few cases.

Requires emergency referral due to risk of pulmonary embolism.

Bibliography

Baum PL: Heed the early warning signs of peripheral vascular disease. Nursing 85 15:50–57, 1985.

Birdsall C: How do you interpret pulses? Am J Nurs 85(7):785–786, 1985.

Fahey VA: Vascular Nursing. Philadelphia: WB Saunders, 1988.

Gage AM, Gage AA: Evaluation and treatment of varicose veins. Hosp Med 23(9):93–120, 1987.

Haimovici H: The peripheral vascular system. *In* Rossman I (Ed): Clinical Geriatrics. 3rd ed. Philadelphia, JB Lippincott, 1986.

Herman J: Nursing assessment and nursing diagnosis in patients with peripheral vascular disease. Nurs Clin N Am 21(2):219–231, 1986.

Johnson TR, Moore WM, Jeffries JE: Children Are Different: Developmental Physiology. 2nd ed. Columbus, Ohio: Ross Labs, 1978.

Massey JA: Diagnostic testing for peripheral vascular disease. Nurs Clin N Am 21(2):207–217, 1986.

Mathewson M: Fact or myth: A Homan's sign is an effective method of diagnosing thrombophlebitis in bedridden patients . . . fact or myth? Crit Care Nurs 4:64, 1983.

Nardone DA, McAfee JH: Causes of peripheral edema. Hosp Med 23(9):162–179, 1987.

Peterson FY: Assessing peripheral vascular disease at the bedside. Am J Nurs 83:1549–1551, 1983.

CHAPTER

19 Musculoskeletal System

STRUCTURE AND FUNCTION

The musculoskeletal system consists of the body's bones, joints, and muscles. Humans need this system for *support* to stand erect and for *movement.* The musculoskeletal system also functions to encase and *protect* the inner vital organs (e.g., brain, spinal cord, heart), to *produce* the red blood cells in the bone marrow (hematopoiesis), and for *storage* of minerals, such as calcium and phosphorus in the bones.

COMPONENTS OF THE MUSCULOSKELETAL SYSTEM

The skeleton is the bony framework of the body. It has 206 bones, which support the body, like the posts and beams of a building. The joint (or articulation) is the place of union of two or more bones. Joints are the functional units of the musculoskeletal system because they permit the mobility needed for activities of daily living.

Joints can be nonsynovial or synovial. In *nonsynovial* joints, the bones are united by fibrous tissue or cartilage, and are immovable (e.g., sutures in the skull) or only slightly movable (e.g., the vertebrae). *Synovial* joints are freely movable because they have bones that are separated from each other and are enclosed in a joint cavity (Fig. 19–1). This cavity is filled with a lubricant, or synovial fluid. Just like grease on gears, synovial fluid allows sliding of opposing surfaces, and this sliding permits movement.

In synovial joints, a layer of resilient *cartilage* covers the surface of opposing bones. This cartilage cushions the bones and gives a smooth surface to facilitate movement. The joint is surrounded by a fibrous capsule and is supported by ligaments. *Ligaments* are fibrous bands running directly from one bone to another that strengthen the joint and help prevent movement in undesirable directions. A *bursa* is an enclosed sac filled with viscous synovial fluid, much like a joint. Bursae are located in areas of potential friction (e.g., subacromial

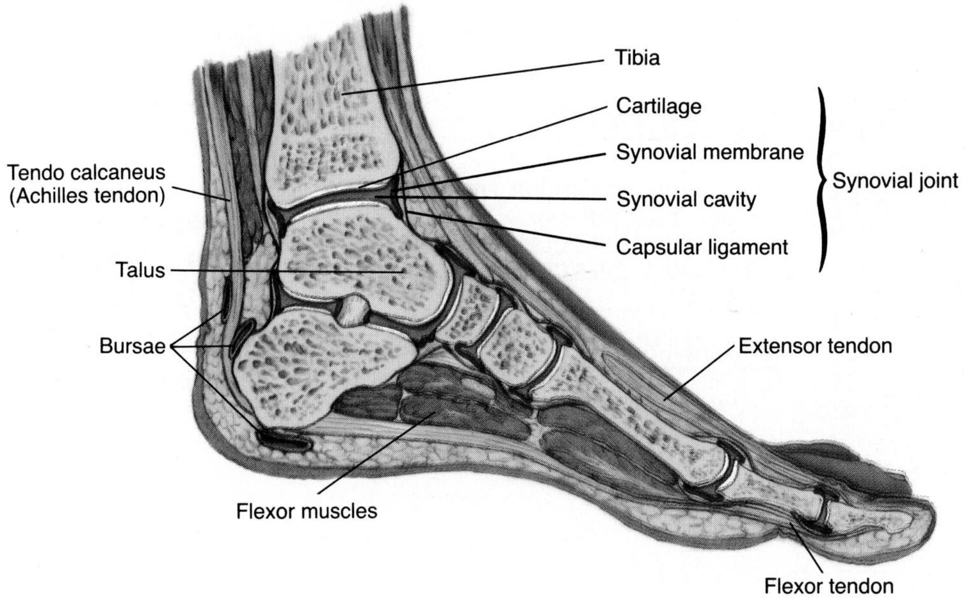

► **Figure 19–1**

bursa of the shoulder, prepatellar bursa of the knee) and help muscles and tendons glide smoothly over bone.

Muscles account for 40 to 50 percent of the body's weight. When they contract, they produce movement. Muscles are of three types: skeletal, smooth, and cardiac. This chapter is concerned with skeletal or voluntary muscles, those under conscious control.

Each skeletal muscle is composed of bundles of muscle fibers, or *fasciculi.* The skeletal muscle is attached to bone by a *tendon*—a strong fibrous cord. Skeletal muscles produce the following movements (Fig. 19–2):

1. flexion—bending a limb at a joint
2. extension—straightening a limb at a joint
3. abduction—moving a limb away from the midline of the body
4. adduction—moving a limb toward the midline of the body
5. pronation—turning the forearm so that the palm is down
6. supination—turning the forearm so that the palm is up
7. circumduction—moving the arm in a circle around the shoulder
8. inversion—moving the sole of the foot inward at the ankle
9. eversion—moving the sole of the foot outward at the ankle
10. rotation—moving the head around a central axis
11. protraction—moving a body part forward and parallel to the ground
12. retraction—moving a body part backward and parallel to the ground
13. elevation—raising a body part
14. depression—lowering a body part

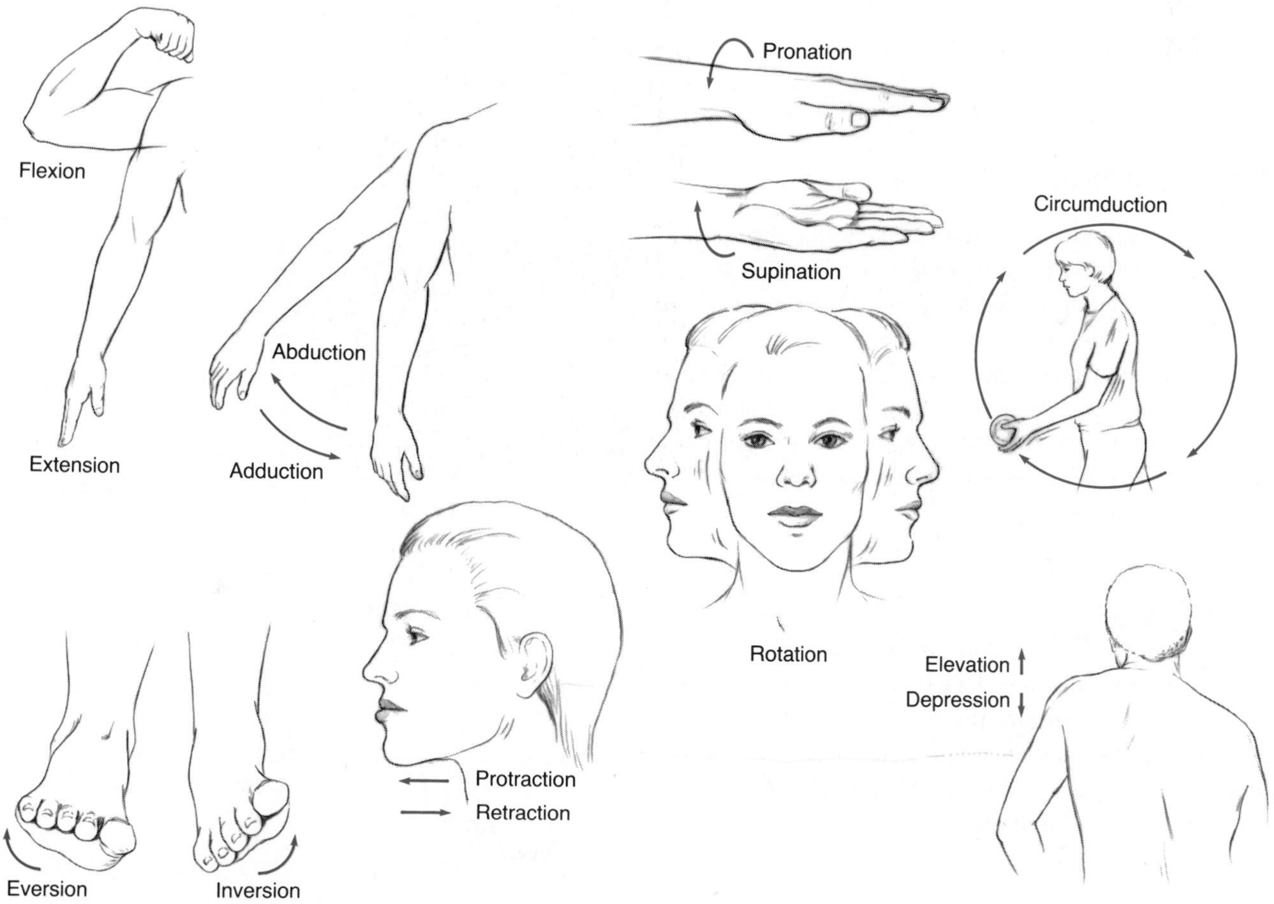

► **Figure 19–2**

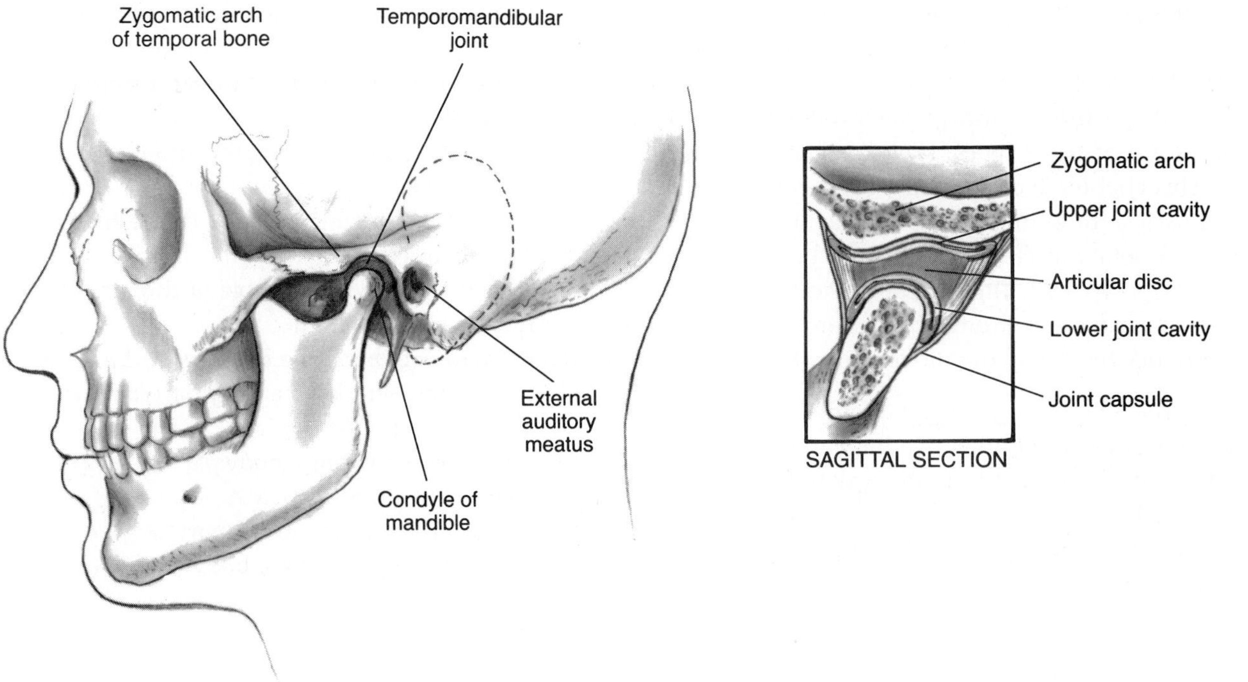

► **Figure 19–3**

Temporomandibular Joint

The temporomandibular joint (TMJ) is the articulation of the mandible and the temporal bone (Fig. 19–3). You can feel it in the depression anterior to the tragus of the ear. The temporomandibular joint permits jaw function for speaking and chewing. The joint allows three motions: (1) hinge action to open and close the jaws, (2) gliding action for protrusion and retraction, and (3) gliding for side to side movement of the lower jaw.

Spine

The vertebrae are 33 connecting bones stacked in a vertical column (Fig. 19–4). You can feel their spinous processes in a furrow down the midline of the back. The furrow has paravertebral muscles mounded on either side down to the sacrum, where it flattens. There are 7 cervical, 12 thoracic, 5 lumbar, 5 sacral, and 3 to 4 coccygeal vertebrae. The following surface landmarks will orient you to their levels:

- The spinous processes of C7 and T1 are prominent at the base of the neck.
- The inferior angle of the scapula normally is at the level of the interspace between T7 and T8.
- An imaginary line connecting the highest point on each iliac crest crosses L4.

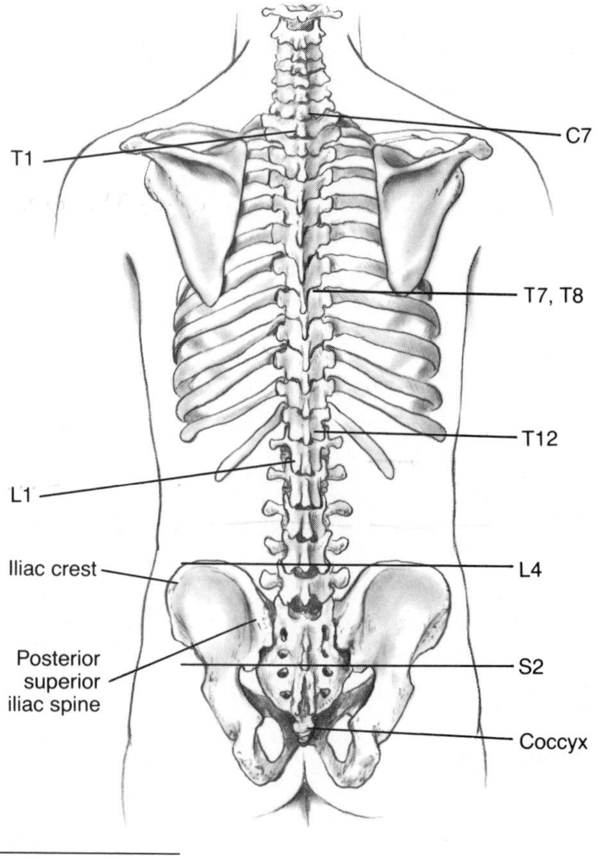

► **Figure 19–4**

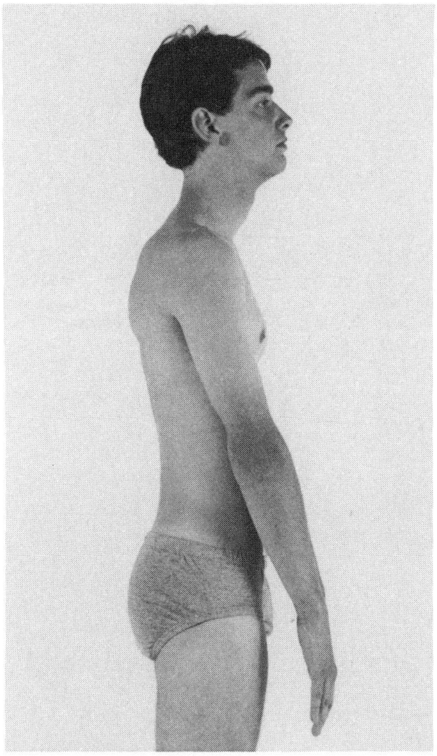

► Figure 19-5

- An imaginary line joining the two symmetric dimples that overlie the posterior superior iliac spines crosses S2.

A lateral view shows that the vertebral column has four curves (a double S shape) (Fig. 19-5). The cervical and lumbar curves are concave (inward), and the thoracic and sacrococcygeal curves are convex. The balanced or compensatory nature of these curves, together with the resilient intervertebral discs, allows the spine to absorb a great deal of shock.

The *intervertebral discs* are elastic fibrocartilaginous plates that constitute one-quarter the length of the column (Fig. 19-6). Each disc center has a *nucleus pulposus,* made of soft mucoid material. The discs cushion the spine like a shock absorber and help it move. As the spine moves, the elasticity of the discs allows compression on one side, with compensatory expansion on the other.

The unique structure of the spine enables both upright posture and flexibility for motion. The motions of the vertebral column are flexion (bending forward), extension (bending back), abduction (to either side), and rotation.

Upper Extremity

Shoulder

The *glenohumoral joint* is the articulation of the humerus with the glenoid fossa of the scapula (Fig. 19-7). Its ball and socket action allows great mobility of the arm on many axes. The joint is enclosed by a group of four powerful muscles and tendons that support and stabilize it. Together these are called the *rotator cuff* of the shoulder. The large *subacromial bursa* helps during abduction of the arm, so that the greater tubercle of the humerus moves easily under the acromion process of the scapula.

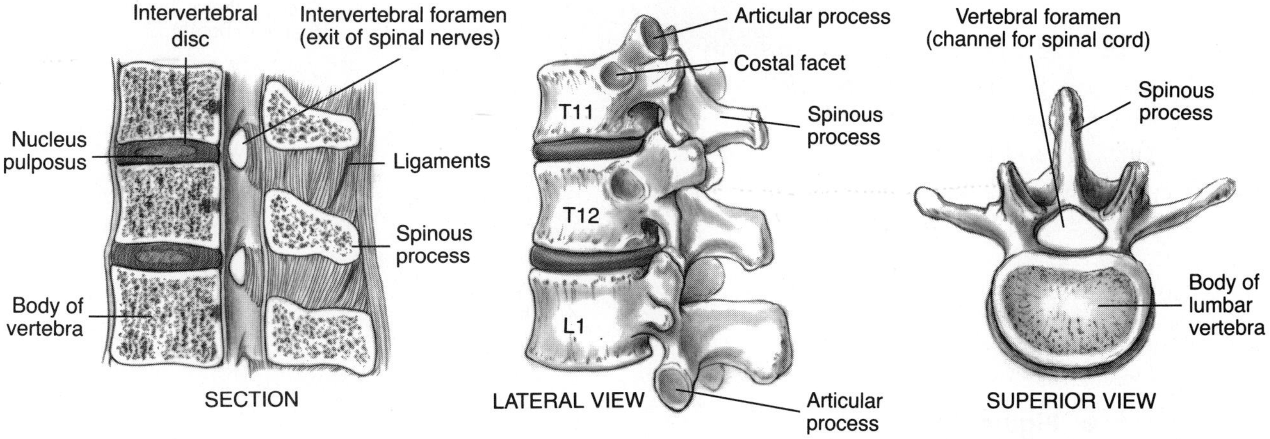

► Figure 19-6

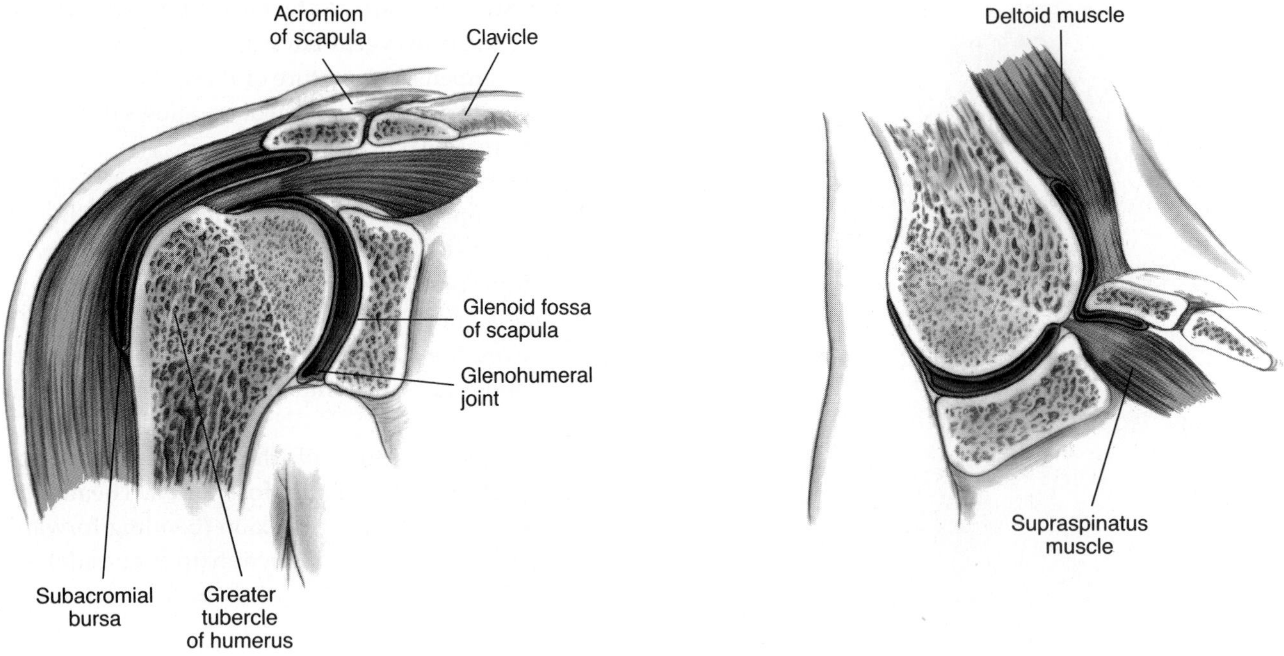

► **Figure 19–7**

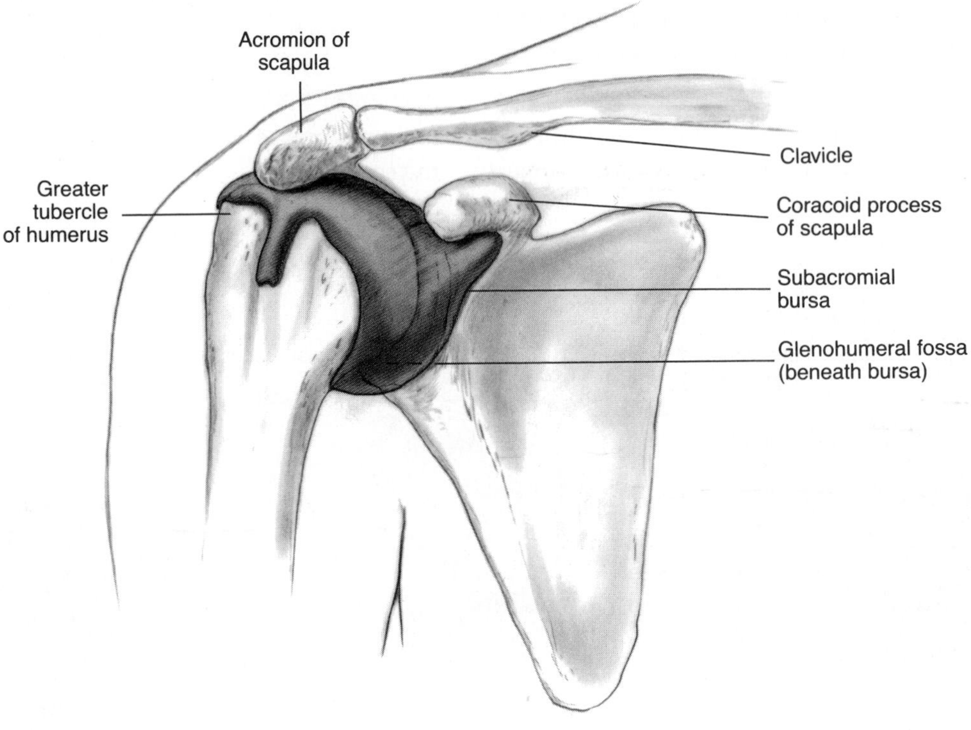

► **Figure 19–8**

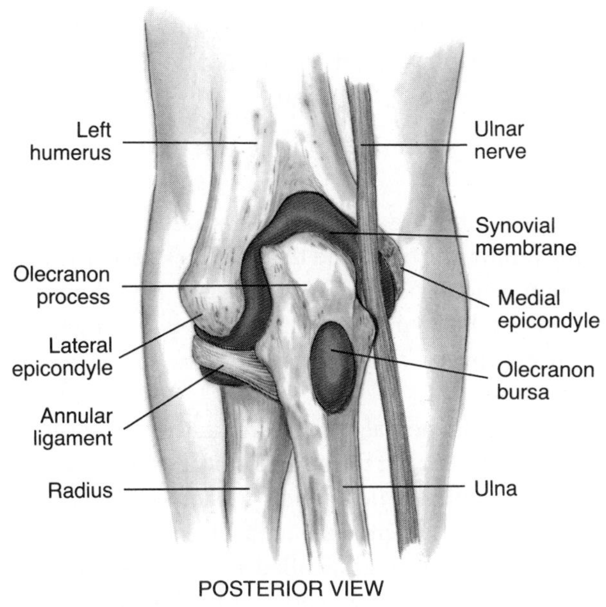

► **Figure 19-9**

The bones of the shoulder have palpable landmarks to guide your examination (Fig. 19-8). The scapula and the clavicle connect to form the shoulder girdle. You can feel the bump of the scapula's *acromion process* at the very top of the shoulder. Move your fingers in a small circle outward, down, and around. The next bump is the *greater tubercle* of the humerus a few centimeters down and laterally, and from that the *coracoid process* of the scapula is a few centimeters medially. These surround the deeply situated joint.

Elbow

The elbow joint contains the three bony articulations of the humerus, radius, and ulna of the forearm (Fig. 19-9). Its hinge action moves the forearm (radius and ulna) on one plane, allowing flexion and extension. The olecranon bursa lies between the olecranon process and the skin.

Palpable landmarks are the medial and lateral epicondyles of the humerus, and the large olecranon process of the ulna in between them. The sensitive ulnar nerve runs between the olecranon process and the medial epicondyle.

The radius and ulna articulate with each other at two radioulnar joints, one at the elbow and one at the wrist. These move together to permit pronation and supination of the hand and forearm.

Wrist and Carpals

The wrist or *radiocarpal joint* is the articulation of the radius (on the thumb side) and a row of carpal bones (Fig. 19-10). Its condyloid action permits movement in two planes at right angles: flexion and extension, and side to side deviation. You can feel the groove of this joint on the dorsum on the wrist.

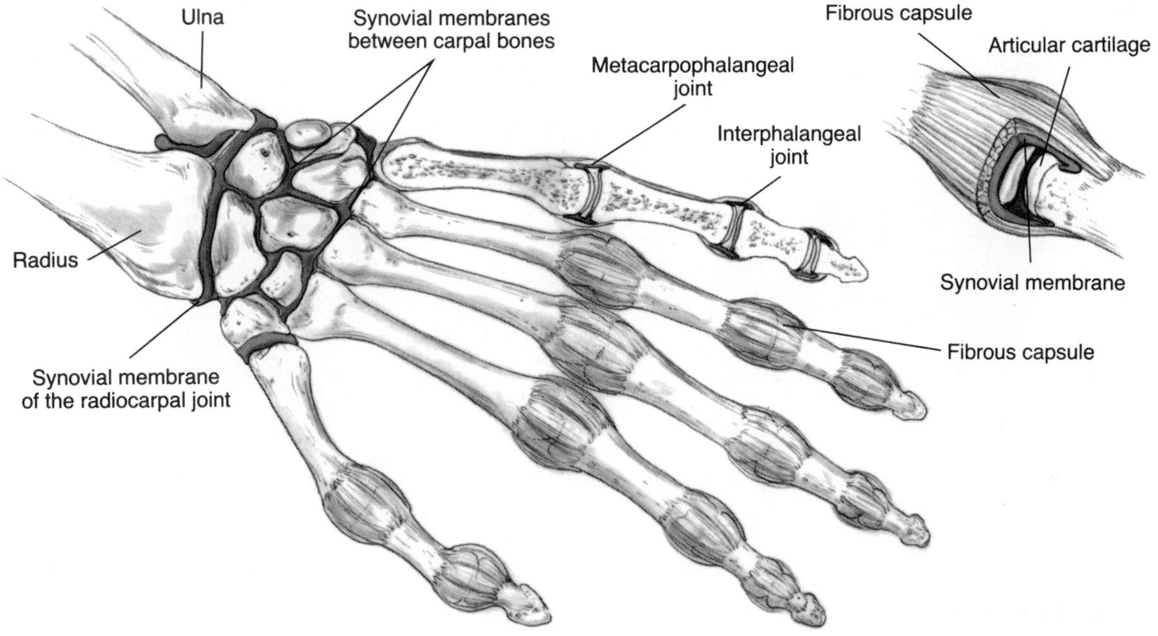

► **Figure 19-10**

The *midcarpal* joint is the articulation between the two parallel rows of carpal bones. It allows flexion, extension, and some rotation. The *metacarpophalangeal* and the *interphalangeal* joints permit finger flexion and extension. The flexor tendons of the wrist and hand are enclosed in synovial sheaths.

Lower Extremity

Hip

The hip joint is the articulation between the acetabulum and the head of the femur (Fig. 19–11). Like the shoulder, its ball and socket action permits a wide range of motion on many axes. The hip has somewhat less range of motion (ROM) than the shoulder, but it has more stability as befits its weight-bearing function. Hip stability is due to powerful muscles that spread over the joint, a strong fibrous articular capsule, and the very deep insertion of the head of the femur. Three bursae facilitate movement.

Palpation of these bony landmarks will guide your examination. You can feel the entire iliac crest, from the *anterior superior iliac* spine to the posterior. The *ischial tuberosity* lies under the gluteus maximus muscle, and is palpable when the hip is flexed. The *greater trochanter* of the femur is normally the width of the person's palm below the iliac crest, and halfway between the anterior superior iliac spine and the ischial tuberiosity. Feel it when the person is standing, in a flat depression on the upper lateral side of the thigh.

Knee

The knee joint is the articulation of three bones, including the femur, the tibia, and the patella (kneecap), in one common articular cavity (Fig. 19–12). It is the largest joint in the body and is complex. It is a hinge joint, permitting flexion and extension of the lower leg on a single plane.

The knee's synovial membrane is the largest in the body. It forms a sac at the superior border of the patella, called the *suprapatellar pouch,* which extends up as much as 6 cm behind the quadriceps muscle. Two wedge-shaped cartilages, called the *medial* and *lateral menisci,* cushion the tibia and femur. The joint is stabilized by two sets of ligaments. The *cruciate ligaments* (not shown) crisscross within the knee; they give anterior and posterior stability and help control rotation. The *collateral ligaments* connect the joint at both sides; they give medial and lateral stability and prevent dislocation. Numerous bursae prevent friction. One, the *prepatellar bursa,* lies between the patella and the skin. The *infrapatellar fat pad* is a small, triangular fat pad below the patella and behind the patellar ligament.

Landmarks of the knee joint start with the large *quad-*

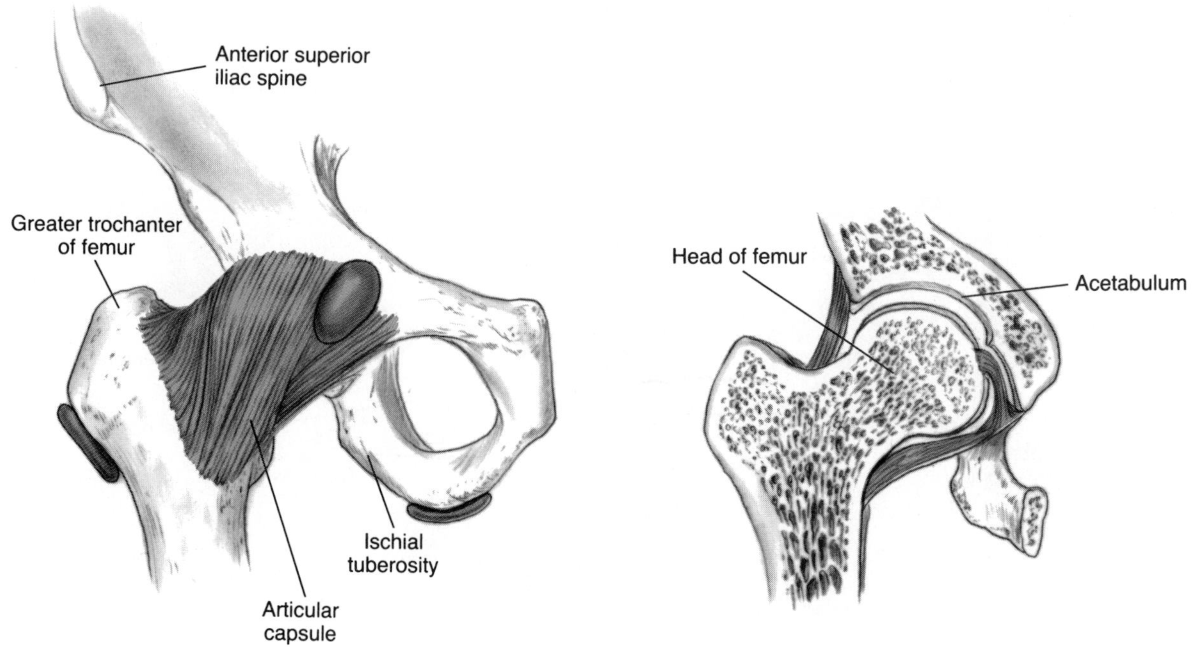

► **Figure 19–11**

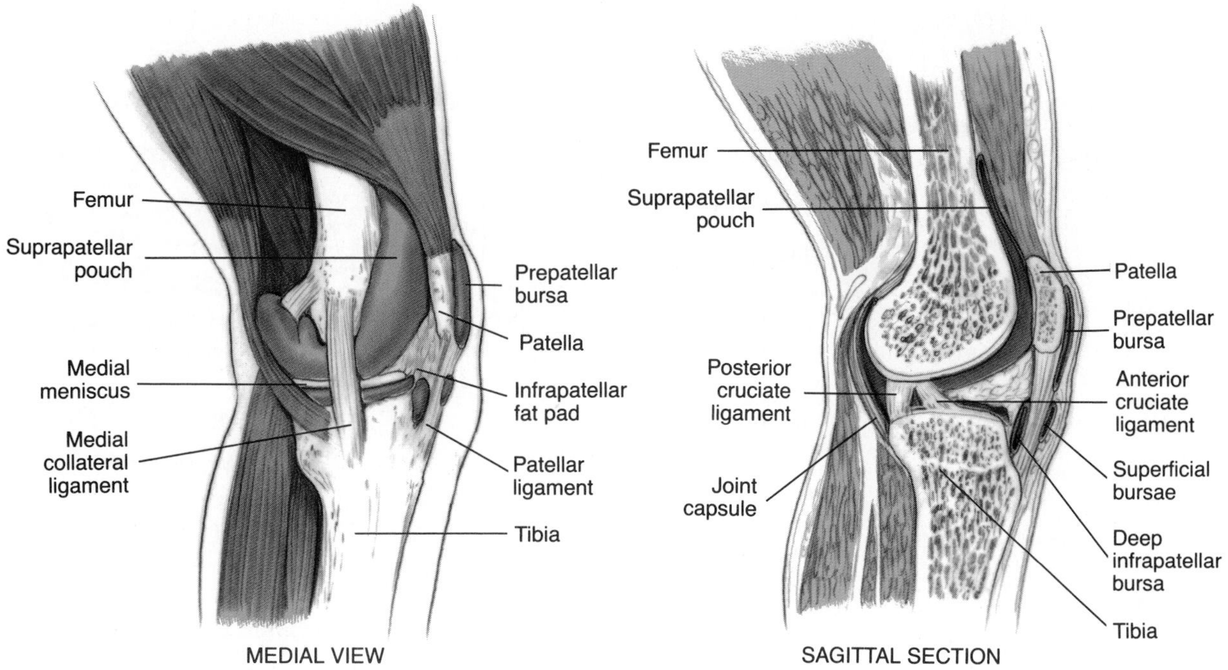

► **Figure 19 – 12**

riceps muscle, which you can feel on your anterior and lateral thigh (Fig. 19 – 13). The muscle's four heads merge into a common tendon that continues down to enclose the round bony patella. Then the tendon inserts down on the *tibial tuberosity,* which is felt as a bony prominence in the midline. Move to the sides and a bit superiorly and note the lateral and medial condyles of the tibia. Superior to those on either side of the patella are the medial and lateral epicondyles of the femur.

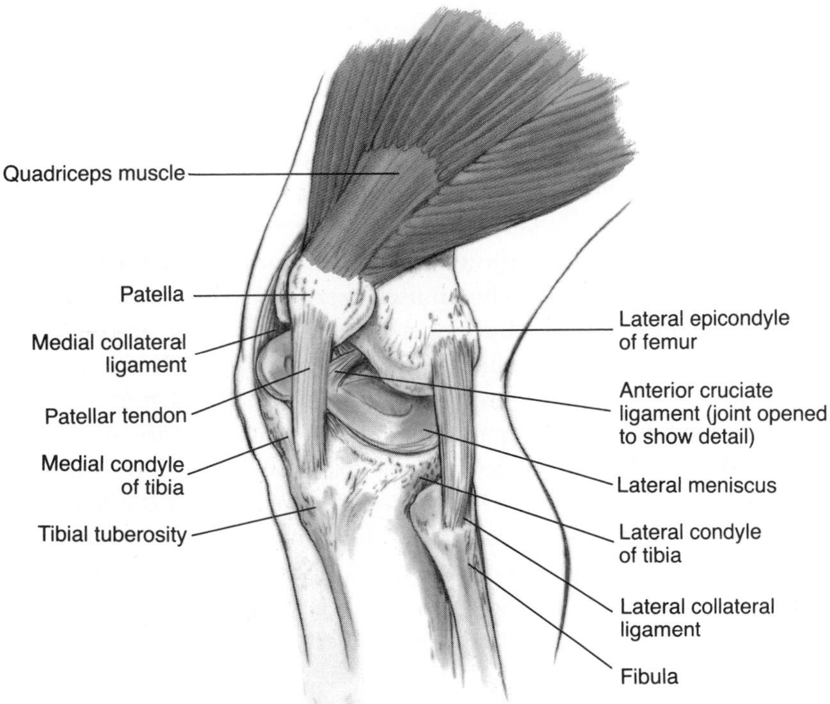

► **Figure 19 – 13**

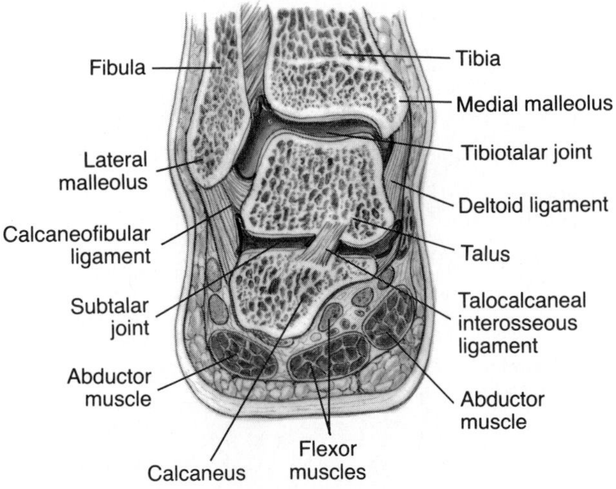

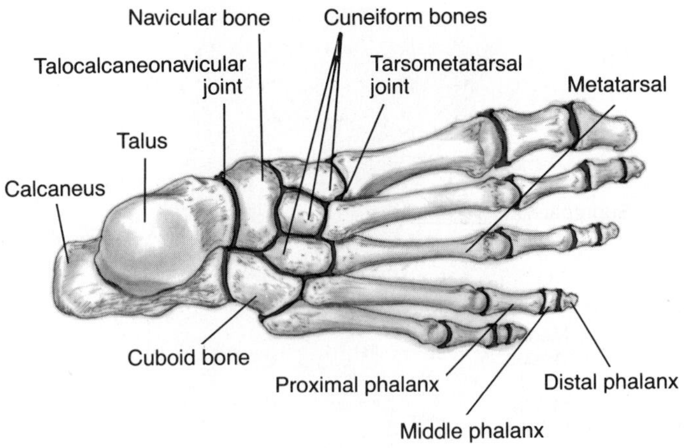

▶ **Figure 19-14**

Ankle and Foot

The ankle or *tibiotalar joint* is the articulation of the tibia, fibula, and talus (Fig. 19-14). It is a hinge joint, limited to flexion (dorsiflexion) and extension (plantar flexion) on one plane. Landmarks are two bony prominences on either side—the *medial malleolus* and the *lateral malleolus.* Strong tight medial and lateral ligaments extend from each malleolus onto the foot. These help the lateral stability of the ankle joint, although they may be torn in eversion or inversion sprains of the ankle.

Joints distal to the ankle give additional mobility to the foot. The subtalar joint permits inversion and eversion of the foot. The foot has a longitudinal arch with weight-bearing distributed between the parts that touch the ground—the heads of the metatarsals and the calcaneus (heel).

DEVELOPMENTAL CONSIDERATIONS

Infants and Children

By 3 months' gestation, the fetus has formed a "scale model" of the skeleton made up of cartilage. During succeeding months in utero, the cartilage ossifies into true bone and starts to grow. Bone growth continues after birth—rapidly during infancy and then steadily during childhood—until adolescence, when both boys and girls experience a rapid growth spurt.

Long bones grow in two dimensions. They increase in width or diameter by deposition of new bony tissue around the shafts. Lengthening occurs at the *epiphyses,* or growth plates. These specialized growth centers are transverse discs located at the ends of long bone. Any trauma or infection at this location puts the growing child at risk for bone deformity. This longitudinal growth continues until closure of the epiphyses; the last closure occurs at about age 20.

Skeletal contour changes are apparent at the vertebral column. At birth, the spine has a single C-shaped curve. At 3-4 months, raising of the head from prone position develops the anterior curve in the cervical neck region. From 1 year to 18 months, standing erect develops the anterior curve in the lumbar region.

Whereas the skeleton contributes to linear growth, muscles and fat are significant for weight increase. Individual muscle fibers grow through childhood, but growth is marked during the adolescent growth spurt. Then muscles respond to increased secretion of growth hormone, adrenal androgens, and in boys, to further stimulation by testosterone. Muscles vary in size and strength in different people. This is due to genetic programming, nutrition, and exercise. All through life, muscles increase with use and atrophy with disuse.

Fat accumulates rapidly for the first 6 months, then the infant "slims down" after 1 year of age. Fat accumulates again at 6 to 8 years, but this time more slowly. The first signs of obesity may show at this age in some children. Until puberty, boys and girls have the same accumulation and distribution of fat. During the adolescent growth spurt in boys, the amount of fat decreases because body energy focuses on bone and muscle. Fat accumulation does not reappear until early adulthood. In girls, fat accumulation continues at adolescence but the distribution shifts to the mature female shape.

The Pregnant Female

Increased levels of circulating hormones (estrogen, relaxin from the corpus luteum, and corticosteroids) presumably cause increased mobility in the joints. Increased mobility in the sacroiliac, sacrococcygeal, and symphysis pubis joints in the pelvis may contribute to the noticeable changes in maternal posture. The most characteristic change in posture is progressive *lordosis.* Lordosis compensates for the enlarging fetus, which would shift the center of balance forward. Lordosis compensates by shifting the weight farther back on the lower extremities. This shift in balance in turn creates strain on the low back muscles, felt as low back pain during late pregnancy in some women.

Anterior flexion of the neck and slumping of the shoulder girdle are other postural changes that compensate for the lordosis. These upper back changes may put pressure on the ulnar and median nerves during the third trimester. Nerve pressure creates aching, numbness, and weakness in the upper extremities in some women.

The Aging Adult

With aging, loss of bone matrix (resorption) occurs more rapidly than new bone growth (deposition). The net effect is a loss of bone density, or *osteoporosis.* Although some degree of osteoporosis is nearly universal, females experience it more than males, and whites more than blacks.

Postural changes are evident with aging, and decreased height is the most noticeable. Long bones do not shorten with age. Decreased height is due to shortening of the vertebral column. This is caused by thinning of the intervertebral discs, which occurs more in the middle years, and a decrease in height of individual vertebrae, which occurs in later years from osteoporosis. Both men and women can expect a progressive decrease averaging 2 inches in the 50-year span from 20s through 70s (Rossman, 1986). There is a greater decrease in the 8th and 9th decades owing to osteoporotic collapse of the vertebrae. The result is a shortening of the trunk and comparatively long extremities. Other postural changes are kyphosis, and a backward head tilt to compensate for kyphosis, and a slight flexion of hips and knees.

The distribution of subcutaneous fat changes through life. Usually, men and women gain weight in their 40s and 50s. The contour is different, even if the weight is the same as when younger. They begin to lose fat in the face and deposit it in abdomen and hips. In the 80s and 90s, fat further decreases in periphery, especially noticeable in the forearms, although it is still apparent over the abdomen and hips.

Loss of subcutaneous fat leaves bony prominences more marked (e.g., tips of vertebrae, ribs, iliac crests), and body hollows deeper (e.g., cheeks, axillae). There is an absolute loss in muscle mass; some muscles decrease in size and some atrophy, producing weakness. The contour of muscles becomes more prominent, and muscle bundles and tendons feel more distinct.

It has become more apparent that lifestyle affects musculoskeletal changes. A sedentary lifestyle hastens musculoskeletal changes of aging. However, physical exercise increases skeletal mass. This helps prevent or delay osteoporosis. Physical activity delays or prevents bone loss in postmenopausal and older women (Spencer et al, 1986).

TRANSCULTURAL CONSIDERATIONS

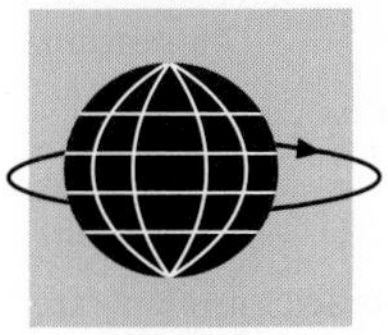

The long bones of blacks are significantly longer, narrower, and denser than those of whites (Farrally and Moore, 1975). Bone density measured by race and sex reveal that black males have the densest bones, thus accounting for the relatively low incidence of osteoporosis in this population. Bone density in the Chinese, Japanese, and Eskimos is below that of white Americans (Garn, 1964).

Curvature of the long bones varies widely among culturally diverse groups. Native Americans have anteriorly convex femurs, blacks have markedly straight femurs, and in whites the femoral curvature is intermediate. This characteristic is related to both genetics and body weight. Thin blacks and whites have less curvature than average, whereas obese blacks and whites display increased curvatures. It is possible that the heavier density of the bones of blacks helps to protect them from increased curvature due to obesity.

Table 19–1 summarizes reported biocultural variations occurring in the musculoskeletal system.

Table 19–1 ▶ Biocultural Variations in the Musculoskeletal System

	VARIATIONS
Bone	
Frontal	Thicker in black males than in white males
Parietal occiput	Thicker in white males than in black males
Palate	Tori (protuberances) along the suture line of the hard palate
	Problematic for denture wearers
	Incidence:
	Blacks — 20 percent
	Whites — 24 percent
	Asians — Up to 50 percent
	Native Americans — Up to 50 percent
Mandible	Tori (protuberances) on the lingual surface of the mandible near the canine and premolar teeth
	Problematic for denture wearers
	Most common in Asians and Native Americans; incidence exceeds 50 percent in some Eskimo groups
Humerus	Torsion or rotation of proximal end with muscle pull
	Whites have a greater incidence than blacks
	Torsion in blacks is symmetric; torsion in whites greater on the right side than on the left side
Radius	Length at the wrist variable
Ulna	Ulna or radius may be longer
	Equal length
	Swedes — 61 percent
	Chinese — 16 percent
	Ulna longer than radius
	Swedes — 16 percent
	Chinese — 48 percent
	Radius longer than ulna
	Swedes — 23 percent
	Chinese — 10 percent
Vertebrae	24 vertebrae (cervical, thoracic, lumbar) are found in 85 to 93 percent of all people. Racial and sex differences reveal 23 or 25 vertebrae in select groups
	Vertebrae — Population
	23 — 11 percent of black females
	25 — 12 percent of Eskimo and Native American males
	Increased number is related to lower back pain and lordosis
Pelvis	Hip width is 1.6 cm (0.6 in) smaller in black women than in white women; Asian women have significantly smaller pelvises
Femur	Curvature — Population
	Convex anterior — Native American
	Straight — Black
	Intermediate — White
Second tarsal	Second toe longer than the great toe
	Incidence:
	Whites — 8 to 34 percent
	Blacks — 8 to 12 percent
	Vietnamese — 31 percent
	Melanesians — 21 to 57 percent
	Clinical significance for joggers and athletes, who reported increased foot problems

Table 19-1 ▶ Biocultural Variations in the Musculoskeletal System *Continued*

	VARIATIONS
Height	White males are 1.27 cm (0.5 in) taller than black males and 7.6 cm (2.9 in) taller than Asian males White females have the same height as black females Asian females are 4.14 cm (1.6 in) shorter than white or black females
Composition of long bones	Longer, narrower, and denser in blacks than whites; bone density in whites is greater than in Chinese, Japanese, and Eskimos Osteoporosis incidence is lowest in black males; highest in white females
Muscle	
Peroneus tertius	Responsible for dorsiflexion of foot Muscle absent: Asians, Native Americans, and whites — 3 to 10 percent Blacks — 10 to 15 percent Berbers (Sahara desert) — 24 percent No clinical significance because the tibialis anterior also dorsiflexes the foot
Palmaris longus	Responsible for wrist flexion Muscle absent: Whites — 12 to 20 percent Native Americans — 2 to 12 percent Blacks — 5 percent Asians — 3 percent No clinical significance because three other muscles are also responsible for flexion

(Table based on data reported by: Overfield T: Biologic Variation in Health and Illness: Race, Age, and Sex Differences. Menlo Park, CA, Addison Wesley Publishing; Boyle JS, Andrews MM (Eds): Transcultural Concepts in Nursing Care. Glenview, IL, Scott, Foresman & Co., 1989.)

SUBJECTIVE DATA

Joints
- pain
- stiffness
- swelling, heat
- limitation of movement

Muscles
- pain (cramps)
- weakness

Bones
- pain
- deformity
- trauma (fractures, sprains, dislocations)

Functional assessment (ADL)

Self-care behaviors

EXAMINER ASKS:	RATIONALE:
1. Do you have any problems with your joints? Any pain?	**Joint pain** and loss of function are the most common musculoskeletal concerns that prompt a person to seek care.
What is the location—which joints? Is it on one side or both sides?	Rheumatoid arthritis (RA) involves symmetric joints; other musculoskeletal illnesses involve isolated or unilateral joints.
Quality—what does the pain feel like: aching, stiff, sharp or dull, shooting? Severity—how strong is the pain?	Exquisitely tender with acute inflammation.
Onset—when did this pain start?	
Timing—what time of day does the pain occur? How long does it last? How often does it occur?	RA pain is worse in morning when the person gets up; osteoarthritis—worse later on in the day; tendinitis—worse in morning, improves during the day.
Is the pain aggravated by: movement, rest, position, weather? Is the pain relieved by: rest, medications, application of heat or ice?	Movement increases most joint pain except in RA, in which movement decreases pain.
Is the pain associated with: chills, fever, recent sore throat, trauma, repetitive activity?	Joint pain occurring 10 to 14 days after a sore throat suggests rheumatic fever. Joint injury occurs from trauma, repetitive motion.
2. Do you have any **stiffness in your joints?**	RA stiffness occurs in morning and after rest periods.
3. Is there any **swelling, heat, redness** in the joints?	Suggests acute inflammation.
4. Is there any **limitation of movement** in any joint? Which joint? Which activities give you problems? (see functional assessment below)	Decreased ROM may be due to joint problems (injury to cartilage or capsule) or to muscle contracture.
5. Do you have any problems in the muscles, such as any **pain or cramping?** Which muscles have this pain?	**Muscle pain** usually is felt as cramping or aching.
If in calf muscles: Is the pain with walking? Does it go away with rest?	Suggests intermittent claudication (see Chapter 18).
Are your muscle aches associated with: fever, chills, the "flu"?	Viral illness often includes muscle aches (myalgia).
6. Do you have any **weakness in muscles?**	
Location—Where is the weakness? How long have you noticed weakness?	Weakness may involve musculoskeletal or neurologic systems (see also Chapter 20).
Do the muscles look smaller there?	Atrophy
Does the weakness interfere with daily activities? Which ones? (Note functional assessment below)	
7. Have you noticed any problems with any bones, such as **bone pain?** Is the pain affected by movement?	A fracture causes sharp pain that increases with movement. Other bone pain usually feels "dull" and "deep" and is unrelated to movement.
8. Do you have any **deformity** of any bone or joint? Is the deformity due to injury or trauma? Does the deformity affect ROM?	
9. Have you ever had any **accidents or trauma** affecting the bones or joints: fractures, joint strain, sprain, dislocation? Which ones?	

EXAMINER ASKS:	RATIONALE:

When did this occur? What treatment was given? Do you have any problems or limitations now as a result?

Do you have a history of back pain? In which part of your back is the pain located? Is pain felt anywhere else, e.g., shooting down leg?

Do you have any numbness and tingling? Do you have any problem with walking, e.g., limping?

10. Do your joint (muscle, bone) problems create any limits on your usual daily activities? Which ones? (Note: Ask about each category; if the person answers "yes," ask specifically about each activity in category.)

Functional assessment.

Bathing—getting in and out of the tub, turning faucets?

Assess any self-care deficit.

Toileting—urinating, moving bowels, able to get self on/off toilet, wipe self?

Dressing—doing buttons, zipper, fasten opening behind neck, pulling dress or sweater over head, pulling up pants, tying shoes, getting shoes that fit?

Grooming—shaving, brushing teeth, brushing or fixing hair, applying makeup?

Eating—preparing meals, pouring liquids, cutting up foods, bringing food to mouth, drinking?

Mobility—walking, walking up or down stairs, getting in/out of bed, getting out of house?

Impaired physical mobility

Communicating—talking, using phone, writing?

Impaired verbal communication

11. Do you have any lifestyle factors that could affect the muscles and joints? Any occupational hazards? Does your work involve heavy lifting? Does your work include any repetitive motion or chronic stress to joints?

Self-care behaviors

Tell me about your exercise program. Describe the type of exercise, frequency, the warm-up program.

Do you have any pain during exercise? How do you treat it?

Have you had any recent weight gain? Please describe your usual daily diet. (Note the person's usual caloric intake, all four food groups, daily amount of protein, calcium.)

Are you taking any medications for musculoskeletal system: aspirin, anti-inflammatory, muscle relaxant?

12. (If person has chronic disability or crippling illness) How has your illness affected:

your interaction with family,
your interaction with friends,
the way you view yourself?

Assess for:

self-esteem disturbance
loss of independence
body image disturbance
role performance disturbance
social isolation

ADDITIONAL QUESTIONS FOR INFANTS AND CHILDREN

Were you told about any trauma to infant during labor and delivery? Did the baby come head first? Was there a need for forceps?

Traumatic delivery increases risk for fractures, e.g., humerus, clavicle.

Did the baby need resuscitation?

Period of anoxia may result in hypotonia of muscles.

EXAMINER ASKS:	RATIONALE:

Were the baby's motor milestones achieved at about the same time as siblings or age-mates?

Has your child ever broken any bones? Any dislocations? How were these treated?

Have you ever noticed any bone deformity? Spinal curvature? Unusual shape of toes or feet? At what age did you notice any of these? Have you ever sought treatment for any of these?

ADDITIONAL QUESTIONS FOR ADOLESCENTS

Are you involved in any sports at school or after school? How frequently (times per week) do you participate in or practice this sport?

Assess safety of sport for child. Note if child's height and weight are adequate for the particular sport, e.g., football.

Do you use any special equipment? Is there any training program for your sport?

Use of safety equipment and presence of adult supervision decreases risk of sports injuries.

What is the nature of your daily warm-up?

Lack of adequate warm-up increases risk of sports injury.

What do you do if you get hurt?

Some students will not report injury or pain for fear of limiting participation in sport.

How does your sport fit in with other school demands and other activities?

ADDITIONAL QUESTIONS FOR THE AGING ADULT

Use the Functional Assessment history questions to elicit any loss of function, self-care deficit, or safety risk that may occur as a process of aging or musculoskeletal illness. (If needed, review the section on functional assessment in Chapter 4 for further detail.)

Have you noticed any change in weakness over the past months, or years?

Have you noticed any increase in falls or stumbling over the past months, or years?

Do you use any mobility aids to help you get around: cane, walker?

OBJECTIVE DATA

Equipment Needed

Tape measure
Goniometer, to measure joint angles
Skin marking pen

Preparation

The purpose of the musculoskeletal examination is to assess function for ADL, as well as to screen for any abnormalities. You already will have considerable data regarding ADL through the history. Note additional ADL data as the person goes through the motions necessary for an examination: gait, posture, how the person sits in a chair, raises from chair, takes off jacket, manipulates small object such as a pen, raises from supine.

A *screening* musculoskeletal examination suffices for most people:

- Inspection and palpation of joints integrated with each body region
- Observation of ROM as person proceeds through motions described earlier
- Age-specific screening measures, e.g., Ortolani's sign for infants, or scoliosis screening for adolescents

A *complete* musculoskeletal examination, as described in this chapter, is appropriate for persons with articular disease, or a history of musculoskeletal symptoms, or any problems with ADL.

Make the person comfortable before and throughout the examination. Drape for full visualization of the body part you are examining, without needlessly exposing the person.

Take an orderly approach—head to toe, proximal to distal.

The joint to be examined should be supported at rest. Muscles must be soft and relaxed in order to assess the joints under them accurately. Take care when examining any inflamed area where rough manipulation could cause pain and muscle spasm. To avoid this use firm support, gentle movement, and gentle return to a relaxed state.

Compare corresponding paired joints. Expect symmetry of structure and function, as well as normal parameters for that joint.

ORDER OF THE EXAMINATION

Use the following order for each specific joint.

Inspection

Note the *size* and *contour* of the joint. Inspect the skin and tissues over the joints for *color, swelling,* any *masses or deformity.* Presence of swelling is significant and signals joint irritation. Swelling may be due to excess joint fluid (effusion), thickening of the synovial lining, inflammation of surrounding soft tissue (bursae, tendons), or bony enlargement. Deformities include *dislocation* (one or more bones in a joint being out of position), *subluxation* (partial dislocation of a joint), *contracture* (shortening of a muscle leading to limited ROM of joint), or *ankylosis* (stiffness or fixation of a joint).

Palpation

Palpate each joint, including its skin for temperature, its muscles, bony articulations, and area of joint capsule. Notice any heat, tenderness, swelling, or masses. Joints normally are not tender to palpation. If any tenderness does occur, try to localize it to specific anatomic structures (e.g., skin, muscles, bursae, ligaments, tendons, fat pads, or joint capsule).

The synovial membrane normally is not palpable. When thickened, it feels "doughy" or "boggy." A small amount of fluid is present in the normal joint, but it is not palpable. Palpable fluid is abnormal. Because fluid is contained in an enclosed sac, if you push on one side of the sac, the fluid will shift and cause a visible bulging on another side.

Range of Motion (ROM)

Ask for *active* range of motion while stabilizing the body area proximal to that being moved. Familiarize yourself with the type of each joint and its normal range of motion so that you can recognize limitations. If you see a limitation, gently attempt *passive* motion. Anchor the joint with one hand while your other hand slowly moves it to its limit. The normal ranges of active and passive motion should be the same.

If any limitation or any increase in ROM occurs, use a goniometer to measure the angles precisely (Fig. 19–15). First extend the joint to neutral or 0 degrees. Center the 0 point of the goniometer on the joint. Keep the fixed arm of the goniometer on the 0 line and use the movable arm to measure; then flex the joint and measure through the goniometer to determine the angle of greatest flexion.

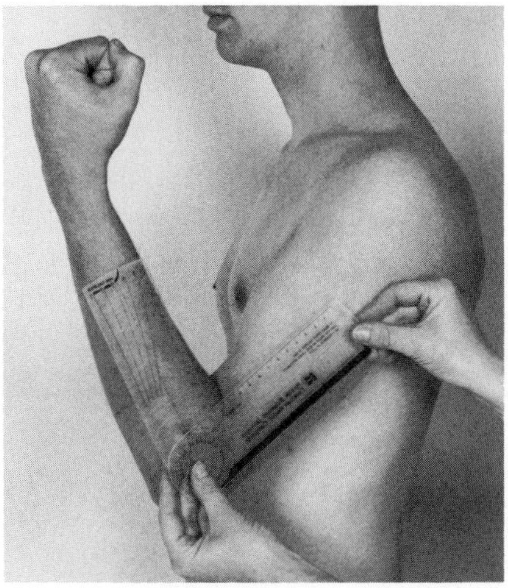

► **Figure 19–15**

Joint motion normally causes no tenderness, pain, or crepitation. Crepitation is an audible and palpable crunching or grating that accompanies movement. It occurs when the articular surfaces in the joints are roughened, as with rheumatoid arthritis. Do not confuse crepitation with the normal discrete "crack" heard as a tendon or ligament slips over bone during motion, such as when you do a knee bend.

Muscle Testing

Test the strength of the prime mover muscle groups for each joint. Repeat the motions you elicited for active ROM. Now ask the person to flex and hold as you apply opposing force. Muscle strength should be equal bilaterally and should fully resist your opposing force. (Note: Muscle status and joint status are interdependent and should be interpreted together. Chapter 20 discusses the examination of muscles for size and development, tone, and presence of tenderness.)

Table 19-2 ▶ Grading Muscle Strength

GRADE	DESCRIPTION	PERCENT NORMAL	ASSESSMENT
5	Full ROM against gravity, full resistance	100	Normal
4	Full ROM against gravity, some resistance	75	Good
3	Full ROM with gravity	50	Fair
2	Full ROM with gravity eliminated (passive motion)	25	Poor
1	Slight contraction	10	Trace
0	No contraction	0	Zero

There is a wide variability of strength among people. You may wish to use a grading system from no voluntary movement to full strength, as shown in Table 19-2.

METHOD OF EXAMINATION

NORMAL RANGE OF FINDINGS

TEMPOROMANDIBULAR JOINT

With the person seated, inspect the area just anterior to the ear. Place the tips of your first two fingers in front of each ear and ask the person to open and close the mouth. Drop your fingers into the depressed area over the joint, and note smooth motion of the mandible. An audible and palpable snap or click occurs in many normal people as the mouth opens (Fig. 19-16).

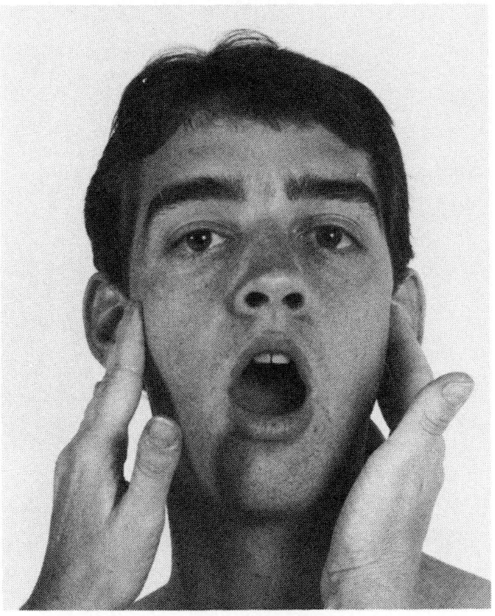

▶ **Figure 19-16**

ABNORMAL FINDINGS

Swelling looks like a round bulge over the joint, although it must be moderate or marked to be visible.

Crepitus

Pain

NORMAL RANGE OF FINDINGS	ABNORMAL FINDINGS

Ask the person to perform these motions (Fig. 19–17):

INSTRUCTIONS TO PERSON	MOTION AND EXPECTED RANGE	ABNORMAL FINDINGS
• Open mouth maximally	Vertical motion. You can measure the space between the upper and lower incisors. Normal is 3 to 6 cm, or three fingers inserted sideways.	
• Partially open mouth, protrude lower jaw and move it side to side.	Lateral motion. Normal extent is 1 to 2 cm.	Lateral motion may be lost earlier and more significantly than vertical.
• Stick out lower jaw.	Protrude without deviation.	

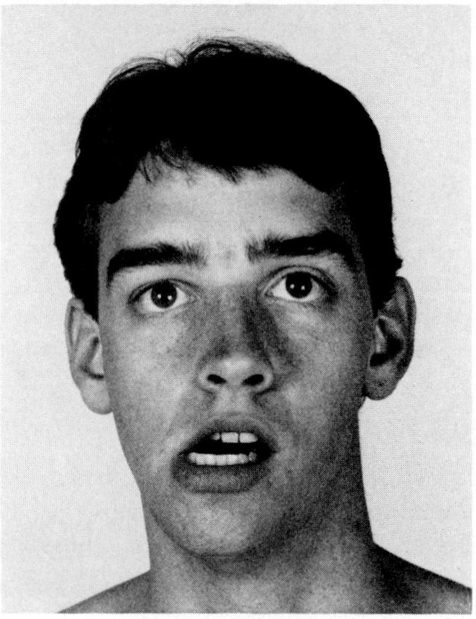

► **Figure 19–17**

Palpate the contracted temporalis and masseter muscles as the person clenches the teeth. Compare right and left sides for size, firmness, and strength. Ask the person to move the jaw forward and laterally against your resistance, open mouth against your resistance. This also tests the integrity of cranial nerve V.

CERVICAL SPINE

Inspect the alignment of head and neck. The spine should be straight and the head erect. Palpate the spinous processes and the sternomastoid, trapezius, and paravertebral muscles. They should feel firm, with no muscle spasm or tenderness.

Abnormal findings: Head tilted to one side. Asymmetry of muscles. Tenderness. Hard muscles with muscle spasm.

Ask the person to follow these motions (Fig. 19–18):*

* DO NOT ATTEMPT IF YOU SUSPECT NECK TRAUMA.

NORMAL RANGE OF FINDINGS

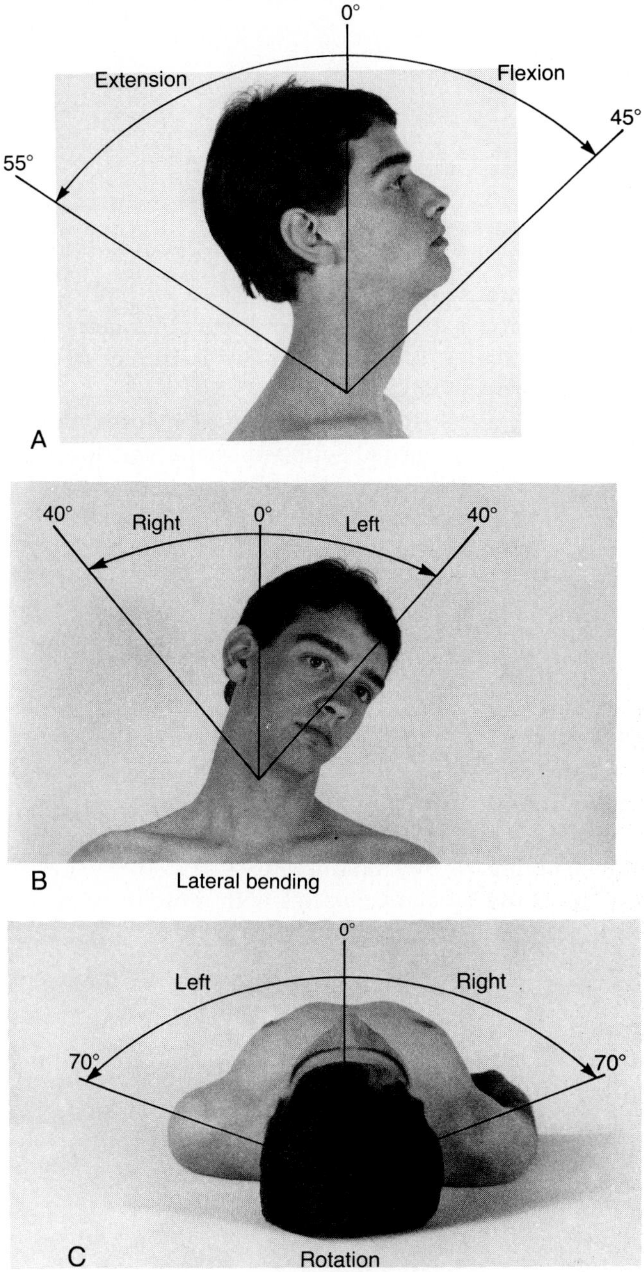

► **Figure 19–18**

INSTRUCTIONS TO PERSON	MOTION AND EXPECTED RANGE
• Touch chin to chest.	Flexion of 45 degrees.
• Lift the chin toward the ceiling.	Hyperextension of 55 degrees.
• Touch each ear toward the corresponding shoulder. Do not lift up the shoulder.	Lateral bending of 40 degrees.
• Turn the chin toward each shoulder.	Rotation of 70 degrees.

ABNORMAL FINDINGS

Limited ROM.
Pain with movement.

NORMAL RANGE OF FINDINGS	ABNORMAL FINDINGS
Repeat the motions while applying opposing force. The person normally can maintain flexion against your full resistance. This also tests integrity of cranial nerve XI.	The person cannot hold flexion.

UPPER EXTREMITY

Shoulders

Inspect and compare both shoulders posteriorly and anteriorly. Check the size and contour of the joint and compare shoulders for equality of bony landmarks. Normally, there is no redness, muscular atrophy, deformity, or swelling. Check the anterior aspect of the joint capsule and the subacromial bursa for abnormal swelling.

Abnormal findings: Redness.
Inequality of bony landmarks.
Atrophy, shows as lack of fullness.
Dislocated shoulder loses the normal rounded shape and looks flattened laterally.
Swelling from excess fluid is best seen anteriorly. There must be considerable fluid to cause a visible distention because the capsule normally is so loose.
Swelling of subacromial bursa is localized under deltoid muscle, and may be accentuated when the person tries to abduct the arm.

If the person reports any shoulder pain, ask that he or she point to the spot with the hand of the unaffected side. Be aware that shoulder pain may be from local causes, or it may be referred pain due to a hiatal hernia or a cardiac or pleural condition, which could be potentially serious. Pain from a local cause is reproducible during the examination by palpation or motion.

While standing in front of the person, palpate both shoulders, noting any muscular spasm or atrophy, swelling, heat, or tenderness. Start at the clavicle and methodically explore the acromioclavicular joint, scapula, greater tubercle of the humerus, area of the subacromial bursa, the biceps groove, and the anterior aspect of the glenohumeral joint. Palpate the pyramid-shaped axilla; there should be no adenopathy or masses.

Abnormal findings: Swelling.
Hard muscles with muscle spasm.
Tenderness or pain.

Test ROM by asking the person to perform four motions (Fig. 19–19). Cup one hand over the shoulder during ROM to note any crepitation; normally there is none.

INSTRUCTIONS TO PERSON	MOTION AND EXPECTED RANGE
1. With arms at sides and elbows extended, move both arms forward and up in wide vertical arcs. Then move them back.	Forward flexion of 180 degrees. Hyperextension up to 50 degrees.
2. Rotate arms internally behind back, place back of hands as high as possible toward the scapulae.	Internal rotation of 90 degrees.
3. With arms at sides and elbows extended, raise both arms in wide arcs in the coronal plane. Touch palms together above head.	Abduction of 180 degrees. Adduction of 50 degrees.
4. Touch both hands behind the head, with elbows flexed and rotated posteriorly.	External rotation of 90 degrees.

Abnormal findings: Limited ROM.
Asymmetry.
Pain with motion.
Crepitus with motion.

Rotator cuff lesions may cause limited ROM and pain and muscle spasm during abduction, whereas forward flexion stays fairly normal.

NORMAL RANGE OF FINDINGS | **ABNORMAL FINDINGS**

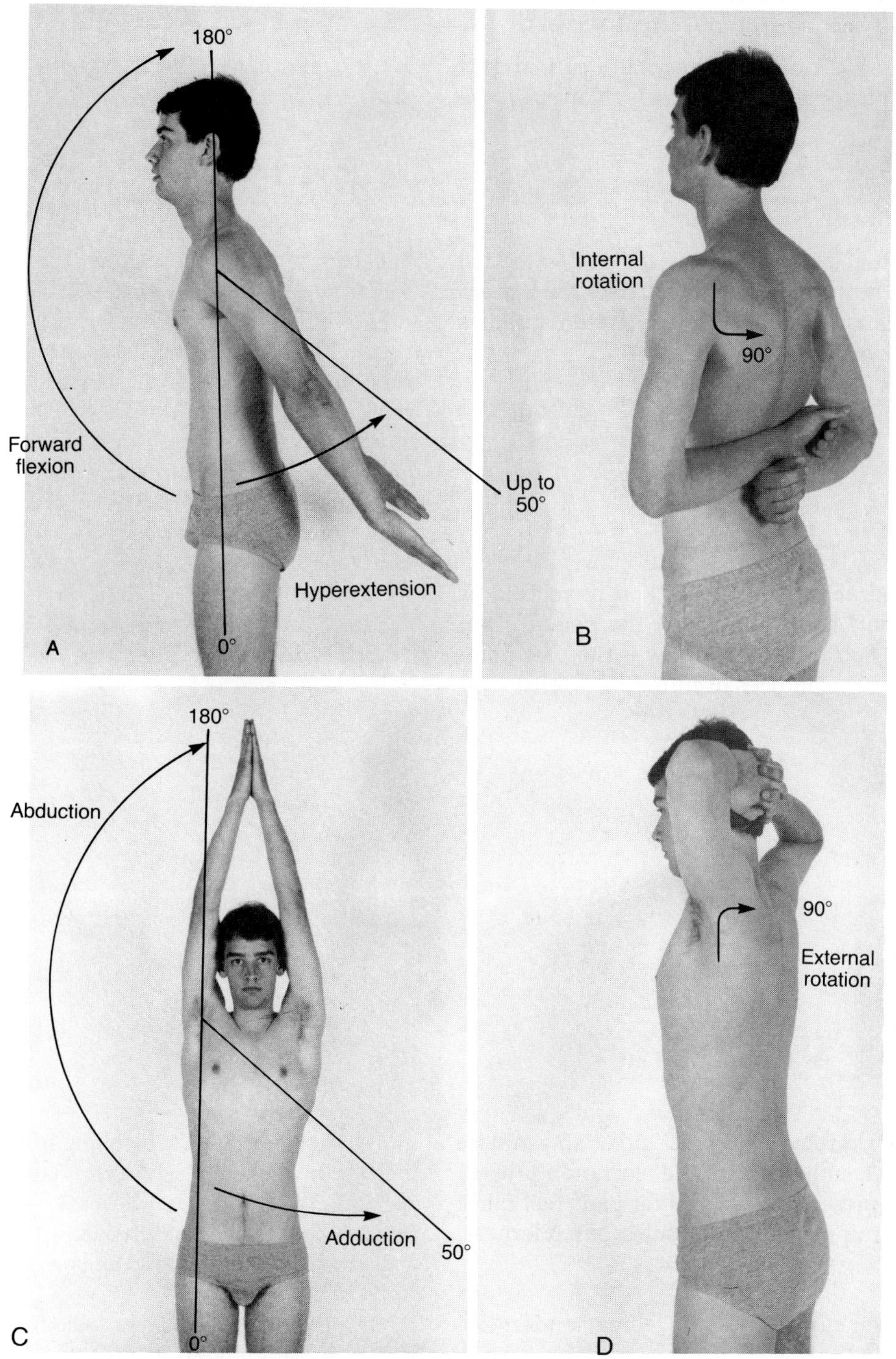

▶ **Figure 19-19**

If you note any limitation in ROM, further test the ROM of the glenohumeral joint while immobilizing the scapula with one hand. (See Polley and Hunder, 1978, or another orthopedic text for details.)

Test the strength of the shoulder muscles by asking the person to

NORMAL RANGE OF FINDINGS | **ABNORMAL FINDINGS**

shrug the shoulders, flex forward and up, and abduct against your resistance. The shoulder shrug also tests the integrity of cranial nerve XII.

Drop Arm Test. If you suspect muscle damage in the rotator cuff, abduct the person's arm and then ask the person to lower it slowly. Normally, the arm lowers smoothly.

If the arm drops suddenly, it indicates a rotator cuff tear.

Elbow

Inspect the size and contour of the elbow in both flexed and extended positions. Look for any deformity, redness, or swelling. Check these areas for abnormal swelling: olecranon bursa, and the normally present hollows on either side of the olecranon process.

Subluxation of the elbow shows the forearm dislocated posteriorly.

Swelling and redness of olecranon bursa are localized and easy to observe because of the close proximity of the bursa to skin.

Effusion or synovial thickening shows first as a bulge or fullness in groove on either side of the olecranon process, and it occurs with gouty arthritis.

Palpate with the elbow flexed about 70 degrees and as relaxed as possible (Fig. 19–20). Use your left hand to support the person's left forearm and palpate the extensor surface of the elbow—the olecranon process, and the medial and lateral epicondyles of humerus—with your right thumb and fingers.

Epicondyles, head of radius, and tendons are common sites of inflamation and local tenderness, or "tennis elbow."

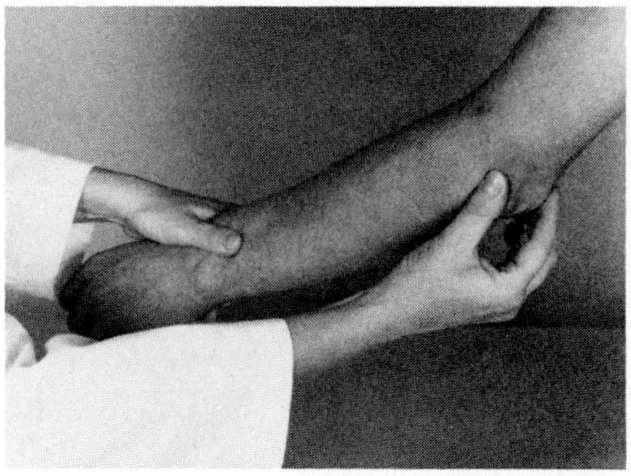

► Figure 19–20

With your thumb in the lateral groove and your index and middle fingers in the medial groove, palpate either side of the olecranon process using varying pressure. Normally present tissues and fat pads feel fairly solid. Check for any synovial thickening, swelling, nodules, or tenderness.

Soft boggy or fluctuant swelling in both grooves occurs with synovial thickening or effusion.

Local heat or redness (signs of inflammation) can extend beyond synovial membrane.

Palpate the area of the olecranon bursa for heat, swelling, tenderness, consistency, or nodules.

Subcutaneous nodules are raised, firm, and nontender, and overlying skin moves freely. Common sites are in the olecranon bursa and along extensor surface of the ulna. These nodules occur with rheumatoid arthritis (see Table 19–5).

Test ROM (Fig. 19–21) by asking the person to:

NORMAL RANGE OF FINDINGS

ABNORMAL FINDINGS

INSTRUCTIONS TO PERSON	MOTION AND EXPECTED RANGE
• Bend and straighten the elbow.	Flexion of 150 to 160 degrees, extension at 0. Some normal people lack 5 to 10 degrees of full extension, and others have 5 to 10 degrees of hyperextension.
• Hold the hand midway, then touch front and back sides of hand to table.	Movement of 90 degrees in pronation and supination (Fig. 19–22).

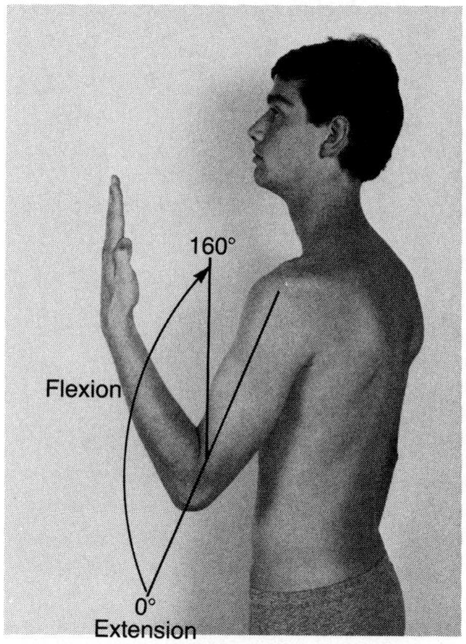

► **Figure 19–21**

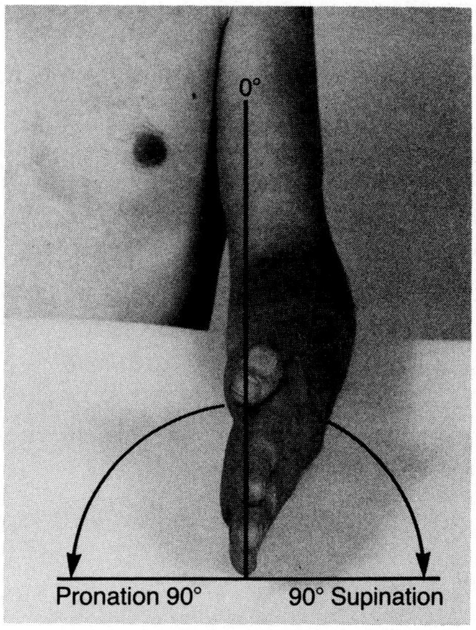

► **Figure 19–22**

While testing muscle strength, stabilize the person's arm with one hand (Fig. 19–23). Have the person flex the elbow against your resistance applied just proximal to the wrist. Then ask the person to extend the elbow against your resistance.

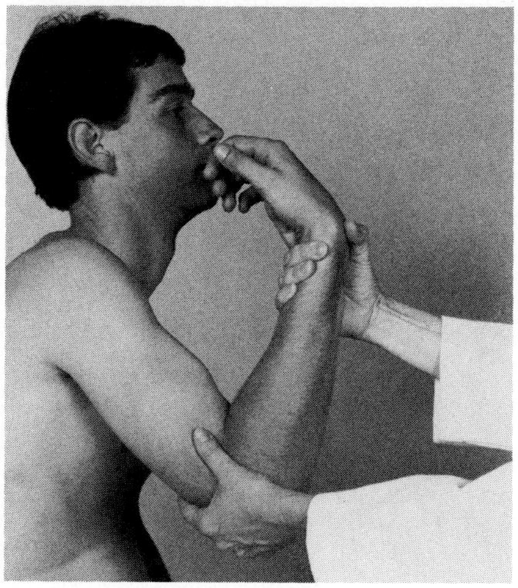

► **Figure 19–23**

NORMAL RANGE OF FINDINGS	ABNORMAL FINDINGS

Wrist and Hand

Inspect the hands and wrists on the dorsal and palmar sides, noting position, contour, and shape. The normal functional position of the hand shows the wrist in slight extension. This way the fingers can flex efficiently, and the thumb can oppose them for grip and manipulation. The fingers lie straight in the same axis as the forearm. Normally, there is no swelling or redness, deformity, or nodules.

The skin looks smooth with knuckle wrinkles present, and no swelling or lesions. Muscles are full, with the palm showing a rounded mound proximal to the thumb (the *thenar eminence*), and a smaller rounded mound proximal to the little finger.

Subluxation of wrist.

Ulnar deviation; fingers list to ulnar side.

Ankylosis; wrist in extreme flexion.

Dupuytren's contracture; flexion contracture of finger(s).

Swan neck or boutonnière deformity in fingers.

Atrophy of the thenar eminence (see Table 19–6, Abnormalities of the Wrist and Hand).

Palpate each joint in the wrist and hands. Facing the person, support the hand with your fingers under it and palpate the wrist firmly with both your thumbs on its dorsum (Fig. 19–24). Make sure the person's wrist is relaxed and in straight alignment. Move your palpating thumbs side to side to identify the normal depressed areas that overlie the joint space. Use gentle but firm pressure. Normally, the joint surfaces feel smooth, with no swelling, bogginess, nodules, or tenderness.

Ganglion in wrist.
Synovial swelling on dorsum.
Generalized swelling.
Tenderness.

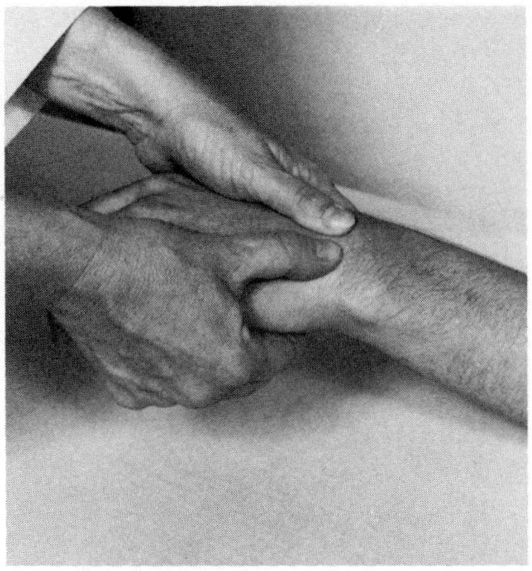

▶ **Figure 19–24**

Palpate the metacarpophalangeal joints with your thumbs, just distal to and on either side of the knuckle (Fig. 19–25).

NORMAL RANGE OF FINDINGS

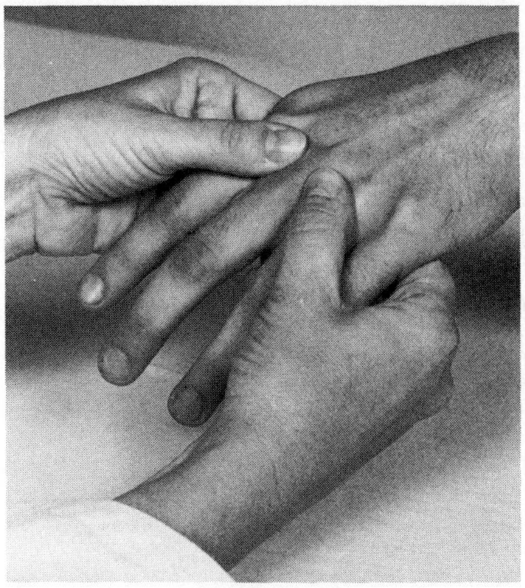

▶ **Figure 19–25**

Use your thumb and index finger in a pinching motion to palpate the sides of the interphalangeal joints (Fig. 19–26). Normally, there is no synovial thickening, tenderness, warmth, or nodules.

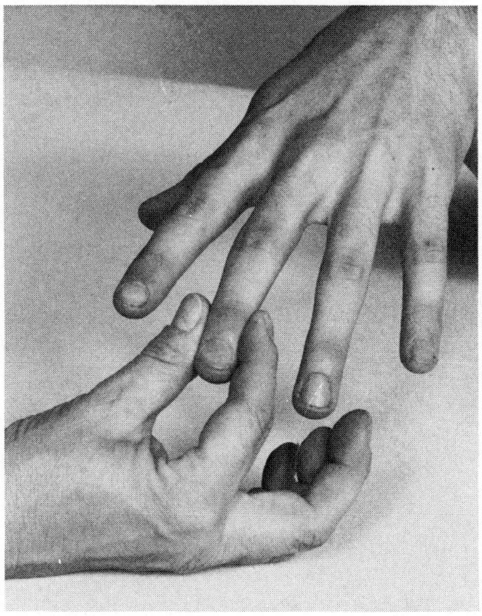

▶ **Figure 19–26**

ABNORMAL FINDINGS

Heberden's and Bouchard's nodules are hard and nontender and occur with osteoarthritis (see Table 19–6).

NORMAL RANGE OF FINDINGS

Test ROM (Fig. 19–27) by asking the person to:

INSTRUCTIONS TO PERSON	MOTION AND EXPECTED RANGE
• Bend the hand up at the wrist.	Hyperextension of 70 degrees.
• Bend hand down at the wrist.	Palmar flexion of 90 degrees.
• Bend the fingers up and down at metacarpophalangeal joints.	Flexion of 90 degrees. Hyperextension of 30 degrees.
• With palms flat on table, turn them outward and in.	Ulnar deviation of 50–60 degrees, and radial deviation of 20 degrees.
• Spread fingers apart; make a fist.	Abduction of 20 degrees; fist tight. The responses should be equal bilaterally.
• Touch the thumb to each finger and to the base of little finger.	The person is able to perform, and the responses are equal bilaterally.

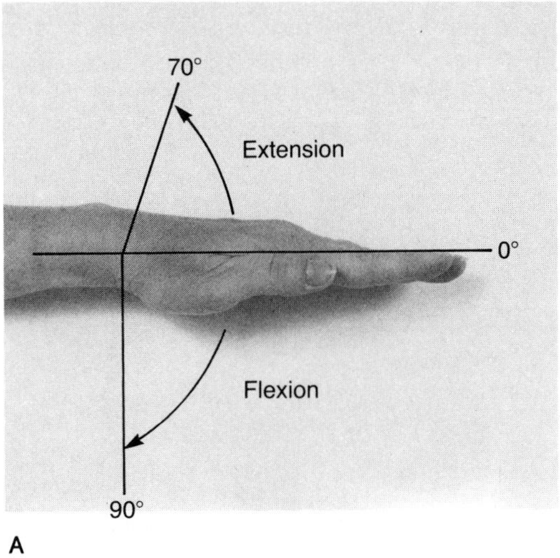

A

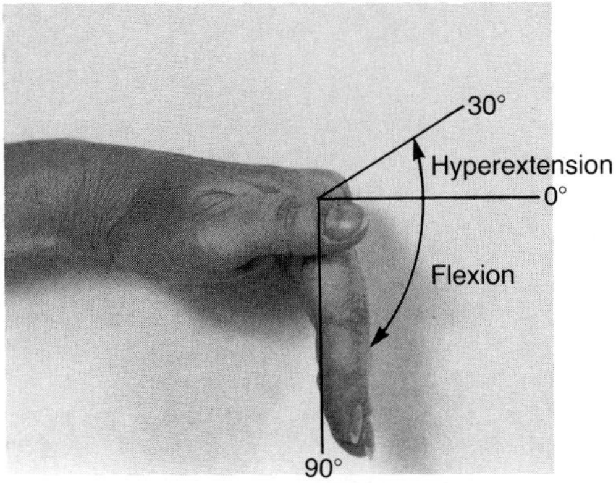

B

► **Figure 19–27**

ABNORMAL FINDINGS

Loss of ROM here is the most common and the most significant type of functional loss of the wrist.

Limited motion.

Pain on movement.

NORMAL RANGE OF FINDINGS | **ABNORMAL FINDINGS**

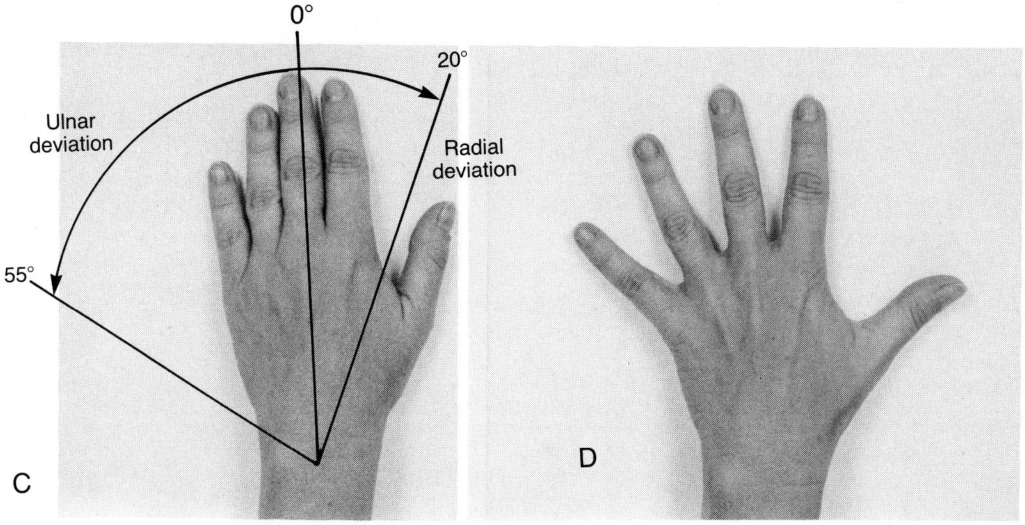

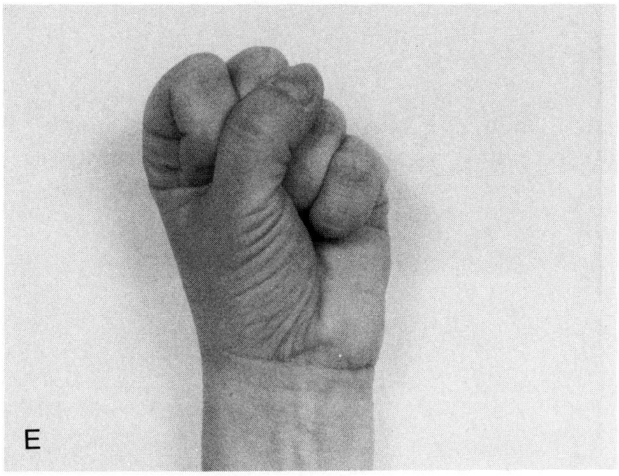

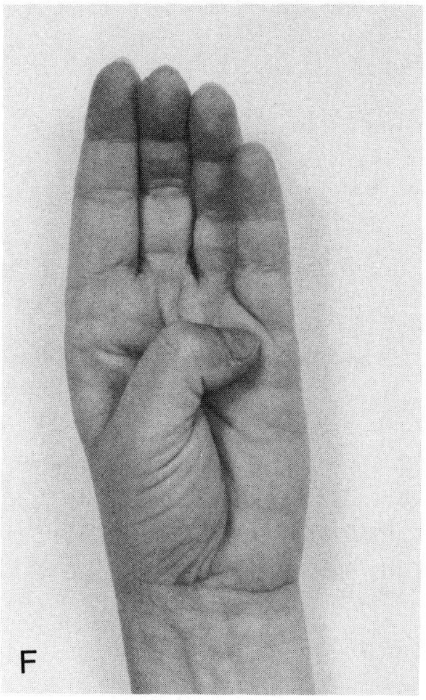

► **Figure 19–27** *Continued*

NORMAL RANGE OF FINDINGS	ABNORMAL FINDINGS

For muscle testing, position the person's forearm supinated (palm up) and resting on a table (Fig. 19–28). Stabilize by holding your hand at the person's mid forearm. Ask the person to flex the wrist against your resistance at the palm.

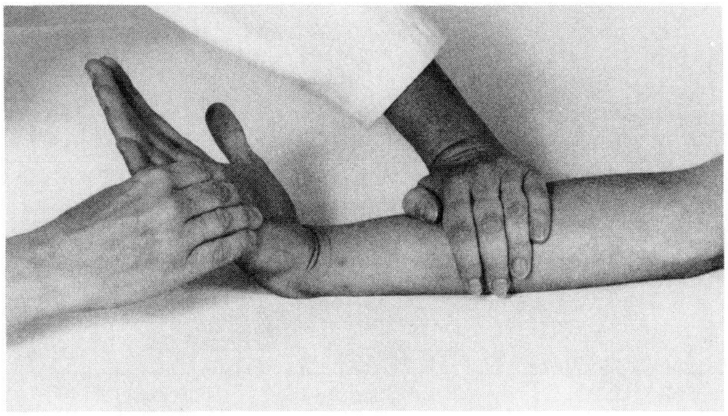

▶ **Figure 19–28**

Phalen's Test. Ask the person to hold both hands back to back while flexing the wrists 90 degrees. Acute flexion of the wrist for 60 seconds produces no symptoms in the normal hand (Fig. 19–29).

Phalen's test reproduces numbness and burning in a person with carpal tunnel syndrome (see Table 19–6).

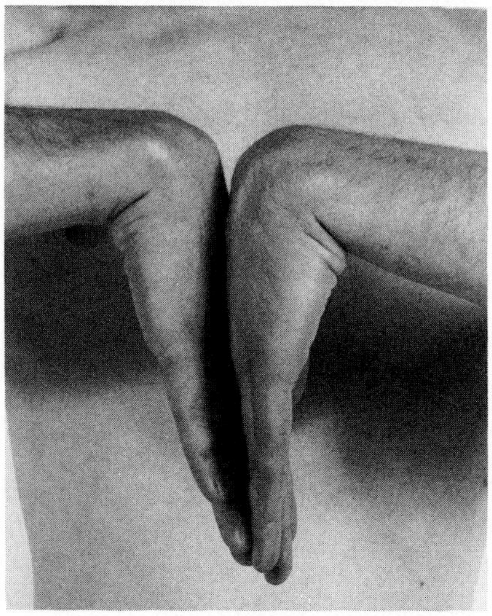

▶ **Figure 19–29**

Tinel's Sign. Direct percussion of the location of the median nerve at the wrist produces no symptoms in the normal hand (Fig. 19–30).

In carpal tunnel syndrome, percussion of the median nerve produces burning and tingling along its distribution, which is a positive indication of Tinel's sign.

NORMAL RANGE OF FINDINGS | **ABNORMAL FINDINGS**

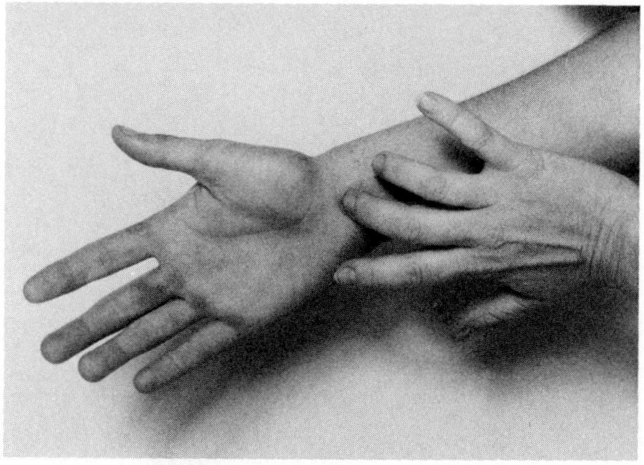

► **Figure 19–30**

LOWER EXTREMITY

Hip

Wait to inspect the hip joint together with the spine a bit later in the examination as the person stands. At that time, note symmetric levels of iliac crests, gluteal folds, and equally sized buttocks. A smooth even gait reflects equal leg lengths and functional hip motion.

Help the person into a supine position, and palpate the hip joints. The joints should feel stable and symmetric, with no tenderness or crepitance.

Abnormal: Pain with palpation. Crepitation.

Assess ROM (Fig. 19–31) by asking the person to:

INSTRUCTIONS TO PERSON	MOTION AND EXPECTED RANGE	ABNORMAL FINDINGS
• Raise each leg with knee extended.	Hip flexion of 90 degrees.	Limited motion. Pain with motion.
• Bend each knee up to the chest while keeping the other leg straight.	Hip flexion of 120 degrees. The opposite thigh should remain on the table.	Flexion flattens the lumbar spine; if this reveals a flexion deformity in the opposite hip, it represents a positive *Thomas test.*
• Flex knee and hip to 90 degrees. Stabilize by holding the thigh with one hand and the ankle with the other hand. Swing the foot outward. Swing the foot inward. (Foot and thigh move in opposite directions.)	Internal rotation of 40 degrees. External rotation of 45 degrees (Fig. 19–32).	Limited internal rotation of hip is an early and reliable sign of hip disease.
• Swing leg laterally, then medially, with knee straight. Stabilize pelvis by pushing down on the opposite anterior superior iliac spine.	Abduction of 40 to 45 degrees. Adduction of 20 to 30 degrees (Fig. 19–33).	Limitation of abduction of the hip while supine is the most common motion dysfunction found in hip disease.
• When standing (later in examination), swing straight leg back behind body. Stabilize pelvis to eliminate exaggerated lumbar lordosis. The most efficient way is to ask person to bend over the table and to support the trunk on the table. Or, the person can lie prone on the table.	Hyperextension of 15 degrees when stabilized (Fig. 19–34).	

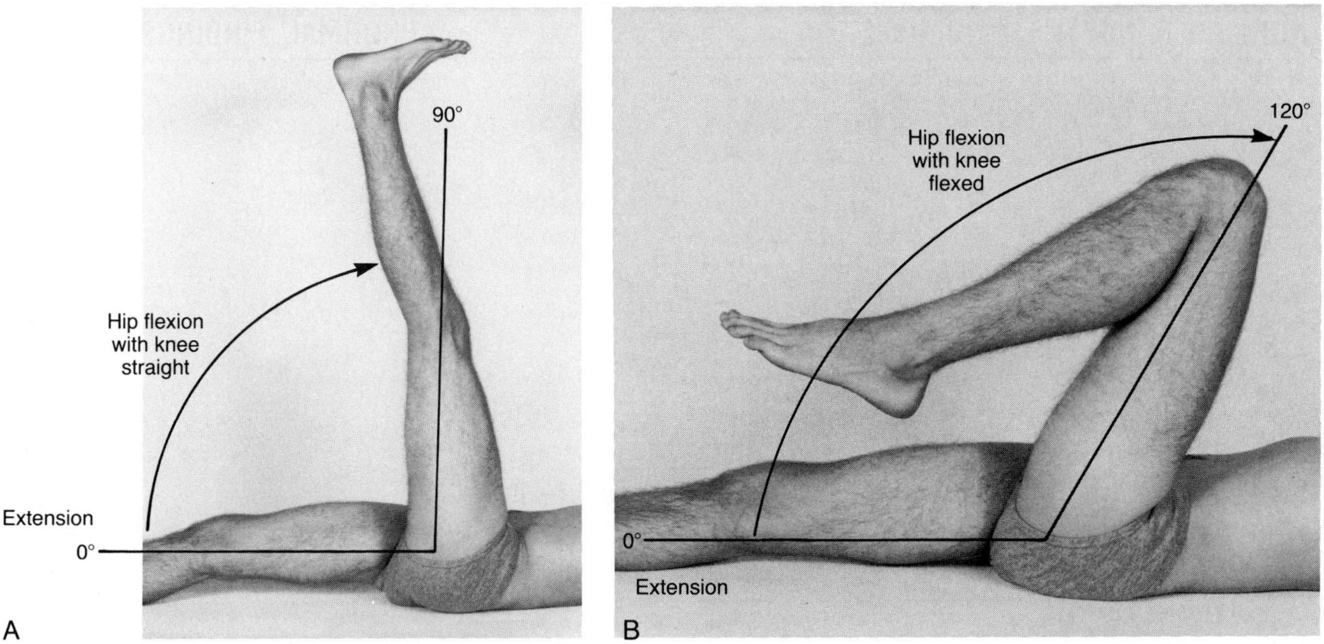

► **Figure 19-31**

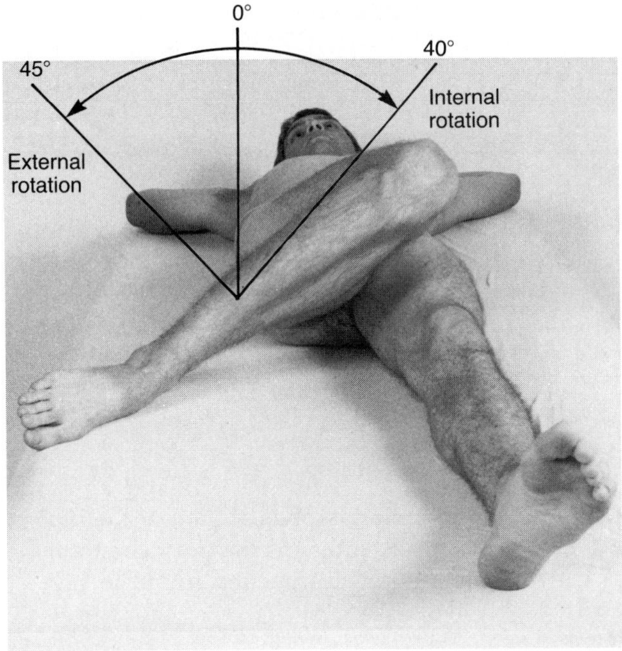

► **Figure 19-32**

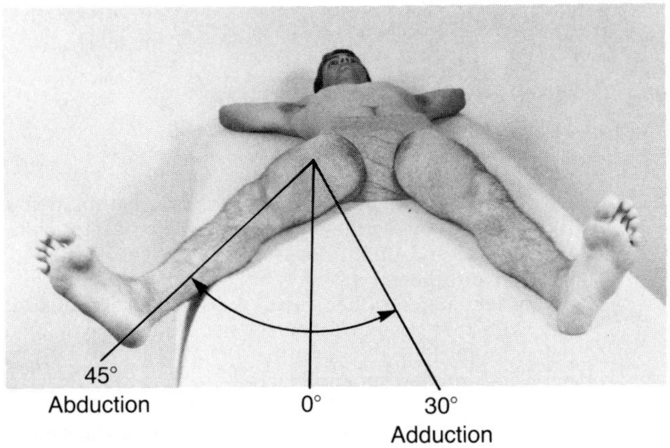

► **Figure 19-33**

NORMAL RANGE OF FINDINGS	ABNORMAL FINDINGS

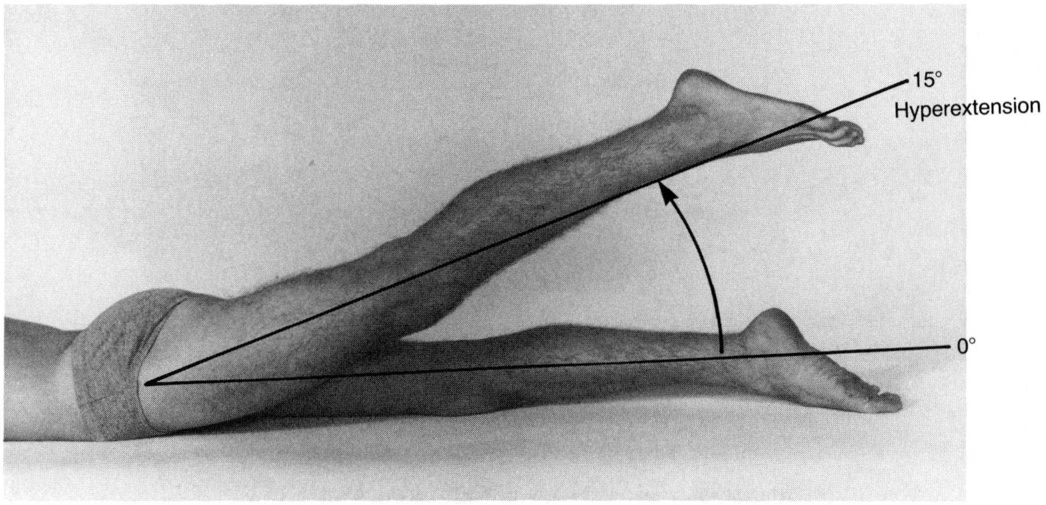

► Figure 19–34

Knee

The person should remain supine with legs extended, although some examiners prefer the knees to be flexed and dangling for inspection. The skin normally looks smooth, with even coloring and free of lesions.

Calluses.
Shiny and atrophic skin.
Inflammation.
Lesions, e.g., psoriasis.

Inspect lower leg alignment. The lower leg should extend in the same axis as the thigh.

Angulation deformity:
- genu varum
- genu valgum
- flexion contracture

(See Table 19–7).

Inspect the knee's shape and contour. Normally, there are distinct concavities, or hollows, on either side of the patella. Check them for any sign of fullness or swelling. Note other locations, such as the prepatellar bursa and the suprapatellar pouch, for any abnormal swelling.

Hollows disappear, then they may bulge with synovial thickening or effusion.

Check the quadriceps muscle in the anterior thigh for any atrophy. Since it is the prime mover of knee extension, this muscle is important for joint stability during weight-bearing.

Atrophy occurs with disuse or chronic disorders. First, it appears in the medial part of the muscle, although it is difficult to note because the vastis medialis is relatively small.

Enhance palpation with the knee in the supine position with complete relaxation of the quadriceps muscle. Start high on the anterior thigh, about 10 cm above the patella. Palpate with your left thumb and fingers in a grasping fashion (Fig. 19–35). Proceed down toward the knee, exploring the region of the suprapatellar pouch. Note the consistency of the tissues. The muscles and soft tissues should feel solid and the joint should feel smooth, with no warmth, tenderness, thickening, or nodularity.

Feels fluctuant or boggy with synovitis of suprapatellar pouch.

NORMAL RANGE OF FINDINGS

ABNORMAL FINDINGS

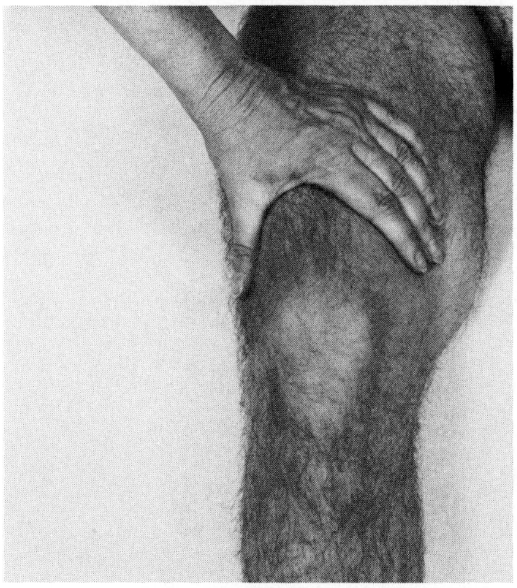

► **Figure 19-35**

When swelling occurs, you need to distinguish whether it is due to soft tissue swelling or increased fluid in the joint. The tests for the bulge sign and ballottement of the patella aid this assessment.

Bulge Sign. For swelling in the suprapatellar pouch, the bulge sign confirms the presence of fluid. Firmly stroke up on the medial aspect of the knee two or three times to displace any fluid (Fig. 19-36*A*). Tap the lateral aspect (Fig. 19-36*B*). Watch the medial side in the hollow for a distinct bulge from a fluid wave. Normally, there is none.

The bulge sign occurs with very small amounts of effusion, 4 to 8 ml.

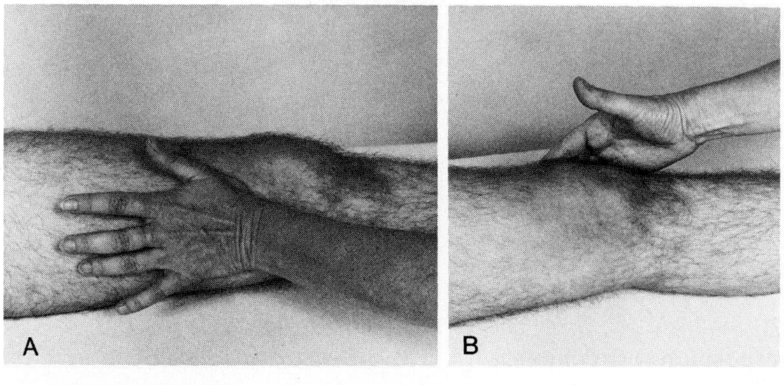

► **Figure 19-36**

NORMAL RANGE OF FINDINGS	ABNORMAL FINDINGS

Ballottement of the Patella. This test is reliable when larger amounts of fluid are present. Use your left hand to compress the suprapatellar pouch. With your right hand, push the patella sharply against the femur. If no fluid is present, the patella already is snug against the femur (Fig. 19–37).

If fluid has collected, your tap on the patella displaces the fluid, and you will hear a tap as the patella bumps up on the femur.

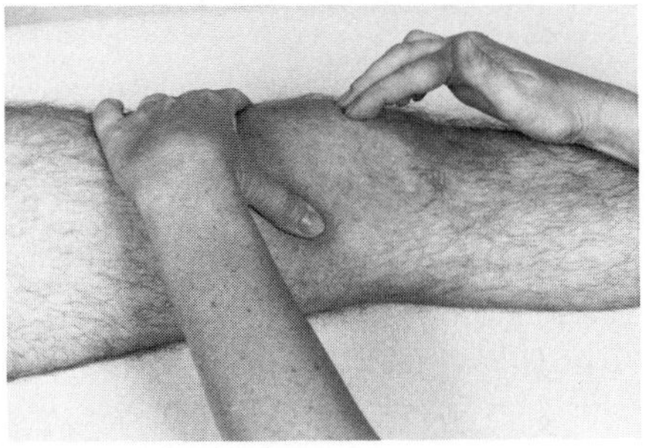

► **Figure 19–37**

Continue palpation and explore the tibiofemoral joint (Fig. 19–38). Note smooth joint margins and absence of pain. Palpate the infrapatellar fat pad and the patella. Check for crepitus by holding your hand on the patella as the knee is flexed and extended. Some crepitus in an otherwise asymptomatic knee is not uncommon.

Irregular bony margins, occur with osteoarthritis.

Pain at joint line.

Pronounced crepitus is significant, and it occurs with degenerative diseases of the knee.

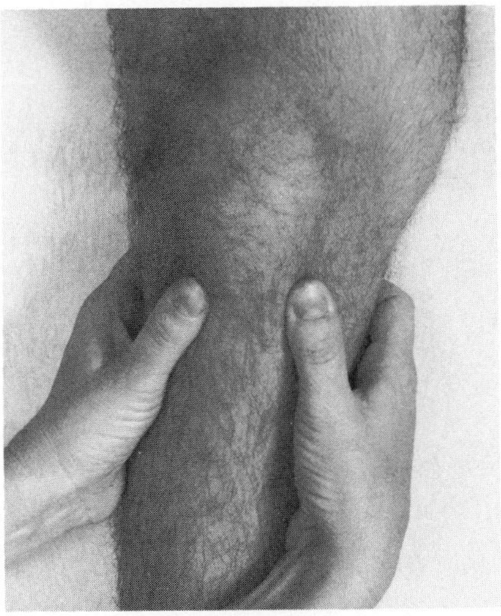

► **Figure 19–38**

NORMAL RANGE OF FINDINGS | ABNORMAL FINDINGS

Check ROM (Fig. 19–39) by asking the person to:

INSTRUCTIONS TO PERSON	MOTION AND EXPECTED RANGE
• Bend each knee.	Flexion of 130 to 150 degrees.
• Extend each knee.	A straight line of 0 degrees, in some persons; a hyperextension of 15 degrees in others.
• Check knee ROM during ambulation.	

Limited ROM.
Contracture.
Pain with motion.

Limp.

Sudden locking—the person is unable to extend the knee fully. This usually occurs with a painful and audible "pop" or "click." Sudden buckling, or "giving way," occurs with ligament injury, which causes weakness and instability.

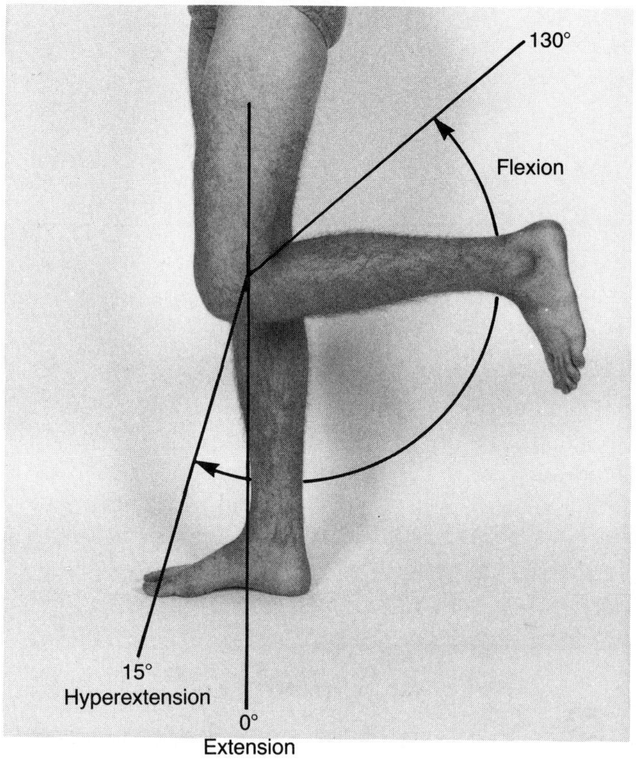

► **Figure 19–39**

Check muscle strength by asking the person to maintain knee flexion while you oppose by trying to pull the leg forward. Muscle extension is demonstrated by the person's success in rising from a seated position in a low chair or by rising from a squat without using the hands for support.

Special Tests for Meniscal Tears

McMurray's Test. Perform this test when the person has reported a history of trauma, followed by locking, giving way, or local pain in the knee. Position the person supine, as you stand on the affected side. Hold the heel and flex the knee and hip. Place your other hand on the knee with fingers on the medial side. Rotate the leg in and out to loosen the joint. Externally rotate the leg and push a valgus (inward) stress on the knee. Then, slowly extend the knee. Normally the leg extends smoothly with no pain (Fig. 19–40).

If you hear or feel a "click," the McMurray test is positive for a torn meniscus.

NORMAL RANGE OF FINDINGS	ABNORMAL FINDINGS

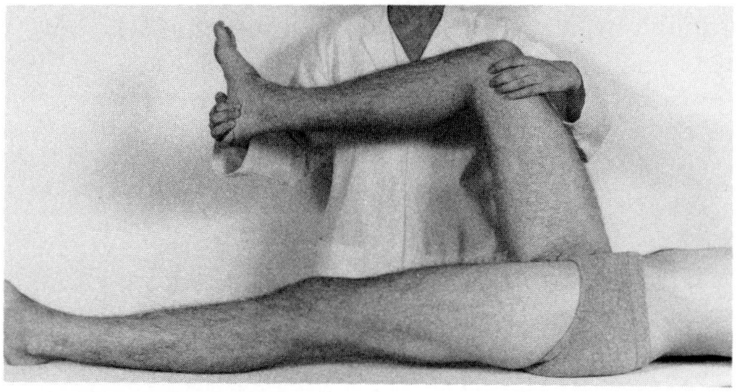

► Figure 19–40

Ankle and Foot

Inspect while the person is in a sitting, non-weight-bearing position, as well as when standing and walking. Compare both feet, noting position of feet and toes, contour of joints, and skin characteristics. The foot should align with the long axis of the lower leg; an imaginary line would fall from midpatella to between the first and second toes.

Weight-bearing should fall on the middle of the foot, from the heel, along the mid-foot, to between the second and third toes. Most feet have a longitudinal arch, though that can vary normally from "flat feet" to a high instep.

The toes point straight forward and lie flat. The ankles (malleoli) are smooth bony prominences. Normally, the skin is smooth, with even coloring and no lesions. Note the locations of any calluses or bursal reactions because they reveal areas of abnormal friction. Examining well-worn shoes helps assess areas of wear and accommodation.

Hallux valgus (see Table 19–8).
Hammer toes.
Claw toes.
Swelling or inflammation.
Calluses.
Ulcers.

Support the ankle by grasping the heel with your fingers while palpating with your thumbs (Fig. 19–41). Explore the joint spaces. They should feel smooth and depressed, with no fullness, swelling, or tenderness.

Swelling or inflammation.
Tenderness.

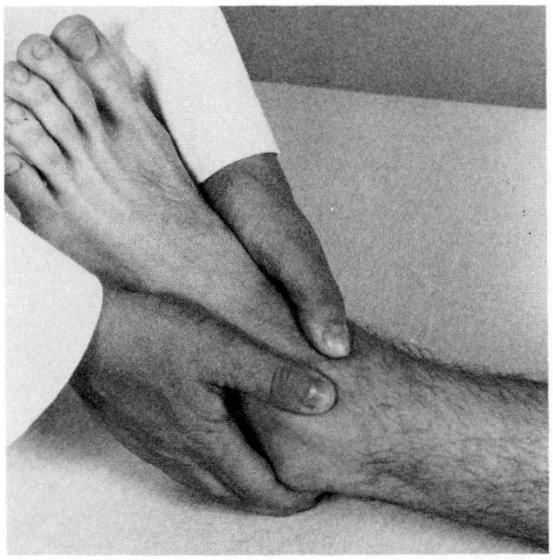

► Figure 19–41

NORMAL RANGE OF FINDINGS	ABNORMAL FINDINGS
Palpate the metatarsophalangeal joints between your thumb on the dorsum and your fingers on the plantar surface (Fig. 19–42).	Swelling or inflammation. Tenderness.

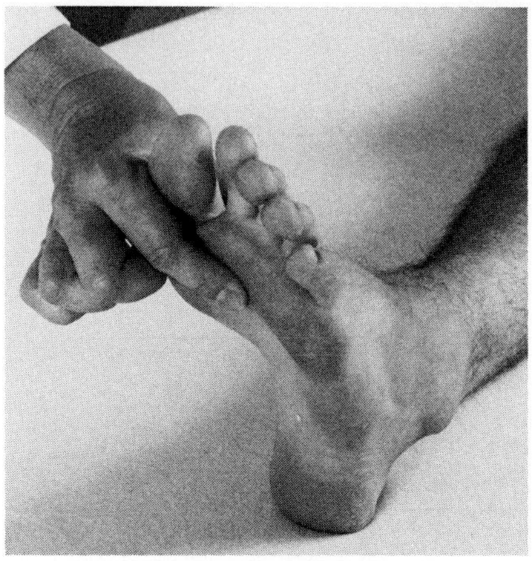

▶ **Figure 19–42**

NORMAL RANGE OF FINDINGS	ABNORMAL FINDINGS
Using a pinching motion of your thumb and forefinger, palpate the interphalangeal joints on the medial and lateral sides of the toes.	Swelling. Inflammation. Tenderness.
Test ROM (Fig. 19–43) by asking the person to:	

INSTRUCTIONS TO PERSON	MOTION AND EXPECTED FINDINGS
• Point toes toward the floor.	Plantar flexion of 45 degrees.
• Point toes toward your nose.	Dorsiflexion of 20 degrees.
• Turn soles of feet out, then in. (Stabilize the ankle with one hand, hold heel with the other to test the subtalar joint.)	Eversion of 20 degrees. Inversion of 30 degrees.
• Flex and straighten toes.	

ABNORMAL FINDINGS: Limited ROM.
Pain with motion.

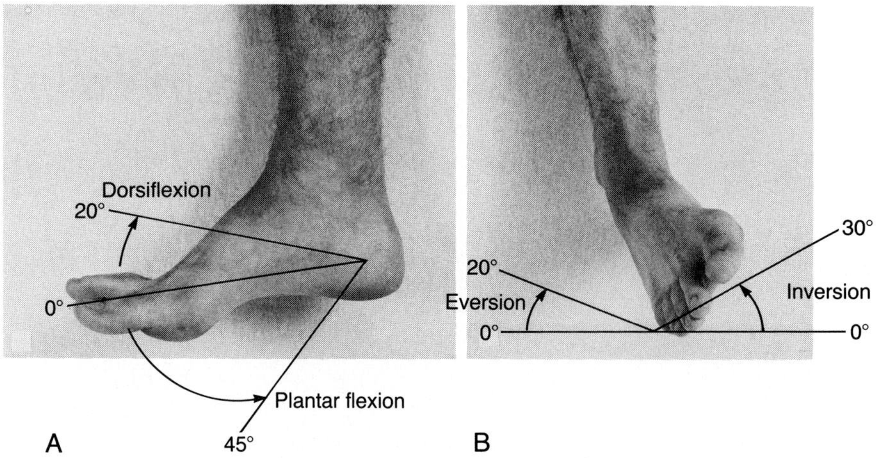

▶ **Figure 19–43**

NORMAL RANGE OF FINDINGS	ABNORMAL FINDINGS

Assess muscle strength by asking the person to maintain dorsiflexion and plantar flexion against your resistance.

Unable to hold flexion.

SPINE

The person should be standing, draped in a gown open at the back. Place yourself far enough back so that you can see the entire back. Note if the spine is straight by following an imaginary vertical line from the head through the spinous processes and down through the gluteal cleft, and by noting equal horizontal positions for the shoulders, scapulae, iliac crests, and gluteal folds, and equal spaces between arm and lateral thorax on the two sides (Fig. 19–44*A*). The person's knees and feet should be aligned with the trunk and should be pointing forward.

A difference in shoulder elevation and in level of scapulae and iliac crests occurs with scoliosis (see Table 19–9).

Lateral tilting and forward bending occur with a herniated nucleus pulposus (see Table 19–9).

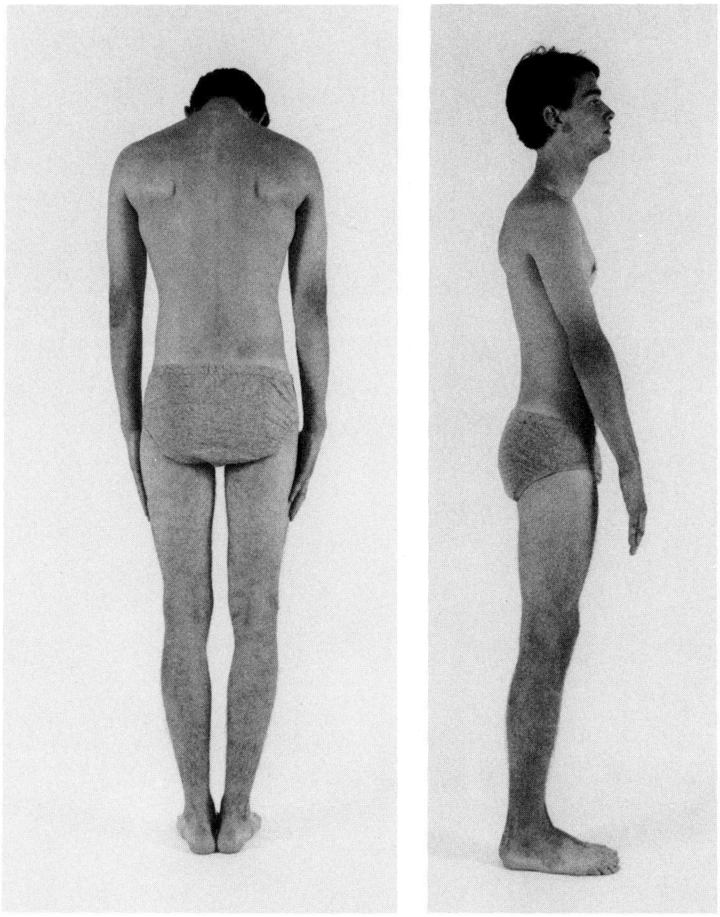

A B

▶ **Figure 19–44**

NORMAL RANGE OF FINDINGS

From the side, note the normal convex thoracic curve and concave lumbar curve (Fig. 19–44*B*). An enhanced thoracic curve, or kyphosis, is common in aging people. A pronounced lumbar curve, or lordosis, is common in obese people.

Palpate the spinous processes. Normally, they are straight and not tender. Palpate the paravertebral muscles; they should feel firm with no tenderness or spasm.

Check ROM of the spine by asking the person to bend forward and touch the toes (Fig. 19–45). Look for flexion of 75 to 90 degrees and smoothness and symmetry of movement. Note that the concave lumbar curve should disappear with this motion, and the back should have a single convex C-shaped curve.

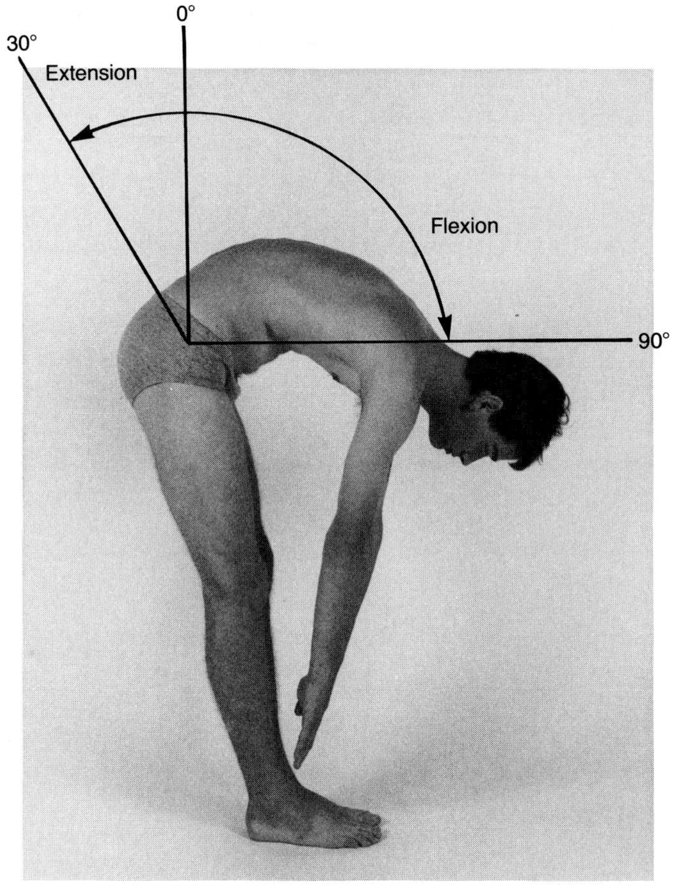

► **Figure 19–45**

If you suspect a spinal curvature during inspection, this may be more clearly seen when the person touches the toes. While the person is bending

ABNORMAL FINDINGS

Spinal curvature
Tenderness
Spasm of paravertebral muscles

NORMAL RANGE OF FINDINGS

over, mark a dot on each spinous process. When the person resumes standing, the dots should form a straight vertical line.

Stabilize the pelvis with your hands. Check ROM (Fig. 19–46) by asking the person to:

INSTRUCTIONS TO PERSON	MOTION AND EXPECTED RANGE
• Bend sideways.	Lateral bending of 35 degrees.
• Bend backward.	Hyperextension of 30 degrees.
• Twist shoulders to one side, then the other.	Rotation of 30 degrees, bilaterally.

These maneuvers reveal only gross restriction. Movement is still possible, even if some spinal fusion has occurred.

ABNORMAL FINDINGS

Limited ROM
Pain with motion

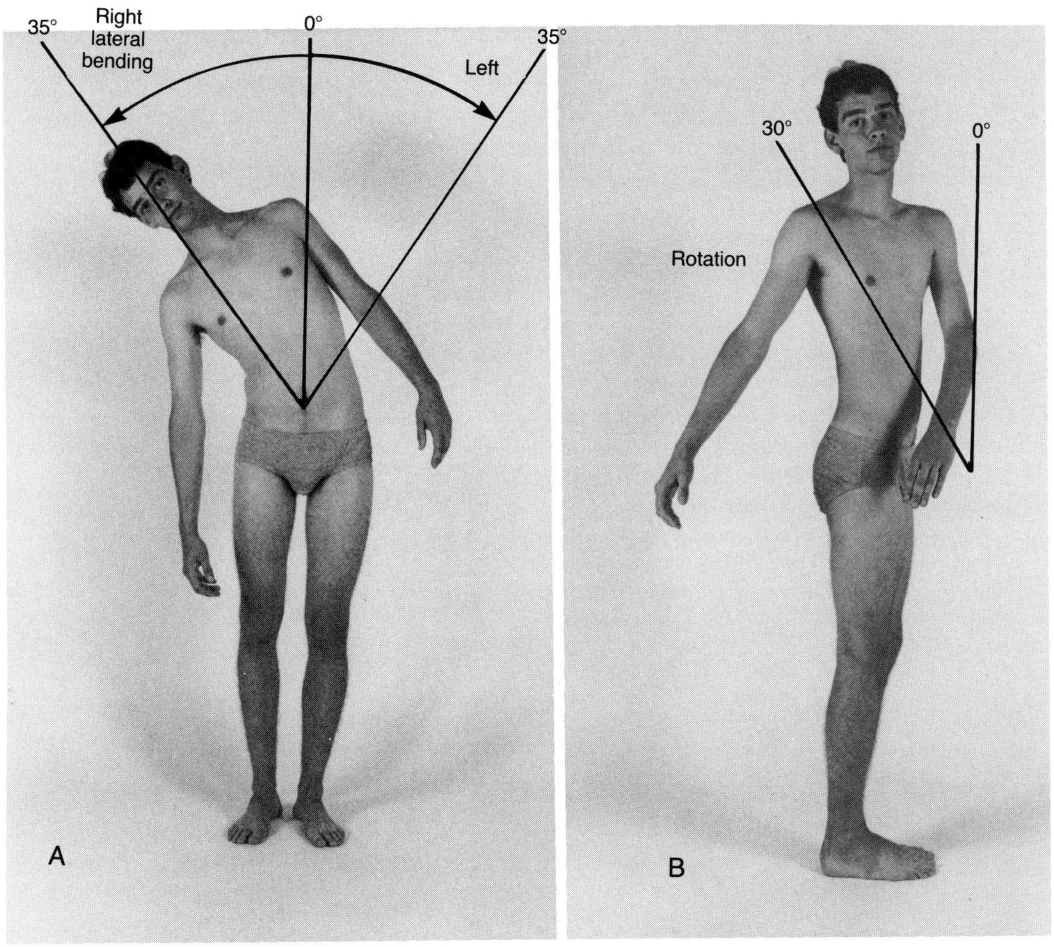

► **Figure 19–46**

NORMAL RANGE OF FINDINGS	ABNORMAL FINDINGS

Straight Leg Raising or LaSegue's Test. These maneuvers reproduce back and leg pain, and help confirm the presence of a herniated nucleus pulposus (Fig. 19–47).

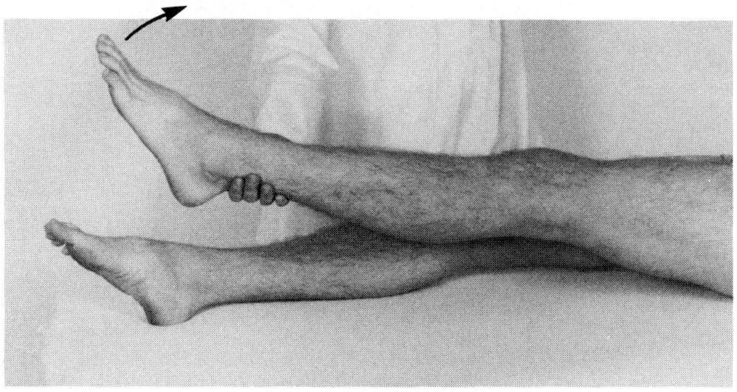

► **Figure 19–47**

Straight leg raising while keeping the knee extended normally produces no pain. Raise the affected leg just short of the point where it produces pain. Then dorsiflex the foot.

Positive if the test reproduces sciatic pain.

If the test reproduces sciatic pain, it confirms the presence of a herniated nucleus pulposus.

Raise the unaffected leg while leaving the other leg flat. Inquire about the involved side.

If the test reproduces sciatic pain on involved side, it strongly suggests a herniated nucleus pulposus.

Measure Leg Length Discrepancy. Perform this measurement if you need to determine if one leg is shorter than the other. For *true leg length,* measure between *fixed* points, from the anterior iliac spine to the medial malleolus, crossing the medial side of the knee (Fig. 19–48). Normally these measurements are equal or within 1 cm, indicating no true bone discrepancy.

Unequal leg lengths

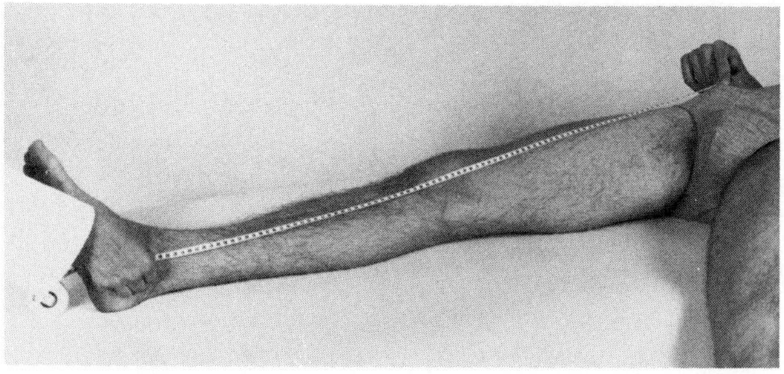

► **Figure 19–48**

Sometimes the true leg length is equal, but the legs still look unequal. For *apparent leg length,* measure from a nonfixed point (the umbilicus) to a fixed point (medial malleolus) on each leg.

True leg lengths are equal, but apparent leg lengths unequal—this condition occurs with pelvic obliquity or adduction or flexion deformity in the hip.

NORMAL RANGE OF FINDINGS | **ABNORMAL FINDINGS**

DEVELOPMENTAL CONSIDERATIONS

Review the developmental milestones discussed in Chapter 2. Keep handy a concise chart of the usual sequence of motor development. You can refer to expected findings for the age of each child you are examining. Use the Denver II to screen the fine and gross motor skills for the child's age.

Since there is some overlap between the musculoskeletal and neurologic examinations, assessment of muscle tone, resting posture, and motor activity are discussed in the next chapter.

Infants

Examine the infant fully undressed and lying on the back. Take care to place the newborn on a warming table to maintain body temperature.

Start with the feet and work your way up the extremities. Note any *positional deformities,* a residual of fetal positioning. Often the newborn's feet are not held straight but in a varus (apart) or valgus (together) position. It is important to distinguish whether this position is flexible (and thus usually self-correctible) or fixed. Scratch the outside of the bottom of the foot. If the deformity is self-correctible, the foot assumes a normal right angle to the lower leg. Or, immobilize the heel with one hand and gently push the forefoot to the neutral position with the other hand. If you can move it to neutral position, it is flexible.

A true deformity is fixed and assumes a right angle only with forced manipulation or not at all.

Note the relationship of the forefoot to the hindfoot. Commonly, the hindfoot is in alignment with lower leg and just the forefoot angles inward. This forefoot adduction is *metatarsus adductus.* It is usually present at birth and usually resolves spontaneously by age 3 years.

Metatarsus varus—adduction and inversion of forefoot.

Talipes equinovarus (see Table 19–10).

Check for *tibial torsion,* a twisting of the tibia. Place both feet flat on the table, and push to flex up the knees. With the patella and the tibial tubercle in a straight line, place your fingers on the malleoli. In an infant, note that a line connecting the four malleoli is parallel to the table.

More than 20 degrees of deviation; or if lateral malleolus is anterior to medial malleolus, it indicates tibial torsion.

Tibial torsion may originate from intrauterine positioning and then may be exacerbated at a later age by continuous sitting in a reverse tailor position, the "TV squat." This is sitting with the buttocks on the floor and the lower legs splayed back and out on either side.

Check the hips for *congenital dislocation.* The most reliable method is the *Ortolani maneuver,* which should be done at every professional visit until the infant is 1 year old (Fig. 19–49). With the infant supine, flex the

With a dislocated hip, the head of the femur is not cupped in the acetabulum but rests posterior to it.

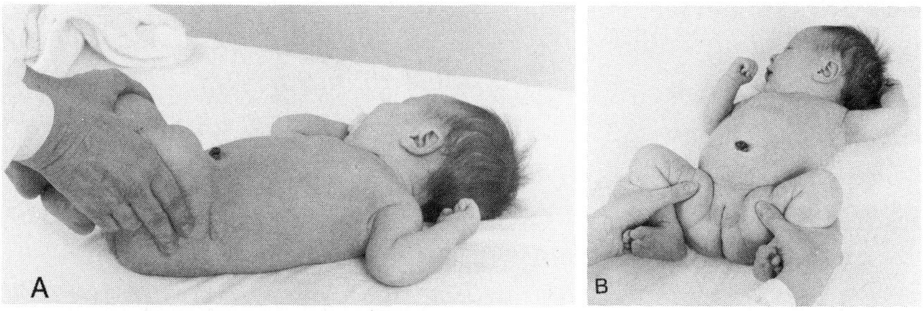

▸ Figure 19–49

NORMAL RANGE OF FINDINGS

knees holding your thumbs on the inner mid-thighs, and your fingers outside on the hips touching the greater trochanters. Adduct the legs until your thumbs touch. Then *abduct,* moving the knees apart and down so their lateral aspects touch the table. This external rotation normally feels smooth and has no sound.

The *Allis test* also is used to check for hip dislocation by comparing leg lengths (Fig. 19–50). Place the baby's feet flat on the table and flex the knees up. Scan the tops of the knees; normally, they are at the same elevation.

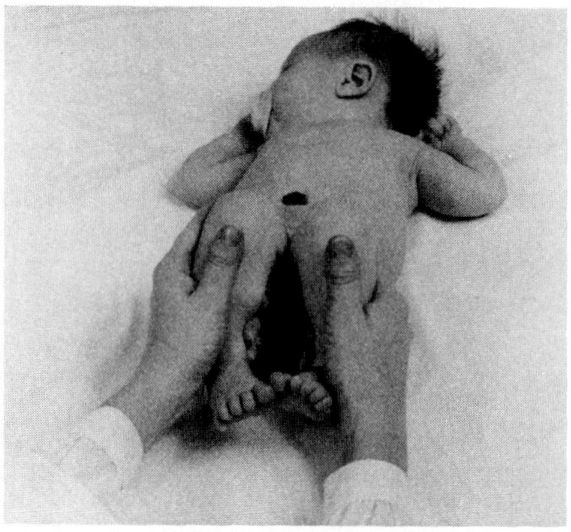

► **Figure 19–50**

Note the gluteal folds. Normally they are equal on both sides. However, some asymmetry may occur in normal children.

Inspect the hands, noting shape, number, and position of fingers and palmar creases.

Palpate the length of the clavicles because the clavicle is the bone most frequently fractured during birth. The clavicles should feel smooth, regular, and without crepitus. Also note equal ROM of arms during the Moro reflex.

Lift up the infant and examine the back. Note the normal single C curve of the newborn's spine (Fig. 19–51). By 2 months of age, the infant can lift the head while prone. This builds the concave cervical spinal curve, and indicates normal forearm strength. Inspect the length of the spine for

ABNORMAL FINDINGS

During external rotation, you will feel and hear a click as the head of the femur pops back into place. This is a *positive Ortolani sign* and warrants referral.

Finding one knee significantly lower than the other is a positive indiction of Allis' sign and suggests hip dislocation.

Unequal gluteal folds may accompany hip dislocation after 2 to 3 months of age.

Polydactyly is the presence of extra fingers or toes.

Syndactyly is webbing between adjacent fingers or toes (see Table 19–6).

A simian crease is a single palmar crease that occurs with Down syndrome, accompanied by short broad fingers, incurving of little fingers and low-set thumbs.

Fractured clavicle—note irregularity at the fracture site, crepitus, and angulation. The site has rapid callus formation with a palpable lump within a few weeks. Observe limited arm ROM and unilateral response to the Moro reflex.

NORMAL RANGE OF FINDINGS

any tuft of hair, dimple in midline, cyst, or mass. Normally, there are none. Transilluminate any mass, and gently check it for tenderness.

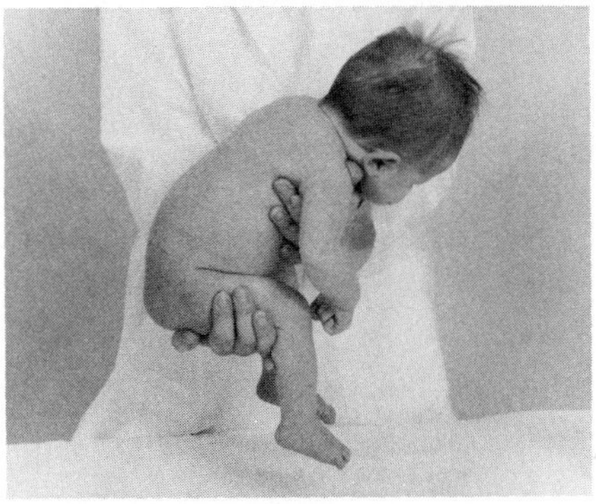

▶ Figure 19–51

Observe ROM through spontaneous movement of extremities.

Test muscle strength by lifting up the infant with your hands under the axillae (Fig. 19–52). A baby with normal muscle strength wedges securely between your hands.

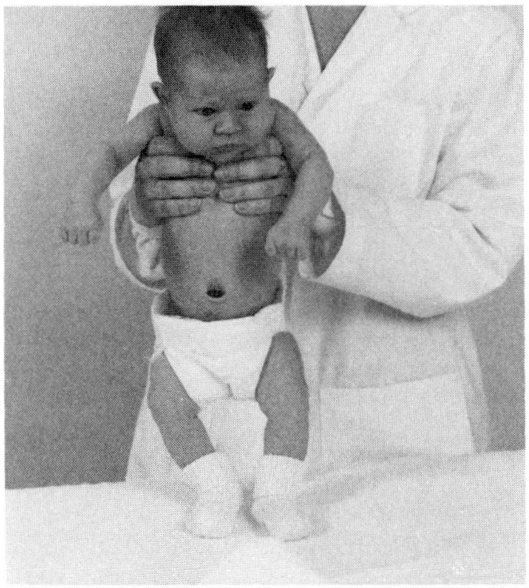

▶ Figure 19–52

Preschool and School-Aged Children

Once the infant learns to crawl and then to walk, the waking hours show perpetual motion. This is convenient for your musculoskeletal assessment —you can observe the muscles and joints during spontaneous play before a table-top examination. Most young children enjoy showing off their physical accomplishments. For specific motions coax the toddler, "Show me how you can walk to Mom," ". . . climb the step stool." Ask the preschooler to hop on one foot or to jump.

While the child is standing, note the posture. From behind, you should note a "plumb line" from the back of the head, along the spine, to the middle of the sacrum. Shoulders are level within 1 cm and scapulae are

ABNORMAL FINDINGS

A tuft of hair over a dimple in the midline may indicate spina bifida.

A small dimple in the midline, anywhere from the head to the coccyx, suggests dermoid sinus.

Mass, e.g., meningocele.

A baby who starts to "slip" between your hands shows weakness of the shoulder muscles.

NORMAL RANGE OF FINDINGS	ABNORMAL FINDINGS

symmetrical. From the side, lordosis is common throughout childhood, appearing more pronounced in children with a protuberant abdomen.

Lordosis is marked with muscular dystrophy and rickets.

Anteriorly, note the leg position. A "bowlegged" stance *(genu varum)* is a lateral bowing of the legs (Fig. 19–53*A*). It is present when you measure a persistent space of more than 2.5 cm between the knees when the medial malleoli are together. Genu varum is normal for 1 year after the child begins walking. "Knock knees" *(genu valgum)* are present when there is more than 2.5 cm between the medial malleoli when the knees are together (Fig. 19–53*B*). It occurs normally between 2 and 3 1/2 years of age.

Genu varum also occurs with rickets.

Genu valgum also occurs with rickets, poliomyelitis, and syphilis.

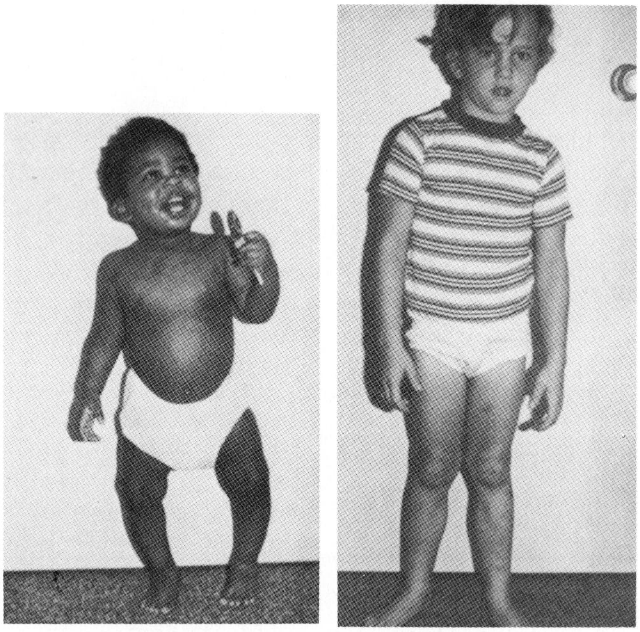

A B

► **Figure 19–53**

Often, parents tell you they are concerned about the child's foot development. The most common questions are about "flatfeet" and "pigeon toes." Flatfoot (pes planus) is pronation, or turning in of the medial side of the foot. The young child may look flatfooted because the normal longitudinal arch is concealed by a fat pad until age 3 years. When standing begins, the child takes a broad-based stance, which causes pronation. Thus, pronation is common between 12 to 30 months. You can see it best from behind the child, where the medial side of the foot drops down and in.

Pronation beyond 30 months.

Pigeon toes, or toeing in, are demonstrated when the child tends to walk on the lateral side of the foot and the longitudinal arch looks higher than normal. It often starts as a forefoot adduction, which usually corrects spontaneously by age 3 years, as long as the foot is flexible.

Toeing in from forefoot adduction that is fixed, or lasts beyond age 3 years.

Toeing in from tibial torsion.

Check the child's gait while walking away from and returning to you. Let the child wear socks, because a cold tile floor will distort the usual gait.

Limp; usually caused by trauma, fatigue, or hip disease.

NORMAL RANGE OF FINDINGS

From 1 to 2 years of age, expect a broad-based gait, with arms out for balance. Weight-bearing falls on the inside of the foot. From 3 years of age, the base narrows and the arms are closer to the sides. Inspect the shoes for spots of greatest wear to aid your judgment of the gait. Normally the shoes wear more on the outside of the heel and the inside of the toe.

Check the *Trendelenburg sign* to screen progressive subluxation of the hip (Fig. 19–54). Watching from behind, ask the child to stand on one leg, then the other. Watch the iliac crests; they should stay level when weight is shifted.

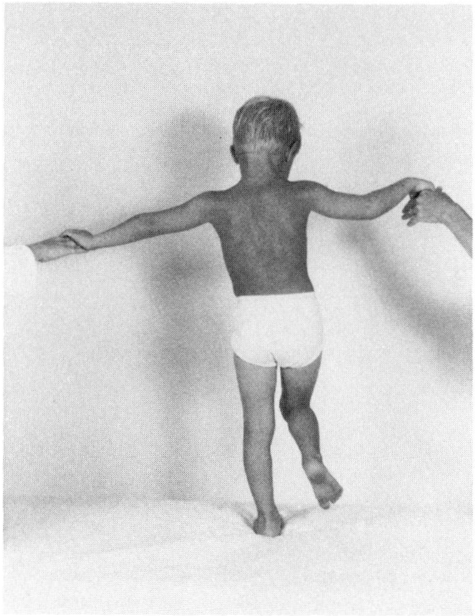

▶ **Figure 19–54**

The child may sit for the remainder of the examination. Start with the feet and hands of the child from 2 to 6 years of age because the child is happy to show these off, and proceed through the examination described earlier.

Particularly, check the arm for full ROM and presence of pain. Look for subluxation of the elbow (head of the radius). This occurs most often between 2 and 4 years of age as a result of forceful removal of clothing or dangling while adults suspend the hands.

Palpate the bones, joints, and muscles of the extremities as described in the adult examination.

ABNORMAL FINDINGS

Abnormal gait patterns (see Chapter 20).

The sign occurs with subluxation of one hip. When the child stands on the good leg, the pelvis looks level. When the child stands on the affected leg, the pelvis drops toward the "good" side.

Inability to supinate the hand while the arm is flexed, together with pain in elbow indicates subluxation of the head of the radius.

Pain or tenderness in extremities usually is caused by trauma or infection.

Fractures are usually due to trauma and are exhibited as an inability to use the area, a deformity, or an excess motion in the involved bone with pain and crepitation.

Enlargement of the tibial tubercles with tenderness suggests Osgood-Schlatter disease, which may be caused by stress on the patellar tendon. This pain may increase with kicking, running, and kneeling. (see Table 19–7).

NORMAL RANGE OF FINDINGS	ABNORMAL FINDINGS

Adolescents

Proceed with the musculoskeletal examination you provide for the adult, except pay special note to spinal posture. Kyphosis is common during adolescence because of chronic poor posture. Screen for *scoliosis* starting at age 12 (Fig. 19–55). Seat yourself behind the standing child, and ask the child to bend forward to touch the toes. Expect a straight vertical spine while standing and also while bending forward. Posterior ribs should be symmetric, with equal elevation of shoulders, scapulae, and iliac crests. You may wish to mark each spinous process with a felt marker. The line-up of ink dots highlights even a subtle curve.

Scoliosis is exhibited as ribs hump up on one side as child bends forward, and with unequal landmark elevation (see Table 19–9).

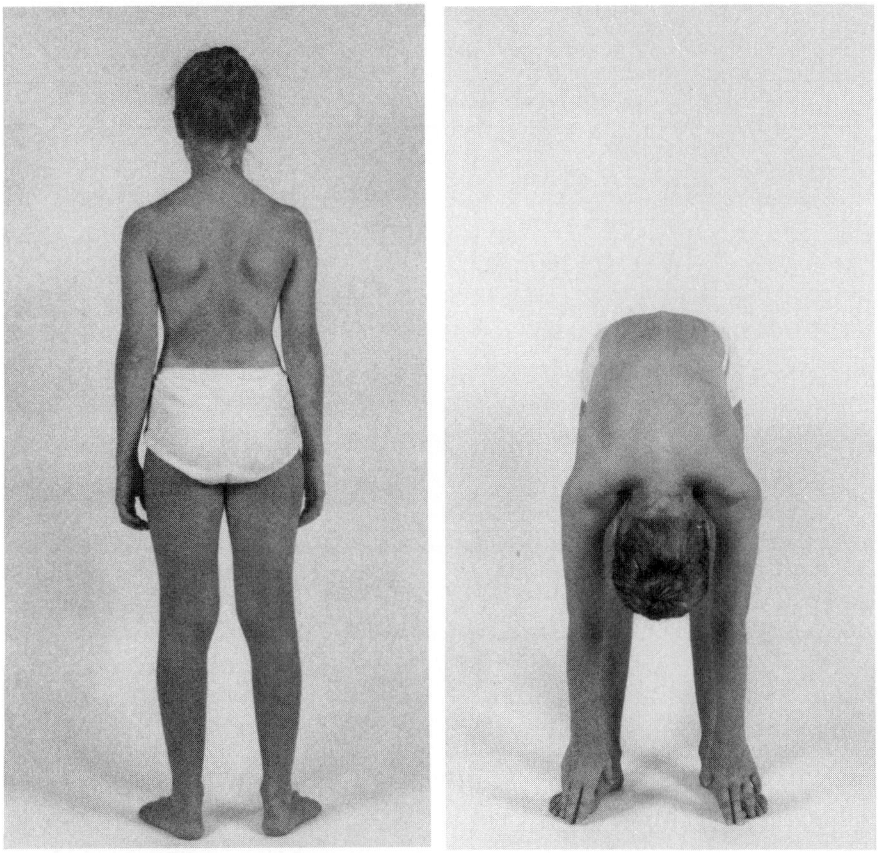

A B

▶ **Figure 19–55**

Be aware of the risk of sports-related injuries with the adolescent, because sports participation and competition reach a height with this age group.

The Pregnant Female

Proceed through the examination described in the adult section. Expected postural changes in pregnancy include progressive lordosis and, toward

NORMAL RANGE OF FINDINGS | **ABNORMAL FINDINGS**

the third trimester, anterior cervical flexion, kyphosis, and slumped shoulders. When the pregnancy is at term, the protuberant abdomen and the relaxed mobility in the joints create the characteristic "waddling" gait.

The Aging Adult

Postural changes include a decrease in height, more apparent in the eighth and ninth decades (Fig. 19–56). "Lengthening of the arm-trunk axis" describes this shortening of the trunk with comparatively long extremities. Kyphosis is common, with a backward head tilt to compensate. This creates the outline of a figure 3 when you view this older adult from the left side. Slight flexion of hips and knees also is common.

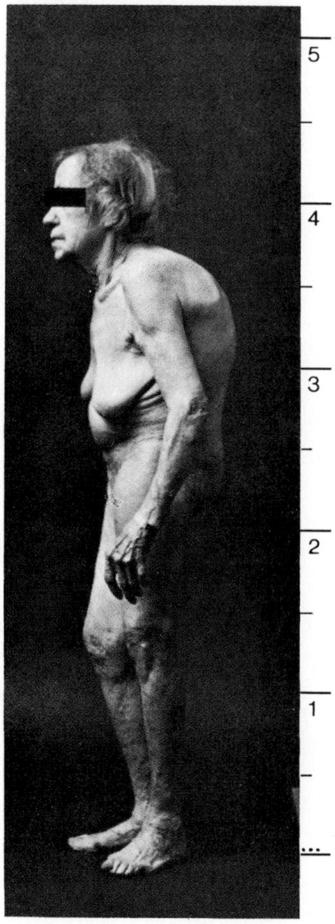

► **Figure 19–56**

Contour changes include a decrease of fat in the body periphery, and fat deposition over the abdomen and hips. The bony prominences become more marked.

For most older adults, ROM testing proceeds as described earlier. ROM and muscle strength are much the same as with the younger adult, provided there are no musculoskeletal illnesses or arthritic changes.

NORMAL RANGE OF FINDINGS | ABNORMAL FINDINGS

Functional Assessment

For those with advanced aging changes, arthritic changes, or musculoskeletal disability, perform a functional assessment for ADL. This applies the range of motion and muscle strength assessments to the accomplishment of specific activities. You need to determine adequate and safe performance of functions essential for independent home life.

INSTRUCTIONS TO PERSON	COMMON ADAPTATION FOR AGING CHANGES*
1. Walk (with shoes on)	Shuffling pattern; swaying; arms out to help balance; broader base of support; person may watch feet.
2. Climb up stairs	Person holds hand rail; may haul body up with it; may lead with favored (stronger) leg.
3. Walk down stairs	Holds hand rail, sometimes with both hands. If the person is weak, he or she may descend sideways lowering the weaker leg first. If the person is unsteady, he or she may watch feet.
4. Pick up object from floor	Person often bends at waist instead of bending knees; holds furniture to support while bending and straightening.
5. Rise up from sitting in chair	Person uses arms to push off chair arms, upper trunk leans forward before body straightens, feet planted wide in broad base of support.
6. Rise up from lying in bed	May roll to one side, push with arms to lift up torso, grab bedside table to increase leverage.

* Data from Bowers AC, Thompson JM: Clinical Manual of Health Assessment. 3rd ed. St Louis, CV Mosby, 1988.

☑ SUMMARY CHECKLIST

For each joint to be examined:

1 ▶ Inspection
Size and contour of joint
Skin color and characteristics

2 ▶ Palpation of joint area
Skin
Muscles
Bony articulations
Joint capsule

3 ▶ ROM
Active
Passive (if there is limitation in active ROM)
Measure with goniometer (if there is abnormality in ROM)

4 ▶ Muscle testing

SAMPLE RECORDING

Subjective

► States no joint pain, stiffness, swelling, or limitation. No muscle pain or weakness. No history of bone trauma or deformity. Able to manage all usual daily activities with no physical limitations. Occupation involves no musculoskeletal risk factors. Exercise pattern is brisk walk 1 mile 5 × /week.

Objective

► Joints and muscles symmetric; no swelling, masses, deformity; normal spinal curvature. No tenderness to palpation of joints; no heat, swelling, or masses. Full ROM; movement smooth, no crepitance, no tenderness. Muscle strength—able to maintain flexion against resistance, and without tenderness.

SAMPLE CLINICAL PROBLEM

M.T. is a 45-year-old white female salesperson with a diagnosis of rheumatoid arthritis 3 years PTA, who seeks care now for "swelling and burning pain in my hands" for 1 day.

Subjective

► M.T. was diagnosed as having rheumatoid arthritis at age 41, by staff at this agency. Since that time, her "flare-ups" seem to come every 6 to 8 months. Acute episodes involve hand joints, and are treated with aspirin, which gives relief. Typically experiences morning stiffness, lasting ½ to 1 hour. Joints feel warm, swollen, tender. Has had weight loss of 15 pounds over last 4 years, and feels fatigued much of the time. States should rest more, but "I can't take the time." Daily exercises have been prescribed but doesn't do them regularly. Takes aspirin for acute flare-ups, feels better in a few days, decreases dose by herself.

Objective

► Body joints within normal limits with exception of joints of wrist and hands. Radiocarpal, metacarpophalangeal, and proximal interphalangeal joints are red, swollen, tender to palpation. Spindle-shaped swelling of proximal interphalangeal joints of third digit right hand and second digit left hand; ulnar deviation of metacarpophalangeal joints.

Assessment

► Acute pain R/T inflammation
Impaired physical mobility R/T inflammation
Knowledge deficit about aspirin treatment R/T lack of exposure
Noncompliance with exercise program R/T lack of perceived benefits of treatment
Noncompliance with advised rest periods R/T lack of perceived benefits of treatment

NURSING DIAGNOSES COMMONLY ASSOCIATED WITH THE MUSCULOSKELETAL DISORDERS

Diagnosis	Related Factors (Etiology)	Defining Characteristics (Symptoms and Signs)
Impaired physical mobility	Neuromuscular impairment Sensory-perceptual impairment Fatigue, decreased strength and endurance Intolerance to activity Effects of trauma or surgery Inflammation Pain Obesity Side effects of sedatives, narcotics, or tranquilizers Depression Severe anxiety Fear of movement Architectural barriers Lack of assistive devices	Reluctance to attempt movement Imposed restrictions on movement Limited range of motion Decreased muscle strength, control, or mass Inability to move purposefully within the environment Impaired coordination Falling or stumbling
Potential for disuse syndrome		Presence of risk factors such as: Paralysis Mechanical immobilization Prescribed immobilization Severe pain Altered level of consciousness
Potential for trauma	Balancing difficulties Pain Reduced large, small muscle coordination Reduced mobility of arms, legs Weakness Insufficient finances to purchase safety equipment or to make repairs Lack of safety precautions, safety education Fatigue Visual, hearing impairment History of Previous trauma Substance abuse	

Diagnosis	Related Factors (Etiology)	Defining Characteristics (Symptoms and Signs)
Pain	Inflammation Muscle spasm Effects of surgery or trauma Immobility Pressure points Infectious process Overactivity Obstructive processes	Clutching of painful area Trembling Facial mask of pain Changes in posture or gait Changes in muscle tone: listless to rigid Reports of pain Anxiety Immobilization Positive response to palpation Withdrawal reflex Autonomic responses Increased blood pressure, pulse, respirations Diaphoresis Dilated pupils Crying or moaning Fatigue Distraction behavior—pacing, restlessness Focused on self Depression

Other related nursing diagnoses:

- Activity intolerance (see Chapter 15)
- Body image disturbance
- Chronic pain
- Diversional activity deficit
- Impaired home maintenance management (see Chapter 11)
- Impaired skin integrity (see Chapter 9)
- Self-care deficit
- Sleep pattern disturbance

ABNORMAL CONDITIONS

Table 19–3 ▶ Abnormalities Affecting Multiple Joints

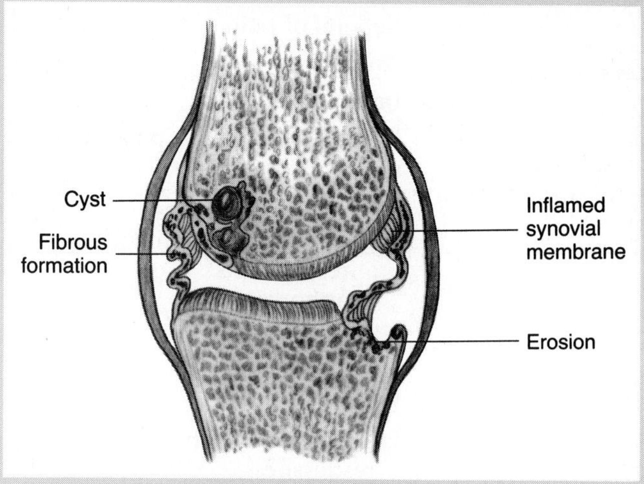

INFLAMMATORY CONDITIONS

Rheumatoid Arthritis

Chronic systemic inflammatory disease of joints and surrounding connective tissue. Inflammation of synovial membrane leads to thickening; then to fibrosis, which limits motion; and finally to bony ankylosis. The disorder is symmetric and bilateral, and is characterized by heat, redness, swelling, and painful motion of the affected joints. Associated signs are described in the following tables, especially Table 19–6.

Table 19–3 ▸ Abnormalities Affecting Multiple Joints *Continued*

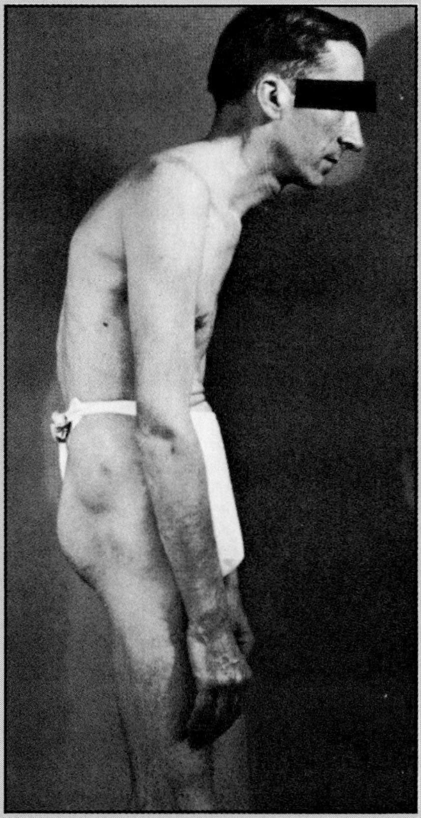

Ankylosing Spondylitis

Chronic progressive inflammation of spine, sacroiliac, and larger joints of the extremities, leading to bony ankylosis and deformity. Affects primarily men by 10 : 1 ratio, in late adolescence or early adulthood. Spasm of paraspinal muscles pulls spine into forward flexion, obliterating cervical and lumbar curves. Thoracic curve exaggerated into single kyphotic rounding. Also includes flexion deformities of hips and knees.

METABOLIC CONDITIONS

Gout (Gouty Arthritis)

Metabolic disorder of disturbed purine metabolism, usually associated with elevated serum uric acid. Deposits of urate crystals in joints lead to inflammation, cartilage damage, and severe crushing pain. Occurs primarily in men over 40 years of age (see Table 19–5 and Table 19–8).

Osteoporosis (not illustrated)

Decrease in skeletal bone mass occurring when rate of bone resorption is greater than that of bone formation. The weakened bone state increases risk for stress fractures, especially at wrist, hip, and vertebrae. Occurs primarily in postmenopausal white women.

DEGENERATIVE CONDITIONS

Degenerative Joint Disease (Osteoarthritis)

Noninflammatory, progressive disorder involving deterioration of articular cartilages and formation of new bone (osteophytes) at joint surfaces. Aging increases incidence; nearly all adults over 60 have some radiographic signs of osteoarthritis. Commonly affects hands, knees, hips, and lumbar and cervical segments of the spine. Affected joints have stiffness, swelling with hard bony protuberances, pain with motion, and limitation of motion (see Table 19–6).

Table 19–4 ▶ Abnormalities of the Shoulder

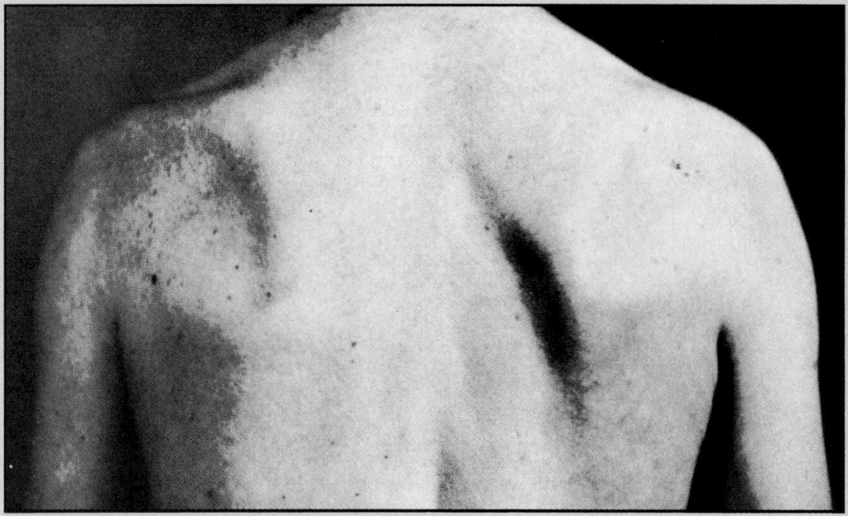

ATROPHY

Loss of muscle mass is exhibited as a lack of fullness surrounding the scapulae, here greater on the left side than on the right. In this case, atrophy is due to cervical radiculitis. Atrophy also occurs from disuse, muscle tissue damage, or motor nerve damage.

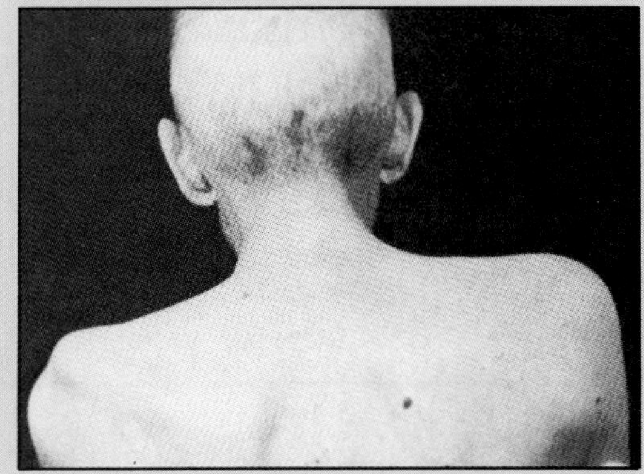

DISLOCATED SHOULDER

Anterior dislocation (95 percent) is exhibited as a hollow where normally it would look rounded. It occurs with trauma involving abduction, extension, and external rotation, e.g., falling on an outstretched arm or diving into a pool.

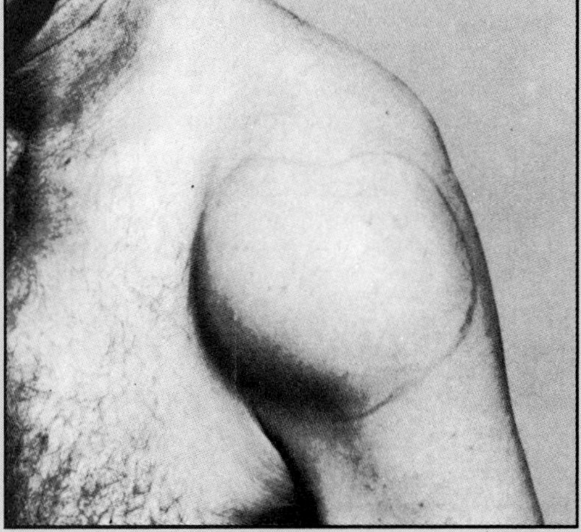

JOINT EFFUSION

Swelling from excess fluid in the joint capsule, here from rheumatoid arthritis. Best observed anteriorly. Fluctuant to palpation. There must be considerable fluid to cause a visible distention because the capsule normally is so loose.

Table 19-4 ▸ Abnormalities of the Shoulder *Continued*

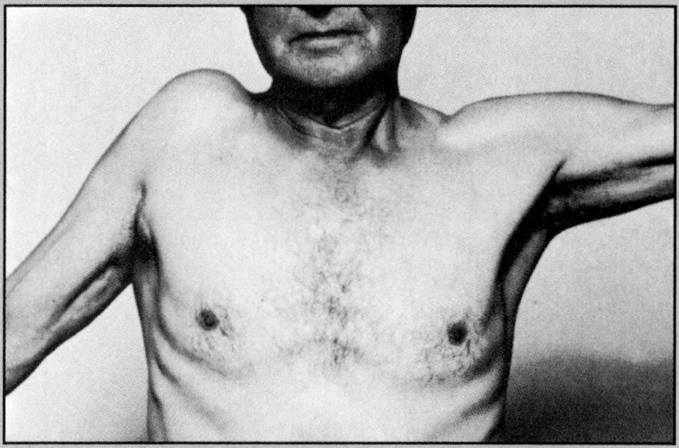

TEAR OF ROTATOR CUFF

Characteristic "hunched" position and limited abduction of arm. Occurs from traumatic adduction while arm is held in abduction, or from fall on shoulder, throwing, or heavy lifting. Positive drop arm test: if the arm is passively abducted at the shoulder, the person is unable to sustain the position and the arm falls to the side.

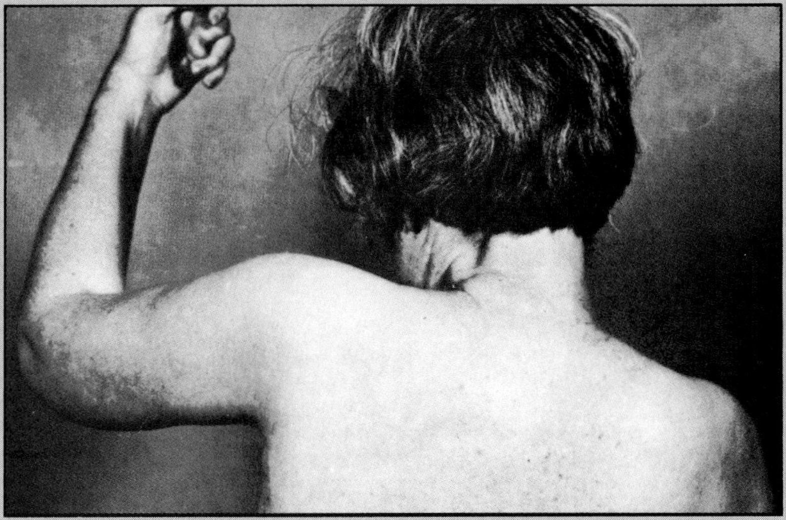

FROZEN SHOULDER—ADHESIVE CAPSULITIS

Fibrous tissues form in the joint capsule, causing progressive limitation of motion and pain. Motion limited in abduction and external rotation. It may lead to atrophy of shoulder girdle muscles. Gradual onset; unknown cause. It is associated with prolonged bed rest or shoulder immobility. May resolve spontaneously.

SUBACROMIAL BURSITIS (not illustrated)

Inflammation and swelling of subacromial bursa causes limited ROM and pain with motion. Localized swelling under deltoid muscle may increase by partial passive abduction of the arm. Caused by direct trauma, strain during sports, local or systemic inflammatory process, or repetitive motion with injury.

Table 19-5 ▸ Abnormalities of the Elbow

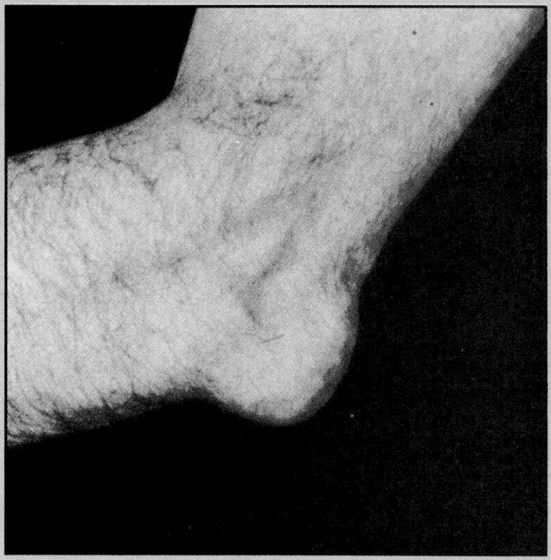

OLECRANON BURSITIS

Large knob, or "goose egg," and redness due to inflammation of olecranon bursa. Localized and easy to see because bursa lies just under skin.

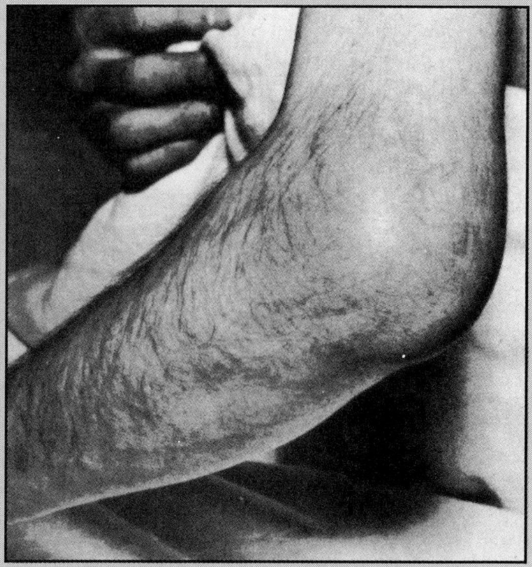

GOUTY ARTHRITIS

Joint effusion or synovial thickening, seen first as bulge or fullness in grooves on either side of olecranon process. Redness and heat can extend beyond area of synovial membrane. Soft, boggy, or fluctuant fullness to palpation.

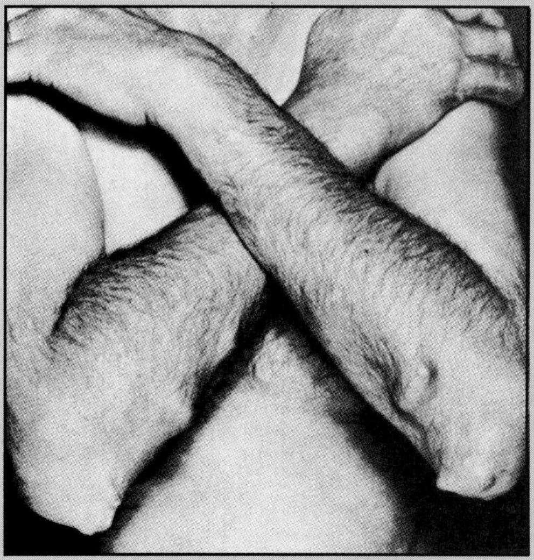

SUBCUTANEOUS NODULES

Raised, firm nontender nodules. These nodules occur with RA. Common sites are in the olecranon bursa and along extensor surface of ulna. Skin slides freely over the nodules.

EPICONDYLITIS—TENNIS ELBOW (not illustrated)

Chronic disabling pain at lateral epicondyle of humerus, radiates down extensor surface of forearm. Due to activities combining excessive pronation and supination of forearm with an extended wrist, e.g., racquet sports, or using a screwdriver.

Medial epicondylitis is more rare and is due to activity of forced palmar flexion of wrist against resistance.

Table 19-6 ▸ Abnormalities of the Wrist and Hand

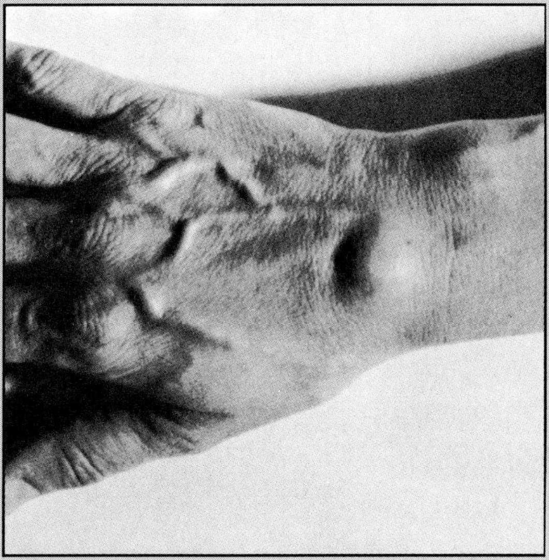

GANGLION

Round, cystic, nontender nodule overlying a tendon sheath or joint capsule, usually on dorsum of wrist. Flexion makes it more prominent. A common benign tumor; it does not become malignant.

COLLES' FRACTURE (not illustrated)

Nonarticular fracture of distal radius, with or without fracture of ulna at styloid process. Usually from a fall on an outstretched hand; occurs more often in older women. Wrist looks puffy, with "silver fork" deformity, a characteristic hump when viewed from the side.

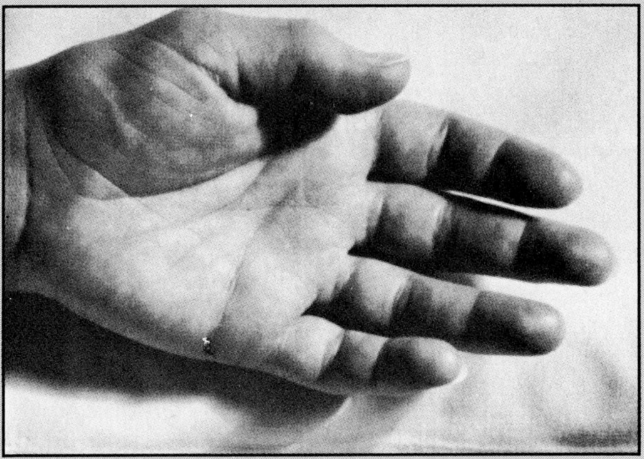

ATROPHY OF THENAR EMINENCE WITH CARPAL TUNNEL SYNDROME

Atrophy occurs from interference with motor function, due to compression of the median nerve inside the carpal tunnel. Occurs between 30 to 60 years of age and is five times more common in women than in men. Symptoms of carpal tunnel syndrome include pain, burning and numbness, positive findings on Phalen's test, positive indication of Tinel's sign, and often atrophy of thenar muscles.

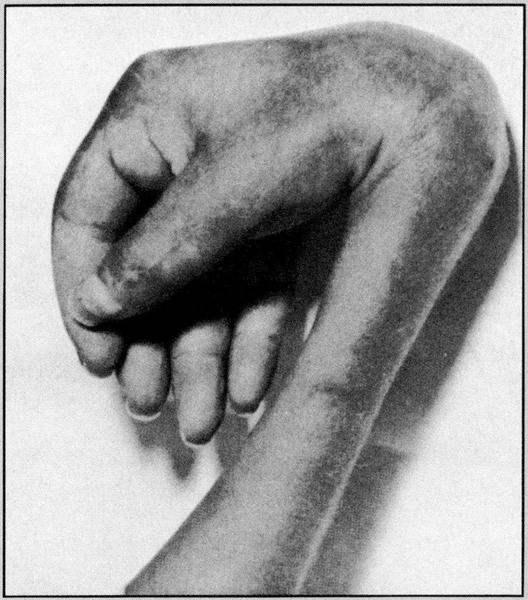

ANKYLOSIS

Wrist in extreme flexion, due to severe rheumatoid arthritis. This is a functionally useless hand, because when the wrist is palmar flexed, a good deal of power is lost from the fingers, and the thumb cannot oppose the fingers.

Table continued on following page

Table 19-6 ▸ Abnormalities of the Wrist and Hand *Continued*

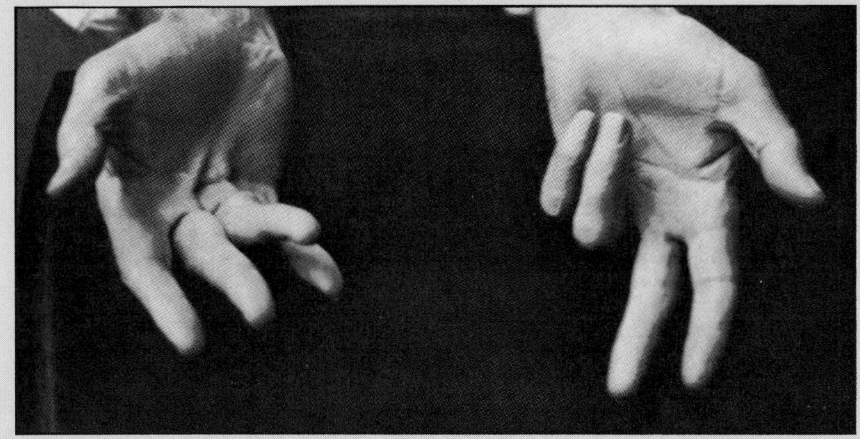

DUPUYTREN'S CONTRACTURE

Chronic hyperplasia of the palmar fascia causes flexion contractures of the digits, first in the fourth digit, then the fifth digit, and then the third digit. Note the bands that extend from the mid-palm to the digits, and the puckering of palmar skin. The condition occurs commonly in men past 40 years of age, and is usually bilateral. Its cause is unknown. The contracture is painless but impairs hand function.

CONDITIONS CAUSED BY CHRONIC RHEUMATOID ARTHRITIS

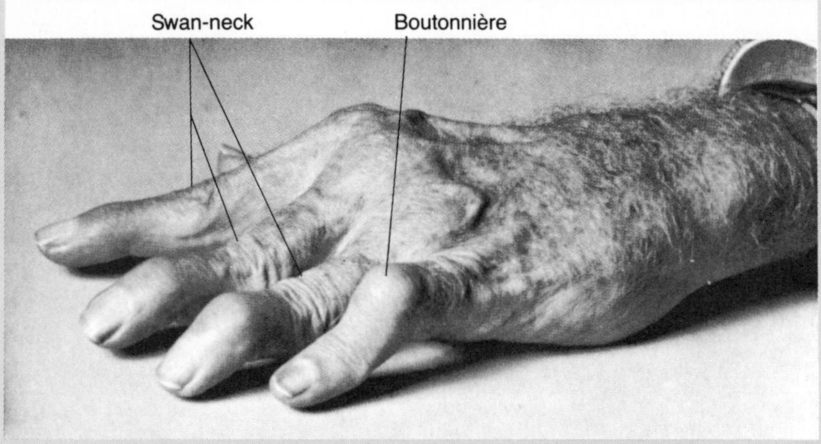

Swan Neck Deformity. Flexion contracture resembles curve of a swan's neck. Note flexion contracture of metacarpophalangeal joint, then hyperextension of the proximal interphalangeal joint, and flexion of the distal interphalangeal joint. It is often accompanied by ulnar drift of the fingers.

Boutonnière Deformity. In this condition the knuckle looks as if it were being pushed through a buttonhole. It is a relatively common deformity and includes flexion of proximal interphalangeal joint with compensatory hyperextension of distal interphalangeal joint.

Table 19-6 ▸ Abnormalities of the Wrist and Hand *Continued*

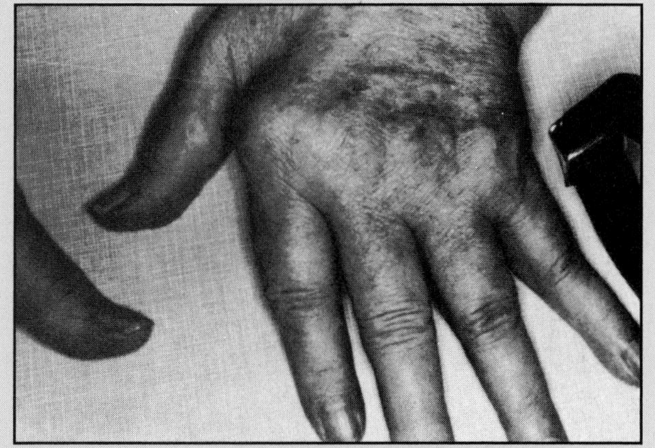

Ulnar Deviation or Drift. Fingers drift to the ulnar side because of stretching of the articular capsule and muscle imbalance. This is caused by chronic rheumatoid arthritis.

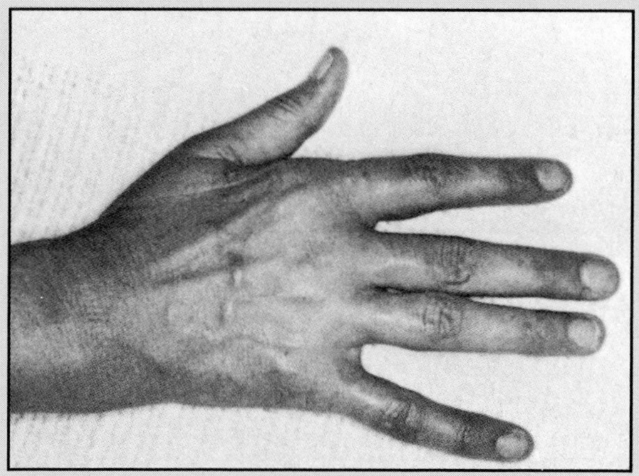

ACUTE RHEUMATOID ARTHRITIS

Painful swelling and stiffness of joints, with fusiform or spindle-shaped swelling of proximal interphalangeal joints. Fusiform swelling is usually symmetric, the hands are warm, and the veins are engorged.

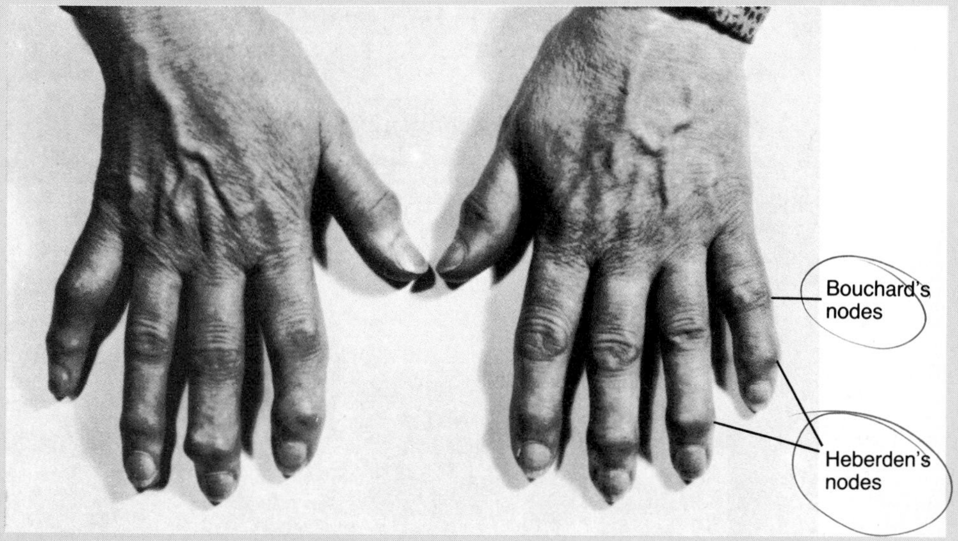

DEGENERATIVE JOINT DISEASE (OSTEOARTHRITIS)

Characterized by hard, nontender nodules, 2 to 3 mm or more. These bony overgrowths of the distal interphalangeal joints are called Heberden's nodes, and those of the proximal interphalangeal joints are called Bouchard's nodes.

Table continued on following page

Table 19–6 ▸ Abnormalities of the Wrist and Hand *Continued*

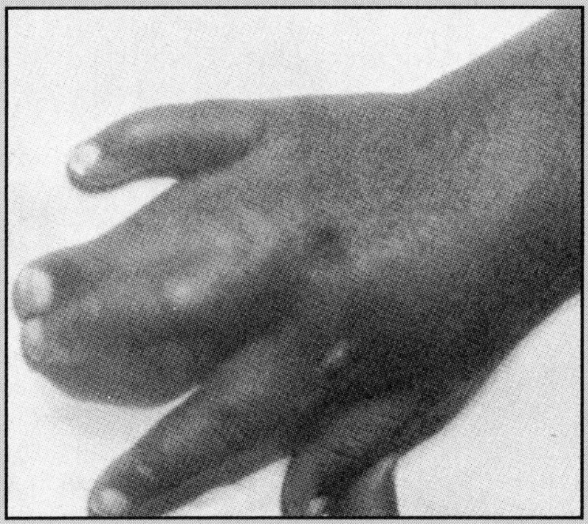

SYNDACTYLY

Webbed fingers are a congenital deformity, usually requiring surgical separation. The metacarpals and phalanges or the webbed fingers are different lengths and the joints do not line up. To leave the fingers fused would thus limit their flexion and extension.

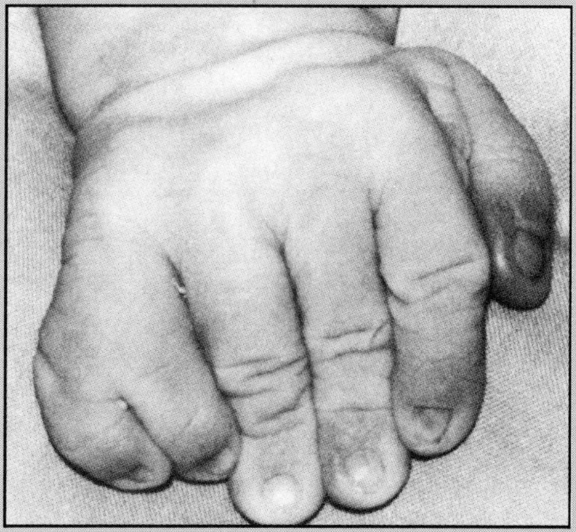

POLYDACTYLY

Extra digits are a congenital deformity, usually occurring at the fifth finger or the thumb. Surgical removal is needed.

Table 19–7 ▸ Abnormalities of the Knee

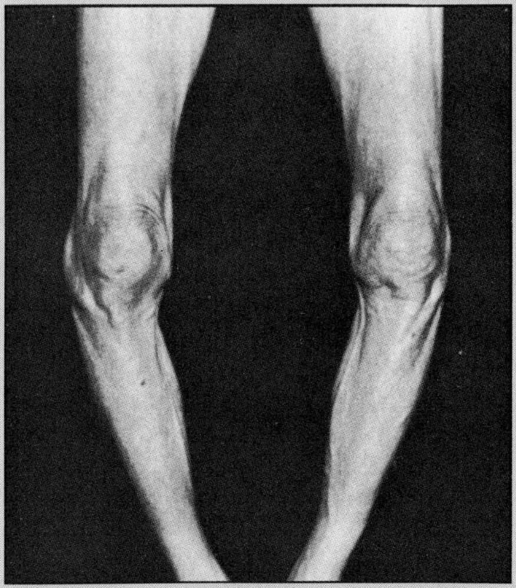

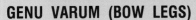

GENU VARUM (BOW LEGS)

Lateral angulation deformity (knees apart), here from degenerative disease. Accompanied by joint instability and medial tenderness at the tibiofemoral joint.

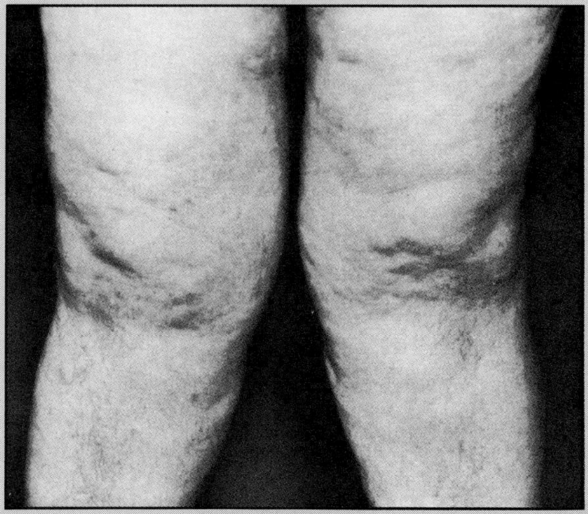

GENU VALGUM (KNOCK KNEES)

Medial angulation deformity (knees together), from degenerative disease. Tibiofemoral joint has tenderness laterally.

Table 19-7 ▸ Abnormalities of the Knee *Continued*

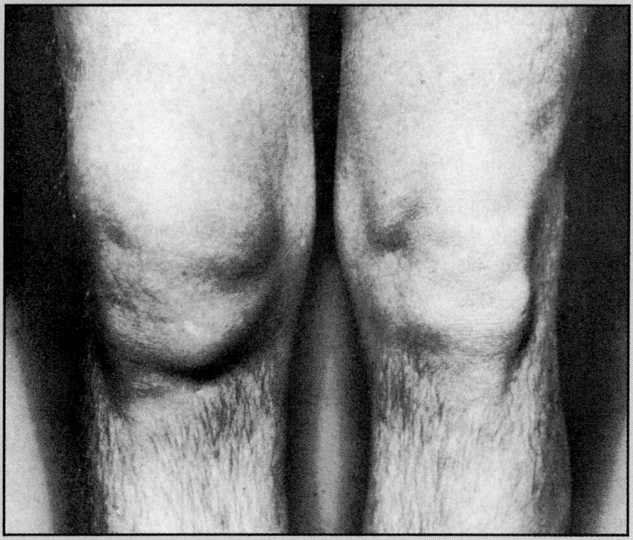

MILD SYNOVITIS

Loss of normal hollows on either side of the patella, which are replaced by mild distention. Occurs with synovial thickening or effusion (excess fluid). Also note mild distention of the suprapatellar pouch.

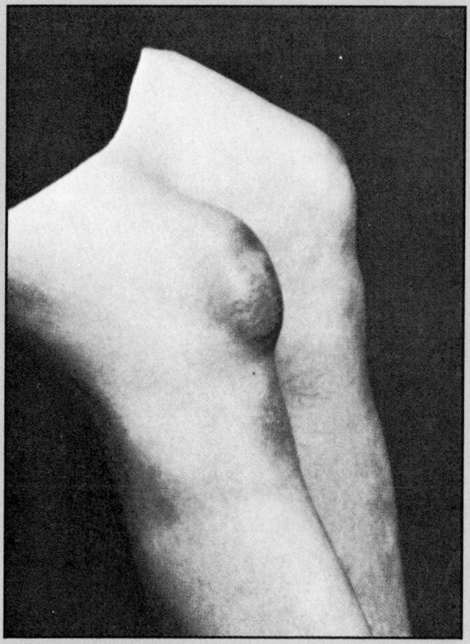

PREPATELLAR BURSITIS

Localized swelling on anterior knee between patella and skin. You will palpate a fluctuant mass with sharp border demarcations indicating swelling. The condition is limited to the bursa, and the knee joint itself is not involved. Overlying skin may be red, shiny, atrophic, or coarse and thickened.

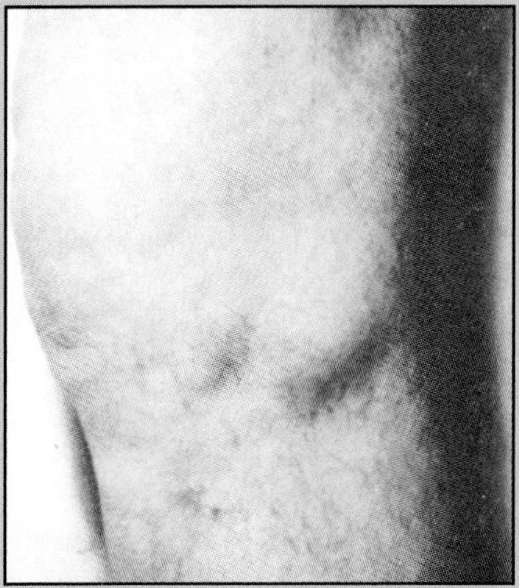

SWELLING OF MENISCI

Localized soft swelling due to cyst in medial meniscus shows at the midpoint of the anteromedial joint line. Flexion of the knee makes swelling more prominent.

OSGOOD-SCHLATTER DISEASE (not illustrated)

Painful swelling of the tibial tubercle just below the knee, probably due to repeated stress on the patellar tendon. Occurs most in puberty during rapid growth, and most often in males. Pain increases with kicking, running, bike riding, stair climbing, or kneeling. The condition is usually self-limited, and symptoms resolve with rest.

CHONDROMALACIA PATELLAE (not illustrated)

Degeneration of articular surface of patellae. The condition occurs most often in females, and its cause is unknown. May produce mild effusion. Joint motion is painless but crepitus may be present. Pain starts with kneeling.

Table 19-8 ▸ Abnormalities of the Ankle and Foot

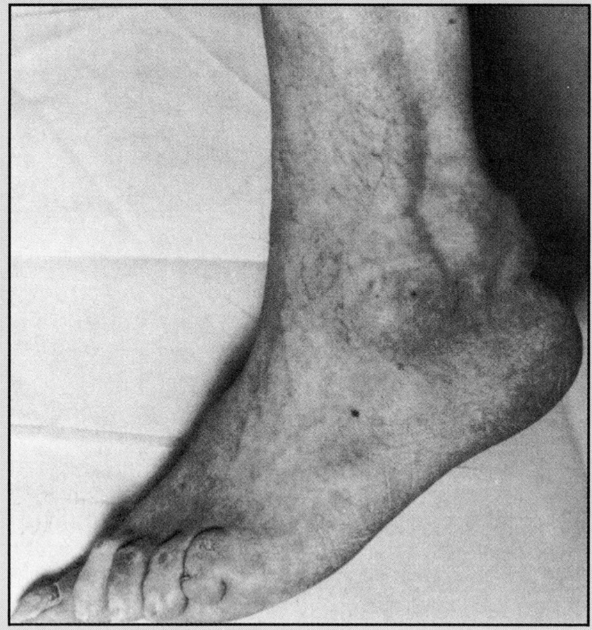

ACHILLES TENOSYNOVITIS

Inflammation of a tendon sheath near the ankle (here the Achilles tendon) produces a superficial linear swelling and a localized tenderness along the route of the sheath. Movement of the involved tendon usually causes pain.

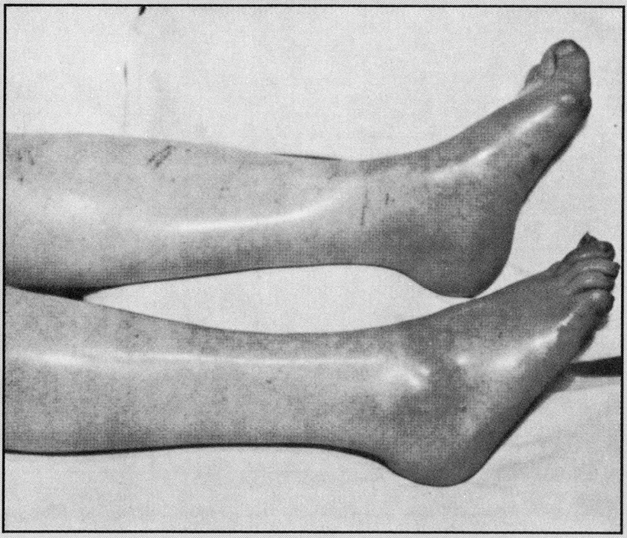

ACHILLES TENDON CONTRACTURES

Contractures due to prolonged bed rest in a person with rheumatoid arthritis. Shiny atrophic skin also is due to disuse.

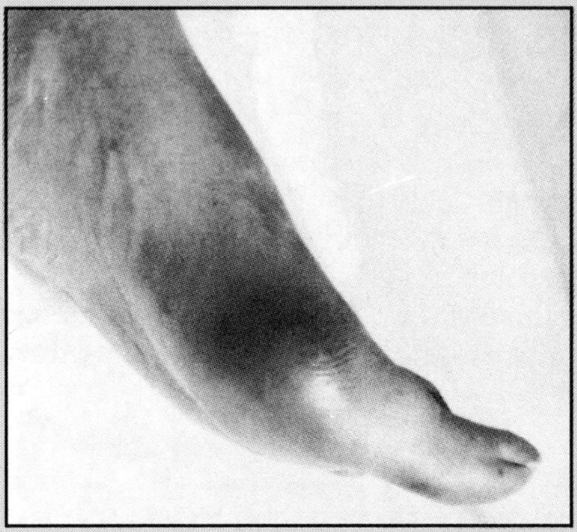

ACUTE GOUTY ARTHRITIS

Episode of gout here involves first the metatarsophalangeal joint. Clinical findings consist of redness, swelling, heat, and extreme tenderness.

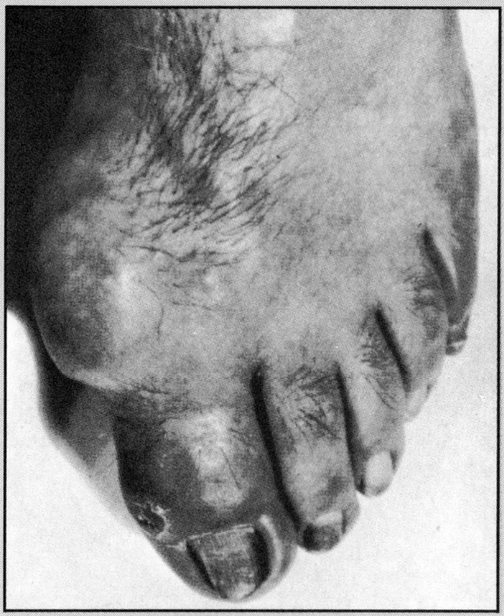

TOPHI WITH CHRONIC GOUT

Hard, painless nodules (tophi) over metatarsophalangeal joint of first toe. Tophi are collections of sodium urate crystals due to chronic gout. They sometimes burst with a chalky discharge.

Table 19-8 ▸ Abnormalities of the Ankle and Foot *Continued*

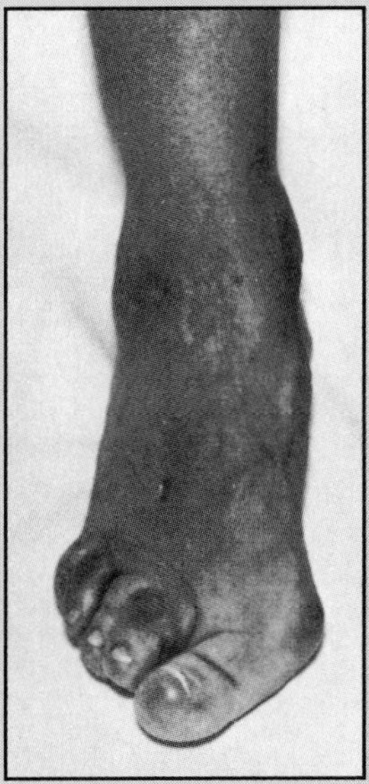

HALLUX VALGUS WITH BUNION AND HAMMER TOES

This common deformity is a lateral or outward deviation of the toe with medial prominence of the head of the first metatarsal. The bunion is the inflamed bursa that forms at the pressure point. The great toe loses power to push off while walking; this stresses the second and third metatarsal heads and they develop calluses and pain. Chronic sequelae include corns, calluses, hammer toes, and joint subluxation.

Note the *hammer toe* deformities in the second, third, fourth, and fifth toes. Often associated with hallux valgus, it includes hyperextension of the metatarsophalangeal joint and flexion of the proximal interphalangeal joint.

Corns (thickening of soft tissue) develop on the dorsum over the bony prominence owing to prolonged pressure from shoes.

CALLUS (not illustrated)

Hypertrophy of the epithelium develops because of prolonged pressure, commonly on the plantar surface of the first metatarsal head in the hallux valgus deformity. The condition is not painful.

PLANTAR WART (not illustrated)

Vascular papillomatous growth probably due to a virus, occurring on the sole of the foot, commonly at the ball. The condition is extremely painful.

INGROWN TOENAIL (not illustrated)

A misnomer; the nail does not grow in, but the soft tissue grows over the nail and obliterates the groove. It occurs almost always on the great toe, on the medial or lateral side. It is due to trimming the nail too short or toe crowding in tight shoes. The area becomes infected when the nail grows and its corner penetrates the soft tissue.

Table 19-9 ▶ Abnormalities of the Spine

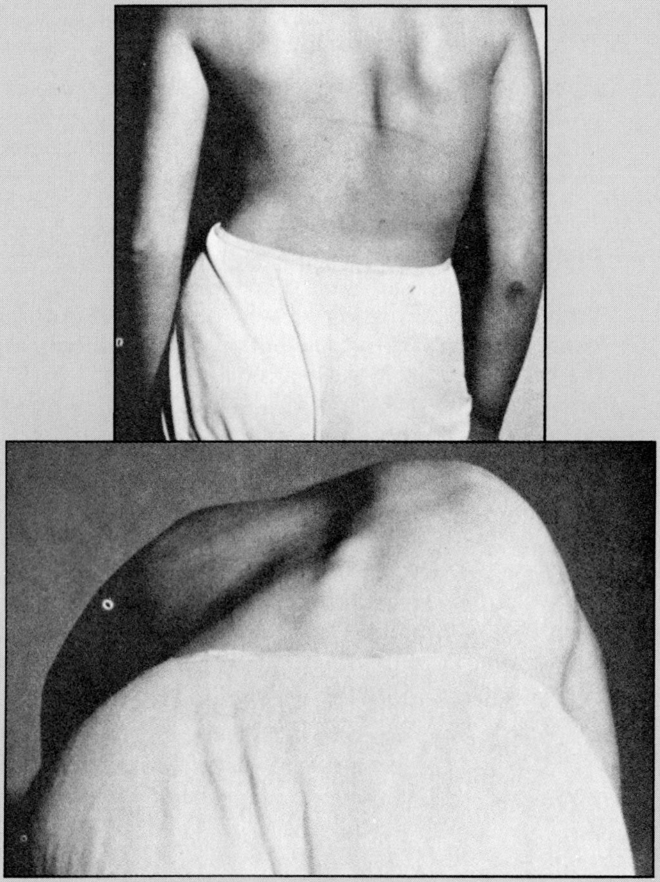

A

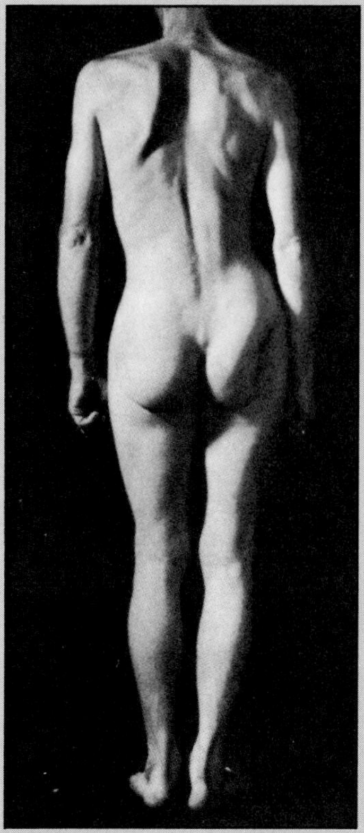

B

SCOLIOSIS

Lateral curvature of thoracic and lumbar segments of the spine, usually with some rotation of involved vertebral bodies.

Functional scoliosis is flexible; it is apparent with standing and disappears with forward bending. It may be compensatory for other abnormalities such as leg length discrepancy.

Structural scoliosis is fixed; the curvature shows both on standing and on bending forward. Note rib hump with forward flexion. When the person is standing note unequal shoulder elevation, unequal scapulae, obvious curvature, unequal elbow level, and unequal hip level. At greatest risk are females aged 10 through adolescence.

HERNIATED NUCLEUS PULPOSUS

The nucleus pulposus (at the center of the intervertebral disc) ruptures into the spinal canal and puts pressure on the local spinal nerve root. Usually occurs from stress, e.g., lifting, twisting, continuous flexion with lifting, or fall on buttocks. Occurs mostly in men 20 to 45 years of age. Lumbar herniations occur mainly in interspaces L4 to L5 and L5 to S1. Note: sciatic pain, numbness, and paresthesia of involved dermatome; listing away from affected side; decreased mobility; low back tenderness; and decreased motor and sensory function in leg. Straight leg raising tests reproduce sciatic pain.

Table 19-10 ▸ Common Congenital or Pediatric Abnormalities

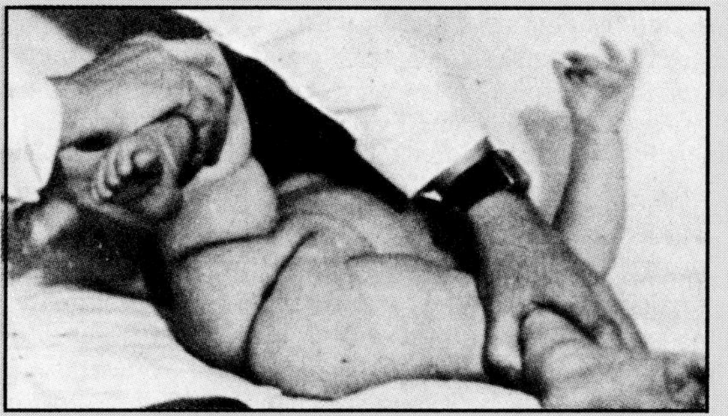

CONGENITAL DISLOCATED HIP

Head of the femur is displaced out of the cup-shaped acetabulum.

The degree of the condition varies; subluxation may occur as stretched ligaments allow partial displacement of femoral head, and acetabular dysplasia may develop because of excessive laxity of hip joint capsule.

Occurrence is 1:500 to 1:1000 births, more frequently in girls by 7:1 ratio. Signs include limited abduction of flexed thigh, positive indications of Ortolani's and Barlow's signs, asymmetric skin creases or gluteal folds, limb length discrepancy, and positive indication of Trendelenburg's sign in older children.

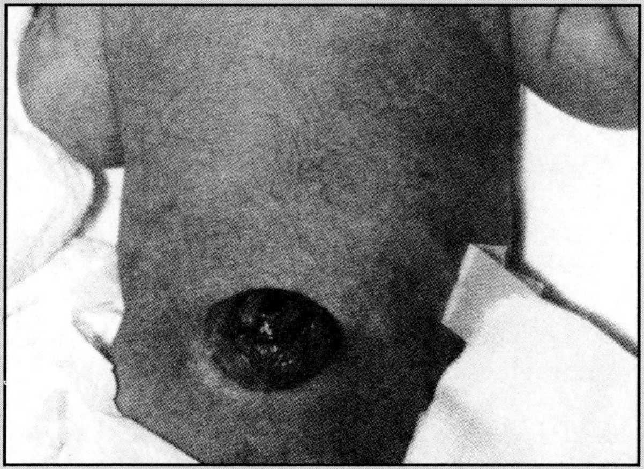

SPINA BIFIDA

Incomplete closure of posterior part of vertebrae results in a neural tube defect. Seriousness varies from skin defect along the spine to protrusion of the sac containing meninges, spinal fluid, or malformed spinal cord. The most serious type is myelomeningocele (shown here), in which the meninges and neural tissue protrude. In these cases, the child is usually paralyzed below the level of the lesion.

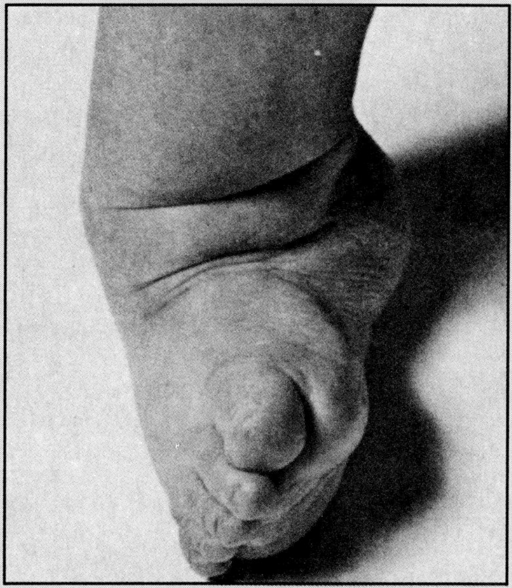

TALIPES EQUINOVARUS (CLUBFOOT)

Congenital, rigid and fixed malposition of foot including (1) inversion, (2) forefoot adduction, and (3) foot pointing downward (equinus). A common birth defect, with an incidence of 1:1000 to 3:1000 live births. Males are affected twice as frequently as females.

COXA PLANA (LEGG-CALVÉ-PERTHES SYNDROME) (not illustrated)

Avascular necrosis of the femoral head, occurring primarily in males between 3 to 12 years of age, with peak at age 6 years. In initial inflammatory stage there is interruption of blood supply to femoral epiphysis, halting growth. Revascularization and healing occur later, but there may be significant residual deformity and dysfunction.

Bibliography

American Nurses' Association and National Association of Orthopaedic Nurses: Orthopaedic Nursing Practice—Process and Outcome Criteria for Selected Diagnoses. Kansas City, MO, American Nurses' Association, 1986.

Ausenhus MK: Osteoporosis: Prevention during the adolescent and young adult years. Nurs Pract 13(a):42–48, 1988.

Barness LA: Manual of Pediatric Physical Diagnosis. Chicago, Year Book Medical Publishers, 1981.

Behrman RE, Vaughan VC (Eds): Nelson Textbook of Pediatrics. 13th ed. Philadelphia, WB Saunders, 1987.

Bluestone R: Symptoms and signs of articular disease. *In* Resnik D, Niwayama G (Eds): Diagnosis of Bone and Joint Disorders, Vol. 1. Philadelphia, WB Saunders, 1981.

Bourne Collo MC, Johnson JL, Finch WR, Felicetta JV: Evaluating arthritic complaints. Nurs Pract 16(2)9–20, 1991.

Bowers AC, Thompson JM: Clinical Manual of Health Assessment. 3rd ed. St. Louis, CV Mosby, 1988.

Debrunner HV: Orthopaedic Diagnosis. Chicago, Year Book Medical Publishers, 1982.

Farrally MR, Moore WJ: Anatomical differences in the femur and tibia between Negroes and Caucasians and their effect on locomotion. Am J Phys Anthropol 43(1):63–69, 1975.

Garn SM: Compact bone in Chinese and Japanese. Science 143(3613):1439–1441, 1964.

Hamerman D: Rheumatic disorders. *In* Rossman I (Ed): Clinical Geriatrics. Philadelphia, JB Lippincott, 1986.

Hoehn JG, Nalebuff EA, Wright PE: Common hand problems in primary care. Patient Care 25(1):72–118, 1991.

Hoppenfeld S: Physical Examination of the Spine and Extremities. New York, Appleton-Century-Crofts, 1976.

Jahss M: Geriatric aspects of the foot and ankle. *In* Rossman I (Ed): Clinical Geriatrics. Philadelphia, JB Lippincott, 1986.

Johnson TR, Moore WM, Jeffries JE (Eds): Children Are Different: Developmental Physiology. 2nd ed. Columbus, OH, Ross Laboratories, 1978.

Kelley WN, Harris ED, Ruddy S, Sledge CB: Textbook of Rheumatology, 2nd ed. Philadelphia, WB Saunders, 1985.

Killam PE: Orthopedic assessment of young children: Developmental variations. Nurs Pract 14(7):27–36.

Linley JF: Screening children for common orthopaedic problems. Am J Nurs 87:1312–1316, 1987.

McCullough FL: Skeletal trauma in children. Orthopaedic Nursing 8(2):41–46, 1989.

McMillan JA, Nieburg PI, Oski FA: The Whole Pediatrician Catalog. Philadelphia, WB Saunders, 1977.

Milde FK: Impaired physical mobility. J Gerontol Nurs 14(3):20–24, 1988.

Pellino TA, et al (Eds): Core Curriculum for Orthopaedic Nursing. Pitman NJ, A Jannette, 1986.

Polley HF, Hunder GG: Rheumatologic Interviewing and Physical Examination of the Joints. Philadelphia, WB Saunders, 1978.

Rodnan GP, Schumacher HR (Eds): Primer on the Rheumatic Diseases. 8th ed. Atlanta, GA, Arthritis Foundation, 1983.

Rossman I (Ed): Clinical Geriatrics. 3rd ed. Philadelphia, JB Lippincott, 1986.

Schoen DC: The Nursing Process in Orthopaedics. Norwalk, CT, Appleton-Century-Crofts, 1986.

Scullo TP (Ed): Orthopaedic Care of the Geriatric Patient. St. Louis, MO, CV Mosby, 1985.

Spencer H, et al: Disorders of the skeletal system. *In* Rossman I (Ed): Clinical Geriatrics. Philadelphia, JB Lippincott, 1986.

CHAPTER

20 Neurologic System

STRUCTURE AND FUNCTION

The nervous system can be divided into two parts—central and peripheral. The *central nervous system* (CNS) includes the brain and spinal cord. The *peripheral nervous system* includes the 12 pairs of cranial nerves, the 31 pairs of spinal nerves, and all their branches. The peripheral nervous system carries messages *to* the CNS from sensory receptors and *from* the CNS out to muscles and glands.

THE CENTRAL NERVOUS SYSTEM (CNS)

Components of the CNS

Cerebral Cortex

The cerebral cortex is the cerebrum's outer layer of nerve cell bodies, also called gray matter. The cerebral cortex is the center for human's highest functions, governing thought, memory, reasoning, sensation, and voluntary movement (Fig. 20–1). Each half of the cerebrum is a *hemisphere;* the left hemisphere is dominant in most (95 percent) people, including those who are left-handed.

Each hemisphere is divided into four *lobes:* frontal, parietal, temporal, and occipital. The lobes have certain areas that mediate specific functions.

- The *frontal* lobe has areas concerned with personality, behavior, emotions, and intellectual function.
- The precentral gyrus of the frontal lobe initiates voluntary movement.
- The *parietal* lobe's postcentral gyrus is the primary center for sensation.
- The *occipital* lobe is the primary visual receptor center.
- The *temporal* lobe behind the ear has the primary auditory reception center.
- *Wernicke's area* in the temporal lobe also is associated with auditory reception. When damaged in the person's dominant hemisphere, aphasia results. The person hears sound, but it has no meaning, like hearing a foreign language.
- *Broca's area* in the frontal lobe mediates speech formation. When injured in the dominant hemisphere, another type of aphasia results; the person cannot talk. The person knows what he or she wants to say, but only a garbled sound is produced.

Damage to any of these specific cortical areas produces a corresponding loss of function: motor deficit, paralysis, loss of sensation, or impaired ability to understand and process language. Damage occurs when the highly specialized neurologic cells are deprived of their blood supply, such as when a cerebral artery becomes plugged, or when vascular bleeding or vasospasm occurs.

Basal Ganglia

The basal ganglia are bands of gray matter buried deep within the two cerebral hemispheres that form the subcortical or "primitive" motor areas (Fig. 20–2). They control automatic associated movements of the body, e.g., the arm swing alternating with the legs during walking.

Thalamus

The thalamus is the main relay station for the nervous system. Sensory pathways of the spinal cord and brain stem form *synapses* (sites of contact between two neurons) on their way to the cerebral cortex.

Hypothalamus

The hypothalamus is a vital area with many important functions: temperature control, sleep center, anterior and posterior pituitary gland regulator, coordinator of autonomic nervous system activity, and emotional status.

Cerebellum

The cerebellum is a coiled structure located under the occipital lobe that is concerned with motor coordination

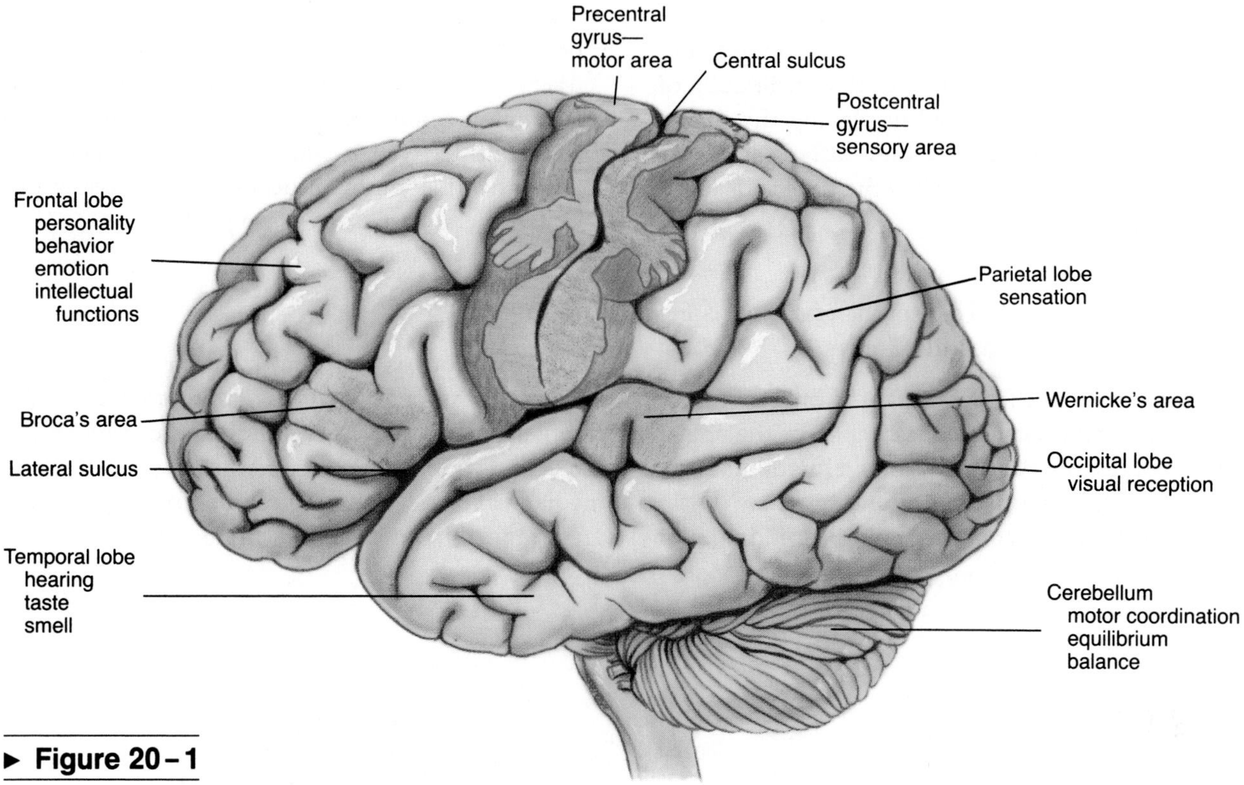

► **Figure 20–1**

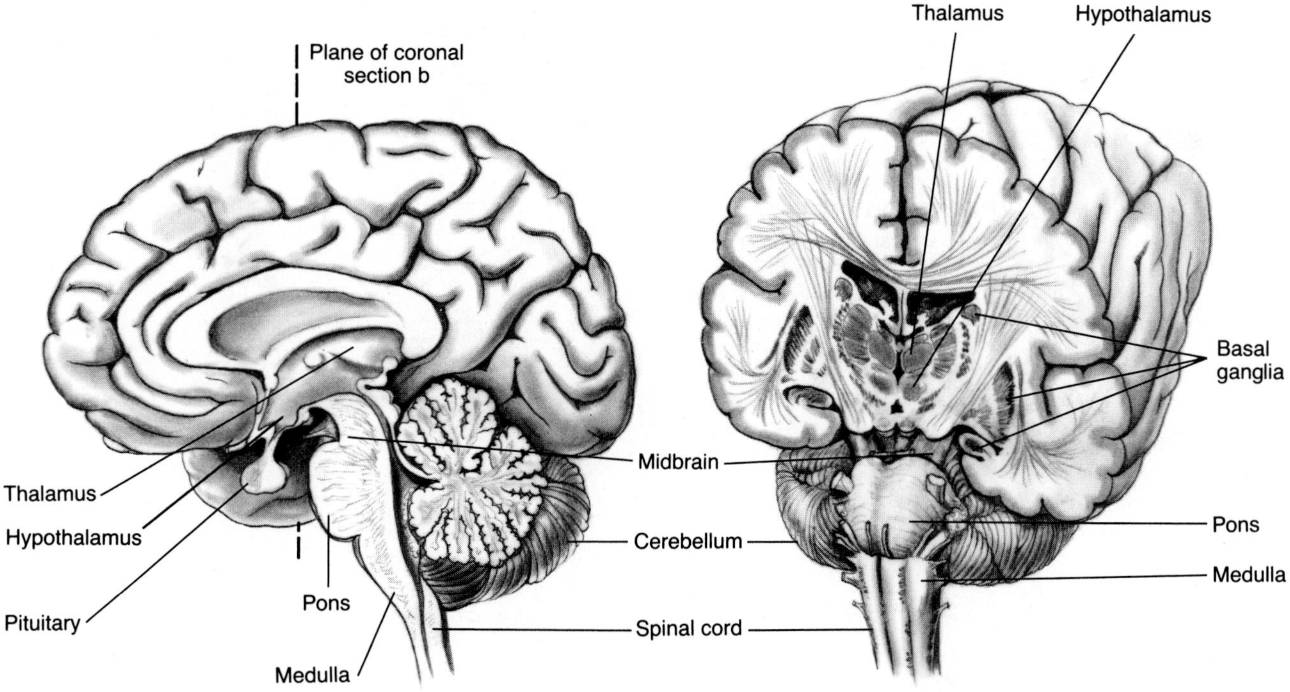

A Medial view of right hemisphere

B Coronal section

► **Figure 20–2**

of voluntary movements, equilibrium, and muscle tone. It does not initiate movement but coordinates and smooths it, e.g., the complex and quick coordination of many different muscles needed in playing the piano, swimming, or juggling. Called the "little brain," the cerebellum operates entirely below the conscious level.

Brain Stem

The brain stem is the central core of the brain consisting of mostly nerve fibers. It has three areas:

- **Midbrain**—the most anterior part of the brain stem that still has the basic tubular structure of the spinal cord. It merges into the thalamus and hypothalamus. It contains many motor neurons and tracts.
- **Pons**—the enlarged area containing ascending and descending fiber tracts.
- **Medulla**—continuation of the spinal cord in the brain that contains all ascending and descending fiber tracts connecting the brain and spinal cord. It has vital autonomic centers (respiration, heart, gastrointestinal function), as well as nuclei for cranial nerves VIII through XII. Pyramidal decussation (crossing of the motor fibers) occurs here (see p. 733).

Spinal Cord

The spinal cord is the long cylindrical structure that occupies the upper two thirds of the vertebral canal. It is the main highway for ascending and descending fiber tracts that connect the brain to the spinal nerves, and it mediates reflexes. Its nerve cell bodies, or gray matter, are arranged in an H shape with anterior and posterior "horns."

► **Figure 20-3**

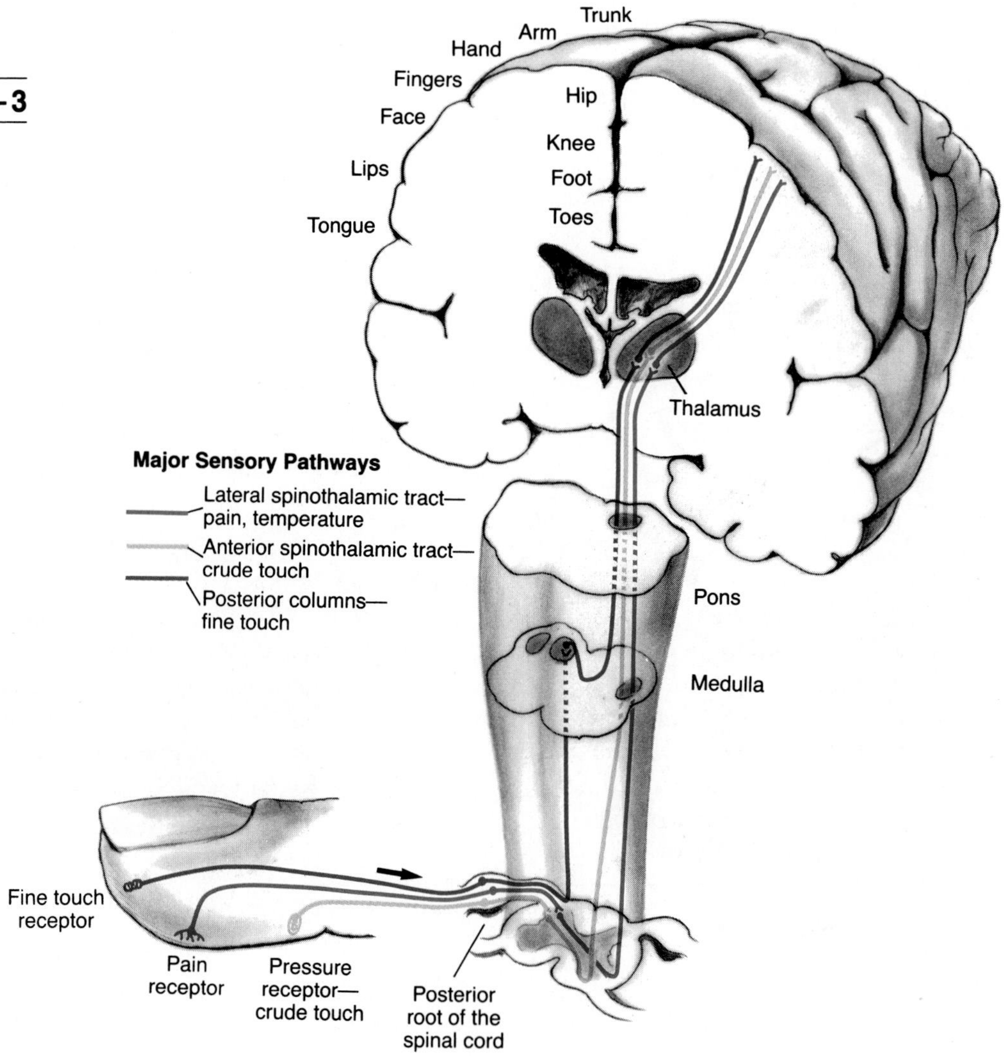

Motor and Sensory Pathways of the CNS

Major Sensory Pathways

Millions of sensory receptors are embroidered into the skin, mucous membranes, muscles, tendons, and viscera. They are important for conscious sensation and reflexes. Sensation travels in the afferent fibers in the peripheral nerve, then through the posterior (dorsal) root, and then into the spinal cord. There, it may take one of two routes — the spinothalamic tract or the posterior columns (Fig. 20 – 3).

Spinothalamic Tract. The spinothalamic tract contains sensory fibers that transmit the sensations of pain, temperature, and crude or light touch. The fibers enter the dorsal root of the spinal cord, synapse with a second sensory neuron, cross to the opposite side, and ascend up the spinothalamic tract to the thalamus. Fibers carrying pain and temperature sensations ascend the *lateral* spinothalamic tract, whereas those of crude touch form the *anterior* spinothalamic tract. At the thalamus, the fibers synapse with another sensory neuron, which carries the message to the sensory cortex for full interpretation.

Posterior Columns. These fibers conduct position, vibration, and finely localized touch.

Position (proprioception) — without looking, you know where your body parts are in space and in relation to each other

Vibration — feeling vibrating objects

Finely localized touch (stereognosis) — without looking, you can identify familiar objects by touch

These fibers enter the dorsal root and proceed immediately up the spinal cord to the brain stem. There, they synapse with a second sensory neuron and cross over. They travel to the thalamus, synapse again, and proceed to the sensory cortex, which localizes the sensation and makes full discrimination.

The sensory cortex is arranged in a specific pattern forming a corresponding "map" of the body. Pain in the right hand is perceived at its specific spot on the map. Some organs are absent from the brain map, such as the heart, liver, or spleen. You know you have one but there is no "felt image" of it (Miller, 1978). Pain originating in these organs is referred, because there is no felt image in which to have pain. Pain is felt "by proxy" by another body part that does have a felt image. For example, pain in the heart is referred to the chest, shoulder, and left arm, which were its neighbors in fetal development. Pain originating in the spleen is felt on the top of the left shoulder.

Major Motor Pathways

Corticospinal or Pyramidal Tract (Fig. 20 – 4). The area has been named "pyramidal" because many of its cell bodies in the cortex have a pyramidal shape. Motor nerve fibers originate in the motor cortex and travel to the brain stem, where they cross to the opposite side (*pyramidal decussation*) and then pass down the spinal cord. At each cord level, they synapse with a lower motor neuron contained in the spinal nerve. Corticospinal fibers mediate voluntary movement, particularly very skilled, discrete, purposeful movements, such as writing.

The corticospinal tract is a newer, "higher," motor system that humans have that permits very skilled and purposeful movements. The tract's origin in the motor cortex is arranged in a specific pattern. It is another body map, this one of a person hanging "upside down." Body parts are not equally represented on the map. It is more like an electoral map than a geographical map (Miller, 1978). That is, body parts whose movements are relatively more important to humans, for example the hand, occupy more space on the brain map.

Extrapyramidal Tract. The extrapyramidal tract includes all the motor nerve fibers originating in the motor cortex, basal ganglia, brain stem, and spinal cord that are *outside* the pyramidal tract. This is an older, "lower," more primitive motor system. These motor fibers maintain muscle tone and control body movements, especially gross automatic movements, such as walking.

Cerebellar System. This motor system coordinates movement, maintains equilibrium, and helps maintain posture. The cerebellum receives information about the position of muscles and joints, the body's equilibrium, and what kind of motor messages are being sent from the cortex to the muscles. The information is integrated, and the cerebellum uses feedback pathways to exert its control back on the cortex or down to lower motor neurons in the spinal cord. This entire process occurs on an unconscious level.

Upper and Lower Motor Neurons

Upper motor neurons are all the descending fibers that can influence or modify the lower motor neurons. Upper motor neurons are located completely within the

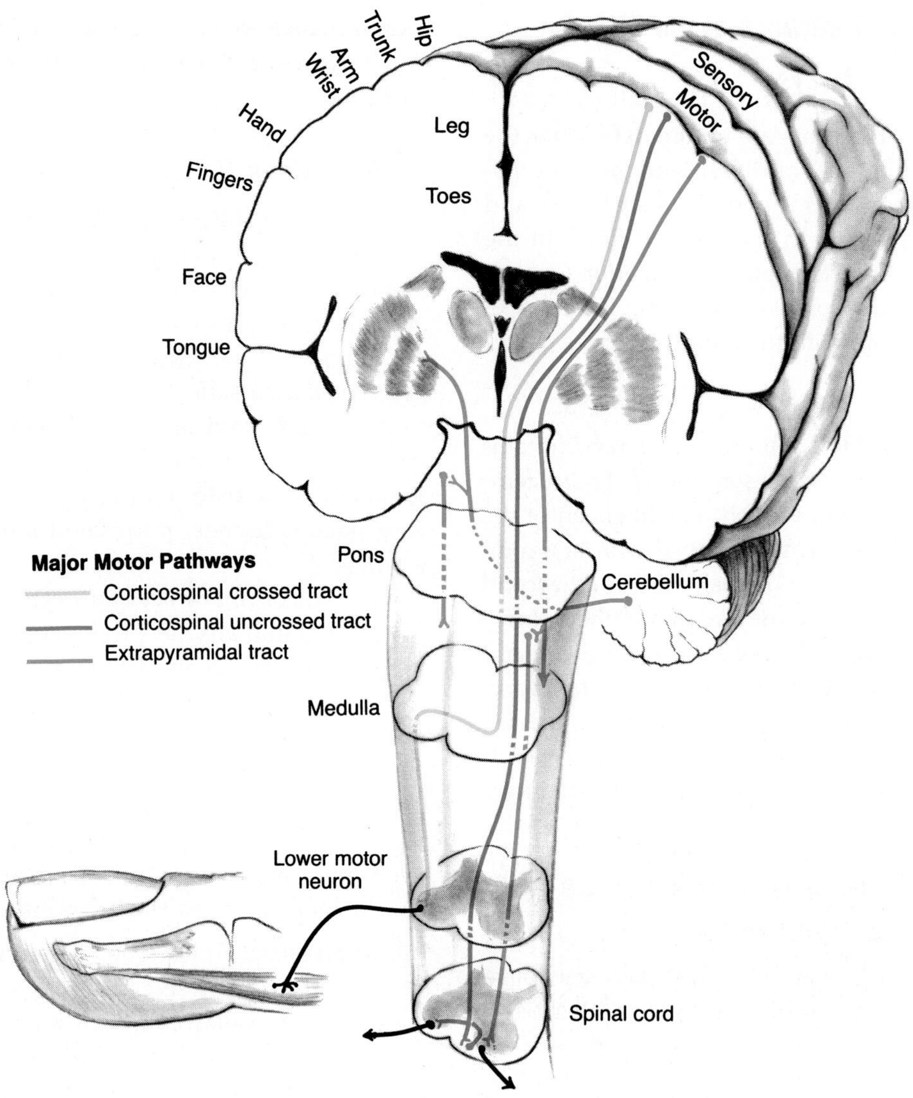

► **Figure 20-4**

CNS. The neurons convey impulses from motor areas of the cerebral cortex to the lower motor neuron to effect muscle action. Examples of upper motor neurons are corticospinal and extrapyramidal tracts. Examples of upper motor neuron diseases are cerebrovascular accident, cerebral palsy, and multiple sclerosis.

The cell body of the lower motor neuron is located in the anterior gray column of the spinal cord, but the nerve fiber extends from here to the muscle. The lower motor neuron is the "final common pathway," which provides the final direct contact with the muscles. Any movement must be translated into action by lower motor neuron fibers. Examples of lower motor neurons are cranial nerves and spinal nerves of the peripheral nervous system. Examples of lower motor neuron diseases are spinal cord lesions or poliomyelitis.

THE PERIPHERAL NERVOUS SYSTEM

A *nerve* is a bundle of fibers *outside* the CNS. The peripheral nerves carry input to the CNS via their sensory afferent fibers, and deliver output from the CNS via the efferent fibers.

Cranial Nerves

Cranial nerves enter and exit the brain rather than the spinal cord (Fig. 20–5 and Table 20–1). The 12 pairs of cranial nerves supply primarily the head and neck, except the vagus nerve (L. vagus, or wanderer as in "vagabond"), which travels to the heart, respiratory muscles, stomach, and gallbladder.

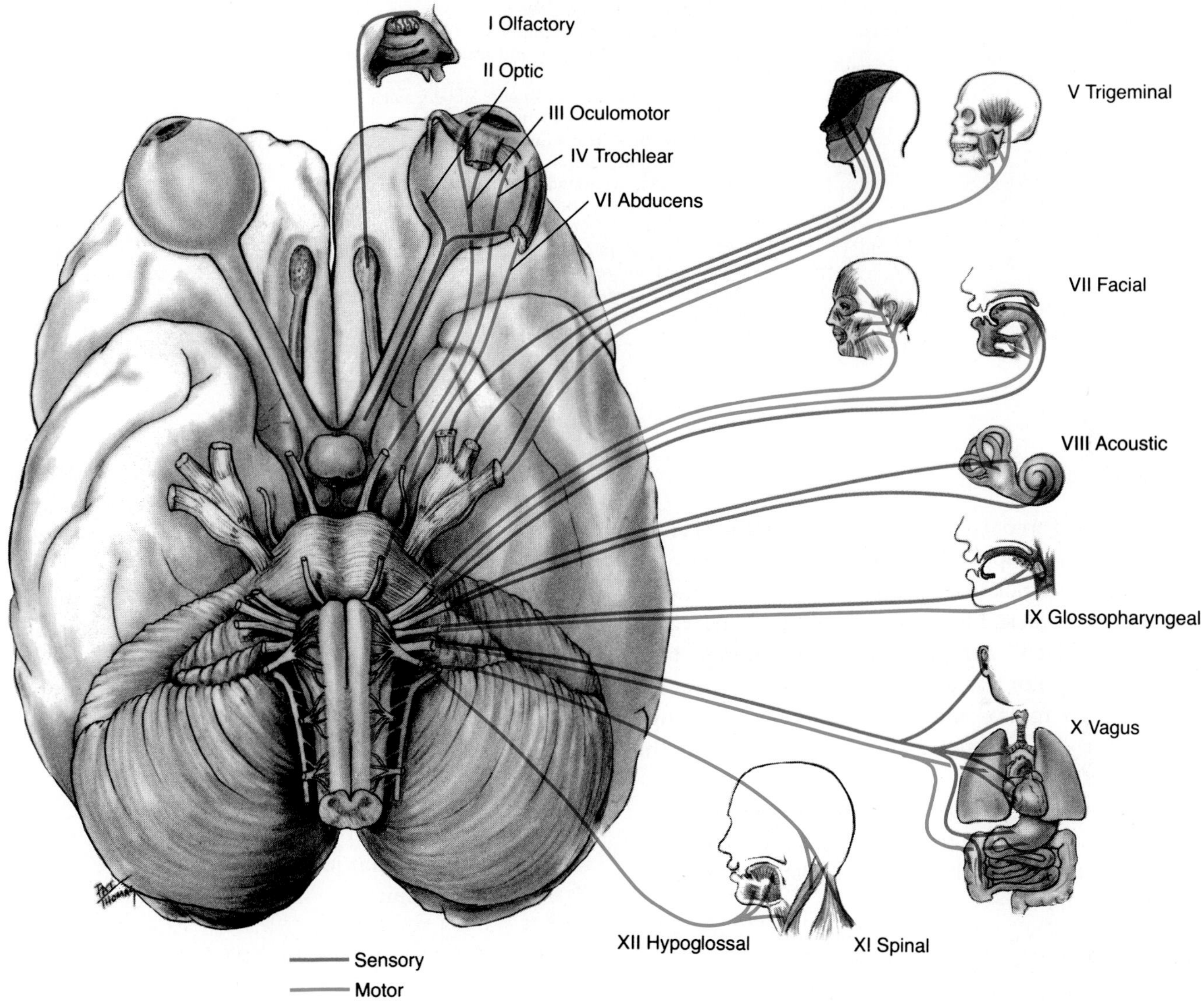

► **Figure 20–5**

Table 20-1 ▶ Cranial Nerves

CRANIAL NERVE	TYPE	FUNCTION
I Olfactory	Sensory	Smell
II Optic	Sensory	Vision
III Oculomotor	Mixed	Motor—most EOM movement, raise eyelids Parasympathetic—pupil constriction, lens shape
IV Trochlear	Motor	Down and inward movement of eye
V Trigeminal	Mixed	Motor—muscles of mastication Sensory—sensation of face and scalp, cornea, mucous membranes of mouth and nose
VI Abducens	Motor	Lateral movement of eye
VII Facial	Mixed	Motor—facial muscles, close eye, labial speech Sensory—taste on anterior two-thirds of tongue Parasympathetic—saliva and tear secretion
VIII Acoustic	Sensory	Hearing and equilibrium
IX Glossopharyngeal	Mixed	Motor—pharynx (phonation and swallowing) Sensory—taste posterior one-third of tongue, pharynx (gag reflex) Parasympathetic—parotid gland, carotid reflex
X Vagus	Mixed	Motor—pharynx and larynx (talking and swallowing) Sensory—general sensation from carotid body, carotid sinus, pharynx, viscera Parasympathetic—carotid reflex
XI Spinal	Motor	Movement of trapezius and sternomastoid muscles
XII Hypoglossal	Motor	Movement of tongue

Spinal Nerves

The 31 pairs of spinal nerves arise from the length of the spinal cord and supply the rest of the body. They are named for the region of the spine from which they exit: 8 cervical, 12 thoracic, 5 lumbar, 5 sacral, and 1 coccygeal. They are "mixed" nerves because they contain both sensory and motor fibers. The nerves enter and exit the cord through roots—sensory afferent fibers through the dorsal roots, and motor efferent fibers through the ventral roots.

The nerves exit the spinal cord in an orderly ladder. Each nerve innervates a particular segment of the body. *Dermal segmentation* is the cutaneous distribution of the various spinal nerves.

A *dermatome* is a circumscribed skin area that is supplied mainly from one spinal cord segment through a particular spinal nerve (Fig. 20–6). The dermatomes overlap, so if one nerve is severed most of the sensations can be transmitted by the one above and the one below. This overlap is a form of biologic insurance (Liebman, 1983).

Reflex Arc

A reflex is a defense mechanism of the nervous system. It operates below the level of conscious control and permits a quick reaction to potentially painful or damaging situations.

The fibers that mediate the reflex are carried by a specific spinal nerve. In the most simple reflex, the sensory afferent fibers carry the message from the receptor and travel through the dorsal root into the spinal cord (Fig. 20–7). They synapse in the cord with the motor neuron in the anterior horn. Motor efferent fibers leave via the ventral root and travel to the muscle.

The deep tendon or stretch reflex has five components:

1. An intact sensory nerve (afferent)
2. A functional synapse in the cord
3. An intact motor nerve fiber (efferent)
4. The neuromuscular junction
5. A competent muscle

Autonomic Nervous System

The peripheral nervous system is composed of cranial nerves and spinal nerves. These nerves carry fibers that can be divided functionally into two parts—somatic and autonomic. The somatic fibers innervate the skeletal (voluntary) muscles; the autonomic fibers innervate smooth (involuntary) muscles, cardiac muscle, and glands. The autonomic system mediates unconscious activity. Although a description of the autonomic system is beyond the scope of this book, its overall function is to maintain homeostasis of the body.

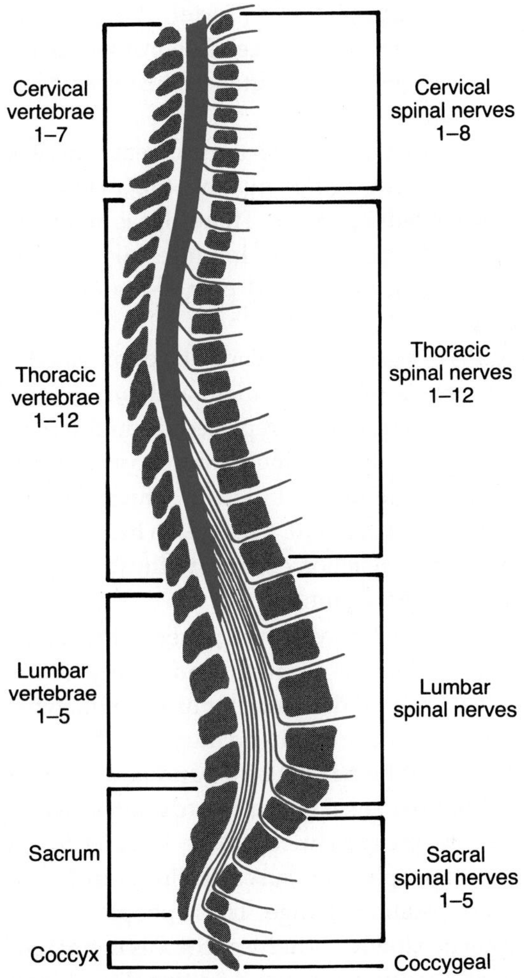

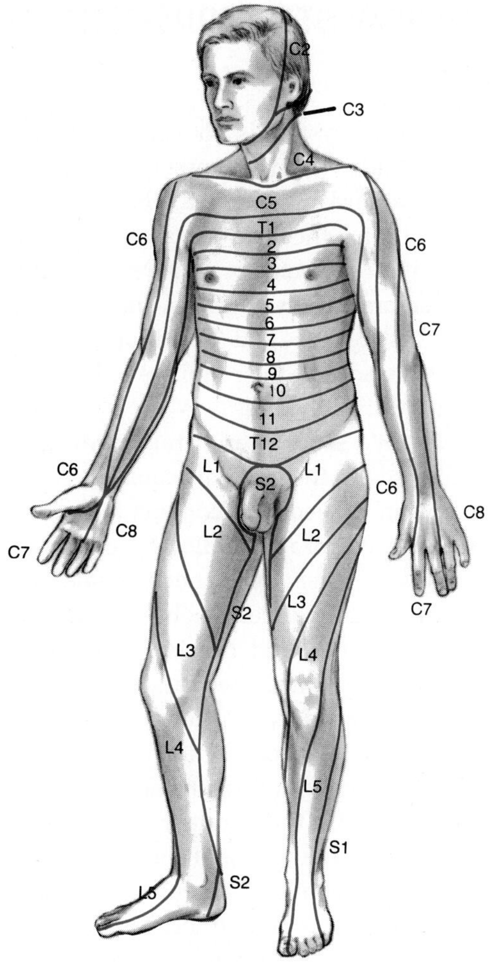

▶ Figure 20 – 6

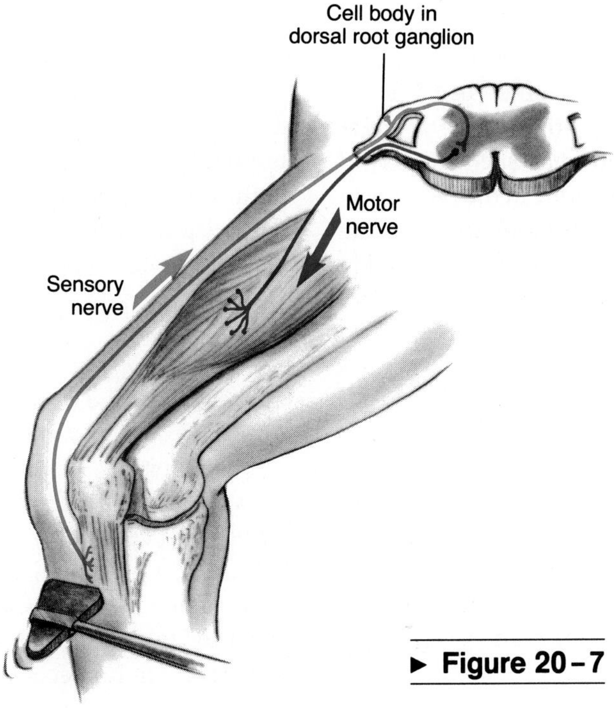

▶ Figure 20 – 7

DEVELOPMENTAL CONSIDERATIONS

Infants

The neurologic system is not completely developed at birth. Motor activity in the newborn is under the control of the spinal cord and medulla. There is very little cortical control, and the neurons are not yet myelinated. Movements are directed primarily by primitive reflexes. As the cerebral cortex develops during the first year, it inhibits these reflexes and they disappear at predictable times. Persistence of the primitive reflexes is an indication of CNS dysfunction.

The infant's sensory and motor development proceeds along with the gradual acquisition of myelin, because myelin is needed to conduct most impulses. The process of myelinization follows a cephalocaudal and proximodistal order (head, neck, trunk, and extremities). This is just the order we observe the infant gaining motor control (lifts head, lifts head and shoulders, rolls over, moves whole arm, uses hands, walks). As the milestones are achieved, each is more complex and coordinated. Milestones occur in an orderly sequence, although the exact age of occurrence may vary.

Sensation also is rudimentary at birth. The newborn needs a strong stimulus, and then responds by crying and with whole body movements. As myelinization develops, the infant is able to localize the stimulus more precisely and to make a more accurate motor response.

The Aging Adult

The aging process causes a steady loss of neurons. Neuron loss occurs in the brain and spinal cord. It leads many people over 65 to show signs that, in the younger adult, would be considered abnormal, such as general loss of muscle bulk, loss of muscle tone in the face, neck, and around the spine, loss of vibratory sense at the ankle, loss of position sense at the big toe, loss of ankle jerk, and irregular pupil shape (Carter, 1986). As long as no other symptoms or evidence of neurologic disease is present, these signs are attributed to the expected aging process.

The velocity of nerve conduction decreases between 5 to 10 percent with aging, making the reaction time slower in some older persons. There also is an increased delay at the synapse, so the impulse takes longer to travel. As a result, touch and pain sensation may be diminished.

Sensations of taste and smell may be diminished. Any change in taste is relatively small, and current studies show tastebuds actually are replaced throughout adulthood. What probably contributes more to any change in eating habits is the deficit in smell, which does occur with aging (Storandt, 1986). Changes in hearing, vision, and pupil size and reaction occur, and these changes are described in earlier chapters.

The motor system may show a general slowing down of movement. Muscle strength and agility decrease. There is a generalized decrease in muscle bulk, which is most apparent in the dorsal hand muscles. Muscle tremors may occur in the hands, head, and jaw, along with possible repetitive facial grimacing (dyskinesias).

Aging has a progressive decrease in cerebral blood flow. In some people this causes dizziness and a loss of balance with position change. These people need to be taught to get up slowly. Otherwise there is increased risk for falls and resulting injuries. Additionally, older people may forget they fell, which makes it hard to diagnose the cause of the injury.

When they are in good health, aging people walk about as well as they did during their middle and younger years, except more slowly and more deliberately. Some survey the ground for obstacles or uneven terrain. Some show a hesitation and a slightly wayward path. More severe gait dysfunction is due to problems with vision, skeletal, or joint changes or conditions affecting the neurologic system (Carter, 1986).

SUBJECTIVE DATA

Headache	Weakness or incoordination
Head injury	Numbness or tingling
Dizziness/vertigo	Difficulty swallowing
Seizures	Difficulty speaking
Tremors	Significant past history

EXAMINER ASKS: / **RATIONALE:**

1. **Headaches**—Do you experience any unusually frequent or severe headaches?

When did this type of headache start? How often do the headaches occur?

Where in your head do you feel the headaches? Do the headaches seem to be associated with anything? (Headache history fully discussed in Chapter 10.)

[Pain in body part. Although pain is a neurologic phenomenon, it usually does not come up during the history in relation to the neurologic system. Pain is usually mentioned in relation to the body system in which it occurs. Pain arising from neurologic dysfunction is usually mentioned during the review of systems for the head, back, or extremities.]

2. Have you ever had any **head injury?** Please describe what happened. What part of the head was hit?

Did you have a loss of consciousness? For how long?

3. **Dizziness**—Do you ever feel lightheaded, a swimming sensation, like feeling faint?

When have you noticed this? How often does it occur? Does it occur with: activity, change in position?

Do you ever feel a sensation called **vertigo,** a rotational spinning sensation? (Note—distinguish vertigo from dizziness.) Do you feel as if the room spins (objective vertigo)? or, do you feel that you are spinning (subjective vertigo)? Did this come on suddenly or gradually?

Rationale: Syncope is a sudden loss of strength, a temporary loss of consciousness due to lack of cerebral blood flow, a faint.

True vertigo is rotational spinning caused by neurologic dysfunction or a problem in the vestibular apparatus or the vestibular nuclei in brain stem.

4. Have you ever had any convulsions? When did they start? How often do they occur?

Rationale: **Seizure** is an attack of epilepsy. Epilepsy is a paroxysmal disease characterized by altered or loss of consciousness, involuntary muscle movements, and sensory disturbances.

EXAMINER ASKS:	RATIONALE:
Course and Duration — When a seizure starts, do you have any warning sign? What type of sign?	Obtain sequence. Aura is a subjective sensation that precedes a seizure; it could be auditory, visual, or motor.
Motor activity — Where in body do the seizures begin? Do the seizures travel through body? On one side or both? Does your muscle tone seem tense or limp? Do you have any associated signs: color change in face or lips, loss of consciousness, for how long, automatisms (eyelid fluttering, eyes roll, lip smacking), incontinence? Postictal phase — After the seizure, are you told you spend time sleeping or have any confusion, weakness, headache, or muscle ache? Precipitating factors — Does anything seem to bring on the seizures: activity, discontinuing medication, fatigue, stress? Are you on any medication? Coping strategies — How have the seizures affected daily life, occupation?	
5. Have you noticed any shakes or **tremors** in the hands or face? When did these start? Do they seem to grow worse with anxiety, intention, or rest? Are they relieved with rest, activity, alcohol? Do they affect daily activities? Have you experienced any sudden jerks or twitches? Where? When did you first notice this?	Tremor is an involuntary shaking, vibrating, or trembling.
6. Do you have any **weakness** or problem moving any body part? Is this generalized or local? Does it occur with anything?	Paresis is a slight paralysis. Paralysis is a loss of motor function due to a lesion in the neurologic or muscular system, or of sensory innervation.
7. Do you have any problem with **coordination?** Do you have any problem with balance when walking? Do you list to one side? Have you experienced any falling? Which way? Do your legs seem to give way? Do you have any clumsy movement?	Dysmetria is the inability to control range of motion of muscles.
8. Have you noted any **numbness or tingling** in any body part? Does it feel like pins and needles? When did this start? Where do you feel it? Does it occur with activity?	Paresthesia is an abnormal sensation, e.g., burning, tingling.
9. Do you have any problem **swallowing?** Does this occur with solids or liquids? Have you experienced excessive saliva, drooling?	
10. Have you experienced any problem **speaking:** with forming words, or with saying what you intended to say? When did you first notice this? How long did it last?	
11. Do you have a **past history** of stroke (cerebrovascular accident)? Are there any aftereffects from this stroke? Do you have a past history of: spinal cord injury, meningitis or encephalitis, congenital defect, or alcoholism?	
12. Are you exposed to any environmental/occupational hazards: insecticides, organic solvents, lead? Are you taking any medications now?	Review especially anticonvulsants, anti-tremor, anti-vertigo, pain medication.

EXAMINER ASKS:	RATIONALE:

How much alcohol do you drink? Each week? Each day?

How about other drugs: marijuana, cocaine, barbiturates, tranquilizers, any other mood-altering drugs?

ADDITIONAL QUESTIONS FOR INFANTS AND CHILDREN

Did you (the mother) have any health problems during the pregnancy: any infections or illnesses, medications taken, toxemia, hypertension, alcohol or drug use, diabetes?

Prenatal history may affect infant's neurologic development.

Please tell me about this baby's birth. Was the baby at term or premature? What was the birth weight?

Was there any birth trauma? Did the baby breathe immediately? Were you told the baby's Apgar scores? Did the baby have any congenital defects?

Reflexes — What have you noticed about the baby's behavior? Do the baby's sucking and swallowing seem coordinated? When you touch the cheek, does the baby turn his or her head toward touch? Does the baby startle with a loud noise or shake of crib? Does the baby grasp your finger?

Does the child seem to have any problem with balance? Have you noted any unexplained falling, clumsy or unsteady gait, progressive muscular weakness, problem with going up or down stairs, problem with getting up from lying position?

If occurs, may not be noticed until starts to walk in late infancy.

Screens for muscular dystrophy.

Has this child had any seizures? Please describe. Did the seizure occur with a high fever? Was there any loss of consciousness — how long? How many seizures occured with this same illness (if occur with high fever)?

Seizures may occur with high fever in infants and toddlers.

Or, seizures may be sign of neurologic disease.

Did this child's motor or developmental milestones seem to come at about the right age? Does this child seem to be growing and maturing normally to you? How does this child's development compare to siblings, or to age mates?

Do you know if your child has had any environmental exposure to lead?

Chronically elevated lead levels may cause a developmental delay, a loss of a newly acquired skill, or there may be no clinical signs.

Have you been told about any learning problems in school: problems with attention span, cannot concentrate, hyperactive?

Is there any family history: seizure disorder, cerebral palsy, muscular dystrophy?

ADDITIONAL QUESTIONS FOR THE AGING ADULT

Have you noticed any problem with dizziness? Does this occur when you first sit or stand up, when you move your head, when you get up and walk just after eating?

Diminished cerebral blood flow and diminished vestibular response may produce staggering with position change, which increases risk of falls.

(For men) Do you ever get up at night and then feel faint while standing to urinate?

Micturition syncope.

EXAMINER ASKS:	RATIONALE:
How does dizziness affect your daily activities? Are you able to drive safely and to maneuver within your house safely?	
What safety modifications have you applied at home?	
Have you noticed any decrease in memory, change in mental function? Have you felt any confusion? Did this seem to come on suddenly or gradually?	
Have you noticed any muscle weakness? Is this all over or in one local body part? Does the weakness occur with any activities?	
Have you ever noticed any tremor? Is this in your hands or face? Is this worse with: anxiety, activity, rest? Does the tremor seem to be relieved with: alcohol, activity, rest? Does the tremor interfere with daily or social activities?	Senile tremor is relieved by alcohol, although this is not a recommended treatment. Assess if the person is abusing alcohol in effort to relieve tremor.
Have you ever had any sudden vision change, fleeting blindness? Did this occur along with weakness? Did you have any loss of consciousness?	Screen symptoms of stroke.

OBJECTIVE DATA

Equipment Needed:

- Penlight
- Tongue blade
- Sterile needle
- Cotton ball
- Tuning fork (128 Hz)
- Percussion hammer
- (Possibly) familiar aromatic substances

Preparation

Perform a *screening* neurologic examination (items identified in following sections) on seemingly well persons who have no significant subjective findings from the history.

Perform a *complete* neurologic examination on persons who have neurologic concerns (e.g., headache, weakness, loss of coordination) or who have shown signs of neurologic dysfunction.

Perform a *neurologic recheck* examination on persons with demonstrated neurologic deficits who require periodic assessments (e.g., hospitalized persons or those in extended care), using the exam sequence beginning on page 774.

Integrate the steps of the neurologic examination with the examination of each particular part of the body, as much as you are able. For example, test cranial nerves while assessing the head and neck (recall Chapters 10 through 13) and superficial abdominal reflexes while assessing the abdomen. When recording your findings, however, consider all neurologic data as a functional unit, and record them all together.

Use the following sequence for the complete neurologic examination.

1. Mental status (see Chapter 5)
2. Cranial nerves.
3. Motor system
4. Sensory system
5. Reflexes

Position the person sitting up with the head at your eye level.

METHOD OF EXAMINATION

NORMAL RANGE OF FINDINGS	ABNORMAL FINDINGS

CRANIAL NERVES

Test cranial nerves.

Cranial Nerve I — Olfactory Nerve

Do not test routinely. Test the sense of smell in those who report loss of smell and when the presence of an intracranial lesion is suspected. First, assess patency by occluding one nostril at a time and asking the person to sniff. Then, with the person's eyes closed, occlude one nostril and present an aromatic substance. Use familiar, conveniently obtainable and non-noxious smells, such as coffee, toothpaste, orange, vanilla, soap, peppermint, or tobacco. Alcohol swabs smell familiar and are easy to find but are irritating. Normally, a person can identify an odor on each side of the nose. Smell normally is decreased bilaterally with aging. Any asymmetry in the sense of smell is important.

The examiner cannot test smell when air passages are occluded with upper respiratory infection or with sinusitis.

Anosmia — decrease or loss of smell occurs bilaterally with tobacco smoking, allergic rhinitis, and cocaine use.

Unilateral loss in the absence of nasal disease is termed neurogenic anosmia (see Table 20–3).

Cranial Nerve II — Optic Nerve

Test visual acuity and test visual fields by confrontation (see Chapter 11). Using the ophthalmoscope, examine the ocular fundus (see Chapter 11).

Visual field loss (see Table 11–2). Papilledema with increased intracranial pressure; optic atrophy (see Table 11–11).

Cranial Nerves III, IV, and VI — Oculomotor, Trochlear, and Abducens Nerves

Palpebral fissures are usually equal in width or nearly so.

Ptosis (drooping), with myasthenia gravis, dysfunction of cranial nerve III, or Horner's syndrome (see Table 11–4, p. 351).

NORMAL RANGE OF FINDINGS

Check pupils for size, regularity, equality, light reaction, and accommodation (see Chapter 11).

Assess extraocular movements by the cardinal positions of gaze (see Chapter 11).

Nystagmus is a back-and-forth oscillation of the eyes. End-point nystagmus, a few beats of horizontal nystagmus at extreme lateral gaze, occurs normally. Assess any other nystagmus carefully, noting:

- presence of the condition in one or both eyes
- *pendular* movement (oscillations move equally left to right) or *jerk* (a quick phase in one direction then a slow phase in the other). Classify the jerk nystagmus in the direction of the quick phase.
- amplitude. Judge whether the degree of movement is fine, medium, or coarse.
- frequency. Is it constant, or does it fade after a few beats?
- plane of movement: horizontal, vertical, rotary, or a combination of the two (Condi, 1983).

Cranial Nerve V—Trigeminal Nerve

Motor Function. Assess the muscles of mastication by palpating the temporal and masseter muscles as the person clenches the teeth (Figs. 20–8 and 20–9). Muscles should feel equally strong on both sides.

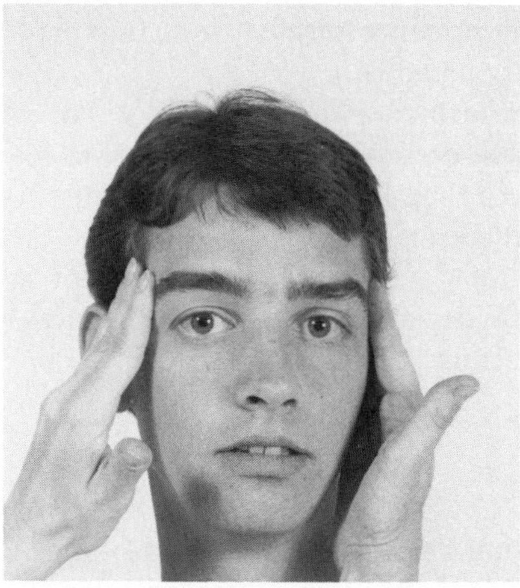

▶ **Figure 20–8**

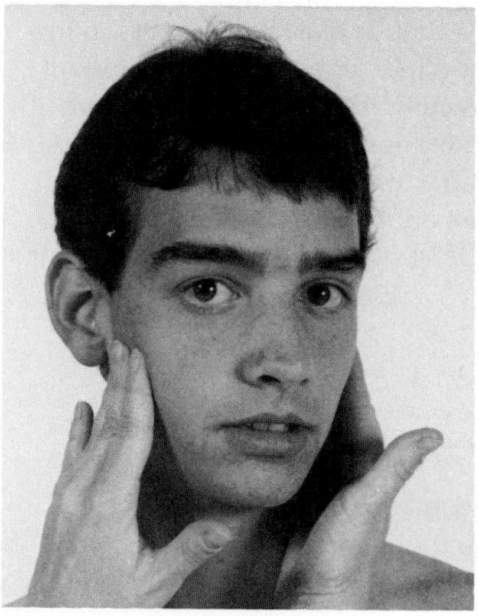

▶ **Figure 20–9**

Try to separate the jaws by pushing down on the chin; normally you cannot.

Sensory Function. With the person's eyes closed, test light touch sensation by touching a cotton wisp to these designated areas on person's face: forehead, cheeks, and chin (Fig. 20–10). Ask the person to say "Now,"

ABNORMAL FINDINGS

See Table 11–9, p. 356.

Deviated gaze or limited movement (see Table 11–3).

Decreased strength on one or both sides.
Asymmetry in jaw movement.
Pain with clenching of teeth.

NORMAL RANGE OF FINDINGS

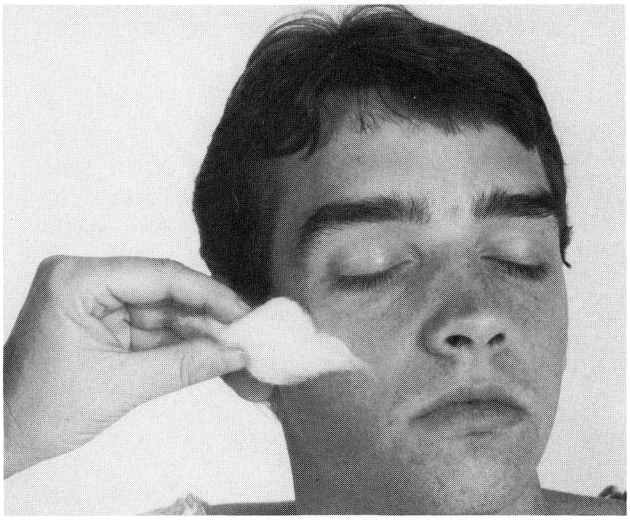

▶ **Figure 20–10**

whenever the touch is felt. This tests all three divisions of the nerve: (1) ophthalmic, (2) maxillary, and (3) mandibular.

Corneal Reflex. (This test is often omitted during the screening examination.) Remove any contact lenses. With the person looking forward, bring a wisp of cotton in from the side (to minimize defensive blinking) and lightly touch the cornea, not the conjunctiva (Fig. 20–11). Normally, the person will blink bilaterally. The corneal reflex may be decreased or absent in those who have worn contact lenses. This procedure tests the sensory afferent in cranial nerve V and the motor efferent in cranial nerve VII.

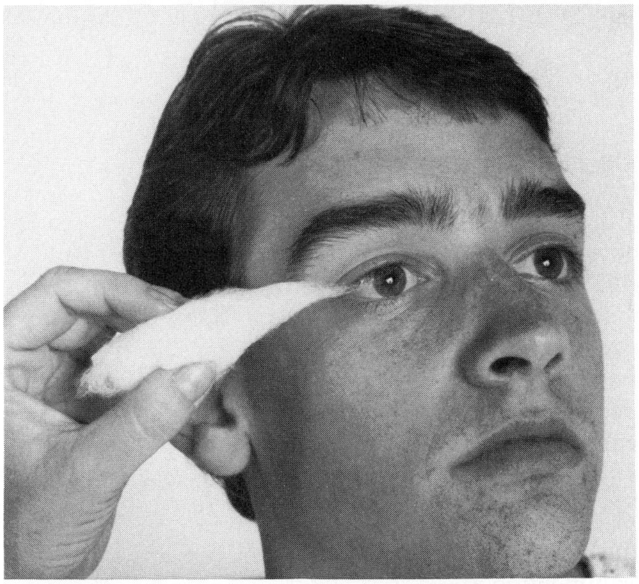

▶ **Figure 20–11**

ABNORMAL FINDINGS

Decreased or unequal sensation.

No blink, occurs with a lesion of cranial nerve V or cranial nerve paralysis.

NORMAL RANGE OF FINDINGS | **ABNORMAL FINDINGS**

Cranial Nerve VII—Facial Nerve

Motor Function. Note mobility and facial symmetry as the person responds to these requests: smile, frown, close eyes tightly (against your attempt to open them), lift eyebrows, show teeth, and puff cheeks (Fig. 20–12). Then, press the person's puffed cheeks in, and note that the air should escape equally from both sides.

Abnormal findings: Muscle weakness is shown by loss of the nasolabial fold, drooping of one side of the face, lower eyelid sagging, and escape of air from only one cheek that is pressed in.

Loss of movement and asymmetry of movement occur with both upper and lower motor neuron lesions.

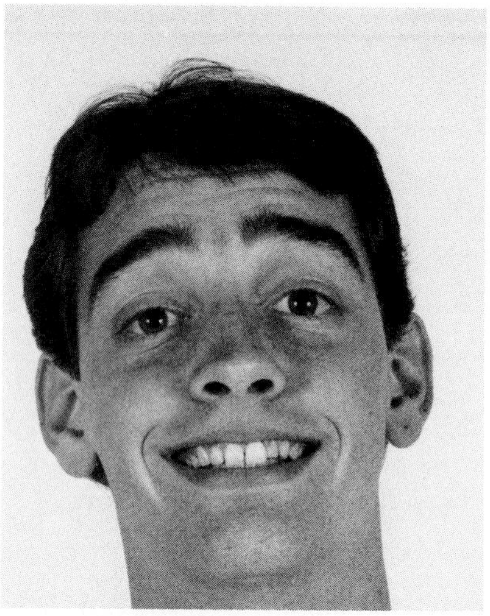

▶ Figure 20–12

Sensory Function. Do not test routinely. When indicated, test sense of taste by applying to the tongue a cotton applicator covered with a small amount of solution of sugar, salt, or lemon juice (sour). Ask the person to identify the taste.

Cranial Nerve VIII—Acoustic (Vestibulocochlear) Nerve

Test hearing acuity (see Chapter 12).

Cranial Nerves IX and X—Glossopharyngeal and Vagus Nerves

Motor Function. Depress the tongue with a tongue blade, and note pharyngeal movement as the person says "ahhh" or yawns; the uvula and soft palate should rise in the midline, and the tonsillar pillars should move medially.

Abnormal findings: Absence or asymmetry of soft palate movement.
Uvula deviates to side.
Asymmetry of tonsillar pillar movement.

Touch the posterior pharyngeal wall with a tongue blade, and note the gag reflex. Also note that the voice sounds smooth and not strained.

Abnormal findings: Hoarse or brassy voice occurs with vocal cord dysfunction; nasal twang occurs with weakness of soft palate.

Sensory Function. Cranial nerve IX does mediate taste on the posterior one third of the tongue, but technically this sensensation is too difficult to test.

NORMAL RANGE OF FINDINGS	ABNORMAL FINDINGS

Cranial Nerve XI — Spinal Accessory Nerve

Examine the sternomastoid and trapezius muscles for equal size. Check equal strength by asking the person to rotate the head forcibly against resistance applied to the side of the chin (Fig. 20 – 13). Then ask the person to shrug the shoulders against resistance (Fig. 20 – 14). These movements should feel equally strong on both sides.

Atrophy.
Muscle weakness or paralysis.

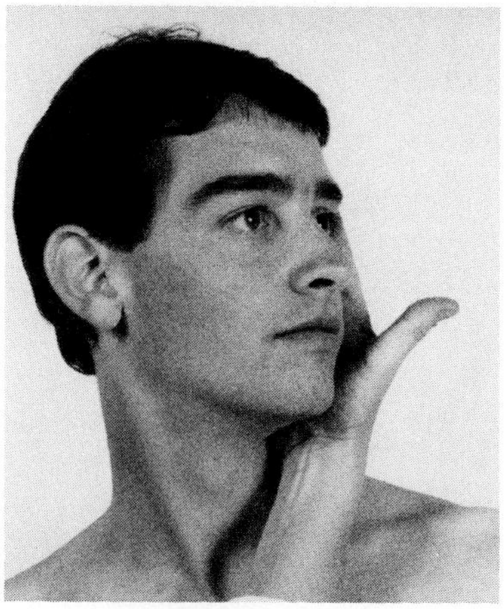

► Figure 20 – 13

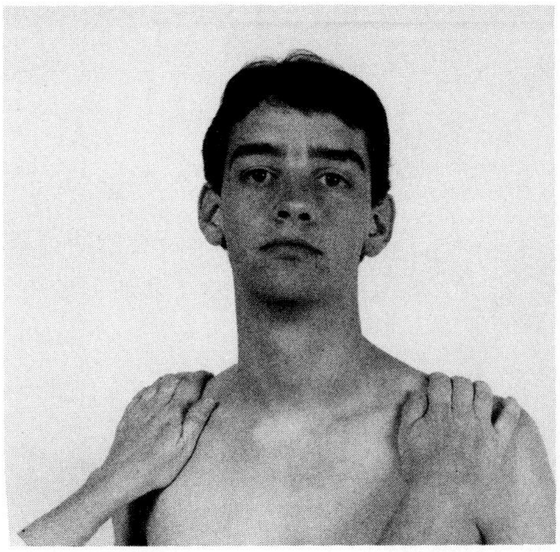

► Figure 20 – 14

Cranial Nerve XII — Hypoglossal Nerve

Inspect the tongue. There should be no wasting or tremors. Note the forward thrust in the midline as the person protrudes the tongue. Also ask the person to say "light, tight, dynamite," and note that lingual speech (sounds of letters l, t, d, n) is clear and distinct.

Atrophy.
Fasciculations.

Tongue deviates to side (when this occurs, deviation is toward the paralyzed side).

THE MOTOR SYSTEM

Inspect and palpate the motor system.

Muscles

Size. As you proceed through the examination, inspect all muscle groups for size. Compare one side to the other. Muscle groups should be within the normal size limits for age and should be symmetric bilaterally. When muscles in the extremities look asymmetric, measure each in centimeters and record the difference. A difference of 1 cm or less is not significant. Note that it is difficult to assess muscle mass in very obese people.

Atrophy — abnormally small muscle with a wasted appearance; occurs with disuse, injury, lower motor neuron disease, and muscle disease.

Hypertrophy — increased size and strength; occurs with isometric exercise.

Strength. (See Chapter 19, Assessing the Musculoskeletal System) Test homologous muscles simultaneously.

NORMAL RANGE OF FINDINGS	ABNORMAL FINDINGS

Tone. Tone is the normal degree of tension (contraction) in voluntarily relaxed muscles. It shows as a mild resistance to passive stretch. To test muscle tone, move the extremities through a passive range of motion. First, persuade the person to relax completely, to "go loose like a rag doll." Move each extremity smoothly through a full range of motion. Support the arm at the elbow and the leg at the knee (Fig. 20–15). Normally, you will note a mild, even resistance to movement.

Limited range of motion.

Pain with motion.

Flaccidity—decreased resistance, hypotonic.

Spasticity and rigidity—types of increased resistance (see Table 20–4).

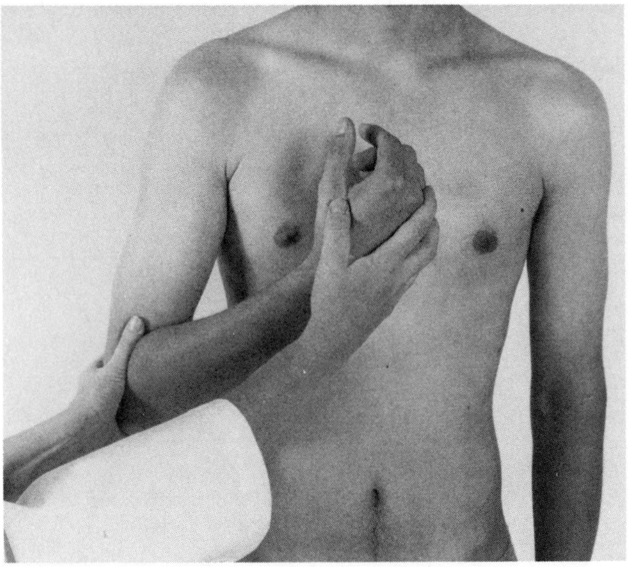

▶ **Figure 20–15**

Involuntary Movements. Normally, there are no involuntary movements. If they are present, note their location, frequency, rate, and amplitude. Note if the movements can be controlled at will.

Tic, tremor, and fasciculation (see Table 20–5).

Cerebellar Function

Balance Tests

Gait. Observe as the person walks 10 to 20 feet, turns, and returns to the starting point. Normally, the person moves with a sense of freedom. The gait is smooth, rhythmic, and effortless; the opposing arm swing is coordinated; the turns are smooth. The step length is about 15 inches from heel to heel.

Stiff, immobile posture.
Staggering or reeling.
Wide base of support.
Lack of arm swing or rigid arms.
Unequal rhythm of steps.
Slapping of foot.
Scraping of toe of shoe.

Ataxia—uncoordinated or unsteady gait (see Table 20–6).

NORMAL RANGE OF FINDINGS

Ask the person to walk a straight line in a heel-to-toe fashion (tandem walking) (Fig. 20 – 16). This decreases the base of support and will accentuate any problem with coordination. Normally, the person can walk straight and stay balanced.

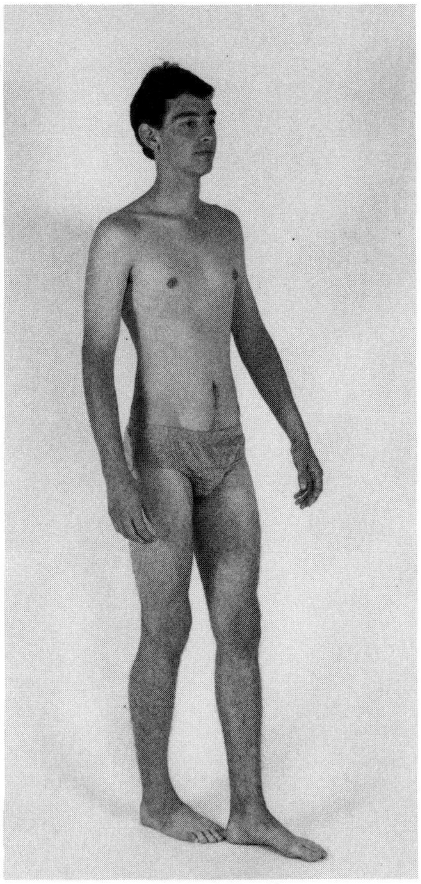

► **Figure 20 – 16**

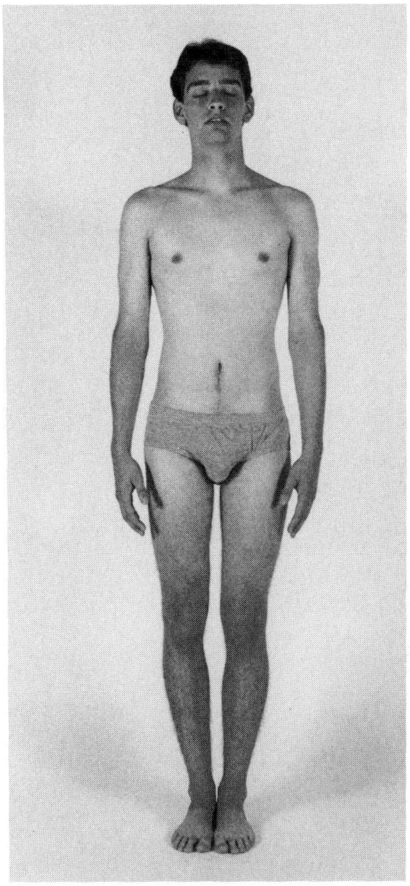

► **Figure 20 – 17**

Romberg's Test. Ask the person to stand up with feet together and arms at the sides. Once in a stable position, ask the person to close the eyes and to hold the position (Fig. 20 – 17). Wait about 20 seconds. Normally, a person can maintain posture and balance, although there may be slight swaying. (Stand close to catch the person in case he or she falls.)

ABNORMAL FINDINGS

Crooked line of walk.

Widens base to maintain balance.

Staggering, reeling, loss of balance.

An ataxia that did not appear with regular gait may appear now.

Sways; falls; widens base of feet to avoid falling.

Positive Romberg's sign is loss of balance that is increased by closing of the eyes. You eliminate the advantage of orientation with the eyes, which had compensated for sensory loss. A positive Romberg's sign occurs with cerebellar ataxia (multiple sclerosis, alcohol intoxication), loss of proprioception, and loss of vestibular function.

NORMAL RANGE OF FINDINGS	ABNORMAL FINDINGS

Ask the person to perform a shallow knee bend, or to hop in place, first on one leg, then the other (Fig. 20–18). This demonstrates normal position sense, muscle strength, and cerebellar function. Note that some individuals cannot hop owing to aging or obesity.

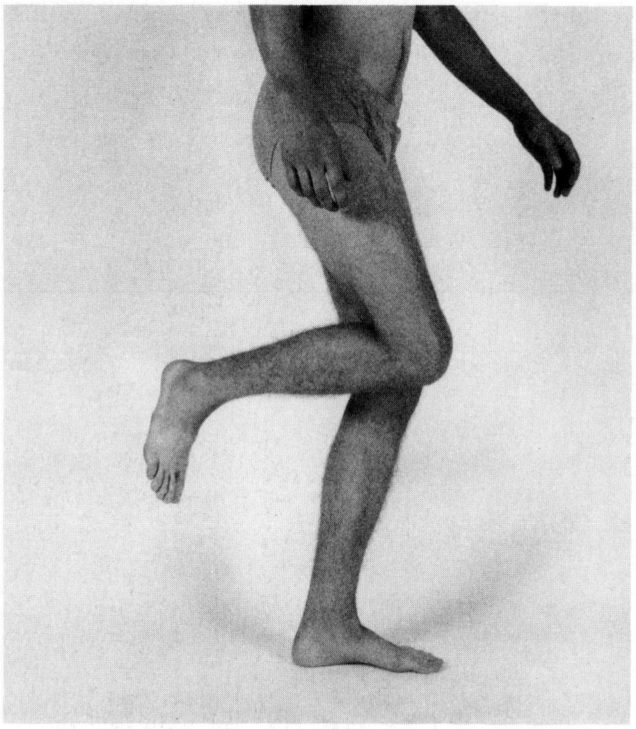

▶ **Figure 20–18**

Coordination and Skilled Movements

Rapid Alternating Movements (RAM). Ask the person to pat the knees with both hands, lift up, turn hands over, and pat the knees with the backs of the hands (Fig. 20–19). Then ask the person to do this faster. Normally, this is done with equal turning and a quick rhythmic pace.

Lack of coordination.

Slow, clumsy, and sloppy response occurs with cerebellar disease.

Alternatively, ask the person to touch the thumb to each finger on the same hand, starting with the index finger, then reverse direction (Fig. 20–20). Normally, this can be done quickly and accurately.

Lack of coordination.

NORMAL RANGE OF FINDINGS

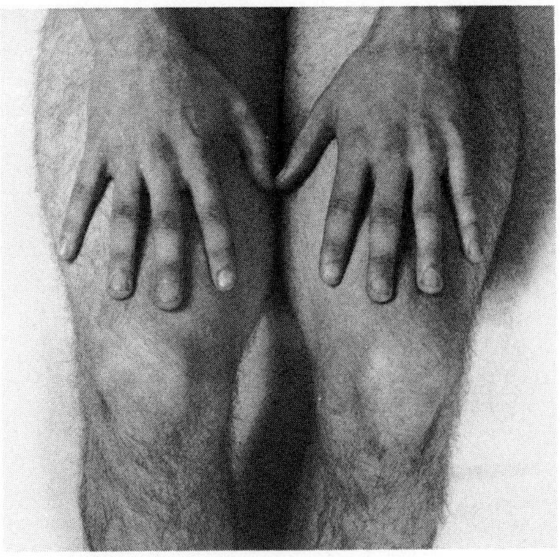

► **Figure 20–19**

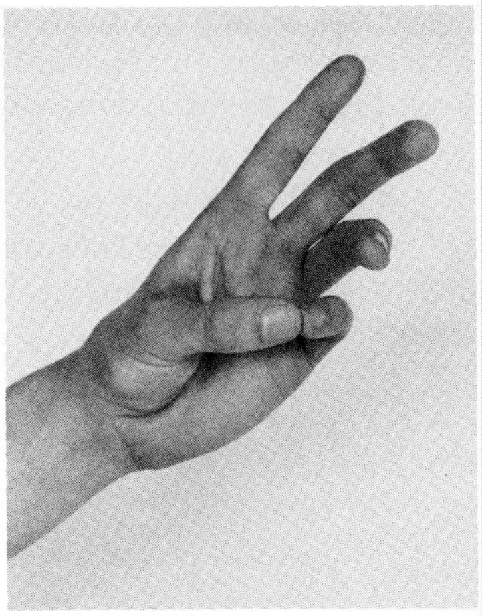

► **Figure 20–20**

Finger-to-Finger Test. With the person's eyes open, ask that he or she use the index finger to touch your finger, then the person's own nose (Fig. 20–21). After a few times move your finger to a different spot. The person's movement should be smooth and accurate.

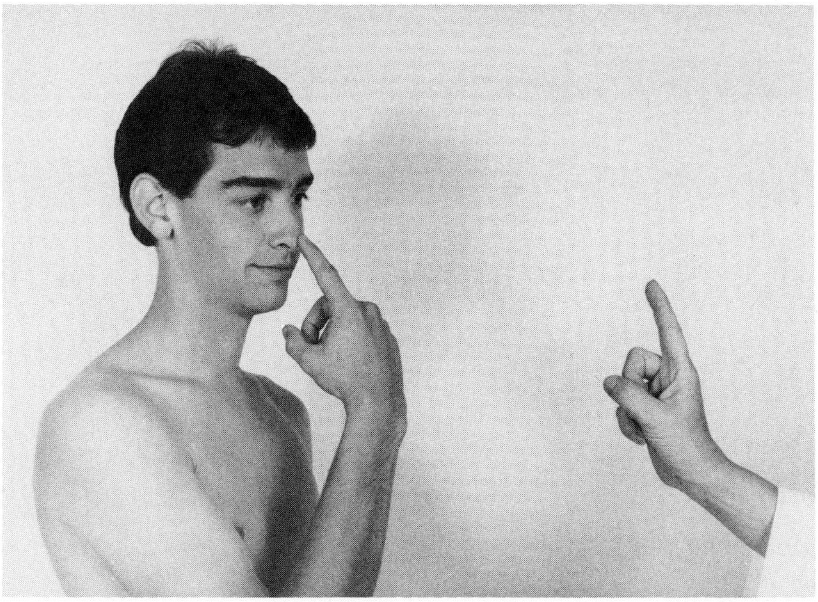

► **Figure 20–21**

ABNORMAL FINDINGS

Misses the mark.

NORMAL RANGE OF FINDINGS	ABNORMAL FINDINGS
Finger-to-Nose Test. Ask the person to close the eyes and to stretch out the arms. Ask the person to touch the tip of his or her nose with each index finger, alternating hands and increasing speed. Normally this is done with accurate and smooth movement.	Misses nose.
Heel-to-Shin Test. Test lower extremity coordination by asking the person, who is in a supine position, to place the heel on the opposite knee, and run it down the shin from the knee to the ankle (Fig. 20–22). Normally, the person moves the heel in a straight line down the shin.	Lack of coordination. Heel falls off shin.

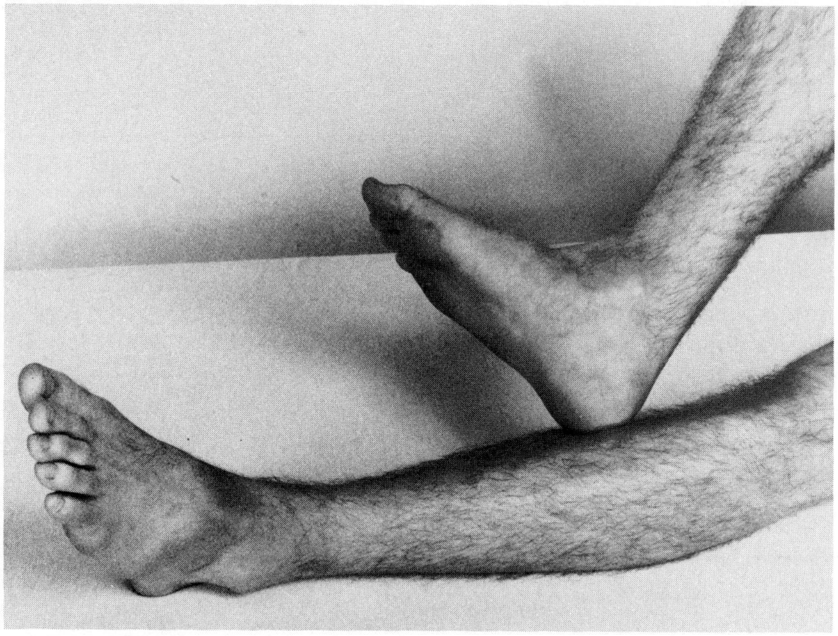

► **Figure 20–22**

THE SENSORY SYSTEM

Assess the sensory system.

Asking the person to identify various sensory stimuli tests the intactness of the peripheral nerve fibers, the sensory tracts, and higher cortical discrimination.

Ensure validity of sensory system testing by making sure the person is alert, cooperative, and comfortable and has an adequate attention span. Otherwise, you may get misleading and invalid results. Testing of the sensory system can be fatiguing. You may need to repeat the examination later or to break it into parts when the person is tired.

You do not need to test the entire skin surface for every sensation. Routine screening procedures include testing superficial pain, light touch, and vibration in a few distal locations, and testing stereognosis. This will

NORMAL RANGE OF FINDINGS

suffice for all who have not demonstrated any neurologic symptoms or signs. Complete testing of the sensory system is warranted in those with neurologic symptoms (e.g., localized pain, numbness, and tingling) or when you discover abnormalities (e.g., motor deficit). Then, test all sensory modalities and cover most dermatomes of the body.

Compare sensations on symmetric parts of the body. When you find a definite decrease in sensation, map it out by systematic testing in that area. Proceed from the point of decreased sensation toward the sensitive area. By asking the person to tell you where the sensation changes, you can map the exact borders of the deficient area. Draw your results on a diagram.

Avoid asking leading questions, "Can you feel this pin prick?" This creates an expectation of how the person should feel the sensation, which is called *suggestion.* Instead, use unbiased directions.

The person's eyes should be closed during each of the tests. Take time to explain what will be happening and exactly how you expect the person to respond.

Spinothalamic Tract

Pain. Pain is tested by the person's ability to perceive a pin prick. Using a sterile needle, lightly apply the sharp point or the dull hub to the person's body in a random, unpredictable order (Fig. 20–23). Ask the person to say "sharp" or "dull," depending on the sensation felt. (Note that the sharp edge is used to test for pain; the dull edge is used to as a general test of the person's responses.) Alternatively, break a tongue blade lengthwise, forming a sharp point at the fractured end, and using the dull spot at the rounded end.*

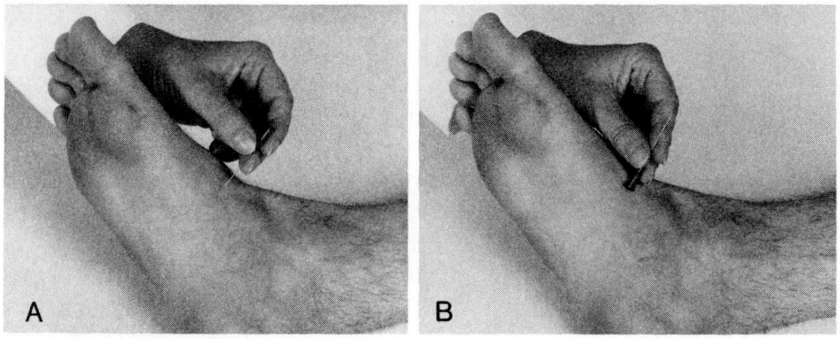

► **Figure 20–23**

Let at least 2 seconds elapse between each stimulus to avoid *summation.* With summation, frequent consecutive stimuli are perceived as one strong stimulus.

* To prevent any possible contagion, do not reuse a needle or sharp tool on another person. Dispose of needles or any sharp tool in a special impenetrable container.

ABNORMAL FINDINGS

Hypalgesia—decreased pain sensation.

Analgesia—absent pain sensation.

Hyperalgesia—increased pain sensation.

NORMAL RANGE OF FINDINGS	ABNORMAL FINDINGS

Temperature. Apply a hot or cold element to the skin. Test temperature sensation only when pain sensation is abnormal; otherwise you may omit it because the fiber tracts are much the same. Fill two test tubes, one with hot water and one with cold water, and apply the bottom ends to the person's skin in a random order. Ask the person to say which temperature is felt.

Light Touch. Apply a wisp of cotton to the skin. Stretch a cotton ball to make a long end and brush it over the skin in a random order of sites and at irregular intervals (Fig. 20 – 24). This prevents the person from responding just from repetition. Include the arms, forearms, hands, chest, thighs, and legs. Ask the person to say "now" or "yes" when touch is felt. Compare symmetric points.

Hypesthesia — decreased touch sensation.

Anesthesia — absent touch sensation.

Hyperesthesia — increased touch sensation.

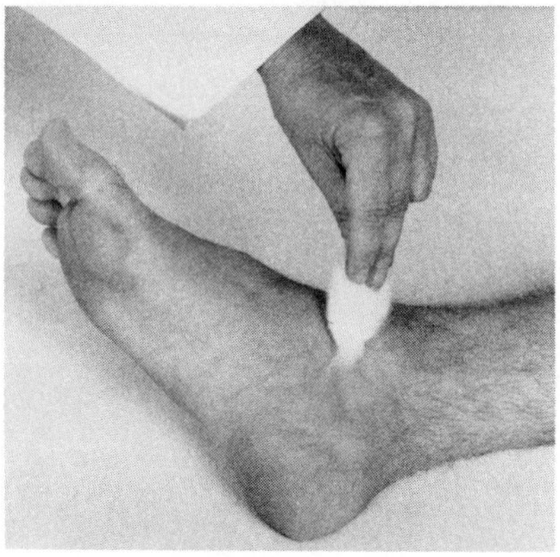

► **Figure 20 – 24**

Posterior Column Tract

Vibration. Test the person's ability to feel vibrations of a tuning fork over bony prominences. Strike a low pitch tuning fork on the heel of your hand, and hold the base on a bony surface of the fingers and great toe (Fig. 20 – 25). Ask the person to indicate when the vibration starts and stops. If the person feels the normal vibration or buzzing sensation on these distal areas, you may assume proximal spots are normal and proceed no further. If no vibrations are felt, move proximally and test ulnar processes, and ankles, patellae, and iliac crests. Compare the right side to the left side. If you find a deficit, note whether it is gradual or abrupt.

Unable to feel vibration. States vibration stops when fork is still vibrating.

Loss of vibration sense occurs with peripheral neuropathy, e.g., diabetes and alcoholism. Often, this is the first sensation lost.

Peripheral neuropathy is worse at the feet and gradually improves as you move up leg, as opposed to a specific nerve lesion, which has a clear zone of deficit for its dermatome.

NORMAL RANGE OF FINDINGS

ABNORMAL FINDINGS

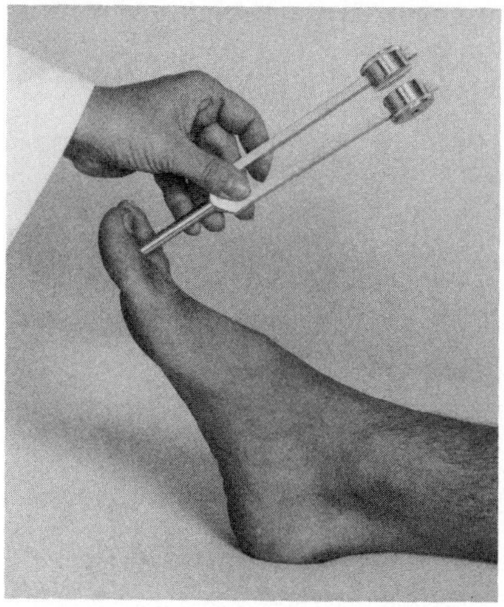

► Figure 20-25

Position (Kinesthesia). Test the person's ability to perceive passive movements of the extremities. Move a finger or the big toe up and down, and ask the person to tell you which way it is moved (Fig. 20-26). The test is done with the eyes closed; but to be sure it is understood, have the person watch a few trials first. Vary the order of movement up or down. Hold the digit by the sides, since upward or downward pressure on the skin may provide a clue as to how it has been moved. Normally, a person can detect movement of a few millimeters.

Loss of position sense.

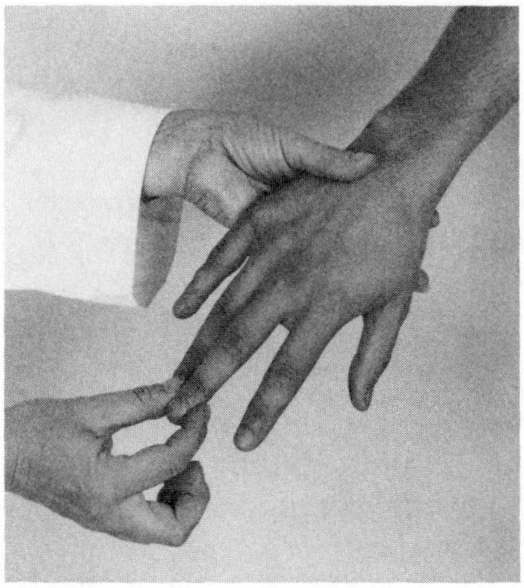

► Figure 20-26

Tactile Discrimination (Fine Touch). The following tests also measure the discrimination ability of the sensory cortex. As a prerequisite, the person needs a normal or near-normal sense of touch and position sense.

Problems with tactile discrimination occur with lesions of the sensory cortex or posterior column.

NORMAL RANGE OF FINDINGS	ABNORMAL FINDINGS

Stereognosis. Test the person's ability to recognize objects by feeling their forms, sizes, and weights. With the eyes closed, place a familiar object (paper clip, key, coin, cotton ball, or pencil) in the person's hand and ask the person to identify it (Fig. 20–27). Normally, a person will explore it with the fingers and correctly name it. Test a different object in each hand; testing the left hand assesses right parietal lobe functioning.

Astereognosis — unable to identify object correctly. Occurs in sensory cortex lesions.

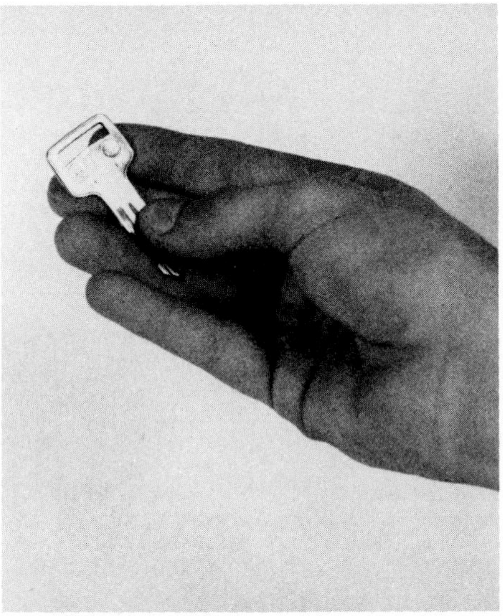

► **Figure 20–27**

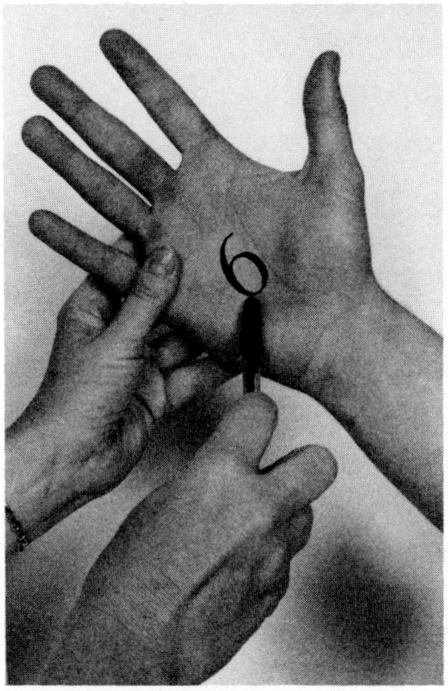

► **Figure 20–28**

Graphesthesia. Graphesthesia is the ability to "read" a number by having it traced on the skin. With the person's eyes closed, use a blunt instrument to trace a single digit number or a letter on the palm (Fig. 20–28). Ask the person to tell you what it is. Graphesthesia is a good measure of sensory loss if the person cannot make the hand movements needed for stereognosis, as occurs in arthritis.

Inability to distinguish number occurs with lesions of the sensory cortex.

Two-Point Discrimination. Test the person's ability to distinguish the separation of two simultaneous pin pricks on the skin. Apply two sterile needles lightly to the skin in ever-closing distances. Note the distance at which the person no longer perceives two separate points. The level of perception varies considerably with the region tested; it is most sensitive in the fingertips (2 to 8 mm) (Fig. 20–29) and least sensitive on the upper arms, thighs, and back (40 to 75 mm).

An increase in the distance it normally takes to identify two separate points occurs with sensory cortex lesions.

NORMAL RANGE OF FINDINGS | **ABNORMAL FINDINGS**

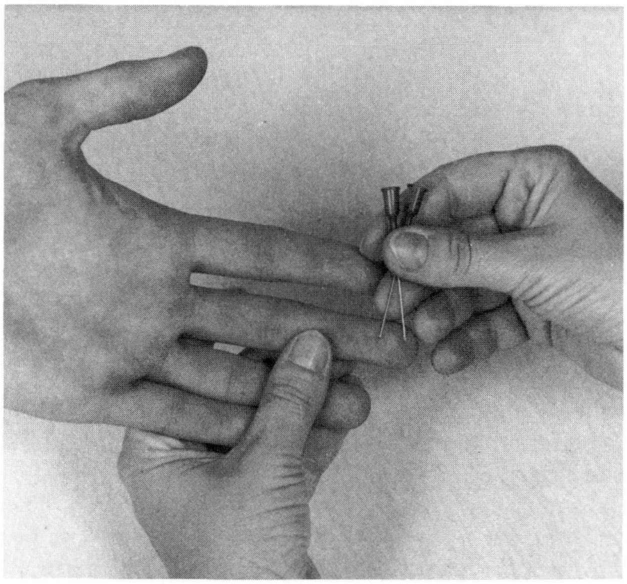

► Figure 20-29

Extinction. Simultaneously touch both sides of the body at the same point. Ask the person to state how many sensations are felt and where they are. Normally both sensations are felt.

The ability to recognize only one of the stimuli occurs with sensory cortex lesion; the stimulus is extinguished on the side *opposite* the lesion.

Point Location. Touch the skin, and withdraw the stimulus promptly. Tell the person, "Put your finger where I touched you." You can perform this test simultaneously with light touch sensation.

With a sensory cortex lesion, the person cannot localize the sensation accurately, even though light touch sensation may be retained.

REFLEXES

Test the reflexes.

Stretch, or Deep Tendon Reflexes (DTRs)

Measurement of the stretch reflexes reveals the intactness of the reflex arc at specific spinal levels as well as the normal override on the reflex of the higher cortical levels.

For an adequate response, the limb should be relaxed and the muscle partially stretched. Stimulate the reflex by directing a short snappy blow of the reflex hammer onto the muscle's insertion tendon. Use a relaxed hold on the hammer. As with the percussion technique, the action takes place at the wrist. Strike a brief well-aimed blow, and bounce up promptly; do not let the hammer rest on the tendon. Use the pointed end of the reflex hammer when aiming at a smaller target such as your thumb on the tendon site; use the flat end when the target is wider or to diffuse the impact and prevent pain.

NORMAL RANGE OF FINDINGS

Use just enough force to get a response. Compare right and left sides — the responses should be equal. The reflex response is graded on a 4-point scale:

4+	very brisk, hyperactive with clonus, indicative of disease
3+	brisker than average, may indicate disease
2+	average, normal
1+	diminished, low normal
0	no response

This is a subjective scale and requires some clinical practice before results can be judged with assurance.

Sometimes the reflex response fails to appear. Try further encouragement of relaxation, varying the person's position or increasing the strength of the blow. *Reinforcement* is another technique to relax the muscles and enhance the response (Fig. 20–30). Ask the person to perform an isometric exercise in a muscle group somewhat away from the one being tested. For example, to enhance a patellar reflex, ask the person to lock the fingers together and "pull." To enhance a biceps response, ask the person to clench the teeth, or to grasp the thigh with the opposite hand.

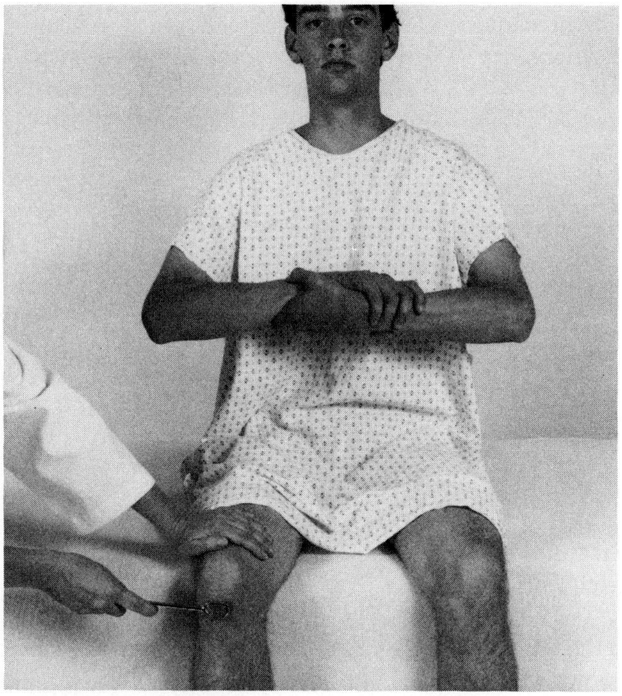

► **Figure 20–30**

Biceps Reflex (C5 to C6). Support the person's forearm on yours; this position relaxes, as well as partially flexes, the person's arm. Place your thumb on the biceps tendon and strike a blow on your thumb. You can feel

ABNORMAL FINDINGS

Clonus is a set of short jerking contractions of the same muscle.

NORMAL RANGE OF FINDINGS

as well as see the normal response, which is flexion of the forearm (Fig. 20–31).

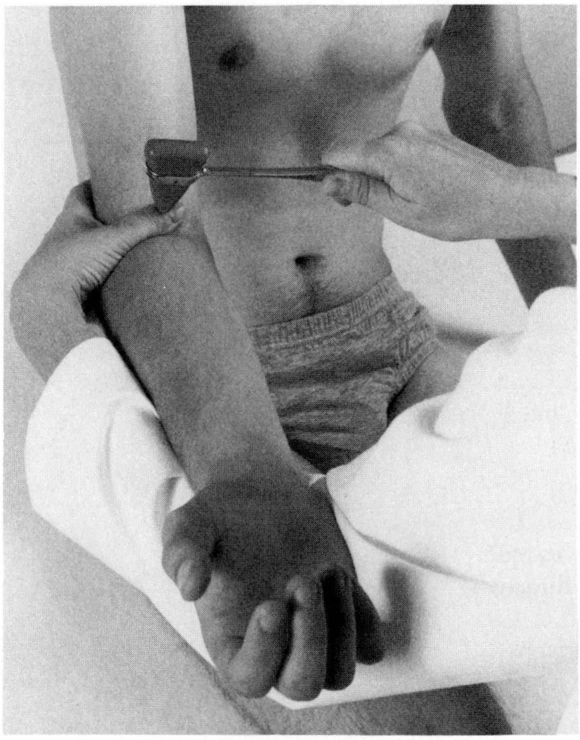

► Figure 20–31

Triceps Reflex (C7 to C8). Tell the person to let the arm "just go dead" as you suspend it by holding the upper arm. Strike the triceps tendon directly just above the elbow (Fig. 20–32). The normal response is extension of the forearm. Alternately, hold the person's wrist across the chest to flex the arm at the elbow, and tap the tendon.

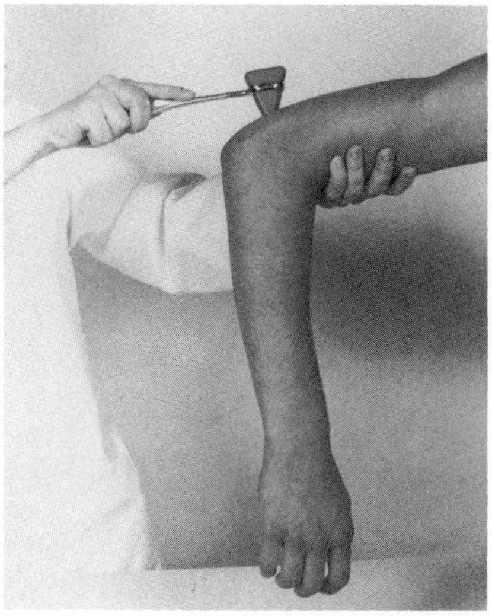

► Figure 20–32

ABNORMAL FINDINGS

Hyperreflexia is the exaggerated reflex seen when the monosynaptic reflex arc is released from the influence of higher cortical levels. This occurs with upper motor neuron lesions, e.g., a cerebrovascular accident.

Hyporeflexia, which is the absence of a reflex, is a lower motor neuron problem. It occurs with interruption of sensory afferents or destruction of motor efferents and anterior horn cells, e.g., spinal cord injury.

NORMAL RANGE OF FINDINGS	ABNORMAL FINDINGS

Brachioradialis Reflex (C5 to C6). Hold the person's thumbs to suspend the forearms in relaxation. Strike the forearm directly, about 2 to 3 cm above the radial styloid process (Fig. 20–33). The normal response is flexion and supination of the forearm.

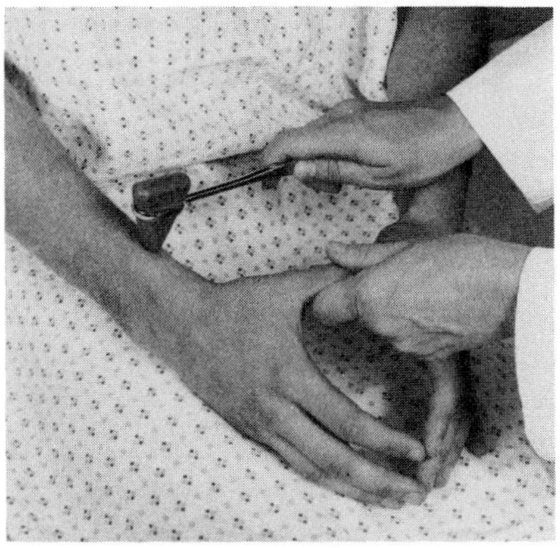

▸ Figure 20–33

Quadriceps Reflex ("Knee Jerk") (L2 to L4). Let the lower legs dangle freely to flex the knee and stretch the tendons. Strike the tendon directly just below the patella (Fig. 20–34). Extension of the lower leg is the expected response. You also will palpate contraction of the quadriceps.

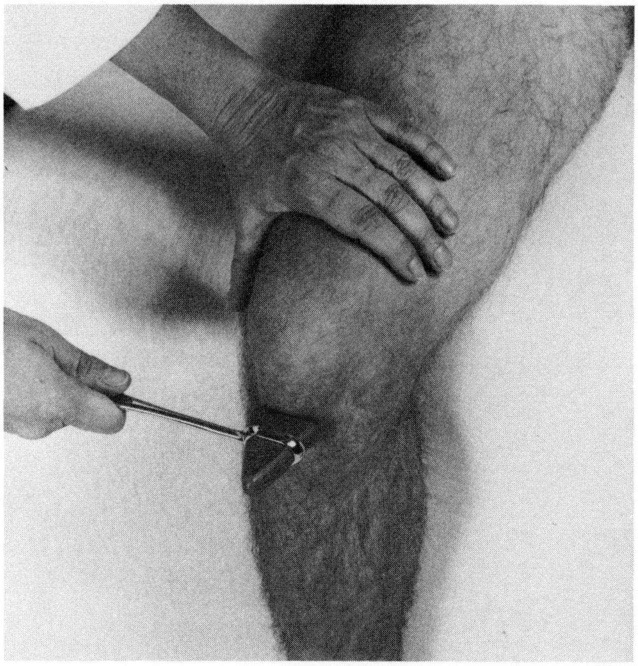

▸ Figure 20–34

NORMAL RANGE OF FINDINGS

ABNORMAL FINDINGS

For the person in the supine position, use your own arm as a lever to support the weight of one leg against the other leg (Fig. 20–35). This maneuver also flexes the knee.

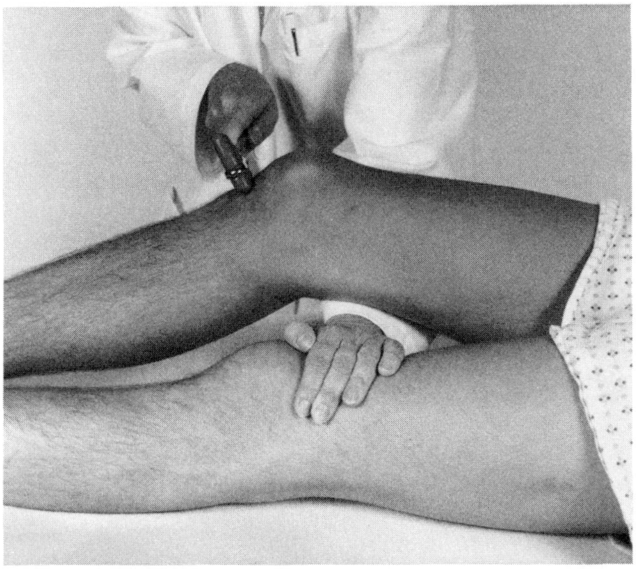

► **Figure 20–35**

Achilles Reflex ("Ankle Jerk") (L5 to S2). Position the person with the knee flexed and the hip externally rotated. Hold the foot in dorsiflexion, and strike the Achilles tendon directly (Fig. 20–36). Feel the normal response as the foot plantar flexes against your hand.

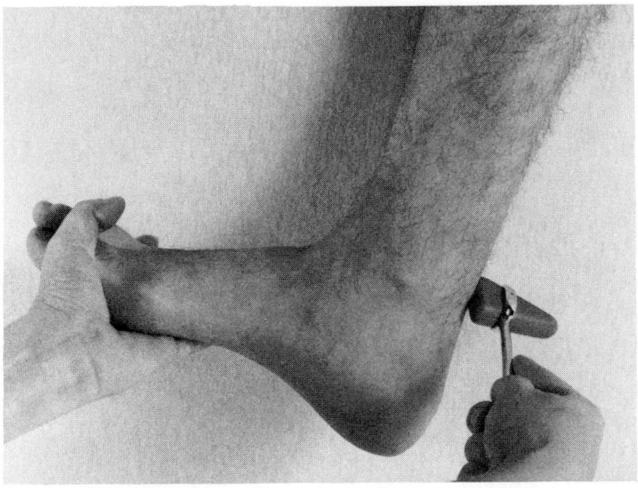

► **Figure 20–36**

NORMAL RANGE OF FINDINGS	ABNORMAL FINDINGS

For the person in the supine position, flex one knee and support that lower leg against the other leg so that it falls "open." Dorsiflex the foot and tap the tendon (Fig. 20–37).

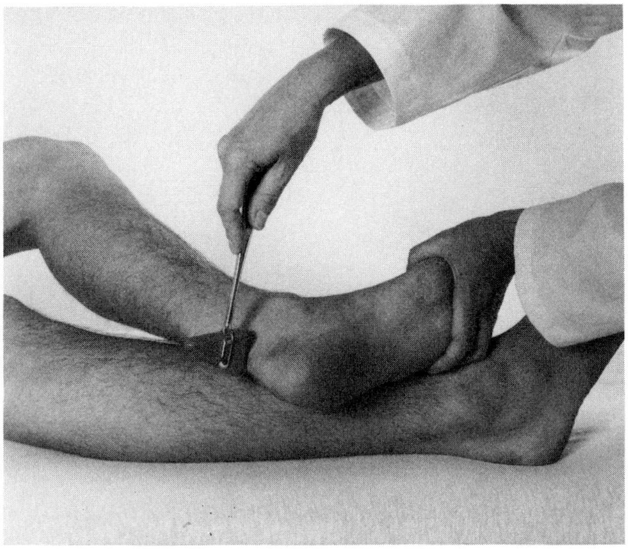

▶ **Figure 20–37**

Clonus. Test for clonus, particularly when the reflexes are hyperactive. Support the lower leg in one hand. With your other hand, stretch the muscle by briskly dorsiflexing the foot. Hold the stretch (Fig. 20–38). With a normal response, you feel no further movement. When clonus is present, you will feel and see rapid rhythmic contractions of the foot.

A hyperactive reflex with sustained clonus (lasting as long as the stretch is held) occurs with upper motor neuron disease.

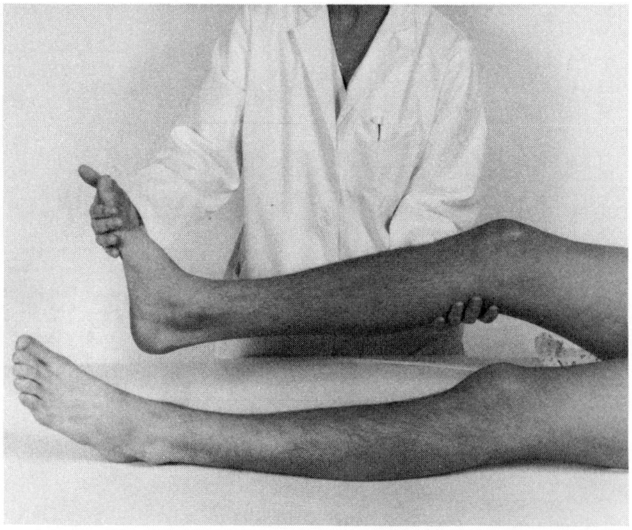

▶ **Figure 20–38**

NORMAL RANGE OF FINDINGS | **ABNORMAL FINDINGS**

Superficial Reflexes

Here, the receptors are in the skin rather than the muscles.

Abdominal Reflexes. Upper (T8 to T10) Lower (T10 to T12). Have the person assume a supine position, with the knees slightly bent. Use the handle end of the reflex hammer, a wood applicator tip, or the end of a split tongue blade to stroke the skin. Move from the side of the abdomen toward the midline at both the upper and lower abdominal level (Fig. 20–39). The normal response is ipsilateral contraction of the abdominal muscle with an observed deviation of the umbilicus toward the stroke. When the abdominal wall is very obese, pull the skin to the opposite side, and feel it contract toward the stimulus.

Abnormal findings: Superficial reflexes are absent with diseases of the pyramidal tract, e.g., they are absent on the contralateral side with cerebrovascular accident.

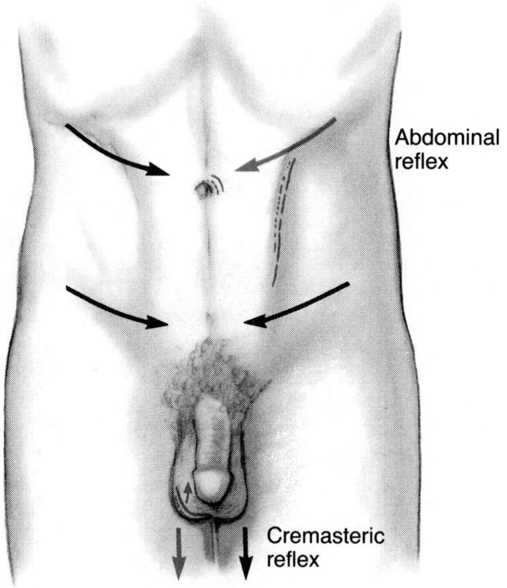

► **Figure 20–39**

Cremasteric Reflex (L1 to L2). On the male, lightly stroke the inner aspect of the thigh with the reflex hammer or tongue blade. Note elevation of the ipsilateral testicle.

Plantar Reflex (L4 to S2). With the same instrument, draw a light stroke up the lateral side of the sole of the foot and across the ball of the foot, like an upside-down "J" (Fig. 20–40). The normal response is plantar flexion of the toes and sometimes of the whole foot.

Abnormal findings: Except in infancy, the abnormal response is dorsiflexion of the big toe and fanning of all toes, which is a *positive Babinski sign*. This occurs with upper motor neuron disease of the pyramidal tract.

NORMAL RANGE OF FINDINGS | **ABNORMAL FINDINGS**

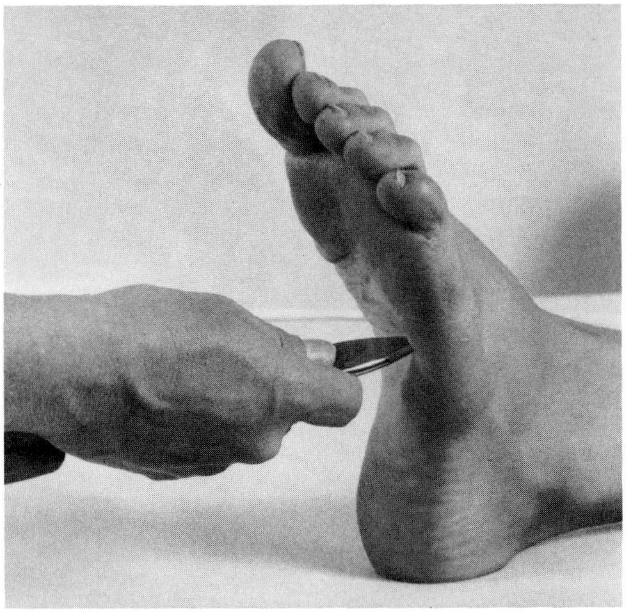

► **Figure 20–40**

DEVELOPMENTAL CONSIDERATIONS

Infants (Birth to 12 Months)

The neurologic system shows dramatic growth and development during the first year of life. Assessment includes noting that milestones you normally would expect for each month have indeed been achieved, and that the early, more primitive reflexes are eliminated from the baby's repertory when they are supposed to.

Failure to attain a skill by expected time.

Persistence of reflex behavior beyond the normal time.

At birth, the newborn is very alert, with the eyes open, and demonstrates strong, urgent sucking. The normal cry is loud, lusty, and even angry. The next 2 or 3 days may be spent mostly sleeping as the baby recovers from the birth process. After that, the pattern of sleep and waking activity is highly variable; it depends on the baby's individual body rhythm as well as external stimuli.

A high-pitched shrill cry or cat-sounding screech occurs with CNS damage.

A weak, groaning cry or expiratory grunt occurs with respiratory distress.

The behavioral assessment should include your observations of the infant's waking activity, responses to environmental stimuli, and social interaction with the parents and others.

Lethargy, hyporeactivity, hyperirritability, and parent's report of significant change in behavior all warrant referral.

By 2 months of age, the baby smiles responsively and recognizes the parent's face. Babbling occurs at 4 months, and one or two words (mama, dada) are used nonspecifically after 9 months.

The cranial nerves cannot be tested directly, but you can infer their proper functioning by the maneuvers shown in Table 20–2.

NORMAL RANGE OF FINDINGS

Table 20-2 ▶ Testing Cranial Nerve Function of Infants

II, III, IV, VI	Optical blink reflex—shine light in open eyes, note rapid closure.
	Regards face or close object.
	Eyes follow movement.
V	Rooting reflex, sucking reflex.
VII	Facial movements (e.g., wrinkling forehead and nasolabial folds) symmetric when crying or smiling.
VIII	Loud noise yields Moro reflex (until 4 months).
	Acoustic blink reflex—infant blinks in response to a loud hand clap 30 cm (12 in) from head. (Avoid making air current.)
	Eyes follow direction of sound.
IX, X	Swallowing, gag reflex.
XII	Coordinated sucking and swallowing.
	Pinch nose, infant's mouth will open and tongue rise in midline.

The Motor System

Observe spontaneous motor activity for smoothness and symmetry. Smoothness of movement suggests proper cerebellar function, as does the coordination involved in sucking and swallowing. To screen gross and fine motor coordination, use the Denver II with its age-specific developmental milestones. You also can assess movement by testing the reflexes listed in the following section. Note their smoothness of response and symmetry. Also, note whether their presence or absence is appropriate for the infant's age.

Assess muscle tone by first observing resting posture. The newborn favors a flexed position; extremities are symmetrically folded inward, the hips are slightly abducted, and the fists are tightly flexed. Infants born by breech delivery, however, do not have flexion in the lower extremities.

After 2 months of age, flexion gives way to gradual extension, beginning with the head and continuing in a cephalocaudal direction. Now is the time to check for spasticity; there should be none. Test for spasticity by flexing the infant's knees onto the abdomen and then quickly releasing them. They will unfold but not too quickly. Also, gently push the head forward—the baby should comply.

The fists normally are held in tight flexion for the first 3 months. Then the fists open for part of the time. There is a purposeful reach for an object with both hands around 4 months of age, a transfer of an object from hand to hand at 7 months of age, a grasp using fingers and apposing thumb at 9 months of age, and a purposeful release at 10 months of age. Babies are normally ambidextrous for the first 18 months.

ABNORMAL FINDINGS

Delay in motor activity occurs with brain damage, mental retardation, peripheral neuromuscular damage, prolonged illness, and parental neglect.

Abnormal postures:

Frog position—hips abducted and almost flat against the table, externally rotated (only normal after breech delivery).

Opisthotonos—head arched back, stiffness of neck, and extension of arms and legs; occurs with meningeal or brain stem irritation (see Table 20-10).

Any type of continual asymmetry.

Spasticity is an early sign of cerebral palsy. After releasing flexed knees, legs will quickly extend and adduct, even to a "scissoring" motion when spasticity is present. Also, the baby often resists head flexion and extends back against your hand when spasticity is present.

Note persistent one-hand preference in children younger than 18 months of age. The condition may indicate a motor deficit on the opposite side.

NORMAL RANGE OF FINDINGS

Head control is an important milestone in motor development. You can incorporate the following two movements into every infant assessment to check the muscle tone necessary for head control.

First, with the baby supine, pull to a sit holding the wrists and note head control (Fig. 20–41). The newborn will hold the head almost in the same plane as the body, and it will balance briefly when the baby reaches a sitting position, then flop forward. (Even a premature infant shows some head flexion.) At 4 months of age, the head stays in line with the body and does not flop.

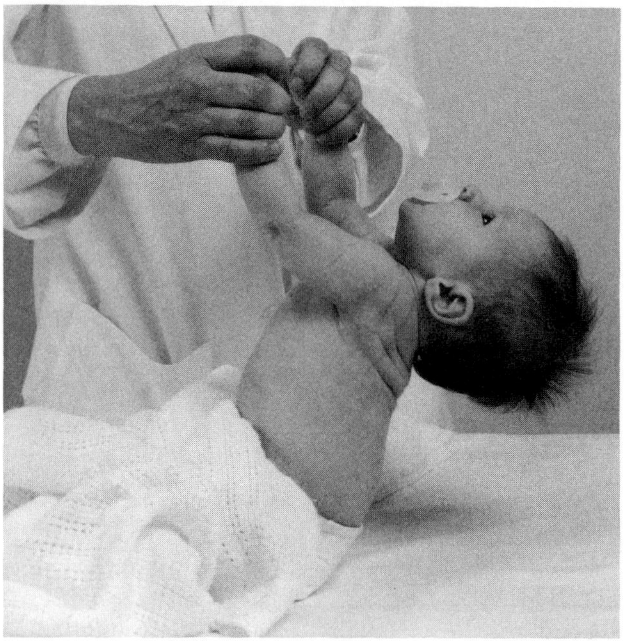

► **Figure 20–41**

Second, lift up the baby in a prone position, with one hand supporting the chest (Fig. 20–42). The term newborn holds the head at an angle of 45 degrees or less from horizontal, the back is straight or slightly arched, and the elbows and knees are partly flexed. At 3 months of age, the baby raises the head and arches the back. This is the *Landau reflex,* which persists until 1 1/2 years of age.

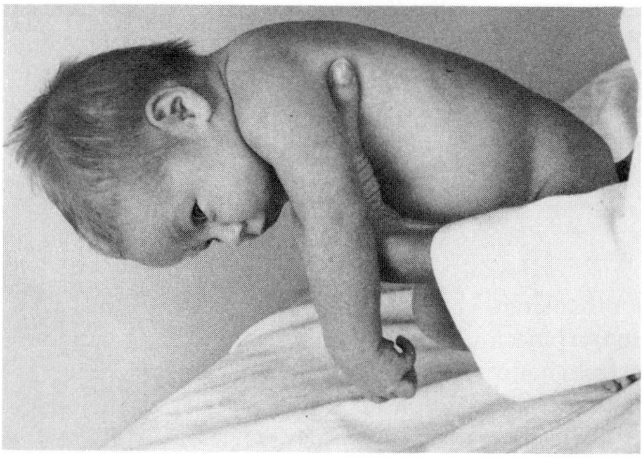

► **Figure 20–42**

ABNORMAL FINDINGS

Because development progresses in a cephalocaudal direction, head lag is an early sign of brain damage.

After 6 months of age, refer any baby with failure to hold head in midline when sitting.

Head lag; a limp, floppy trunk; and dangling arms and legs.

Absence of the reflex indicates motor weakness, upper motor neuron disease, or mental retardation.

NORMAL RANGE OF FINDINGS | **ABNORMAL FINDINGS**

Assess muscle strength by noting the strength of sucking and of spontaneous motor activity. Normally, there are no tremors or any continual overshooting of the mark when reaching.

Recall that the newborn's neuromuscular development can be tested by the Dubowitz Clinical Assessment for gestational age (see Chapter 8).

The Sensory System

You will perform very little sensory testing with infants and toddlers. The newborn normally has hypesthesia and requires a strong stimulus to elicit a response. The baby responds to pain by crying and a general reflex withdrawal of all limbs. By 7 to 9 months of age, the infant can localize the stimulus and shows more specific signs of withdrawal. Other sensory modalities are not tested.

Unusually rapid withdrawal is hyperesthesia, which occurs with spinal cord lesions, CNS infections, increased intracranial pressure, peritonitis.

No withdrawal is decreased sensation, and occurs with decreased consciousness, mental deficiency, spinal cord or peripheral nerve lesions.

Reflexes

Infantile automatisms are reflexes that have a predictable timetable of appearance and departure. The reflexes most commonly tested are listed in the following section. For the screening examination, you can just check the rooting, grasp, tonic neck, and Moro reflexes.

Rooting Reflex. Brush the infant's cheek near the mouth. Note whether the infant turns the head toward that side and opens the mouth (Fig. 20–43). Appears at birth, and disappears 3 to 4 months.

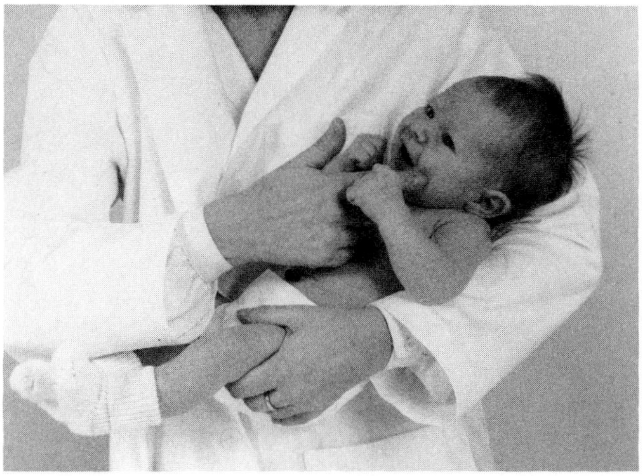

► **Figure 20–43**

NORMAL RANGE OF FINDINGS	ABNORMAL FINDINGS

Sucking Reflex. Touch the lips, and offer your finger to suck. Note strong sucking reflex. The reflex is present at birth and disappears 10 to 12 months.

Palmar Grasp. Place the baby's head midline to ensure symmetric response. Offer your finger from the baby's ulnar side, away from the thumb. Note tight grasp of all the baby's fingers (Fig. 20–44). Sucking enhances grasp. Often, you can pull baby to a sit from grasp. The reflex is present at birth, is strongest at 1 to 2 months, and disappears at 3 to 4 months.

Abnormal findings: The reflex is absent with brain damage and with local muscle or nerve injury.

Persistence of the reflex after 4 months of age occurs with frontal lobe lesion.

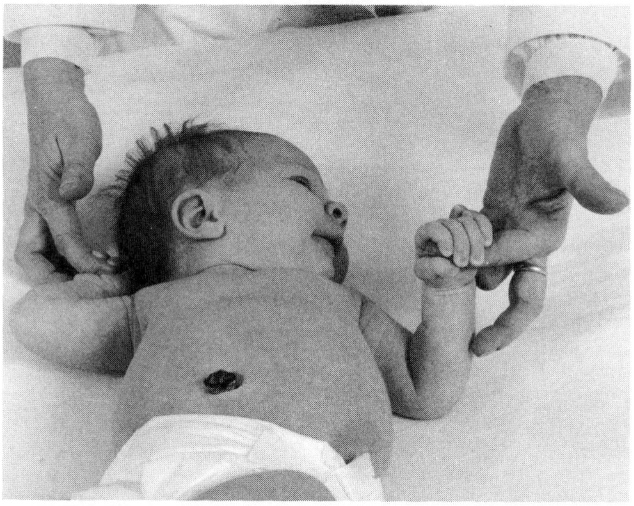

► Figure 20–44

Plantar Grasp. Touch thumb at the ball of the baby's foot. Note that the toes curl down tightly (Fig. 20–45). The reflex is present at birth, and disappears 8 to 10 months.

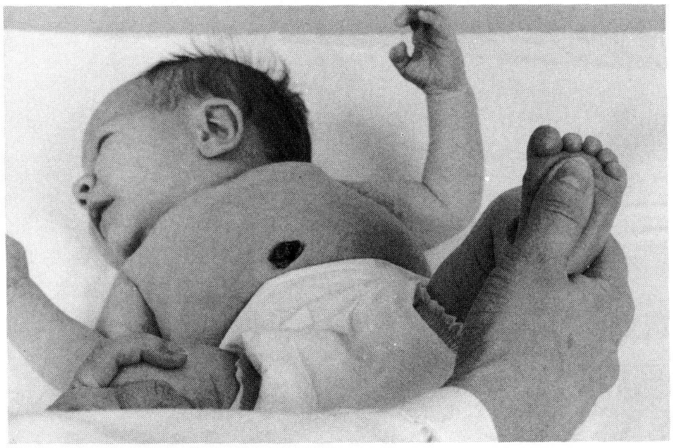

► Figure 20–45

NORMAL RANGE OF FINDINGS

Babinski's Reflex. Stroke your finger up the lateral edge and across the ball of the infant's foot. Note fanning of toes (positive Babinski's reflex) (Fig. 20–46). The reflex is present at birth and disappears (changes to the adult response) by 24 months of age (variable).

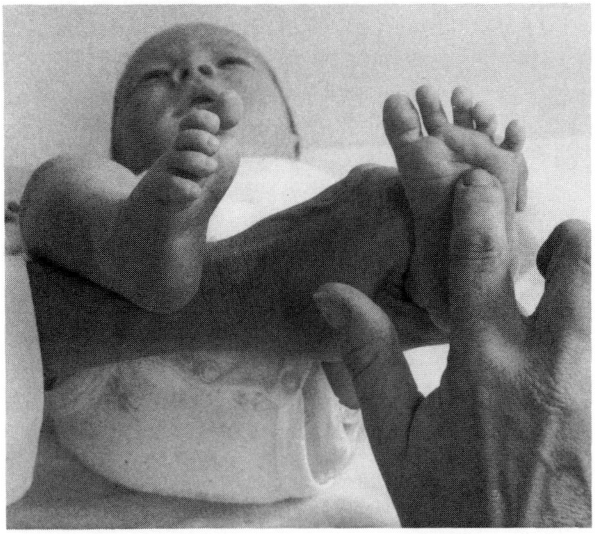

► **Figure 20–46**

Tonic Neck Reflex. With the baby supine, relaxed, or sleeping, turn the head to one side with the chin over shoulder. Note ipsilateral extension of the arm and leg, and flexion of the opposite arm and leg; this is the "fencing" position. If you turn the infant's head to the opposite side, positions will reverse (Fig. 20–47). The reflex appears by 2 to 3 months, decreases at 3 to 4 months, and disappears by 4 to 6 months.

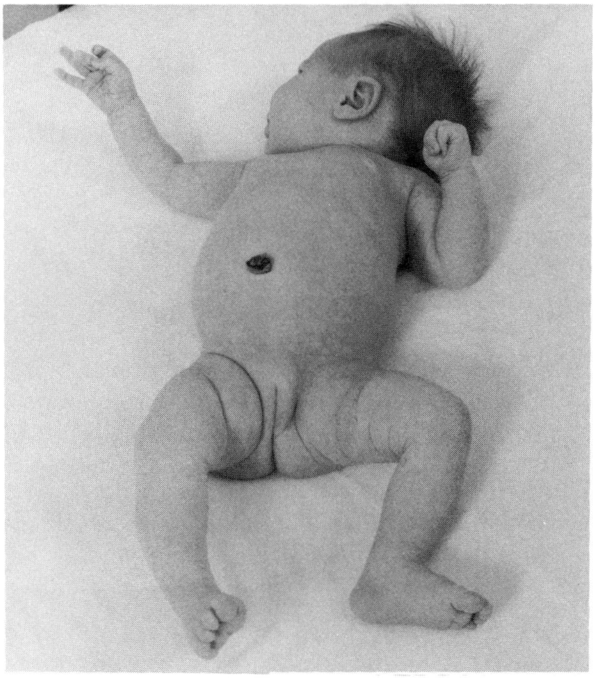

► **Figure 20–47**

ABNORMAL FINDINGS

Positive Babinski's reflex after 2 or 2 1/2 years of age occurs with pyramidal tract disease.

Persistence later in infancy occurs with brain damage.

NORMAL RANGE OF FINDINGS	ABNORMAL FINDINGS

Moro Reflex. Startle the infant by jarring the crib, making a loud noise or supporting the head and back in a semi-sitting position and quickly drop the infant to 30 degrees. The baby looks as if he or she is "grasping a tree" (Barness, 1981). That is, there is symmetric abduction and extension of the arms and legs, fanning fingers, and curling of the index finger and thumb to C position. The infant then brings in both arms and legs (Fig. 20–48). The reflex is present at birth, and disappears at 1 to 4 months.

Absence in the newborn or persistence after 5 months of age indicates severe CNS injury.

Absence of movement in one arm occurs with fracture of the humerus or clavicle, and brachial nerve palsy.

Absence in one leg occurs with a lower spinal cord problem or a dislocated hip.

A hyperactive Moro reflex occurs with tetany or CNS infection.

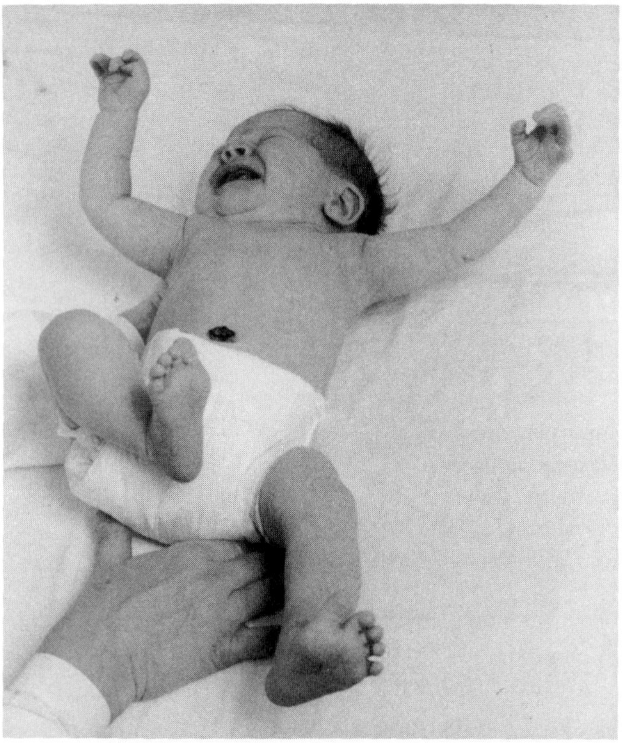

► **Figure 20–48**

Placing Reflex. Hold the infant upright under the arms, close to a table. Let the dorsal "top" of foot touch the under side of table (Fig. 20–49). Note flexing of hip and knee to place foot on table. Reflex appears at 4 days after birth.

Stepping Reflex. Hold the infant upright under the arms, with the feet on a flat surface. Note regular alternating steps (Fig. 20–50). The reflex disappears before voluntary walking.

Extensor thrust, or "scissoring"; crossing of lower extremities.

Landau's Reflex. This reflex is discussed in the section on Motor Function.

NORMAL RANGE OF FINDINGS | ABNORMAL FINDINGS

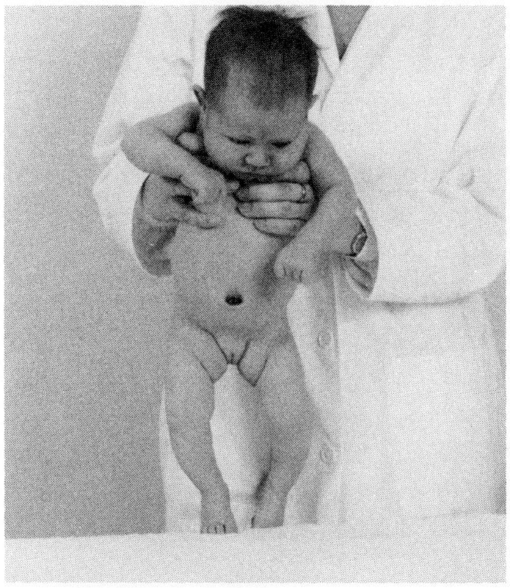

► Figure 20-49

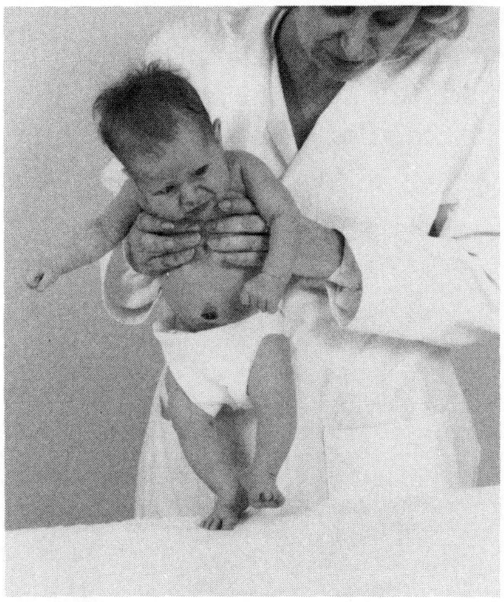

► Figure 20-50

Preschool and School-Aged Children

Use the same sequence of neurologic assessment as with the adult, with the omissions or modifications mentioned in the following section.

Assess the child's general behavior during play activities, reaction to parent, and cooperation with parent and with you. Complete details are described in Chapter 5, Mental Health Assessment.

Smell and taste are almost never tested, but if you need to test the child's sense of smell (cranial nerve I), use a scent familiar to the child such as peanut butter or orange peel. When testing visual fields (cranial nerve II) and cardinal positions of gaze (cranial nerves III, IV, VI), you often need to gently immobilize the head or the child will track with the whole head. Make a game out of asking the child to imitate your funny "faces" (cranial nerve VII); thus, the child has fun and you win a friend.

Much of the motor assessment can be derived from watching the child undress and dress and manipulate buttons. This indicates muscle strength, symmetry, joint range of motion, and fine motor skills. Use the Denver II to screen gross and fine motor skills that are appropriate for the child's specific age. Be familiar with developmental milestones described in Chapter 2 for each age.

Note the child's gait, during both walking and running. Allow for the normal wide-based gate of the toddler and the normal knock-kneed walk of the preschooler. Normally, the child can balance on one foot for about 5 seconds by 4 years of age, for 8 to 10 seconds at 5 years of age, and can hop at 4 years. Children enjoy performing these tests.

Muscle hypertrophy or atrophy occurs with muscular dystrophy.
Muscle weakness.
Incoordination.

Causes of motor delay are listed earlier in the infant section.

Staggering, falling.

Weakness climbing up or down stairs occurs with muscular dystrophy.

Broad-based gait beyond toddlerhood, scissor gait (see Table 20-6).

Failure to hop after 5 years of age indicates incoordination of gross motor skill.

NORMAL RANGE OF FINDINGS | **ABNORMAL FINDINGS**

Observe the child as he or she rises from the floor in a supine position then to a sitting position, and then to a stand. Note the muscles of the neck, abdomen, arms, and legs. Normally, the child curls up in the midline to sit up, then pushes off with both hands against the floor to stand (Fig. 20–51*A*).

Weak pelvic muscles are a sign of muscular dystrophy; from the supine position, the child will roll to one side, bend forward to all four extremities, plant hands on legs, and literally "climb" up himself. This is *Gower's sign* (Fig. 20–51*B*).

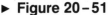

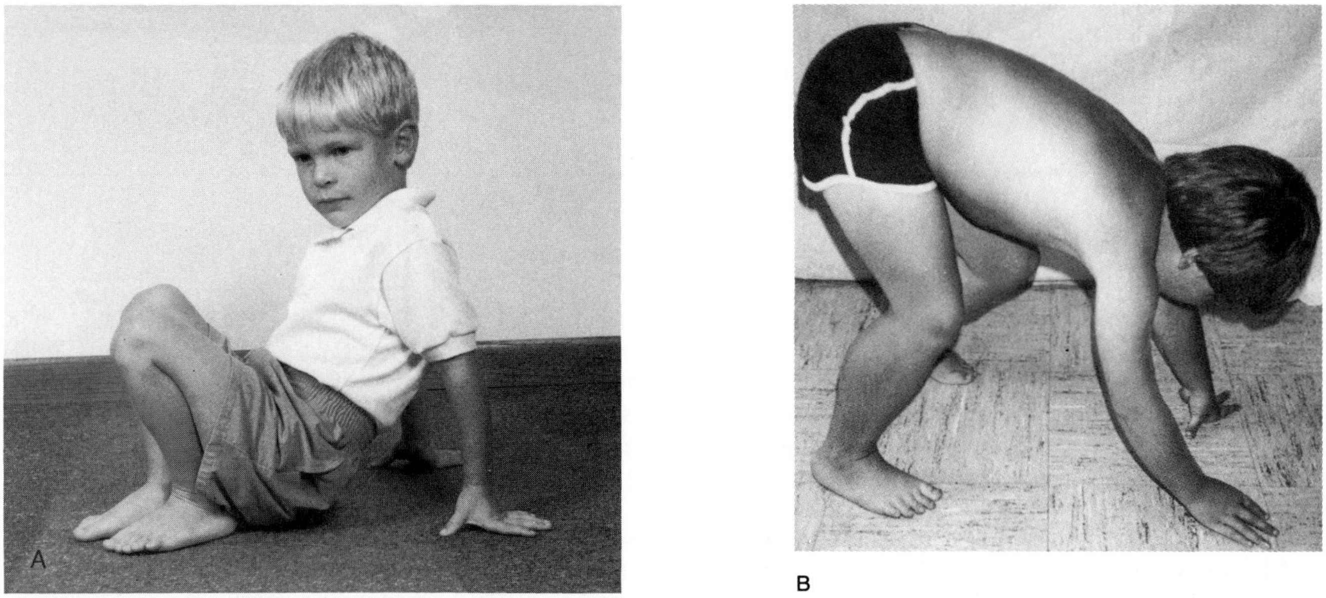

▶ **Figure 20–51**

Assess fine coordination by using the finger-to-nose test if you can be sure the young child understands your directions. Demonstrate the procedure first, then ask the child to do the test with the eyes open, then with the eyes closed. Fine coordination is not fully developed until the child has reached 4 or 6 years of age. Consider it normal if a younger child can bring the finger to within 2 to 5 cm (1 to 2 in) of the nose.

Testing sensation is very unreliable on toddlers and preschoolers. You may test light touch by asking the child to close the eyes and then to point to the spot where you touch or tickle. Testing of vibration, position, stereognosis, graphesthesia, or two-point discrimination usually is not done on a child younger than 6 years of age. Also, do not test for perception of superficial pain because the child has a natural fear of needles. In children older than 6 years of age, you may perform sensory testing as with adults. Use a fractured tongue blade instead of a needle if you need to test superficial pain.

Failure of the finger-to-nose test with the eyes open indicates gross incoordination; failure of the test with the eyes closed indicates minor incoordination or lack of position sense.

Sensory loss occurs with decreased consciousness, mental deficiency, or spinal cord or peripheral nerve dysfunction.

NORMAL RANGE OF FINDINGS

The deep tendon reflexes usually are not tested in children younger than 5 years of age due to lack of cooperation in relaxation. When you need to test DTRs in a young child, use your finger to percuss the tendon. Use a reflex hammer only with an older child. Coax the child to relax, or distract and percuss discretely when the child is not paying attention. The knee jerk is present at birth, then the ankle jerk and brachial reflex appear, and the triceps reflex is present at 6 months.

The Aging Adult

Use the same examination as used with the younger adult. Be aware that some aging adults show a slower response to your requests, especially to those calling for coordination of movements. The conditions discussed in the following sections are normal variants due to aging.

Although the cranial nerves mediating taste and smell are not usually tested, they may show some decline in function.

Any decrease in muscle bulk is most apparent in the hand, as seen by guttering between the metacarpals. These dorsal hand muscles often look wasted, even with no apparent arthropathy. The grip strength remains relatively good.

Senile tremors occasionally occur. These benign tremors include an intention tremor of the hands, head nodding (as if saying yes or no), and tongue protrusion. *Dyskinesias* are the repetitive stereotyped movements in the jaw, lips, or tongue that may accompany senile tremors. There is no associated rigidity.

The gait may be slower, more deliberate, and may deviate slightly from a midline path than that in the younger person.

The rapid alternating movements, e.g., pronating and supinating the hands on the thigh, may be more difficult to perform by the aging adult.

After 65 years of age, loss of the sensation of vibration at the ankle malleolus is common and is usually accompanied by loss of the ankle jerk. Position sense in the big toe may be lost, although this is less common than vibration loss. Tactile sensation may be impaired. The aging person may need stronger stimuli for light touch and especially pain.

The DTRs are less brisk. Those in the upper extremities are usually present, but the ankle jerks are commonly lost. Knee jerks may be lost, but this occurs less often. Because aging people find it difficult to relax their limbs, always use reinforcement when eliciting the DTRs.

The plantar reflex may be absent or difficult to interpret. Often, you will not see a definite normal flexor response. However, you still should consider a definite extensor response to be abnormal.

The superficial abdominal reflexes may be absent, probably due to stretching of the musculature through pregnancy or obesity.

ABNORMAL FINDINGS

Hyperactivity of DTRs occurs with upper motor neuron lesion, hypocalcemia, hyperthyroidism, and with muscle spasm associated with early poliomyelitis.

Decreased or absent reflexes occur with a lower motor neuron lesion, muscular dystrophy, and flaccidity or flaccid paralysis.

Clonus may occur with fatigue, but it usually indicates hyperreflexia.

Hand muscle atrophy is worsened with disuse and degenerative arthropathy.

Distinguish senile tremors from tremors of parkinsonism. The latter includes rigidity, and slowness and weakness of voluntary movement.

Absence of a rhythmic reciprocal gait pattern is seen in parkinsonism and hemiparesis (see Table 20 – 6).

Note any difference in sensation between right and left sides, which may indicate a neurologic deficit.

NORMAL RANGE OF FINDINGS	ABNORMAL FINDINGS

NEUROLOGIC RECHECK

Some hospitalized persons have head trauma or a neurologic deficit due to a systemic disease process. These people must be monitored closely for any improvement or deterioration in neurologic status and for any indication of increasing intracranial pressure. Signs of increasing intracranial pressure signal impending cerebral disaster and death, and require early and prompt intervention.

Use an abbreviation of the neurologic examination in the following sequence:

1. Level of consciousness
2. Motor function
3. Pupillary response
4. Vital signs

Level of Consciousness. A *change* in the level of consciousness is the single most important factor in this examination. It is the earliest and most sensitive index of change in neurologic status. Note the ease of *arousal* and the state of awareness, or *orientation.* Assess orientation by asking questions about:

person — own name, occupation, names of workers around person, their occupation

place — where person is, nature of building, city, state

time — day of week, month, year

Abnormal findings: A change in consciousness may be subtle. Note any decreasing level of consciousness, disorientation, memory loss, uncooperative behavior, or even complacency in a previously combative person.

Vary the questions during repeat assessments so that the person is not merely memorizing answers. Note the quality and the content of the verbal response; articulation, fluency, manner of thinking, and any deficit in language comprehension or production (see Chapter 5).

When the person is intubated and cannot speak, you will have to ask questions that require a nod or shake of the head, "Is this a hospital?" "Are you at home?" "Are we in Texas?"

A person is fully alert when his or her eyes open at your approach or spontaneously; when he or she is oriented to person, place, and time; and when he or she is able to follow verbal commands appropriately.

Abnormal findings: Review Table 5–3, Levels of Consciousness, Chapter 5.

If the person is not fully alert, increase the amount of stimulus used in this order:

name called

light touch on person's arm

vigorous shake of shoulder

pain applied (pinch nail bed, pinch trapezius muscle, rub your knuckles on the person's sternum)

Record the stimulus used as well as the person's response to it.

Motor Function. Check the voluntary movement of each extremity by giving the person specific commands. (This procedure also tests level of consciousness by noting the person's ability to follow commands.)

Ask the person to lift the eyebrows, frown, bare teeth. Note symmetric facial movements and bilateral nasolabial folds (cranial nerve VII).

NORMAL RANGE OF FINDINGS

ABNORMAL FINDINGS

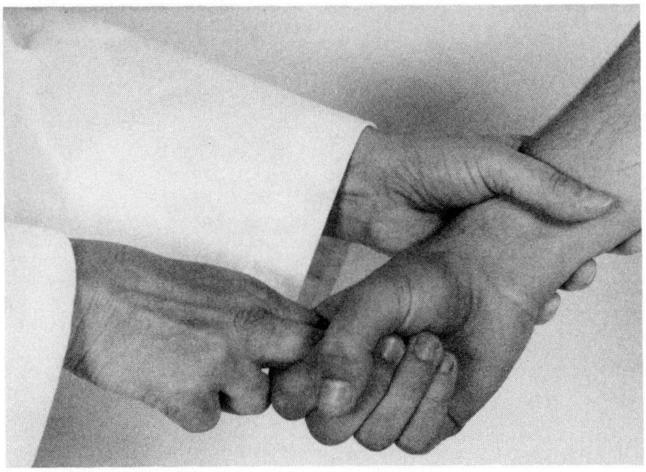

► **Figure 20–52**

You can check upper arm strength by checking hand grasps. Ask the person to squeeze your fingers. Offer your two fingers, one on top of the other, so that a strong hand grasp does not hurt your knuckles (Fig. 20–52). Be judicious about asking the person to squeeze your hands; some persons with diffuse brain damage, especially frontal lobe injury, have a grasp that is a reflex only. Alternatively, ask the person to lift each hand or to hold up one finger. You also can check upper extremity strength by palmar drift. Ask the person to extend both arms forward or halfway up, palms up, eyes closed, and hold for 10 to 20 seconds (Fig. 20–53). Normally, the arms stay steady with no downward drift.

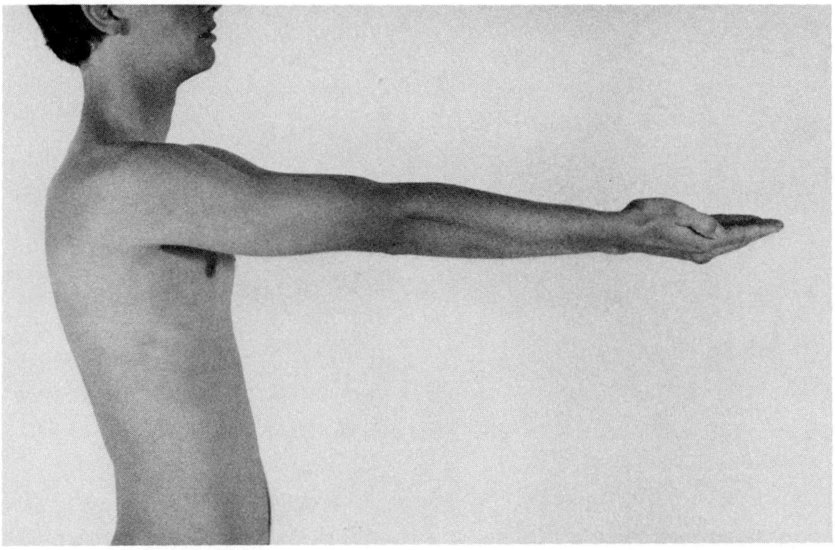

► **Figure 20–53**

NORMAL RANGE OF FINDINGS

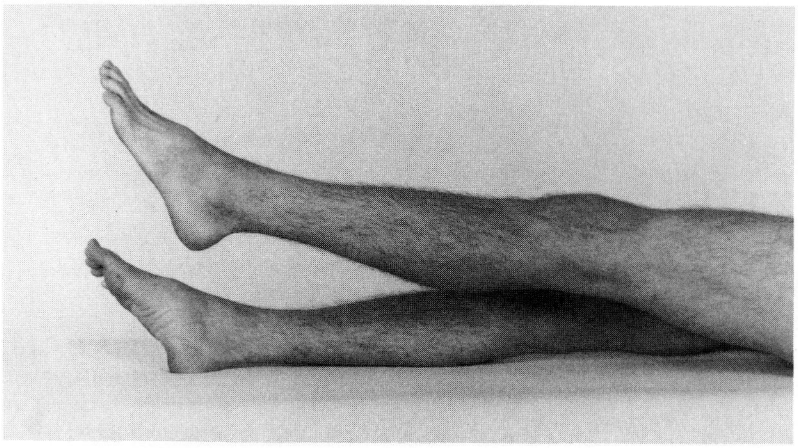

► **Figure 20-54**

Check lower extremities by asking the person to do straight leg raises. Ask the person to lift one leg at a time straight up off the bed (Fig. 20-54). Full strength allows the leg to be lifted 90 degrees. If multiple trauma, pain, or equipment preclude this motion, ask the person to push one foot at a time against your hand's resistance, "like putting your foot on the gas pedal of your car" (Fig. 20-55).

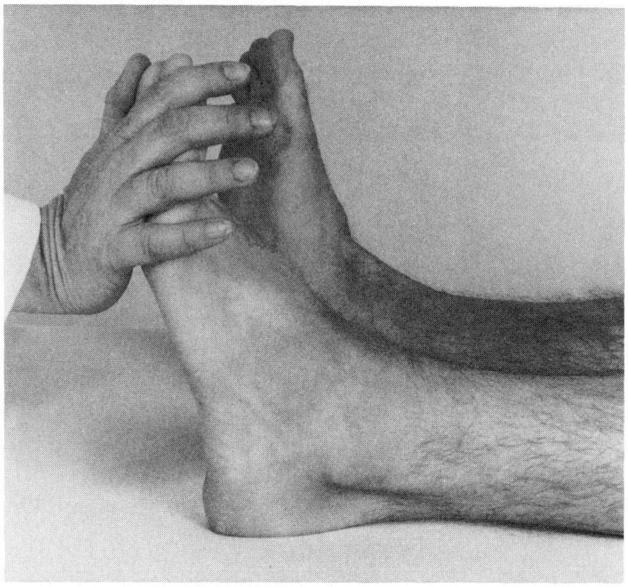

► **Figure 20-55**

For the person with decreased level of consciousness, note if movement occurs spontaneously, and as a result of noxious stimuli such as pain or suctioning. An attempt to push away your hand after such stimuli is called *localizing* and is characterized as purposeful movement.

ABNORMAL FINDINGS

Any abnormal posturing, decorticate rigidity, or decerebrate rigidity indicates diffuse brain injury (see Table 20-10).

NORMAL RANGE OF FINDINGS

Pupillary Response. Note the size, shape, and symmetry of both pupils. Shine a light into each pupil and note the direct and consensual light reflex. Both pupils should constrict briskly. (Allow for the effects of any medication that could affect pupil size and reactivity.) When recording, pupil size is best expressed in millimeters. Tape a millimeter scale onto a tongue blade and hold it next to the person's eyes for the most accurate measurement (Fig. 20–56).

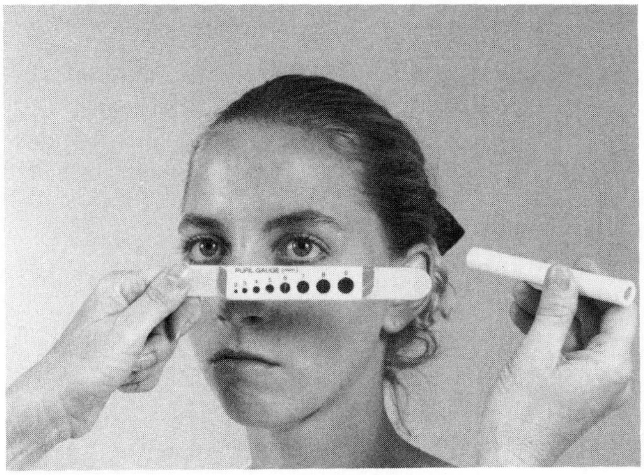

► **Figure 20–56**

Vital Signs. Measure the temperature, pulse, respiration, and blood pressure as often as the person's condition warrants. Although they are vital to the overall assessment of the critically ill person, pulse and blood pressure are notoriously unreliable parameters of CNS deficit. Any changes are late consequences of rising intracranial pressure.

The Glasgow Coma Scale (GCS). Since the terms describing levels of consciousness are ambiguous, the Glasgow Coma Scale was developed as an accurate and reliable *quantitative* tool (Teasdale and Jennett, 1974) (Fig. 20–57). The GCS is an objective assessment that defines the level of consciousness by giving it a numerical value.

The scale is divided into three areas: eye opening, verbal response, and motor response. Each area is rated separately, and a number is given for the person's best response. The three numbers are added; the total score reflects the brain's functional level. A fully alert, normal person has a score of 15, whereas a score of 7 or less reflects coma. Serial assessments can be plotted on a graph to illustrate visually whether the person is stable, improving, or deteriorating.

The GCS assesses the functional state of the brain as a whole, not of any particular site in the brain (Teasdale, 1975). The scale is easy to learn and master, is reliable, and enhances interprofessional communication by a common language.

ABNORMAL FINDINGS

In a brain-injured person, a sudden, unilateral, dilated and nonreactive pupil is ominous. Cranial nerve III runs parallel to the brain stem. When increasing intracranial pressure pushes the brain stem down (uncal herniation), it puts pressure on cranial nerve III, causing pupil dilatation.

Signs of increasing intracranial pressure, the *Cushing reflex:*

Blood pressure—sudden elevation with widening pulse pressure;

Pulse—decreased rate, slow and bounding

NORMAL RANGE OF FINDINGS | **ABNORMAL FINDINGS**

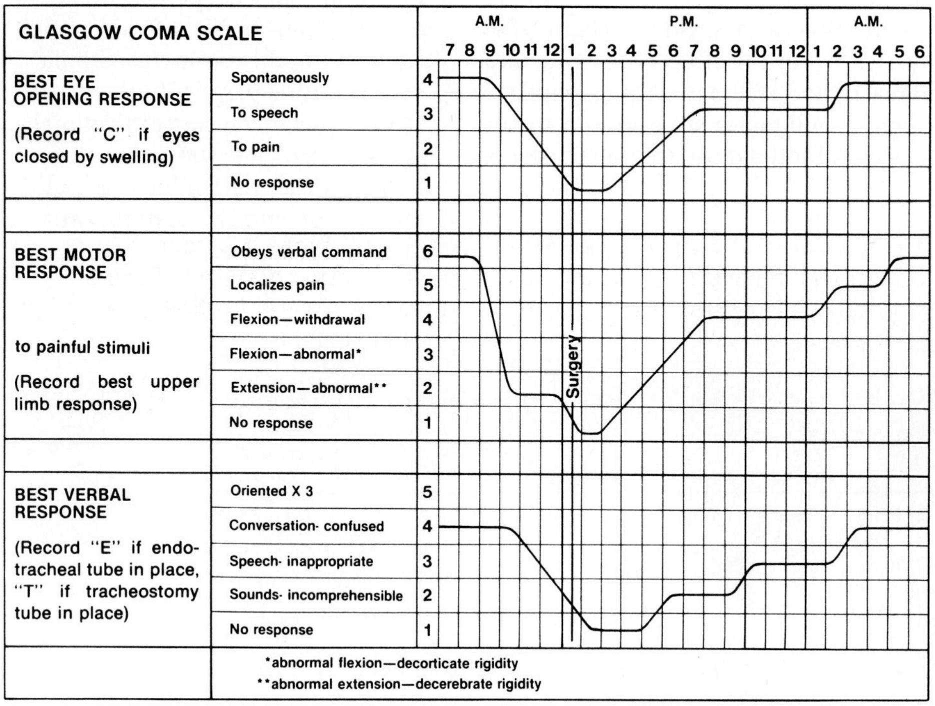

GLASGOW COMA SCALE
A.M.
P.M.
A.M.
7 8 9 10 11 12 1 2 3 4 5 6 7 8 9 10 11 12 1 2 3 4 5 6
BEST EYE OPENING RESPONSE
(Record "C" if eyes closed by swelling)
Spontaneously 4
To speech 3
To pain 2
No response 1
BEST MOTOR RESPONSE
to painful stimuli
(Record best upper limb response)
Obeys verbal command 6
Localizes pain 5
Flexion—withdrawal 4
Flexion—abnormal* 3
Extension—abnormal** 2
No response 1
Surgery
BEST VERBAL RESPONSE
(Record "E" if endotracheal tube in place, "T" if tracheostomy tube in place)
Oriented X 3 5
Conversation- confused 4
Speech- inappropriate 3
Sounds- incomprehensible 2
No response 1
*abnormal flexion—decorticate rigidity
**abnormal extension—decerebrate rigidity

▶ **Figure 20-57**

☑ SUMMARY CHECKLIST

Neurologic Screening Examination

1 ▶ Mental Status

2 ▶ Cranial Nerves
- II Optic
- III, IV, VI—Extraocular muscles
- V
- VII Facial mobility

3 ▶ Motor function
- Gait and balance
- Knee flexion—hop or shallow knee bend

4 ▶ Sensory function
- Superficial pain and light touch—arms and legs
- Vibration—arms and legs

5 ▶ Reflexes
- Biceps
- Triceps
- Patellar
- Achilles

Neurologic Complete Examination

1 ▶ Mental Status

2 ▶ Cranial Nerves, II through XII

3 ▶ Motor System
- Muscle size, strength, tone
- Gait and balance
- Rapid alternating movements

4 ▶ Sensory function
- Superficial pain and light touch
- Vibration
- Position sense
- Stereognosis, graphesthesia, two-point discrimination

5 ▶ Reflexes
- DTRs: biceps, triceps, brachioradialis, patellar, Achilles
- Superficial: abdominal, plantar

SAMPLE RECORDING

Subjective

- States has had no unusually frequent or severe headaches, no head injury, dizziness or vertigo, seizures or tremors. No weakness, numbness or tingling, difficulty swallowing or speaking. Has no past history of stroke, spinal cord injury, meningitis, or alcoholism.

Objective

- *Mental status:* appearance, behavior, & speech appropriate; alert & oriented × 3; recent and remote memory intact.

Cranial nerves:
I identifies coffee and tobacco
II vision 20/20 OS, 20/20 OD, peripheral fields intact by confrontation, fundi normal
III, IV, VI EOMs intact, no ptosis or nystagmus, PERRLA*
V sensation intact & = bilaterally, jaw strength = bilaterally
VII facial muscles intact & symmetric
VIII hearing—whispered words heard bilaterally, Weber midline
IX, X swallowing intact, gag reflex present, uvula rises in midline on phonation
XI shoulder shrug, head movement intact & = bilaterally
XII tongue protrudes midline, no tremors

Motor: No atrophy, weakness or tremors. Gait normal, able to tandem walk, no Romberg's sign. RAM—finger-to-nose smoothly intact.

Sensory: Pin prick, light touch, vibration intact. Stereognosis—able to identify key.

Reflexes: Normal abdominal, no Babinski's sign.

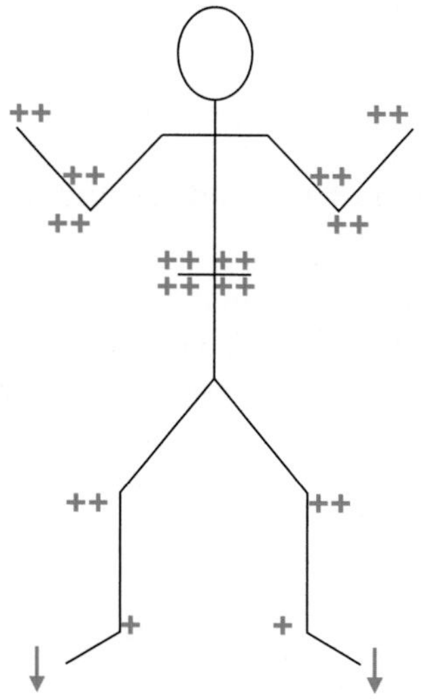

* PERRLA: pupils equal, round, react to light and accommodation.

SAMPLE CLINICAL PROBLEM

J.T. is a 61-year-old white male carpenter with a large building firm, who is admitted to the Rehabilitation Institute with a diagnosis of right hemiplegia and aphasia following a CVA 4 weeks PTA.

Subjective

▶ Because of J.T.'s speech dysfunction, history provided by wife.
4 weeks PTA—Complaint of severe headache, then sudden onset of collapse and loss of consciousness while at work. Did not strike head as fell. Transported by ambulance to Memorial Hospital where admitting physician said J.T. "probably had a stroke." Right arm and leg were limp and he remained unconscious. Admitted to Critical Care Unit. Regained consciousness day 3 after admission, unable to move right side, unable to speak clearly or write. Remained in ICU 4 more days until "doctors were sure heart and breathing were steady."
3 weeks PTA—Transferred to medical floor where care included physical therapy twice per day, and passive ROM 4 x/day.
Now—Some improvement in right motor function. Bowel control achieved with use of commode same time each day (after breakfast). Bladder control improved with some occasional incontinence, usually when cannot tell people he needs to urinate.

Objective

▶ *Mental status:* Dressed in jogging suit, sitting in wheel chair, appears alert with appropriate eye contact, listening intently to history. Speech is slow, requires great effort, able to give one-word answers that are appropriate but lack normal tone. Seems to understand all language spoken to him. Follows requests appropriately, within limits of motor weakness.

Cranial nerves:
II: Acuity normal, fields by confrontation—right homonymous hemianopsia, fundi normal.
III, IV, VI: EOMs intact, no ptosis or nystagmus, PERRLA
V: Sensation intact to pin prick and light touch. Jaw strength weak on right.
VII: Flat nasolabial fold on right, motor weakness on right lower face. Able to wrinkle forehead bilaterally, but unable to smile or bare teeth on right.
VIII: Hearing intact.
IX, X: Swallowing intact, gag reflex present, uvula rises midline on phonation.
XI: Shoulder shrug, head movement weaker on right.
XII: Tongue protrudes midline, no tremors

Sensory:
Pin prick and light touch present but diminished on right arm and leg. Vibration intact. Position sense impaired on right side. Stereognosis intact.

Motor: Right hand grip weak, right arm drifts, right leg weak, unable to support weight. Spasticity in right arm and leg muscles, limited range of motion on passive motion. Unable to stand up and walk unassisted. Unable to perform finger-to-nose or heel-to-shin on right side, left side smoothly intact.

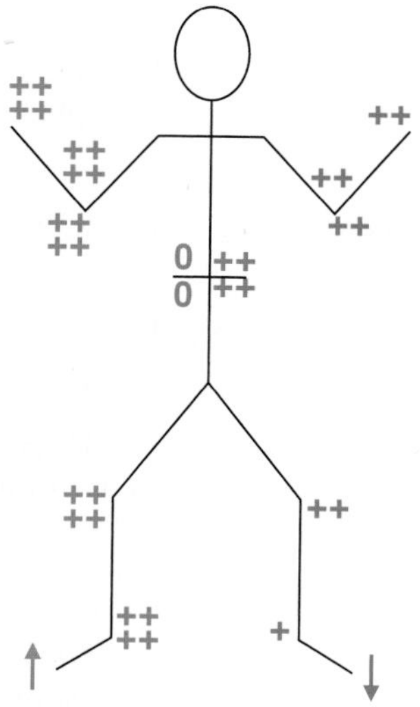

Abdominal and cremasteric reflexes absent on right

Assessment

- ▶ Impaired verbal communication R/T effects of CVA
  Impaired physical mobility R/T neuromuscular impairment
  Body image disturbance R/T effects of loss of body function
  Self-care deficits: feeding, bathing, toileting, dressing/grooming R/T muscular weakness
  Sensory-perceptual alteration (absent right visual fields) R/T neurologic impairment
  Potential for injury R/T visual field deficit

NURSING DIAGNOSES COMMONLY ASSOCIATED WITH NERVOUS SYSTEM—NEUROLOGIC DISORDERS

Diagnosis	Related Factors (Etiology)	Defining Characteristics (Symptoms and Signs)
Sensory perceptual alteration: kinesthetic	Effects of inner ear inflammation Neurologic impairment Side effects of tranquilizers, sedatives, muscle relaxants, or antihistamines Sleep deprivation	Falling Vertigo Stumbling Nausea Motion sickness Motor incoordination Alteration in posture Inability to sit or stand

Table continued on following page

Diagnosis	Related Factors (Etiology)	Defining Characteristics (Symptoms and Signs)

Impaired verbal communication	Altered thought processes
	Auditory impairment
	Decreased circulation to the brain
	Effects of surgery or trauma
	Physical barriers of
	  Intubation
	  Tracheostomy
	Inability to read or write
	Language barrier
	Psychological barriers
	  Anxiety
	  Fear
	Inflammation
	Mental retardation
	Oral deformities
	Respiratory embarrassment
	Speech pattern dysfunction
		Difficulty with phonation
		Disorientation
		Dyspnea
		Flight of ideas
		Impaired articulation
		Inability to
		  Find words
		  Identify objects
		  Modulate speech
		  Name words
		Incessant verbalization
		Lack of desire to speak
		Loose association of ideas
		Stuttering or slurring

Reflex incontinence	Neurologic impairment
	  Cerebral loss
	  Interruption of spinal nerve impulse above the level of S_3
		Lack of awareness of
		  Being incontinent
		  Bladder filling
		Lack of urge to void or feelings of fullness
		Somewhat unpredictable voiding pattern
		Uninhibited bladder contractions and spasms at regular intervals
		Voiding in large amounts

Unilateral neglect	Effects of disturbed perceptual abilities, e.g., hemianopsia, One-sided blindness Effects of neurologic illness or trauma	Does not look toward affected side Consistent inattention to stimuli on affected side Leaves food on plate on the affected side Inadequate self-care, positioning, and/or safety precautions in regard to affected side

Other related nursing diagnoses:
- Activity intolerance (see Chapter 15)
- Body image disturbance
- Diversional activity deficit
- Dysreflexia

Diagnosis	Related Factors (Etiology)	Defining Characteristics (Symptoms and Signs)
Fear		
Home maintenance management		
Impaired physical mobility (see Chapter 19)		
Potential for trauma (see Chapter 19)		
Sensory perceptual alteration: tactile, visual		
Skin integrity, potential impaired (see Chapter 9)		
Total incontinence		
Urinary elimination, altered patterns of		

ABNORMAL FINDINGS

Table 20–3 ► Abnormalities in Cranial Nerves

NERVE	TEST	ABNORMAL FINDINGS	POSSIBLE CAUSES
I Olfactory	Identify familiar odors	Anosmia	Upper respiratory infection (temporary); tobacco or cocaine use; fracture of cribriform plate or ethmoid area; frontal lobe lesion; tumor in olfactory bulb or tract
II Optic	Visual acuity	Defect or absent central vision	Congenital blindness, refractive error, acquired vision loss from numerous diseases (e.g., cerebrovascular accident, diabetes), trauma to globe or orbit (see discussion of cranial nerve III)
	Visual fields	Defect in peripheral vision, hemianopsia	
	Shine light in eye	Absent light reflex	
	Direct inspection	Papilledema	Increased intracranial pressure
		Optic atrophy	Glaucoma
		Retinal lesions	Diabetes
III Oculomotor	Inspection	Dilated pupil, ptosis, eye turns out and slightly down	Paralysis in cranial nerve III from internal carotid aneurysm, tumor, inflammatory lesions, uncal herniation with increased intracranial pressure
	Extraocular muscle movement	Failure to move eye up, in, down	Ptosis from myasthenia gravis, oculomotor nerve palsy, Horner's syndrome
	Shine light in eye	Absent light reflex	Blindness, drug influence, increased intracranial pressure, CNS injury, circulatory arrest, CNS syphilis

Table continued on following page

Table 20-3 ► Abnormalities in Cranial Nerves *Continued*

NERVE	TEST	ABNORMAL FINDINGS	POSSIBLE CAUSES
IV Trochlear	Extraocular muscle movement	Failure to turn eye down or out	Fracture of orbit, brain stem tumor
V Trigeminal	Superficial touch—three divisions Corneal reflex	Absent touch and pain, paresthesias No blink	Trauma, tumor, pressure from aneurysm, inflammation, sequelae of alcohol injection for trigeminal neuralgia
	Clench teeth	Weakness of masseter or temporalis muscles	Unilateral weakness with cranial nerve V lesion; bilateral weakness with upper or lower motor neuron or LMN disorder
VI Abducens	Extraocular muscle movement to right and left side	Failure to move laterally, diplopia on lateral gaze	Brain stem tumor or trauma, fracture of orbit
VII Facial	Wrinkle forehead, close eyes tightly. Smile, puff cheeks	Absent or asymmetric facial movement	Bell's palsy (lower motor neuron lesion) causes paralysis entire half of face
	Identify tastes	Loss of taste	Upper motor neuron lesions (cerebrovascular accident, tumor, inflammatory) cause paralysis lower half of face, leaving forehead intact Other lower motor neuron causes of paralysis: swelling from ear or meningeal infections
VIII Acoustic	Hearing acuity	Decrease or loss of hearing	Inflammation, occluded ear canal, otosclerosis, presbycusis, drug toxicity, tumor
IX Glossopharyngeal	Gag reflex	See cranial nerve X	
X Vagus	Phonates "ahh" Gag reflex	Uvula deviates to side, No gag reflex	Brain stem tumor, neck injury, cranial nerve X lesion
	Note voice quality	Hoarse or brassy Nasal twang Husky	Vocal cord weakness Soft palate weakness Unilateral cranial nerve X lesion
	Note swallowing	Dysphagia, fluids regurgitate through nose	Bilateral cranial nerve X lesion
XI Spinal Accessory	Turn head, shrug shoulders against resistance	Absent movement of sternomastoid or trapezius muscles	Neck injury, torticollis
XII Hypoglossal	Protrude tongue Wiggle tongue from side to side	Deviates to side Slowed rate of movement	Lower motor neuron lesion Bilateral upper motor neuron lesion

Table 20-4 ▸ Abnormalities in Muscle Tone

CONDITION	DESCRIPTION	ASSOCIATED WITH
Flaccidity	Decreased muscle tone or hypotonia; muscle feels limp, soft, and flabby; muscle is weak and easily fatigued	Lower motor neuron injury (peripheral neuritis, poliomyelitis), and early cerebrovascular accident
Spasticity	Increased tone; increased resistance to passive lengthening; then may suddenly give way (clasp-knife phenomenon)	Injury to corticospinal motor tract, e.g., paralysis with cerebrovascular accident
Rigidity	Constant state of resistance; resists passive movement in any direction; dystonia	Injury to extrapyramidal motor tract, e.g., parkinsonism
Cogwheel rigidity	Type of rigidity in which the increased tone is released by degrees during passive range of motion so it feels like small, regular jerks	Parkinsonism

Table 20-5 ▸ Abnormalities in Muscle Movement

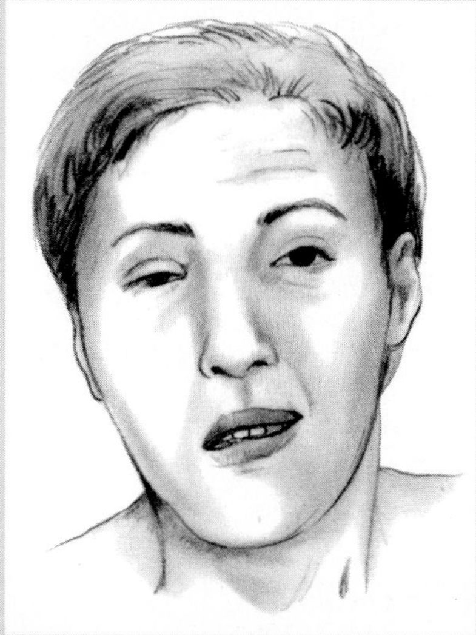

PARALYSIS

Decreased or loss of motor power, due to problem with motor nerve or muscle fibers. Causes: acute—trauma, poliomyelitis, polyneuritis, Bell's palsy; chronic—muscular dystrophy, diabetic neuropathy, multiple sclerosis; episodic—myasthenia gravis.

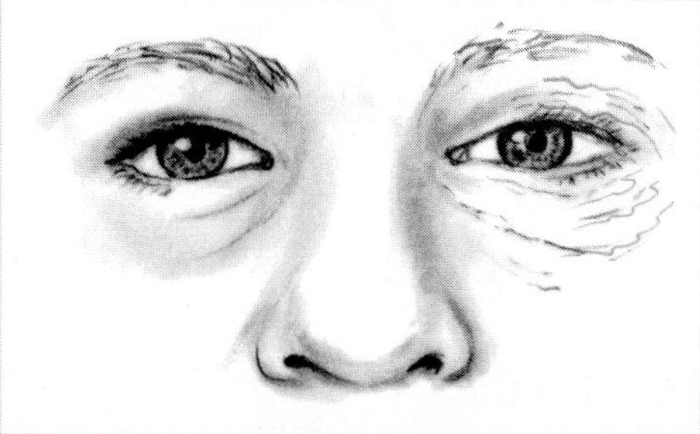

FASCICULATION

Rapid continuous twitching of resting muscle or part of muscle, without movement of limb. Types: fine—occurs with lower motor neuron disease, associated with atrophy and weakness; coarse—occurs with cold exposure or fatigue, and is not significant.

Table continued on following page

Table 20-5 ▸ Abnormalities in Muscle Movement *Continued*

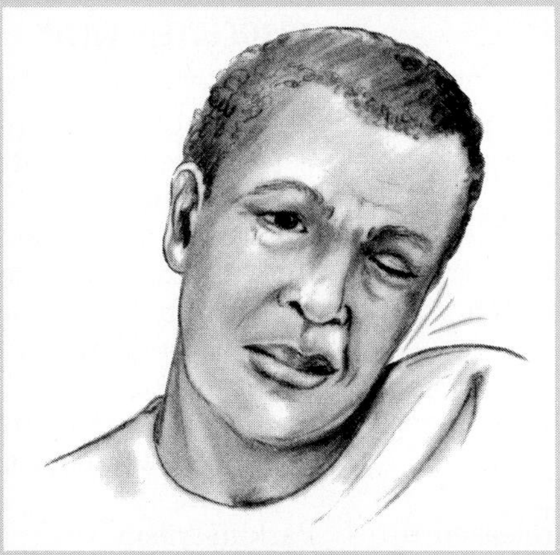

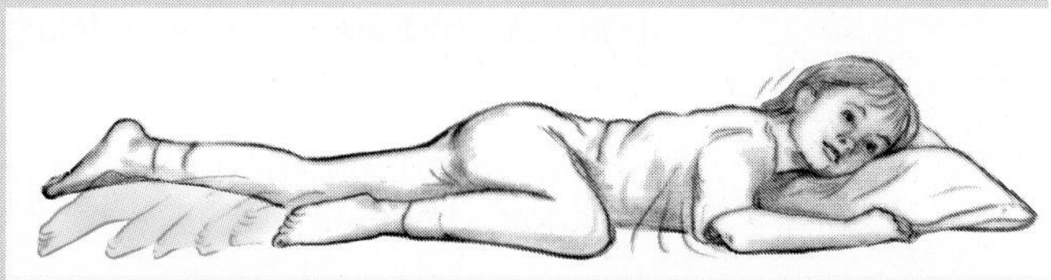

TIC

Repetitive twitching of a muscle group at inappropriate times, e.g., wink, grimace, head movement, shoulder shrug; due to a neurologic or emotional cause; may be under voluntary control.

MYOCLONUS

Rapid, sudden, single jerk or a short series of jerks at fairly regular intervals. A hiccup is a myoclonus of diaphragm. Single myoclonic arm or leg jerk is normal when the person is falling asleep; myoclonic jerks are severe with grand mal seizures.

TREMOR

Involuntary contraction of opposing muscle groups. Results in rhythmic, back-and-forth movement of one or more joints. May occur at rest or with voluntary movement. All tremors disappear while sleeping. Tremors may be slow (3 to 6 per second) or rapid (10 to 20 per second).

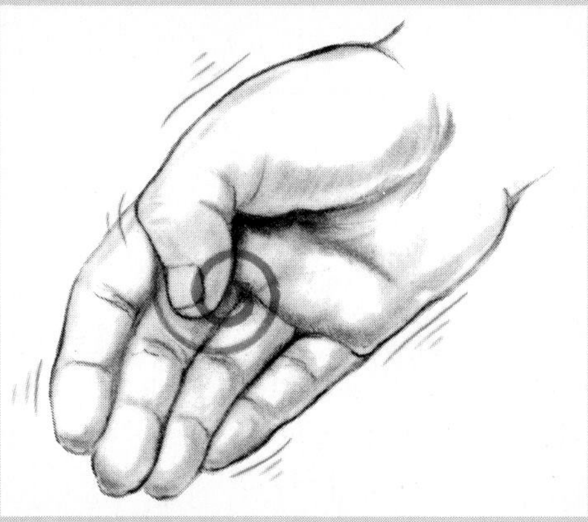

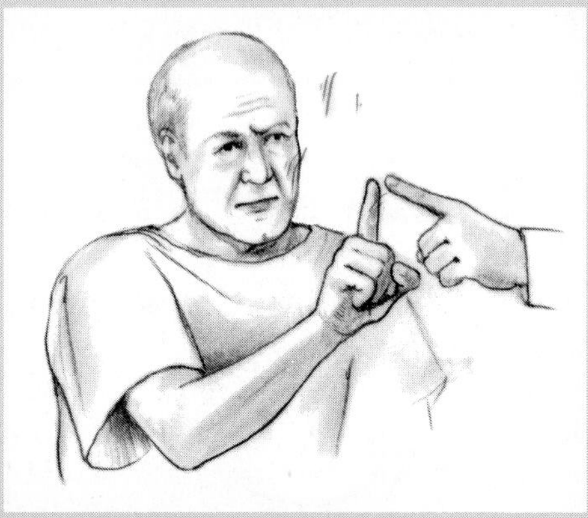

REST TREMOR

Coarse and slow (3 to 6 per second); partly or completely disappears with voluntary movement, e.g., "pill rolling" tremor of parkinsonism, with thumb and opposing fingers.

INTENTION TREMOR

Rate varies; worse with voluntary movement. Occurs with cerebellar disease and multiple sclerosis.

Essential tremor (familial)—A type of intention tremor; most common tremor with older people. Benign (no associated disease) but causes emotional stress in business or social situations. Improves with the administration of sedatives, propranalol, alcohol; but use of alcohol is discouraged because of the risk of addiction.

Table 20-5 ▸ Abnormalities in Muscle Movement *Continued*

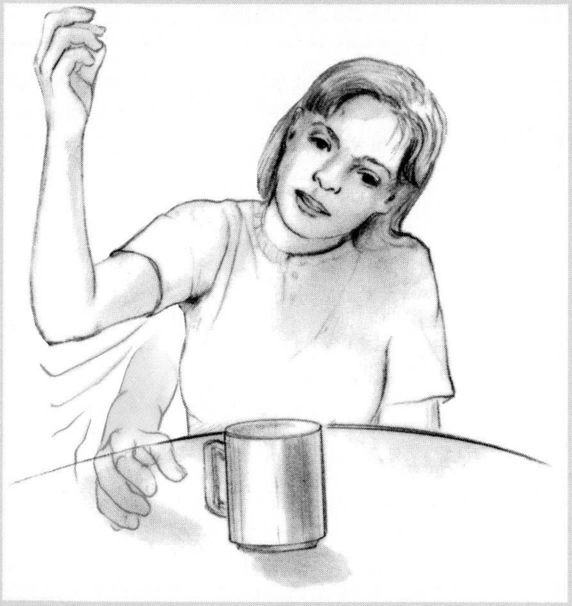

CHOREA

Sudden, rapid, jerky, purposeless movement, involving limbs, trunk, or face.

Occurs at irregular intervals, not rhythmic or repetitive, more convulsive than a tic. Some are spontaneous, and some are initiated; all are accentuated by voluntary acts. Disappears with sleep. Common with Sydenham's and Huntington's chorea.

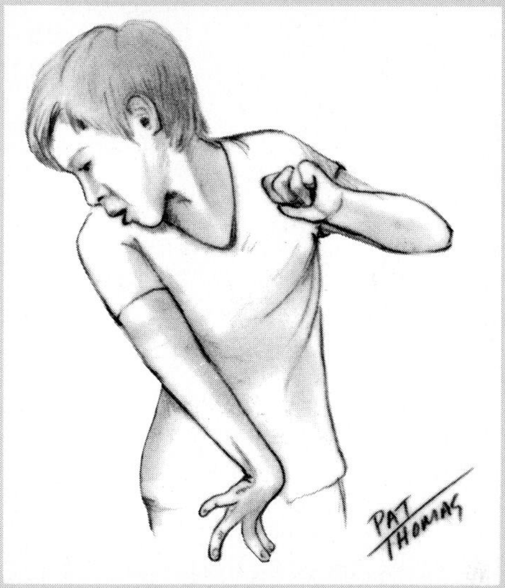

ATHETOSIS

Slow, twisting, writhing, continuous movement, resembling a snake or worm. Involves distal part of limb more than the proximal part. Occurs with cerebral palsy. Disappears with sleep. "Athetoid" hand —some fingers are flexed and some are extended.

Table 20-6 ▸ Abnormal Gaits

TYPE	CHARACTERISTIC APPEARANCE	POSSIBLE CAUSE
Spastic hemiparesis 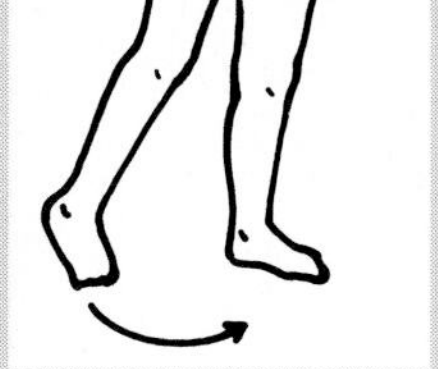	Arm is immobile against the body, with flexion of the shoulder, elbow, wrist, fingers, and adduction of shoulder. The leg is stiff and extended, and circumducts with each step (drags toe in a semicircle).	Upper motor neuron lesion of the corticospinal tract, e.g., cerebrovascular accident, trauma.

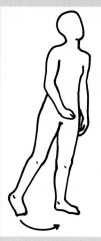

Table continued on following page

Table 20-6 ▸ Abnormal Gaits *Continued*

TYPE	CHARACTERISTIC APPEARANCE	POSSIBLE CAUSE
Cerebellar ataxia 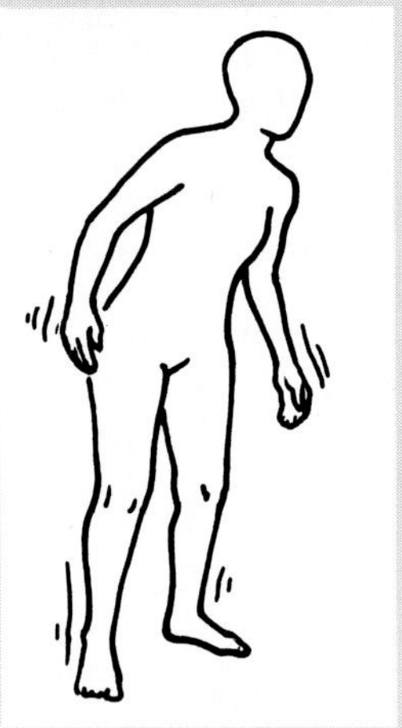	Staggering, wide-based gait; difficulty with turns; uncoordinated movement with positive Romberg's sign.	Alcohol or barbiturate effect on cerebellum; cerebellar tumor; multiple sclerosis.
Parkinsonian (festinating) 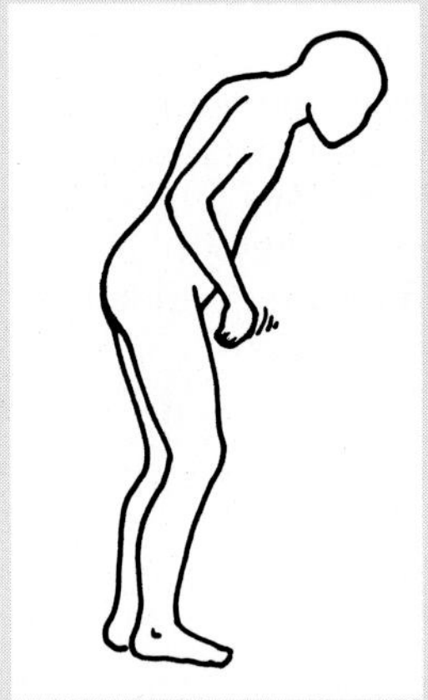	Posture is stooped; trunk is pitched forward; elbows, hips, and knees are flexed. Steps are short and shuffling. Hesitation to begin walking, and difficult to stop suddenly. The person holds the body rigid. Walks and turns body as one fixed unit. Difficulty with any change in direction.	Parkinsonism.
Scissors 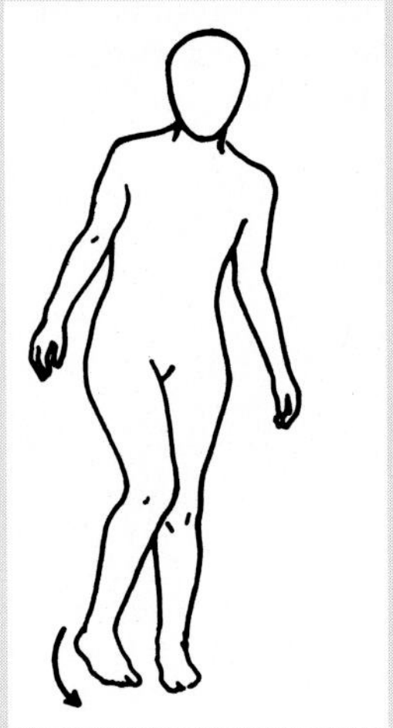	Knees cross or are in contact, like holding an orange between the thighs. The person uses short steps, and walking requires effort.	Paraparesis of legs, multiple sclerosis.

Table 20-6 ▸ Abnormal Gaits *Continued*

TYPE	CHARACTERISTIC APPEARANCE	POSSIBLE CAUSE
Steppage or footdrop 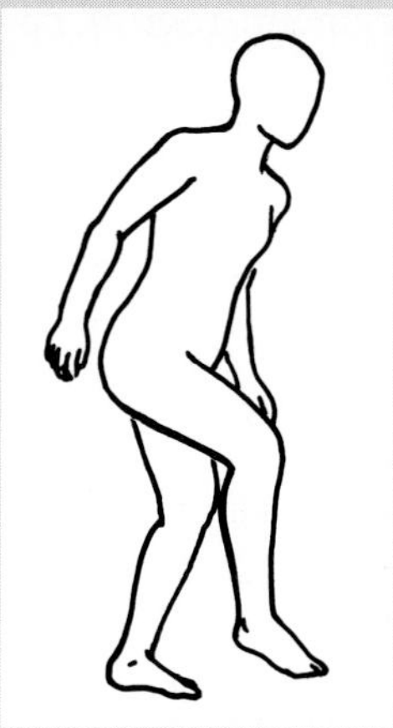	Slapping quality—looks as if walking up stairs and finds no stair there. Lifts knee and foot high and slaps it down hard and flat to compensate for footdrop.	Weakness of peroneal and anterior tibial muscles; due to lower motor neuron lesion at the spinal cord, e.g., poliomyelitis, Charcot-Marie-Tooth disease.
Waddling 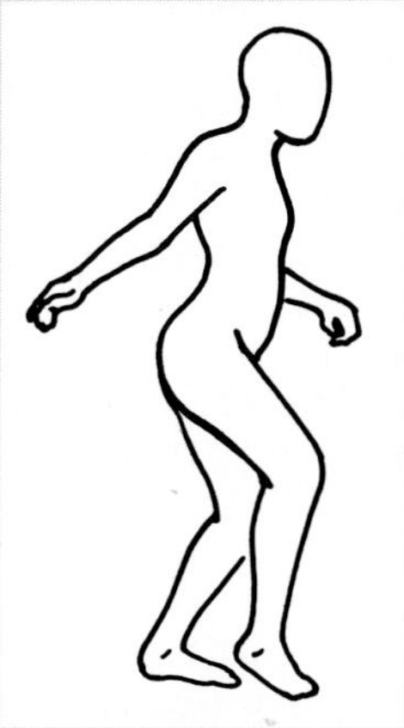	Weak hip muscles—when the person takes a step, the opposite hip drops, which allows compensatory lateral movement of pelvis. Often, the person also has marked lumbar lordosis and a protruding abdomen.	Hip girdle muscle weakness due to muscular dystrophy, dislocation of hips.
Short leg 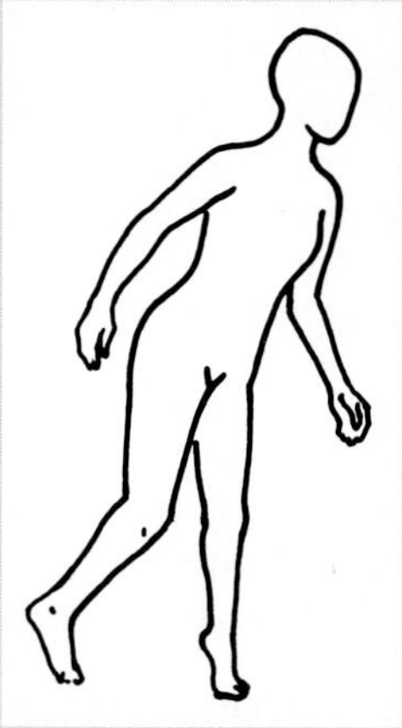	Leg length discrepancy > 2.5 cm (1 inch). Vertical telescoping of affected side, which dips as the person walks. Appearance of gait varies depending on amount of accompanying muscle dysfunction.	Congenital dislocated hip; acquired shortening due to disease, trauma.

Table 20-7 ▸ Characteristics of Upper and Lower Motor Neuron Lesions

	UPPER MOTOR NEURON LESION	LOWER MOTOR NEURON LESION
Weakness/paralysis	In muscles corresponding to distribution of damage in pyramidal tract lesion; usually in hand grip, arm extensors, leg flexors	In specific muscles served by damaged spinal segment, root or peripheral nerve
Example	Cerebrovascular accident	Poliomyelitis
Muscle tone	Increased; spasticity	Loss of tone, flaccidity
Bulk	May have some atrophy from disuse; otherwise normal	Atrophy (wasting)
Abnormal movements	None	Fasciculations
Reflexes	Hyperreflexia, ankle clonus; positive Babinski's sign	Hyporeflexia or areflexia; negative Babinski's sign
Possible nursing diagnoses	Potential for contractures; impaired physical mobility	Impaired physical mobility

Table 20-8 ▸ Common Patterns of Motor System Dysfunction

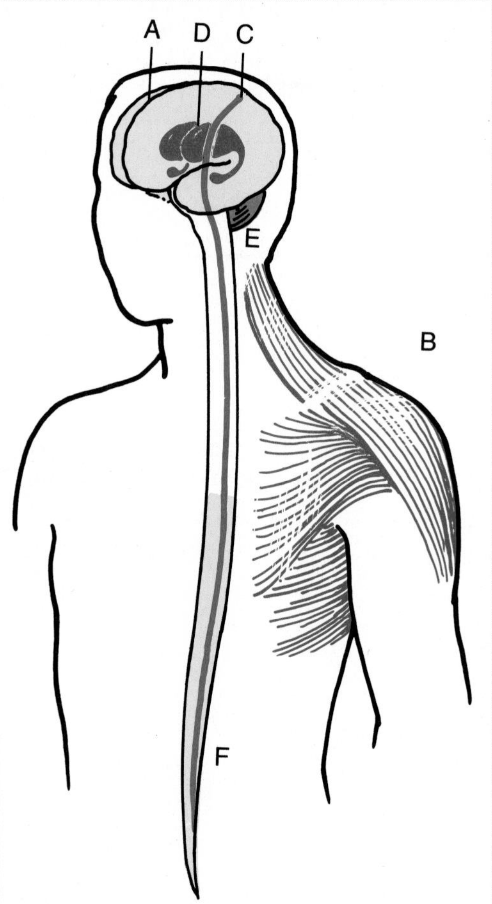

A Cerebral palsy Mixed group of paralytic neuromotor disorders of infancy and childhood; due to brain lesions caused by a developmental defect, intrauterine meningitis or encephalitis, birth trauma, anoxia, or kernicterus.

B Muscular dystrophy Chronic, progressive wasting of skeletal musculature, which produces weakness, contractures, and in severe cases, respiratory dysfunction and death. Onset of symptoms occurs in childhood. There are many types; the most severe is Duchenne's dystrophy, characterized by the waddling gait described on p. 789.

C Hemiplegia Damage to corticospinal tract. Initially flaccid when the lesion is acute; later, the muscles become spastic, and abnormal reflexes appear. Characteristic posture: arm — shoulder adducted, elbow flexed, wrist pronated; leg extended; face — weakness only in lower muscles. Hyperreflexia and possible clonus occur on the involved side; loss of corneal, abdominal, and cremasteric reflexes; positive Babinski's and Hoffman's reflexes.

D Parkinsonism Defect of extrapyramidal tract, especially in the region of the basal ganglia. Body tends to stay immobile; facial expression is flat, staring, expressionless; excessive salivation occurs; reduced eye blinking. Posture is stooped; equilibrium is impaired; loses balance easily; gait is described on p. 788. Parkinsonian tremor; cogwheel rigidity on passive range of motion.

E Cerebellar A lesion in one hemisphere produces motor abnormalities on the ipsilateral side. Characterized by ataxia, lurching forward of affected side while walking, rapid alternating movements are slow and arrhythmic, finger-to-nose test reveals ataxia and tremor, and eyes display coarse nystagmus.

F Paraplegia Caused by spinal cord injury. A severe injury or complete transection initially produces "spinal shock," which is defined as no movement or reflex activity below the level of the lesion. Gradually, DTRs reappear and become increased, flexor spasms of legs occur, and finally, extensor spasms of legs occur, which leads to prevailing extensor tone.

Table 20–9 ▶ Common Patterns of Sensory Loss

TYPE	CHARACTERISTICS	POSSIBLE CAUSES
Peripheral neuropathy 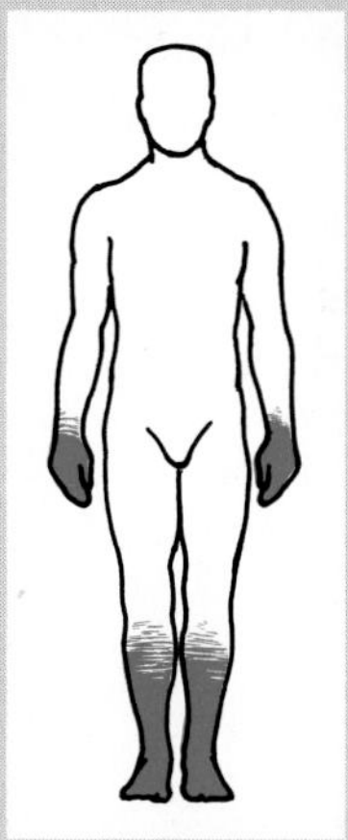	Loss of sensation involves all modalities. Loss is most severe distally (feet and hands), response improves as stimulus is moved proximally (glove-and-stocking anesthesia). Anesthesia zone gradually merges into a hypesthesia zone, then gradually becomes normal.	Metabolic disease, nutritional deficiency
Individual nerves or roots 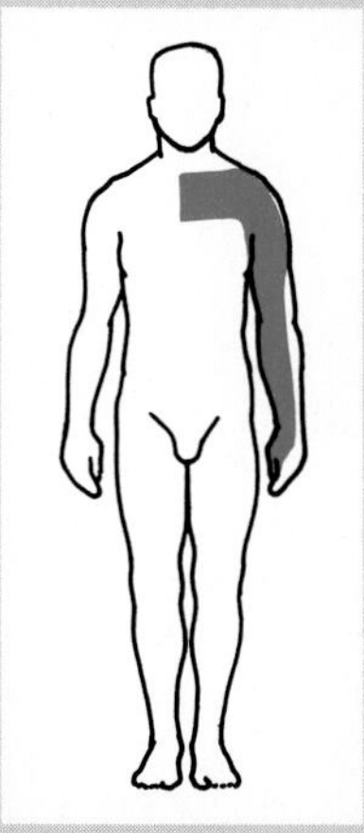	Decrease or loss of all sensory modalities. Area of sensory loss corresponds to distribution of the involved nerve.	Trauma, vascular occlusion
Spinal cord hemisection (Brown-Séquard syndrome) 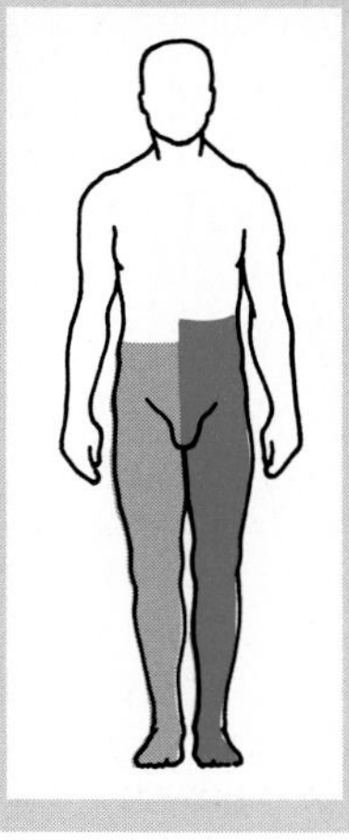	Loss of pain and temperature, contralateral side, starting 1 to 2 segments below the level of the lesion. Loss of vibration and position discrimination on the ipsilateral side, below the level of the lesion.	Meningioma, neurofibroma, cervical spondylosis, multiple sclerosis

Table continued on following page

Table 20-9 ▶ Common Patterns of Sensory Loss *Continued*

TYPE	CHARACTERISTICS	POSSIBLE CAUSES
Complete transection of the spinal cord 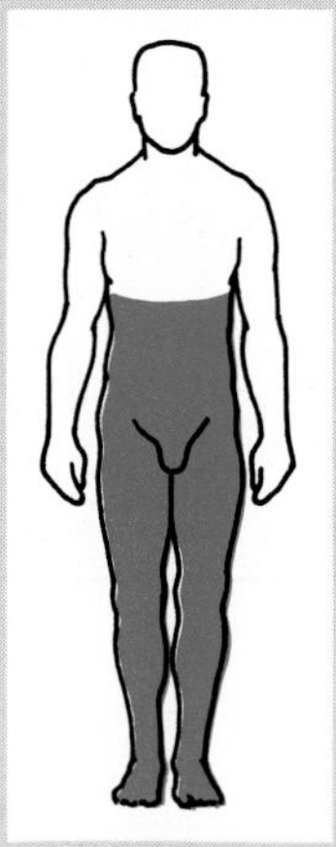	Complete loss of all sensory modalities below the level of the lesion. Condition is associated with motor paralysis and loss of sphincter control.	Trauma, demyelinating disorders, tumor
Thalamus 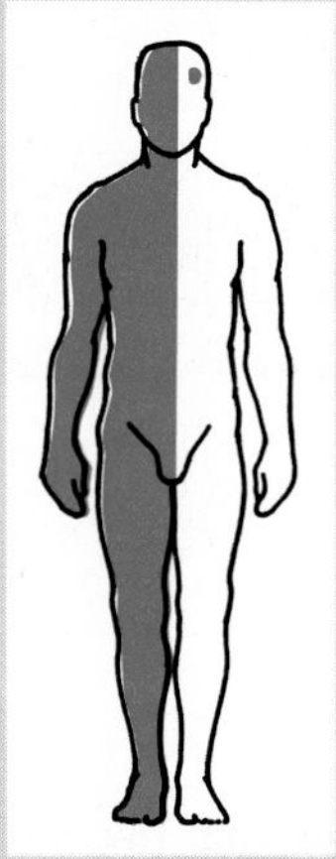	Loss of all sensory modalities on the face, arm, and leg on the side contralateral to the lesion.	Vascular occlusion
Cortex 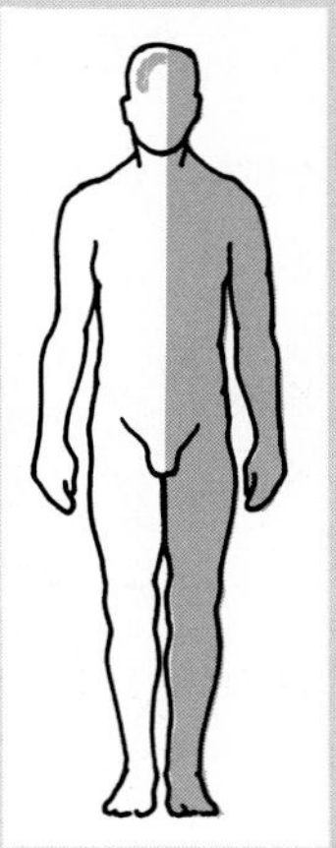	Since pain, vibration, and crude touch are mediated by thalamus, there is little loss of these sensory functions with a cortex lesion. There is loss of discrimination on the contralateral side. Loss of graphesthesia, stereognosis, recognition of shapes and weights, finger finding.	Parietal lobe lesion

Table 20-10 ► Abnormal Postures

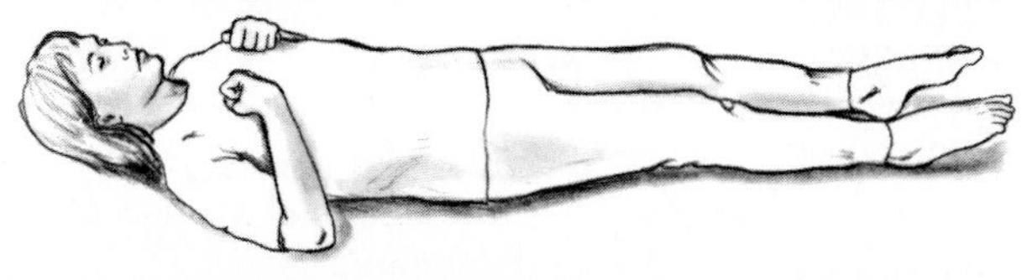

DECORTICATE RIGIDITY

Upper extremities—flexion of arm, wrist, and fingers; adduction of arm. Lower extremities—extension, internal rotation, plantar flexion. This indicates hemispheric lesion of cerebral cortex.

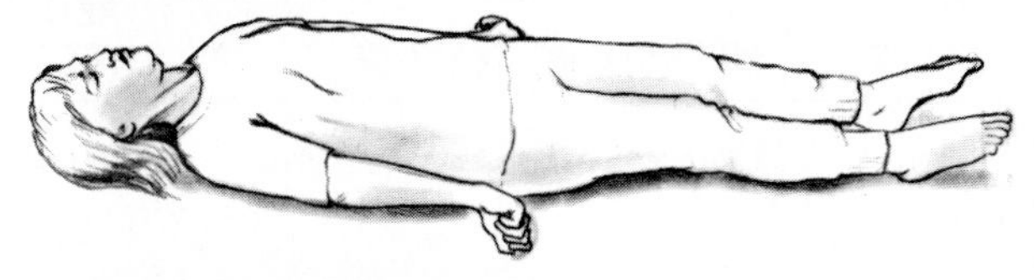

DECEREBRATE RIGIDITY

Upper extremities stiffly extended, adducted, internal rotation, palms pronated. Lower extremities stiffly extended, plantar flexion; teeth clenched. More ominous than decorticate rigidity; indicates lesion in brain stem at midbrain or upper pons.

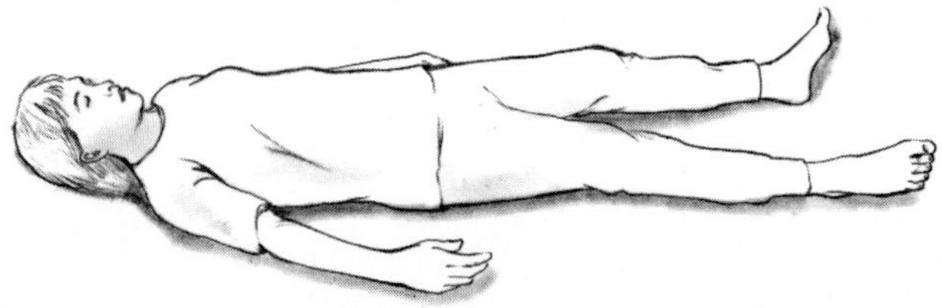

FLACCID QUADRIPLEGIA

Complete loss of muscle tone, indicating completely nonfunctional brain stem.

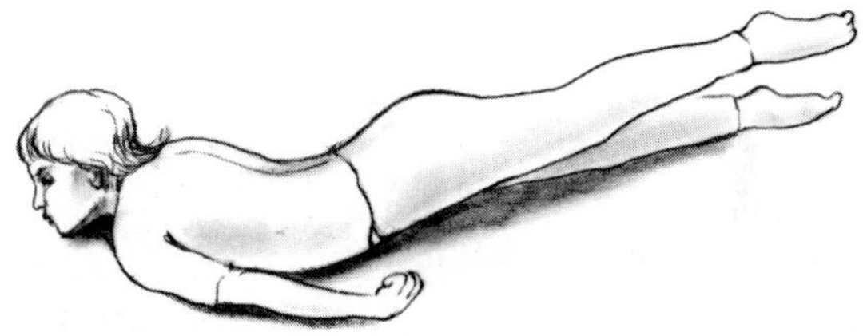

OPISTHOTONOS

Prolonged arching of the back, with head and heels bent backward. This indicates meningeal irritation.

Table 20-11 ► Pathologic Reflexes

REFLEX	METHOD OF TESTING	ABNORMAL RESPONSE (REFLEX IS PRESENT)	INDICATIONS
Babinski	Stroke lateral aspect and across ball of foot	Extension of great toe, fanning of toes	Pyramidal tract disease
Oppenheim	Stroke anterior medial tibial muscle	Same as above	Same
Gordon	Firmly squeeze calf muscles	Same as above	Same
Hoffmann	Flick distal phalanx of middle or index finger	Clawing of fingers and thumb	Same
Kernig	Raise leg straight or flex thigh on abdomen and extend knee	Resistance to straightening, pain down posterior thigh	Meningeal irritation
Brudzinski	Flex chin on chest	Resistance and pain	Meningeal irritation

Table 20-12 ► Frontal Release Signs

REFLEX	METHOD OF TESTING	ABNORMAL RESPONSE (REFLEX IS PRESENT)	INDICATIONS
Snout 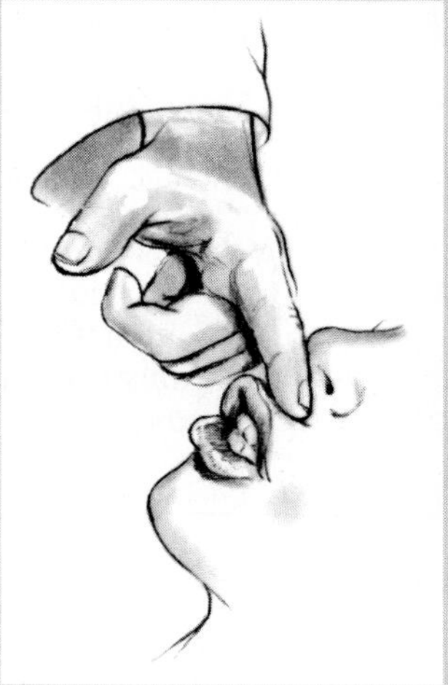	Gently percuss oral region	Puckers lips	Frontal lobe disease, cerebral degenerative disease (Alzheimer's)
Sucking 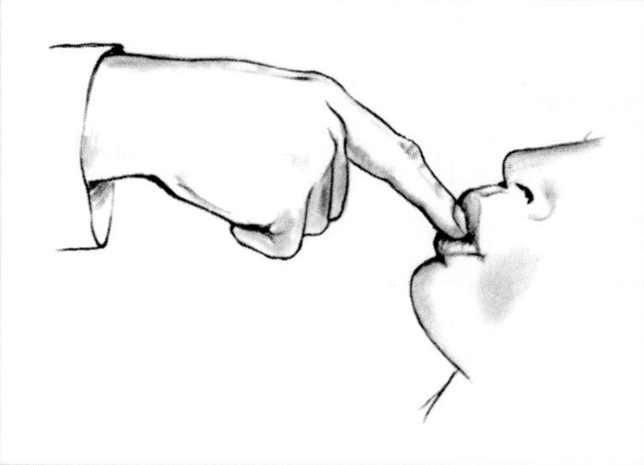	Touch oral region	Sucking movements of lips, tongue, jaw	Same
Grasp 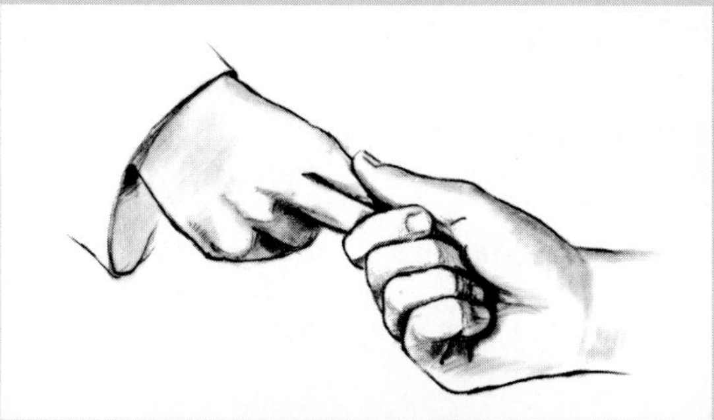	Touch palm with your finger (Grasp is usually last of these signs to appear, so its presence indicates severe disease)	Uncontrolled, forced grasping	Same

Bibliography

Barness LA: Manual of pediatric physical diagnosis. Chicago, Year Book Medical Publishers, 1981.

Barker PO, Lewis DA: The management of lead exposure in pediatric populations. Nurs Pract 15(12):8–16, 1990.

Carter AB: The neurologic aspects of aging. *In* Rossman, I (Ed): Clinical Geriatrics. Philadelphia, JB Lippincott, 1986.

Chusid JG: Correlative neuroanatomy and functional neurology. Los Altos, CA, Lange Medical Publications, 1985.

Condi, JK: Types and causes of nystagmus in the neurosurgical patient. J Neurosurg Nurs 15(2):56–64, 1983.

Fenichel GM: Clinical Pediatric Neurology. Philadelphia, WB Saunders, 1988.

Hickey JV: Neurological and neurosurgical nursing. 2nd ed. Philadelphia, JB Lippincott, 1986.

Kallman H, Kay AD, Zuckerman JD: Gait evaluation in the elderly. Patient Care 24(11):129–144, 1990.

Knight RL: The Glasgow Coma Scale: Ten years after. Crit Care Nurse 6(3):65–71, 1986.

Konikow NS: Alterations in movement: Nursing assessment and implications. J Neurosurg Nurs 17(1):61–65, 1985.

Lehman LB: Preventing nervous system sports injuries. Nurs Pract 14(3):42–46, 1989.

Leibman M: Neuroanatomy made easy and understandable. 2nd ed. Rockville, MD, Aspen Systems Corporation, 1983.

Lord-Feroli K, Maguire-McGinty M: Toward a more objective approach to pupil assessment. J Neurosurg Nurs 17(5):309–312, 1985.

Mayo Clinic: Clinical examinations in neurology. Philadelphia, WB Saunders, 1981.

Miller J: The Body in Question. New York, Random House, 1978.

Ozuna J: Alterations in mentation: Nursing assessment and intervention. J Neurosurg Nurs, 17(1):66–70, 1985.

Rudy EB: Advanced Neurological and Neurosurgical Nursing. St. Louis, CV Mosby, 1984.

Rusinski PS: Neurological assessment of the hemiplegic patient. Nurse Pract 4:26–32, 1979.

Sphritz DW: Emergency neurologic assessment. Crit Care Nurse 5(5):66–68, 1985.

Snyder M: A Guide to Neurological and Neurosurgical Nursing. New York, John Wiley & Sons, 1983.

Storandt M: Psychological aspects of aging. *In* Rossman, I (Ed): Clinical Geriatrics. Philadelphia, JB Lippincott, 1986.

Teasdale G: Acute impairment of brain function. Nurs Times, 71:914–917, 1975.

Teasdale G, Jennett, B: Assessment of coma and impaired consciousness; A practical coma scale. Lancet 20:81–83, 1974.

Tedder JL: Using the Brazelton neonatal assessment scale to facilitate the parent-child relationship in a primary care setting. Nurs Pract 16(3):26–36, 1991.

Weisberg LA, Strub RL, Garcia CA: Essentials of Clinical Neurology. Baltimore: University Park Press, 1983.

Wyness MA: Perceptual dysfunction: Nursing assessment and management. J Neurosurg Nurs 17(2):105–110, 1985.

CHAPTER

21 Male Genitalia

STRUCTURE AND FUNCTION

The male genital structures include the penis and scrotum externally, and the testis, epididymis and vas deferens internally. Glandular structures accessory to the genital organs (the prostate, seminal vesicles and bulbourethral glands) are discussed in Chapter 23.

The penis is composed of three cylindrical columns of erectile tissue: the two corpora cavernosa on the dorsal side and the corpus spongiosum ventrally (Fig. 21 – 1). At the distal end of the shaft, the corpus spongiosum expands into a cone of erectile tissue, the *glans.* The shoulder where the glans joins the shaft is the *corona.* The urethra transverses the corpus spongiosum, and its meatus forms a slit at the glans tip. Over the glans, the skin folds in and back on itself forming a hood or flap. This is the *foreskin* or *prepuce.* Often, it is surgically removed shortly after birth by circumcision. The *frenulum* is a fold of the foreskin extending from the urethral meatus ventrally.

The scrotum is a loose sac, which is a continuation of the abdominal wall (Fig. 21 – 2). After adolescence, the scrotal skin is deeply pigmented and has large sebaceous follicles. The scrotal wall consists of thin skin lying in folds or *rugae* and the underlying cremaster muscle. The cremaster muscle controls the size of the scrotum by responding to ambient temperature. When it is cold, the muscle contracts raising the sac and bringing the testes closer to the body to absorb heat necessary for sperm viability. As a result, the scrotal skin looks corrugated.

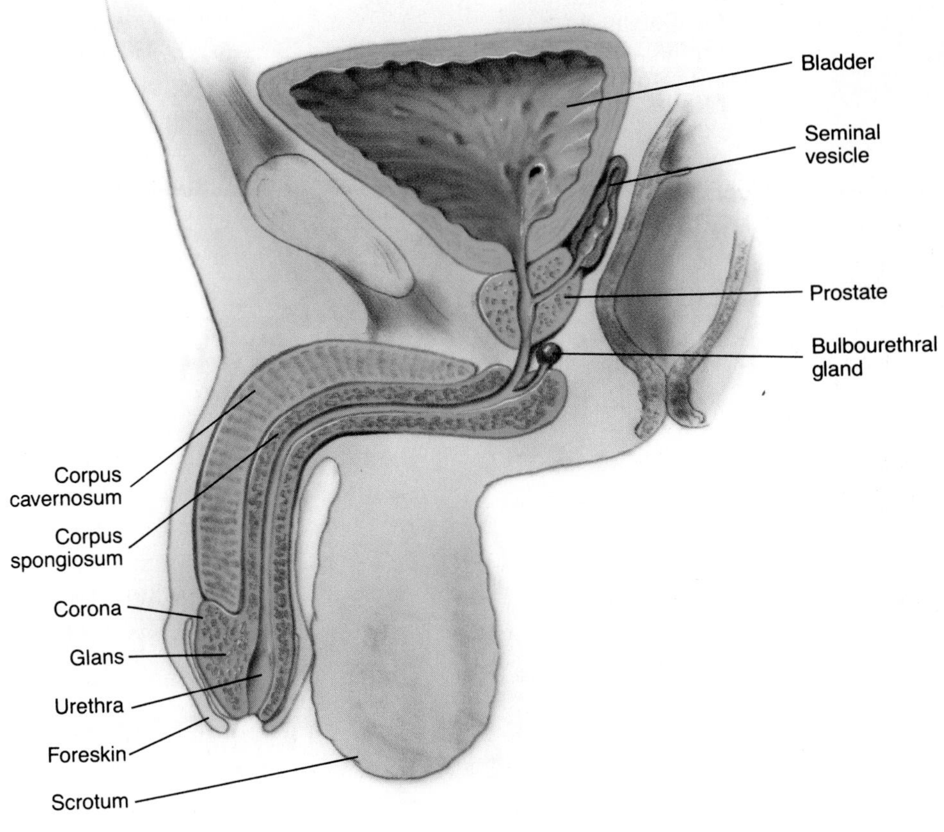

► **Figure 21 – 1**

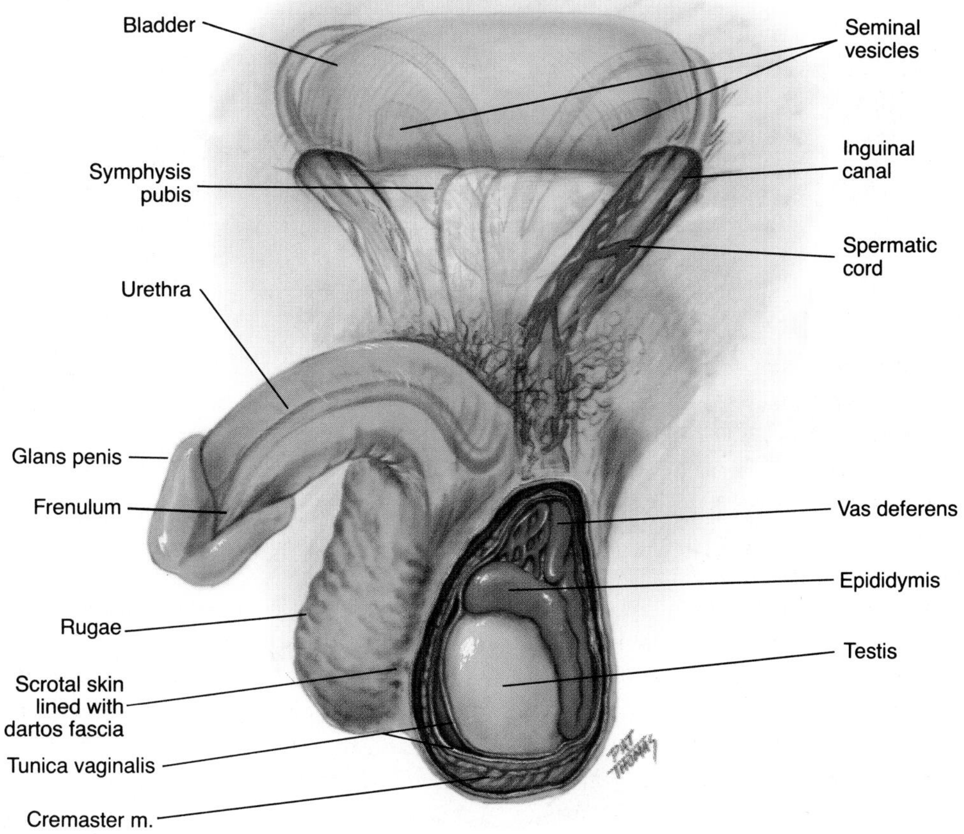

▶ Figure 21 – 2

When it is warmer, the muscle relaxes, the scrotum lowers, and the skin looks smoother.

Inside, a septum separates the sac into two halves. In each scrotal half is a testis, which produces sperm. The testis has a solid oval shape, which is compressed laterally and measures 4 to 5 cm long by 3 cm wide in the adult. The testis is suspended vertically by the spermatic cord. The left testis is lower than the right because the left spermatic cord is longer. Each testis is covered by a double-layered membrane, the tunica vaginalis, which separates it from the scrotal wall.

The testis is capped by the epididymis, which is a markedly coiled duct system. It is a comma-shaped structure, curved over the top and the posterior surface of the testis. Occasionally (in 6 to 7 percent of males), the epididymis is anterior to the testis.

The lower part of the epididymis is continuous with the vas deferens. This duct approximates with other vessels (arteries and veins, lymphatics, nerves) to form the *spermatic cord.* The spermatic cord ascends along the posterior border of the testis and runs through the inguinal canal into the abdomen. Here, the vas deferens continues back and down behind the bladder, where it joins the duct of the seminal vesicle to form the ejaculatory duct. This duct empties into the urethra.

The lymphatics of the penis and scrotal surface drain into the inguinal lymph nodes, whereas those of the testes drain into the abdomen.

The inguinal area, or groin, is the juncture of the lower abdominal wall and the thigh (Fig. 21 – 3). Its diagonal borders are the anterior superior iliac spine and the symphysis pubis. Between these landmarks lies the *inguinal ligament* (Poupart's ligament). Superior to the ligament lies the *inguinal canal,* a narrow tunnel passing obliquely between layers of abdominal muscle. It is 4 to 6 cm long in the adult. Its openings are an internal ring, located 1 to 2 cm above the midpoint of the inguinal ligament, and an external ring, located just above and lateral to the pubis.

Inferior to the inguinal ligament is the *femoral canal.* It is a potential space located 3 cm medial to and parallel with the femoral artery. You can use the artery as a landmark to find this space.

Knowledge of these anatomic areas in the groin is

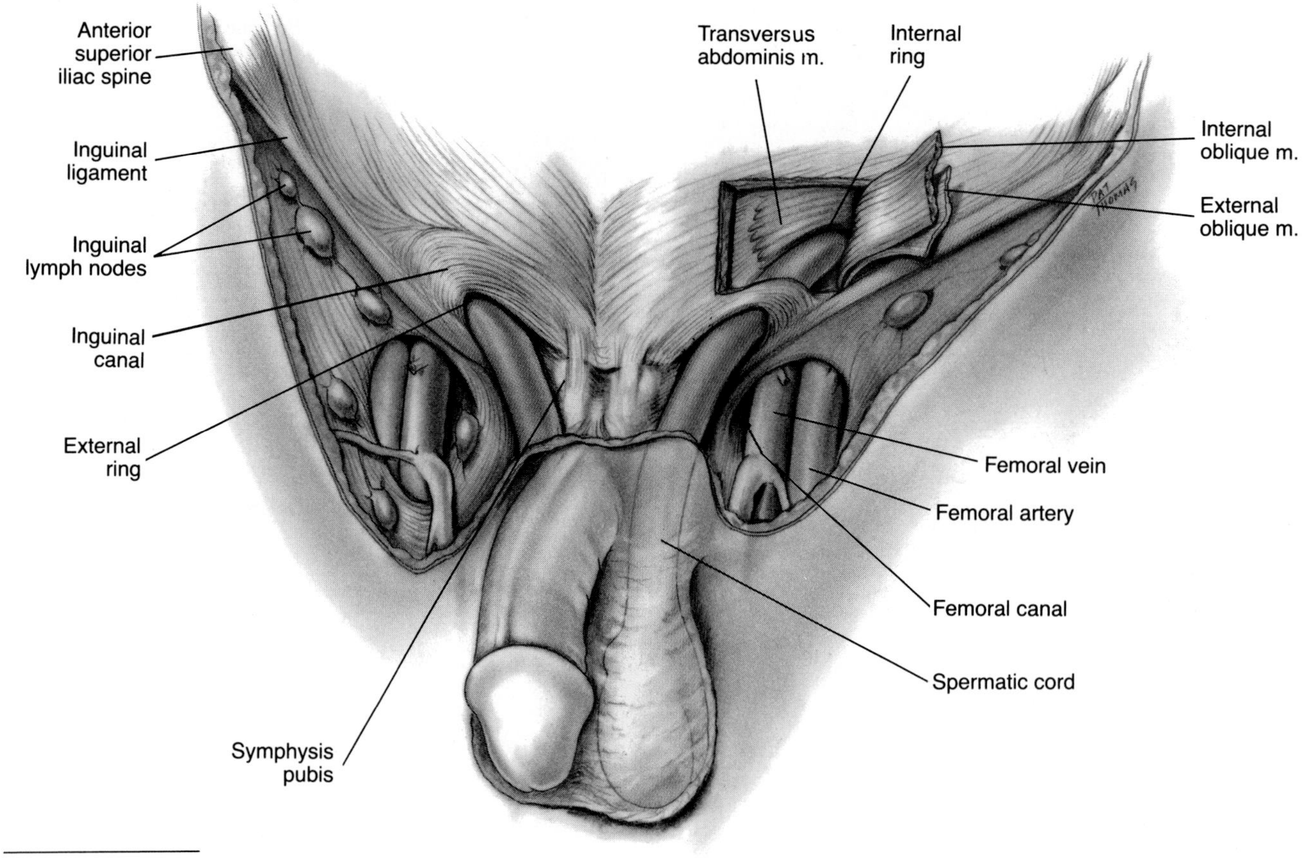

▶ **Figure 21-3**

useful because they are potential sites for a hernia, which is a loop of bowel protruding through a weak spot in the musculature.

DEVELOPMENTAL CONSIDERATIONS

Prenatally the testes develop in the abdominal cavity. They descend along the inguinal canal into the scrotum before birth. At birth, each testis measures 1.5 to 2 cm long and 1 cm wide. There is only a slight increase in size during the prepubertal years.

Puberty begins sometime between the ages of 9 1/2 and 13 1/2. The first sign is enlargement of the testes. Next, pubic hair appears, then penis size increases. The stages of development are documented in Tanner's sexual maturity ratings (SMR) (Table 21-1).

The complete change in development from a preadolescent to an adult takes around 3 years, although the normal range is 2 to 5 years (Fig. 21-4). The chart shown in Figure 21-4 is useful in teaching a boy the expected sequence of events, and in reasuring him about the wide range of normal ages when these events are experienced.

Although Tanner's studies were based on data from post World War II British youth, Tanner's results are corroborated by the U.S. Health Examination Survey, which studied close to 7000 youths from 1966 to 1970

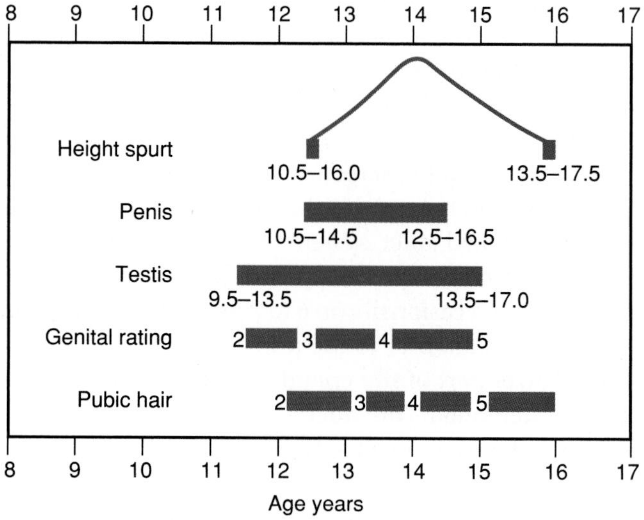

▶ **Figure 21-4**

Table 21-1 ► Sex Maturity Ratings (SMR) in Boys

DEVELOPMENTAL STAGE	PUBIC HAIR	PENIS	SCROTUM
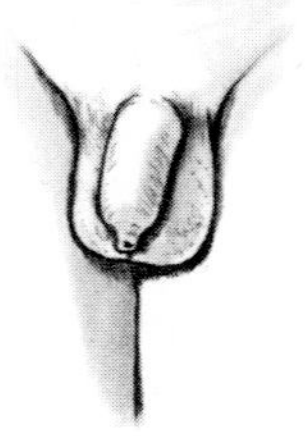	No pubic hair. Fine body hair on abdomen (vellus hair), continues over pubic area	Preadolescent, size and proportion the same as during childhood	Preadolescent, size and proportion the same as during childhood
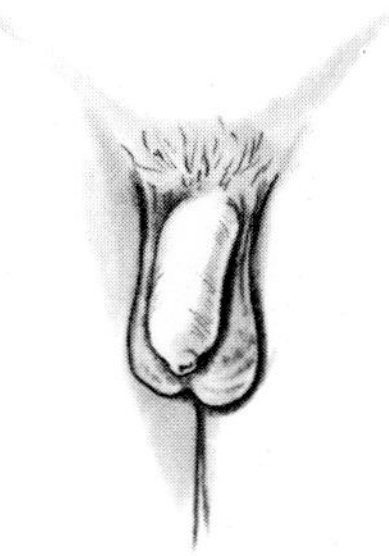	Few straight slightly darker hairs at base of penis. Hair is long and downy	Little or no enlargement	Testes and scrotum begin to enlarge. Scrotal skin reddens and changes in texture
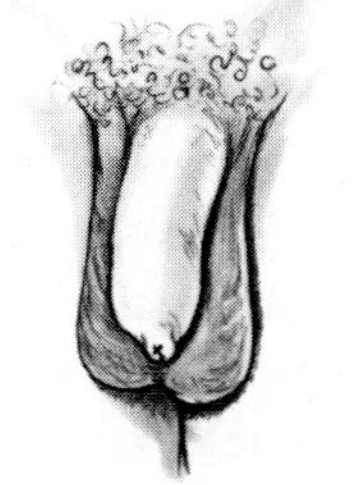	Sparse growth over entire pubis. Hair darker, coarser and curly	Penis begins to enlarge, especially in length	Further enlarged
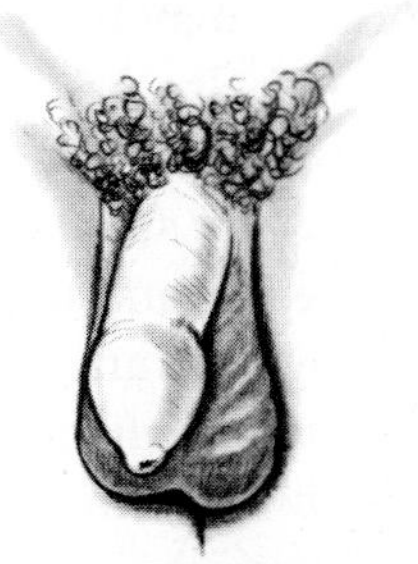	Thick growth over pubic area but not on thighs. Hair coarse and curly as in adult	Penis grows in length and diameter, with development of glans	Testes almost fully grown, scrotum darker
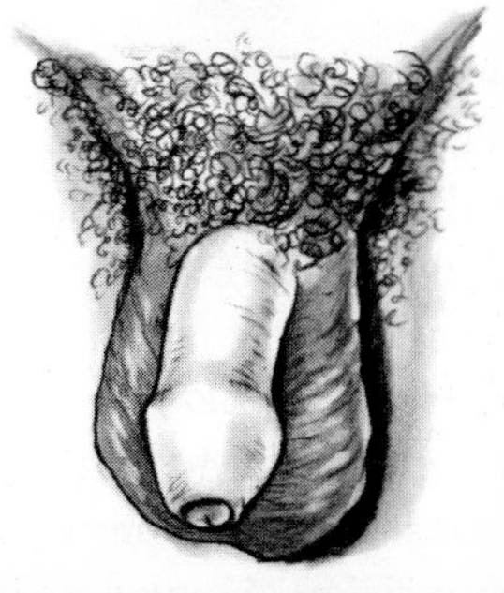	Growth spread over medial thighs, although not yet up toward umbilicus*	Adult size and shape	Adult size and shape

(Adapted from Tanner JM: Growth at Adolescence. Oxford, England, Blackwell Scientific, 1962.)
* After puberty, pubic hair growth continues until the mid-20s, extending up the abdomen toward the umbilicus.

(Harlan et al, 1979). This study found concordance between Tanner's stages for pubic hair and genitalia. It also found that sexual characteristics developed similarly for black and white boys, and that development was not influenced by socioeconomic status.

The level of sexual development at the end of puberty remains constant through young and middle adulthood, with no further genital growth and no change in circulating sex hormone.

The male does not experience a definite end to fertility as the female does. Around age 40 years, the production of sperm begins to decrease, although it continues into the 80s and 90s. After age 55 to 60 years, testosterone production declines (Masters et al, 1982). This decline proceeds very gradually so that resulting physical changes are not evident until later in life. Aging changes also are due to decreased muscle tone, decreased subcutaneous fat, and decreased cellular metabolism.

In the aging male, the amount of pubic hair decreases and the remaining hair turns gray. Penis size decreases. Due to decreased tone of the dartos muscle, the scrotal contents hang lower, the rugae decrease and the scrotum looks pendulous. The testes decrease in size and are less firm to palpation. There is increased connective tissue in the tubules, so these become thickened and produce less sperm.

In general, declining testosterone production leaves the older male with a slower and less intense sexual response. Although there is a wide range of individual differences, the older male may find that an erection takes longer to develop and that it is less full or firm. Once obtained, the erection may be maintained for longer periods without ejaculation. Ejaculation is shorter and less forceful, and the volume of seminal fluid is less than when the man was younger. After ejaculation, there is rapid detumescence (return to the flaccid state), especially after 60 years of age. This occurs in a few seconds as compared with minutes or hours in the younger male. The refractory state (when the male is physiologically unable to ejaculate) lasts longer, from 12 to 24 hours as compared with 2 minutes in the younger male.

Sexual Expression in Later Life. Chronologic age by itself should not mean a halt in sexual activity. The above-mentioned physical changes need not interfere with the libido and pleasure from sexual intercourse. The older male is capable of sexual function as long as he is in reasonably good health and has an interested willing partner. Even chronic illness does not mean a complete end to sexual desire or activity.

The danger is in the male misinterpreting normal age changes as a sexual failure. Once this idea occurs, it may demoralize the man and place undue emphasis on performance rather than pleasure. In the absence of disease, a withdrawal from sexual activity may be due to:

- Loss of spouse
- Depression
- Preoccupation with work
- Marital or family conflict
- Side effects of medications such as anti-hypertensives, psychotropics, anti-depressants, anti-spasmodics, sedatives, tranquilizers or narcotics, and estrogens
- Heavy use of alcohol
- Lack of privacy (living with adult children, or in a nursing home)
- Economic or emotional stress
- Poor nutrition
- Fatigue

TRANSCULTURAL CONSIDERATIONS

Occasionally, during pregnancy or the immediate neonatal period, parents will ask the health professional about whether or not to circumcise the male infant. There are no medical indications for routine male circumcision (Behrman and Vaughan, 1987). Some may believe that circumcision enhances hygiene and helps prevent disease later in life, but there is no scientific basis for this belief. Indeed, circumcision carries a very small but possible risk of complications, such as sepsis, amputation of the distal edge of the glans, removal of an excessive amount of foreskin, and urethrocutaneous fistula about which the parents should know (Behrman and Vaughan, 1987).

The decision to circumcise is culturally based (Harris, 1986). In the United States, 80 to 90 percent of newborn males are circumcised, a rate that is much higher than in countries such as Canada, England, and Sweden, where circumcision is considered unnecessary (Wirth, 1980). Some groups practice circumcision as part of their religious value system, such as Jews and Muslims. Other groups such as Native Americans and Hispanics have no tradition to practice circumcision. However, many parents in the United States who are not part of these groups also believe in circumcision because it conforms to dominant American cultural values.

SUBJECTIVE DATA

Frequency, urgency, and nocturia	Penis—pain, lesion, discharge
Dysuria	Scrotum—pain, lumps
Hesitancy and straining	Self-care behaviors
Urine color (cloudy or hematuria)	Sexual relationship
Past genitourinary history	Sexually transmitted disease (STD) contact

EXAMINER ASKS:	RATIONALE:
1. Are you urinating more often than usual now?	**Frequency.** Average adult voids 5 to 6 times per day, varying with fluid intake, individual habits. Polyuria—excessive quantity. Oliguria—diminished quantity, <400 ml/24 hours.
Do you ever feel as if you cannot wait to urinate?	**Urgency.**
Do you awaken during the night because you need to urinate? How often? Is this a recent change?	**Nocturia** occurs together with frequency and urgency in urinary tract disorders. Other origins: cardiovascular, habitual, diuretic medication.
2. Do you have any pain or burning with urinating?	**Dysuria.** Burning is common with acute cystitis, prostatitis, urethritis.
3. Do you have any trouble starting the urine stream?	**Hesitancy.**
Do you have to strain to start or maintain stream?	Straining.
Has there been any change in force of stream: narrowing, becoming weaker?	Loss of force and decreased caliber.
Do you experience dribbling, such that you must stand closer to the toilet?	Terminal dribbling.
Afterward, do you still feel you need to urinate?	Sense of residual urine.
Have you ever had any urinary tract infections?	Recurrent episodes of acute cystitis. Above-mentioned symptoms (i.e., hesitancy, and so on) suggest progressive prostatic obstruction (Smith, 1978).
4. Is the usual **urine** clear or discolored, cloudy, foul-smelling, bloody?	As in urinary tract infection. Hematuria—a danger sign that warrants further workup.
5. Do you have any difficulty controlling your urine?	True incontinence—loss of urine without warning. Urgency incontinence—sudden loss, as with acute cystitis.

EXAMINER ASKS:	RATIONALE:
Do you accidentally urinate when you sneeze, laugh, cough, or bear down?	Stress incontinence—loss of urine with physical strain due to weakness of sphincters.
6. Do you have any **history** of kidney disease, kidney stones, flank pain, urinary tract infections, prostate trouble?	
7. Do you have any problem with your penis—**pain, lesions?**	
Do you have any discharge? How much? Has that increased or decreased since start?	Urethral discharge.
What is the color? Is there any odor? Is the discharge associated with pain or with urination?	
8. Do you have any problem with the scrotum or testicles?	
Do you perform testicular self-examination?	**Self-care behaviors.**
Have you noticed any **lump or swelling** on testes?	
Have you noted any change in size of the scrotum?	
Have you noted any bulge or swelling in the scrotum? How long have you had it? Have you ever been told you have a hernia? Have you a dragging, heavy feeling in scrotum?	Possible hernia.
9. Are you in a relationship involving sexual intercourse now? Are aspects of sex satisfactory to you and your partner? Are you satisfied with the way you and your partner communicate about sex? Occasionally a man notices a change in erection when aroused. Have you noticed any changes?* Do you and your partner use a contraceptive? Which method? Is this satisfactory? Do you have any questions about this method? How many sexual partners have you had in the last 6 months?	Questions about **sexual activity** should be routine in review of body systems for these reasons: • communicates that you accept individual's sexual activity and believe it is important • your comfort with discussion prompts person's interest and possibly relief that topic has been introduced • establishes a data base for comparison with any future sexual activities • provides opportunity to screen sexual problems Your questions should be objective and matter-of-fact.
What is your sexual preference—relationship with a woman, a man, both?	Gay and lesbian people need to feel acceptance to discuss their health concerns.
10. Are you aware of any sexual contact with a partner having a **sexually transmitted disease,** such as gonorrhea, herpes, AIDS, chlamydia, venereal warts, syphilis? When was this contact? Did you get the disease? How was it treated? Were there any complications? Do you use condoms to prevent STD? Do you have any questions or concerns about any of these diseases?	

* At times, phrase your questions so that it is all right for the person to acknowledge a problem.

EXAMINER ASKS:	RATIONALE:

ADDITIONAL QUESTIONS FOR INFANTS AND CHILDREN

Does your child have any problem urinating? Does the urine stream look straight?

Does your child have any pain with urinating, crying, or holding the genitals? Has he ever had a urinary tract infection?

(If child older than 2 to 2 1/2 years of age) Has toilet training started? How is it progressing?

Does your child wet the bed at night? Is this a problem for child or for you (parents)? What have you done? How does the child feel about it?

Have you noticed any problem with child's penis or scrotum: sores, swelling, discoloration?

Have you been told if his testes are descended?

Has your child ever had a hernia or hydrocele? Have you ever noticed swelling in his scrotum during crying or coughing?

(Ask directly to preschooler or young school age) Has anyone ever touched your penis or in between your legs and you did not want them to?

Screen for sexual abuse.

Sometimes that happens to children. They should remember that they have not been bad. They should try to tell an adult about it.

ADDITIONAL QUESTIONS FOR PREADOLESCENTS AND ADOLESCENTS

Ask the questions for symptoms and signs of the genitourinary tract as described in the adult section.

Use the following questions regarding sexual growth and development and sexual behavior. First, note:

- Ask questions that seem appropriate for boy's age but be aware that norms vary widely. When you are in doubt, it is better to ask too many questions than to omit something. Children obtain information, often misinformation, from the media and from peers at surprisingly early ages. You may be sure your information will be more thoughtful and accurate.
- Ask direct, matter-of-fact questions. Avoid sounding judgmental.
- Start with a *permission statement,* "Often boys your age experience . . ." This conveys that it is normal and all right to think or feel a certain way.
- Try the *ubiquity approach,* "When did you . . ." rather than "Do you . . ." (Mitchell, 1980). This method is less threatening because it implies that the topic is normal and unexceptional.
- Do not be concerned if a boy will not discuss sexuality with you or respond to your offers for more information. He may not wish to let on he needs or wants more information. You do well to "open the door." The adolescent may come back at a future time.

Has your body changed physically during the last 2 years? What do you think about the changes?

Around age 12 to 13 years, but sometimes earlier, boys start to change and grow around the penis and scrotum. What changes have you noticed?

EXAMINER ASKS:	RATIONALE:
Most boys compare their body changes with those of other boys around them. Have you ever seen charts and pictures of normal growth patterns for boys? Let us go over these now.	
Who can you talk to about your body changes and about sex information? How do these talks go? Do you think you get enough information? What about sex education classes at school? How about your parents? Is there a favorite teacher, nurse, doctor, minister, or counselor whom you can talk to?	
Boys around age 12–13 years (SMR3) have a normal experience of fluid coming out of the penis at night, called nocturnal emissions, or "wet dreams." Have you had this?	An occasional boy confuses this with a sign of sexually transmitted disease, or feels guilty.
Teenage boys have other normal experiences and wonder if they are the only ones who ever had them, like having an erection at embarrassing times, having sexual fantasies, or masturbating. Also, a boy might have a thought about touching another boy's genitals and wonder if this thought means he might be homosexual. Would you like to talk about any of these things?	A boy may feel guilty about experiencing these things if not informed that they are normal.
Often boys your age have questions about sexual activity. What questions do you have? How about things like birth control, or STDs such as gonorrhea or herpes. Any questions about these?	Assess level of knowledge. Many boys will not admit they need more knowledge.
Are you dating? Someone steady? Have you had intercourse? Are you using birth control? What kind?	Avoid the term "having sex." It is ambiguous and teens can take it to mean anything from foreplay to intercourse.
What kind of birth control did you use the *last* time you had intercourse?	This particular question often reveals that the teen is not using any method of birth control.
Has a nurse or doctor ever taught you how to examine your own testicles to make sure they are healthy?	Assess knowledge of testicular self-examination.
Has anyone ever touched your genitals and you did not want them to? Another boy, or an adult, even a relative? Sometimes that happens to teenagers. They should remember it is not their fault. They should tell another adult about it.	

ADDITIONAL QUESTIONS FOR THE AGING ADULT

Ask the same questions as for the younger male adult, with the following special emphases.

EXAMINER ASKS:	RATIONALE:
Are you having any difficulty urinating? Do you have any hesitancy and straining? Have you noticed a weakened force of stream? Do you feel any dribbling? Or, any incomplete emptying?	Early symptoms of enlarging prostate may be tolerated or ignored. Later symptoms are more dramatic: hematuria, urinary tract infection.
Do you need to get up at night to urinate? What medications are you taking? What fluids do you drink in the evening?	Nocturia may be due to diuretic medication, habit, or fluid ingestion 3 hours before bedtime, especially coffee and alcohol, which have a specific diuretic effect. Also fluid retention from mild heart failure or varicose veins produces nocturia; recumbency at night mobilizes fluid.

EXAMINER ASKS:	RATIONALE:
A man in his 70s, 80s, or 90s may notice changes in his sexual relationship or in his sexual response and wonder if it is normal. For example, it is normal for an erection to develop slowly at this age. This is not a sign of impotence, but a man might wonder if it is.	Excluding physical illness, an older man is fully capable of sexual function. But some men assume normal changes mean that they are "old men" and voluntarily withdraw from sexual activity. The older person is not reluctant to discuss sexual activity, and most welcome the opportunity. Depressants to sexual desire and function: anti-hypertensives, sedatives, tranquilizers, estrogens, alcohol. Alcohol decreases the sexual response even more dramatically in the older person.

OBJECTIVE DATA

Equipment Needed:

Gloves — Wear gloves during every male genitalia examination.
Occasionally: glass slide for urethral specimen
flashlight

Preparation

Position the male standing with undershorts down and appropriate draping. The examiner should be sitting. Alternatively, the male may be supine for the first part of the examination and stand to check for a hernia.

It is normal for a male to feel apprehensive about having his genitalia examined, especially by a female examiner. Among adolescents, the younger the boy is, the greater the level of concern (Mitchell, 1980). But any male may have difficulty dissociating a necessary matter-of-fact step in the physical examination from the feeling this is an invasion of his privacy. His concerns are similar to those experienced by the female during the examination of the genitalia: modesty, fear of pain or negative judgment, or memory of previously uncomfortable examinations. Additionally, he may fear having an erection during the examination and that this would be misinterpreted by the examiner.

This normal apprehension becomes manifested in different behaviors. Many act resigned and embarrassed and avoid eye contact. An occasional man will laugh and make jokes to cover embarrassment. Also, a man may refuse examination by a female and insist on a male examiner.

Take time to consider these feelings, as well as to explore your own. It is normal for you to feel embarrassed and apprehensive, too. You may worry about your age, lack of clinical experience, causing pain, or even that your movements might "cause" an erection. Some examiners feel guilty when this occurs. You need to accept these feelings and work through them in order to examine the male in a professional way. Discussing these concerns in a group with other beginning examiners works best. Your demeanor is important. Your unresolved discomfort magnifies any discomfort the man may have.

Your demeanor should be *confident* and relaxed, unhurried yet business-like. Do not discuss genitourinary history or sexual practices while you are performing the examination. This may be perceived as judgmental. Use a firm deliberate touch, not a soft, stroking one. If an erection does occur, do *not* stop the examination or leave the room. This only focuses more attention on the erection and increases embarrassment. Reassure the male that this is only a normal physiologic response to touch, just as when the knee jerks when tapped with the reflex hammer, or the pupil constricts in response to bright light (Chard, 1976). Proceed with the rest of the examination.

METHOD OF EXAMINATION

NORMAL RANGE OF FINDINGS	ABNORMAL FINDINGS
PENIS	
Inspect and palpate the penis.	
The skin normally looks wrinkled, hairless, and without lesions. The dorsal vein may be apparent (Fig. 21–5).	Generalized swelling. Inflammation. Lesions: nodules, solitary ulcer (chancre), grouped vesicles or superficial ulcers, wartlike papules (see Table 21–2).
The glans looks smooth and without lesions. Ask the uncircumcised male to retract the foreskin, or you retract it. It should move easily. Some cheesy smegma may have collected under the foreskin. After inspection, slide the foreskin back to the original position.	Inflammation. Lesions on glans or corona. Phimosis—unable to retract the foreskin. Paraphimosis—unable to return foreskin to original position.
The urethral meatus is positioned just about centrally.	Hypospadias—ventral location of meatus. Epispadias—dorsal location of meatus (see Table 21–3).
At the base of the penis, pubic hair distribution is consistent with age. Hair is without pest inhabitants.	Pubic lice or nits. Excoriated skin usually accompanies.

NORMAL RANGE OF FINDINGS | **ABNORMAL FINDINGS**

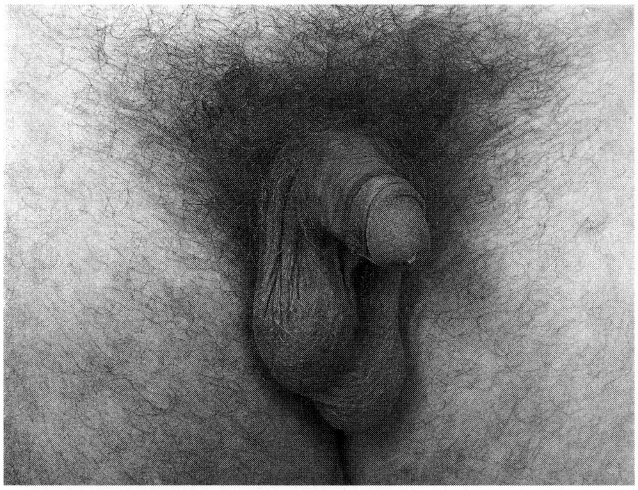

► **Figure 21–5**

Compress the glans anteroposteriorly between your thumb and forefinger (Fig. 21–6). The meatus edge should appear pink, smooth, and without discharge.

Stricture — narrowed opening.

Edges that are red, everted, edematous, along with purulent discharge, suggest urethritis (see Table 21–4).

If you note urethral discharge, collect a smear for microscopic examination and a culture. If no discharge shows but the person gives a history of it, ask him to milk the shaft of the penis. This should produce a drop of discharge.

Palpate the shaft of the penis between your thumb and first two fingers. Normally the penis feels smooth, semifirm, and nontender.

Nodule.
Induration.
Hard subcutaneous plaque.
Tenderness.

See discussion of stricture and Peyronie's disease, Table 21–4.

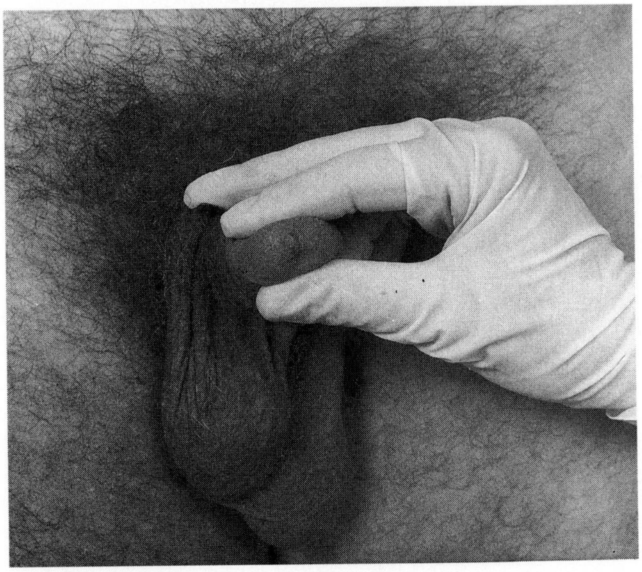

► **Figure 21–6**

NORMAL RANGE OF FINDINGS | **ABNORMAL FINDINGS**

SCROTUM

Inspect and palpate the scrotum.

Inspect the scrotum as male holds the penis out of the way. Alternatively, you hold the penis out of the way with the back of your hand (Fig. 21–7). Scrotal size varies with ambient room temperature. Asymmetry is normal, with the left scrotal half lower than the right.

Scrotal swelling (edema) may be taut and pitting. This occurs with congestive heart failure, renal failure, or local inflammation.

Lesions.

Inflammation.

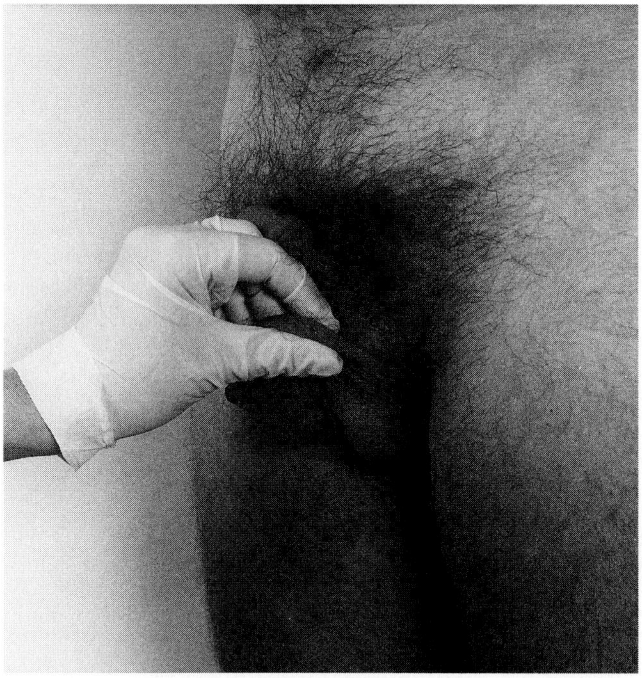

▶ **Figure 21–7**

Spread rugae out between your fingers. Lift the sac to inspect the posterior surface. Normally, there are no scrotal lesions, except for the commonly found sebaceous cysts. These are yellowish, 1-cm nodules and are firm, nontender and often multiple.

Palpate each scrotal half between your thumb and first two fingers (Fig. 21–8). The scrotal contents should slide easily. Testes normally feel oval, firm and rubbery, smooth, and equal bilaterally and are freely movable and slightly tender to moderate pressure. Each epididymis normally feels discrete, softer than the testis, smooth, and nontender.

Absent testis—may be a temporary migration or true cryptorchidism (see Table 21–5).

Atrophied testes—small and soft.

Fixed testes.

Nodules on testes or epididymides.

Marked tenderness.

An indurated, swollen, and tender epididymis indicates epididymitis.

NORMAL RANGE OF FINDINGS | **ABNORMAL FINDINGS**

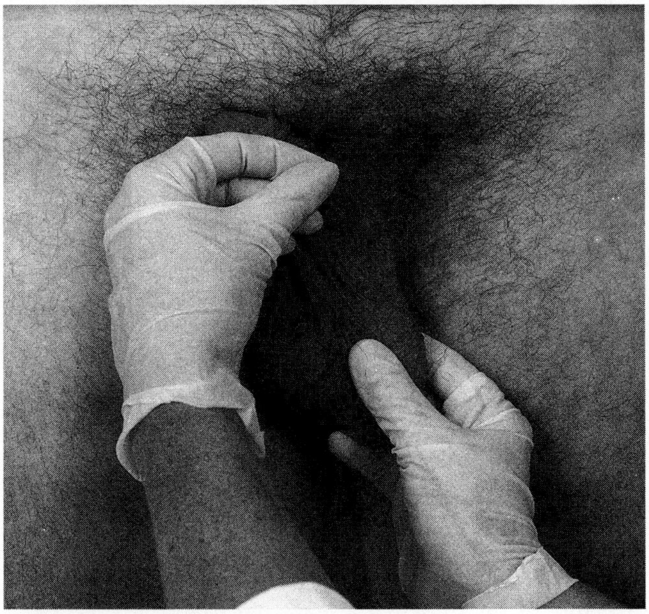

► **Figure 21-8**

Palpate each spermatic cord between your thumb and forefinger, along its length from the epididymis up to the external inguinal ring (Fig. 21-9). You should feel a smooth nontender cord.

Abnormal findings: Thickened.
Soft, swollen, and tortuous—see the discussion of varicocele, Table 21-5.

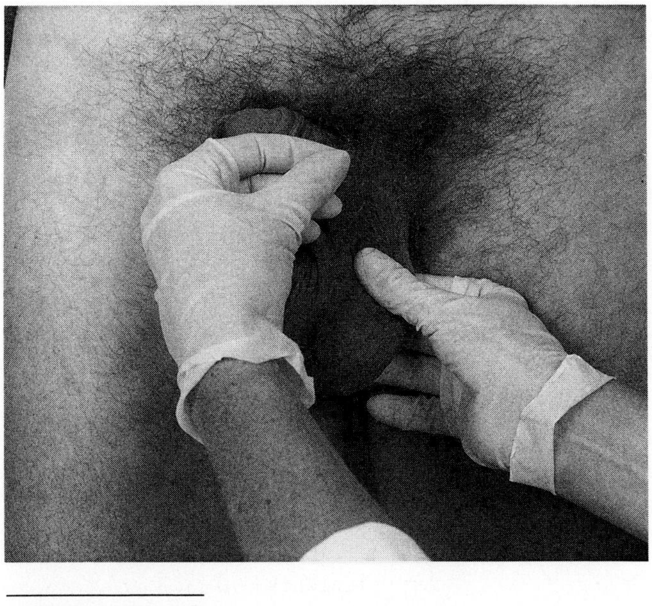

► **Figure 21-9**

NORMAL RANGE OF FINDINGS	ABNORMAL FINDINGS

Normally, there are no other scrotal contents. If you do find a mass, note:

- Is there any tenderness?
- Is the mass distal or proximal to testis?
- Can you place your fingers over it?
- Does it reduce when person lies down?
- Can you auscultate bowel sounds over it?

Abnormalities in the scrotum: hernia, tumor, orchitis, epididymitis, hydrocele, spermatocele, varicocele (see Table 21–5).

Transillumination. Perform this maneuver if you note a swelling or mass. Darken the room. Shine a strong flashlight from behind the scrotal contents. Normal scrotal contents do not transilluminate.

Serous fluid does transilluminate and shows as a red glow, e.g., hydrocele, or spermatocele. Solid tissue and blood do not transilluminate, e.g., hernia, epididymitis, or tumor (see Table 21–5).

HERNIA

Inspect and palpate for hernia.

Inspect the inguinal region for a bulge as the person stands and as he strains down. Normally there is none.

Bulge at external inguinal ring, or femoral canal. (A hernia may be present but easily reduced and appear only intermittently with an increase in intra-abdominal pressure.)

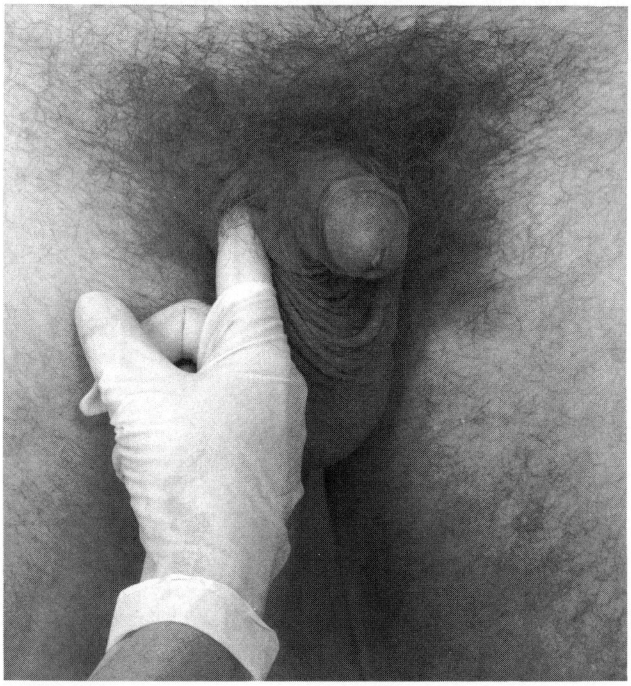

► **Figure 21–10**

NORMAL RANGE OF FINDINGS | **ABNORMAL FINDINGS**

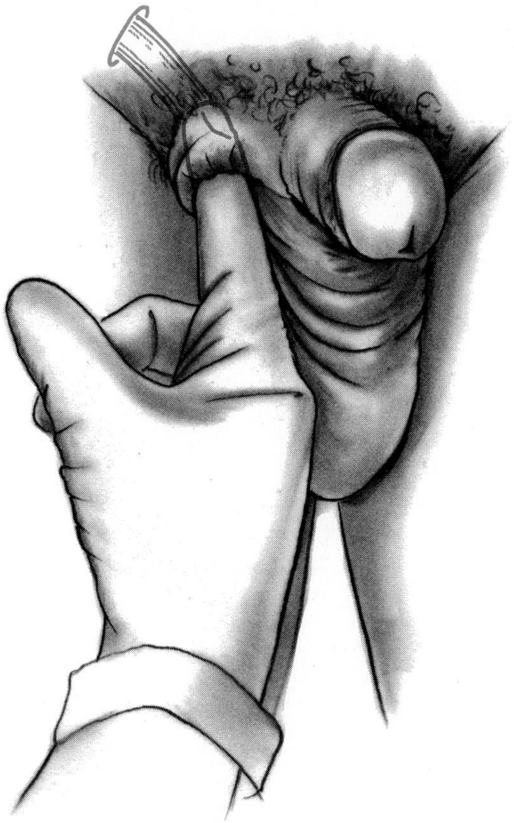

▶ **Figure 21-11**

Palpate the inguinal canal (Figs. 21-10 and 21-11). For the right side, ask the male to shift his weight onto the left (unexamined) leg. Place your right index finger low on the right scrotal half. Palpate up the length of the spermatic cord, invaginating the scrotal skin as you go, to the external inguinal ring. It feels like a triangular slitlike opening, and it may or may not admit your finger. If it will admit your finger, gently insert it into the canal and ask the person to bear down. Normally you feel no change. Repeat the procedure on the left side.

Abnormal: Palpable herniating mass bumps your fingertip or pushes against the side of your finger (see Table 21-6).

Palpate the femoral area for a bulge. Normally you feel none.

INGUINAL LYMPH NODES

Palpate the horizontal chain along the groin inferior to the inguinal ligament, and the vertical chain along the upper inner thigh.

NORMAL RANGE OF FINDINGS | **ABNORMAL FINDINGS**

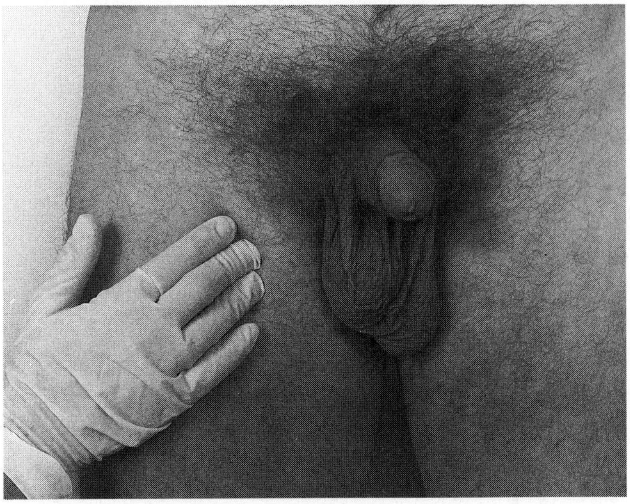

► **Figure 21 - 12**

It is normal to palpate an isolated node on occasion; it then feels small (<1 cm), soft, discrete, and movable (Fig. 21 - 12).

Enlarged, hard, matted, fixed nodes.

SELF-CARE—TESTICULAR SELF-EXAMINATION (TSE)

Encourage self-care behaviors by instructing each male (from adolescence to adulthood) how to examine his own testicles every month. The incidence of testicular cancer is not high, but such a tumor has no early symptoms. If detected early by palpation and treated, the prognosis is much improved. Early detection is enhanced if the person is familiar with his normal consistency. Phrase your teaching something like this:

A good time to examine the testicles is during the shower or bath, when your hands and scrotum are warm. Cold hands stimulate a muscle (cremasteric) reflex, retracting the scrotal contents. The procedure is simple. Hold the scrotum in the palm of your hand, and gently feel each testicle using your thumb and first two fingers. If it hurts, you are using too much pressure. The testicle is egg-shaped and movable. It feels rubbery with a smooth surface. The epididymis is on top and behind the testicle; it feels a bit softer. If you ever notice a firm painless lump, a hard area, or an overall enlarged testicle, call your physician for a further check.

DEVELOPMENTAL CONSIDERATIONS

Infants and Children

For an infant or toddler, perform this procedure right after the abdominal examination. In a preschool to young school-aged child (3 to 8 years of age), leave underpants on until just before the examination. Reassure parents of normal findings. In an older school-aged child or adolescent, offer an extra drape, as with the adult. Reassure child and parents of normal findings.

NORMAL RANGE OF FINDINGS

Inspect the penis and scrotum. Penis size is usually small in infants (2 to 3 cm) (Fig. 21 – 13) and in young boys until puberty. In the obese boy, the penis looks even smaller because of folds of skin covering the base.

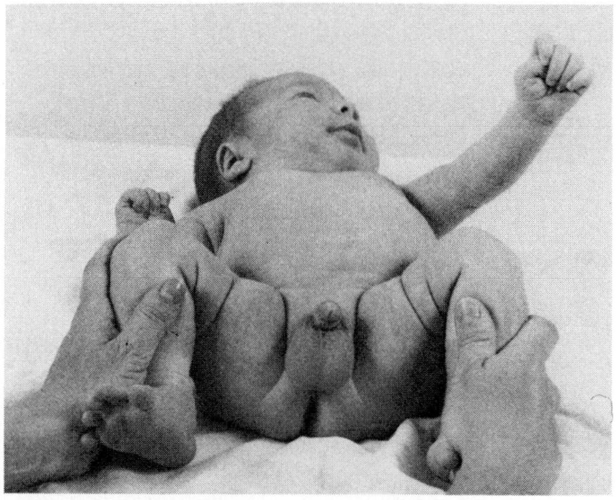

▸ **Figure 21 – 13**

In the circumcised infant, the glans looks smooth with the meatus centered at the tip. While the child wears diapers, the meatus may become ulcerated from ammonia irritation. This is more common in circumcised infants.

If possible, observe the newborn's first voiding to assess strength and direction of stream.

If uncircumcised, the foreskin is normally tight during the first 3 months, and should not be retracted because of the risk of tearing the membrane attaching the foreskin to the shaft. This leads to scarring and, possibly, to adhesions later in life. In infants older than 3 months of age, retract the foreskin gently to check the glans and meatus. It should return to its original position easily.

The scrotum looks pink in white infants and dark brown in dark-skinned infants. Rugae are well formed in the full-term infant. Size varies with ambient temperature, but overall, the infant's scrotum looks large in relation to the penis. There are no bulges, either constant or intermittent.

ABNORMAL FINDINGS

Rarely, a very small penis may be an enlarged clitoris in a genetically female infant.

Enlarged penis — precocious puberty.

Redness, swelling, lesions.

Redness, swelling, lesions.

Hypospadias, epispadias (see Table 21 – 3).

Stricture — narrowed opening.

Discharge.

Occasionally, ulceration may produce a stricture, shown by a pinpoint meatus and a narrow stream. This increases the risk of urine obstruction.

Poor stream is significant, because it may indicate a stricture or neurogenic bladder.

Phimosis — unable to retract the foreskin.

Paraphimosis — the foreskin cannot be slipped forward once it is retracted.

Pinpoint meatus.

Dirt and smegma collecting under foreskin.

NORMAL RANGE OF FINDINGS

Palpate the scrotum and testes. The cremasteric reflex is strong in the infant, pulling the testes up into the inguinal canal and abdomen from exposure to cold, touch, exercise, or emotion. Take care not to elicit the reflex. (1) Keep your hands warm and palpate from the external inguinal ring down. (2) Block the inguinal canals with the thumb and forefinger of your other hand to prevent the testes from retracting (Fig. 21–14).

Normally the testes are descended and are equal in size bilaterally (1.5 to 2 cm until puberty). It is important to document that you have palpated the testes. Once palpated they are considered descended, even if they have retracted momentarily at the next visit.

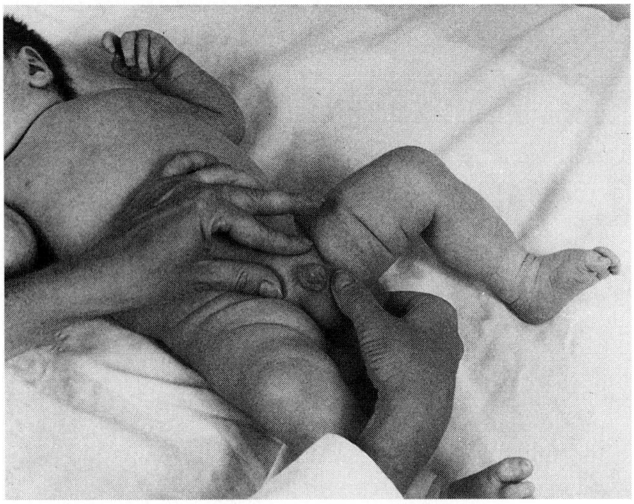

▶ Figure 21–14

If the scrotal half feels empty, search for the testes along the inguinal canal and try to milk them down. Ask the toddler or child to squat with the knees flexed up; this pressure may force the testes down. Or, have the young child sit cross-legged to relax the reflex (Fig. 21–15).

Migratory testes (physiologic cryptorchidism) are common because of the strength of the cremasteric reflex and the small mass of the prepubertal testes. Note that the affected side has a normally developed scrotum (with true cryptorchidism, the scrotum is atrophic) and that the testis can be milked down. These testes descend at puberty and are normal.

Palpate the epididymis and spermatic cord as described in the adult section. A common scrotal finding in the boy under 2 years of age is a *hydrocele*, or fluid in the scrotum. It appears as a large scrotum and transilluminates as a faint pink glow. It usually disappears spontaneously.

Inspect the inguinal area for a bulge. If you do not see a bulge but the parent gives a positive history of one, try to elicit it by increasing intra-abdominal pressure. Ask the boy to hold his breath and strain down, or have him blow up a balloon.

If a hernia is suspected, palpate the inguinal area. Use your little finger to reach the external inguinal ring.

ABNORMAL FINDINGS

Cryptorchidism — undescended testes (those that have never descended). Undescended testes are common in premature infants. They occur in 3 to 4 percent of term infants, although most have descended by 3 months of age. Age at which child should be referred differs among physicians (see Table 21–5).

(See Table 21–5.)

NORMAL RANGE OF FINDINGS | **ABNORMAL FINDINGS**

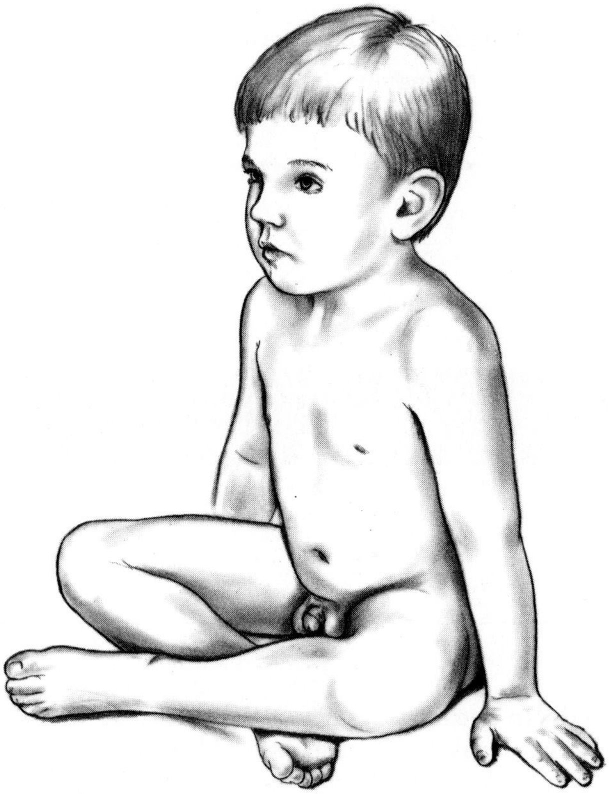

▶ **Figure 21 – 15**

The Adolescent

The adolescent shows a wide variation in normal development of the genitals. Using the SMR charts, note:

1. Enlargement of the testes and scrotum
2. Pubic hair growth
3. Darkening of scrotal color
4. Roughening of scrotal skin
5. Increase in penis length and width
6. Axillary hair growth

Be familiar with the normal sequence of growth.

The Aging Adult

In the older male, you may note thinner, graying pubic hair and the decreased size of the penis. The size of the testes may be decreased and feel less firm. The scrotal sac is pendulous with less rugae. The scrotal skin may become excoriated if the man continually sits on it.

☑ SUMMARY CHECKLIST

1 ▶ Inspect and palpate the penis.

2 ▶ Inspect and palpate the scrotum.

3 ▶ If a mass exists, transilluminate it.

4 ▶ Palpate for an inguinal hernia.

5 ▶ Palpate the inguinal lymph nodes.

SAMPLE RECORDING

Subjective

▶ Urinates 4 to 5 times/day, clear, straw-colored. No nocturia, dysuria or hesitancy. No pain, lesions, or discharge from penis. Does not do testicular self-examination. No history of genitourinary disease. Sexually active in a monogamous relationship. Sexual life satisfactory to self and partner. Uses birth control via barrier method (partner uses diaphragm). No known STD contact.

Objective

▶ No lesions, inflammation or discharge from penis. Scrotum — testes descended, symmetric, no masses. No inguinal hernia.

SAMPLE CLINICAL PROBLEM

Subjective

▶ R.C. is a 19-year-old student who 2 days PTA noted acute onset of painful urination, frequency, and urgency. Noted some thick penile discharge. States has no side pain, no abdominal pain, no fever, or genital skin rash. R.C. is concerned he has an STD because of episode of unprotected intercourse with a new partner 6 days PTA. Has no known allergies.

Objective

- Vital signs 37°C-72-16. No lesions or inflammation around penis or scrotum. Urethral meatus has mild edema with purulent urethral discharge. No pain on palpation of genitalia. Testes symmetric with no masses. No lymphadenopathy.

Assessment

- Urethral discharge
  Knowledge deficit about STD prevention R/T lack of information recall

NURSING DIAGNOSES COMMONLY ASSOCIATED WITH THE MALE GENITALIA AND RELATED DISORDERS

Diagnosis	Related Factors (Etiology)	Defining Characteristics (Symptoms and Signs)
Altered sexuality patterns	Effects of illness or medical treatment Drugs Radiation Anomalies Extreme fatigue Obesity Pain Performance anxiety Knowledge/skill deficit about alternative responses to health-related transitions Pregnancy Surgery Recent childbirth Trauma Menopause Impaired relationship with a significant other Fear of pregnancy or of acquiring a sexually transmitted disease Conflicts with sexual orientation or variant preferences Ineffective or absent role models Loss of job or ability to work Separation from or loss of significant other	Identification of sexual difficulties, limitations, or changes

Table continued on following page

Diagnosis	Related Factors (Etiology)	Defining Characteristics (Symptoms and Signs)
Urinary retention	Diminished or absent sensory and/or motor impulses Effects of medications Anesthetics Opiates Psychotropics Strong sphincter Urethral blockage associated with fecal impaction Prostate hypertrophy Surgical swelling Postpartum edema Anxiety (fear of postoperative pain)	Bladder distention Diminished force of urinary stream Dribbling Dysuria Hesitancy High residual urine Nocturia Sensation of bladder fullness Small, frequent voiding or absence of urine output
Impaired skin integrity	Infection Allergy Chemical substances on skin Autoimmune dysfunction Decreased circulation Edema Effects of aging or medications Excretions/secretions Immobility Insect bites Parasites Pressure Radiation Shearing force Stress Surgery	Blisters Chafing Disruption of skin surface or layers Lesions Pruritus Bruising Cyanosis Denuded skin Erythema Induration

Other related nursing diagnoses:
- Sexual dysfunction (see Chapter 22)
- Rape trauma response (see Chapter 22)
- Rape trauma syndrome: Compound reaction
- Rape trauma syndrome: Silent reaction

ABNORMAL CONDITIONS

Table 21-2 ► Genital Skin Lesions

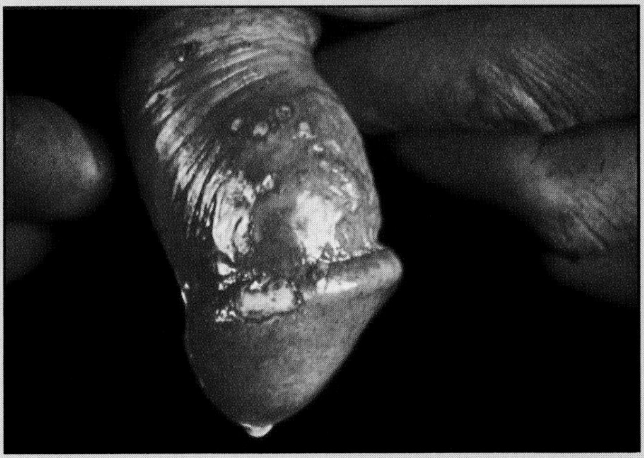

HERPES PROGENITALIS

Clusters of small vesicles with surrounding erythema, which are often painful, erupt on the glans or foreskin. These rupture to form superficial ulcers. An STD, the initial infection lasts 7 to 10 days. The virus remains dormant indefinitely; recurrent infections last 3 to 10 days with milder symptoms.

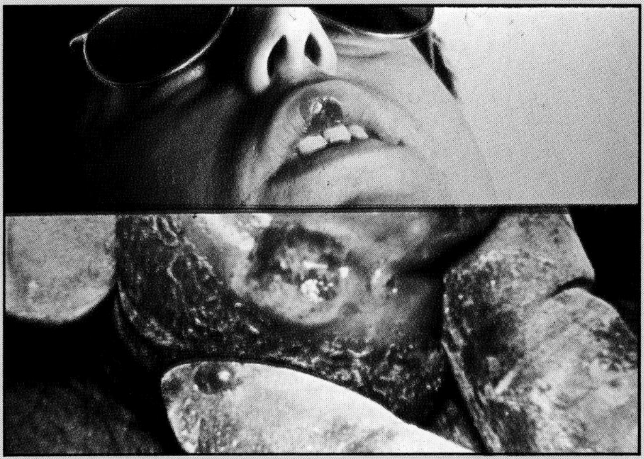

SYPHILITIC CHANCRE

Begins as a small, solitary, silvery papule that erodes to a red, round or oval, superficial ulcer with a yellowish serous discharge. Palpation reveals a nontender indurated base that can be lifted like a button between the thumb and the finger. Lymph nodes enlarge early but are nontender. This is an STD.

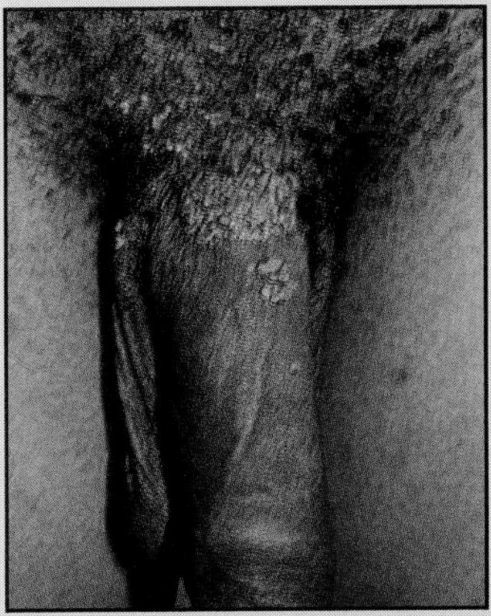

CONDYLOMATA ACUMINATA (VENEREAL WART)

Soft, pointed, moist, wartlike papules may be single or multiple in a cauliflower-like patch. Occur on shaft of penis or behind corona or around anus. This is an STD.

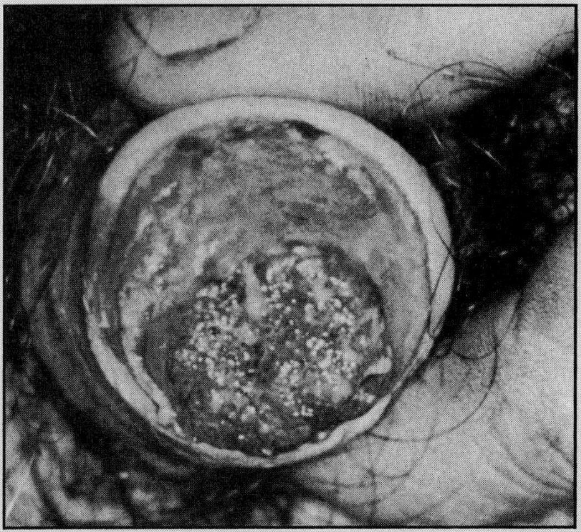

CARCINOMA

Begins as red, raised warty growth or as an ulcer, with watery discharge. As it grows, may necrose and slough. Usually painless. Almost always on glans or inner lip of foreskin, and follows chronic inflammation. Enlarged lymph nodes are common.

Table 21-3 ▶ Structural Abnormalities on Penis

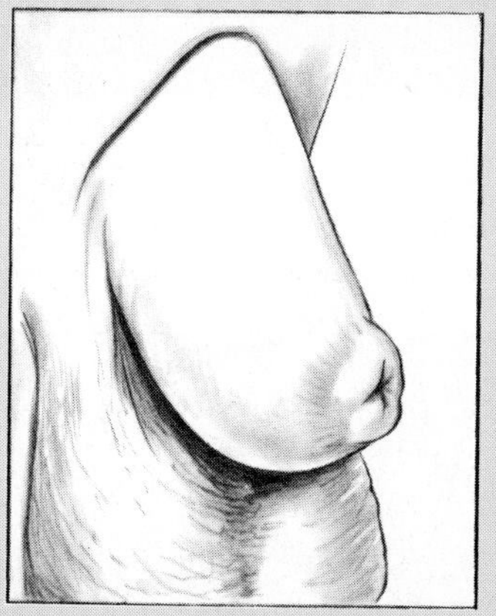

PHIMOSIS

Foreskin is advanced and fixed; so tight it is impossible to retract over glans. May be congenital or acquired from adhesions secondary to infection. Poor hygiene leads to retained dirt and smegma, which increases risk of inflammation or calculus formation.

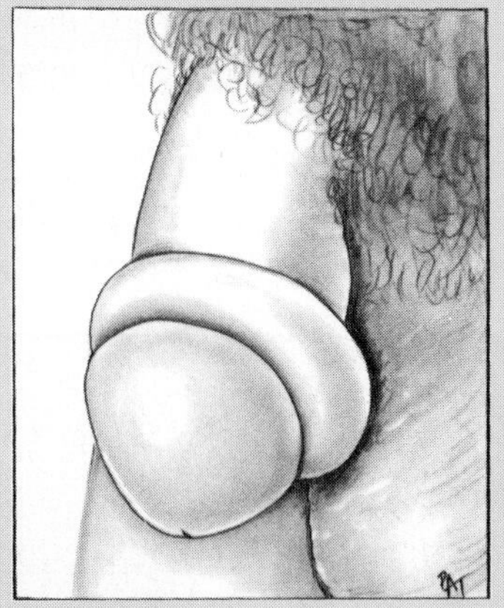

PARAPHIMOSIS

Foreskin is retracted and fixed. Once retracted behind glans, a tight or inflamed foreskin cannot return to its original position. Constriction impedes circulation so glans swells. If untreated, it may compromise arterial circulation.

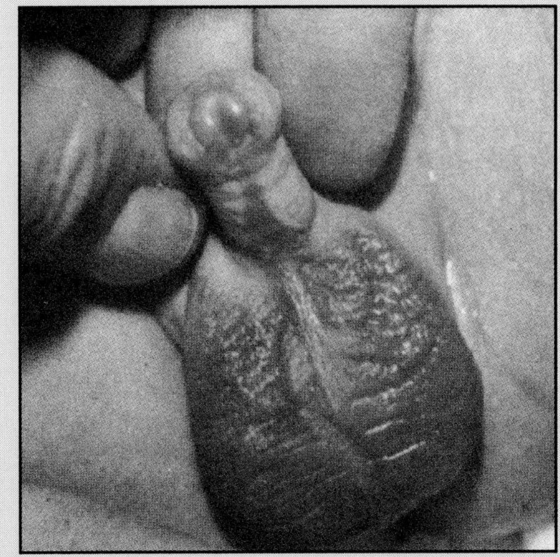

HYPOSPADIAS

Meatus opens on the ventral (under) side of glans, shaft, or at the penoscrotal junction. A groove extends from the meatus to the normal location at the tip. This is a congenital defect.

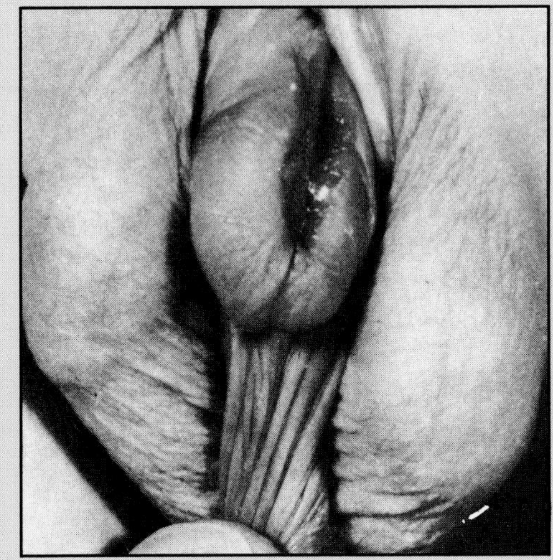

EPISPADIAS

Meatus opens on the dorsal (upper) side of glans or shaft. Rare; less common than hypospadias but more disabling because of associated urinary incontinence and separation of pubic bones.

Table 21-4 ▶ Abnormalities of the Penis

URETHRAL STRICTURE (not illustrated)

Pinpoint, constricted opening at meatus or inside along urethra. Occurs congenitally or secondary to urethral injury. Gradual decrease in force and caliber of urine stream is most common symptom. Shaft feels indurated along ventral aspect at the site of the stricture.

URETHRITIS (URETHRAL DISCHARGE AND DYSURIA)

Infection of urethra causes painful burning urination. Meatus edges are reddened, everted, and swollen. Purulent urethral discharge present. Urine is cloudy with discharge and mucous shreds. Cause determined by culture: (1) gonococcal urethritis has thick, profuse, yellow or gray-brown discharge; (2) nonspecific urethritis (NSU) may have similar discharge but often has scanty, mucoid discharge. Of these, about 50 percent are caused by chlamydia infection. This is important to differentiate because antibiotic treatment is different.

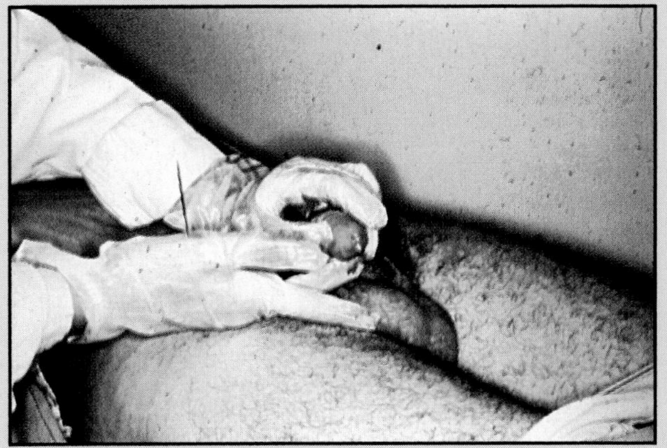

PEYRONIE'S DISEASE (not illustrated)

Hard, nontender, subcutaneous plaques palpated on dorsal or lateral surface of penis. May be single or multiple and asymmetric. They are associated with painful bending of the penis during erection. Plaques are fibrosis of covering of corpora cavernosa. Usually occurs after 45 years. Its cause is unknown.

PRIAPISM (not illustrated)

Prolonged painful erection of penis without sexual desire. Rare condition occurs with sickle cell trait or disease; leukemia where increased numbers of white blood cells produce engorgement; malignancy; or local trauma or spinal cord injuries with autonomic nervous system dysfunction.

Table 21-5 ► Abnormalities in the Scrotum

	CLINICAL FINDINGS	DISCUSSION
Absent testis Cryptorchidism 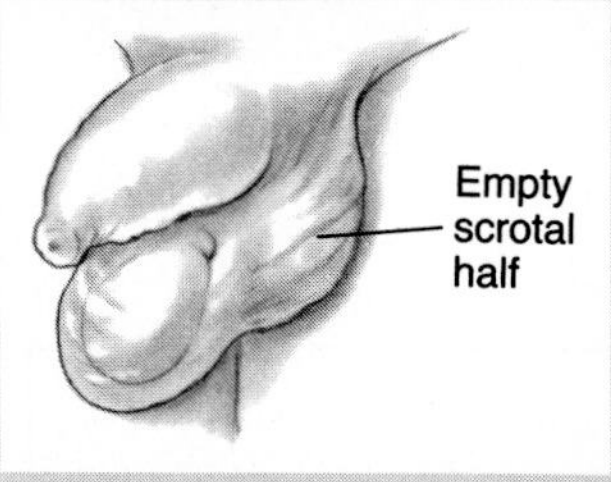	S: Empty scrotal half O: Inspection—In true maldescent, atrophic scrotum on affected side Palpation—No testis A: Absent testis	True cryptorchidism—testes that have never descended. Incidence at birth is 3 to 4 percent, one-half of these descend in first month. Incidence with premature infants is 30 percent; in the adult 0.7 to 0.8 percent. True undescended testes have a histologic change by 6 years, causing decreased spermatogenesis and infertility
Small Testis 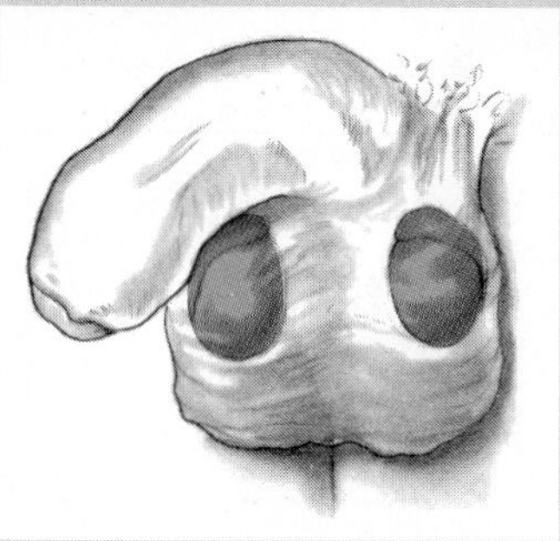	S: (None) O: Palpation—Small and soft (rarely may firm) A: Small testis	Small and soft (<3.5 cm) indicates atrophy as with cirrhosis, hypopituitarism, following estrogen therapy, or as a sequelae of orchitis. Small and firm (<2 cm) occurs with Klinefelter's syndrome (hypogonadism)
Scrotal edema 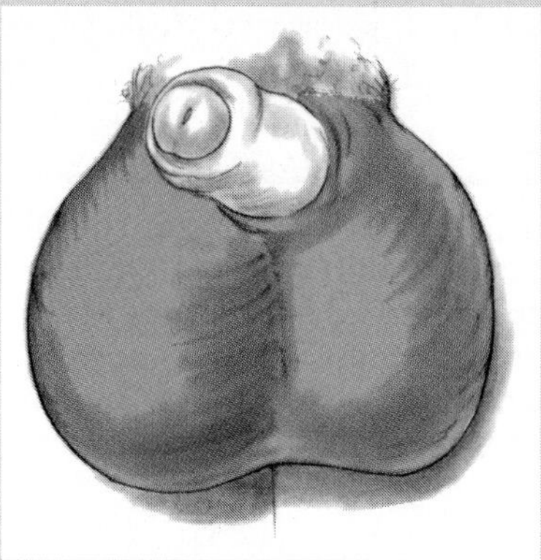	S: Tenderness O: Inspection—Enlarged, may be reddened (with local irritation) Palpation—Taut with pitting. Probably unable to feel scrotal contents. A: Scrotal edema	Accompanies marked edema in lower half of body, e.g., congestive heart failure, renal failure, and portal vein obstruction. Occurs with local inflammation: epididymitis, torsion of spermatic cord. Also obstruction of inguinal lymphatics produces lymphedema of scrotum
Hydrocele 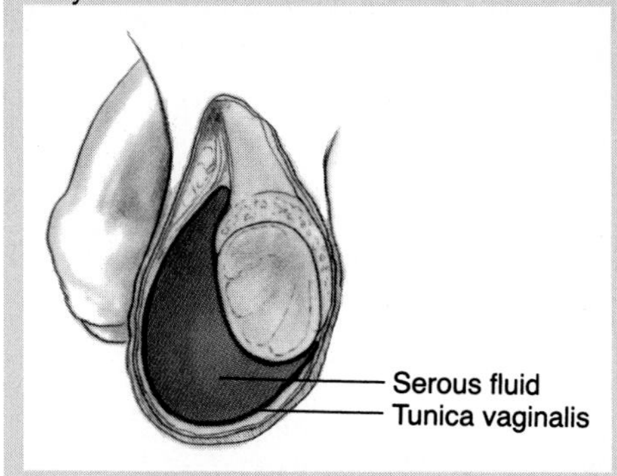	S: Painless swelling, although person may complain of weight and bulk in scrotum O: Inspection—Enlarged, mass does transilluminate Palpation—Nontender mass, able to get fingers above mass (in contrast to scrotal hernia) A: Nontender swelling of testis	Cystic. Circumscribed collection of serous fluid in tunica vaginalis, surrounding testis. May occur following epididymitis, trauma, hernia, tumor of testis, or spontaneously in the newborn

S, subjective; O, objective; A, assessment.

Table 21-5 ► Abnormalities in the Scrotum *Continued*

	CLINICAL FINDINGS	DISCUSSION
Scrotal hernia 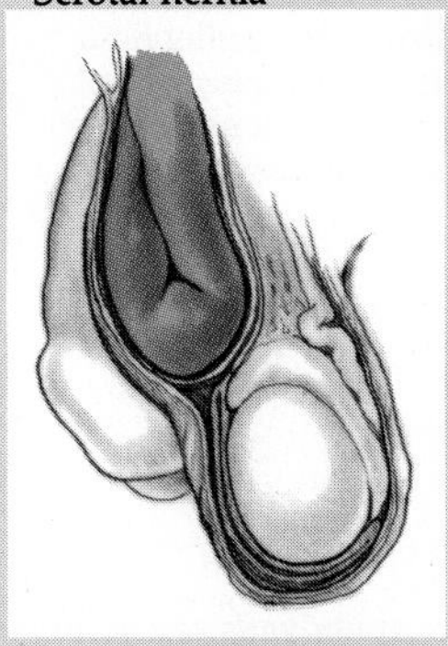	S: Swelling, may have pain with straining O: Inspection—Enlarged, may reduce when supine, does not transilluminate Palpation—Soft mushy mass, palpating fingers cannot get above mass. Mass is distinct from testicle that is normal A: Nontender swelling of scrotum	Scrotal hernia usually due to indirect inguinal hernia (see Table 21-6)
Early testicular tumor 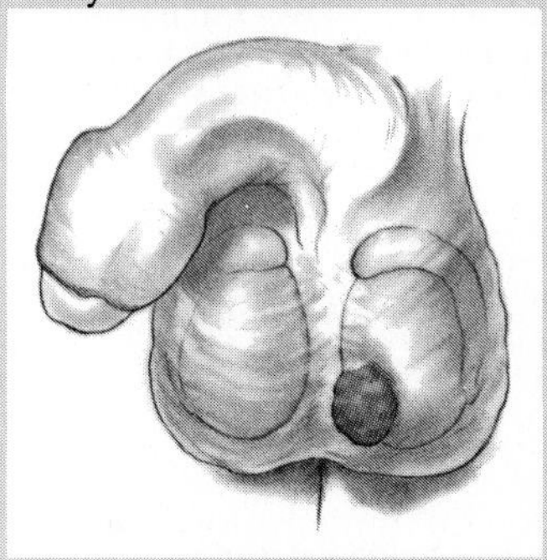	S: Painless, found on examination O: Palpation—Firm nodule, or harder than normal section of testicle A: Solitary nodule	Most testicular tumors occur between the ages of 18 and 35. Practically all are malignant. Occurs in whites; relatively rare in blacks, Mexican-Americans, and Asians. Must biopsy to confirm. Most important risk factor is undescended testis, even those surgically corrected. Early detection important in prognosis, but practice of testicular self-examination is currently low
Diffuse tumor 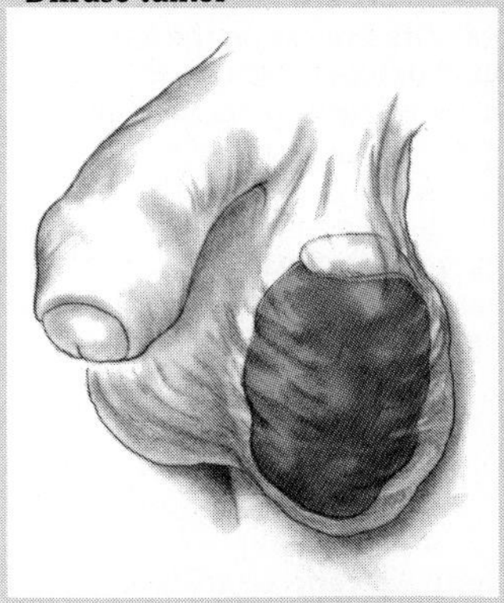	S: Enlarging testis (most common symptom). When enlarges, has feel of increased weight O: Inspection—Enlarged, does not transilluminate Palpation—Enlarged, smooth, ovoid, firm. Important—firm palpation does *not* cause usual sickening discomfort as with normal testis A: Nontender swelling of testis	Diffuse tumor maintains shape of testis
Orchitis 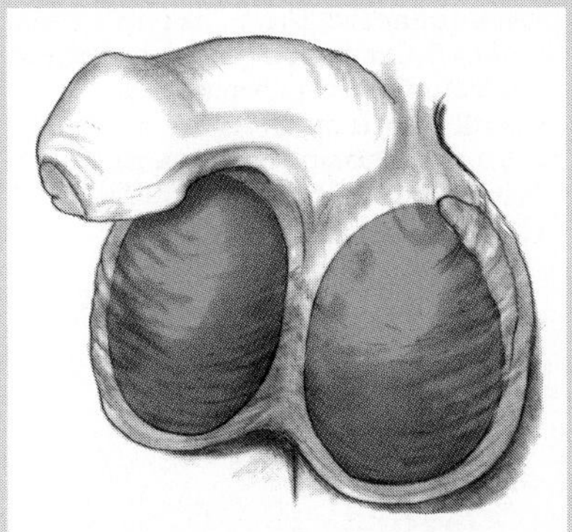	S: Acute or moderate pain of sudden onset, swollen testis, feeling of weight, fever O: Inspection—Enlarged, edematous, reddened; does not transilluminate Palpation—Swollen, congested, tense, and tender; hard to distinguish testis from epididymis A: Tender swelling of testis	Acute inflammation of testis. Most common cause is mumps; can occur with any infectious disease May have associated hydrocele that does transilluminate

S, subjective; O, objective; A, assessment.

Table continued on following page

Table 21-5 ► Abnormalities in the Scrotum *Continued*

	CLINICAL FINDINGS	DISCUSSION
Spermatocele 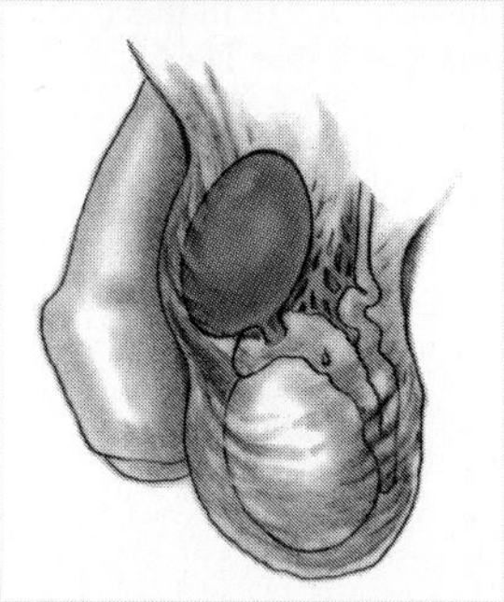	S: Painless, usually found on examination O: Inspection—Does transilluminate Palpation—Round, freely movable mass lying above and behind testis. If large, feels like a third testis A: Free cystic mass on epididymis	Retention cyst in epididymis. Cause unclear but may be obstruction of tubules. Filled with thin, milky fluid-containing sperm. Most spermatoceles are small (<1 cm); occasionally, they may be larger and then mistaken for hydrocele
Epididymitis 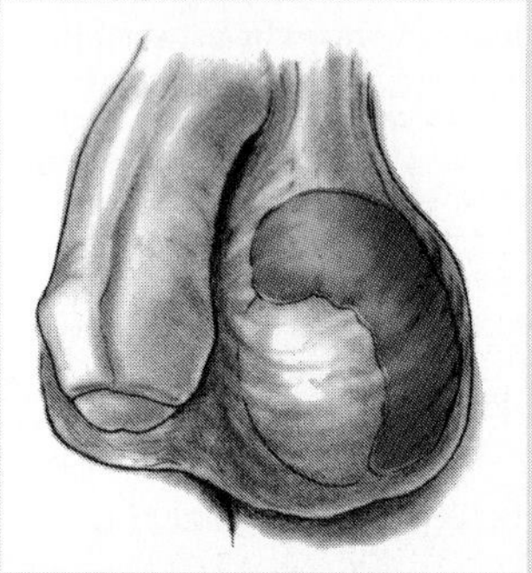	S: Severe pain of sudden onset in scrotum, somewhat relieved by elevation; also rapid swelling, fever O: Inspection—Enlarged scrotum; reddened Palpation—Exquisitely tender; epididymis enlarged, indurated; may be hard to distinguish from testis A: Tender swelling of epididymis	Acute infection of epididymis commonly caused by prostatitis, after prostatectomy because of trauma of urethral instrumentation, or due to chlamydial or other bacterial infection
Testicular torsion 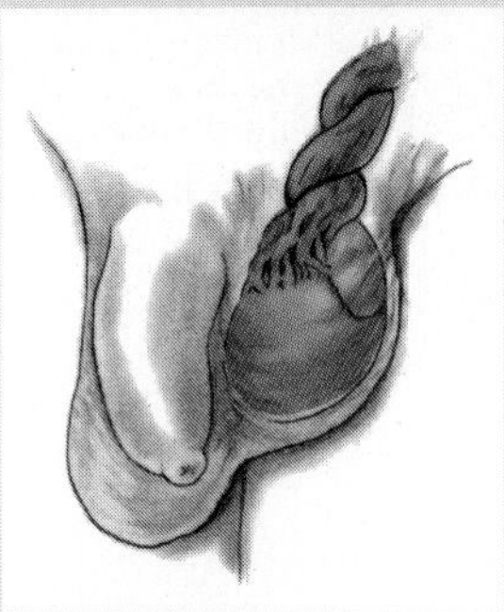	S: Excruciating pain of sudden onset, often during sleep. May also have lower abdominal pain, nausea and vomiting, no fever O: Inspection—red, swollen scrotum, one testis (usually left) higher owing to rotation and shortening Palpation—cord feels thick, swollen, tender	Occurs in late childhood, early adolescence, rare after age of 20 years. Torsion occurs usually on the left side. Faulty anchoring of testis on wall of scrotum allows testis to rotate. The anterior part of the testis rotates medially toward the other testis. Blood supply is cut off, resulting in ischemia and engorgement. This is an emergency requiring surgery; testis can become gangrenous in a few hours
Spermatic cord Varicocele 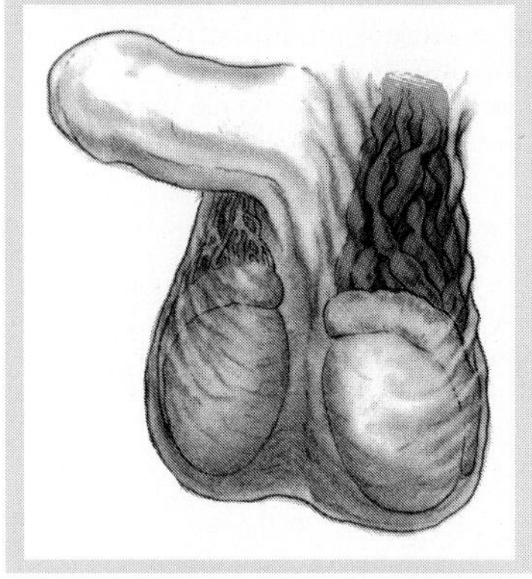	S: Dull pain; constant pulling or dragging feeling; or may be asymptomatic O: Inspection—Usually no sign. May show bluish color through light scrotal skin Palpation—When standing, feel soft, irregular mass posterior to and above testis; collapses when supine, refills when upright A: Soft mass on spermatic cord	Dilated, tortuous varicose veins in spermatic cord, most often on left side. Feels distinctive, like a "bag of worms." Common in young males; not treated unless it contributes to infertility or is painful The testis on the side of the varicocele may be smaller owing to impaired circulation

S, subjective; O, objective; A, assessment.

Table 21-6 ▶ Inguinal and Femoral Hernias

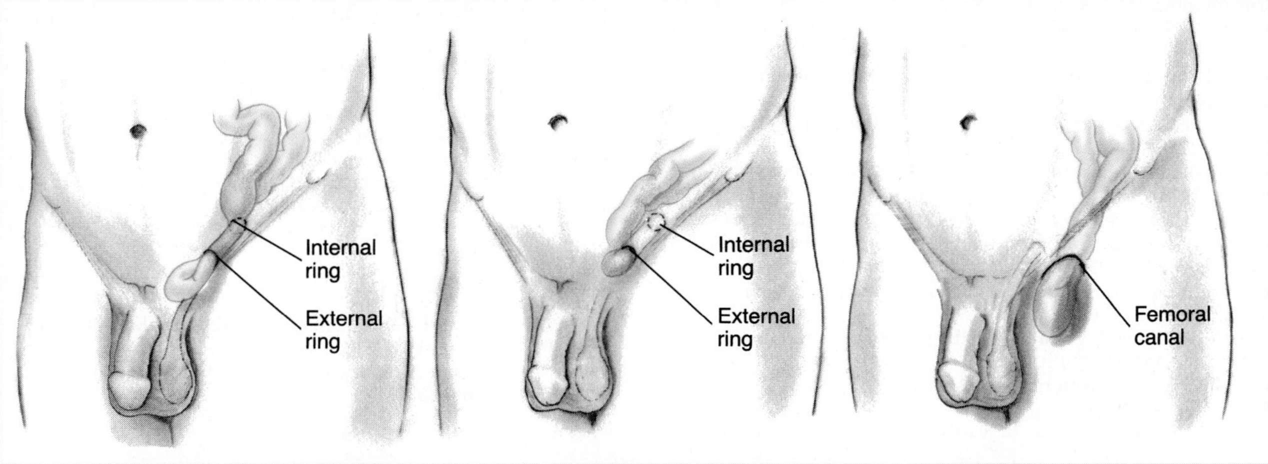

	INDIRECT INGUINAL	DIRECT INGUINAL	FEMORAL
Course	Sac herniates through internal inguinal ring; can remain in canal or pass into scrotum	Directly behind and through external inguinal ring, above inguinal ligament; rarely enters scrotum	Through femoral ring and canal, below inguinal ligament, more often on right side
Clinical symptoms and signs	Pain with straining; soft swelling that increases with increased intra-abdominal pressure; may decrease when lying down	Usually painless; round swelling close to the pubis in area of internal inguinal ring; easily reduced when supine*	Pain may be severe, may become strangulated
Frequency	Most common; 60 percent of all hernias. More common in infants <1 year and in males 16 to 20 years of age	Less common, occurs most often in men >40, rare in women	Least common, 4 percent of all hernias; more common in women
Cause	Congenital or acquired	Acquired weakness; brought on by heavy lifting, muscle atrophy, obesity, chronic cough, or ascites	Acquired; due to increased abdominal pressure, muscle weakness, or frequent stooping

* Reducible—Contents will return to abdominal cavity by lying down or gentle pressure. Incarcerated—Herniated bowel cannot be returned to abdominal cavity. Strangulated—Blood supply to hernia is shut off. Accompanied by nausea, vomiting, and tenderness.

Bibliography

Behrman RE, Vaughan VC: Nelson Textbook of Pediatrics. 13th ed. Philadelphia, W.B. Saunders, 1987.

Boyarsky R: Sexuality and the aged. *In* Steinberg F (Ed): Care of the Geriatric Patient. St. Louis, C.V. Mosby, 1983, pp 501–508.

Chard M: An approach to examining the adolescent male. Matern Child Nurs J 1(1): 41–43, 1976.

Cohen S: Patient assessment: Examination of the male genitalia. Am J Nurs 79:689–712, 1979.

Haggerty B: Prevention and differential of scrotal cancer. Nurse Pract 8:45–52, 1983.

Harlan W, Grillo GP, Corroni-Huntley J, et al: Secondary sex characteristics of boys 12 to 17 years of age. The U.S. Health Examination Survey. J Pediatr 95:293, 1979.

Harris CC: Cultural values and the decision to circumcise. Image 18(3):98–104, 1986.

Marshall W, Tanner J: Variations in the pattern of pubertal changes in boys. Arch Dis Child 45:13, 1970.

Mason DR: Erectile dysfunctions: Assessment and care. Nurs Pract 14(12):23–34, 1989.

Masters WH, Johnson VE, Kolodyn RC: Human Sexuality. Boston, Little, Brown, 1982.

Mitchell J: Male adolescents; concern about a physical examination conducted by a female. Nurs Res 29:165–169, 1980.

Muscari ME: Obtaining the adolescent sexual history. Pediatric Nurs 13(5):307–310, 1987.

Nettina SL, Kauffman FH: Diagnosis and management of sexually transmitted genital lesions. Nurs Pract 15(1):20–39, 1990.

Pfeiffer E: Sexuality and aging. *In* Rossman I (Ed): Clinical Geriatrics. Philadelphia, J.B. Lippincott, 1979.

Reno DR: Men's knowledge and health beliefs about testicular cancer and testicular self-examination. Cancer Nurs 11(2):112–117, 1988.

Shen J: Adolescent sexual behavior. Postgrad Med 71:46–55, 1982.

Smith D: General Urology. 9th ed. Los Altos, CA, Lange Medical Publications, 1978.

Tanner J: Growth at Adolescence. 2nd ed. Oxford, Blackwell Scientific Publications, 1962.

Walsh PC, Perlmutter AD, Gittes RF, et al: Campbell's Urology. 5th ed. Philadelphia, W.B. Saunders, 1986.

Wirth J: Current circumcision practices: Canada. Pediatrics 66(5):705–708, 1980.

CHAPTER

22 Female Genitalia

STRUCTURE AND FUNCTION

EXTERNAL GENITALIA

The external genitalia are called the *vulva* or pudendum (Fig. 22–1). The *mons pubis* is a round firm pad of adipose tissue covering the symphysis pubis. After puberty, it is covered with hair in the pattern of an inverted triangle. The *labia majora* are two rounded folds of adipose tissue extending from the mons pubis down and around to the perineum. After puberty, hair covers the outer surfaces of the labia while the inner folds are smooth, moist, and contain sebaceous follicles.

Inside the labia majora are two smaller, darker folds of skin, the *labia minora.* These are joined anteriorly at the clitoris where they form a hood, or prepuce. The labia minora are joined posteriorly by a transverse fold, the *frenulum* or fourchette. The *clitoris* is a small, pea-shaped erectile body, homologous with the male penis and highly sensitive to tactile stimulation.

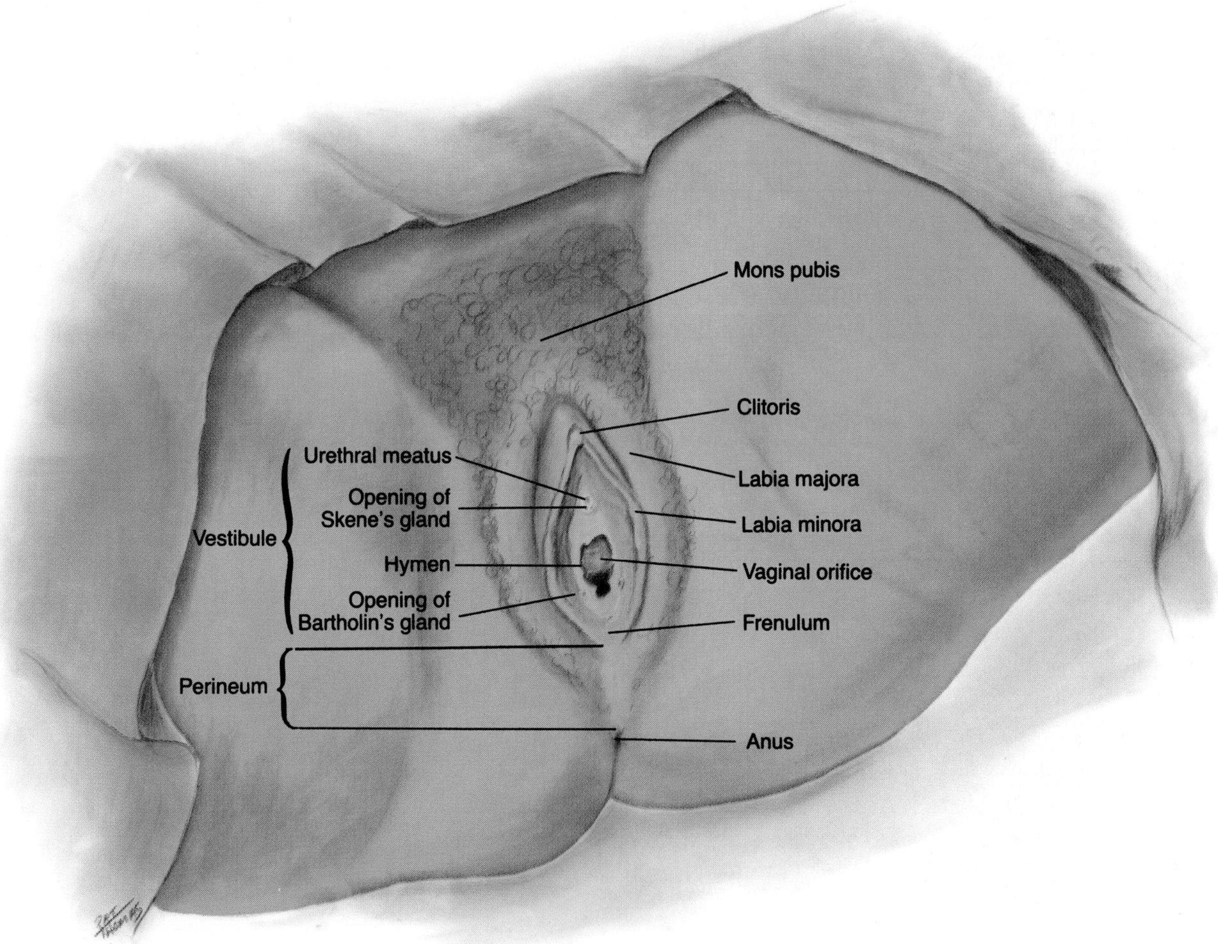

► **Figure 22–1**

The labial structures encircle a boat-shaped space, or cleft, termed the *vestibule.* Within it are numerous openings. The *urethral meatus* appears as a dimple 2.5 cm posterior to the clitoris. Surrounding the urethral meatus are the tiny, multiple *paraurethral (Skene's) glands.* Their ducts are not visible but open posterior to the urethra at the 5 and 7 o'clock positions.

The *vaginal orifice* is posterior to the urethral meatus. It appears either as a thin median split or as a large opening with irregular edges, depending on the presentation of the membranous *hymen.* The hymen is a thin, circular or crescent-shaped fold that may cover part of the vaginal orifice or may be absent completely. On either side and posterior to the vaginal orifice are two *vestibular (Bartholin's) glands,* which secrete a clear lubricating mucus during intercourse. Their ducts are not visible but open in the groove between the labia minora and the hymen.

INTERNAL GENITALIA

The internal genitalia include the *vagina,* a flattened, tubular canal extending from the orifice up and backward into the pelvis (Fig. 22–2). It is 9 cm long and sits between the rectum posteriorly and the bladder and urethra anteriorly. Its walls are in thick transverse folds, or *rugae,* enabling the vagina to dilate widely during childbirth.

At the end of the canal, the uterine *cervix* projects into the vagina. In the nulliparous female, the cervix appears as a smooth doughnut-shaped area with a small circular hole or *os.* After childbirth, the os is slightly enlarged and irregular. The cervical epithelium is of two distinct types. The vagina and cervix are covered with smooth, pink, stratified squamous epithelium. Inside the os, the endocervical canal is lined with columnar epithelium that looks red and rough. The point where these two

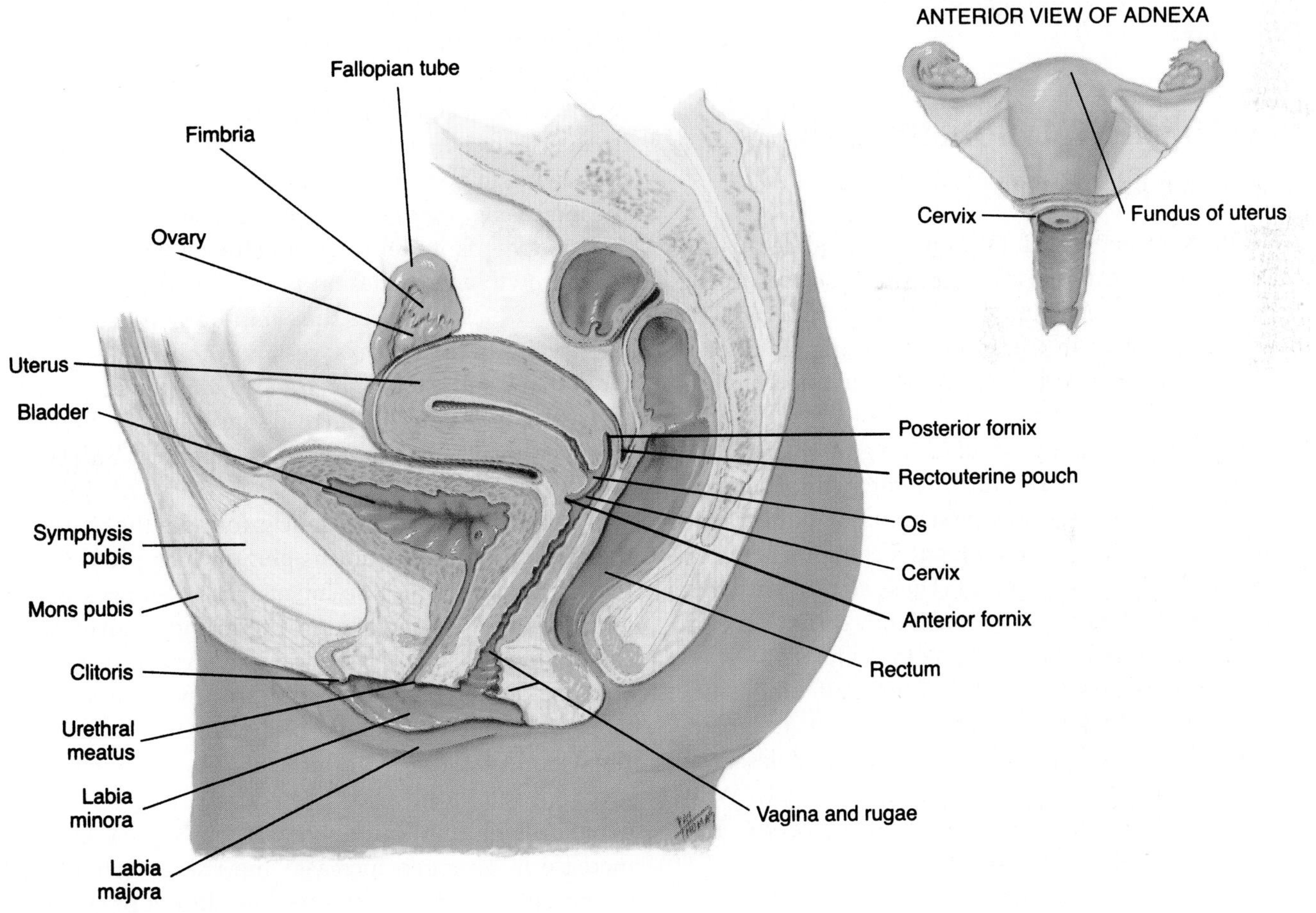

▶ **Figure 22–2**

tissues meet is the squamocolumnar junction and is not visible.

There is a continuous recess around the cervix, termed the *anterior fornix* in front and the *posterior fornix* behind. Behind the posterior fornix, another deep recess is formed by the peritoneum. It dips down between the rectum and cervix to form the *rectouterine pouch* or *cul-de-sac of Douglas.*

The *uterus* is a pear-shaped, thick-walled, muscular organ. It is flattened anteroposteriorly, measuring 5.5 to 8 cm long by 3.5 to 4 cm wide and 2 to 2.5 cm thick. It is freely movable, not fixed, and usually tilts forward and superior to the bladder (a position labeled as anteverted and anteflexed, see p. 852).

The *fallopian tubes* are two pliable, trumpet-shaped tubes, 10 cm in length, extending from the uterine fundus laterally to the brim of the pelvis. There, they curve posteriorly, their fimbriated ends located near the *ovaries.* The two ovaries are located one on each side of the uterus at the level of the anterior superior iliac spine. Each is oval shaped, 3 cm long by 2 cm wide by 1 cm thick, and serves to develop ova (eggs) as well as the female hormones.

DEVELOPMENTAL CONSIDERATIONS

Infants and Adolescents

At birth, the external genitalia are engorged because of the presence of maternal estrogen. The structures recede in a few weeks, remaining small until puberty. The ovaries are located in the abdomen during childhood. The uterus is small with a straight axis and no anteflexion.

At puberty, estrogens stimulate the growth of cells in the reproductive tract and the development of secondary sex characteristics. The first signs of puberty are breast and pubic hair development, beginning between the ages of 8 1/2 and 13 years. These signs are usually concurrent, but it is not abnormal if they do not develop together. They take about 3 years to complete.

Menarche occurs during the latter half of this sequence, just after the peak of growth velocity. Irregularity of the menstrual cycle is common during adolescence because of the girl's occasional failure to ovulate. With menarche, the uterine body flexes on the cervix. The ovaries now are in the pelvic cavity.

Tanner's table on the five stages of pubic hair development is helpful in teaching girls the expected sequence of sexual development (Table 22–1).

These data are derived from Tanner's study of white British females and may not necessarily generalize to all other racial groups. For example, mature Asian women normally have fine sparse pubic hair. However, the U.S. Health Examination Survey (Harlan, 1980) studied girls representative of the contemporary United States population. Its findings correlate closely with Tanner's results. One significant difference is that black girls tend to develop breast and pubic hair earlier than white girls of the same age.

The Pregnant Female

Shortly after the first missed menstrual period, the female genitalia show signs of the growing fetus. The cervix softens (*Goodell's sign*) at 4 to 6 weeks, and the vaginal mucosa and cervix look cyanotic (*Chadwick's sign*) at 8 to 12 weeks. These changes occur because of increased vascularity and edema of the cervix, and hypertrophy and hyperplasia of the cervical glands. The isthmus of the uterus softens (*Hegar's sign*) at 6 to 8 weeks.

The greatest change is in the uterus itself. It increases in capacity by 500 to 1000 times its nonpregnant state, at first owing to hormone stimulation, and then owing to the increasing size of its contents (Pritchard et al, 1985). The nonpregnant uterus has a flattened pear shape. Its early growth encroaches on the space occupied by the bladder, which produces the symptoms of urinary frequency. By 10 to 12 weeks' gestation, it becomes globular in shape and is too large to stay in the pelvis. At 20 to 24 weeks, the uterus has an oval shape. It rises almost to the liver, displacing the intestines superiorly and laterally.

A clot of thick, tenacious mucus forms in the spaces of the cervical canal (the mucus plug), which protects the fetus from infection. The mucus plug dislodges when labor begins at the end of term, producing a sign of labor called "bloody show." Cervical and vaginal secretions increase during pregnancy and are thick, white, and more acidic. The increased acidity occurs because of the action of *Lactobacillus acidophilus,* which changes glycogen into lactic acid. The acidic pH keeps pathogenic bacteria from multiplying in the vagina, but the increase in glycogen increases the risk of candidiasis (commonly called a yeast infection) during pregnancy.

Table 22-1 ▶ Sex Maturity Rating (SMR) in Girls

STAGE	DESCRIPTION	
1	Preadolescent. No pubic hair. Mons and labia covered with fine vellus hair as on abdomen.	
2	Growth sparse and mostly on labia. Long downy hair, slightly pigmented, straight or only slightly curly.	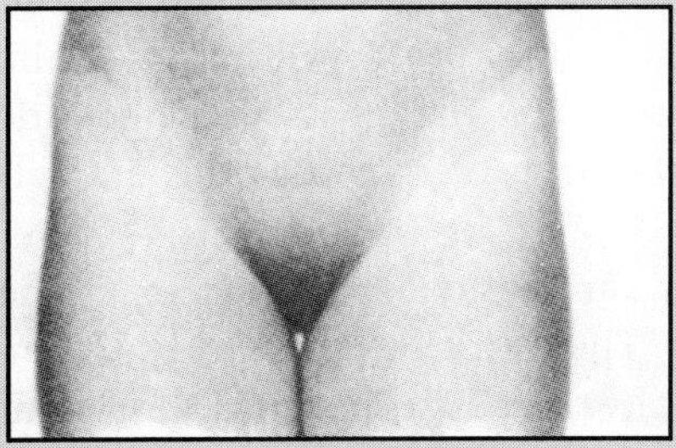 2
3	Growth sparse and spreading over mons pubis. Hair is darker, coarser, curlier.	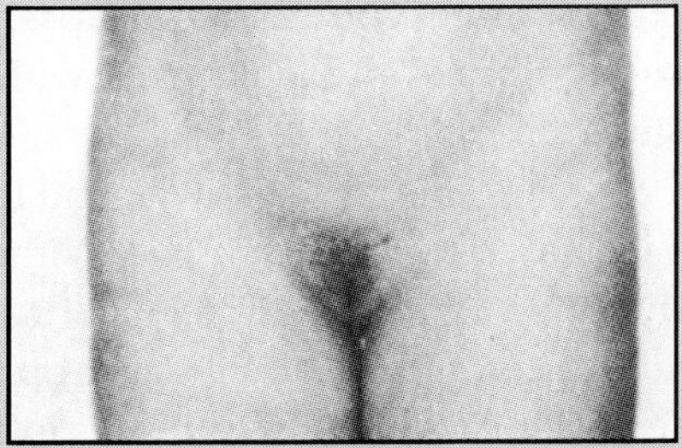 3
4	Hair is adult in type but over smaller area; none on medial thigh.	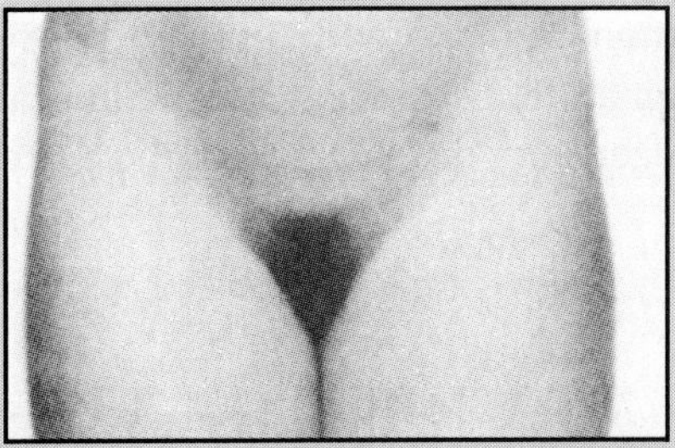 4
5	Adult in type and pattern; inverse triangle. Also on medial thigh surface.	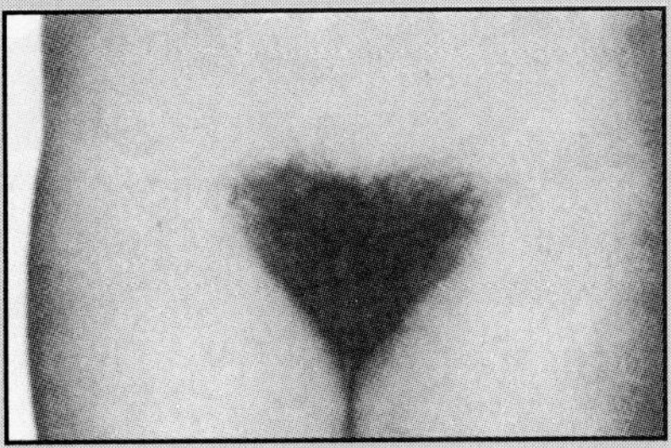 5

The Aging Female

In contrast to the slowly declining hormones in the aging male, the female's hormonal milieu decreases rapidly. *Menopause* is cessation of the menses. Usually this occurs around the ages of 48 to 51 years, although there is a wide normal variation of ages from 35 to 60 years. The stage of menopause includes the preceding 1 to 2 years of decline in ovarian function, shown by irregular menses that gradually become farther apart and produce a lighter flow than usual. The ovaries stop producing progesterone and estrogen. Since cells in the reproductive tract are estrogen dependent, decreased estrogen levels during menopause bring dramatic physical changes.

The uterus shrinks in size because of its decreased myometrium. The ovaries atrophy to 1 to 2 cm and are not palpable after menopause. Ovulation still may occur sporadically after menopause. The sacral ligaments relax, and the pelvic musculature weakens, so the uterus droops. Sometimes it may protrude, or prolapse, into the vagina. The cervix shrinks and looks paler with a thick glistening epithelium.

The vagina becomes shorter, narrower, and less elastic because of increased connective tissue. Without sexual activity, the vagina atrophies to one half its former length and width. The vaginal epithelium atrophies, becoming thinner, drier, and itchy. This results in a fragile mucosal surface that is at risk for bleeding and vaginitis. Decreased vaginal secretions leave the vagina dry and at risk for irritation and pain with intercourse (dyspareunia). The vaginal pH becomes more alkaline, and a decreased glycogen content occurs from the decreased estrogen. These factors also increase the risk of vaginitis because they create a suitable medium for pathogens.

Table 22-2 ▶ Aging Changes in Sexual Response Cycle

PHASE	PHYSIOLOGIC CHANGE
Excitement	Reduced amount of vaginal secretion and lubrication.
Plateau	Less expansion of vagina Labia majora do not elevate against perineum No color change in labia minora (was from pink to cardinal-red or dark red) Size of clitoris decreases after age 60
Orgasm	Shorter duration
Resolution	Occurs more rapidly

Data from Masters WH, Johnson VE: Human Sexual Response. Boston, Little, Brown, and Company, 1966.

Externally, the mons pubis looks smaller because the fat pad atrophies. The labia and clitoris gradually decrease in size. Pubic hair becomes thin and sparse.

Declining estrogen levels produce some physiologic changes in the female sexual response cycle (Table 22-2). However, these changes do not affect sexual pleasure and function. Sexual desire and the need for full sexual expression continue. As with the male, the older female is capable of sexual function given reasonably good health and an interested partner. The problem for many older women is finding a socially acceptable sexual partner. Aging women greatly outnumber their male counterparts. And, aging women are more likely to be single while males their same age are more likely to be married.

SUBJECTIVE DATA

- Menstrual history
- Obstetric history
- Menopause
- Self-care behaviors
- Urinary symptoms
- Vaginal discharge
- Sexual relationships
- Contraceptive use
- Sexually transmitted disease (STD) contact

EXAMINER ASKS:	RATIONALE:
1. Tell me about your menstrual periods:	**Menstrual history** is usually nonthreatening, thus it is a good place to start history.
What was the date of your last menstrual period?	LMP = last menstrual period.
At what age did you start having periods?	Menarche—onset between 12 and 14 years indicates normal growth; onset between 16 and 17 years suggests an endocrine problem.
How often do your periods come?	Cycle—normally varies every 18 to 45 days. Amenorrhea—absent menses.
How many days does your period usually last?	Duration—average 3 to 7 days.
What is your usual amount of flow: light, medium, heavy? How many pads or tampons do you use each day or hour?	Menorrhagia—heavy menses.
Do you have any clotting?	Clotting indicates heavy flow or vaginal pooling.
Do you have any pain or cramps before or during period? How do you treat it? Do the cramps interfere with daily activities? Do you have any other associated symptoms: bloating, cramping, breast tenderness, moodiness? Do you have any spotting between periods?	Dysmenorrhea.
2. Have you ever been pregnant?	**Obstetric history.**
How many times?	Gravida—number of pregnancies.
How many babies did you have?	Para—number of births.
Did you have a miscarriage or an abortion?	Abortions—interrupted pregnancies, including elective abortions and spontaneous miscarriages.
For each pregnancy, describe: duration, any complication, labor and delivery, baby's sex, birth weight, condition.	
Do you think you may be pregnant now? What symptoms have you noticed that suggest pregnancy?	
3. Have your periods slowed down or stopped?	**Menopause**—cessation of menstruation.
Do you have any associated symptoms of menopause, e.g., hot flash, numbness and tingling, headache, palpitations, drenching sweats, mood swings, vaginal dryness, itching? Are you on any treatment for these symptoms?	Perimenopausal period, from 40 to 55 years of age, has hormone shifts, resulting in vasomotor instability.
If you are on estrogen replacement, how much do you take? How is the treatment working? Do you have any side effects?	Side effects of ERT include fluid retention, breast pain or enlargement, vaginal bleeding.
How do you feel about going through menopause?	Although this is a normal life stage, reaction varies from acceptance to feelings of loss.
4. How often do you have a gynecologic check-up? When was your last Papanicolaou's test? What were the results?	Assess **self-care behaviors.**
Has your mother ever mentioned taking hormones while pregnant with you?	Maternal ingestion of DES (diethylstilbestrol) causes cervical and vaginal abnormalities in female offspring.
5. Do you have any problems with urinating?	**Urinary symptoms.**
Do you urinate frequently and small amounts?	Frequency.
Do you feel as if you cannot wait to urinate?	Urgency.

EXAMINER ASKS:	RATIONALE:
Do you have any burning or pain on urinating?	Dysuria.
Do you awaken during night to urinate?	Nocturia.
Is there blood in the urine?	Hematuria.
Is your urine dark, cloudy, foul smelling?	Bile in urine or urinary tract infection (UTI).
Do you have any difficulty controlling urine or wetting yourself?	True incontinence—loss of urine without warning. Urgency incontinence—sudden loss, as with acute cystitis.
Do you urinate with sneeze, laugh, cough, bear down?	Stress incontinence—loss of urine with physical strain due to muscle weakness.
6. Do you have any unusual **vaginal discharge?** Is there an increased amount?	Normal discharge is small, clear or cloudy, nonirritating.
What is the character or color: white, yellow-green, gray, curd-like, foul smelling?	Suggests vaginal infection; character of discharge often suggests causative organism.
When did this begin?	Acute versus chronic problem.
Is the discharge associated with vaginal itching, rash, pain with intercourse?	Occurs secondary to irritation from discharge. Dyspareunia occurs with vaginitis of any cause.
Are you taking any medications?	Factors that increase the risk of vaginitis: • Oral contraceptives increase glycogen content of vaginal epithelium, providing fertile medium for some organisms. • Broad-spectrum antibiotics alter balance of normal flora.
Do you have a family history of diabetes?	• Increased glycogen content.
What part of your menstrual cycle are you in now?	• Menses, postpartum, menopause have a more alkaline vaginal pH.
Do you use a vaginal douche? How often?	• Frequent douching alters pH.
Do you use feminine hygiene spray?	• Risk of contact dermatitis.
Do you wear nonventilating underpants, pantyhose?	• Local irritation.
Have you treated the discharge with anything?	
What was the result?	
7. Do you have any other problems in the genital area? Do you have any sores or lesions—now or in the past? How were these treated?	
Do you have any abdominal pain?	
Have you had any past surgery on uterus, ovaries, vagina?	Assess feelings about surgery. Some fear loss of sexual response following hysterectomy. This belief may cause problems in intimate relationship.

EXAMINER ASKS:	RATIONALE:

8. Often women have a question about their **sexual relationship** and how it affects their health. Do you?

Are you in a relationship involving sex now?

Are aspects of sex satisfactory to you and your partner?

Are you satisfied with the way you and partner communicate about sex?

Are you satisfied with your ability to respond sexually?

Do you have more than one sexual partner?

Begin with open-ended question to assess individual needs. Include appropriate questions as a routine part of history:

- Communicates that you accept individual's sexual activity and believe it is important.
- Your comfort with discussion prompts person's interest and possibly relief that the topic has been introduced.
- Establishes a data base for comparison with any future sexual activities.
- Provides opportunity to screen sexual problems.

What is your sexual preference: relationship with a man, with a woman, both?

Gay and lesbian people need to feel acceptance to discuss their health concerns.

9. Are you currently planning a pregnancy, or avoiding pregnancy?

Do you and your partner use a **contraceptive?** Which method? Is this satisfactory? Do you have any questions about method?

If oral contraceptives are used, assess smoking history. Cigarettes increase cardiovascular side effects of oral contraceptives.

Which methods have you used in the past? Have you and partner discussed having children?

Have you ever had any problems becoming pregnant?

Infertility.

10. Are you aware of any sexual contact with partner having a **sexually transmitted disease,** such as gonorrhea, herpes, AIDS, chlamydial infection, venereal warts, syphilis? When? How was this treated? Were there any complications?

Do you use any precautions to prevent the transmission of STDs?

Do you have any questions or concerns about any of these matters?

ADDITIONAL QUESTIONS FOR INFANTS AND CHILDREN

Does your child have any problem urinating? Does she have any pain with urinating, crying, holding genitals? Has she ever had a urinary tract infection?

(If the child is older than 2 to 2 1/2 years of age.) Has toilet training started? How is it progressing?

Does the child wet bed at night? Is this a problem for child or you (parents)? What have you (parents) done? How does your child feel about it?

Does she have any problem with genital area: itching, rash, vaginal discharge?

Occurs with poor perineal hygiene, or insertion of foreign body in vagina.

(To child) Has anyone ever touched you in between your legs and you did not want them to? Sometimes that happens to children. They should remember they have not been bad. They should try to tell an adult about it.

Screen for sexual abuse.

EXAMINER ASKS:	RATIONALE:

ADDITIONAL QUESTIONS FOR PREADOLESCENTS AND ADOLESCENTS

Ask the questions about genitourinary symptoms as described in the adult section.

Use the following questions, as appropriate, to assess sexual growth and development and sexual behavior. First, note:

- Ask questions that seem appropriate for girl's age but be aware that norms vary widely. When you are in doubt, it is better to ask too many questions than to omit something. Children obtain information, often misinformation, from the media and from peers at surprisingly early ages. You can be sure your information will be more thoughtful and accurate.
- Ask direct, matter-of-fact questions. Avoid sounding judgmental.
- Start with a *permission statement,* "Often girls your age experience . . ." This conveys that it is normal to think or feel a certain way.
- Try the *ubiquity approach,* "When did you . . ." rather than "Do you . . ." (Mitchell, 1980). This is less threatening because it implies that the topic is normal and unexceptional.

Has your body changed since 2 years ago? What do you like about the changes? What do you not like?

Around age 11, but sometimes earlier, girls start to develop breasts and pubic hair. Have you ever seen charts and pictures of normal growth patterns for girls? Let us go over these now.

Have your periods started? How did you feel? Were you prepared or surprised?

Assess attitude of girl and parents. Note inadequate preparation or attitude of distaste.

Who in your family do you talk to about your body changes and about sex information? How do these talks go? Do you think you get enough information? What about sex education classes at school? Is there a teacher, a nurse or doctor, a minister, a counselor whom you can talk to?

Often girls your age have questions about sexual activity. Have you? Are you dating? Someone steady?

Do you and your boyfriend have intercourse? Are you using birth control? What questions do you have?

Has anyone ever talked to you about sexually transmitted diseases, such as herpes or gonorrhea? What questions do you have?

Sometimes it happens that a person touches a girl in a way that she does not want them to. Has that ever happened to you? If that happens, the girl should remember it is not her fault. She should tell another adult about it.

ADDITIONAL QUESTIONS FOR THE AGING ADULT

(Use the questions listed for the younger adult, with the following additions.)

After menopause, have you ever noted any vaginal bleeding?

Postmenopausal bleeding warrants further workup and referral.

EXAMINER ASKS:	RATIONALE:
Do you have any vaginal itching, discharge, pain with intercourse?	Associated with atrophic vaginitis.
Do you feel any pressure in genital area, loss of urine with cough or sneeze, back pain, constipation?	Occurs with weakened pelvic musculature and uterine prolapse.
Are you in a relationship involving sex now? Are aspects of sex satisfactory to you and your partner? Is there adequate privacy for a sexual relationship?	

OBJECTIVE DATA

Equipment Needed:

Assemble these items before helping the woman into position. Arrange within easy reach.

- Gloves
- Goose-necked lamp with a strong light
- Vaginal speculum of appropriate size (Fig. 22–3)
  - Graves' speculum—useful for most adult women, available in varying lengths and widths
  - Pederson speculum—narrow blades, useful for virginal or postmenopausal women with a narrowed introitus
- Large cotton-tipped applicators (rectal swabs)
- Materials for cytologic study:
  - Glass slide
  - Sterile cotton-tipped applicator
  - Ayre's spatula
  - Spray fixative
  - A small bottle of normal saline
  - A small bottle of potassium hydroxide (KOH)
  - A bottle of acetic acid (white vinegar)
- Lubricant

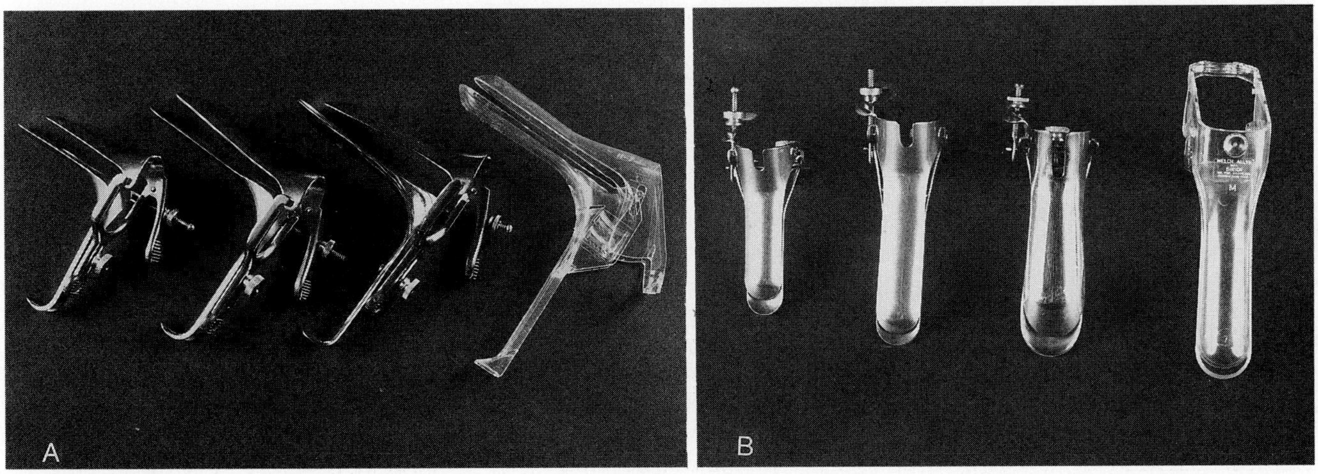

► Figure 22–3

Preparation

Familiarize yourself with the vaginal speculum before the examination. Practice opening and closing the blades, locking them into position, and releasing them. Try both metal and plastic types. Note that the plastic speculum locks and unlocks with a resounding click that can be alarming to the uninformed client.

POSITION

Initially, the woman should be sitting up. An equal status position is important to establish trust and rapport before the vaginal examination.

For the examination, the woman should be placed in the lithotomy position, with the examiner sitting on a stool. Help the woman into lithotomy position, with the body supine, feet in stirrups and knees apart, and buttocks at edge of examining table (Fig. 22–4). Ask the woman to lift her hips as you guide them to the edge of the table. Some women prefer to leave their shoes or socks on. The arms should be at the woman's sides or across the chest, not over the head, because this position only tightens the abdominal muscles. The traditional mode is to drape the woman fully, covering the stomach, knees, and legs, exposing only the vulva to your view. Be sure to push down the drape between the woman's legs so that you can see her face.

The lithotomy position leaves many women feeling helpless and vulnerable. Indeed, many women tolerate the pelvic examination because they consider it basic for health care, yet they find it embarrassing and uncomfortable. Previous examinations may have been painful, or the previous examiner's attitude hurried and patronizing.

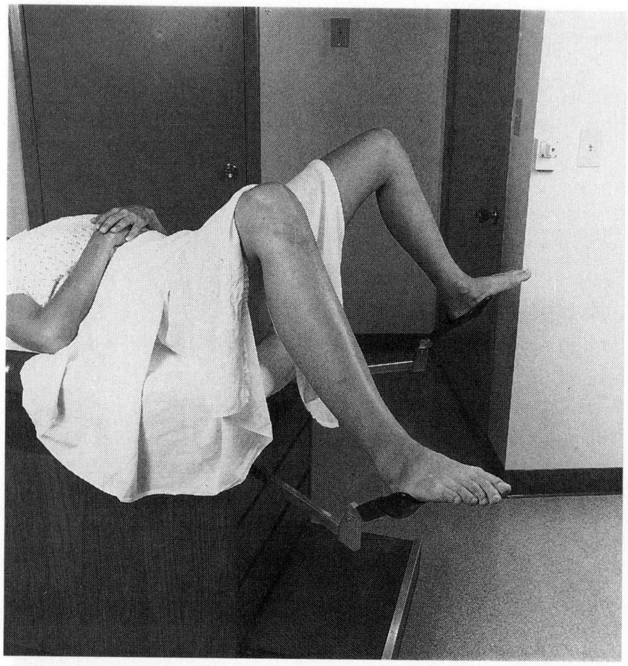

► **Figure 22–4**

The examination need not be this way. You can help the woman relax, decrease her anxiety, and retain a sense of control by employing these measures.

- Have her empty the bladder before the examination.
- Elevate her head and shoulders to maintain eye contact.
- Pull out the stirrups so the legs are not abducted too far.
- Explain each step in the examination before you do it.
- Assure the woman she can stop the examination at any point should she feel any discomfort.
- Touch the inner thigh before you touch the vulva.
- Communicate throughout the examination. Maintain a dialogue to share information.
- Use the techniques of the *educational* or *mirror pelvic examination* (Fig. 22–5) (Latta and Wiesmeier, 1982; Liston, 1978; Wells, 1977). This is a routine examination with some modifications in attitude, position, and communication. First, the woman is considered an active participant, one who is interested in learning and in sharing decisions about her own health care. Some practitioners do not use drapes in order to communicate comfort with one's own body. The woman props herself up on one elbow, or the head of the table is raised. Her other hand holds a mirror between her legs, above the examiner's hands. The woman can see all that the examiner is doing and has a full view of her genitalia.

The mirror works well for teaching normal anatomy and its relation to sexual behavior. Even women who are in sexual relationships or who have had children may be surprisingly uninformed about their own anatomy. You will find the woman's enthusiasm on seeing her own cervix is rewarding too.

The mirror pelvic examination also works well when abnormalities arise because the woman can see the rationale for treatment and can monitor progress at the next appointment. She is more willing to comply with treatment when she shares in the decision.

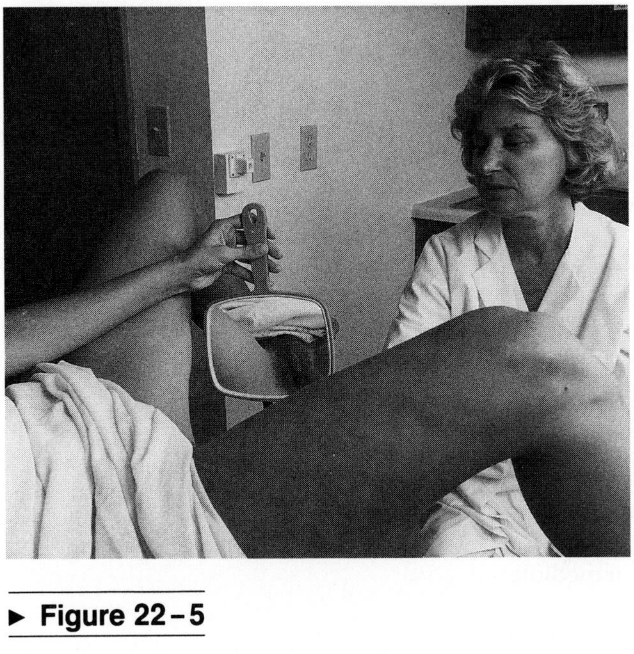

► **Figure 22–5**

METHOD OF EXAMINATION

NORMAL RANGE OF FINDINGS	ABNORMAL FINDINGS

EXTERNAL GENITALIA

Inspect the external genitalia noting:

- Skin color (Fig. 22–6).
- Hair distribution is in the usual female pattern of inverted triangle, although it normally may trail up the abdomen toward the umbilicus.

Consider delayed puberty if no pubic hair or breast development has occurred by age 13.

Nits or lice at the base of pubic hair.

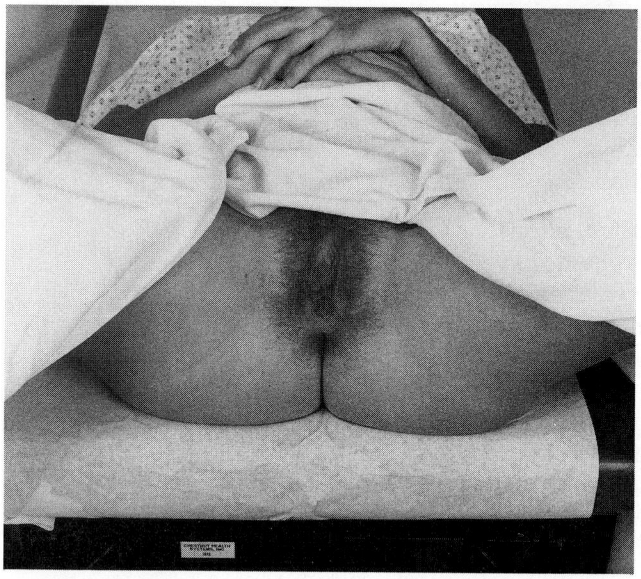

▶ **Figure 22–6**

- Labia majora normally are symmetric, plump, and well formed. In the nulliparous woman, labia meet in the midline; following a vaginal delivery, the labia are gaping, and slightly shriveled.

Swelling.

- There should be no lesions, except for occasional sebaceous cysts. These are yellowish, 1-cm nodules that are firm, nontender, and often multiple.

Excoriation.
Nodules.
Rash or lesions (Table 22–3).

With your gloved hand, separate the labia majora to inspect:

- Clitoris.
- Labia minora are dark pink and moist, usually symmetric.
- Urethral opening appears stellate or slitlike and is midline.
- Vaginal opening, or introitus, may appear as a narrow vertical slit or as a larger opening.
- Perineum is smooth. A well-healed episiotomy scar, midline or mediolateral, may be present following a vaginal birth.
- Anus has coarse skin of increased pigmentation (see Chapter 23 for assessment).

Enlarged clitoris.
Inflammation.
Polyp.
Rash or lesions.
Foul-smelling, irritating discharge.

NORMAL RANGE OF FINDINGS	ABNORMAL FINDINGS

Palpate glands.

Assess urethra and Skene's glands (Fig. 22–7). Insert your index finger into the vagina, and gently milk the urethra by applying pressure up and out. This procedure should produce no pain. If any discharge appears, culture it.

Tenderness.
Induration along urethra.
Urethral discharge.

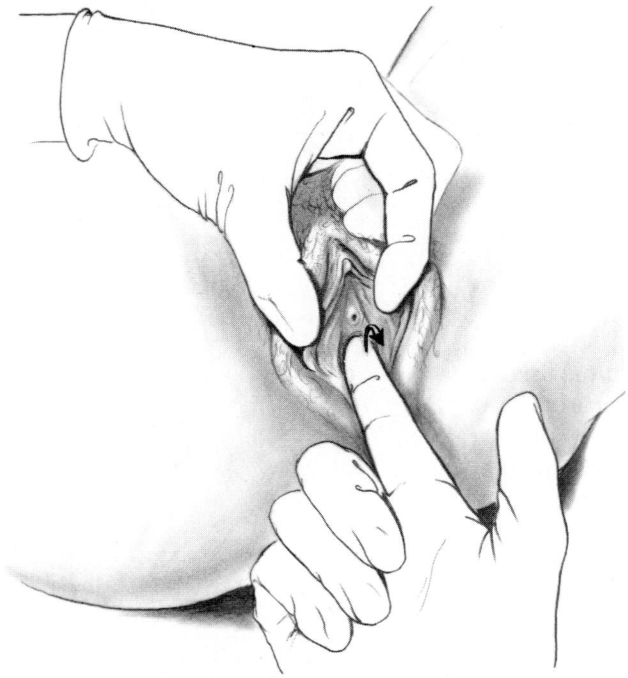

► Figure 22–7

Assess Bartholin's glands. Palpate the posterior parts of the labia majora with your index finger in the vagina and your thumb outside (Fig. 22–8). Normally, the labia feel soft and homogeneous.

Swelling (see Table 22–3).
Induration.
Pain with palpation.
Discharge from duct opening.

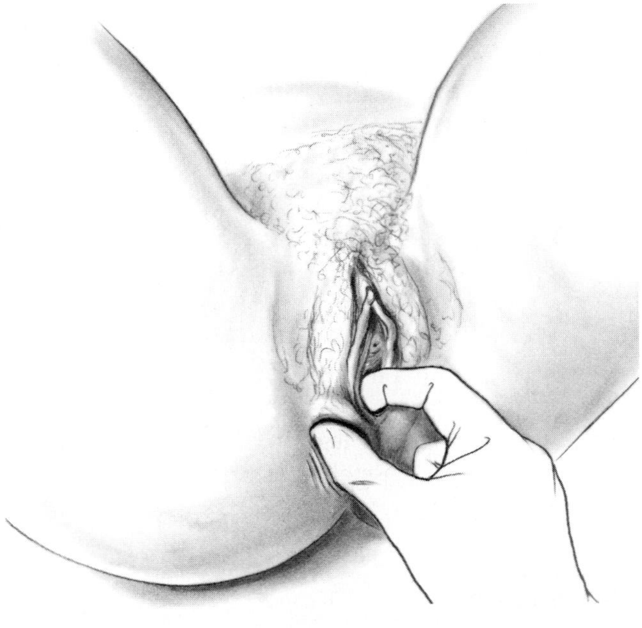

► Figure 22–8

NORMAL RANGE OF FINDINGS	ABNORMAL FINDINGS
Assess the support of pelvic musculature by using these maneuvers:	
1. Palpate the perineum. Normally, it feels thick, smooth, and muscular in the nulliparous woman, and thin and rigid in the multiparous woman.	Tenderness. Paper-thin perineum.
2. Ask the woman to squeeze the vaginal opening around your fingers; it should feel tight in the nulliparous woman and have less tone in the multiparous woman.	Absent or decreased tone may diminish sexual satisfaction.
3. Using your index and middle fingers, separate the vaginal orifice and ask the woman to strain down. Normally, there is no bulging of vaginal walls or urinary incontinence.	Bulging of the vaginal wall indicates cystocele, rectocele, or uterine prolapse (see Table 22-4). Urinary incontinence.

INTERNAL GENITALIA

Speculum Examination

Select the proper-sized speculum. Warm and lubricate the speculum under warm running water. Avoid gell lubricant at this point because it is bacteriostatic and would distort cells in the cytology specimen you will collect.

Hold the speculum in your right hand with the index and the middle fingers surrounding the blades and your thumb under the thumbscrew. This prevents the blades from opening painfully during insertion. With your left index and middle fingers, push the introitus down and open (Fig. 22-9). Tilt the width of the blades obliquely and insert the speculum past your left fingers, applying any pressure downward. This avoids pressure on the anterior vaginal wall and on the sensitive urethra above it.

Ease insertion by asking the woman to bear down. This method relaxes the perineal muscles and opens the introitus. (With experience, you can combine speculum insertion with assessing the support of the vaginal

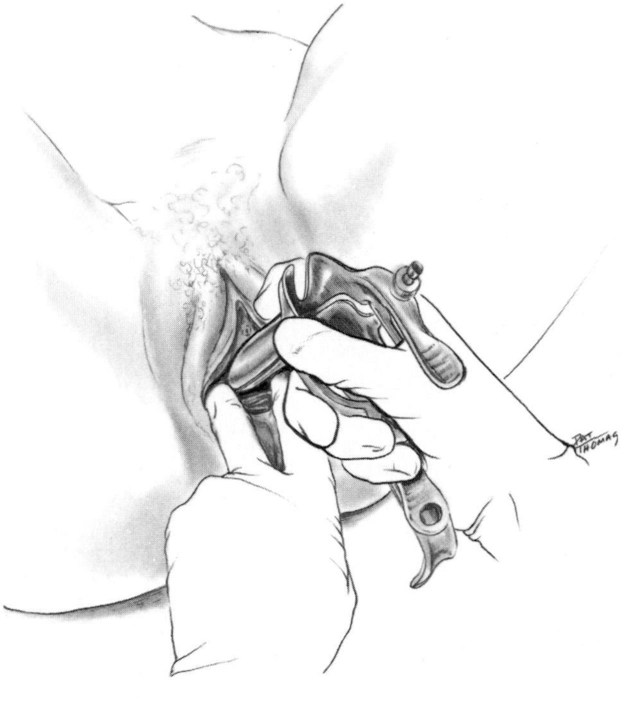

► Figure 22-9

NORMAL RANGE OF FINDINGS

ABNORMAL FINDINGS

muscles.) As the blades pass your left fingers, withdraw your fingers. Now turn the width of the blades horizontally, and continue to insert in a 45-degree angle downward toward the small of the woman's back (Fig. 22–10). This matches the natural slope of the vagina.

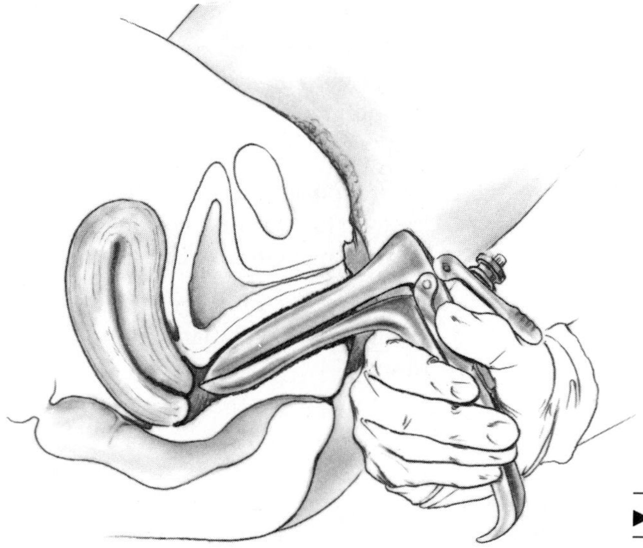

► Figure 22–10

After the blades are fully inserted, open them by squeezing the handles together (Fig. 22–11). The cervix should be in full view. Sometimes this does not occur (especially with beginning examiners). Usually, the

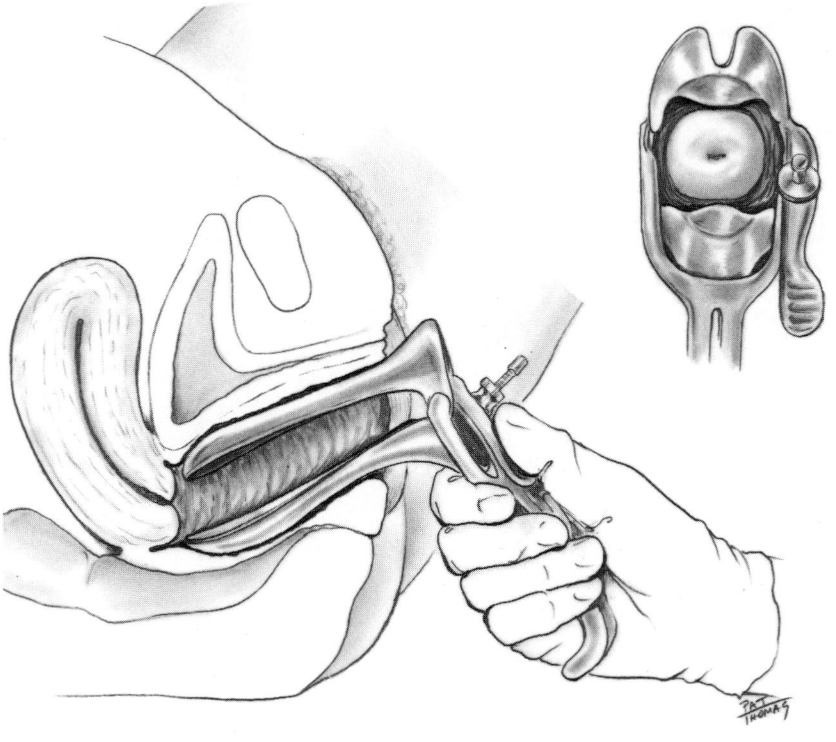

► Figure 22–11

NORMAL RANGE OF FINDINGS	ABNORMAL FINDINGS
blades are angled above the location of the cervix. Try closing the blades, withdrawing about halfway, and reinserting in a more downward plane. Once you have the cervix in full view, lock the blades open by tightening the thumbscrew.	
Inspect the cervix and its os. Note:	
1. Color. Normally the cervical mucosa is pink and even. During the second month of pregnancy it looks blue (Chadwick's sign), and after menopause it is pale.	Redness, inflammation. Pallor with anemia. Cyanotic other than with pregnancy (see Table 22–5).
2. Position. Midline, either anterior or posterior. Projects 1 to 3 cm into the vagina.	Lateral position may be due to adhesion or tumor. Projection of more than 3 cm may be a prolapse.
3. Size. Diameter is 2.5 cm (1 inch).	Hypertrophy of more than 4 cm occurs with inflammation or tumor.

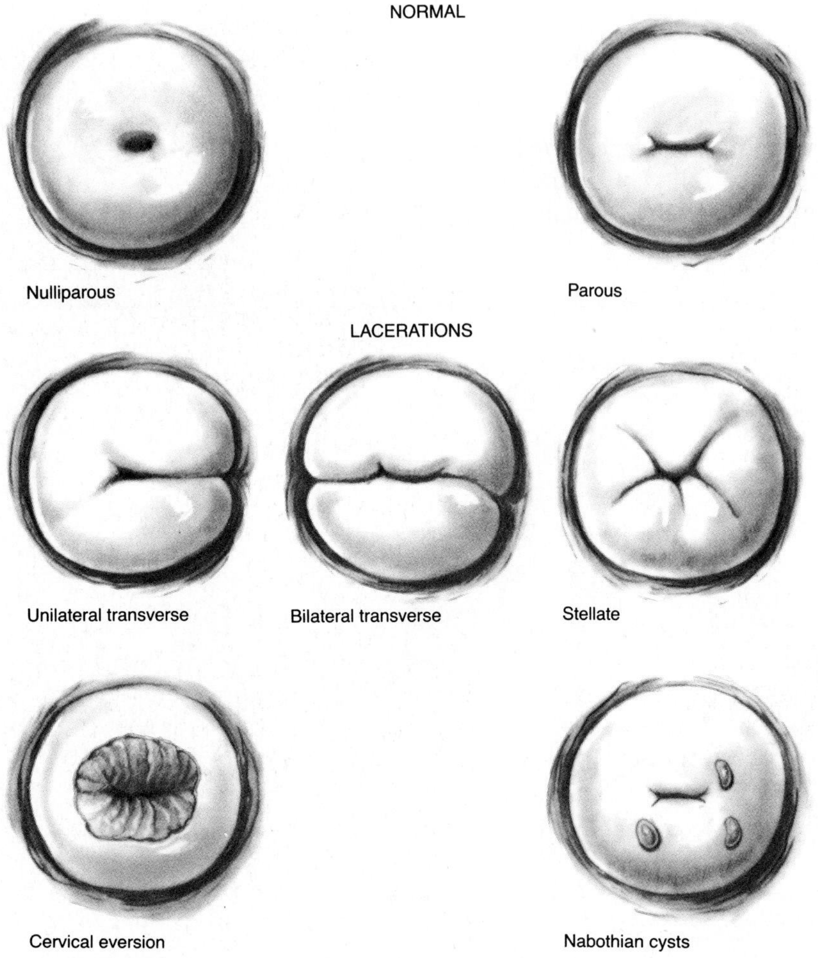

▶ **Figure 22–12**

NORMAL RANGE OF FINDINGS

ABNORMAL FINDINGS

4. Os. This is small and round in the nulliparous woman. In the parous woman, it is a horizontal irregular slit and also may show healed lacerations on the sides (Fig. 22–12).
5. Surface. This is normally smooth but *cervical eversion,* or ectropion, may occur normally after vaginal deliveries. The endocervical canal is everted or "rolled out." It looks like a red, beefy halo inside the pink cervix surrounding the os. It is difficult to distinguish this normal variation from an abnormal condition (e.g., erosion, or carcinoma) and biopsy may be needed.

Surface reddened, granular, and asymmetric, particularly around os.
Friable, bleeds easily.
White patch on cervix.
Strawberry spot.
See erosion, ulceration, and carcinoma (Table 22–5).

Nabothian cysts are benign growths that commonly appear on the cervix after childbirth. They are small, smooth, yellow nodules that may be single or multiple. Less than 1 cm, they are retention cysts due to obstruction of cervical glands.

Cervical polyp—bright red growth protruding from the os (see Table 22–5).

6. Note the cervical secretions. Depending on the day of the menstrual cycle, secretions may be clear and thin, or thick, opaque, and stringy. Always they are odorless and nonirritating.
   If secretions are copious, swab the area with a thick-tipped rectal swab. This method sponges away secretions, and you have a better view of the structures.

Foul-smelling, irritating, with yellow, green, white, or gray discharge (see Table 22–6).

Obtain cervical smears and cultures.

The Papanicolaou, or Pap, smear screens for cervical cancer. Instruct the woman not to douche within 24 hours before collecting the specimens. Laboratories may vary in method, so compare the following procedure with that of your agency. The test consists of three specimens:

Endocervical Swab (Fig. 22–13). Insert a premoistened* cotton applicator into the os, and rotate it 360 degrees. Roll the swab gently on a glass slide to deposit all the cells. Avoid leaving a thick specimen that would be hard to read under the microscope. Immediately spray the slide with fixative to avoid drying.

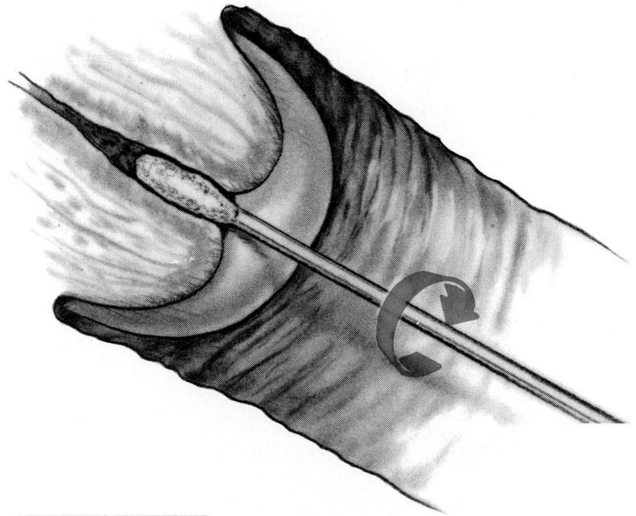

► **Figure 22–13**

* Premoistening the applicator with normal saline prevents the sample cells from being absorbed into the cotton, and it prevents cotton threads from distorting the specimen.

NORMAL RANGE OF FINDINGS

Some examiners use a wire with a small thin brush at the end because it collects a better specimen of endocervical cells (Helderman et al, 1990). The woman may feel a slight pinch when the brush is inserted into the os, and the cervix may respond with scant bleeding.

Cervical Scrape (Fig. 22–14). Insert the bifid end of an Ayre spatula into the vagina with the more pointed bump into the cervical os. Rotate it 360 degrees. The rounded cervix fits snugly into the spatula's groove. The spatula scrapes the surface of the squamocolumnar junction and cervix as you turn the instrument. Spread the specimen from both sides of the spatula onto a glass slide. Use a single stroke to thin out the specimen, not a back-and-forth motion.

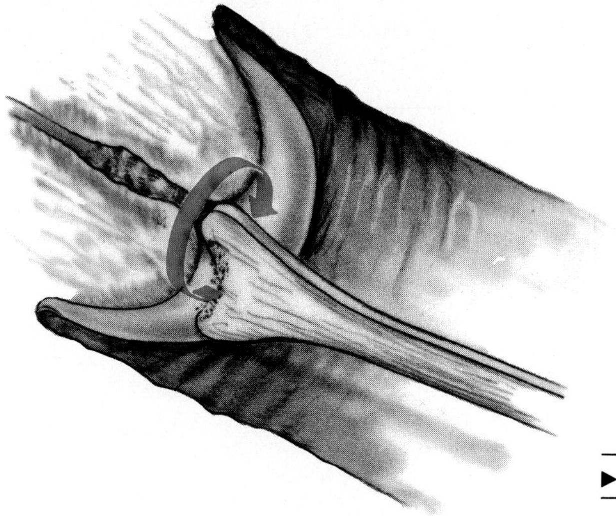

► **Figure 22–14**

Vaginal Pool. Reverse the spatula, and gently rub the blunt end over the vaginal wall under and lateral to the cervix (Fig. 22–15). Wipe the specimen on a slide. If the mucosa is very dry (as in a postmenopausal woman), moisten a sterile swab with normal saline to collect this specimen.

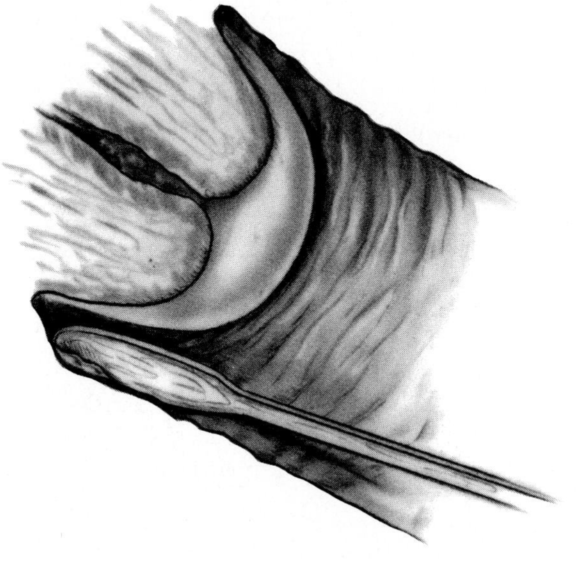

► **Figure 22–15**

ABNORMAL FINDINGS

NORMAL RANGE OF FINDINGS

(For the woman whose cervix has been removed, do a scrape from the end of the vagina and a vaginal pool.)

Immediately (within 15 to 30 seconds) spray the slides with fixative solution or place them in a container of fixative. Label the specimens. Send them to the laboratory with the following necessary data: age of the woman, date of last menstrual period, hormone administration, known infections, previous abnormal cytology. These data are important for accurate interpretation; e.g., a specimen may be interpreted as positive unless the laboratory technicians know the woman has had prior radiation treatment.

If the woman's history indicates, or if you note any abnormal vaginal discharge, obtain a sample to study under the microscope.

Saline Mount, or "Wet Prep." Spread a sample of the discharge onto a glass slide, add one drop of normal saline, and a coverslip.

KOH Prep. To a sample of the discharge on a glass slide, add one drop potassium hydroxide and a coverslip.

Gonorrhea ("GC") Culture. Insert a sterile cotton applicator into the os, rotate it 360 degrees, and leave it in place 10 to 20 seconds for complete saturation. So that all swab surfaces contact the culture medium, gently roll the swab while simultaneously spreading it in a Z pattern onto a Thayer-Martin culture plate (Fig. 22–16). Cover, label, and incubate immediately.

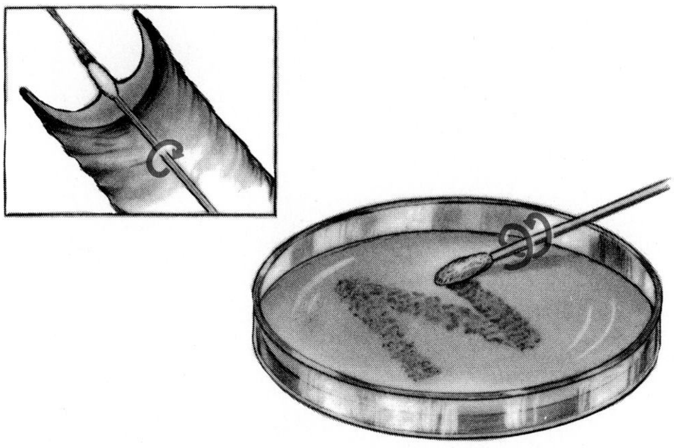

► **Figure 22–16**

Anal Culture. Insert a sterile cotton swab into the anal canal about 1 cm. Rotate it, and move it side to side. Leave in place 10 to 20 seconds. If the swab collects feces, discard it and begin again. Inoculate a culture plate in the Z pattern described above.

Five-Percent Acetic Acid Wash. Acetic acid wash screens for asymptomatic human papilloma virus (HPV), which causes genital warts. After all other specimens are gathered, soak a thick-tipped cotton rectal swab with acetic acid and "paint" the cervix. A normal response (indicating no HPV infection) is no change in the cervical epithelium.

ABNORMAL FINDINGS

Rapid acetowhitening or blanching, especially with irregular borders, suggests HPV infection.

NORMAL RANGE OF FINDINGS	ABNORMAL FINDINGS

Inspect the vaginal wall.

Loosen the thumbscrew but continue to hold the speculum blades open. Slowly withdraw the speculum, rotating it as you go, to fully inspect the vaginal wall. Normally, the wall looks pink, deeply rugated, moist and smooth, and is free of inflammation or lesions. Normal discharge is thin and clear, or opaque and stringy, but always odorless.

Reddened.
Pallor prior to menopause.
Lesions.

Leukoplakia, appears as spot of dried white paint.

Vaginal discharge: Thick, white, and curdlike with candidiasis; profuse, watery, gray-green, and frothy with trichomoniasis; or any gray, green-yellow, white, or foul-smelling discharge (see Table 22–6).

When the blade ends near the vaginal opening, let them close, but be careful not to pinch the mucosa or catch any hairs. Turn the blades obliquely to avoid stretching the opening. Clean the metal speculum and place it in a soaking solution; discard the plastic variety.

Bimanual Examination

Use both hands to palpate the internal genitalia to assess their location, size, and mobility, and to screen for any tenderness or mass. One hand is on the abdomen while the other (often the dominant, more sensitive hand) inserts two fingers into the vagina (Fig. 22–17). It does not matter which you choose as the intravaginal hand; try each way, and settle on the most comfortable method for you.

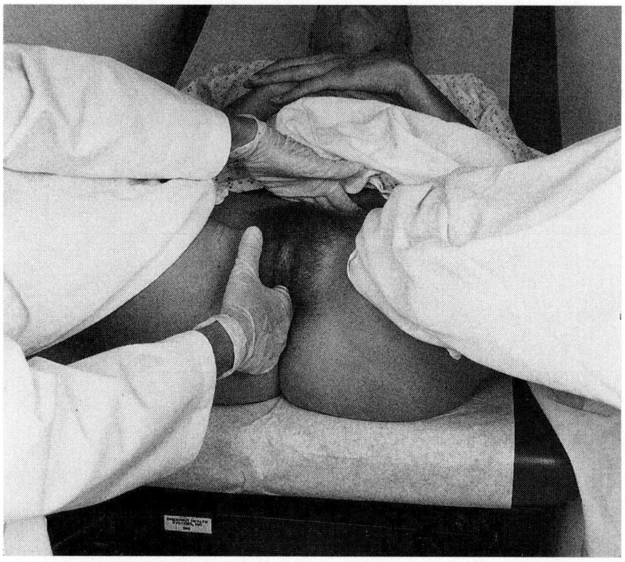

► **Figure 22–17**

Rise to a stand, and have the woman remain in lithotomy position. Glove and lubricate the first two fingers of your intravaginal hand. As-

NORMAL RANGE OF FINDINGS	ABNORMAL FINDINGS
sume the "obstetric" position with the first two fingers extended, the last two flexed onto the palm, and the thumb abducted. Insert your fingers into the vagina, with any pressure directed posteriorly. Wait till the vaginal walls relax, then insert your fingers fully.	
Palpate the vaginal wall. Normally, it feels smooth and has no area of induration or tenderness.	Nodule. Tenderness.
Locate the cervix in the midline, often near the anterior vaginal wall. The cervix points in the opposite direction of the fundus of the uterus. Palpate using the palmar surface of the fingers. Note these characteristics of a normal cervix:	
• Consistency — feels smooth and firm, as the consistency of the tip of the nose. It softens and feels velvety at 5 to 6 weeks of pregnancy (Goodell's sign).	Hard with malignancy. Nodular.
• Contour — evenly rounded.	Irregular.
• Mobility — With a finger on either side, move the cervix gently from side to side. Normally, this produces no pain (Fig. 22–18).	Immobile with malignancy. Painful with inflammation or ectopic pregnancy.
Palpate all around the fornices; the wall should feel smooth.	Nodular. Irregular.

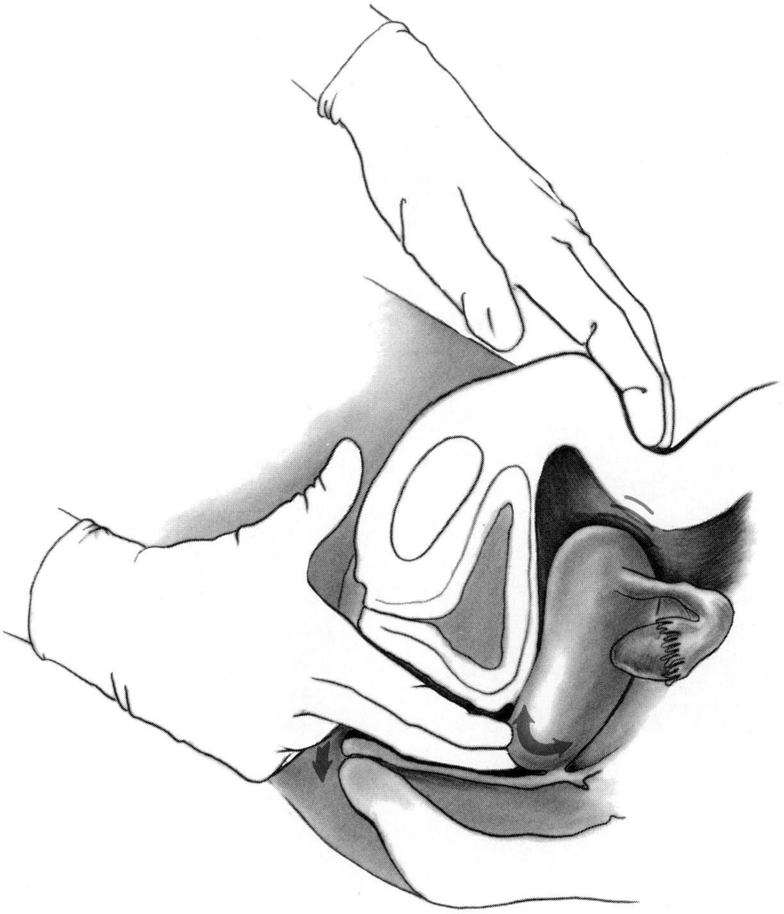

► **Figure 22–18**

NORMAL RANGE OF FINDINGS	ABNORMAL FINDINGS
Next, use your abdominal hand to push the pelvic organs closer for your intravaginal fingers to palpate. Place your hand midway between the umbilicus and the symphysis; push down in a slow, firm manner, fingers together and slightly flexed. Brace the elbow of your pelvic arm against your hip, and keep it horizontal. The woman must be relaxed.	
With your intravaginal fingers in the anterior fornix, assess the uterus. Determine the position, or *version,* of the uterus (Fig. 22–19). This compares the long axis of the uterus with the long axis of the body. In many women, the uterus is anteverted; you palpate it at the level of the pubis with the cervix pointing posteriorly. Two other positions occur normally (midposition and retroverted), as well as two aspects of flexion, where the long axis of the uterus is not straight but is flexed.	
Palpate the uterine wall with your fingers in the fornices. Normally, it feels firm and smooth, with the contour of the fundus rounded. It softens	Enlarged uterus. Lateral displacement.

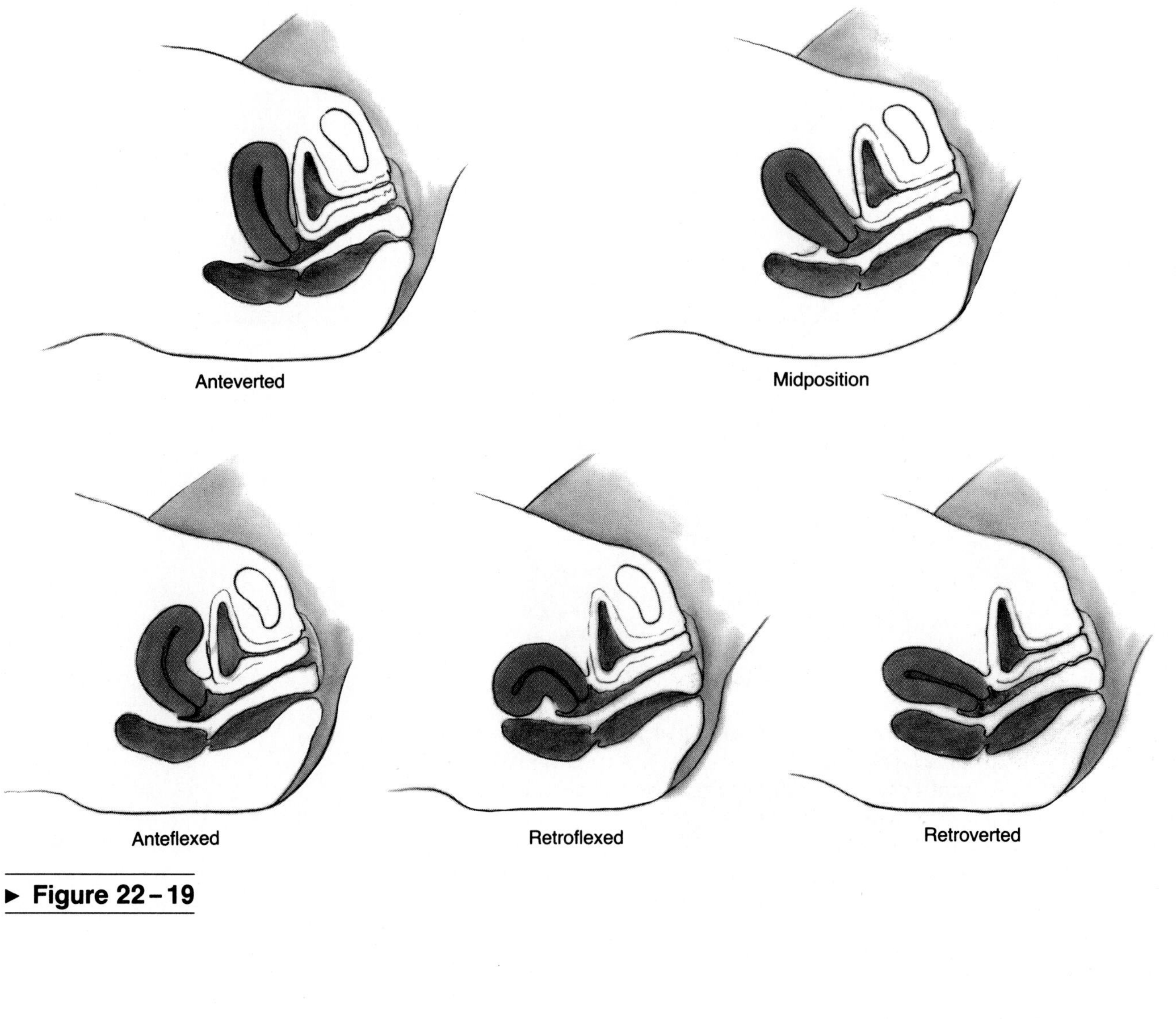

► **Figure 22–19**

NORMAL RANGE OF FINDINGS

during pregnancy. Bounce the uterus gently between your abdominal and intravaginal hand. It should be freely movable and nontender.

Move both hands to the right to explore the adnexa. Place your abdominal hand on the lower quadrant just inside the anterior iliac spine and your intravaginal fingers in the lateral fornix (Fig. 22–20). Push the abdominal hand in and try to capture the ovary. Often, you cannot feel the ovary. When you can, it normally feels smooth, firm, almond shaped, and is highly movable, sliding through the fingers. It is slightly sensitive but not painful. The fallopian tube is not palpable normally. There should be no other mass or pulsation.

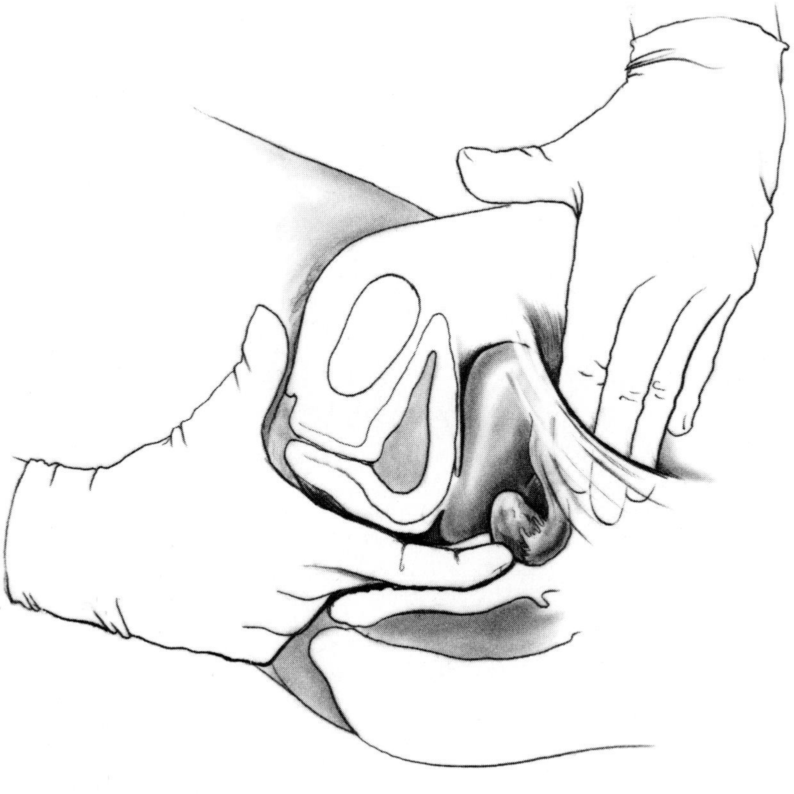

► **Figure 22–20**

A note of caution — normal adnexal structures often are not palpable. Be careful not to mistake an abnormality for a normal structure. To be safe, any mass that you cannot *positively* identify as a normal structure, consider it abnormal and refer the woman for further study.

Move to the left to palpate the other side. Then, withdraw your hand and check secretions on the fingers before discarding the glove. Normal secretions are clear or cloudy and odorless.

ABNORMAL FINDINGS

Nodular mass.
Irregular, asymmetric.
Fixed.
Tenderness.
Enlarged adnexa.
Nodular.
Immobile.
Markedly tender.
Mass.

Pulsation or palpable fallopian tube suggests ectopic pregnancy. Warrants immediate referral.

NORMAL RANGE OF FINDINGS	ABNORMAL FINDINGS

Rectovaginal Examination

Use this technique to assess the rectovaginal septum, posterior uterine wall, cul-de-sac, and rectum. Change gloves to avoid spreading any possible infection. Lubricate the first two fingers. Instruct the woman that this may feel uncomfortable and will mimic the feeling of moving her bowels. Ask her to bear down as you insert your index finger into the vagina and your middle finger gently into the rectum (Fig. 22–21).

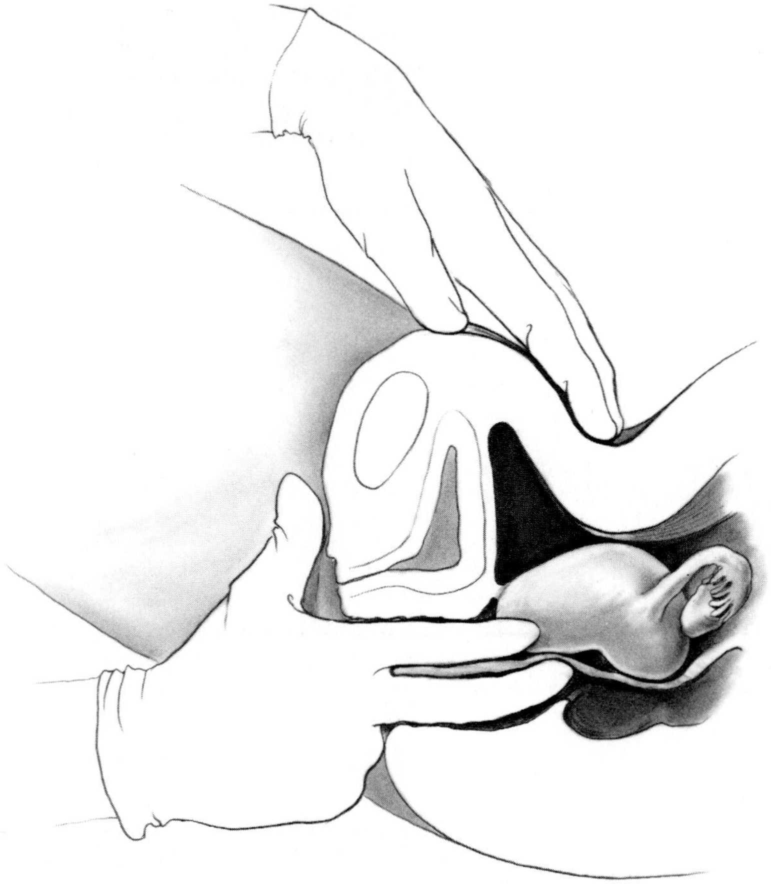

▶ **Figure 22–21**

While pushing with the abdominal hand, repeat the steps of the bimanual examination. Try to keep the intravaginal finger on the cervix so the intrarectal finger does not mistake the cervix for a mass. Note:

- Rectovaginal septum should feel smooth, thin, firm, and pliable.

  Abnormal findings: Nodular; Thickened

- Rectovaginal pouch, or cul-de-sac, is a potential space and usually not palpated.
- Uterine wall and fundus feel firm and smooth.

Rotate the intrarectal finger to check the rectal wall and anal sphincter tone. (See Chapter 23 for Assessment of Anus and Rectum.) Check your gloved finger as you withdraw; test any adherent stool for occult blood.

NORMAL RANGE OF FINDINGS

Give the woman tissues to wipe the area and help her up. Remind her to slide her hips back from the edge before sitting up so she will not fall.

DEVELOPMENTAL CONSIDERATIONS

Infants and Children

Preparation

Infant — place on examination table.

Toddler/Preschooler — place on parent's lap.

Frog-leg position — hips flexed, soles of feet together and up to bottom.

Preschool child may want to separate her own labia.

No drapes — the young girl wants to see what you are doing.

School-aged child — place on examination table, frog-leg position, no drapes.

Adolescent — place on examination table, frog-leg position for examination of external genitalia.

Lithotomy position should be used if internal pelvic examination is warranted.

Drape — see discussion, p. 840.

During childhood, a routine screening is limited to inspection of the external genitalia to determine that (1) the structures are intact, (2) the vagina is present, and (3) the hymen is patent.

The newborn's genitalia are somewhat engorged. The labia majora are swollen, the labia minora are prominent and protrude beyond the labia majora, the clitoris looks relatively large, and the hymen appears thick. Because of transient engorgement, the vaginal opening is more difficult to see now than it will be later. Place your thumbs on the labia majora. Push laterally while pushing the perineum down, and try to note the vaginal opening above the hymenal ring. Do not palpate the clitoris because it is very sensitive.

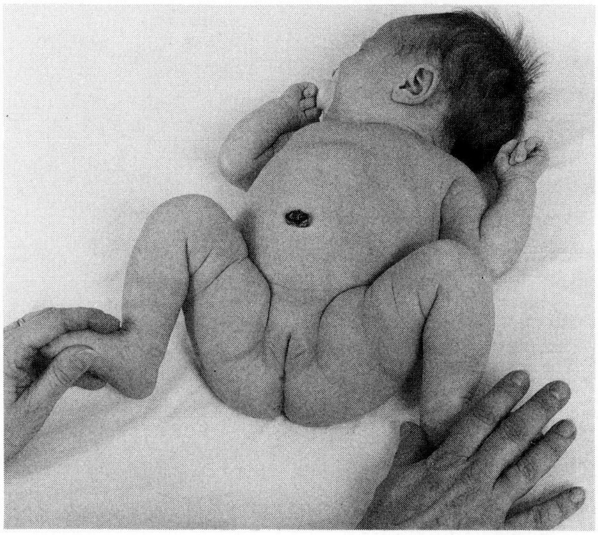

► **Figure 22-22**

ABNORMAL FINDINGS

Ambiguous genitalia are rare but are suggested by a markedly enlarged clitoris, fusion of the labia (resembling scrotum), palpable mass in fused labia (resembling testes).

Imperforate hymen warrants referral.

NORMAL RANGE OF FINDINGS	ABNORMAL FINDINGS
A sanguineous vaginal discharge and/or leukorrhea (mucoid discharge) are normal during the first few weeks because of the maternal estrogen effect. (This also may cause transient breast engorgement and secretion.) During the early weeks, the genital engorgement resolves, and the labia minora atrophy and remain small until puberty (Fig. 22–22).	Lesions, rash.
Between the ages of 2 months and 7 years, the labia majora are flat, the labia minora are thin, the clitoris is relatively small, and the hymen is tissue-paper thin. Normally, there is no irritation or foul-smelling discharge.	Poor perineal hygiene. Pest inhabitants. Excoriations. During and after toddler age, foul-smelling discharge occurs with lodging of foreign body, pinworms, or infection.
In the young school-age girl (7 to 10 years), the mons pubis thickens, the labia majora thicken, and the labia minora become slightly rounded. Pubic hair appears beginning around age 11, although sparse pubic hair may occur as early as age 8 years. Normally, the hymen is perforate.	Absence of pubic hair by 13 years indicates delayed puberty. Amenorrhea in adolescent, together with bluish and bulging hymen, indicates imperforate hymen and warrants referral.
Almost always in these age groups, an external examination will suffice. If needed, an internal pelvic examination is best performed by a pediatric gynecologist using specialized instruments.	

Adolescent

The adolescent girl has special needs during the genitalia examination. Examine her alone, without the mother present. Assure her of privacy and confidentiality. Allow plenty of time for health education and discussion of pubertal progress. Assess her growth velocity, menstrual history, and use the sex maturity rating (SMR) charts to teach breast and pubic hair development. Assure her that increased vaginal fluid (physiologic *leukorrhea*) is normal because of the estrogen effect.

A pelvic examination is indicated when contraception is desired, when the girl's sexual activity includes intercourse, or at age 18 years in virgins. Periodic Papanicolaou smears also are started when intercourse begins. Although the techniques of the examination are listed in the adult section earlier, you will need to provide additional time and psychological support for the adolescent having her first pelvic examination.

The experience of the first pelvic examination determines how the adolescent will approach future care. Your accepting attitude and gentle, unhurried approach are important. You have a unique teaching opportunity here. Take the time to teach, using the girl's own body as illustration. Your frank discussion of anatomy and sexual behavior communicates that these topics are acceptable to discuss and not taboo with health care providers. This affirms the girl's self-concept.

During the bimanual examination, note that the adnexa are not palpable in the adolescent.

Abnormal finding: Pelvic or adnexal mass.

The Pregnant Female

Depending on the week of gestation of the pregnancy, inspection shows the enlarging abdomen (Fig. 22–23). The height of the fundus ascends

NORMAL RANGE OF FINDINGS

ABNORMAL FINDINGS

gradually as the fetus grows. At 16 weeks, the fundus is palpable halfway between the symphysis and umbilicus; at 20 weeks, at the lower edge of the umbilicus; at 28 weeks, halfway between the umbilicus and the xiphoid; and at 34 to 36 weeks, almost to the xiphoid. Then close to term, the fundus drops as the fetal head engages in the pelvis.

The external genitalia show hyperemia of the perineum and vulva because of increased vascularity. Varicose veins may be visible in the labia

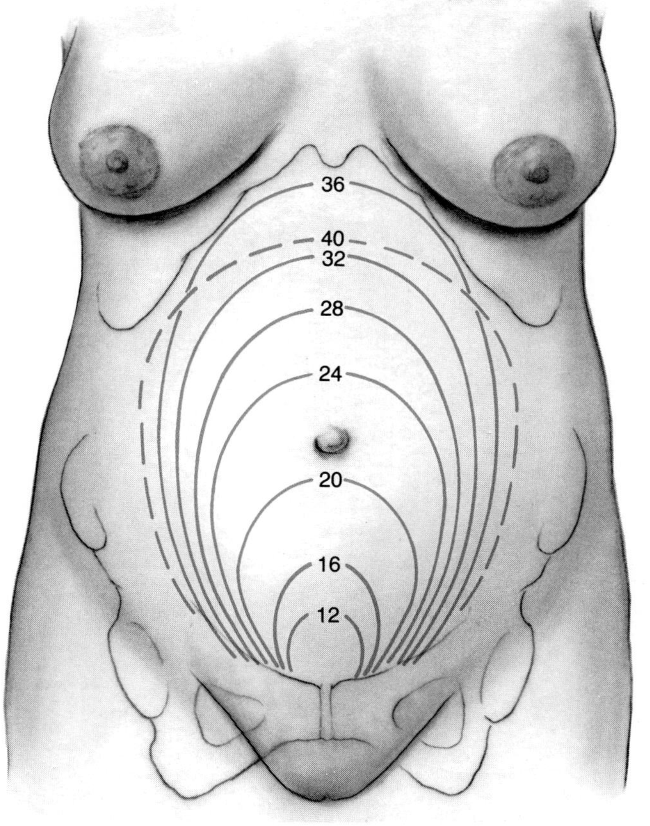

▶ **Figure 22-23**

or legs. Hemorrhoids may show around the anus. Both are caused by interruption in venous return from the pressure of the fetus.

Internally, the walls of the vagina appear violet or blue (Chadwick's sign) owing to hyperemia. The vaginal walls are deeply rugated and the vaginal mucosa thickens. The cervix looks blue, feels velvety, and feels softer than in the nonpregnant state, making it a bit more difficult to differentiate from the vaginal walls.

During bimanual examination, the isthmus of the uterus feels softer and is more easily compressed between your two hands (Hegar's sign). The fundus balloons between your two hands; it feels connected to, but distinct from, the cervix because the isthmus is so soft.

NORMAL RANGE OF FINDINGS	ABNORMAL FINDINGS
Search the adnexal area carefully during early pregnancy. Normally, the adnexal structures are not palpable.	An ectopic pregnancy has serious consequences (see Table 22–8).

The Aging Adult

Natural lubrication is decreased; to avoid a painful examination, take care to lubricate instruments and the examining hand adequately.

Menopause and the resulting decrease in estrogen production shows numerous physical changes. Pubic hair gradually decreases, becoming thin and sparse in later years. Fat deposits decrease, leaving the mons pubis smaller and the labia flatter. Clitoris size also decreases after age 60.

Internally, the rugae of the vaginal walls decrease, and the walls look pale pink because of the thinned epithelium. The cervix shrinks and looks pale and glistening. It may retract, appearing to be flush with the vaginal wall. In some, it is hard to distinguish the cervix from the surrounding vaginal mucosa. Alternately, the cervix may protrude into the vagina if the uterus has prolapsed.

With the bimanual examination, the uterus feels smaller and firmer, and the ovaries are not palpable normally.

☑ SUMMARY CHECKLIST

1 ▶ Inspect external genitalia.
2 ▶ Palpate labia, Skene's and Bartholin's glands.
3 ▶ Using vaginal speculum, inspect cervix and vagina.
4 ▶ Obtain specimens for cytologic study.
5 ▶ Perform bimanual examination: cervix, uterus, adnexa.
6 ▶ Perform rectovaginal examination.
7 ▶ Test stool for occult blood.

SAMPLE RECORDING

Subjective

- Menarche age 12, cycle usually q 28 days, duration 5 days, flow moderate, no dysmenorrhea, LMP April 3. Gravida 0/Para 0/Abortion 0. Gyne checkups yearly. Last Pap test 1 year PTA, negative. No urinary problems, no irritating or foul-smelling vaginal discharge, no sores or lesions, no history pelvic surgery. Satisfied with sexual relationship with husband, uses vaginal diaphragm for birth control, no plans for pregnancy at this time. Aware of no STD contact to self or husband.

Objective

- External genitalia — no swelling, lesions or discharge. No urethral swelling or discharge. Internal — vaginal walls have no bulging or lesions, cervix pink with no lesions, scant clear mucoid discharge. Bimanual — no pain on moving cervix, uterus anteflexed and anteverted, no enlargement or irregularity. Adnexa — ovaries not enlarged. Rectal — no hemorrhoids, fissure or lesions, no masses or tenderness, stool brown with guaiac test negative.

SAMPLE CLINICAL PROBLEM 1

J.K, 27-year-old, white, married, newspaper reporter, Grav 0/Para 0/Ab 0. Presents at clinic with "urinary burning, vaginal itching, and discharge × 4 days."

Subjective

- 3 weeks PTA: Treated at clinic for bronchitis with erythromycin. Improved within 5 days. 4 to 5 days PTA: noted burning on urination, intense vaginal itching, thick, white, "smelly" discharge. Warm water douche — no relief.
  No previous history vaginal infection, urinary tract infection, or pelvic surgery. Monogamous sexual relationship, has used low-estrogen birth control pills for 3 years with no side effects.

Objective

- Vulva and vagina erythematous and edematous. Thick, white, curdlike discharge clinging to vaginal walls. Cervix pink, no lesions. Bimanual examination — no pain on palpating cervix, uterus not enlarged, ovaries not enlarged.
  Specimens: Pap smear, *Chlamydia* to lab. KOH prep shows mycelia and spores of *Candida albicans.*

Assessment

- Candida vaginitis
  Pain R/T infectious process

SAMPLE CLINICAL PROBLEM 2

Brenda, 17-year-old, white, high school student, comes to clinic for pelvic examination.

Subjective

- Menarche 12 years, cycle q. 30 days, duration 6 days, mild cramps relieved by acetaminophen. LMP March 10. No dysuria, vaginal discharge, vaginal itching. Relationship involving intercourse with one boyfriend for 8 months PTA. For birth control boyfriend uses condoms "sometimes." Wants to start birth control pills. Never had pelvic examination. No knowledge of breast self-examination. No knowledge of STDs except AIDS. Smokes cigarettes, 1/2 PPD, started age 11.

Objective

- Breasts—symmetric, no lesions or discharge, palpation reveals no mass or tenderness. External genitalia—No redness, lesions or discharge. Internal genitalia—vaginal walls and cervix pink with no lesions or discharge. Specimens obtained. Acetic acid wash shows no acetowhitening. Bimanual—no tenderness to palpation, uterus anteverted with no enlargement, ovaries not enlarged. Rectum—no masses, fissure, or tenderness. Stool brown and guaiac test negative.
  Specimens—GC, *Chlamydia,* Pap smear to lab.

Assessment

- Normal breast and pelvic examination.
  Knowledge deficit regarding: breast self-examination; birth control measures; STD prevention; cigarette smoking R/T lack of exposure.

NURSING DIAGNOSES COMMONLY ASSOCIATED WITH THE FEMALE GENITALIA AND RELATED DISORDERS

Diagnosis	Related Factors (Etiology)	Defining Characteristics (Symptoms and Signs)
Sexual dysfunction	Depression Disturbance in self-esteem or body image Lack of significant other Lack of privacy Effects of actual or perceived limitation imposed by disease and/or therapy Substance abuse	Decreased or absent sexual desire Impotence Delayed development of secondary sex characteristics Sexual promiscuity Exhibitionism Guilt Alterations in achieving perceived sex role or sexual satisfaction

Diagnosis	Related Factors (Etiology)	Defining Characteristics (Symptoms and Signs)
	Physical or psychosocial abuse Dysfunctional interpersonal relationships Ineffective or absent role models Failure to identify satisfactorily with same-sex parent Cultural norms regarding male/female roles Values conflict Knowledge deficit	Verbalization about the problem Conflicts involving values Change in interest in self and others Seeking confirmation of desirability Voyeurism Transsexualism Transvestism Masochism/sadism
Functional incontinence	Deficits Cognitive Motor Sensory Altered environment	Unpredictable voiding pattern Unrecognized signals of bladder fullness Urge to void or bladder contractions sufficiently strong to result in loss of urine before reaching an appropriate site or receptacle
Rape-trauma response	Rape event	ACUTE PHASE Emotional reactions Anger Crying Overcontrol Panic Denial Self-blame Emotional shock Embarrassment Fear of being alone Humiliation Fear of physical violence and death Mistrust of the opposite sex Desire for revenge Change in sexual behavior

Diagnosis	Related Factors (Etiology)	Defining Characteristics (Symptoms and Signs)

		Multiple physical symptoms
		  Muscle tension
		  Pain
		  Sleep pattern disturbance
		  Gastrointestinal irritability
		  Genitourinary discomfort
		LONG-TERM PHASE
		Mentally reliving rape
		Depression
		Loss of self-confidence
		Changes in lifestyle
		  Changes in residence
		  Dealing with repetitive nightmares and phobias
		Anxiety
		Ambivalence about own sexuality

Other related nursing diagnoses
  Impaired skin integrity (see Chapters 9 and 21)
  Altered sexuality patterns (see Chapter 21)
  Stress incontinence
  Reflex incontinence
  Total incontinence
  Urge incontinence		

ABNORMAL FINDINGS

Table 22-3 ► Abnormalities of the External Genitalia

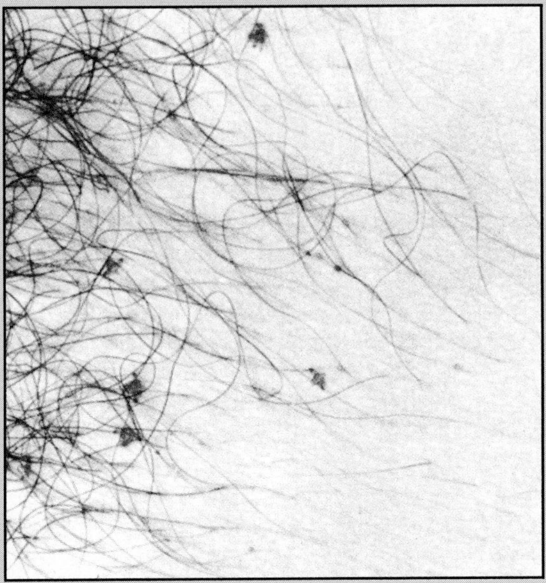

PEDICULOSIS PUBIS (CRAB LICE)

S: Severe perineal itching.
O: Excoriations and erythematous areas. May see little dark spots (lice are small), nits (eggs) adherent to pubic hair near roots. Usually localized in pubic hair, occasionally in eyebrows or eyelashes.

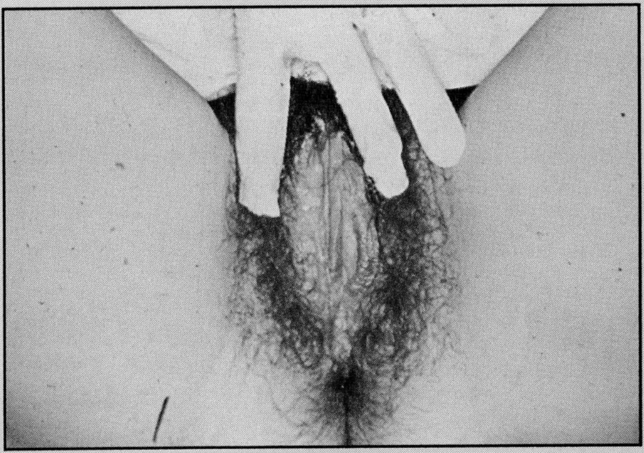

HERPES PROGENITALIS*

S: Episodes of local pain, dysuria, fever.
O: Clusters of small, shallow vesicles with surrounding erythema; erupt on genital areas and inner thigh. Also, inguinal adenopathy, edema. Initial infection lasts 7–10 days. Virus remains dormant indefinitely; recurrent infections last 3 to 10 days with milder symptoms.

S, subjective data; O, objective data.

Table continued on following page

Table 22-3 ▸ Abnormalities of the External Genitalia *Continued*

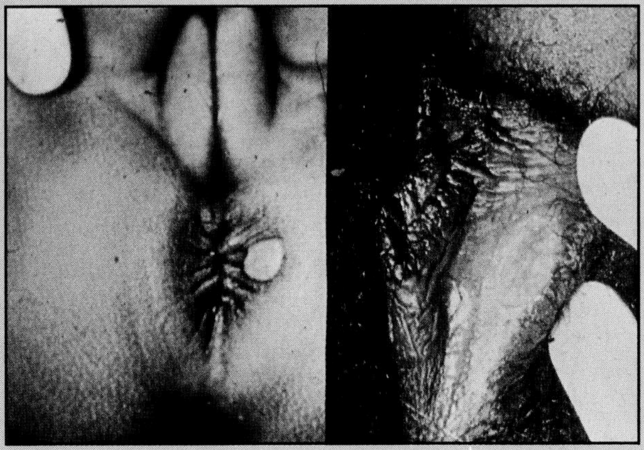

SYPHILITIC CHANCRE*

O: Begins as a small, solitary silvery papule that erodes to a red, round or oval, superficial ulcer with a yellowish serous discharge. Palpation—nontender indurated base; can be lifted like a button between thumb and finger. Nontender inguinal lymphadenopathy.

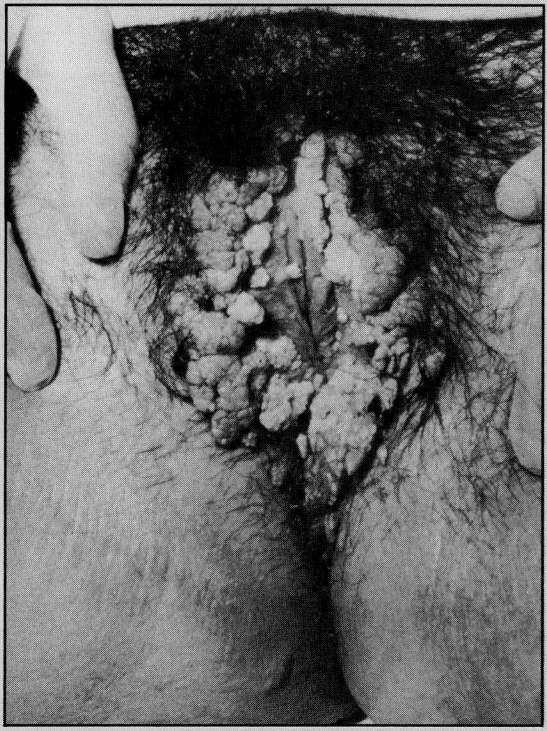

CONDYLOMATA ACUMINATA (VENEREAL WARTS)*

O: Pink or flesh-colored, soft, pointed, moist, warty papules. Single or multiple in a cauliflower-like patch. Occur around vulva, introitus, anus, vagina, cervix.

URETHRAL CARUNCLE (not illustrated)

S: Tender, painful with urination, dyspareunia.
O: Small, deep red mass protruding from meatus; usually secondary to urethritis or skenitis; lesion may bleed on contact.

URETHRITIS (not illustrated)

S: Dysuria.
O: Palpation of anterior vaginal wall shows tenderness, induration along urethra, purulent discharge from meatus. Caused by gonococcal or nongonococcal infection.

S, subjective data; O, objective data.

Table 22-3 ► Abnormalities of the External Genitalia *Continued*

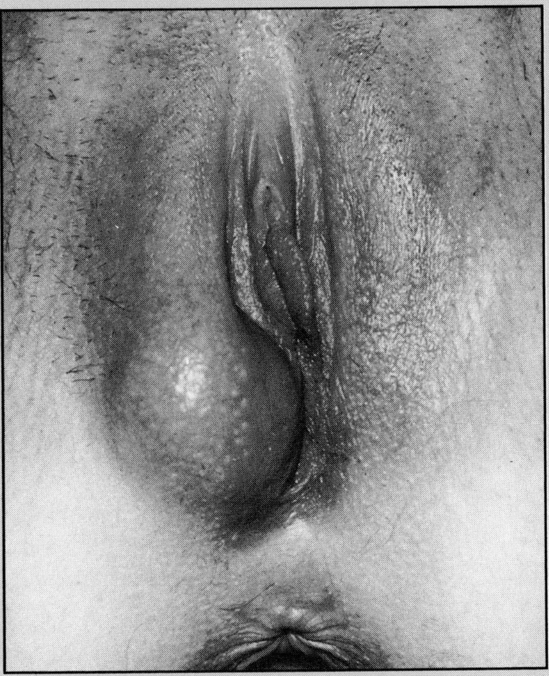

ABSCESS OF BARTHOLIN'S GLAND

S: Local pain, can be severe.
O: Overlying skin red and hot. Posterior part of labia swollen; palpable fluctuant mass and tenderness. Mucosa shows red spot at site of duct opening; can express purulent discharge. Often secondary to gonococcal infection.*

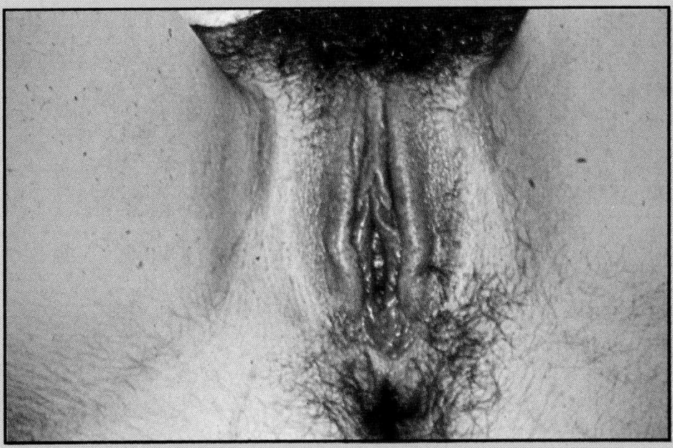

RED RASH—CONTACT DERMATITIS

S: History of skin contact with allergenic substance in environment, intense pruritus.
O: Primary lesion—red, swollen, vesicles. Then may have weeping of lesions, crusts, scales, thickening of skin, excoriations from scratching. May result from reaction to feminine hygiene spray or synthetic underclothing.

---

* This condition is a sexually transmitted disease (STD). The classic term, *venereal disease,* a disease transmitted only by sexual intercourse, now is obsolete. A broader category, sexually transmitted diseases, includes all conditions that are *usually* or *can be* transmitted during sexual intercourse or intimate sexual contact with an infected partner. Although not inclusive of all STDs, the conditions described in this table encompass more common conditions.

S, subjective data; O, objective data.

Table 22-4 ▸ Abnormalities of Pelvic Musculature

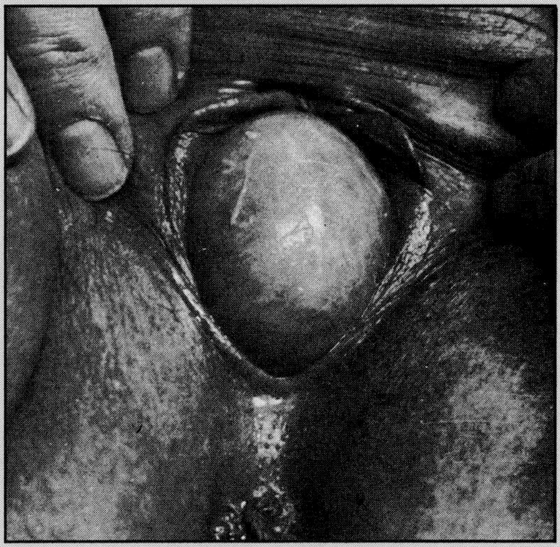

CYSTOCELE

S: Feeling of pressure in vagina, stress incontinence.
O: With straining or standing, note introitus widening and the presence of a soft, round anterior bulge. The bladder, covered by vaginal mucosa, prolapses into vagina.

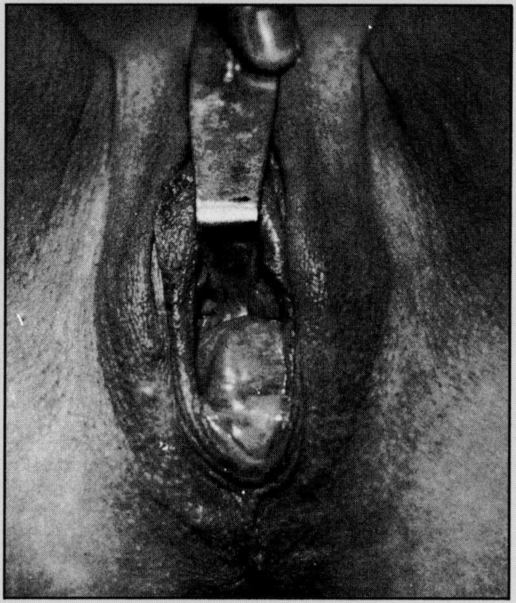

RECTOCELE

S: Feeling of pressure in vagina, possibly constipation.
O: With straining or standing, note introitus widening and the presence of a soft, round bulge from posterior. Here, part of the rectum, covered by vaginal mucosa, prolapses into vagina.

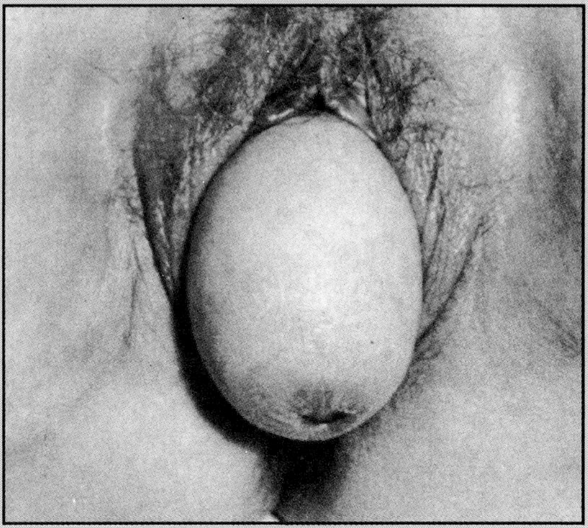

UTERINE PROLAPSE

O: With straining or standing, uterus protrudes into vagina. Prolapse is graded: first degree, cervix appears at introitus with straining; second degree, cervix bulges outside introitus with straining; third degree, whole uterus protrudes even without straining, essentially uterus is inside out.

ENTEROCELE (not illustrated)

O: With straining a bulge appears from posterior fornix, as cul-de-sac (pouch of Douglas) protrudes into the vagina.

S, subjective data; O, objective data.

Table 22-5 ▶ Abnormalities of the Cervix

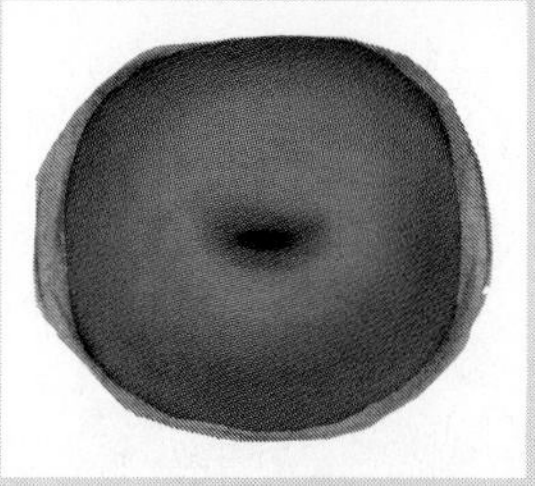

BLUISH CERVIX—CYANOSIS

O: Bluish discoloration of the mucosa occurs normally in pregnancy (Chadwick's sign at 6 to 8 weeks' gestation), and with any other condition causing hypoxia or venous congestion, e.g., congestive heart failure, pelvic tumor.

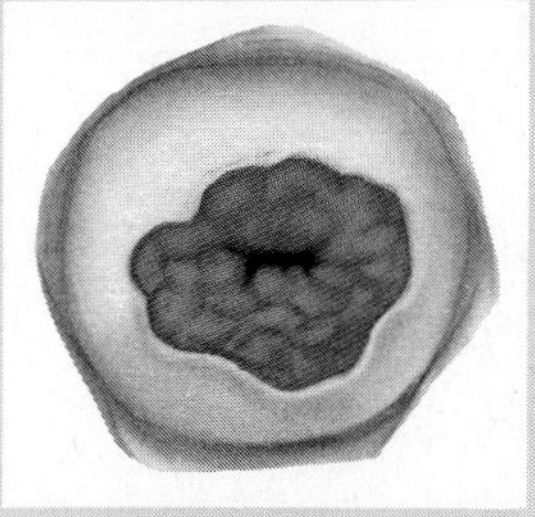

EROSION

O: Cervical lips inflamed and eroded. Reddened granular surface is superficial inflammation, with no ulceration (loss of tissue). Usually secondary to purulent or mucopurulent cervical discharge. Biopsy needed to distinguish erosion from carcinoma; cannot rely on inspection.

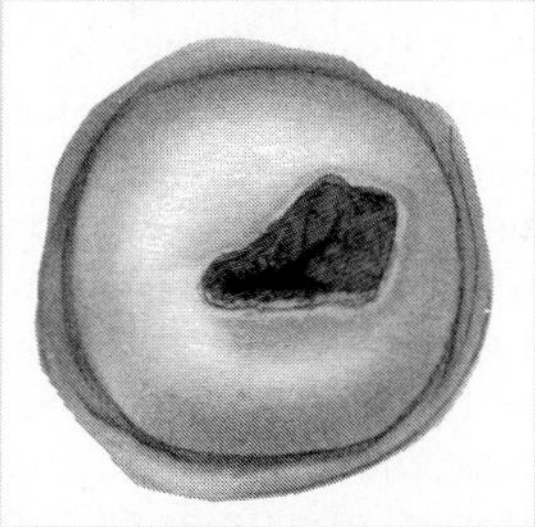

ULCERATION

O: Reddened ulcerated area with loss of both epithelium and underlying tissue. Due to local trauma, syphilis, tuberculosis, carcinoma.

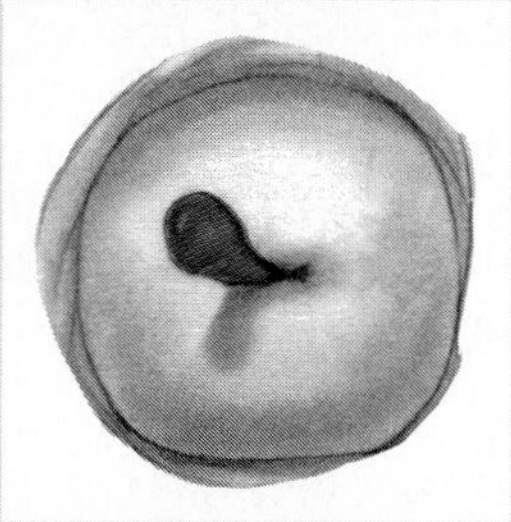

POLYP

S: May have mucoid discharge or bleeding.
O: Bright red, soft, pedunculated growth emerges from os. It is a benign lesion.

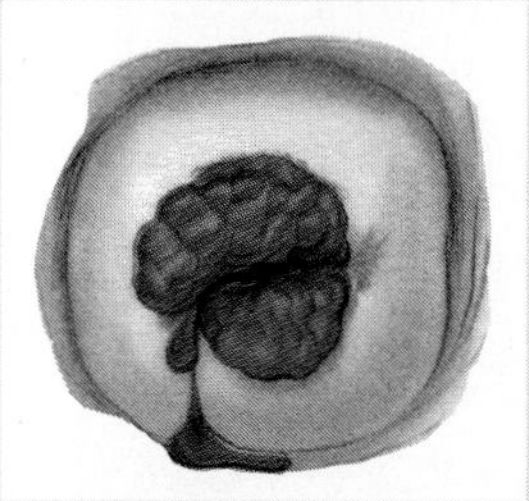

CARCINOMA

S: Bleeding between menstrual periods or after menopause, unusual vaginal discharge.
O: Chronic ulcer and induration are early signs of carcinoma, although the lesion may or may not show on the exocervix. Diagnosed by Papanicolaou smear and biopsy. Risk factors for cervical cancer are early age at first intercourse, multiple sex partners, cigarette smoking, certain STDs.

DIETHYLSTILBESTROL (DES) SYNDROME

S: Prenatal exposure to DES causes cervical and vaginal abnormalities.
O: Red, granular patches of columnar epithelium extend beyond normal squamocolumnar junction onto cervix, and into fornices (vaginal adenosis). Also cervical abnormalities: circular groove, transverse ridge, protuberant anterior lip, "cockscomb" formation. Warrants monitoring by physician.

S, subjective data; O, objective data.

Table 22-6 ► Vulvovaginal Inflammations

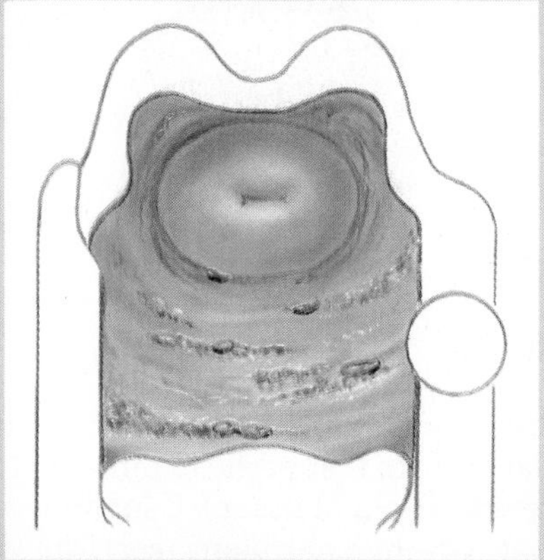

ATROPHIC VAGINITIS

S: Postmenopausal vaginal itching, dryness, burning sensation, dyspareunia, mucoid discharge (may be flecked with blood).

O: Pale mucosa with abraded areas that bleed easily; may have bloody discharge. Related to chronic estrogen deficiency.

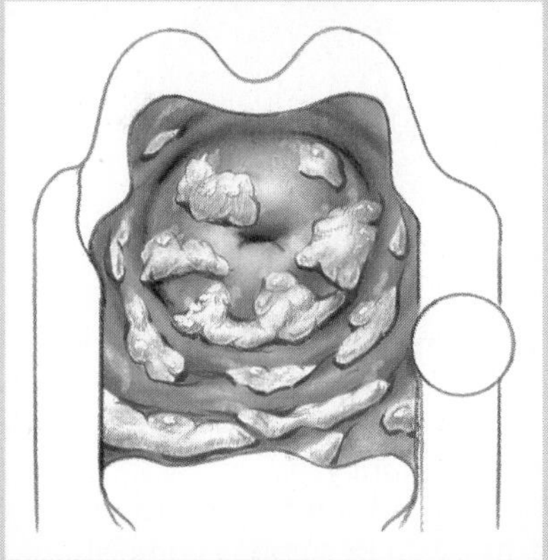

CANDIDIASIS (MONILIASIS)

S: Intense pruritus, thick whitish discharge.

O: Vulva and vagina are erythematous and edematous. Discharge is usually thick, white, curdy, like "cottage cheese." Diagnose by microscopic examination of discharge on KOH wet mount.

Predisposing causes—use of oral contraceptives or antibiotics, more alkaline vaginal pH (as with menstrual periods, post partum, menopause), also pregnancy from increased glycogen and diabetes.

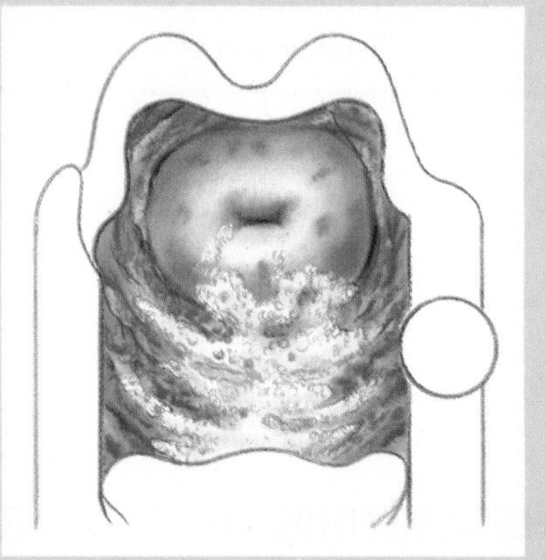

TRICHOMONIASIS*

S: Pruritus, watery and often malodorous vaginal discharge, urinary frequency, terminal dysuria.

O: Vulva may be erythematous. Vagina diffusely red, granular, occasionally with red raised papules and petechiae ("strawberry" appearance). Frothy, yellow-green, foul-smelling discharge. Microscopic examination of saline wet mount specimen shows characteristic flagellated cells.

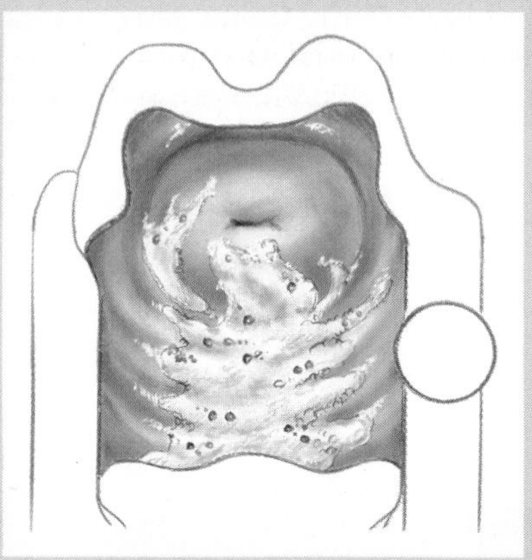

BACTERIAL VAGINOSIS *(GARDNERELLA VAGINALIS* or *HAEMOPHILUS VAGINALIS)**

S: Profuse discharge, "constant wetness" with "foul, fishy, rotten" odor.

O: Thin, creamy, gray-white, malodorous discharge. No inflammation on vaginal wall or cervix because this is a surface parasite. Microscopic view of saline wet mount specimen shows typical "clue cells."

Table 22-6 ▸ Vulvovaginal Inflammations *Continued*

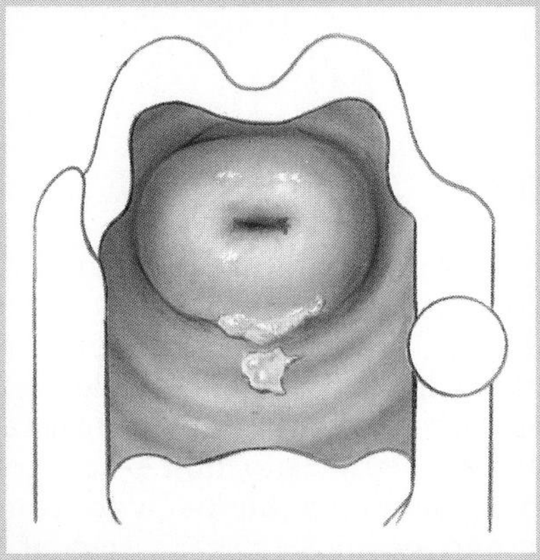

CHLAMYDIA*

S: (Mimics gonorrhea) Urinary frequency, dysuria in some, vaginal discharge, often mild or asymptomatic.

O: Signs are subtle, easily mistaken for gonorrhea. Important to distinguish because antibiotic treatment is different; if wrong drug is given or if the condition is untreated, chlamydia can spread through the reproductive tract causing sterility. Disease is widespread; it is the most prevalent of all STDs.

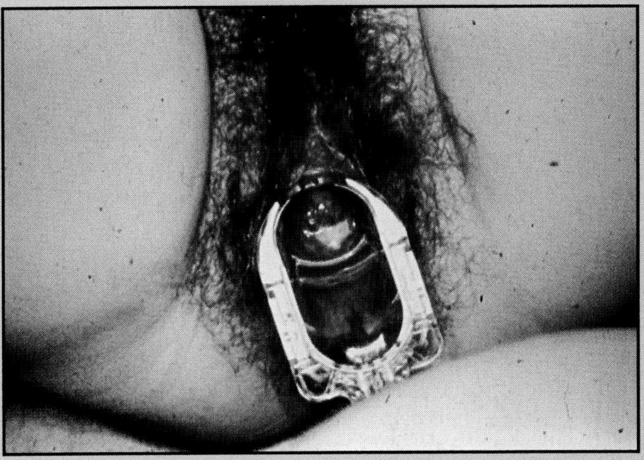

GONORRHEA*

S: Variable: vaginal discharge, dysuria, abscess in Bartholin's or Skene's glands; the majority are asymptomatic.

O: Often no signs are apparent. May have purulent vaginal discharge. Diagnose by positive culture of organism. If the condition is untreated, it may progress to acute salpingitis, pelvic inflammatory disease (PID).

---

* This condition is considered an *STD*.

S, subjective data; O, objective data.

Table 22-7 ▸ Conditions of Uterine Enlargement

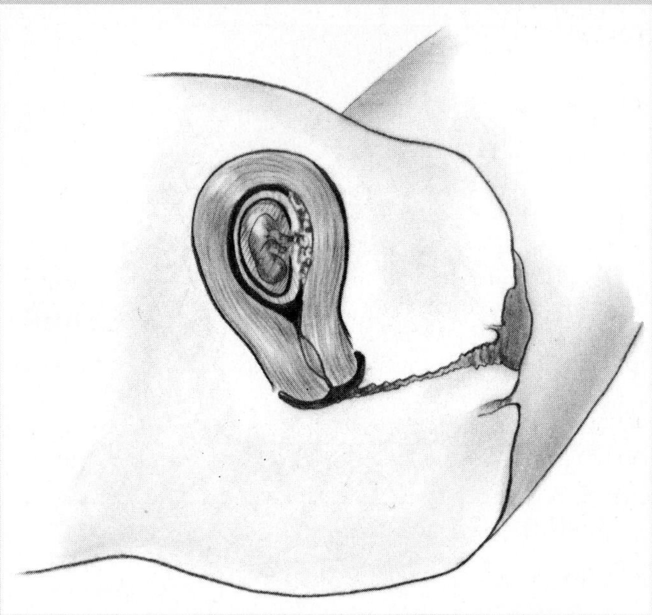

PREGNANCY

Obviously a normal condition, pregnancy is included here for comparison.

S: Amenorrhea, fatigue, breast engorgement, nausea, change in food tolerance, weight gain.

O: Early signs: cyanosis of vaginal mucosa and cervix (Chadwick's sign). Palpation—soft consistency of cervix, enlarging uterus with compressible fundus and isthmus (Hegar's sign at 10 to 12 weeks).

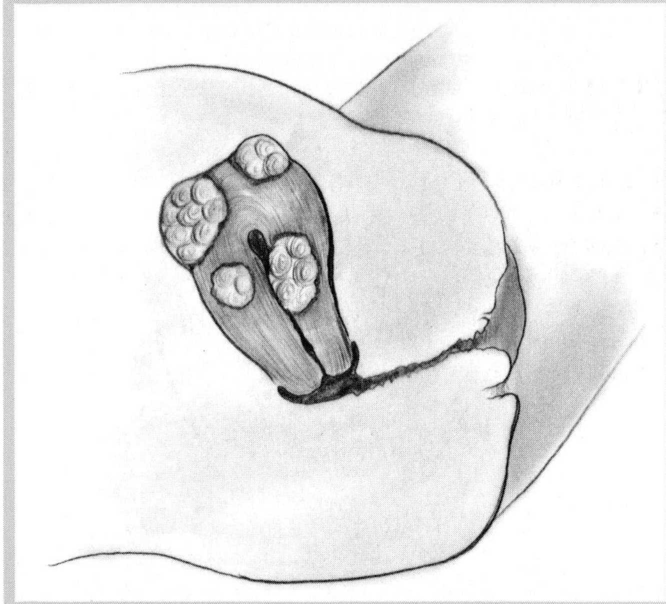

MYOMAS—FIBROIDS

S: Varies, depending on size and location. Often no symptoms. Or, hypermenorrhea if myoma disturbs endometrium.

O: Uterus enlarged, firm, mobile, and nodular with hard painless nodules in the uterine wall. They are usually benign. Highest incidence between the ages of 30 and 45 years and in blacks. After menopause, the lesions usually regress but do not disappear.

S, subjective data; O, objective data.

Table 22-7 ▸ Conditions of Uterine Enlargement *Continued*

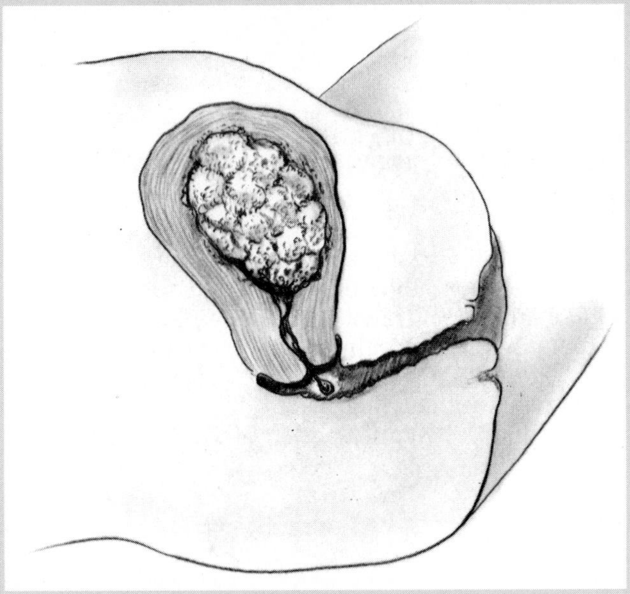

CARCINOMA OF THE ENDOMETRIUM

S: Abnormal and intermenstrual bleeding before menopause; postmenopausal bleeding or mucosanguineous discharge.

O: Uterus may be enlarged. The Pap smear is only partly effective in detecting endometrial cancer. Women at high risk should have an endometrial tissue sample evaluated at menopause (American Cancer Society, 1991). Risk factors for endometrial cancer are history of infertility, failure to ovulate, prolonged estrogen therapy, obesity.

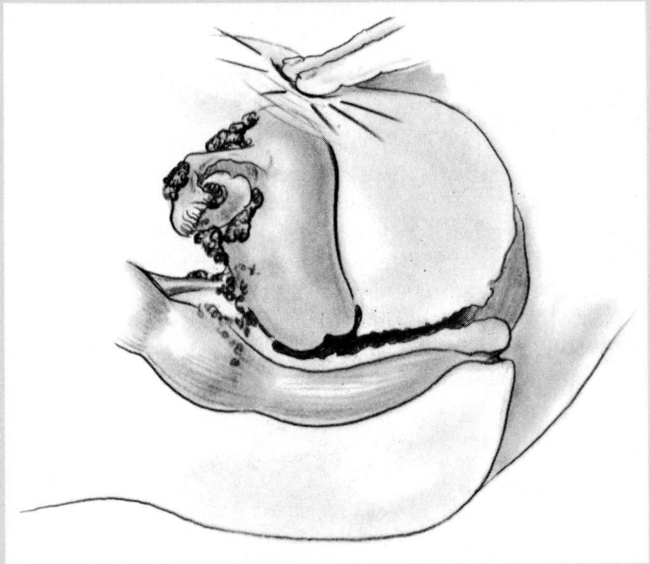

ENDOMETRIOSIS

S: May have irregular uterine bleeding or hypermenorrhea or may be asymptomatic. Dysmenorrhea, may be progressive.

O: Uterus fixed, tender to movement. Small, firm nodular masses tender to palpation on posterior aspect of fundus, uterosacral ligaments, ovaries, sigmoid colon. Ovaries often enlarged. Masses are aberrant growths of endometrial tissue scattered throughout pelvis. May cause sterility due to pelvic adhesions, tubal obstruction, decreased ovarian function.

Table 22-8 ▸ Adnexal Enlargement

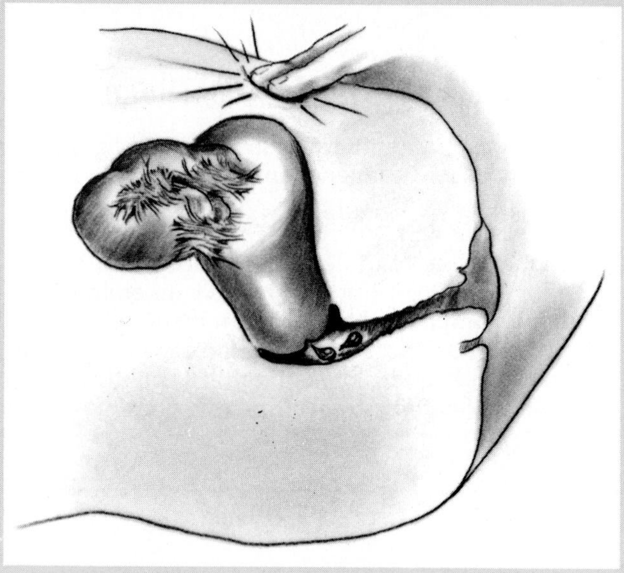

FALLOPIAN TUBE MASS—ACUTE SALPINGITIS (PELVIC INFLAMMATORY DISEASE [PID])

S: Sudden fever, suprapubic pain and tenderness
O: Acute—rigid boardlike lower abdominal musculature. Movement of uterus and cervix causes intense pain. Pain in lateral fornices and adnexa. Bilateral adnexal masses difficult to palpate owing to pain and muscle spasm.
Chronic—bilateral, tender, fixed adnexal masses.

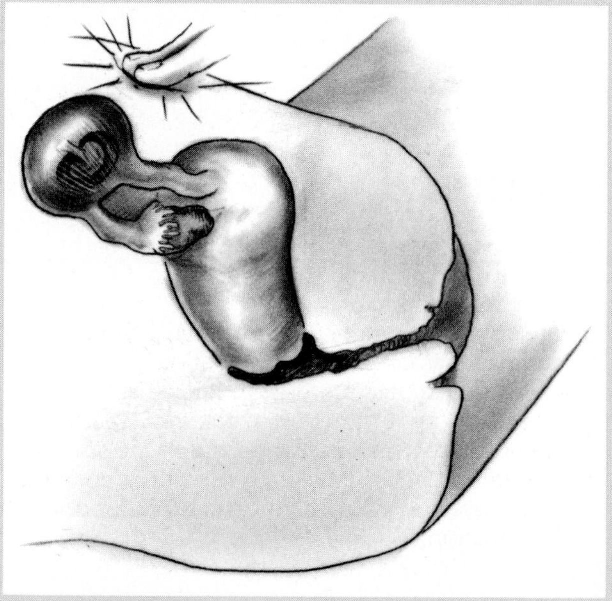

FALLOPIAN TUBE MASS—ECTOPIC PREGNANCY

S: Amenorrhea or irregular vaginal bleeding, pelvic pain
O: Softening of cervix and fundus; movement of cervix and uterus causes pain; palpable tender pelvic mass, which is solid, mobile, unilateral. This has potential for serious sequelae; seek gynecologic consultation immediately if the mass ruptures, shows signs of acute peritonitis.

S, subjective data; O, objective data.

Table 22-8 ► Adnexal Enlargement *Continued*

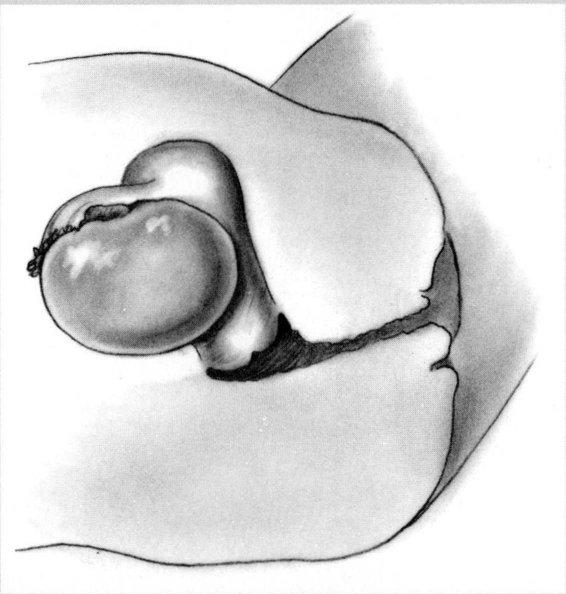

FLUCTUANT OVARIAN MASS—OVARIAN CYST

S: Usually asymptomatic
O: Smooth, round, fluctuant, mobile, nontender mass on ovary. Some cysts resolve spontaneously within 60 days but must be followed closely.

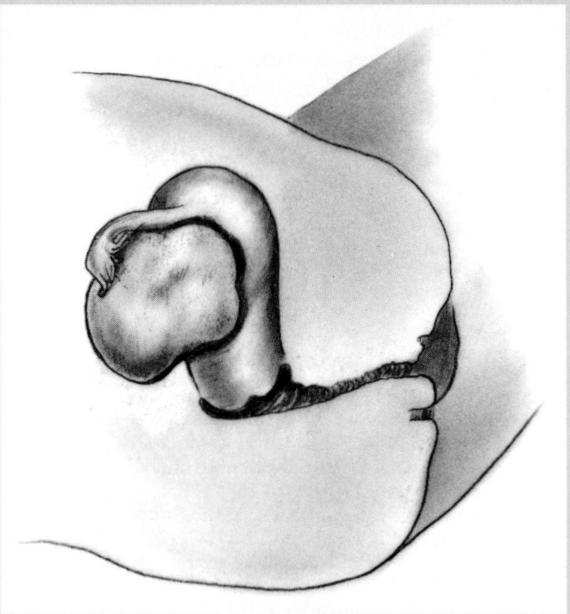

SOLID OVARIAN MASS—OVARIAN CANCER

S: Usually asymptomatic. May have abdominal enlargement from fluid accumulation.
O: Solid tumor palpated on ovary. Heavy, solid, fixed, poorly defined mass suggests malignancy; benign mass may feel mobile and solid. Biopsy necessary to distinguish the two types of masses. The Pap smear does not detect ovarian cancer. Women over age 40 should have a thorough pelvic examination every year.

Table 22-9 ▸ Abnormalities in Pediatric Genitalia

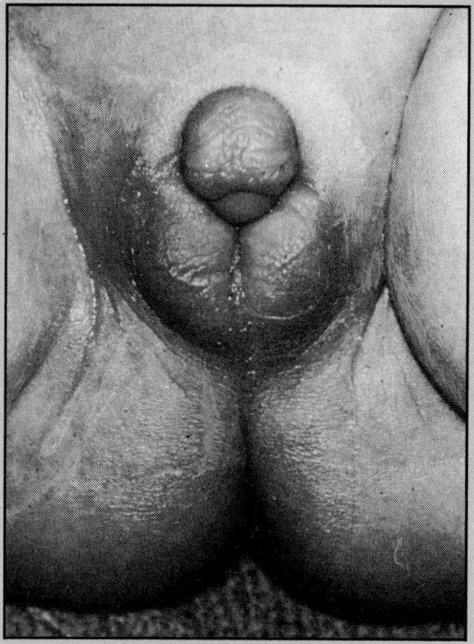

AMBIGUOUS GENITALIA

Masculinized external genitalia of a female infant showing enlargement of clitoris and labial fusion. Ambiguous means genitalia may look like an enlarged clitoris or a small penis with hypospadias, and may look like fused labia or an incompletely formed scrotum with absent testes. Refer for diagnostic evaluation.

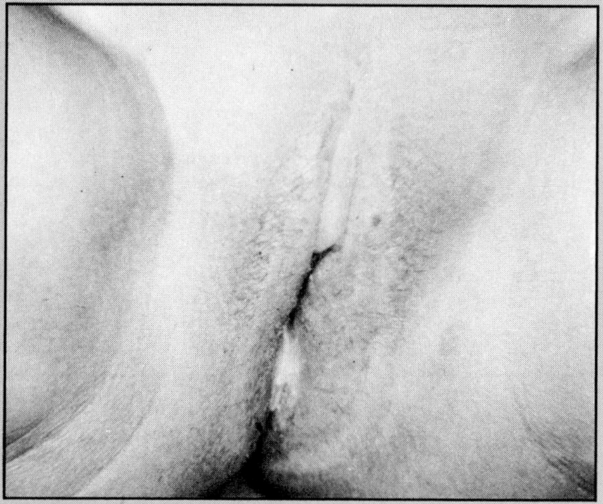

VULVOVAGINITIS IN CHILD

This infection is caused by *Candida albicans* in a diabetic child. Symptoms include pruritus and burning when urine touches excoriated area. Examination shows red, shiny, edematous vulva, vaginal discharge, excoriated area from scratching.

Bibliography

American Cancer Society: Cancer Facts & Figures—1991. Atlanta, GA, American Cancer Society, 1991.

Benson RC: Current Obstetric and Gynecologic Diagnoses and Treatment. 3rd ed. Los Altos, CA, Lange Medical Publications, 1980.

Cowell CA (Ed): Pediatric and adolescent gynecology. Pediatric Clin North Am 28(2):247–530, 1981.

Draye MA: An approach to infertility investigation. Nurse Pract 10:13–22, 1985.

Enterline JA, Leonardo JP: Condylomata acuminata (venereal warts). Nurse Pract 14:8–16, 1989.

Frank DI, Lang, AR: Alcohol use and sexual arousal research: Application of the health belief model. Nurs Pract 15(5):32–35, 1990.

Harlan WR, Harlan EA, Grillo GP: Secondary sex characteristics of girls 12 to 17 years of age—The U.S. health examination survey. J Pediatr 96:1074–1078, 1980.

Helderman G, Graham L, Cannon D, et al: Comparing two sampling techniques for endocervical cell recovery on Papanicolaou smears. Nurs Pract 15(11):30–32, 1990.

Jarrett ME, Lethbridge DJ: The contraceptive needs of midlife women. Nurs Pract 15(12):34–39, 1990.

Kaplan HS: The Evaluation of Sexual Disorders—Psychological and Medical Aspects. New York, Brunner/Mazel, 1983.

Kelley SJ: Interviewing the sexually abused child: Principles and techniques. J Emerg Nurs 11(5):234–241, 1985.

Latta W, Wiesmeier E: Effects of an educational gynecological exam on women's attitudes. JOGN Nurs 11:242–245, 1982.

Liston J, Liston E: The mirror pelvic examination—assessment in clinic setting. JOGN Nurs 7:47–49, 1978.

Loucks A: Chlamydia, an unheralded epidemic. AJN 87:920–922, 1987.

Marshall WA, Tanner JM: Variations in pattern of pubertal changes in girls. Arch Dis Child 44:291–303, 1969.

Martin LL: Health Care of Women. Philadelphia, JB Lippincott, 1978.

Masters WH, Johnson VE: Human Sexual Response. Boston, Little Brown, 1966.

Mitchell JR: Male adolescents' concern about a physical examination conducted by a female. Nurs Res 29(3):165–169, 1980.

Morrison-Beedy D, Robbins L: Sexual assessment and the aging female. Nurs Pract 14(12):35–45, 1989.

Nolan JW: Developmental concerns and the health of midlife women. Nurs Clin North Am 21(1):151–159, 1986.
Olsson HM, Gullberg MT: Role of the woman patient and fear of the pelvic examination. Western J Nurs Res 9(3):357–367, 1987.
Pfeiffer E: Sexuality and aging. *In* Rossman I: Clinical Geriatrics. Philadelphia, JB Lippincott, 1979, pp 568–575.
Primrose RB: Taking the tension out of pelvic exams. Am J Nurs 84:72–74, 1984.
Pritchard JA, MacDonald PC, Gant NF: Williams' Obstetrics. 17th ed. Norwalk, CT, Appleton-Century-Crofts, 1985.
Quilligan EJ, Zuspan FP: Current Therapy in Obstetrics and Gynecology. 3rd ed. Philadelphia, WB Saunders, 1990.
Sheahan SL: Identifying female sexual dysfunctions. Nurse Pract 14:25–34, 1989.
Steinke EE: Older adults' knowledge and attitudes about sexuality and aging. Image 20(2):93–95, 1988.
Szydlo VL: Approaching an adolescent about a pelvic exam. AJN 88:1502–1506, 1988.
Vieiraloes-Wiltgen C, Engle V: Identification and management of DES-exposed women. Nurse Pract 13(11):15–27, 1988.
Wells G: Reducing the threat of a first pelvic exam. Matern Child Nurs 2(5):304–306, 1977.
Worth AM, Dougherty MC, McKey PL: Development and testing of the circumvaginal muscles rating scale. Nurs Res 35(3):166–168, 1986.

CHAPTER

23 Anus, Rectum, and Prostate

STRUCTURE AND FUNCTION

The anal canal is the outlet of the gastrointestinal tract, and it is about 3.8 cm long in the adult. It is lined with modified skin (having no hair or sebaceous glands) that merges with rectal mucosa at the anorectal junction. The canal slants forward toward the umbilicus, forming a distinct right angle with the rectum, which rests back in the hollow of the sacrum. Although the rectum contains only autonomic nerves, there are numerous somatic sensory nerves in the anal canal and external skin, so a person feels sharp pain from any trauma to the anal area.

The anal canal is surrounded by two concentric layers of muscle, the *sphincters* (Fig. 23–1). The internal sphincter is under involuntary control by the autonomic nervous system. The external sphincter surrounds the internal sphincter but also has a small section overriding

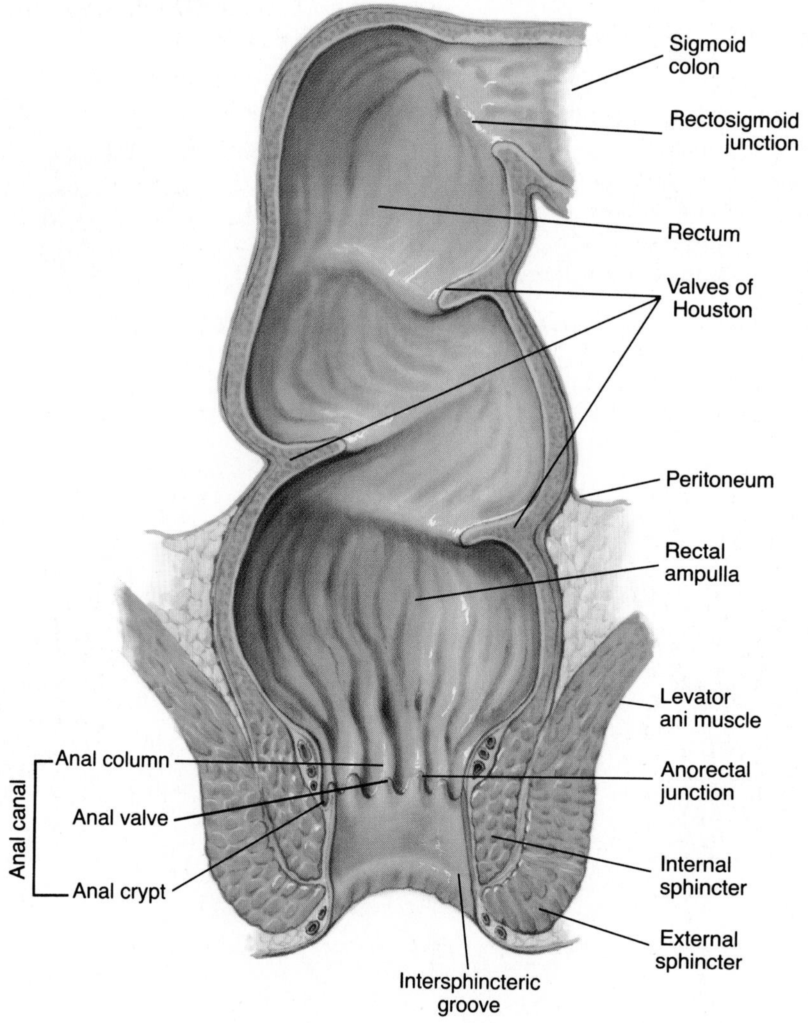

▶ **Figure 23–1**

the tip of the internal sphincter at the opening. It is under voluntary control. Except for the passing of feces and gas, the sphincters keep the anal canal tightly closed. The *intersphincteric groove* separates the internal and external sphincters, and is palpable.

The *anal columns* (or columns of Morgagni) are folds of mucosa. These extend vertically down from the rectum and end in the *anorectal junction* (also called the mucocutaneous junction, pectinate, or dentate line). This junction is not palpable, but it is visible on proctoscopy. Each anal column contains an artery and a vein. Under conditions of chronic increased venous pressure, the vein may enlarge forming a hemorrhoid. At the lower end of each column is a small crescent fold of mucous membrane, the *anal valve.* The space above the anal valve (between the columns) is a small recess, the *anal crypt.*

The rectum, which is 12 cm long, is the distal portion of the large intestine. It extends from the sigmoid colon, at the level of the third sacral vertebra and ends at the anal canal. Just above the anal canal, the rectum dilates and turns posteriorly, forming the rectal ampulla. The rectal interior has three semilunar transverse folds called the *valves of Houston.* These cross one-half the circumference of the rectal lumen. Their function is unclear, but they may serve to hold feces as the flatus passes. The lowest is within reach of palpation, usually on the person's left side, and must not be mistaken for an intrarectal mass.

Peritoneal Reflection. The peritoneum covers only the upper two-thirds of the rectum. In the male, the anterior part of the peritoneum reflects down to within 7.5 cm of the anal opening, forming the *rectovesical pouch* (Fig. 23–2) and then covers the bladder. In the female, this is termed the *rectouterine pouch,* and extends down to within 5.5 cm of the anal opening.

In the male, the *prostate gland* lies in front of the anterior wall of the rectum. It surrounds the bladder neck and the urethra, and it secretes a thin milky alkaline fluid that helps sperm viability. It is a bilobed structure with a round or heart shape. It measures 2.5 cm long and 4 cm in diameter. The two lateral lobes are separated by a shallow groove called the *median sulcus.* The two seminal vesicles project like rabbit ears above the prostate. The two bulbourethral (Cowper's) glands

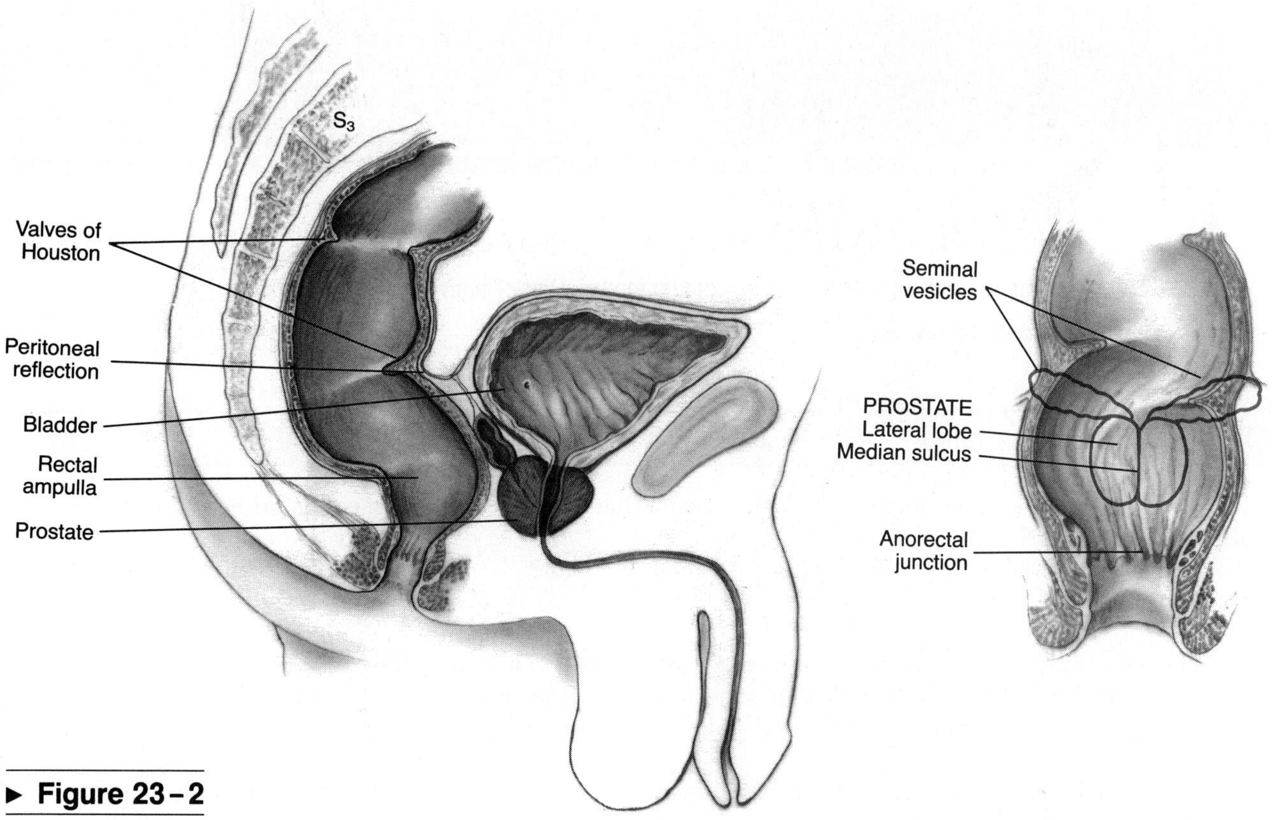

► **Figure 23–2**

are each the size of a pea and are located inferior to the prostate on either side of the urethra (see Fig. 23–5).

In the female, the uterine cervix lies in front of the anterior rectal wall and may be palpated through it.

The combined length of the anal canal and the rectum is about 16 cm in the adult. The average length of the examining finger is from 6 cm to 10 cm, bringing many rectal structures within reach.

The sigmoid colon is named from its S-shaped course in the pelvic cavity. It extends from the iliac flexure of the descending colon and ends at the rectum. It is 40 cm long, and is accessible to examination only through the sigmoidoscope. The flexible fiberoptic scope (60 cm) in current use provides a view of the entire mucosal surface of the sigmoid, as well as parts of the proximal colon.

DEVELOPMENTAL CONSIDERATIONS

The first stool passed by the newborn is dark green meconium and occurs within 24 to 48 hours of birth, indicating anal patency. From that time on, the infant usually has a stool after each feeding. This response to eating is a wave of peristalsis called the gastrocolic reflex. It continues throughout life, although children and adults usually produce no more than one or two stools per day.

The infant passes stools by reflex. Voluntary control of the external anal sphincter cannot occur until the nerves supplying the area have become fully myelinated, usually around 1 1/2 to 2 years of age. Toilet training usually starts after age 2 years.

At puberty, the prostate gland has a very rapid increase to more than twice its prepubertal size. During young adulthood its size remains fairly constant. It commonly starts to enlarge during the middle adult years. This *benign prostatic hypertrophy* (BPH) is present in 1 out of 10 males at the age of 40 years and increases with age. It is thought that the hypertrophy is caused by hormonal imbalance that leads to the proliferation of benign adenomas, which gradually impede urine output.

SUBJECTIVE DATA

Usual bowel routine: frequency, stool color
Change in bowel habits: diarrhea, constipation
Medications: laxatives
Rectal conditions (pruritus, hemorrhoids, fissure, fistula)
Diet of high-fiber foods

EXAMINER ASKS:	RATIONALE:
1. Do your bowels move regularly? How often? What color is the stool? Is it hard or soft?	Assess **usual bowel routine.**
Do you ever have pain while passing a bowel movement?	Dyschezia. Pain may be due to a local condition (hemorrhoid, fissure) or constipation.
2. Have you noticed any **change** in your usual **bowel habits?** Do you have loose stools, or diarrhea? When did this start? Is the diarrhea associated with nausea and vomiting, abdominal pain, something you ate recently?	Diarrhea occurs with gastroenteritis, colitis, irritable colon syndrome.
Have you eaten at a restaurant recently? Does anyone else in your group or family have the same symptoms?	Consider food poisoning.

EXAMINER ASKS:	RATIONALE:
Have you traveled to a foreign country during the last 6 months?	Consider parasitic infection.
Do your stools have a hard consistency? When did this start?	Constipation.
Have you ever had black or bloody stools? When did you first notice blood in the stools? What is the color, bright red or dark red-black? How much blood would you say there is: spotting on the toilet paper or outright passing of blood with the stool? Do the bloody stools have a particular smell?	Melena. Black stools may be tarry due to occult blood (melena) from gastrointestinal bleeding, or nontarry from ingestion of iron medications. Red blood in stools occurs with gastrointestinal bleeding or localized bleeding around the anus.
Have you ever had clay-colored stools?	Clay color indicates absent bile pigment.
Have you ever had mucus or pus in stool?	
Have you ever had frothy stool?	Steatorrhea is excessive fat in the stool as in malabsorption of fat.
Do you need to pass gas frequently?	Flatulence.
3. What **medications** do you take—prescription and over-the-counter? Do you use laxatives or stool softeners? Which ones? How often? Do you take iron pills? Do you ever use enemas to move your bowels? How often?	
4. Do you have any problems in rectal area: itching, pain or burning, hemorrhoids? How do you treat these? Do you use any hemorrhoid preparations? Have you ever had a fissure, or fistula? How was this treated?	Pruritus.
Have you ever had a problem controlling your bowels?	Fecal incontinence. Mucoid discharge and soiled underwear occur with prolapsed hemorrhoids.
6. What is the usual amount of **high-fiber foods** in your daily diet: cereals, apples or other fruits, vegetables, whole-grain breads? How many glasses of water do you drink each day?	High-fiber foods of the soluble type have been shown to lower cholesterol (beans, prunes, barley, carrots, broccoli, cabbage), while insoluble fiber foods reduce the risk of colon cancer (cereals, wheat germ). Also, fiber foods help fight obesity, stabilize blood sugar, and may help certain gastrointestinal disorders.

EXAMINER ASKS:	RATIONALE:

ADDITIONAL QUESTIONS FOR INFANTS AND CHILDREN

At what age did you start toilet training for your child? At what age did your child achieve bowel control? How did your child react to toilet training?

Have you ever noticed any irritation in your child's anal area: redness, raised skin, frequent itching?

In children, pinworms are a common cause of intense itching and irritated anal skin.

OBJECTIVE DATA

Equipment Needed:

- Penlight
- Lubricating jelly
- Glove
- Guaiac test reagents

Preparation

Perform a rectal examination on all adults and particularly for those in middle and late years. Help the person assume one of the following positions (Fig. 23–3): Examine the male in the left lateral decubitus or standing position. Place the female in lithotomy position if examining genitalia as well; use the left lateral decubitus position for the rectal area alone.

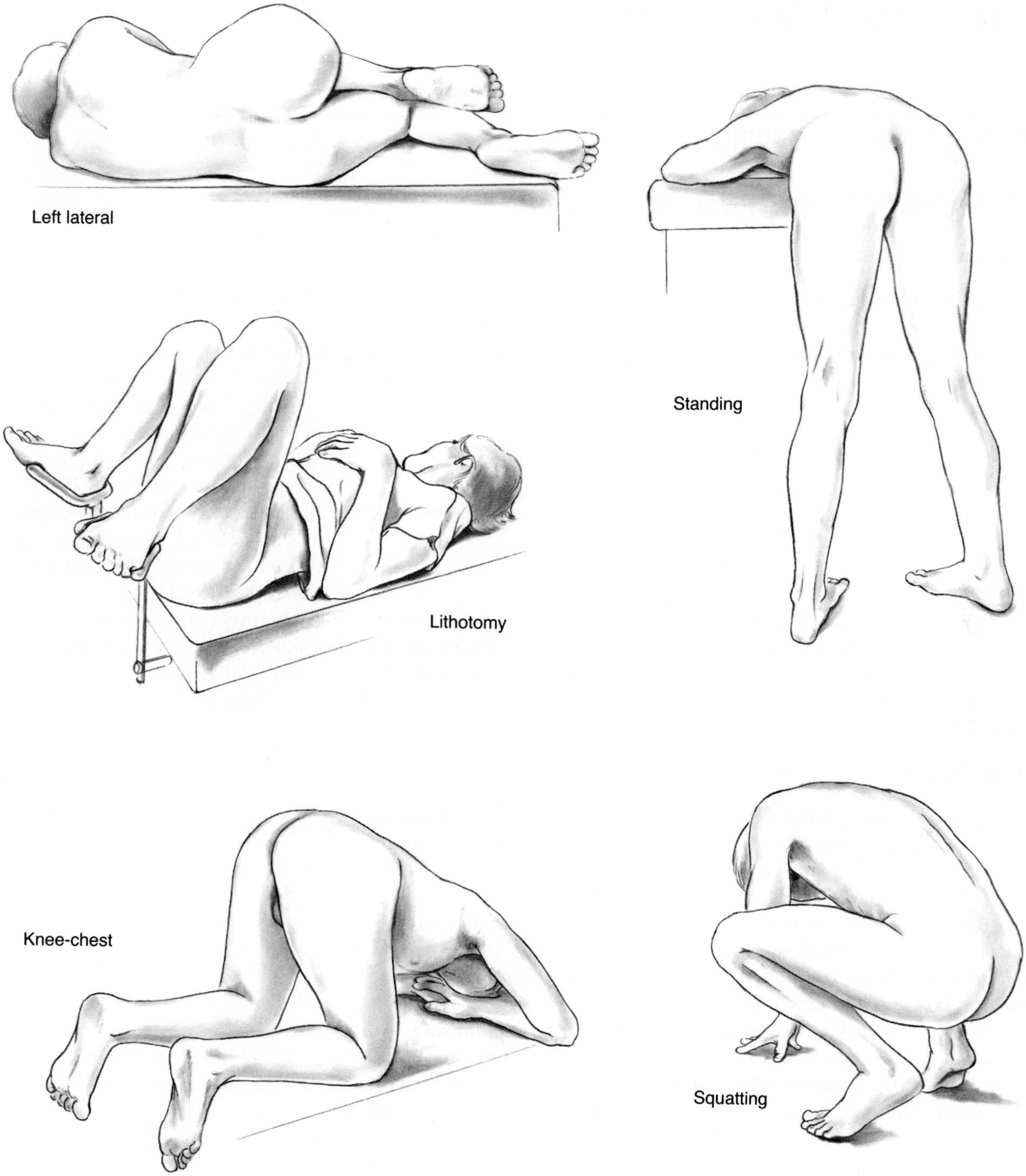

► Figure 23–3

METHOD OF EXAMINATION

NORMAL RANGE OF FINDINGS	ABNORMAL FINDINGS

EXAMINATION OF THE ANAL REGION

Inspect the perianal area.

Spread the buttocks wide apart and observe the perianal region. The anus normally looks moist and hairless, with coarse folded skin that is more pigmented than the perianal skin. The anal opening is tightly closed. There are no lesions.

Inflammation.
Lesions or scars.
Linear split—fissure.
Flabby skin sac—hemorrhoid.
Shiny blue skin sac—thrombosed hemorrhoid.
Small round opening in anal area—fistula (see Table 23–1).

Inspect the sacrococcygeal area. Normally, it appears smooth and even.

Inflammation or tenderness, swelling, tuft of hair, or dimple at tip of coccyx may indicate pilonidal cyst (see Table 23–1).

Instruct the person to hold the breath and bear down by performing a Valsalva maneuver. There should be no break in skin integrity or protrusion through the anal opening. Describe any abnormality in clock-face terms, with 12:00 as the anterior point toward the symphysis pubis and 6:00 toward the coccyx.

Appearance of fissure.
Appearance of hemorrhoids.
Circular red doughnut of tissue—rectal prolapse.

Palpate the anus and rectum.

Don a glove and drop lubricating jelly onto your index finger. Instruct the person that palpation is not painful but may feel like needing to move the bowels. Place the pad of your index finger gently against the anal verge (Fig. 23–4). You will feel the sphincter tighten, then relax. As it relaxes, flex the tip of your finger and slowly insert it into the anal canal in a direction toward the umbilicus. *Never* approach the anus at right angles with your index finger extended. Such a jabbing motion does not promote sphincter relaxation and is painful.

Rotate your examining finger to palpate the entire muscular ring. The canal should feel smooth and even. Note the intersphincteric groove circling the canal wall. To assess tone, ask the person to tighten the muscle. The sphincter should tighten evenly around your finger with no pain to the person.

Decreased tone.
Increased tone occurs with inflammation and anxiety.

Use a bidigital palpation with your thumb against the perianal tissue (Fig. 23–5). Press your examining finger toward it. This maneuver highlights any swelling or tenderness and helps assess the bulbourethral glands.

Tenderness.

Above the anal canal, the rectum turns posteriorly, following the curve of the coccyx and sacrum. Insert your finger farther and explore all around the rectal wall. It normally feels smooth with no nodularity. Promptly report any mass you discover for further examination.

Internal hemorrhoid above anorectal junction is not palpable unless thrombosed.
A soft, slightly movable mass may be a polyp.
A firm or hard mass with irregular shape or rolled edges may signify carcinoma (see Table 23–2).

NORMAL RANGE OF FINDINGS | **ABNORMAL FINDINGS**

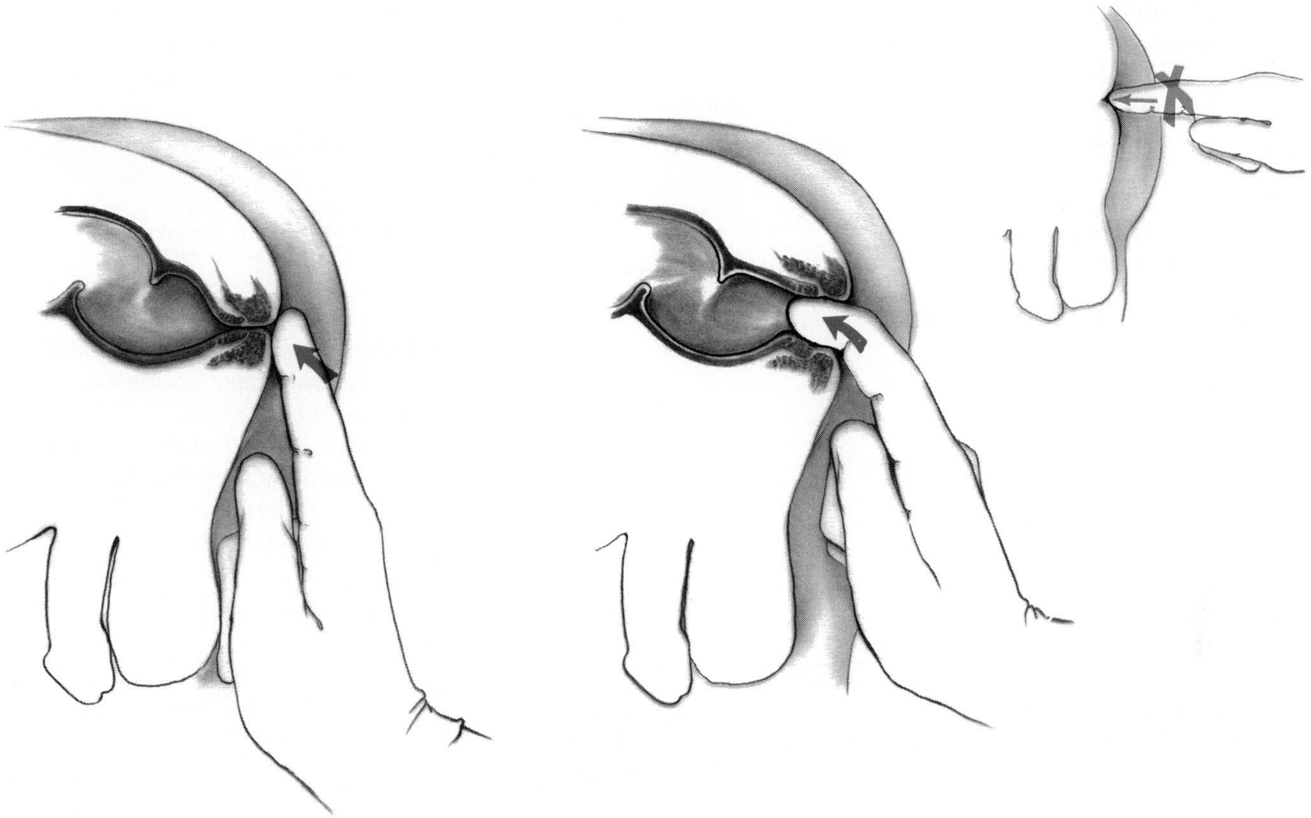

► **Figure 23-4**

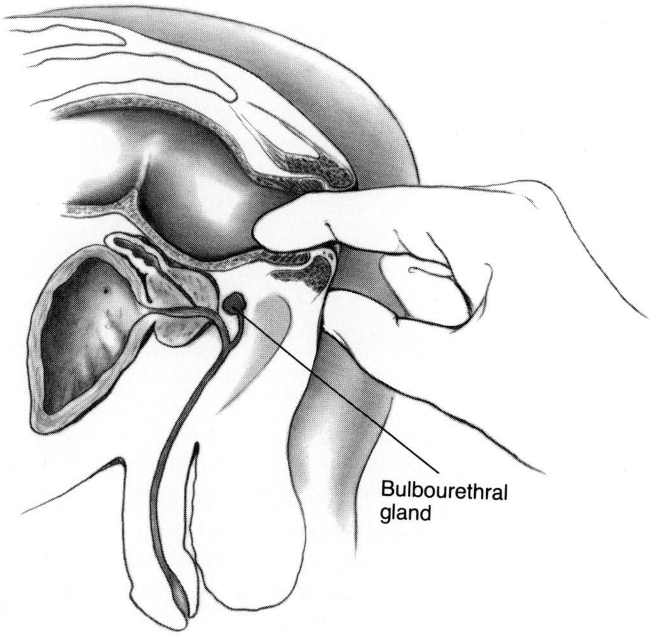

► **Figure 23-5**

NORMAL RANGE OF FINDINGS		ABNORMAL FINDINGS
On the anterior wall in the male, palpate the prostate gland (Fig. 23–6). Note:		
Size	2.5 cm long by 4 cm wide. Should not protrude more than 1 cm into the rectum.	Enlarged or atrophied gland.
Shape	Heart shape, with palpable central groove.	Flat with no groove.
Surface	Smooth.	Nodular.
Consistency	Elastic, rubbery.	Hard, boggy, soft, fluctuant.
Mobility	Slightly movable.	Fixed.
Sensitivity	Nontender to palpation.	Tender.

Enlarged, firm smooth gland with central groove obliterated suggests BPH.

Swollen, exquisitely tender gland accompanies prostatitis.

Any stone-hard, irregular, fixed nodule indicates carcinoma (see Table 23–3).

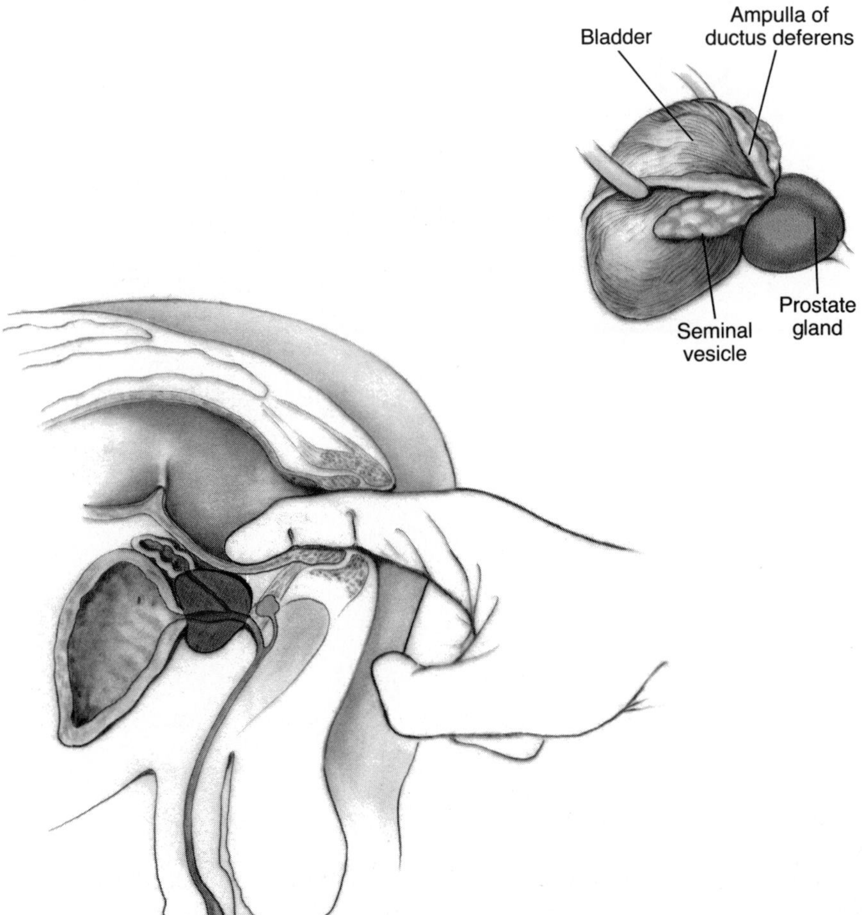

▶ **Figure 23–6**

NORMAL RANGE OF FINDINGS

ABNORMAL FINDINGS

In the female, palpate the cervix through the anterior rectal wall. It normally feels like a small round mass. You also may palpate a retroverted uterus or a tampon in the vagina. Do not mistake the cervix or a tampon for a tumor.

Withdraw your examining finger; normally, there is no bright red blood or mucus on the glove. To complete the examination, offer the person tissues to remove the lubricant and help the person to a more comfortable position.

Examination of Stool. Inspect any feces remaining on the glove. Normally, the color is brown and the consistency is soft.

Jelly-like mucus shreds mixed in stool indicate inflammation.

Bright red blood on stool surface indicates rectal bleeding. Bright red blood mixed with feces indicates possible colonic bleeding.

Test any stool on the glove for *occult blood.* Use the *guaiac test* to detect small quantities of blood. Use the guaiac testing procedure that your agency or hospital directs. A negative response is normal. If the stool is *guaiac positive,* it indicates occult blood. Note that a false-positive finding may occur if the person has ingested significant amounts of red meat within 3 days of the test.

Black tarry stool with distinct malodor indicates upper gastrointestinal bleeding, with blood partially digested. (Must lose more than 50 cc from upper gastrointestinal tract to be considered melena.)

Black stool—also occurs with ingesting iron or bismuth preparations.

Gray, tan stool—absent bile pigment, e.g., obstructive jaundice.

Pale yellow, greasy stool—increased fat content (steatorrhea), as occurs with malabsorption syndrome.

Occult bleeding usually indicates cancer of colon.

DEVELOPMENTAL CONSIDERATIONS

Routinely inspect the anal region in all infants and children. However, do not perform internal palpation routinely unless the history or symptoms indicate.

For the newborn, hold the feet with one hand and flex the knees up onto the abdomen. Note the presence of the anus. Confirm a patent rectum and anus by noting the first meconium stool passed within 24 to 48 hours of birth. To assess sphincter tone, check the *anal reflex.* Gently stroke the anal area and note a quick contraction of the sphincter.

Imperforate anus.

For each infant and child, note that the buttocks are firm and rounded with no masses or lesions. Recall that the *mongolian spot* is a common variation of hyperpigmentation in black, native American, Mediterranean, and Asian newborns (see Chapter 9).

Flattened buttocks in cystic fibrosis or celiac syndrome.
Coccygeal mass.
Meningocele.
Tuft of hair or pilonidal dimple.

NORMAL RANGE OF FINDINGS	ABNORMAL FINDINGS
The perianal skin is free of lesions. However, diaper rash is common in children younger than 1 year of age, and is exhibited as a generalized reddened area with papules or vesicles.	Pustules indicate secondary infection of diaper rash. Signs of physical or sexual abuse. Fissure—common cause of constipation or rectal bleeding in child. (Painful, so the child does not defecate.)
If internal palpation is needed, position the infant or child on the back with the legs flexed, and gently insert a gloved, well-lubricated finger into the rectum. Your fifth finger usually is long enough and its smaller size is more comfortable for the infant or child. However, you may need to use the index finger because of its better control and increased tactile sensitivity. On withdrawing the finger, scant bleeding or protruding rectal mucosa may occur. Inspect the perianal region of the school-aged child and adolescent during examination of the genitalia. Internal palpation is not performed routinely. As an aging person performs the Valsalva maneuver, you may note relaxation of the perianal musculature and decreased sphincter control. Otherwise, the full examination proceeds as that described earlier for the younger adult.	

☑ SUMMARY CHECKLIST

1 ▶ Inspect anus and perianal area.
2 ▶ Inspect during Valsalva maneuver.
3 ▶ Palpate anal canal and rectum on all adults.
4 ▶ Test stool for occult blood.

SAMPLE RECORDING

Subjective

▶ Has 1 BM daily, soft, brown, no pain, no change in bowel routine. On no medications. Has no history of pruritus, hemorrhoids, fissure, or fistula. Diet includes fresh fruits and vegetables but no whole grain cereals or breads.

Objective

- No fissure, hemorrhoids, fistula, or skin lesions in perianal area. Sphincter tone good, no prolapse. Rectal walls smooth, no masses or tenderness. Prostate not enlarged, no masses or tenderness. Stool brown, guaiac negative.

SAMPLE CLINICAL PROBLEM

Subjective

- C.M. is a 62-year-old white male with chronic obstructive pulmonary disease for 15 years, who today has "diarrhea for 3 days."
  7 days PTA: C.M. seen at this agency for acute respiratory infection that was diagnosed as acute bronchitis and treated with oral ampicillin. Took medication as directed.
  3 days PTA: Symptoms of respiratory infection improved. Ingesting usual diet. Onset of four to five loose, unformed, brown stools a day. No abdominal pain or cramping. No nausea.
  Now: Diarrhea continues. No blood or mucus noticed in stool. No new foods or restaurant food in past 3 days. Wife not ill.

Objective

- Vital signs: 37°C-88-18. B/P 142/82.
  Respiratory: Respirations unlabored. Barrel chest. Hyperresonant to percussion. Lung sounds clear but diminished. No crackles or rhonchi today.
  Abdomen: Flat. Bowel sounds normal. No organomegaly or tenderness to palpation.
  Rectal: No lesions in perianal area. Sphincter tone good. Rectal walls smooth, no mass or tenderness. Prostate smooth and firm, no median sulcus palpable, no masses or tenderness. Stool brown, guaiac negative.

Assessment

- Diarrhea R/T effects of medication

NURSING DIAGNOSES COMMONLY ASSOCIATED WITH ANAL AND RECTAL DISORDERS

Diagnosis	Related Factors (Etiology)	Defining Characteristics (Symptoms and Signs)

Constipation	Less than adequate dietary intake and bulk
	Neuromuscular or musculoskeletal impairment
	Pain and discomfort on defecation
	Effects of
	  Diagnostic procedures
	  Pregnancy
	  Aging
	  Medication
	  Stress or anxiety
	Weak abdominal musculature
	Immobility or less than adequate physical activity
	Chronic use of laxatives and enemas
	Ignoring the urge to defecate
	Fear of rectal or cardiac pain
	Gastrointestinal lesions
		Frequency less than usual pattern
		Hard, formed stools
		Palpable mass
		Straining at stool
		Less than usual amount of stool
		Decreased bowel sounds
		Gas pain and flatulence
		Abdominal or back pain
		Reported feeling of abdominal or rectal fullness or pressure
		Impaired appetite
		Headache
		Nausea
		Irritability
		Palpable hard stool on rectal examination

Bowel incontinence	Diarrhea
	Impaction
	Impairment
	  Cognitive
	  Neuromuscular
	  Perceptual
	Large stool volume
	Depression
	Severe anxiety
	Physical or psychological barriers that prevent access to an acceptable toileting area
	Effects of medications
	Excessive use of laxatives
		Involuntary passage of stool
		Lack of awareness of need to defecate
		Lack of awareness of passage of stool
		Rectal oozing of stool
		Urgency

Other related nursing diagnoses:
- Diarrhea (see Chapter 17)
- Perceived constipation
- Colonic constipation

ABNORMAL FINDINGS

Table 23-1 ▶ Abnormalities of the Anus and Perianal Region

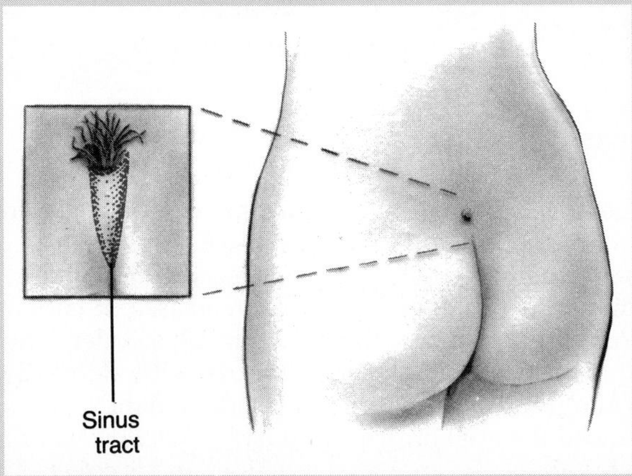

PILONIDAL CYST OR SINUS

A hair-containing cyst or sinus located in the midline over the coccyx or lower sacrum. Often opens as a dimple with visible tuft of hair and, possibly, an erythematous halo. Or, may appear as a palpable cyst. When advanced, has a palpable sinus tract. Although it is a congenital disorder, the lesion is first diagnosed between the ages of 15 and 30 years.

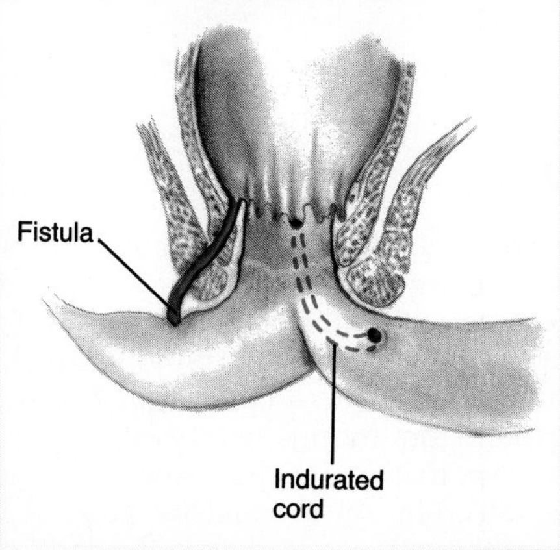

ANORECTAL FISTULA

A chronically inflamed gastrointestinal tract creates an abnormal passage from inner anus or rectum out to skin surrounding anus. Usually originates from a local abscess. The red, raised tract opening may drain serosanguineous or purulent matter when pressure is applied. Bidigital palpation may reveal an indurated cord.

Table continued on following page

Table 23-1 ▶ Abnormalities of the Anus and Perianal Region *Continued*

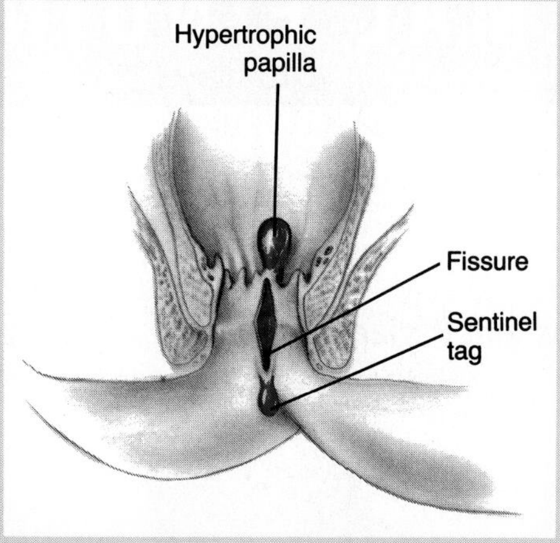

FISSURE

A painful longitudinal tear in the superficial mucosa at the anal margin. Most fissures (>90 percent) occur in the posterior midline area. They are frequently accompanied by a papule of hyperplastic skin, called a *sentinel tag,* on the anal margin below. Fissures often result from trauma, e.g., passing a large, hard stool or from irritant diarrheal stools. The person has itching, bleeding, and exquisite pain. A resulting spasm in the sphincters makes the area painful to examine; local anesthesia may be indicated.

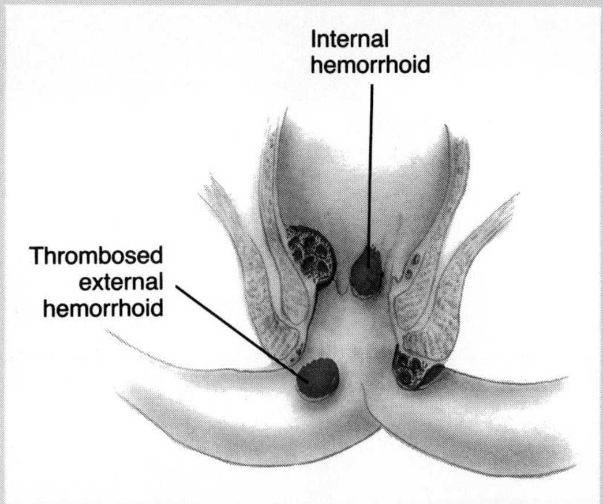

HEMORRHOIDS

These painless flabby papules are due to a varicose vein of the hemorrhoidal plexus. An *external hemorrhoid* originates below the anorectal junction and is covered by anal skin. When *thrombosed,* it contains clotted blood and becomes a painful, swollen, shiny blue mass that itches and bleeds with defecation. When it resolves, it leaves a painless, flabby skin sac around the anal orifice. An *internal hemorrhoid* originates above the anorectal junction, and is covered by mucous membrane. When the person performs a Valsalva maneuver, it may appear as a red mucosal mass. It is not palpable. All hemorrhoids result from increased portal venous pressure, as occurs with straining at stool, chronic constipation, pregnancy, obesity, chronic liver disease, or the low-fiber diet common in Western society.

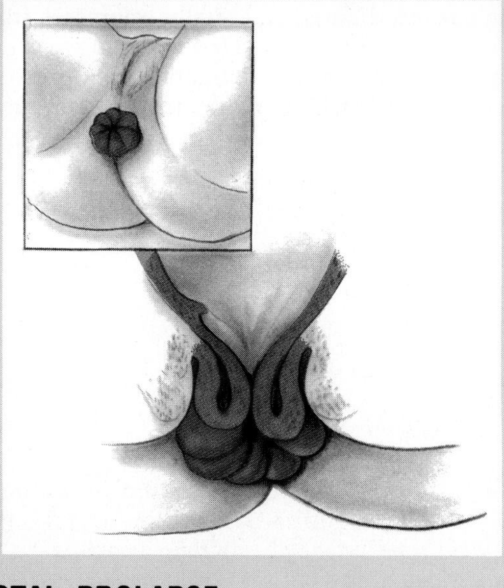

RECTAL PROLAPSE

The rectal mucous membrane protrudes through the anus, appearing as a moist red doughnut with radiating lines. When prolapse is incomplete, only the mucosa bulges. When complete, it includes the anal sphincters. Occurs following a Valsalva maneuver, such as straining at stool, or with exercise.

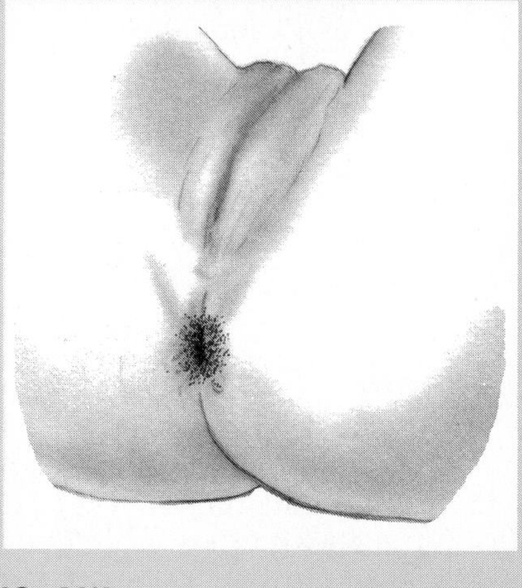

PRURITUS ANI

Intense perianal itching is manifested by red, raised, thickened, excoriated skin around the anus. Common causes are pinworms in children and fungal infections in adults. The area is swollen and moist, and with a fungal infection, it appears dull grayish-pink. The skin is dry and brittle with psychosomatic itching.

Table 23-2 ► Abnormalities of the Rectum

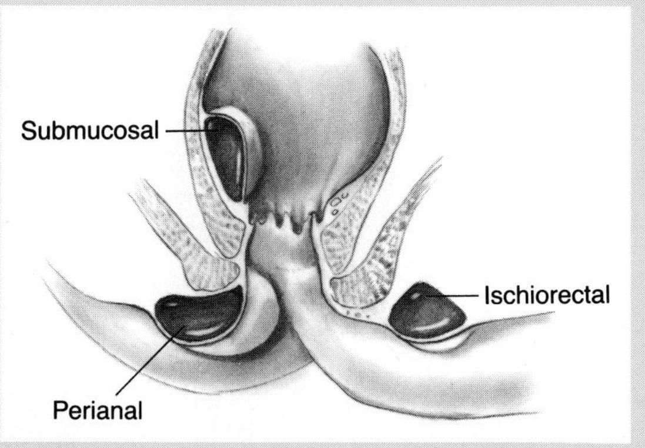

ABSCESS

A localized cavity of pus from infection in a pararectal space. Infection usually extends from an anal crypt. Characterized by persistent throbbing rectal pain. Termed by the space it occupies, e.g., a perianal abscess is superficial around the anal skin, and appears red, hot, swollen, indurated, and tender. An ischiorectal abscess is deep and tender to bidigital palpation. It occurs laterally between the anus and ischial tuberosity, and is uncommon.

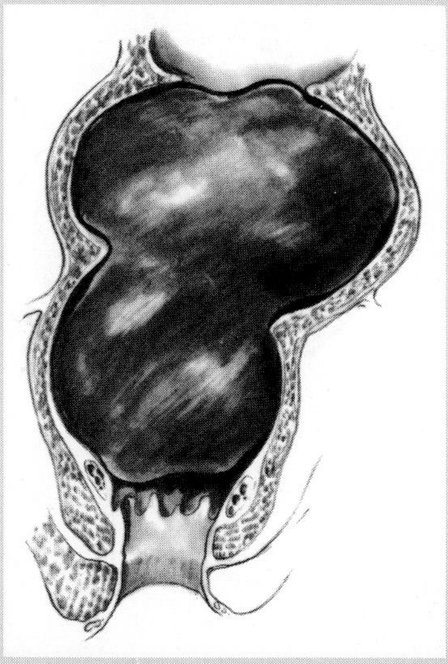

FECAL IMPACTION

A collection of hard desiccated feces in the rectum. The obstruction often results from decreased bowel motility, in which more water is reabsorbed from the stool. Also occurs with retained barium from gastrointestinal x-ray examination. The person may complain of constipation or diarrhea as a fecal stream passes around the impaction.

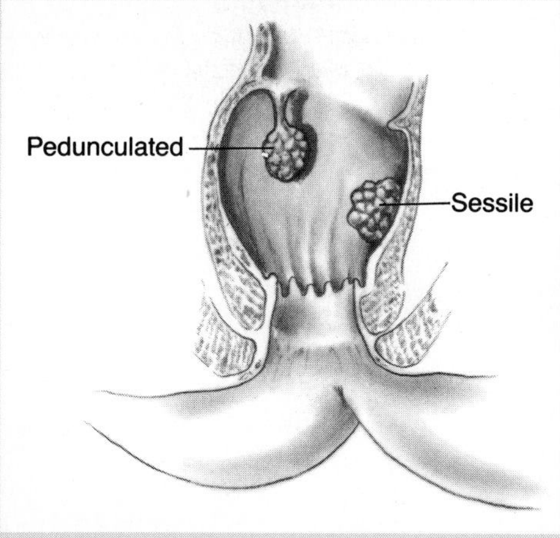

RECTAL POLYP

A protruding growth from the rectal mucous membrane that is fairly common. The polyp may be *pedunculated* (on a stalk), or *sessile* (a mound on the surface, close to the mocosal wall). The soft nodule is difficult to palpate. Proctoscopy is needed as well as biopsy to screen for a malignant growth.

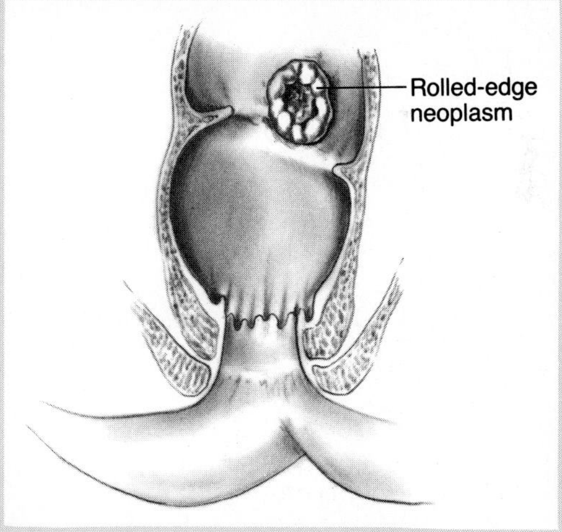

CARCINOMA

A malignant neoplasm in the rectum is asymptomatic, thus the importance of routine rectal palpation. An early lesion may be a single firm nodule. You may palpate an ulcerated center with rolled edges. As the lesion grows, it has an irregular cauliflower shape and is fixed and stone-hard. Refer a person with any rectal lesion for further study because about half are malignant.

Table 23-3 ▶ Abnormalities of the Prostate Gland

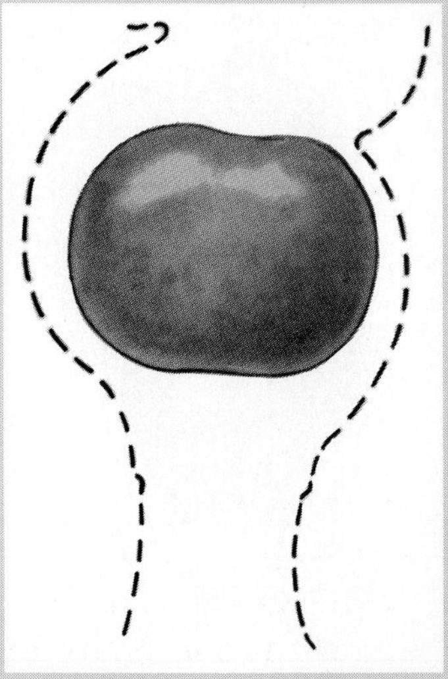

BENIGN PROSTATIC HYPERTROPHY (BPH)

A symmetric nontender enlargement commonly occurs in males beginning in the middle years. The prostate surface feels smooth, rubbery or firm (like the consistency of the nose), with the median sulcus obliterated.

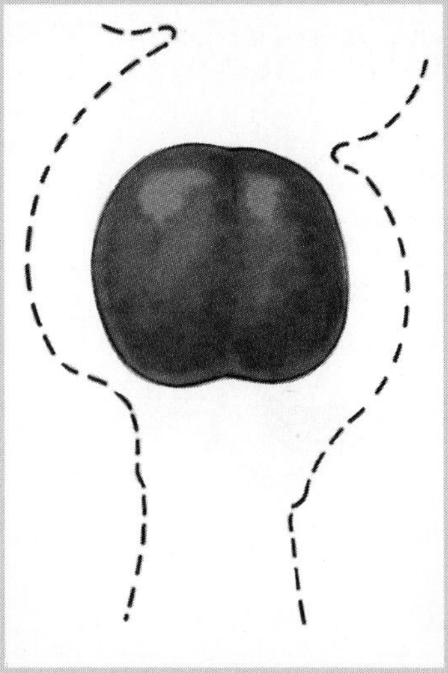

PROSTATITIS

An exquisitely tender enlargement is *acute* inflammation of the prostate gland yielding a swollen, slightly asymmetric gland that is quite tender to palpation.

With a *chronic* inflammation the signs can vary from tender enlargement with a boggy feel, to isolated firm areas due to fibrosis. Or, the gland may feel normal.

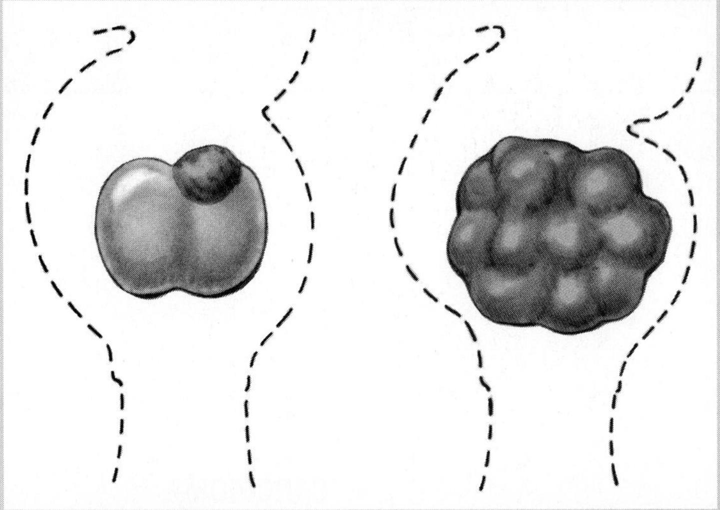

CARCINOMA

A malignant neoplasm often starts as a single hard nodule on the posterior surface, producing asymmetry and a change in consistency. As it invades normal tissue, there are multiple hard nodules or the entire gland feels stone-hard and fixed. The median sulcus is obliterated.

Bibliography

Kratzer GL, Demarest RJ: Colon and Rectal Disease. Philadelphia, WB Saunders, 1985.

Schrock TR: Diseases of the anorectum. *In* Sleisenger, MH, Fordtran JS (Eds): Gastrointestinal Disease. 4th ed. Philadelphia, WB Saunders, 1989.

Spiro HM: Clinical Gastroenterology. 3rd ed. New York, Macmillan Publishing, 1983.

Sprague-McRae JM: Encopresis: Developmental, behavioral and physiological considerations for treatment. Nurs Pract 15(6):8–24, 1990.

UNIT

3 Integration of the Health Assessment

CHAPTER

24 The Complete Health Assessment

The choreography of the complete history and physical examination is the art of arranging all the separate steps you have learned so far. Your first examination may seem awkward and contrived; you may have to pause and think of what comes next rather than just gather data. Repeated rehearsals make the choreography smoother. You will come to the point at which the procedure flows naturally, and even if you forget a step, you will be able to insert it gracefully into the next logical place.

The following examination sequence is one suggested route. It is intended to minimize the number of position changes for the client and for you. With experience, you may wish to adapt this and arrange a sequence that feels natural for you. Perform all the steps listed here for a complete examination. With experience, you will learn to strike a balance between which steps you must retain to be thorough and which corners you may safely cut when time is pressing.

Have all equipment prepared and accessible before the examination. Review Chapter 7, Getting Ready, for the list of necessary equipment, the setting, the client's emotional state, your demeanor, and the preparation of the client considering his or her age.

SEQUENCE	SELECTED PHOTOS

The person walks into the room, sits; the examiner sits facing the person; the person is in street clothes.

THE HEALTH HISTORY

1. Collect the history, complete or limited as visit warrants.

While obtaining the history and throughout the examination, note data on the person's general appearance.

GENERAL APPEARANCE

1. Appears stated age.
2. Level of consciousness.
3. Skin color.
4. Nutritional status.
5. Posture and position comfortably erect.
6. Obvious physical deformities.
7. Mobility.
   Gait
   Use of assistive devices
   Range of motion of joints
   No involuntary movement
8. Facial expression.
9. Mood and affect.
10. Speech: articulation, pattern, content.
    Appropriate, native language
11. Hearing.
12. Personal hygiene.

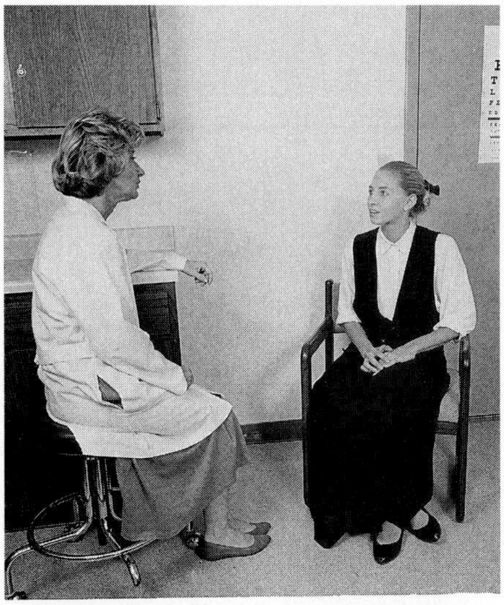

► Figure 24-1

MEASUREMENT

1. Weight.
2. Height.
3. Skinfold thickness, if indicated.
4. Vision using Snellen eye chart.

SEQUENCE	SELECTED PHOTOS

Ask the person to empty the bladder (save specimen, if needed), disrobe except for underpants, and put on a gown. The person sits with legs dangling off side of the bed or table, you stand in front of the person.

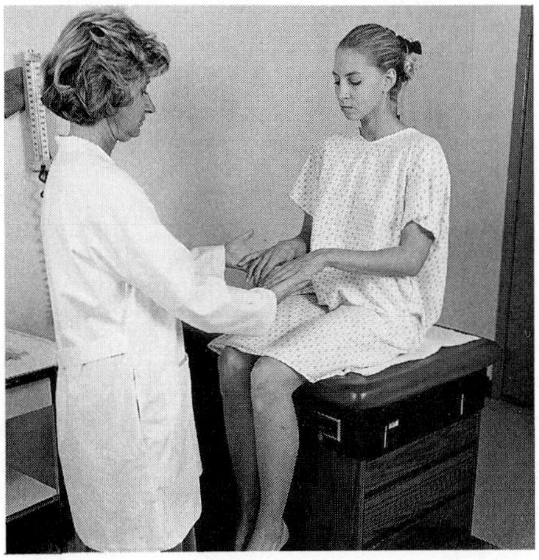

► Figure 24-2

SKIN

1. Examine both hands and inspect the nails.
2. For the rest of the examination, examine skin with corresponding regional examination.

VITAL SIGNS

1. Radial pulse.
2. Respirations.
3. Blood pressure.
4. Temperature (if indicated).

HEAD AND FACE

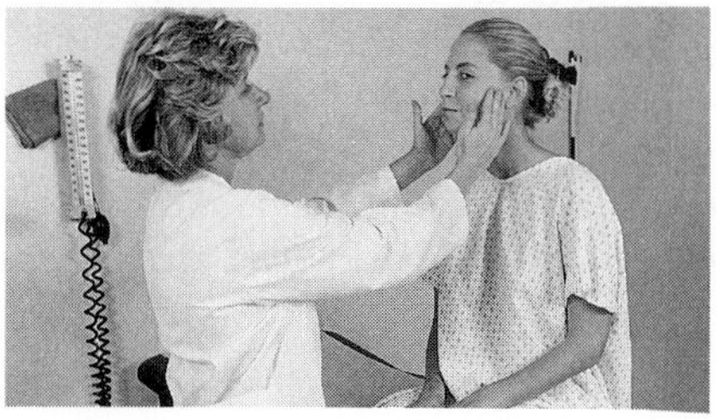

► Figure 24-3

1. Inspect and palpate scalp, hair, and cranium.
2. Inspect face: expression, symmetry (cranial nerve VII).
3. Palpate the temporal artery, then the temporomandibular joint as the person opens and closes the mouth.
4. Palpate the maxillary sinuses and the frontal sinuses; if tender, transilluminate the sinuses.

EYE

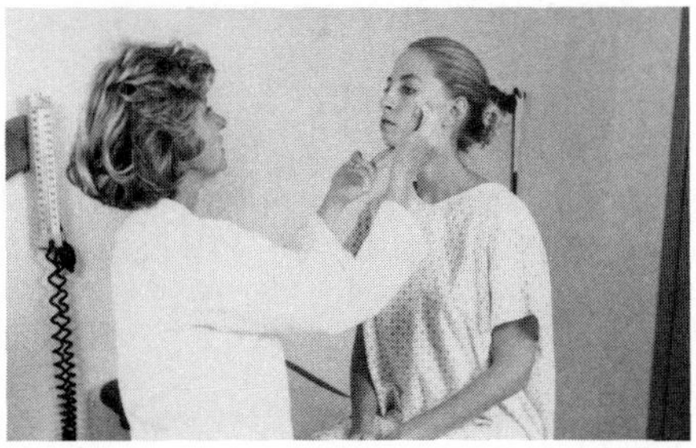

► Figure 24-4

1. Test visual fields by confrontation (cranial nerve II).
2. Test extraocular muscles: corneal light reflex, 6 cardinal positions of gaze (cranial nerves III, IV, VI).
3. Inspect external eye structures.
4. Inspect conjunctivae, scleras, corneas, irides.
5. Test pupil: size, response to light and accommodation.

Darken room

6. Using an ophthalmoscope, inspect ocular fundus: red reflex, disc, vessels, and retinal background.

EAR

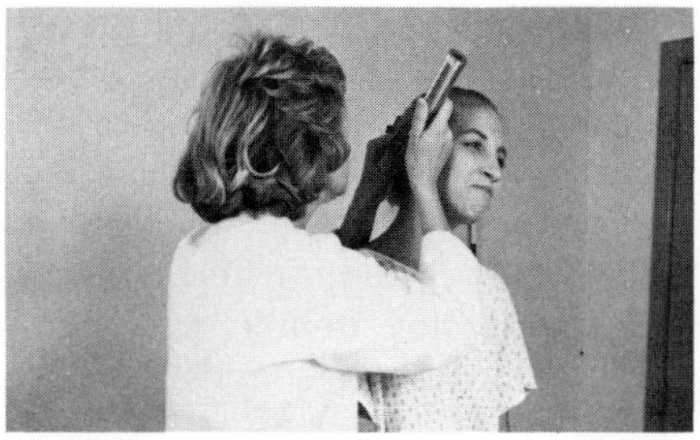

► Figure 24-5

1. Inspect the external ear: position and alignment, skin condition, and auditory meatus.
2. Move auricle and push tragus for tenderness.
3. Using an otoscope inspect the canal, then the tympanic membrane for color, position, landmarks, and integrity.
4. Test hearing: voice test; tuning fork tests—Weber and Rinne.

NOSE

1. Inspect the external nose: symmetry, lesions.
2. Test the patency of each nostril.

SEQUENCE	SELECTED PHOTOS

3. Using a speculum, inspect the nares: nasal mucosa, septum, and turbinates.

MOUTH AND THROAT

1. Using a penlight inspect the mouth: buccal mucosa, teeth and gums, tongue, floor of mouth, palate, and uvula.
2. Grade tonsils, if present.
3. Note mobility of uvula as the person phonates "ahh" and test gag reflex (cranial nerves IX, X).
4. Ask the person to stick out the tongue (cranial nerves XII).
5. Don a glove and bimanually palpate the mouth, if indicated.

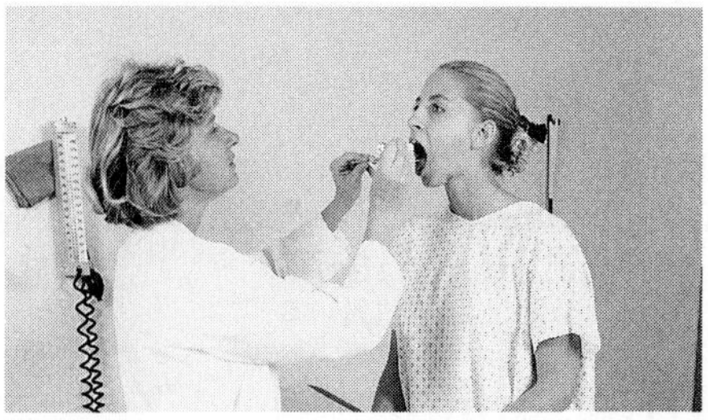

► **Figure 24-6**

NECK

1. Inspect the neck: symmetry, lumps, and pulsations.
2. Palpate the cervical lymph nodes.
3. Inspect and palpate the carotid pulse, one side at a time. If indicated, listen for carotid bruits.
4. Palpate the trachea in midline.
5. Test range of motion and muscle strength against your resistance: head forward and back, head turned to each side, and shoulder shrug (cranial nerve XI).

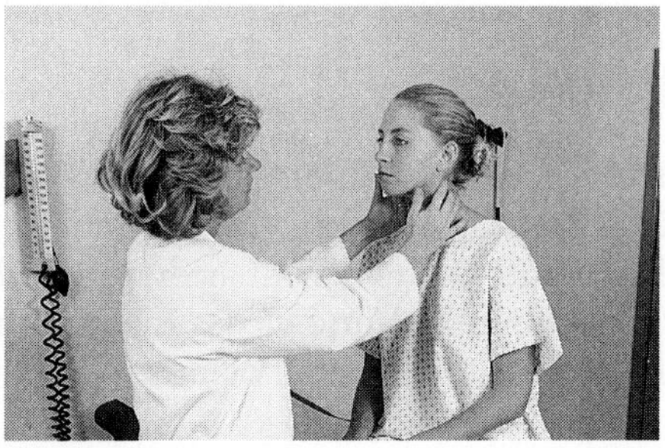

► **Figure 24-7**

Step behind the person, taking your stethoscope, ruler, and marking pen with you.

6. Palpate thyroid gland.

Open the person's gown to expose all of the back, but leave gown on shoulders and anterior chest.

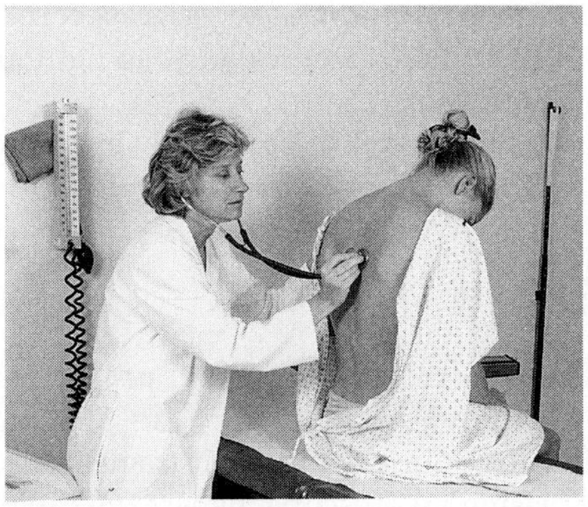

► **Figure 24-8**

CHEST, POSTERIOR AND LATERAL

1. Inspect the posterior chest: configuration of the thoracic cage, skin characteristics, and symmetry of shoulders and muscles.
2. Palpate: symmetric expansion; tactile fremitus, lumps, or tenderness.
3. Palpate length of spinous processes.
4. Percuss over all lung fields, percuss diaphragmatic excursion.
5. Percuss costovertebral angle, noting tenderness.
6. Auscultate breath sounds, note adventitious sounds.

SEQUENCE | **SELECTED PHOTOS**

Move around to face the person; the person remains sitting. For a female breast examination, ask patient's permission to lift gown to drape on the shoulders, exposing the anterior chest; for a male, lower the gown to the lap.

ANTERIOR CHEST

1. Inspect: respirations and skin characteristics.
2. Palpate: tactile fremitus, lumps or tenderness.
3. Percuss lung fields.
4. Auscultate breath sounds.

HEART

1. Ask the person to lean forward and exhale briefly; auscultate base for any murmurs.

UPPER EXTREMITIES

1. Test range of motion and muscle strength of hands, arms, and shoulders.
2. Palpate the epitrochlear nodes.

FEMALE BREASTS

1. Inspect for symmetry, mobility, and dimpling as the woman lifts arms over the head, pushes the hands on the hips, and leans forward.
2. Inspect supraclavicular and infraclavicular areas.

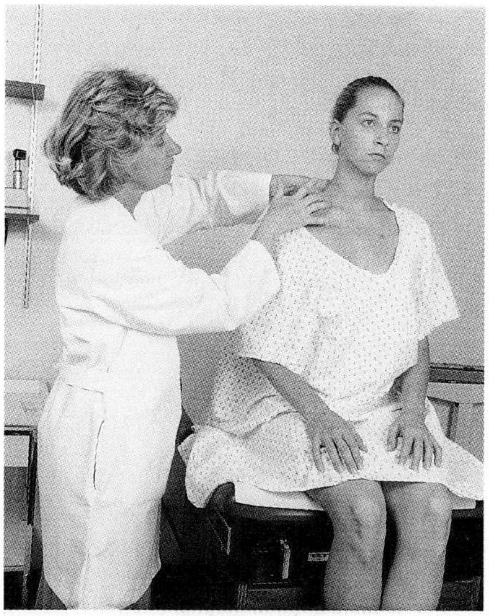

► **Figure 24-9**

Help the person to lie supine with head at a 30- to 45-degree angle. Stand at the person's *right* side. Drape the gown up across shoulders, and place an extra sheet across lower abdomen.

3. Palpate each breast, lifting the same side arm up over head. Include the tail of Spence and areola.
4. Palpate each nipple for discharge.
5. Support the person's arm and palpate axilla and regional lymph nodes.
6. Teach breast self-examination.

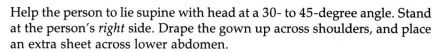

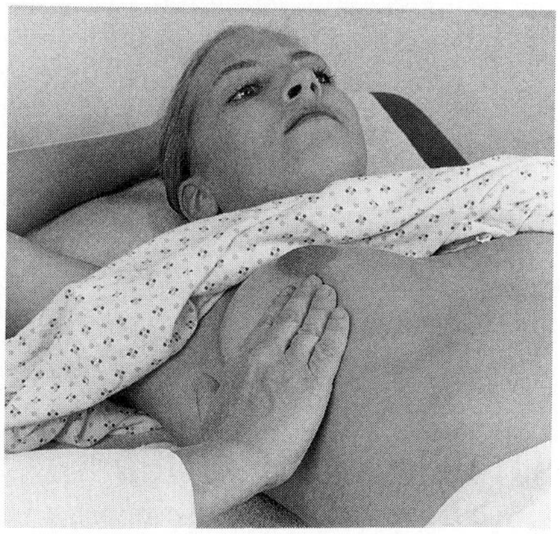

► **Figure 24-10**

MALE BREASTS

1. Inspect and palpate while palpating the anterior chest wall.
2. Supporting each arm, palpate the axilla and regional nodes.

NECK VESSELS

1. Inspect each side of neck for a jugular venous pulse, turning the person's head slightly to the other side.
2. Estimate jugular venous pressure, if indicated.

SEQUENCE	SELECTED PHOTOS

HEART

1. Inspect the precordium for pulsations and heave (lift).
2. Palpate the apical impulse, and note the location.
3. Palpate precordium for thrills.
4. Auscultate apical rate and rhythm.
5. Auscultate with the diaphragm of the stethoscope to study heart sounds, inching from the apex up to the base, or vice versa.
6. Auscultate the heart sounds with the bell of the stethoscope, again inching through all locations.
7. Turn the person over to left side while again auscultating apex with the bell.

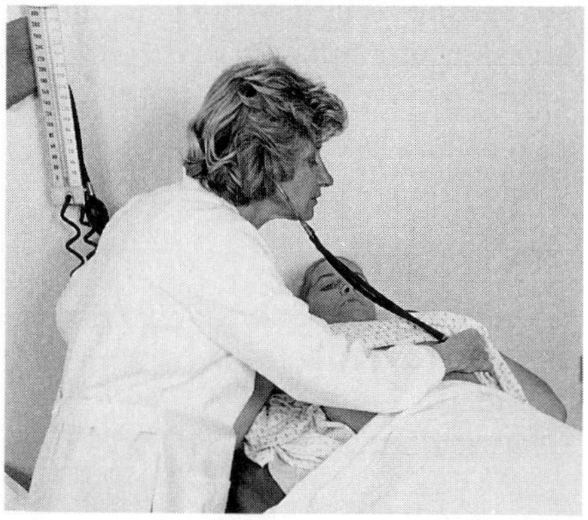

► Figure 24-11

The person should be supine, with the bed or table flat; arrange drapes to expose the abdomen from the chest to the pubis.

ABDOMEN

1. Inspect: contour, symmetry, skin characteristics, umbilicus, and pulsations.
2. Auscultate bowel sounds.
3. Auscultate for vascular sounds over the aorta and renal arteries.
4. Percuss all quadrants.
5. Percuss height of the liver span in right midclavicular line.
6. Percuss the location of the spleen.
7. Palpate: light palpation in all quadrants, then deep palpation in all quadrants.
8. Palpate for liver, for spleen, for kidneys, and for aorta.
9. Test the abdominal reflexes, if indicated.

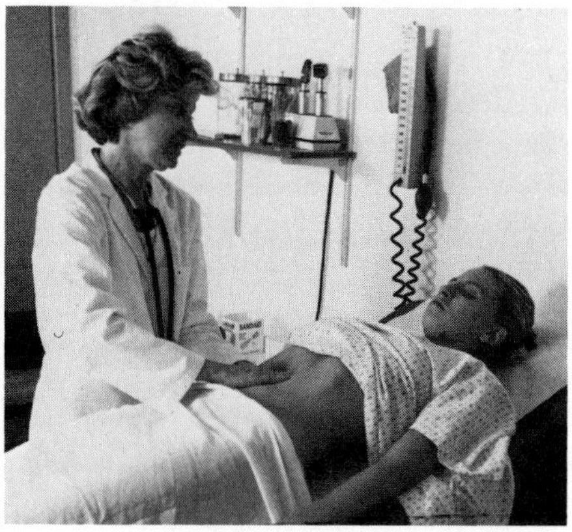

► Figure 24-12

INGUINAL AREA

1. Palpate each groin for the femoral pulse and the inguinal nodes.

Lift the drape to expose the legs.

LOWER EXTREMITIES

1. Inspect: symmetry, skin characteristics, and hair distribution.
2. Palpate pulses: popliteal, posterior tibial, dorsalis pedis.
3. Palpate for temperature and pretibial edema.
4. Separate toes and inspect.
5. Test range of motion and muscle strength of hips, knees, ankles, and feet.

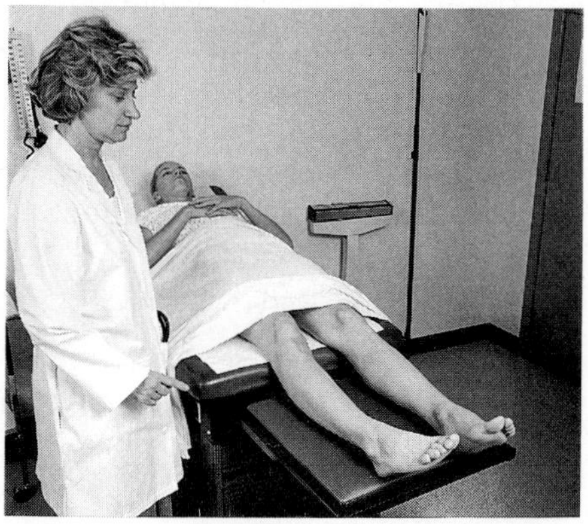

► Figure 24-13

SEQUENCE	SELECTED PHOTOS

Ask the person to sit up and to dangle the legs off the bed or table. Keep the gown on, and the drape over the lap.

MUSCULOSKELETAL

1. Note muscle strength as person performs the sit-up.

NEUROLOGIC

1. Test sensation in selected areas on face, arms, hands, legs, and feet: superficial pain, light touch, and vibration.
2. Test position sense of finger, one hand.
3. Test sterognosis.
4. Test cerebellar function of the upper extremities using finger-to-nose test or rapid-alternating-movements test.
5. Test the cerebellar function of the lower extremities by asking the person to run each heel down the opposite shin.
6. Elicit deep tendon reflexes: biceps, triceps, brachioradialis, patellar, and Achilles.
7. Test the Babinski reflex.

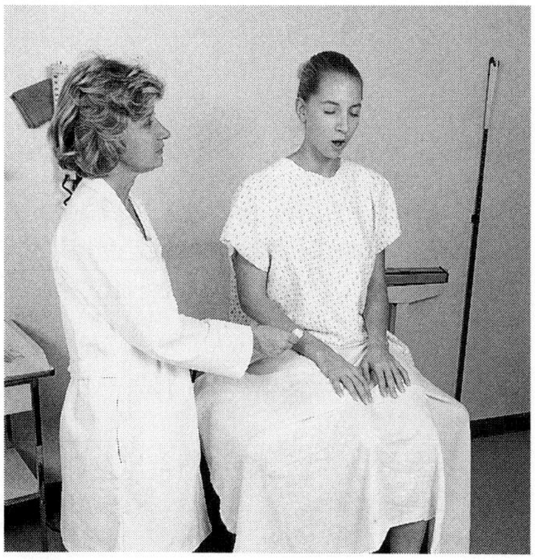

► Figure 24-14

Ask the person to stand with the gown on. Stand close to the person.

LOWER EXTREMITIES

1. Inspect legs for varicose veins.

MUSCULOSKELETAL

1. Ask the person to walk across the room, turn, then walk back toward you, in heel-to-toe fashion.
2. Ask the person to walk on the toes for a few steps, then to walk on the heels for a few steps.
3. Stand close, and check the Romberg sign.
4. Ask the person to hold the edge of the bed and to perform a shallow knee bend, one for each leg.
5. Stand behind, and check the spine as the person touches the toes.
6. Stabilize the pelvis, and test the range of motion of the spine as the person hyperextends, rotates, and laterally bends.

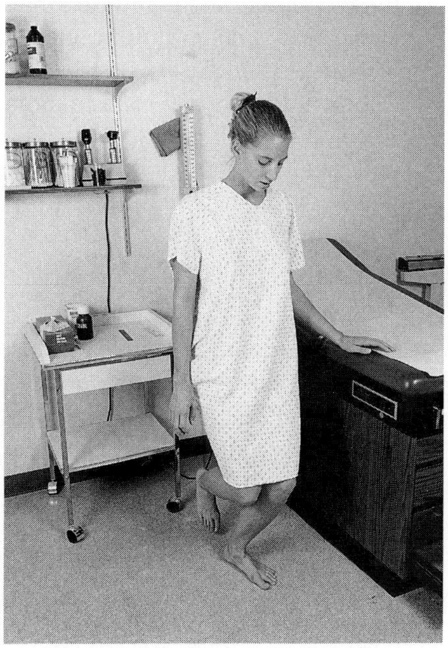

► Figure 24-15

SEQUENCE	SELECTED PHOTOS

Sit on a stool in front of a male. The person stands.

MALE GENITALIA

1. Inspect the penis and scrotum.
2. Palpate the scrotal contents. If a mass exists, transilluminate.
3. Check for inguinal hernia.
4. Teach testicular self-examination.

For an adult male, ask him to bend over the examination table, supporting the torso with forearms on the table. Assist the bedfast male to a left lateral position, with the right leg drawn up.

MALE RECTUM

1. Inspect the perianal area.
2. With a gloved lubricated finger, palpate the rectal walls and prostate gland.
3. Save a stool specimen for a guaiac test.

Assist the female back to the examination table, and help her assume the lithotomy position. Drape her appropriately. You sit on a stool at the foot of the table, then stand.

FEMALE GENITALIA

1. Inspect the perineal and perianal area.
2. Using a vaginal speculum, inspect the cervix and vaginal walls.
3. Procure specimens.
4. Perform a bimanual examination; cervix, uterus, and adnexa.
5. Continue the bimanual examination, checking the rectum and rectovaginal walls.
6. Save a stool specimen for a guaiac test.
7. Wipe the perineal area with tissues, and help the female up to a sitting position.

Tell the person you are finished with the examination and that you will leave the room as he or she gets dressed. Return to discuss the examination and further plans, and answer any questions. Thank the person for his or her time.

For the hospitalized person, return the bed and any room equipment to the way you found it. Make sure the call light and telephone are in easy reach.

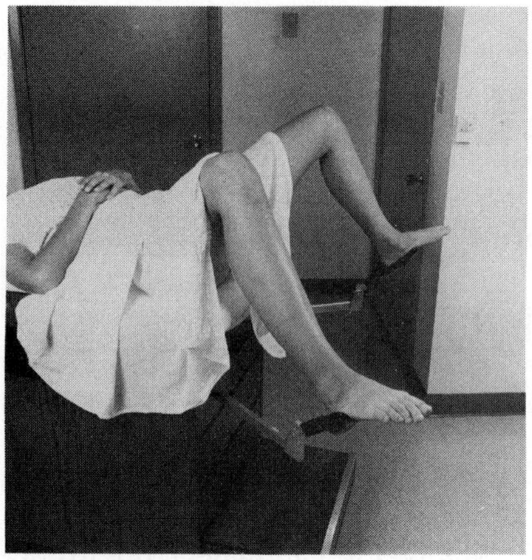

► **Figure 24–16**

THE NEONATE AND INFANT

Review Chapter 7, Getting Ready, for the steps on preparation and positioning, and developmental principles of the infant. The 1-minute and 5-minute Apgar results will give important data on the neonate's immediate response to extrauterine life. The following sequence will expand this data. You may reorder this sequence as the infant's sleep and wakefulness state or physical condition warrants.

SEQUENCE	SELECTED PHOTOS

The infant is supine on a warming table or examination table with an overhead heating element. The infant may be nude except for a diaper over a boy.

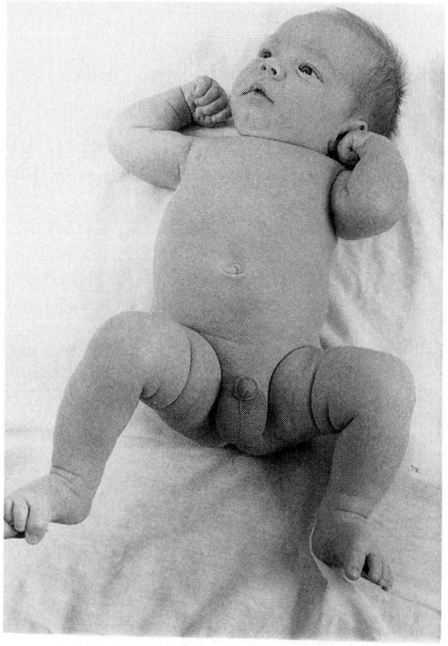

► Figure 24-17

Vital Signs

Note pulse, respirations, and temperature.

Measurement

Weight, length, head circumference are measured and plotted on growth curves for the infant's age.

General Appearance

1. Body symmetry, spontaneous position, flexion of head and extremities, and spontaneous movement.
2. Skin color and characteristics, any obvious deformities.
3. Symmetry and positioning of the facial features.
4. Alert responsive affect.
5. Strong lusty cry.

Chest and Heart

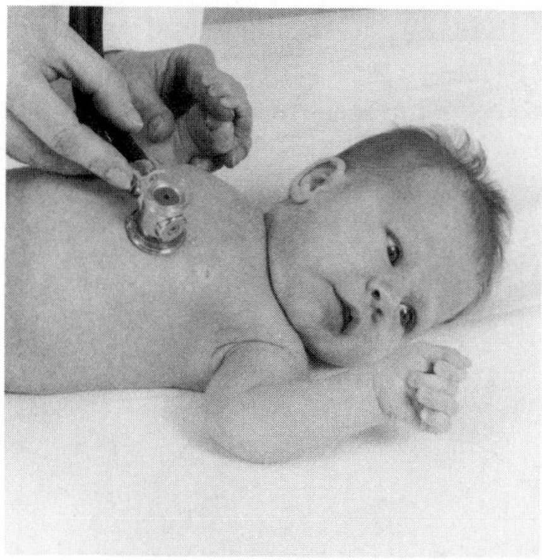

► Figure 24-18

1. If the infant is not crying, auscultate at this time: breath sounds, heart sounds in all locations, and bowel sounds in the abdomen and in the chest.
2. Inspect the skin condition over the chest and abdomen, chest configuration, and nipples and breast tissue.
3. Note movement of the abdomen with respirations, and any chest retraction.
4. Palpate: apical impulse and note location, chest wall for thrills, tactile fremitus if the infant is crying.

Abdomen

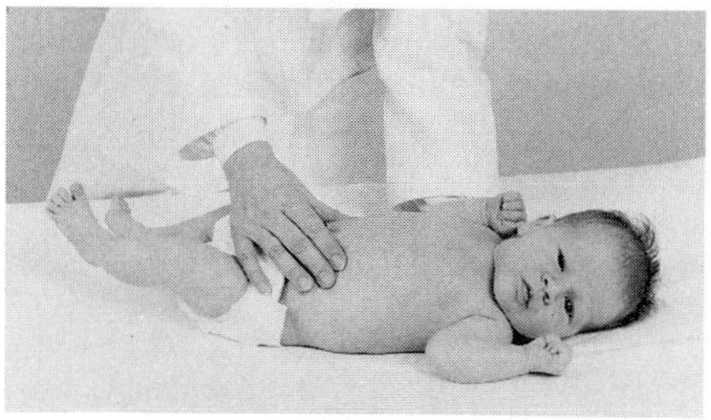

► Figure 24-19

1. Inspect the shape of the abdomen and skin condition.
2. Inspect the umbilicus; count vessels; note condition of cord or stump; any hernia.
3. Palpate skin turgor.
4. Palpate lightly for muscle tone, liver, spleen tip, and bladder.
5. Palpate deeply for kidneys, any mass.
6. Palpate femoral pulses, inguinal lymph nodes.
7. Percuss all quadrants.

SEQUENCE	SELECTED PHOTOS

Head and Face

1. Note molding following delivery; any swelling on cranium, bulging of fontanel with crying or at rest.
2. Palpate fontanels, suture lines, and any swellings.
3. Inspect positioning and symmetry of facial features at rest and while the infant is crying.

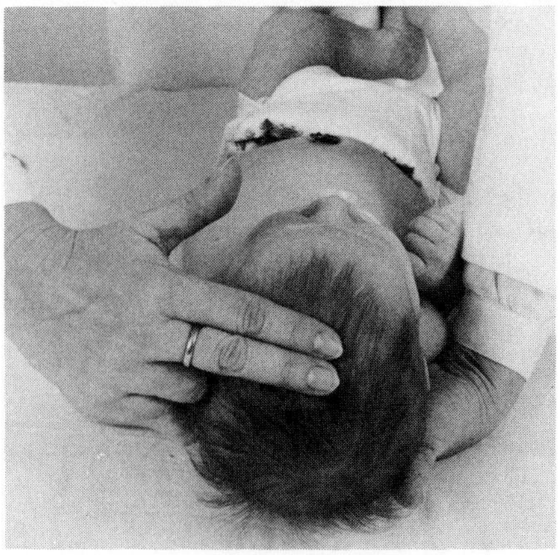

To open the neonate's eyes, support the head and shoulders and gently lower the baby backward, or ask the parent to hold the baby over his or her shoulder while you stand behind the parent.

Eyes

1. Inspect the lids (edematous in the neonate), palpebral slant, conjunctivae, any nystagmus, and any discharge.
2. Using a penlight: elicit the pupillary reflex, blink reflex and corneal light reflex; assess tracking of moving light.
3. Using an ophthalmoscope, elicit the red reflex.

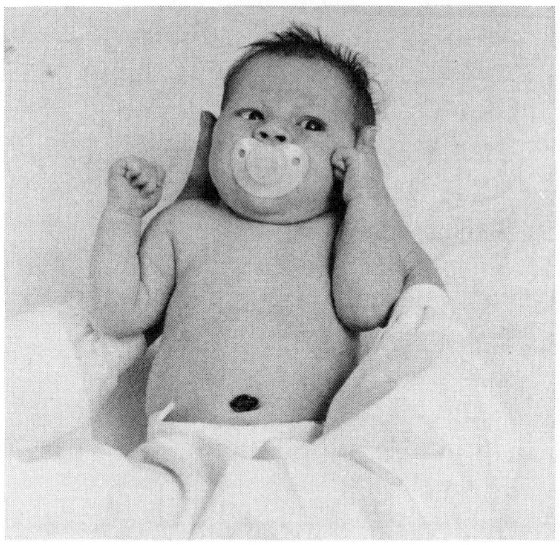

► Figure 24-20

Ears

1. Inspect size, shape, alignment of auricle, patency of auditory canals, any extra skin tags or pits.
2. Note the startle reflex in response to a loud noise.
3. Palpate flexible auricles.
   (Defer otoscopic examination until the end of the complete examination.)

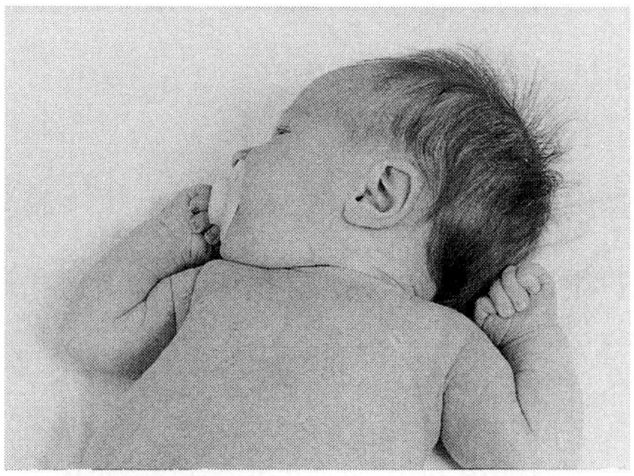

► Figure 24-21

SEQUENCE | **SELECTED PHOTOS**

Nose

1. Determine the patency of the nares.
2. Note the nasal discharge, sneezing, and any flaring with respirations.

Mouth and Throat

1. Inspect the lips and gums, high-arched intact palate, buccal mucosa, tongue size, and frenulum of tongue; note absent or minimal salivation in neonate.
2. Note the rooting reflex.
3. Insert a gloved finger, note the sucking reflex and palpate palate.

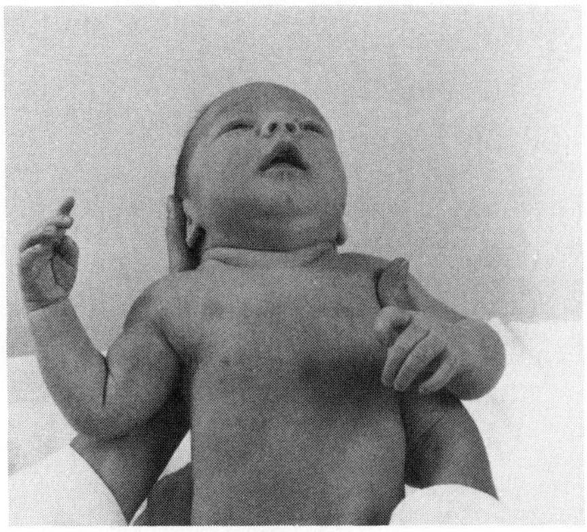

▶ **Figure 24-22**

Neck

1. Lift the shoulders and let the head lag to inspect the neck: note midline trachea, any skin folds, and any lumps.
2. Palpate the lymph nodes, the thyroid, and any masses.
3. While the infant is supine, elicit the tonic neck reflex; note a supple neck with movement.

Hands, Arms, Shoulders

1. Inspect and manipulate noting range of motion, muscle tone, and absence of scarf sign (elbow should not reach midline)
2. Count fingers, count palmar creases, and note color of hands and nail beds.
3. Place your thumbs in the infant's palms to note the grasp reflex, then wrap your hands around infant's hands to pull up and note the head lag.

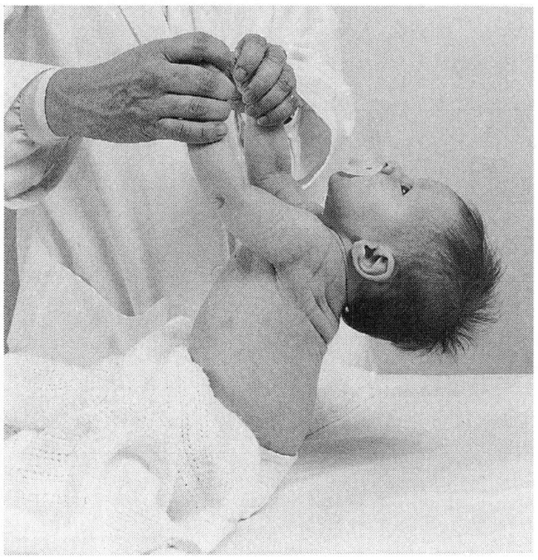

▶ **Figure 24-23**

Legs and Feet

1. Inspect and manipulate the legs and feet, noting range of motion, muscle tone, and skin condition.
2. Note alignment of feet and toes, flat soles, and count toes; note any syndactyly.
3. Test Ortolani's sign for hip stability.

Genitalia

1. Females. Inspect labia and clitoris (edematous in the newborn), vernix caseosa between labia, and patent vagina.
2. Males. Inspect position of urethral meatus (do not retract foreskin), strength of urine stream if possible, and rugae on scrotum.
3. Palpate the testes in the scrotum.

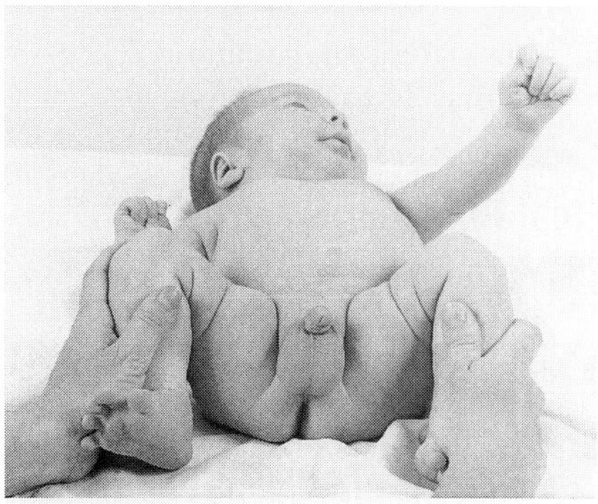

▶ **Figure 24-24**

SEQUENCE	SELECTED PHOTOS

Lift the infant under the axillae, and hold the infant facing you at eye level.

Neuromuscular

1. Note shoulder muscle tone and the infant's ability to stay in your hands without slipping.
2. Rotate the neonate slowly side to side; note the doll's eye reflex.
3. Turn the infant around so his or her back is to you; elicit the stepping reflex and the placing reflex against the edge of the examination table.

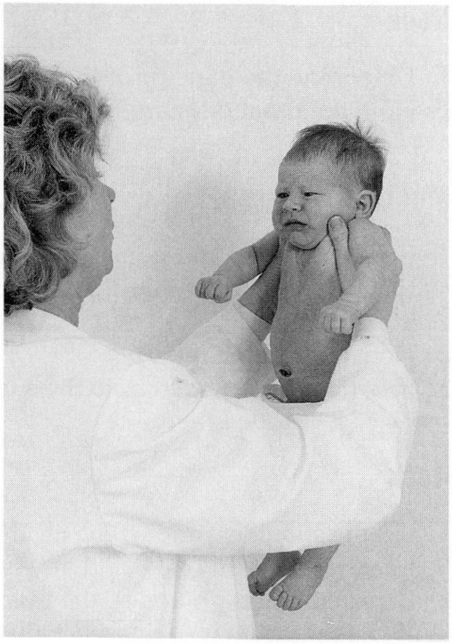

► Figure 24-25

Turn the infant over, and hold him or her prone in your hands, or place the infant prone on the examination table.

Spine and Rectum

1. Inspect the length of the spine, trunk incurvation reflex, and symmetry of gluteal folds.
2. Inspect intact skin; note any sinus openings, protrusions, or tufts of hair.
3. Note patent anal opening. Check for passage of meconium stool during the first 24 to 48 hours.

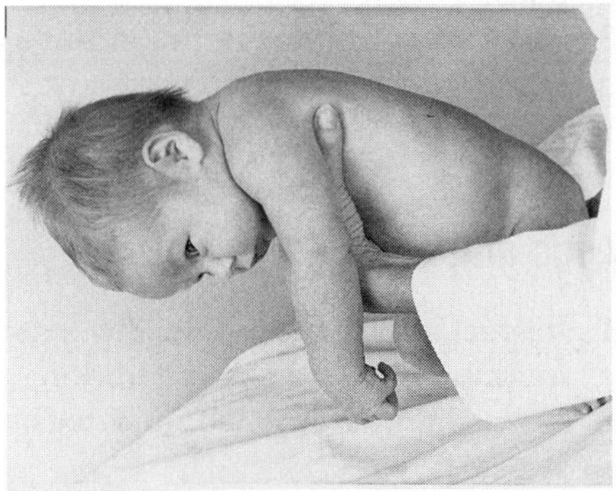

► Figure 24-26

Final Procedures

1. Using an otoscope, inspect the auditory canal and the tympanic membrane.
2. Elicit the Moro reflex by letting the infant's head and trunk drop back a short way, or by jarring crib sides, or making a loud noise.

THE YOUNG CHILD

Review the developmental considerations in preparing for an examination of the toddler and the young child in Chapter 7, Getting Ready. A young child during this time is beset with independence and dependence needs on the parent, is aware of and fearful of a new environment, has a fear of invasive procedures, dislikes being restrained, and may be attached to a security object.

SEQUENCE	SELECTED PHOTOS

Focus on the parent as child plays with a toy at parent's feet.

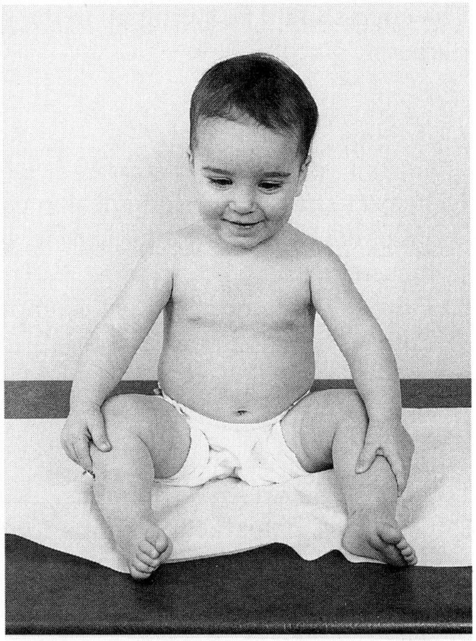

▶ Figure 24-27

The Health History

1. Collect the history, including developmental data.

During the history, note data on general appearance.

General Appearance

1. Note child's ability to amuse himself or herself while the parent speaks.
2. Note parent and child interaction.
3. Note gross motor and fine motor skills as the child plays with toys.

Gradually focus on and involve yourself with the child, at first in a "play" period.

4. Evaluate developmental milestones by using a Denver II test: gait, jumping, hopping, build a tower, and throw a ball.
5. Evaluate posture while the child is sitting and standing. Evaluate alignment of the legs and feet while the child is walking.
6. Evaluate speech acquisition.
7. Evaluate vision, hearing ability.
8. Evaluate social interaction.

Ask the parent to undress the child to the diaper or the underpants. Position the older infant and young child, 6 months to 2 or 3 years, in the parent's lap. Move your chairs to sit knee-to-knee with the parent. A 4- or 5-year old child usually feels comfortable on the examination table.

Measurement

Height, weight, head circumference (may need to defer head circumference until later in the examination).

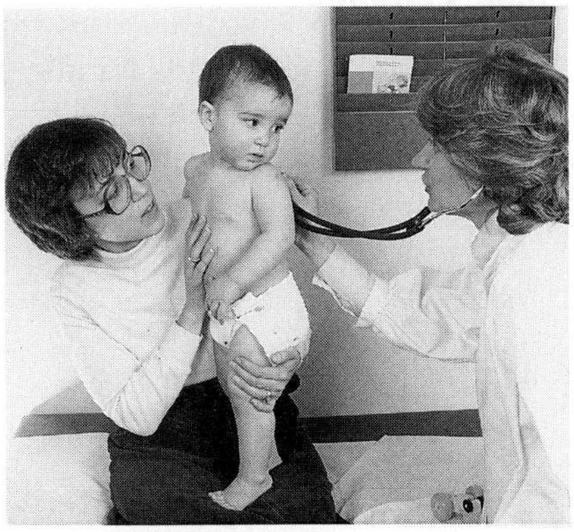

▶ Figure 24-28

Chest and Heart

1. Auscultate breath sounds and heart sounds in all locations, count respiratory rate, count heart rate, and auscultate bowel sounds.
2. Inspect size, shape, and configuration of chest cage. Assess respiratory movement.
3. Inspect pulsations on the precordium. Note nipple and breast development.
4. Palpate: apical impulse and note location, chest wall for thrills, any tactile fremitus.

SEQUENCE	SELECTED PHOTOS

The child should be sitting up in the parent's lap or on examination table, diaper in place.

Abdomen

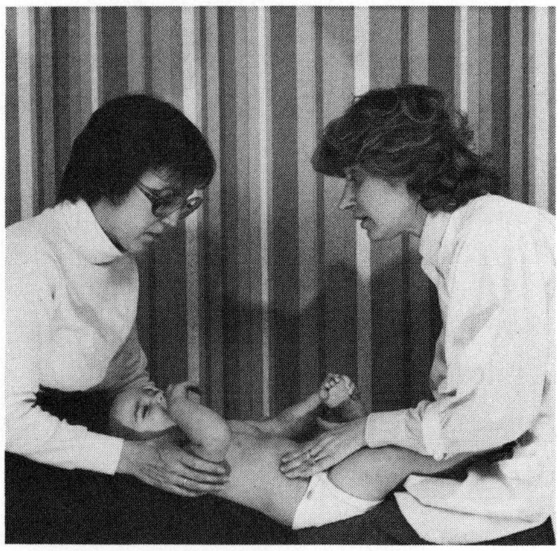

► Figure 24-29

1. Inspect shape of abdomen, skin condition, and periumbilical area.
2. Palpate skin turgor, muscle tone, liver edge, spleen, kidneys, and any masses.
3. Palpate the femoral pulses. Compare strength to radial pulses.
4. Palpate inguinal lymph nodes.

Genitalia

1. Inspect the external genitalia.
2. On males, palpate the scrotum for testes. If masses are present, transilluminate.

Lower Extremities

1. Test Ortolani's sign for hip stability.
2. Note alignment of legs and skin condition.
3. Note alignment of feet. Inspect toes and longitudinal arch.
4. Palpate the dorsalis pedis pulse.
5. Gain cooperation with reflex hammer. Elicit plantar, Achilles, and patellar reflexes.

The child should be sitting up in the parent's lap or on examination table, diaper in place.

Upper Extremities

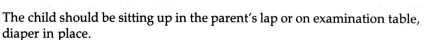

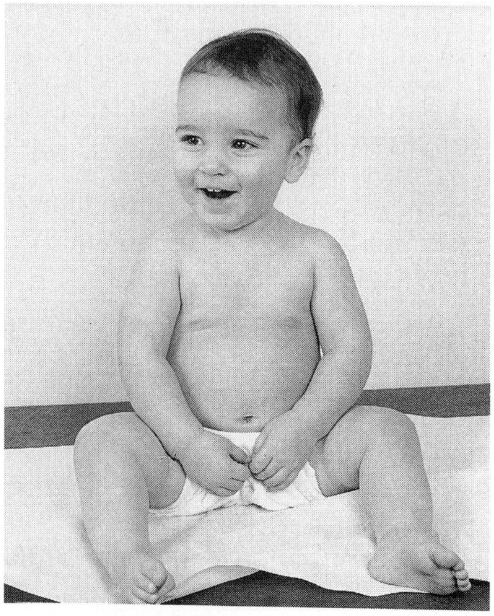

► Figure 24-30

1. Inspect arms and hands for alignment, skin condition; inspect fingers and note palmar creases.
2. Palpate and count the radial pulse.
3. Test biceps and triceps reflexes with a reflex hammer.
4. Measure blood pressure.

SEQUENCE	SELECTED PHOTOS

Head and Neck

1. Inspect the size and shape of the head and symmetry of facies.
2. Palpate the fontanels and cranium. Palpate the cervical lymph nodes, trachea, and thyroid gland.
3. Measure the head circumference.

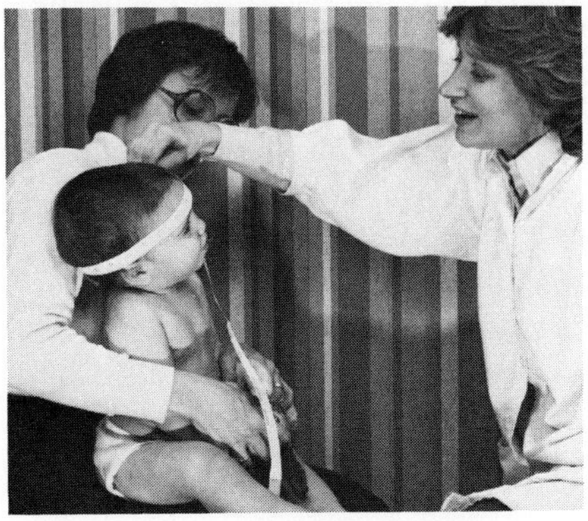

► Figure 24–31

Eyes

1. Inspect the external structures. Note any palpebral slant.
2. Using a penlight, test the corneal light and pupillary light reflexes.
3. Direct a moving penlight for cardinal positions of gaze.
4. If indicated, perform the cover test, covering the eye with your thumb in a young child, or use an index card.
5. Inspect conjunctivae and scleras.
6. Using an ophthalmoscope, check the red reflex. Inspect the fundus as much as possible.

Nose

1. Inspect the external nose and skin condition.
2. Using a penlight, inspect the nares for foreign body, mucosa, septum, and turbinates.

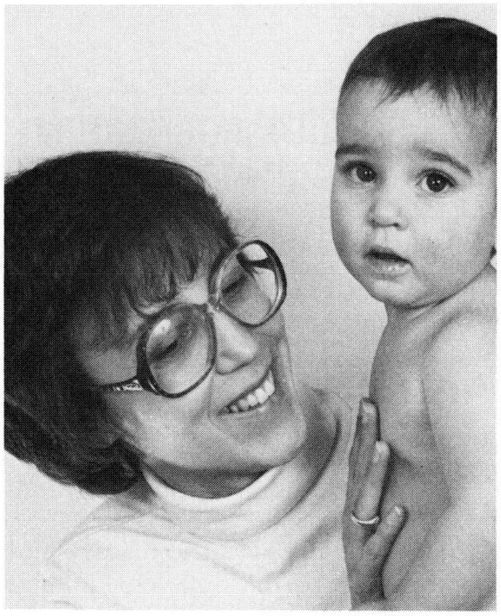

► Figure 24–32

Mouth and Throat

1. Using a penlight, inspect the mouth, buccal mucosa, teeth and gums, tongue, palate, and uvula in midline. Use a tongue blade as the last resort.

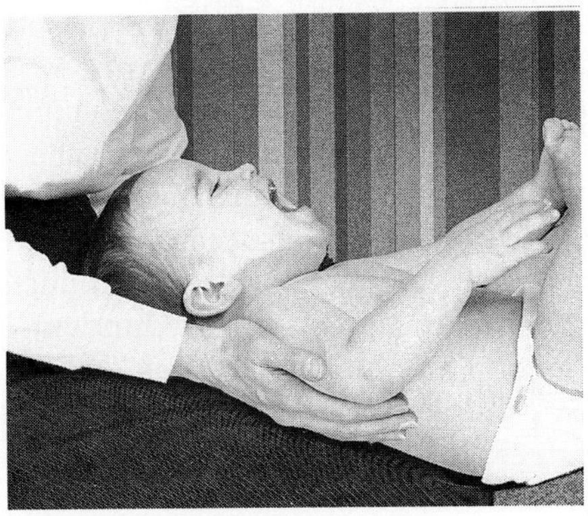

► Figure 24–33

SEQUENCE	SELECTED PHOTOS

Ears

1. Inspect and palpate the auricle. Note any discharge from the auditory meatus. Check for any foreign body.
2. Using an otoscope, inspect the ear canal and tympanic membrane. Gain cooperation through the use of a puppet, encouraging the child to handle the equipment, or to look in the parent's ear as you hold the otoscope. You may need to have the parent help restrain the child.

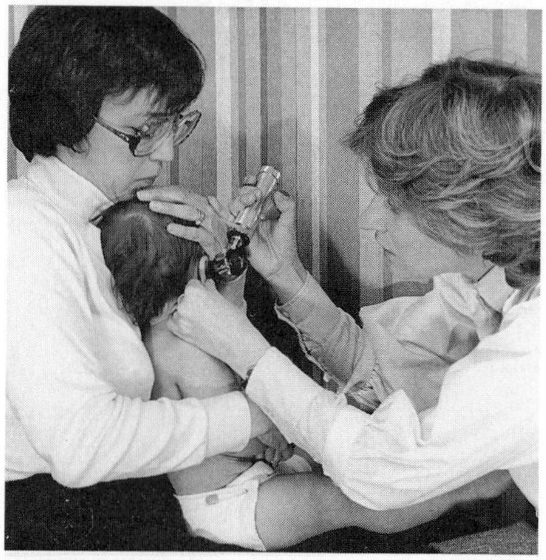

► Figure 24–34

THE SCHOOL-AGED CHILD, THE ADOLESCENT, AND THE AGING ADULT

The sequence of the examination for people in these age groups is the head-to-toe format described in the adult section. However, there are differences in approach and timing, and special developmental considerations. Review Chapter 7, Getting Ready, for a full discussion of these factors.

RECORDING THE DATA

Record the data from the history and physical examination as soon after the event as possible. Memory fades as the day develops, especially when you are responsible for the care of more than one person.

It is difficult to strike a balance between recording too few data and recording too many. It is important to remember that, from a legal perspective, if it is not documented, it was not done. Data important for the diagnosis and treatment of the person's health should be recorded as well as data that contribute to your decision-making process. This includes charting relevant normal or negative findings.

On the other hand, a listing of every assessment parameter described in this text yields an unwieldy, unworkable record. One way to keep your record complete yet succinct is to study your writing style. Use short clear phrases. Avoid redundant introductory phrases such as, "The patient states that . . ." Avoid redundant descriptions such as "no inguinal, femoral, or umbilical hernias." Just write, "no hernias."

Use simple line drawings to describe your findings. You do not need artistic talent; draw a simple sketch of a tympanic membrane, breast, abdomen, or cervix and mark your findings on it. A clear picture is worth many sentences of words.

Study the following complete history and physical examination for a sample write-up. Note that the subject is the same young woman introduced in Chapter 1 of this text.

HEALTH HISTORY

Biographical Data

Name	Ellen K.	*Birthdate*	1/18/
Address	123 Center St.	*Birthplace*	Springfield
Marital Status	Single	*Race*	White

Ellen K. is a 23-year-old, single, white, female cashier at a tavern, presently unemployed for 6 months.

Source. Ellen, seems reliable

Reason for Seeking Care. "I'm coming in for alcohol treatment."

History of Present Illness. First alcoholic drink, age 16. First intoxication, age 17, drinking 1 to 2 times per week, a 6-pack per occasion. Attending high school classes every day, but grades slipping from A−/B+ average, to C− average. At age 20, drinking 2 times per week, 6 to 9 beers per occasion. At age 22, drinking 2 times per week, a 12-pack per occasion, and occasionally a 6-pack the next day to "help with the hangover." During this year, experienced blackouts, failed attempts to cut down on drinking, being physically sick the morning after drinking, and being unable to stop drinking once started. Also, incurred three driving-under-the-influence (DUI) legal offenses. Last DUI 1 month PTA, last alcohol use just before DUI, 18 beers that occasion. Abstinent since that time.

Past Health

Childhood Illnesses. Chicken pox at age 6. No measles, mumps, croup, pertussis. No rheumatic fever, scarlet fever, or polio.

Accidents. 1. Auto accident, age 12, father driving, Ellen thrown from car, right leg crushed. Hospitalized at Memorial, surgery for leg pinning to repair multiple compound fracture. 2. Auto accident, age 21, head hit dashboard, no loss of consciousness, treated and released at Memorial hospital ED. 3. Auto accident, age 23, "car hit median strip," no injuries, not seen at hospital.

Chronic Illnesses. None

Hospitalizations. Age 12, Memorial Hospital, surgery to repair right leg as described, Dr. M J Carlson, surgeon.

Obstetric History. Gravida 0/Para 0/Abortion 0

Immunizations. Childhood immunizations up to date. Last tetanus "probably high school." No Tb skin test.

Last Examinations. Yearly pelvic examinations at Health Department since age 15, told "normal." High school sports physical as sophomore. Last dental examination as high school junior; last vision test for driver's license age 16, never had ECG, chest x-ray study.

Allergies. No known allergies.

Current Medications. Birth control pills, low estrogen type, 1/day, for 5 years. No other prescription or over-the-counter medications.

Family History. Ellen is 2nd and youngest child, parents divorced 8 years, father has chronic alcoholism.

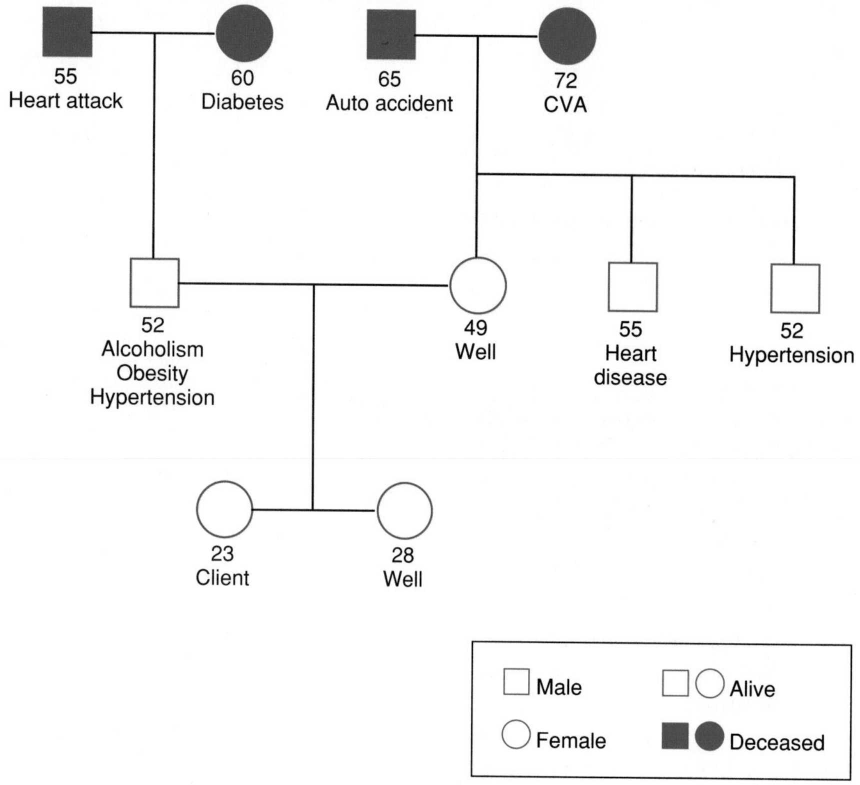

Review of Systems

General Health. Reports usual health "OK." No recent weight change, no fatigue, weakness, fever, sweats.

Skin. No change in skin color, pigmentation, or nevi. No pruritus, rash, lesions. Has bruise now over right eye, struck by boyfriend 1 week PTA. No history skin disease. Hair, no loss, change in texture. Nails, no change. Self-care. Stays in sun "as much as I can." No use of sunscreen. Goes to tanning beds at hair salon 2 × /week during winter.

Head. No unusually frequent or severe headaches, no head injury, dizziness, syncope, or vertigo.

Eyes. No difficulty with vision or double vision. No eye pain, inflammation, discharge, lesions. No history glaucoma or cataracts. Wears no corrective lenses.

Ears. No hearing loss or difficulty. No earaches, infections now or as child, no discharge, tinnitus, or vertigo. Self-care. No exposure to environmental noise, cleans ears with washcloth.

Nose. No discharge, has two to three colds per year, no sinus pain, nasal obstruction, epistaxis, or allergy.

Mouth and Throat. No mouth pain, bleeding gums, toothache, sores or lesions in mouth, dysphagia, hoarseness, or sore throat. Has tonsils. Self-care. Brushes teeth twice/day, no flossing.

Neck. No pain, limitation of motion, lumps, or swollen glands.

Breast. No pain, lump, nipple discharge, rash, swelling, or trauma. No history of breast disease in self, mother, or sister. No surgery. Self-care. Does not do breast self-examination.

Respiratory. No past history lung disease, no chest pain with breathing, wheezing, shortness of breath. Colds sometimes "go to my chest," treats with over-the-counter cough medicine and aspirin. Occasional early morning cough, nonproductive. Smokes cigarettes 2 PPD × 2 years, prior use 1 PPD × 4 years. Never tried to quit. Works in poorly ventilated tavern, "everybody smokes."

Cardiovascular. No chest pain, palpitation, cyanosis, fatigue, dyspnea with exertion, orthopnea, paroxysmal nocturnal dyspnea, nocturia, edema. No history of heart murmur, hypertension, coronary artery disease, or anemia.

Peripheral Vascular. No pain, numbness or tingling, swelling in legs. No coldness, discoloration, varicose veins, infections, or ulcers. Legs are unequal in length as sequelae of accident age 12. Self-care. Usual work as cashier involves standing for 8-hour shifts, no support hose.

Gastrointestinal. Appetite good with no recent change. No food intolerance, heartburn, indigestion, pain in abdomen, no nausea or vomiting. No history of ulcers, liver or gallbladder disease, jaundice, appendicitis, or colitis. Bowel movement 1/day, soft, brown, no rectal bleeding or pain. Self-care. No use of vitamins, antacids, laxatives. Diet recall—see Functional Assessment.

Urinary. No dysuria, frequency, urgency, nocturia, hesitancy, or straining. No pain in flank, groin, suprapubic region. Urine color yellow, no history kidney disease.

Genitalia. Menarche age 11. Last menstrual period April 18. Cycle usually q 28 days, duration 4 to 5 days, flow moderate, no dysmenorrhea. No vaginal itching or discharge, sores, or lesions.

Sexual health. In relationship now that includes intercourse. This boyfriend has been her only sexual partner for 2 years, had one other partner before that. Uses birth control pills to prevent pregnancy, partner uses no condoms. Concerned that boyfriend may be having sex with other women but has not confronted him. Aware of no STD contact. Never been tested for AIDS. Past history of sexual abuse by father from ages 12 to 16 years, abuse did not include intercourse. Ellen is unwilling to discuss further at this time.

Musculoskeletal. No past history arthritis, gout. No joint pain, stiffness, swelling, deformity, limitation of motion. No muscle pain, or weakness. Bone trauma at age 12, has sequela of unequal leg lengths, right leg shorter, walks with limp. Self-care. No walking or running for sport or exercise "because of leg." Able to stand as cashier. Uses lift pad in right shoe to equalize leg length.

Neurologic. No history of seizure disorder, stroke, fainting. Has had blackouts with alcohol use. No weakness, tremor, paralysis, problems with coordination, difficulty speaking or swallowing. No numbness or tingling. Not aware of memory problem, nervousness or mood change, depression.

Had counseling for sexual abuse in the past. Denies any suicidal ideation or intent during adolescent years or now.

Hematologic. No bleeding problems in skin, excessive bruising. Not aware of exposure to toxins, never had blood transfusion, never used needles to shoot drugs.

Endocrine. No family history of diabetes. No increase in hunger, thirst, or unination; no problems with hot or cold environments; no change in skin, appetite, or nervousness.

Functional Assessment

Self-Concept. Graduated from high school. Trained "on-the-job" as bartender, also worked as cashier in tavern. Unemployed now, on public aid, does not perceive she has enough money for daily living. Lives with older sister. Raised as Presbyterian, believes in God, does not attend church. Believes self to be "honest, dependable." Believes limitations are "smoking, weight, drinking."

Activity-Exercise. Typical day: arises 9.00 AM, light chores or TV, spends day looking for work, running errands, with friends, bedtime at 11:00 PM. No sustained physical exercise. Believes self able to perform all ADLs; limp poses no problem in bathing, dressing, cooking, household tasks, mobility, driving a car, or work as cashier. No mobility aids. Hobbies are fishing, boating, snowmobiling, although currently has no finances to engage in most of these.

Sleep-Rest. Bedtime 11:00 PM. Sleeps 8 to 9 hours. No sleep aids.

Nutrition. 24-hour recall: Breakfast, none; Lunch, bologna sandwich, chips, diet soda; Dinner, hamburger, french fries, coffee; Snacks, peanuts, pretzels, potato chips, "bar food." This menu is typical of most days. Eats lunch at home alone. Most dinners at fast-food restaurants or in tavern. Shares household grocery expenses and cooking chores with sister. No food intolerances.

Alcohol. See present illness. Denies use of street drugs. Cigarettes, smokes 2 PPD × 2 years, prior use 1 PPD × 4 years. Never tried to quit. Boyfriend smokes cigarettes.

Interpersonal Relationships. Describes family life growing up as chaotic. Father physically abusive toward mother and sexually abusive toward Ellen. Parents divorced because of father's continual drinking. Few support systems currently. Estranged from mother, "didn't believe me about my father." Father estranged from entire family. Gets along "OK" with sister. Relationship with boyfriend chaotic, has hit her twice in the past. Ellen has never pressed legal charges. No close women friends. Most friends are "drinking buddies" at tavern.

Coping and Stress Management. Believes housing adequate, adequate heat and utilities, and neighborhood safe. Believes home has no safety hazards, does not use seat belts. No travel outside 60 miles of hometown.

Identifies current stresses to be drinking, legal problems with DUIs, unemployment, financial worries. Considers her drinking to be problematic.

Perception of Health. Identifies alcohol as a health problem for herself, feels motivated for treatment. Never been interested in physical health and own body before, "Now I think it's time I learned." Expects health care providers to "Help me with my drinking. I don't know beyond that." Expects to stay at this agency for 6 weeks, "Then, I don't know what."

PHYSICAL EXAMINATION

Height 163 cm (5′ 4″) Weight 68.6 kg (151 lb)
B/P 142/100 right arm, sitting
140/96 right arm, lying
138/98 left arm, lying
Temp 37°C Pulse 76, regular Respirations 16, unlabored

General Survey. Ellen K. is a 23-year-old white female, not currently under the influence of alcohol or other drugs, who articulates clearly, ambulates without difficulty, and is in no distress.

Skin. Uniformly tan-pink in color, warm, dry, intact, turgor good. No lesions, birthmarks, edema. Resolving 2-cm yellow-green hematoma present over right eye, no swelling, ocular structures not involved. Hair, normal distribution and texture, no pest inhabitants. Nails, no clubbing, biting, or discolorations. Nail beds pink and firm with prompt capillary refill.

Head. Normocephalic, no lesions, lumps, scaling, parasites, or tenderness. Face, symmetric, no weakness, no involuntary movements.

Eyes. Acuity by Snellen chart O.D. 20/20, O.S. 20/20 -1. Visual fields full by confrontation. EOMs intact, no nystagmus. No ptosis, lid lag, discharge, or crusting. Corneal light reflex symmetric, no strabismus. Conjunctivae clear. Sclera white, no lesion or redness. PERRLA. Fundi: discs flat with sharp margins. Vessels present in all quadrants without crossing defects. Background has even color, no hemorrhage or exudates.

Ears. Pinna no mass, lesions, scaling, discharge, or tenderness to palpation. Canals clear. Tympanic membrane pearly gray, landmarks intact, no perforation. Whispered words heard bilaterally. Weber midline with lateralization. Rinne AC > BC and = bilaterally.

Nose. No deformities or tenderness to palpation. Nares patent. Mucosa pink, no lesions. Septum midline, no perforation. No sinus tenderness.

Mouth. Mucosa and gingivae pink, no lesions or bleeding. Right lower 1st molar missing, multiple dark spots on most teeth, gums receding on lower incisors. Tongue symmetric, protrudes midline, no tremor. Pharynx pink, no exudate. Uvula rises midline on phonation. Tonsils 1+. Gag reflex present.

Neck. Neck supple with full ROM. Symmetric, no masses, tenderness, lymphadenopathy. Trachea midline. Thyroid nonpalpable, not tender. Jugular veins flat @ 45 degrees. Carotid arteries 2+ and = bilaterally, no bruits.

Spine and Back. Normal spinal profile, no scoliosis. No tenderness over spines, no CVA tenderness.

Thorax and Lungs. AP $<$ transverse diameter. Chest expansion symmetric. Tactile fremitus equal bilaterally. Lung fields resonant. Diaphragmatic excursion 4 cm and = bilaterally. Breath sounds diminished. Expiratory wheeze in posterior chest at both bases, scattered rhonchi in posterior chest at both bases, do not clear with coughing.

Breasts. Symmetric; no retraction, discharge, or lesions. Contour and consistency firm and homogeneous. No masses or tenderness, no lymphadenopathy.

Heart. Precordium, no abnormal pulsations, no heaves. Apical impulse at 5th ics in left MCL, no thrills. S_1-S_2 normal, no S_3 or S_4. Systolic murmur, grade ii/vi, loudest at left lower sternal border, no radiation, present supine and sitting.

Abdomen. Flat, symmetric. Skin smooth with no lesions, scars, or striae. Bowel sounds present, no bruits. Tympany predominates in all quadrants. Liver span 7 cm in right MCL. Abdomen soft, no organomegaly, no masses or tenderness, no inguinal lymphadenopathy.

Extremities. Color tan-pink, no redness, cyanosis, lesions other than surgical scar. Scar right lower leg, anterior, 28 cm × 2 cm wide, well healed. No edema, varicosities. No calf tenderness. All peripheral pulses present, 2+ and = bilaterally. Asymmetric leg length, right leg 3 cm shorter than left.

Musculoskeletal. Temporomandibular joint no slipping or crepitation. Neck full range of motion, no pain. Vertebral column no tenderness, no deformity or curvature. Full extension, lateral bending, rotation. Arms symmetric, legs measure as above, extremities have full ROM, no pain or crepitation. Muscle strength, able to maintain flexion against resistance and without tenderness.

Neurologic. Mental status. Appearance, behavior, speech appropriate. Alert and oriented to person, place, time. Thought coherent. Remote and recent memories intact. Cranial nerves II through XII intact. Sensory: pin prick, light touch, vibration intact. Stereognosis, able to identify key. Motor: no atrophy, weakness, or tremors. Gait has limp, able to tandem walk with shoes on. Negative Romberg's sign. Cerebellar, finger-to-nose smoothly intact.

Genitalia. External genitalia has no lesion, discharge. Internal genitalia: vaginal walls pink, no lesion. Cervix pink, nulliparous os, no lesions, small amount nonodorous clear discharge. Specimens obtained. Bimanual, no pain on moving cervix, uterus midline, no enlargement, masses, or tenderness. Adnexa, ovaries not enlarged, no tenderness. Anus, no hemorrhoids, fissures, or lesions. Rectal wall intact, no masses or tenderness. Stool soft, brown; guaiac negative.

DTRs

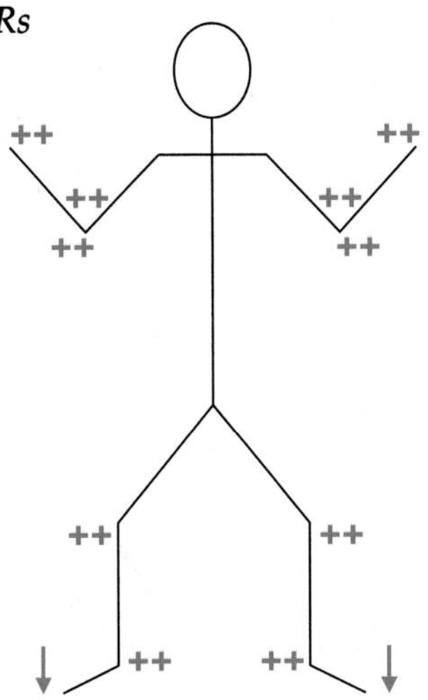

ASSESSMENT

Alcohol dependence, severe

Elevated blood pressure

Systolic murmur

Ineffective airway clearance R/T tracheobronchial secretions and obstruction

Self-care deficit: oral hygiene R/T lack of motivation

Knowledge deficit about alcoholism disease process, treatment options, support systems R/T lack of exposure

Knowledge deficit about balanced diet R/T lack of exposure and substance abuse

Altered family processes R/T effects of alcoholism and unemployment

Low self-esteem R/T effects of alcoholism, sexual abuse, physical abuse

ILLUSTRATION CREDITS

CHAPTER 2

Figure 2-1: From The Seasons of a Man's Life, by Daniel J. Levinson, et al. Copyright 1978 by Daniel J. Levinson. Reprinted by permission of Alfred A. Knopf, Inc.

Figure 2-3: Reprinted with permission from Denver Developmental Materials, Inc., Denver, CO, 1990.

CHAPTER 6

Figures 6-1, 6-2, and 6-3: Reprinted with permission of Ross Laboratories, Columbus, OH 43216, from Guidelines for Anthropometric Measurement, 1987 Ross Laboratories.

Art for Table 6-11: (pellagra) Latham MC, McGandy RB, McCann MB, Stare FJ: Scope Manual on Nutrition. Kalamazoo, MI: The Upjohn Company, 1980, copyright by Thomas Spies, MD: (follicular hyperkeratosis) Taylor KB, Anthony LE: Clinical Nutrition. New York: McGraw-Hill, 1983, copyright by Harold H. Sandstead, MD; (kwashiorkor) Latham MC et al: Scope Manual on Nutrition. Kalamazoo, MI: The Upjohn Company, 1980 copyright by Michael C. Latham, MD: (Bitot's spots) Taylor KB, Anthony LE: Clinical Nutrition. New York: McGraw-Hill, 1983, copyright by Helen Keller International, Inc.; (scorbutic gums) Taylor KB, Anthony LE: Clinical Nutrition. New York: McGraw-Hill, 1983, copyright by The Upjohn Company; (magenta tongue) McLaren DS: Color Atlas of Nutritional Disorders. England: Wolfe Medical, Ltd, copyright by C. E. Butterworth, Jr; (rickets) Latham MC et al: Scope Manual on Nutrition. Kalamazoo, MI: The Upjohn Company, 1980, copyright by Rosa Lee Nemir, MD.

Appendix 6-1: From the Food and Nutrition Board, National Academy of Sciences—National Research Council, Washington, DC, 1980.

Appendix 6-2: Redrawn from Committee on Maternal Nutrition, Food and Nutrition Board, National Research Council, National Academy of Sciences: Maternal Nutrition and the Course of Pregnancy. Washington, DC: Government Printing Office, 1970.

CHAPTER 8

Figure 8-5A-F: 1982 Ross Laboratories (Originally adapted from Hamill PW, Drizd TA, Johnson CL: Physical growth: National Center for Health Statistics percentiles. Am J Clin Nutr 32:607-629, 1979.)

Figure 8-8: From Lubchenco L et al: Intrauterine growth as estimated from liveborn birthweight data at 24 to 42 weeks of gestation. Pediatrics 32:793, 1963. Reproduced by permission of Pediatrics.

Figure 8-9: From Rossman I: Clinical Geriatrics, 3rd ed. Philadelphia, JB Lippincott, 1986, p 6.

Figure 8-18: From Blumenthal S et al: Task Force on BP control in children. Pediatrics 59:797-820, 1977, p 803. Reproduced by permission of Pediatrics.

Figure 8-19: From Master AM, Lasser RP: Blood pressure elevation in the elderly. *In* Brest AM, Moyer JH (Eds): Hypertension: Recent Advances. Philadelphia, Lea & Febiger, 1961.

Art for Table 8-3: A: From Dubowitz LMS, Dubowitz V, Goldberg C: Clinical assessment of gestational age in the newborn infant. J Pediatr 77:1, 1970.

Art for Table 8-9: A: From Wilson JD, Foster DW: Williams' Textbook of Endocrinology. 7th ed. Philadelphia, WB Saunders, 1985, p 599. B: From Jacob SW, Francone CA, Lossow WJ: Structure and Function. 5th ed. Philadelphia, WB Saunders, 1982, p 550. C: From Wilson JD, Foster DW: Williams' Textbook of Endocrinology. 7th ed. Philadelphia, WB Saunders, 1985, p 602. D: From Moore KL: The Developing Human. 4th ed. Philadelphia, WB Saunders, 1988, p 142. E: From Crisp AH: Anorexia Nervosa: Let Me Be. San Diego, Academic Press, 1980, p 55. F: From Delp MH, Manning RT: Major's Physical Diagnosis: An Introduction to the Clinical Process. 9th ed. Philadelphia, WB Saunders, 1981, p 394.

CHAPTER 9

Figure 9-3: From Lookingbill DP, Marks JG: Principles of Dermatology. Philadelphia, WB Saunders, 1986, p 172.

Figure 9-4A: From Hurwitz S: Clinical Pediatric Dermatology: A Textbook of Skin Disorders of Childhood and Adolescence. Philadelphia, WB Saunders, 1981, p 168.

Figure 9-4B: From Hurwitz S: Clinical Pediatric Dermatology: A Textbook of Skin Disorders of Childhood and Adolescence. Philadelphia, WB Saunders, 1981, p 160.

Figure 9-4C: From Lookingbill DP, Marks JG: Principles of Dermatology. Philadelphia, WB Saunders, 1986, p 76.

Figure 9-4D: From Hurwitz S: Clinical Pediatric Dermatology: A Textbook of Skin Disorders of Childhood and Adolescence. Philadelphia, WB Saunders, 1981, p 161.

Figure 9-6: From Domonkos AN, Arnold HL, Odom RB: Andrews' Diseases of the Skin. 7th ed. Philadelphia, WB Saunders, 1982, p 742.

Figure 9-8: From Domonkos AN, Arnold HL, Odom RB: Andrews' Diseases of the Skin. 7th ed. Philadelphia, WB Saunders, 1982, p 979.

Figure 9-9: From Hurwitz S: Clinical Pediatric Dermatology: A Textbook of Skin Disorders of Childhood and Adolescence. Philadelphia, WB Saunders, 1981, p 381.

Figure 9-10: Courtesy of Mead Johnson & Company, Nutritional Division.

Figure 9-11: From Hurwitz A: Clinical Pediatric Dermatology: A Textbook of Skin Disorders of Childhood and Adolescence. Philadelphia, WB Saunders, 1981, p 171.

Figure 9-12: From Hurwitz A: Clinical Pediatric Dermatology: A Textbook of Skin Disorders of Childhood and Adolescence. Philadelphia, WB Saunders, 1981, p 11.

Figure 9-13: From Hurwitz A: Clinical Pediatric Dermatology: A Textbook of Skin Disorders of Childhood and Adolescence. Philadelphia, WB Saunders, 1981, p 8.

Figure 9-14: From Moore M: Realities in Childbearing. 2nd ed. Philadelphia, WB Saunders, 1983, p 632.

Figure 9-15: From Hurwitz A: Clinical Pediatric Dermatology: A Textbook of Skin Disorders of Childhood and Adolescence. Philadelphia, WB Saunders, 1981, p 194.

Figure 9-16: From Hurwitz A: Clinical Pediatric Dermatology: A Textbook of Skin Disorders of Childhood and Adolescence. Philadelphia, WB Saunders, 1981, p 107.

Figure 9-17: From Lookingbill DP, Marks JG: Principles of Dermatology. Philadelphia, WB Saunders, 1986, p 74.

Figure 9-18: From Lookingbill DP, Marks JG: Principles of Dermatology. Philadelphia, WB Saunders, 1986, p 61.

Figure 9-19: From Lookingbill DP, Marks JG: Principles of Dermatology. Philadelphia, WB Saunders, 1986, p 64.

Figure 9-20: From Lookingbill DP, Marks JG: Principles of Dermatology. Philadelphia, WB Saunders, 1986, p 62.

Art for Table 9-6: A: From Hurwitz S: Clinical Pediatric Dermatology: A Textbook of Skin Disorders of Childhood and Adolescence. Philadelphia, WB Saunders, 1981, p 195.

Art for Table 9-7: A: From Hurwitz S: Clinical Pediatric Dermatology: A Textbook of Skin Disorders of Childhood and Adolescence. Philadelphia, WB Saunders, 1981, p 205. B: From Lookingbill DP, Marks JG: Principles of Dermatology. Philadelphia, WB Saunders, 1986, p 203. C: From Hurwitz S: Clinical Pediatric Dermatology: A Textbook of Skin Disorders of Childhood and Adolescence. Philadelphia, WB Saunders, 1981, p 191.

Art for Table 9-8: A: From Hurwitz S: Clinical Pediatric Dermatology: A Textbook of Skin Disorders of Childhood and Adolescence. Philadelphia, WB Saunders, 1981, p 27. B: From Hurwitz S: Clinical Pediatric Dermatology: A Textbook of Skin Disorders of Childhood and Adolescence. Philadelphia, WB Saunders, 1981, p 29. C: From Hurwitz S: Clinical Pediatric Dermatology: A Textbook of Skin Disorders of Childhood and Adolescence. Philadelphia, WB Saunders, 1981, p 216. D: From Hurwitz S: Clinical Pediatric Dermatology: A Textbook of Skin Disorders of Childhood and Adolescence. Philadelphia, WB Saunders, 1981, p 43. E(1): From Feigin RD, Cherry JD: Textbook of Pediatric Infectious Diseases. 2nd ed. Philadelphia, WB Saunders, 1987, p 807. E(2): From Hurwitz S: Clinical Pediatric Dermatology: A Textbook of Skin Disorders of Childhood and Adolescence. Philadelphia, WB Saunders, 1981, p 261. F: From Hurwitz S: Clinical Pediatric Dermatology: A Textbook of Disorders of Childhood and Adolescence. Philadelphia, WB Saunders, 1981, p 265. G: From Feigin RD, Cherry JD: Textbook of Pediatric Infectious Diseases. 2nd ed. Philadelphia, WB Saunders, 1987, p 807.

Art for Table 9-9: A: From Lookingbill DP, Marks JG: Principles of Dermatology. Philadelphia, WB Saunders, 1986, p 38. B: From Lookingbill DP, Marks JG: Principles of Dermatology. Philadelphia, WB Saunders, 1986, p 179. C: From Hurwitz S: Clinical Pediatric Dermatology: A Textbook of Skin Disorders of Childhood and Adolescence. Philadelphia, WB Saunders, 1981, p 283. D: From Feigin RD, Cherry JD: Textbook of Pediatric Infectious Diseases. 2nd ed. Philadelphia, WB Saunders, 1987, p 813. E: From Lookingbill DP, Marks JG: Principles of Dermatology. Philadelphia, WB Saunders, 1986, p 113. F: From Hurwitz S: Clinical Pediatric Dermatology: A Textbook of Skin Disorders of Childhood and Adolescence. Philadelphia, WB Saunders, 1981, p 241. G: From Hurwitz S: Clinical Pediatric Dermatology: A Textbook of Skin Disorders of Childhood and Adolescence. Philadelphia, WB Saunders, 1981, p 244. H: From Lookingbill DP, Marks JG: Principles of Dermatology. Philadelphia, WB Saunders, 1986, p 67. I: From Lookingbill DP, Marks JG: Principles of Dermatology. Philadelphia, WB Saunders, 1986, p 78.

Art for Table 9-10: A: From Hurwitz S: Clinical Pediatric Dermatology: A Textbook of Skin Disorders of Childhood and Adolescence. Philadelphia, WB Saunders, 1981, p 13. B (1 and 2): From Lookingbill DP, Marks JG: Principles of Dermatology. Philadelphia, WB Saunders, 1986, p 227. C: From Hurwitz S: Clinical Pediatric Dermatology: A Textbook of Skin Disorders of Childhood and Adolescence. Philadelphia, WB Saunders, 1981, p 364. D: From Hurwitz S: Clinical Pediatric Dermatology: A Textbook of Skin Disorders of Childhood and Adolescence. Philadelphia, WB Saunders, 1981, p 365. E: From Hurwitz S: Clinical Pediatric Dermatology: A Textbook of Skin Disorders of Childhood and Adolescence. Philadelphia, WB Saunders, 1981, p 368. F: From Hurwitz S: Clinical Pediatric Dermatology: A Textbook of Skin Disorders of Childhood and Adolescence. Philadelphia, WB Saunders, 1981, p 367. G: From Lookingbill DP, Marks JG: Principles of Dermatology. Philadelphia, WB Saunders, 1986, p 191. H: From Hurwitz S: Clinical Pediatric Dermatology: A Textbook of Skin Disorders of Childhood and Adolescence. Philadelphia, WB Saunders, 1981, p 218. I: From Domonkos AN, Arnold HL, Odom RB: Andrews' Diseases of the Skin. 7th ed. Philadelphia, WB Saunders, 1982, p 955.

Art for Table 9-11: E: From Perloff JK: The Clinical Recognition of Congenital Heart Disease, 3rd ed. Philadelphia, WB Saunders, 1987, p 6. F: From Hurwitz S: Clinical Pediatric Dermatology: A Textbook of Skin Disorders of Childhood and Adolescence. Philadelphia, WB Saunders, 1981, p 380. G: From Domonkos AN, Arnold HL, Odom RB: Andrews' Diseases of the Skin. 7th ed. Philadelphia, WB Saunders, 1982, p 980. H: From Lookingbill DP and Marks JG: Principles of Dermatology. Philadelphia, WB Saunders, 1986, p 232.

CHAPTER 10

Figure 10-9: Redrawn from Stratz, modified by Robbins and others: Growth. Yale University Press, 1928.

Figure 10-17: From Tackett JM, Hunsberger M: Family-Centered Care of Children and Adolescents. Philadelphia, WB Saunders, 1981, p 417.

Figure 10-18: From Tackett JM, Hunsberger M: Family-Centered Care of Children and Adolescents. Philadelphia, WB Saunders, 1981, p 417.

Figure 10-20: From Behrman RE, Vaughn VC: Nelson Textbook of Pediatrics. 14th ed. Philadelphia, WB Saunders, 1987, p 1303.

Art for Table 10-1: A: From Jacob SW, Francone CA, Lossow WJ: Structure and Function in Man. 5th ed. Philadelphia, WB Saunders, 1982, p 265. B: From Laurence KM, Weeks R: In Norman AP(ed): Congenital Abnormalities of Infancy, 2nd ed, Oxford, England: Blackwell Scientific Publications Ltd, 1971. C: From Wilson JD, Foster DW: Williams' Textbook of Endocrinology. 7th ed. Philadelphia, WB Saunders, 1985, p 602.

Art for Table 10-2: A: From Domonkos AN, Arnold HL, Odom RB: Andrews' Diseases of the Skin. 7th ed. Philadelphia, WB Saunders, 1982, p 850. B: From Swartz MH: Textbook of Physical Diagnosis. Philadelphia, WB Saunders, 1989, Plate VIIID. C: From Swartz MH: Textbook of Physical Diagnosis. Philadelphia, WB Saunders, 1989, Plate VA. D: From Swartz MH: Textbook of Physical Diagnosis. Philadelphia, WB Saunders, 1989, Plate VB. E: From Behrman RE, Vaughn VC: Nelson Textbook of Pediatrics, 14th ed. Philadelphia, WB Saunders, 1987, p 1338.

Art for Table 10-3: A: From Bartalos M, Baramki TA: Medical Cytogenics. Baltimore: Williams & Wilkins, 1967. B: From Jones KL, Smith DW: Recognition of the fetal alcohol syndrome in early infancy. Lancet 2:999, 1973 and Jones KL et al: Pattern of malformation in offspring of chronic alcoholic mothers. Lancet 1:1267, 1973. C: From Behrman RE, Vaughn VC: Nelson Textbook of Pediatrics, 14th ed. Philadelphia, WB Saunders, 1987, p 1197.

Art for Table 10-4: A: From Bierman CW, Pearlman DS: Allergic Diseases from Infancy to Adulthood. 2nd ed. Philadelphia, WB Saunders, 1988, p 399. B: From Bierman CW, Pearlman DS: Allergic Diseases from Infancy to Adulthood. 2nd ed. Philadelphia, WB Saunders, 1988, p 399.

Art for Table 10-5: B: From Williams RH: Textbook of Endocrinology. 4th ed. Philadelphia, WB Saunders, 1968, p 352. C: From Kelley WN, Harris ED Jr, Ruddy S: Textbook of Rheumatology. 3rd ed. Philadelphia, WB Saunders, 1989, p 1218. D: From Jacob SW, Francone CA, Lossow, WJ: Structure and Function in Man. 5th ed. Philadelphia, WB Saunders, 1982, p 555. E: From Swartz MH: Textbook of Physical Diagnosis. Philadelphia, WB Saunders, 1989, Plate XVC.

CHAPTER 11

Figure 11-23: Courtesy of Heather Boyd-Monk and Wills Eye Hospital, Philadelphia.

Figure 11-24: Courtesy of Heather Boyd-Monk and Wills Eye Hospital, Philadelphia.

Figure 11-28: From Scheie HG, Albert DM: Textbook of Ophthalmology. 9th ed. Philadelphia, WB Saunders, 1977, p 337.

Figure 11-29: From Scheie HG, Albert DM: Textbook of Ophthalmology. 9th ed. Philadelphia, WB Saunders, 1977, p 458.

Figure 11-30: From Scheie HG, Albert DM: Textbook of Ophthalmology. 9th ed. Philadelphia, WB Saunders, 1977, p 458.

Figure 11-31: From Swartz MH: Textbook of Physical Diagnosis. Philadelphia, WB Saunders, 1989, Plate VIA.

Figure 11-32: Courtesy of Heather Boyd-Monk and Wills Eye Hospital, Philadelphia.

Art for Table 11-4: B: From Scheie HG, Albert DM: Textbook of Ophthalmology. 9th ed. Philadelphia, WB Saunders, 1977, p 427. C: Courtesy of Heather Boyd-Monk and Wills Eye Hospital, Philadelphia. E: From Scheie HG, Albert DM: Textbook of Ophthalmology. 9th ed. Philadelphia, WB Saunders, 1977, p 458. F: From Boyd-Monk H: Assessing acquired ocular diseases. Nurs Clin North Am (December): 811-822, 1990. (Originally courtesy of Wills Eye Hospital.) G: From Delp MH, Manning RT: Major's Physical Diagnosis: An Introduction to the Clinical Process. 9th ed. Philadelphia, WB Saunders, 1981, p 171.

Art for Table 11-5: A: From Scheie HG, Albert DM: Textbook of Ophthalmology. 9th ed. Philadelphia, WB Saunders, 1977, p 361. B: Courtesy of Heather Boyd-Monk and Wills Eye Hospital, Philadelphia. C: From Delp MH, Manning RT: Major's Physical Diagnosis: An Introduction to the Clinical Process. 9th ed. Philadelphia, WB Saunders, 1981, p 175. D: From Scheie HG, Albert DM: Textbook of Ophthalmology. 9th ed. Philadelphia, WB Saunders, 1977, p 449. E: From Scheie HG, Albert DM: Textbook of Ophthalmology. 9th ed. Philadelphia, WB Saunders, 1977, p 385.

Art for Table 11-6: A: From Boyd-Monk H: Assessing acquired ocular diseases. Nurs Clin of North Am 25:811-822, 1990. B: From Scheie HG, Albert DM: Textbook of Ophthalmology. 9th ed. Philadelphia, WB Saunders, 1977, p 13. C: Courtesy of Heather Boyd-Monk and Wills Eye Hospital, Philadelphia. D: From Scheie HG, Albert DM: Textbook of Ophthalmology. 9th ed. Philadelphia, WB Saunders, 1977, p 536.

Art for Table 11-7: A: From Scheie HG, Albert DM: Textbook of Ophthalmology. 9th ed. Philadelphia, WB Saunders, 1977, p 459. B: Courtesy of Heather Boyd-Monk and Wills Eye Hospital, Philadelphia.

Art for Table 11-8: B: From Scheie HG, Albert DM: Textbook of Ophthalmology. 9th ed. Philadelphia, WB Saunders, 1977, p 561. C: From Scheie HG, Albert DM: Textbook of Ophthalmology. 9th ed. Philadelphia, WB Saunders, 1977, p 391.

Art for Table 11-10: A: Courtesy of Heather Boyd-Monk and Wills Eye Hospital, Philadelphia.

Art for Table 11-11: A: From Scheie HG, Albert DM: Textbook of Ophthalmology. 9th ed. Philadelphia, WB Saunders, 1977, p 492. B: Courtesy of Heather Boyd-Monk and Wills Eye Hospital, Philadelphia. C: Courtesy of Heather Boyd-Monk and Wills Eye Hospital, Philadelphia.

Art for Table 11-12: A: From Boyd-Monk H: Assessing acquired ocular diseases. Nurs Clin of North Am 25:811-822, 1990.

Art for Table 11-13: A: Courtesy of Heather Boyd-Monk and Wills Eye Hospital, Philadelphia. B: Courtesy of Heather Boyd-Monk and Wills Eye Hospital, Philadelphia.

CHAPTER 12

Figure 12-8: From Adams GL, Boies LR Jr, Hilger PA: Boies Fundamentals of Otolaryngology: A Textbook of Ear, Nose and Throat Diseases. 6th ed. Philadelphia, WB Saunders, 1989, p 6.

Art for Table 12-1: From Sherman JL, Fields SK: Guide to Patient Evaluation, 3rd ed. New York: Medical Examination Publishing Company, 1978.

Art for Table 12-2: A: From Delp MH, Manning RT: Major's Physical Diagnosis: An Introduction to the Clinical Process. 9th ed. Philadelphia, WB Saunders, 1981, p 145. B: From Moore KL: The Developing Human. 4th ed. Philadelphia, WB Saunders, 1988, p 417. C: From Paparella MM, Shumrick DA, Gluckman JL, et al: Otolarnygology. 3rd ed. Philadelphia, WB Saunders, 1991, p 1233. D: From DeWeese DD et al: Otolaryngology—Head and Neck Surgery, 7th ed. St Louis: CV Mosby, 1988, p. 397.

Art for Table 12-3: A: From Paparella MM, Shumrick DA, Gluckman JL, et al: Otolaryngology. 3rd ed. Vol. II. Philadelphia, WB Saunders, 1991, p 1251. B: From Delp MH, Manning RT: Major's Physical Diagnosis: An Introduction to the Clinical Process. 9th ed. Philadelphia, WB Saunders, 1981, p 144. C: From DeWeese DD et al: Otolaryngology—Head and Neck Surgery, 7th ed. St Louis: CV Mosby, 1988, p. 397. D: From Paparella MM, Shumrick DA, Gluckman JL, et al: Otolaryngology. 3rd ed. Philadelphia, WB Saunders, 1991, p 1251. E: From Adams JL, Boies, LR Jr, Hilger PA: Boies Fundamentals of Otolaryngology: A Textbook of Ear, Nose, and Throat Diseases. 6th ed. Philadelphia, WB Saunders, 1989, p 82. F: From Paparella MM, Shumrick DA, Gluckman JL, et al: Otolaryngology, 3rd ed. Philadelphia, WB Saunders, 1991, p 1255.

Art for Table 12-5: A: From Adams JL, Boies, LR Jr, Hilger PA: Boies Fundamentals of Otolaryngology: A Textbook of Ear, Nose, and Throat Diseases. 6th ed. Philadelphia, WB Saunders, 1989, p 6. B: From Swartz MH: Textbook of Physical Diagnosis. Philadelphia, WB Saunders, 1989, Plate VIIIA. C: From Adams JL, Boies LR Jr, Hilger PA: Boies Fundamentals of Otolaryngology: A Textbook of Ear, Nose, and Throat Diseases. 6th ed. Philadelphia, WB Saunders, 1989, p 6. D: From Adams JL, Boies LR Jr, Hilger PA: Boies Fundamentals of Otolaryngology: A Textbook of Ear, Nose, and Throat Disease. 6th ed. Philadelphia, WB Saunders, 1989, p 6. E: From Swartz MH: Textbook of Physical Diagnosis. Philadelphia, WB Saunders, 1989, Plate VIIE. F: From Swartz MH: Textbook of Physical Diagnosis. Philadelphia, WB Saunders, 1989, Plate VIIF.

CHAPTER 13

Figure 13-11: From McCarthy JG: Plastic Surgery. Vol. 3. Philadelphia, WB Saunders, 1990, p 1868.

Figure 13-21: From Regezi JH, Sciubba JJ: Oral Pathology. WB Saunders, 1989, p. 119.

Figure 13-22: From Adams JL, Boies LR Jr, Hilger PA: Boies Fundamentals of Otolaryngology: A Textbook of Ear, Nose, and Throat Diseases. 6th ed. Philadelphia, WB Saunders, 1989, p 282.

Figure 13-27: From Moore ML: Realities in Childbearing. 2nd ed. Philadelphia, WB Saunders, 1983, p 642.

Art for Table 13-2: A: From Adams JL, Boies LR Jr, Hilger PA: Boies Fundamentals of Otolaryngology: A Textbook of Ear, Nose, and Throat Diseases. 6th ed. Philadelphia, WB Saunders, 1989, p 287. B: From Feigin RD, Cherry JD: Textbook of Pediatric Infectious Diseases. Vol 2. 2nd ed. Philadelphia, WB Saunders, 1987, p 1588. C: From Behrman RE, Vaughn VC: Nelson Textbook of Pediatrics. 14th ed. Philadelphia, WB Saunders, 1987, p 80 (bottom).

Art for Table 13-3: A: From Caldwell RC, Stallard RE: A Textbook of Preventive Dentistry. Philadelphia, WB Saunders, 1977. B: From Delp MH, Manning RT: Major's Physical Diagnosis: An Introduction to the Clinical Process. 9th ed. Philadelphia, WB Saunders, 1981, p 150.

C: From Paparella MM , Shumrick DA, Gluckman JL, et al: Otolaryngology, 3rd ed, Vol III. Philadelphia, WB Saunders, 1991, p 2001. D: From Adams JL, Boies LR Jr, Hilger PA: Boies Fundamentals of Otolaryngology. 6th ed. Philadelphia, WB Saunders, 1989, p 298.

Art for Table 13-4: A: From Sleisinger MH, Fordtran JS: Gastrointestinal Diseases: Pathophysiology, Diagnosis, and Management. 4th ed. Philadelphia, WB Saunders, 1989, p xxx (Fig 30-2b). B: From Feigin RD, Cherry JD: Textbook of Pediatric Infectious Diseases. Vol I. 2nd ed. Philadelphia, WB Saunders, 1987, p 309. C: From Sleisinger MH, Fordtran JS: Gastrointestinal Diseases: Pathophysiology, Diagnosis, and Management. 4th ed. Philadelphia, WB Saunders, 1989, p xxx (Fig 30-2a). D: From Adams JL, Boies LR Jr, Hilger PA: Boies Fundamentals of Otolaryngology: A Textbook of Ear, Nose, and Throat Diseases. 6th ed. Philadelphia, WB Saunders, 1989, p 309.

Art for Table 13-5: A: From Adams JL, Boies LR Jr, Hilger PA: Boies Fundamentals of Otolaryngology: A Textbook of Ear, Nose, and Throat Disease. 6th ed. Philadelphia, WB Saunders, 1989, p 286. B: From Adams JL, Boies LR Jr, Hilger PA: Boies Fundamentals of Otolaryngology: A Textbook of Ear, Nose, and Throat Diseases. 6th ed. Philadelphia, WB Saunders, 1989, p 302. C: From Adams JL, Boies LR Jr, Hilger PA: Boies Fundamentals of Otolaryngology: A Textbook of Ear, Nose, and Throat Diseases. 6th ed. Philadelphia, WB Saunders, 1989, p 301. D: From Sleisinger MH, Fordtran JS: Gastrointestinal Diseases: Pathophysiology, Diagnosis, and Management. 4th ed. Philadelphia, WB Saunders, 1989, p xxxv (Fig 30-2d). E: From Adams JL, Boies LR Jr, Hilger PA: Boies Fundamentals of Otolaryngology: A Textbook of Ear, Nose, and Throat Diseases. 6th ed. Philadelphia, WB Saunders, 1989, p 302. F: From Behram RE, Vaughn VC: Nelson Textbook of Pediatrics. 14th ed. Philadelphia, WB Saunders, 1987, p 254. G: From Delp MH, Manning RT: Major's Physical Diagnosis: An Introduction to the Clinical Process. 9th ed. Philadelphia, WB Saunders, 1981, p 152.

Art for Table 13-6: A: From Adams JL, Boies LR Jr, Hilger PA: Boies Fundamentals of Otolaryngology: A Textbook of Ear, Nose, and Throat Diseases. 6th ed. Philadelphia, WB Saunders, 1989, p 287. B: From DeWeese DD et al: Otolaryngology—Head and Neck Surgery, 7th ed. St Louis, CV Mosby, 1988, p 397.

CHAPTER 14

Figure 14-6: Redrawn from Tanner JM: Growth at Adolescence. Oxford, England, Blackwell Scientific, 1962, p 36.

Figure 14-8: From Bland KI, Copeland EM III: The Breast: Comprehensive Management of Benign and Malignant Diseases. Philadelphia, WB Saunders, 1991, p 81.

Figure 14-20: From Bland KI, Copeland EM III: The Breast: Comprehensive Management of Benign and Malignant Diseases. Philadelphia, WB Saunders, 1991, p 152.

Art for Table 14-1: A-J: From Tanner JM: Growth at Adolescence. Oxford, England, Blackwell Scientific, 1962.

Art for Table 14-3: A: From Haagensen CD: Diseases of the Breast. 3rd ed. Philadelphia, WB Saunders, 1986, p 531. B: From Haagensen CD: Diseases of the Breast. 3rd ed. Philadelphia, WB Saunders, 1986, p 529. C: From Haagensen CD: Diseases of the Breast. 3rd ed. Philadelphia, WB Saunders, 1986, p 542. D: From Haagensen CD: Diseases of the Breast. 3rd ed. Philadelphia, WB Saunders, 1986, p 521. E: From Haagensen CD: Diseases of the Breast. 3rd ed. Philadelphia, WB Saunders, 1986, p 529.

Art for Table 14-6: A: From Bland KI, Copeland EM III: The Breast: Comprehensive Management of Benign and Malignant Diseases. Philadelphia, WB Saunders, 1991. B: From Bland KI, Copeland EM III: The Breast: Comprehensive Management of Benign and Malignant Diseases. Philadelphia, WB Saunders, 1991, p 199 (upper left).

Art for Table 14-8: A: From Bland KI, Copeland EM III: The Breast: Comprehensive Management of Benign and Malignant Diseases. Philadelphia, WB Saunders, 1991, p 149. B: From Haagensen CD: Diseases of the Breast. 3rd ed. Philadelphia, WB Saunders, 1986, p 980.

CHAPTER 16

Figure 16-16: From Lakatta EG: Cardiovascular function in later life. Cardiovasc Med 10:37-40, 1985.

Figure 16-17: From Office of Minority Health, Washington, DC, 1990.

CHAPTER 17

Figure 17-9: From Swartz MH: Textbook of Physical Diagnosis. Philadelphia, WB Saunders, 1989, Plate XIIB.

Art for Table 17-3: From Delp MH, Manning RT: Major's Physical Diagnosis: An Introduction to the Clinical Process, 9th ed. Philadelphia, WB Saunders, 1981, p. 326.

CHAPTER 18

Figure 18-8: From Behrman RE, Vaughn VC: Nelson Textbook of Pediatrics. 14th ed. Philadelphia, WB Saunders, 1987, p 7. (After Scammon: The measurement of the body in childhood. *In* Harris et al: The measurement of Man. Minneapolis, University of Minnesota Press, 1930.)

Figure 18-13: From Faibairn JF, Juergens JL, Spittel JA (eds): Peripheral Vascular Disease, 4th ed. Philadelphia, WB Saunders, 1972, p. 27.

Figure 18-20B: From Delp MH, Manning RT: Major's Physical Diagnosis: An Introduction to the Clinical Process. 9th ed. Philadelphia, WB Saunders, 1981, p 327.

Art for Table 18-3: A: From the Clinical Slide Collection on the Rheumatic Diseases, the Arthritis Foundation, 1972. (Reprinted from the Revised Clinical Slide Collection on the Rheumatic Diseases, copyright 1981. Used by permission of the American College of Rheumatology.) B: Mason PB, Allen EV: Congenital familial lymphangiectasis (lymphedema). Am J Dis Child 50:945-953, 1935. Copyright 1935, American Medical Association.

Art for Table 18-4: A: From the Clinical Slide Collection on the Rheumatic Diseases, the Arthritis Foundation, 1972. (Reprinted from the Revised Clinical Slide Collection on the Rheumatic Diseases, copyright 1981. Used by permission of the American College of Rheumatology.) B: From Lookingbill DP, Marks JG: Principles of Dermatology. Philadelphia, WB Saunders, 1986, p 215. C: From Lofgren KA: Varicose veins. *In* Haimovici H (Ed); Vascular Surgery: Principles & Techniques. New York, McGraw-Hill, 1976, pp 799-811. D: From Fahey VA: Deep vein thrombosis. Nursing 84, 14:37, 1984. E: From Fahey VA: Vascular Nursing. Philadelphia, WB Saunders, 1988, p 37.

CHAPTER 19

Figure 19-53: From McDade W: Bow legs and knock knees. Pediatr Clin North Am, 24:830, 1977.

Figure 19-56: Copyright owned by DeWayne Dalrymple.

Art for Table 19-3: B: From Polley HF, Hunder GG: Physical Examination of the Joints. 2nd ed. Philadelphia, WB Saunders, 1978, p 161.

Art for Table 19-4: A: From Polley HF, Hunder GG: Physical Examination of the Joints. 2nd ed. Philadelphia, WB Saunders, 1978, p 66. B: From Rossman I: Clinical Geriatrics. 3rd ed. Philadelphia, JB Lippincott, 1986, p 588. C: From Polley HF, Hunder GG: Physical Examination of the Joints. 2nd ed. Philadelphia, WB Saunders, 1978, p 66. D: From Polley HF, Hunder GG: Physical Examination of the Joints. 2nd ed. Philadelphia, WB Saunders, 1978, p 76. E: From Polley HF,

Hunder GG: Physical Examination of the Joints. 2nd ed. Philadelphia, WB Saunders, 1978, p 71.

Art for Table 19-5: A: From Polley HF, Hunder GG: Physical Examination of the Joints. 2nd ed. Philadelphia, WB Saunders, 1978, p 83. B: From Polley HF, Hunder GG: Physical Examination of the Joints. 2nd ed. Philadelphia, WB Saunders, 1978, p 85. C: From Polley HF, Hunder GG: Physical Examination of the Joints. 2nd ed. Philadelphia, WB Saunders, 1978, p 84.

Art for Table 19-6: A: From Polley HF, Hunder GG: Physical Examination of the Joints. 2nd ed. Philadelphia, WB Saunders, 1978, p 96. B: From Polley HF, Hunder GG: Physical Examination of the Joints. 2nd ed. Philadelphia, WB Saunders, 1978, p 97. C: From Polley HF, Hunder GG: Physical Examination of the Joints. 2nd ed. Philadelphia, WB Saunders, 1978, p 99. D: From Polley HF, Hunder GG: Physical Examination of the Joints. 2nd ed. Philadelphia, WB Saunders, 1978, p 98. E: From Polley HF, Hunder GG: Physical Examination of the Joints. 2nd ed. Philadelphia, WB Saunders, 1978, p 118. F: From Kelley WN, Harris ED Jr, Ruddy S: Textbook of Rheumatology. 3rd ed. Philadelphia, WB Saunders, 1989, p 960. G: From Kelley WN, Harris ED Jr, Ruddy S: Textbook of Rheumatology. 3rd ed. Philadelphia, WB Saunders, 1989, p 934. H: From Polley HF, Hunder GG: Physical Examination of the Joints. 2nd ed. Philadelphia, WB Saunders, 1978, p 120. I: From Perloff JK: Clinical Recognition of Congenital Heart Disease. Philadelphia, WB Saunders, 1987, p 305.

Art for Table 19-7: A: From Polley HF, Hunder GG: Physical Examination of the Joints. 2nd ed. Philadelphia, WB Saunders, 1978, p 213. B: From Polley HF, Hunder GG: Physical Examination of the Joints. 2nd ed. Philadelphia, WB Saunders, 1978, p 214. C: From Polley HF, Hunder GG: Physical Examination of the Joints. 2nd ed. Philadelphia, WB Saunders, 1978, p 215. D: From Polley HF, Hunder GG: Physical Examination of the Joints. 2nd ed. Philadelphia, WB Saunders, 1978, p 216. E: From Polley HF, Hunder GG: Physical Examination of the Joints. 2nd ed. Philadelphia, WB Saunders, 1978, p 217.

Art for Table 19-8: A: From Polley HF, Hunder GG: Physical Examination of the Joints. 2nd ed. Philadelphia, WB Saunders, 1978, p 264. B: From Polley HF, Hunder GG: Physical Examination of the Joints. 2nd ed. Philadelphia, WB Saunders, 1978, p 250. C: From Polley HF, Hunder GG: Physical Examination of the Joints. 2nd ed. Philadelphia, WB Saunders, 1978, p 247. D: From Polley HF, Hunder GG: Physical Examination of the Joints. 2nd ed. Philadelphia, WB Saunders, 1978, p 248. E: From Polley HF, Hunder GG: Physical Examination of the Joints. 2nd ed. Philadelphia, WB Saunders, 1978, p 253.

Art for Table 19-9: A: From Delp MH, Manning RT: Major's Physical Diagnosis: An Introduction to the Clinical Process. 9th ed. Philadelphia, WB Saunders, 1981, p 450. B: From Polley HF, Hunder GG: Physical Examination of the Joints. 2nd ed. Philadelphia, WB Saunders, 1978, p 159.

Art for Table 19-10: A: From Behrman RE, Vaughn VC: Nelson Textbook of Pediatrics. 14th ed. Philadelphia, WB Saunders, 1987, p 1346. B: From Delp MH, Manning RT: Major's Physical Diagnosis: An Introduction to the Clinical Process. 9th ed. Philadelphia, WB Saunders, 1981, p 474. C: From Walsh PC, Gittes RF, Perlmutter AD, et al: Campbell's Urology. 5th ed. Philadelphia, WB Saunders, 1986, p 2194.

CHAPTER 20

Figure 20-51B: From Fenichel GM: Clinical Pediatric Neurology. Philadelphia, WB Saunders, 1988, p 171.

Figure 20-57: From Hickey JV: Neurological and Neurosurgical Nursing. 2nd ed. Philadelphia, JB Lippincott, 1986, p 121.

CHAPTER 21

Figure 21-4: Redrawn from Marshall WA and Tanner JM: Variations in the pattern of pubertal changes in boys. Arch Dis Child 45:22, 1970.

Art for Table 21-1: A: Courtesy of Pfizer Laboratories Division, Pfizer Inc, New York. From "A Close Look at VD: A Slide Presentation Produced as a Public Service." B: Courtesy of Pfizer Laboratories Division, Pfizer Inc, New York. From "A Close Look at VD: A Slide Presentation Produced as a Public Service." C: From Coldiron BM, Jacobson C: Common Penile Lesions. Urol Clin North Am 15:673, 1988. D: From Walsh PC et al: Campbell's Urology, 5th ed. Philadelphia, WB Saunders, 1986, p 1591.

Art for Table 21-3: C: From Hamblin JE, Assimos DG, Kroovand RL: Pediatric urology. Primary Care. Clinics in Office Practice 16:889–904, 1989. D: From Walsh PC, Gittes RF, Perlmutter AD, et al: Campbell's Urology, 5th ed. Philadelphia, WB Saunders, 1986, p 1875.

Art for Table 21-4: A: Courtesy of Pfizer Laboratories Division, Pfizer Inc, New York. From "A Close Look at VD: A Slide Presentation Produced as a Public Service."

CHAPTER 22

Art for Table 22-1: A–D: From Tanner JM: Growth at Adolescence. 2nd ed. Oxford, England, Blackwell Scientific, 1962.

Art for Table 22-3: A: From Domonkos AN, Arnold HL, Odom RB: Andrews' Diseases of the Skin. 7th ed. Philadelphia, WB Saunders, 1982, p 556. B: Courtesy of Pfizer Laboratories Division, Pfizer Inc, New York. From "A Close Look at VD: A Slide Presentation Produced as a Public Service." C: Courtesy of Pfizer Laboratories Division, Pfizer Inc, New York. From "A Close Look at VD: A Slide Presentation Produced as a Public Service." D: From Feigin RD, Cherry JD: Textbook of Pediatric Infectious Diseases. 2nd ed. Philadelphia, WB Saunders, 1987, p 576. E: From Feigin RD, Cherry JD: Textbook of Pediatric Infectious Diseases. 2nd ed. Philadelphia, WB Saunders, 1987, p 566. F: Courtesy of Pfizer Laboratories Division, Pfizer Inc. New York. From "A Close Look at VD: A Slide Presentation Produced as a Public Service."

Art for Table 22-4: A: From Huffman JW: Gynecology and Obstetrics. Philadelphia, WB Saunders, 1962. B: From Huffman JW: Gynecology and Obstetrics. Philadelphia, WB Saunders, 1962. C: From Parsons L, Sommers SC: Gynecology. 2nd ed. Philadelphia, WB Saunders, 1978, p 1443.

Art for Table 22-6: F: Courtesy of Pfizer Laboratories Division, Pfizer Inc, New York. From "A Close Look at VD: A Slide Presentation Produced as a Public Service."

Art for Table 22-9: A: From Moore KL: The Developing Human. 4th ed. Philadelphia, WB Saunders, 1988, p 142. B: From Feigin RD, Cherry JD: Textbook of Pediatric Infectious Diseases. 2nd ed. Philadelphia, WB Saunders, 1987, p 564.

Index

Note: Page numbers in *italics* refer to illustrations; page numbers followed by t refer to tables. See list of Developmental Considerations, and list of Transcultural Considerations on page 952.

Developmental Considerations

Transcultural Considerations